Psychotherapy Research

Omar C.G. Gelo • Alfred Pritz • Bernd Rieken
Editors

Psychotherapy Research

Foundations, Process, and Outcome

Springer

Editors
Omar C.G. Gelo
University of Salento
Lecce, Italy
Sigmund Freud University
Vienna, Austria

Bernd Rieken
Sigmund Freud University
Vienna, Austria

Alfred Pritz
Sigmund Freud University
Vienna, Austria

ISBN 978-3-7091-1945-7 ISBN 978-3-7091-1382-0 (eBook)
DOI 10.1007/978-3-7091-1382-0
Springer Wien Heidelberg New York Dordrecht London

Printed on acid-free paper

Springer is part of Springer Science+Business Media (www.springer.com)

Preface

This book has a long history that can be traced back to 2008, when we—Omar C.G. Gelo, Alfred Pritz, and Bernd Rieken—met in Vienna. Omar C.G Gelo had just finished his experience at the University of Ulm, where he earned his PhD in psychotherapy research under the supervision of Erhard Mergenthaler and where he was introduced by the latter to the Society of Psychotherapy Research (SPR), an international scientific association devoted to research on psychotherapy. At that time, Alfred Pritz and Bernd Rieken were both engaged in starting an international PhD program in psychotherapy science at the Sigmund Freud University, Vienna; their main concern was to develop a curriculum that would bridge clinical practice with scientific investigation by means of a pluralistic approach to inform a comprehensive understanding of psychotherapy practice and research.

It soon became clear to us how much we had in common, despite our somewhat different personal and professional experiences and backgrounds. More specifically, we realized that all three of us were deeply convinced that (a) psychotherapy is an extremely complex phenomenon that nonetheless can be adequately investigated using adequate scientific methods; (b) a self-aware reflection on the foundations of psychotherapy research should necessarily precede its application; (c) scholars should develop a pluralistic attitude toward the sometimes very different existing scientific methods they might rely upon to conduct psychotherapy research; and (d) the process and outcome of psychotherapy represent two of the most important (although not the only) dimensions of the clinical encounter because they primarily address, respectively, what goes on during psychotherapy and its clinical effects.

We thus decided to accept the challenge of putting together a book on psychotherapy research that is informed by these beliefs in an effort to provide the readers with an overview of the basic issues of psychotherapy research and some of its most recent developments and applications. Accordingly, the book focuses on the foundations of psychotherapy research (Part I) and their application to the study of both the process (Part II) and outcome (Part III) of psychotherapy.

Our general aim is to stimulate a reflection on these issues in a way that, at different levels and from different angles and perspectives, might be useful for both researchers and clinicians as well as for undergraduate and graduate students. This is attempted through a balanced mix of chapters that summarize the state of the art of the field from different viewpoints with chapters that present innovative topics and perspectives. The contributors are among the many experts in our national and international professional networks and were invited in order to represent both traditional and emerging approaches in the field across several countries. We hope that this will be a valuable tool for anyone interested in psychotherapy research.

We would like to thank the contributors for their intense and thoughtful work. We are aware of how demanding it can be to write a chapter for a book and to deal with the editors; we really appreciated this. In addition, we are thankful to our extended staff of colleagues and students at our own institutions—the Sigmund Freud University and the University of Salento—as well as to the SPR for all the insightful discussions, debates, and inspiration. Their scientific qualification, passion for knowledge, and open spirit helped us to be adventurous enough to conceive this book and make it happen. Finally, we also want to thank Springer-Verlag for all the support and patience, which such a book needs.

Lecce, Italy — Omar C.G. Gelo
Vienna, Austria — Alfred Pritz
Vienna, Austria — Bernd Rieken

Contents

1 Introduction

Omar Carlo Gioacchino Gelo, Alfred Pritz, and Bernd Rieken

Contents

Abstract

In this chapter, we introduce the subject of the book, whose main aim is to try to answer the following questions: "What is psychotherapy research?," "What should it primarily address?," and "How should it be conducted?" To accomplish this goal, we rely on the following four interrelated basic assumptions: (1) Psychotherapy research and its object of investigation are *social constructions* grounded on the values and beliefs shared by the members of a specific community at a certain time and place. (2) For psychotherapy researchers to be aware not only of what they do but also of why they do it, they should engage in *explicit* and *self-critical reflection* on the foundational assumptions of psychotherapy research. (3) *Pluralism* should be considered not only a valuable stance but also an a priori condition of any scientific account of psychotherapy. (4) Finally, self-reflective and methodologically pluralistic psychotherapy research should be conducted on the *process* and *outcome* of psychotherapy to determine how and why psychotherapy works. With these basic assumptions on the background, in this chapter, we provide a summary of the three main parts of the book; these parts attempt to inform the readers of the foundations of psychotherapy research (Part I) and its applications to the study of the process (Part II) and outcome (Part III) of psychotherapy.

O.C.G. Gelo (✉)
Department of History, Society and Human Studies, University of Salento, Via Stampacchia 45, 73100 Lecce, Italy

Department of Psychotherapy Science, Sigmund Freud University, Freudplatz 1, 1020 Vienna, Austria
e-mail: omar.gelo@unisalento.it; omar.gelo@sfu.ac.at

A. Pritz • B. Rieken
Department of Psychotherapy Science, Sigmund Freud University, Freudplatz 1, 1020 Vienna, Austria

O.C.G. Gelo et al. (eds.), *Psychotherapy Research*,
DOI 10.1007/978-3-7091-1382-0_1, © Springer-Verlag Wien 2015

The *foundations of psychotherapy research* are described with reference to its historical development, philosophical underpinnings, and/or theoretical framework. *Process research* is addressed with reference to both quantitative and qualitative approaches to reflect the increasing relevance that the latter has gained in recent decades. Finally, *outcome research* is described predominantly from the perspective of quantitative approaches, reflecting their predominance in this type of research, although an overview of qualitative approaches is offered as well.

What is psychotherapy research? What should it primarily address? How should it be carried out? In this book, we attempt to answer these basic questions, and we do so by strongly relying on the following four interrelated assumptions: (1) Psychotherapy research as well as its object of investigation are *socially negotiated* and *institutionally legitimated cultural products*, which are grounded on values and beliefs shared by the members of a specific community at a certain time and place. This helps to explain, for example, the historical and contemporary diversity and heterogeneity of the conceptions of the nature of psychotherapy and psychotherapy research (see Frank and Frank 1991; Lambert 2013; Chap. 3). (2) It follows that an *explicit* and *self-critical reflection* on the foundational assumptions of psychotherapy research, far from being trivial, is essential to make psychotherapy researchers aware not only of *what* they do but also of *why* they do it (Gelo 2012; Slife 1998, 2004; see Chaps. 4 and 5). (3) From the first assumption, it also follows that different conceptions and/or theories of scientific investigation in psychotherapy cannot be proven to be absolutely true or false but rather are evaluated as more or less plausible, persuasive, and useful. Thus, *pluralism*—the stance of acknowledging and engaging with diversity (i.e., otherness)—and multiplicity should be considered not only a valuable attitude but also an a priori condition of any scientific account of psychotherapy [see also Kellert, Longino, and Waters (2006) and Teo (2010)]. Specifically regarding methodology, this means that several methods and their underlying principles and philosophies should be allowed to complement one another (Cooper and McLeod 2007; Elliott 2010; Gelo and Gelo 2012; Slife and Gantt 1999, Chap. 4). (4) Finally, to find out how and why psychotherapy works, self-reflective and methodologically pluralistic psychotherapy research should be conducted on both the *process* and *outcome* of psychotherapy. This would enhance the possibility of producing results useful in informing the clinical practice of psychotherapy.

This book, which is organized into three parts, aims to provide the readers with knowledge of the foundations of psychotherapy research (part I) and its applications to the study of the process (part II) and outcome (part III) of psychotherapy.

1.1 Foundations of Psychotherapy Research

The first part of the book addresses some *foundational issues* of psychotherapy research on a historical, philosophical, and theoretical level. Such issues are usually treated in a sporadic and/or isolated way in mainstream psychotherapy research literature; our aim is to try to stimulate a further reflection on them. Chapter 2 focuses on the prehistory of psychotherapy and its implications for psychotherapy science. This issue is very relevant because it shows how what we consider to be the object of our investigation (i.e., psychotherapy) has varied greatly at different times and in different places. We believe that a reflection on the nature of a discipline's object of study is fundamental to better understanding the discipline itself. Chapter 3 offers a review of the history of psychotherapy research, which represents for us an indispensable body of knowledge that researchers and clinicians should be aware of to understand where psychotherapy research comes from and where it can go.

Chapter 4 addresses the extent to which what we consider to be the appropriate way of conducting psychotherapy research is necessarily influenced by our deep and hidden but fundamental philosophical assumptions about the basic aspects of our world. Mainstream and alternative views are discussed. Always from a philosophical perspective, Chap. 5 attempts to provide an epistemological argument for psychotherapy to be considered an academic discipline. This issue, which has been addressed since the birth of modern psychotherapy through Freud's conceptualization of psychoanalysis, is particularly relevant to providing an epistemic status to psychotherapy as science as opposed to psychotherapy as clinical practice. Finally, a philosophical stance is also taken in Chap. 6, where the author attempts to show that interpretation, far from exclusively being an instrument used in clinical practice, may be considered one basic cognitive instrument for the practice of psychotherapy science.

Chapter 7 discusses some of the differences in the regulation of psychotherapy training in different countries. The issue is relevant because different formal requirements for psychotherapy training—which Orlinsky and Howard's (1984) Generic Model of Psychotherapy would ascribe to the domain of input (or antecedents) of psychotherapy—very likely produce different "psychotherapies" with consequences on the nature of the object of our investigation (see also Orlinsky 2009). The implications for psychotherapy research are discussed. The last chapter of this first part, Chap. 8, provides a bridge to the subsequent two parts of the book by innovatively distinguishing three different and alternative purposes of psychotherapy research: theory building, enriching, and fact gathering.

1.2 Psychotherapy Process Research

The second part of this book addresses psychotherapy *process* research, which is very broadly referred here as any research that focuses on the process of psychotherapy and, eventually, its relationship with the outcome. Both quantitative and qualitative approaches are given equal consideration in order to reflect the increasing relevance that qualitative approaches have gained in recent decades. The first three chapters of this part provide a general introduction to both basic and more advanced issues concerning the psychotherapeutic process and its investigation. Chapter 9 unpacks the general meaning of psychotherapy process research by offering an introduction of its aims, typologies, methodology, limitations, and emerging trends. In Chap. 10, the authors outline a general theory of the psychotherapeutic process that is described, from a semiotic and dynamic perspective, in terms of a communicational field. The theoretical considerations that sustain such a view are drawn, and the methodology implications are discussed. Finally, Chap. 11 attempts to provide an evolutionary-based, tripartite model of the relationship to explain how psychotherapy works.

1.2.1 Quantitative Process Research

After these three introductory chapters, a first group of contributions specifically focuses on *quantitative* process research. Chapter 12 provides an introduction to quantitative data analysis in psychotherapy process research. The way psychotherapeutic process data can be organized and structured is described; moreover, an interesting heuristic framework to organize the multitude of basic statistical data-analytic procedures is offered. In Chap. 13, the authors give an overview of three main quantitative approaches that differently focus on the process of psychotherapy and/or its relationship with treatment outcomes: treatment process, change process, and process-outcome research. These are described in terms of research design, data collection, and data analysis. Chapter 14 offers an overview of quantitative process research on group psychotherapy that synthetizes the most recent developments in the field.

Chapter 15 addresses the process of change in psychotherapy by introducing the readers to the debate between common and unique factors.

This debate is discussed with regard to both theoretical and empirical arguments. In the following chapter, Chap. 16, the authors focus on the therapeutic alliance, which over decades of empirical research seems to have gained the status of an empirically supported common therapeutic factor in contemporary literature. After an historical and theoretical introduction and overview, the authors focus on some of the most recent developments in the investigation of alliance ruptures and resolutions. Chapter 17 discusses the contribution of positive psychology to psychotherapy theory, research, and practice. The contribution is interesting because it provides insight into possible change mechanisms that have been largely unexplored up to now. Chapter 18 reviews empirical research on the psychotherapeutic process conducted from the perspective of psychotherapists and discusses therapists' experiences of the process. Finally, in Chap. 19, the authors provide an interesting account of how the traditional psychoanalytic narrative case study has evolved into quantitative single-case research. This latter approach is exemplified by a description of the research conducted by the Ulm Psychoanalytic Process Research Study Group.

1.2.2 Qualitative Process Research

The remaining contributions of the second part of this book focus, on the contrary, on *qualitative* process research. The first two chapters respectively describe the methodology and applications of qualitative process research. Chapter 20 provides a detailed outline of qualitative research methods that may be used to analyze the psychotherapeutic process. Research designs, data collection, and data analysis are reviewed; with regard to the latter two, a dimensional conceptualization is offered that aims to provide a heuristic framework to locate the different existing methods described in the literature. Chapter 21 extensively reviews and discusses applications of qualitative and mixed methods research for the investigation of counseling and psychotherapy.

Finally, the last four contributions describe specific qualitative approaches frequently used in psychotherapy process research. Chapter 22 focuses on Grounded Theory (GT) and develops a detailed compilation of interpretation-driven guidelines for designing and evaluating GT research. Chapter 23 presents a review of Consensual Qualitative Research (CQR) by focusing on its background and methods. Chapter 24 provides a practical overview of the principles of Conversation Analysis (CA) and the main dimensions according to which it may be applied in the investigation of the process of psychotherapy. Lastly, in Chap. 25, the author proposes a pragmatic approach to the study of the therapeutic interaction that integrates theoretical propositions derived from developmental psychology and pragmatics with the methods of CA.

1.3 Psychotherapy Outcome Research

The third and final part of this book addresses psychotherapy *outcome* research, which aims to investigate whether a treatment produces the desired and expected clinical results. Unlike the second part of the book dealing with process research, this part is focused mostly on quantitative approaches, testifying their predominance in this type of research. Two methodological contributions open this part. Chapter 26 reviews the main methodological issues in quantitative psychotherapy outcome research. The main characteristics of Evidence-Based Medicine (EBM) are sketched out along with the research designs' hierarchy of evidence and meta-analysis. The issue of Randomized Controlled Trials (RCTs) is discussed, and other relevant issues such as sampling, treatment manualization, the difference between efficacy and effectiveness, outcome measurement, and statistical data analysis in outcome research are addressed. Chapter 27, on the contrary, reviews the main qualitative methods used in qualitative research with the aim of showing that qualitative methods can complement, enrich, and deepen the more traditional quantitative methods in the study of outcomes.

In Chap. 28, the authors elaborate on research on the outcomes of grief therapy—one class of disorder-specific therapy; discuss its efficacy based on the results of a meta-analysis; and offer recommendations for future outcome research on disorder-specific treatments. Chapter 29 reviews findings concerning the use outcome measures in routine care to provide therapists with patient progress feedback; the extent to which such an approach may enhance therapeutic efficacy is discussed. Finally, in Chap. 30, the authors discuss the use of neuroimaging in investigating the outcome of psychotherapy and review the main empirical results produced in the field.

References

Cooper M, McLeod JA (2007) Pluralistic framework for counselling and psychotherapy: implications for research. Couns Psychother Res 7:135–143

Elliott R (2010) Psychotherapy change process research: realizing the promise. Psychother Res 20(2):123–135. doi:10.1080/10503300903470743

Frank JD, Frank JB (1991) Persuasion and healing: a comparative study of psychotherapy, 3rd edn. Johns Hopkins University Press, Baltimore, MD

Gelo OCG (2012) On research methods and their philosophical assumptions: "Raising the consciousness of researchers" again. Psychother Sozialwiss 14(2): 111–130

Gelo OCG, Gelo C (2012) Dialogical relationship among scientific paradigms in psychotherapy research. Paper presented at the 3rd Joint Meeting of the European and the United Kingdom Chapters of the Society for Psychotherapy Research, Porto, Portugal, October 10–13

Kellert SH, Longino HE, Waters CK (eds) (2006) Scientific pluralism. University of Minnesota Press, Minneapolis, MN

Lambert MJ (ed) (2013) Bergin and Garfield's handbook of psychotherapy and behavior change, 4th edn. Wiley, New York

Orlinsky DE (2009) The "generic model of psychotherapy" after 25 years: evolution of a research-based metatheory. J Psychother Integr 19:319–339

Orlinsky DE, Howard KI (1984) A generic model of psychotherapy. In: Paper presented at the 1st annual meeting of the Society for the Exploration of Psychotherapy Integration (SEPI), Annapolis, MD

Slife BD (1998) Raising the consciousness of researchers: hidden assumptions in the behavioral sciences. Adapt Phys Act Q 15(3):208–221

Slife BD (2004) Theoretical challenges to therapy practice and research: the constraint of naturalism. In: Lambert MJ (ed) Bergin and Garfield's handbook of psychotherapy and behavior change, 5th edn. Wiley, New York, pp 44–83

Slife BD, Gantt E (1999) Methodological pluralism: a framework for psychotherapy research. J Clin Psychol 55(12):1–13

Teo T (2010) Ontology and scientific explanation: pluralism as an *a priori* condition of psychology. New Ideas Psychol 28:235–243. doi:10.1016/j.newideapsych.2009.09.017

Part I

Foundations of Psychotherapy Research

The Prehistory of Psychotherapy and Its Implications for Psychotherapy Science: Shamanism, Folk Medicine, Philosophy, and Religion

2

Bernd Rieken

Contents

Abstract

The individualization of lifestyles as it developed only since the beginning of the twentieth century was accompanied by an increased complexity at the mental level. The downside was that this made people more psychically vulnerable and created a need for specific occupations focused on the psyche, above all psychotherapy. Thus, psychotherapy is a modern phenomenon; it would've been a foreign concept in past epochs. This does not mean that mental illness and its treatment was unknown in the archaic and the premodern period, but that it required different approaches, though those, in their structure, may show similarities with today's methods. This applies equally to the popular healing methods of shamans in archaic cultures and folk healers in the premodern period but also to certain practices of the Christian religion and philosophy shaped in advanced cultures. This chapter will first outline the differences between a modern and a premodern or archaic self-concept; second, the prehistoric precursors of modern psychotherapy will be described; finally, the implications of this outlook for psychotherapy research will be addressed.

It is not an end in itself to start a book on psychotherapy research with a historical part. The intention is to raise awareness that past eras deserve recognition for their serious commitment to physical and emotional health and

B. Rieken (✉)
Department of Psychotherapy Science, Sigmund Freud University, Freudplatz 1, 1020 Vienna, Austria
e-mail: bernd.rieken@sfu.ac.at

O.C.G. Gelo et al. (eds.), *Psychotherapy Research*,
DOI 10.1007/978-3-7091-1382-0_2, © Springer-Verlag Wien 2015

that there are structural similarities between their methods and current treatment techniques that might well give a fresh impetus to current research. In addition, a historical perspective allows us to consider present life in Western countries as a specific form of human existence and reminds us that there were—and are—most definitely alternatives to this way of life. This can help sharpen the gaze for shortcomings and opportunities of the present. Correspondingly, sciences that explore the psyche, too, have time-specific limitations and opportunities. In short and using the words of German poet Kurt Tucholsky: "Who wants to measure the limitations of his home should travel. Who wants to measure the limitations of his time should study history" (Tucholsky 1926).

2.1 Collectivism, Epistemological Egocentrism, and Magic

2.1.1 Collectivism

Psychotherapy is a modern phenomenon that essentially dates back no further than the late nineteenth century, because it is closely linked to an individualization of lifestyles that was not practicable on a broad scale until the twentieth century. This was because individualization puts higher demands on the individual psyche than life in societies that focus strongly on traditions and *collective* patterns of identification (Beck and Beck-Gernsheim 2010; Hernegger 1978, 1982). And since systems theory has long established that systems are more susceptible to interference the more complex they are (Genelot 1992, p. 83; see Schmid GB 2008, Schmid JC 2008), it should not come as a surprise that in present times there are a variety of occupational groups that, as specialists for the "spiritual life," advise the individual and offer their assistance in the form of therapy.

From a sociological and cultural-historical perspective, these developments are associated with, among other things, the increasing intimacy brought on by the transition from large to small family units, with the dynamization and acceleration of living conditions that began in the early modern period and increased once again in present times (Borscheid 2004; Giedion 2009; Schulze 2005), as well as with the multitude of roles and identities that characterize the "saturated self" (Gergen 1991) of western cultures. This is why sociologists talk about a "culture of self-help" (Illouz 2008) or the "advised self" (Maasen et al. 2011) when they refer to the European and North American societies of the present.

The relationship between individualization and "psychotherapeutization" does not imply that psychotherapy has no precedent, but that from a historical perspective, as a defined treatment method and a defined research object, it is an extremely young phenomenon. The origins of individualization, however, date back to the beginning of the European modern period, as historian Jacob Burckhardt pointed out in his famous work *The Civilization of the Renaissance in Italy* when he tried to outline the difference between the medieval and the modern attitude towards life:

> "In the Middle Ages both sides of human consciousness—that which was turned within as that which was turned without—lay dreaming or half awake beneath a common veil. The veil was woven of faith, illusion, and childish prepossession, through which the world and history were seen clad in strange hues. Man was conscious of himself only as a member of a race, people, party, family, or corporation—only through some general category. In Italy this veil first melted into air; an *objective* treatment and consideration of the State and of all the things of this world became possible. The *subjective* side at the same time asserted itself with corresponding emphasis; man became a spiritual *individual*, recognized himself as such" (Burckhardt 1990, p. 98).

That is a pretty pointed formulation, and not a little one sided, because initially and through the centuries, the development of the "spiritual individual" was limited to a few elites and did not include large segments of the population. The quote is still interesting because, on the one hand, it describes the contrast between individualistic and collectivistic or universalistic ideas of man in a pointed way and, on the other hand, points out an apparent paradox, as "subjective" and "objective" are usually considered opposites. Burckhardt, though, postulates a reciprocal set of interdependent conditions. This requires a somewhat more detailed explanation.

The medieval person saw themselves primarily as a member of a community or an estate system that was considered divinely ordained (the following see Rieken 2011b, pp. 10–13). They were mostly a peasant or burgher, a member of a family, a profession, a particular region, or a common and generally binding religion (see Le Goff 1996). It would have been deemed absurd to want to change that by, for example, choosing a different career or switching to a different social class. That would have been a violation of the divinely ordained system, and thus it remained until the seventeenth century. In the great world dramas of the Baroque period, such as the plays by Calderon de la Barca and Andreas Gryphius, there is no individuality in the modern sense, but only roles as assigned by God. A person's only freedom is to play this role prudently and virtuously or fall victim to one's passions and base instincts (Emrich 1981, p. 113). Accordingly, the concept of tragedy is different from our modern understanding. While nowadays it is understood as a conflict situation unresolvable on an individualistic level (Düsing 2007, p. 666)—"Tragedy is where the powers that collide each are true to themselves," writes Karl Jaspers (Jaspers 1947, p. 934)—in the Baroque period, tragedy was defined group specifically as the "drop height": an event was all the more tragic the more extreme the drop height from an upper to a lower social class. This was exemplified in dramas such as Andreas Gryphius' *Catharina of Georgia* (Gryphius 1981) or *Carolus Stuardus* (Gryphius 1972) which depict the falls of great rulers.

The divinely ordained estate system is reflected predominantly in the visual arts. Medieval sculptures often seem barely "realistic" to modern people because they contradict their current ideas of spatial vision. This is due to the *Bedeutungsperspektive* (*hierarchic perspective*) which required that important people, such as God, saints, or secular rulers, were portrayed as taller, regardless of their actual position in the image. Less prominent figures or especially "common" people, however, were depicted as smaller. Nowadays, such images appear "unnatural" because the proportions are not right as figures may be larger in the image background and smaller in the foreground.

In contrast, the transition to an individualizing perspective can hardly be perceived more clearly than in the art of the Italian Renaissance, for it uses the one-point perspective (or central perspective), which does not represent parallel edges in space as parallel to the illustration, but unites them in one imaginary point, the central vanishing point (also called principal vanishing point or center of vision). This is a form of representation roughly equivalent to seeing through the human eye or a camera with a normal lens (50 mm).

This also explains why Burckhardt says that with the discovery of individuality and subjectivity, "an objective consideration of the State and of all things in this world even" was made possible, for the one-point perspective is synonymous with the realization of a subjective "standpoint," and that is exactly what allows a more realistic view of the world.

2.1.2 Epistemological Egocentrism

What this means with regard to psychology was illustrated by Jean Piaget in his famous three mountains task: children aged 4–6 years were shown the model of a landscape with three mountains of different heights and shapes and were asked to describe them from their position. They were then asked how the landscape would look from the perspective of an opposing position, but were not allowed to change location. Their description matched the first one, their current perspective. Only at the age of 7–12 years did the children begin to understand that the model of a landscape looked different from different points of observation, with complete differentiation usually achieved at 9–10 years (Piaget and Inhelder 1956, pp. 210–213).

Due to this lack of "decentering," little children believe that the world is indeed exactly as it presents itself to them. This *epistemological egocentrism* correlates to the "naive" worldview that shaped, or sometimes still shapes, most cultures with their ethnocentrism and uncritical "realism" (in the sense of Piaget) and was curbed only by the discovery of systematic scientific thought. In a psychological context, this means that only when a person is aware of their subjectivity and individuality do they recognize they see the world only from a certain perspective (see Köller 2004). Conversely, however, this means that egocentric thinking stands at the beginning of development, both with regard to the individual and society. This makes sense, because the environment of individuals and groups generally appears to its members as a reasonably ordered, coherent whole. This is not because it actually is so, but because people constitute it in such a way in order to be able to reliably navigate their reality:

> "Inevitably, everyone considers themself the center of their world. If they want circumstances to be meaningful, i.e., meaningful *for them*, they must assume that these circumstances all, directly or indirectly, *relate to them* in some way; it gives them the impression that, ultimately, 'everything revolves around them' as though they had a part in the flow of forces that come into effect in the movements of their environment, as though these forces streamed to them as it were and were redistributed back to their environment by virtue of their actions. Thus, the coherence of their worldview has, primarily at first, always an *egocentric* superstructure" (Müller 1987, p. 198; see Müller 2010, pp. 421–445) and becomes, since the individual can only survive in groups, an ethnocentric structure based on the collective.

2.1.3 Magic

The parallels between individual and collective development can easily be demonstrated by means of magical thinking, because egocentric-animistic and egocentric-finalistic attitudes are of great importance both in childish and in archaic thinking. Thus, as Piaget has shown in his groundbreaking work *The Child's Conception of the World*, any object may have a consciousness at any given time (Piaget 2007, p. 174). For example, if someone bangs against a chair, this is not an accident but intentional, because the chair wanted to hurt the child. And when a bushman stalks his prey and encounters a chameleon with a tucked-in, crooked tail, he knows he has to be careful because this brings about bad luck (Müller 1987, p. 200). In short, the objects of this world are all animated and have it in for people or want to tell them something. These are universal concepts that follow the basic conditions of human existence, namely, the egocentric and ethnocentric view. And they are the reason why the child or the archaic person does not understand themselves as a differentiated individual as we see it, but as someone who is "open" to and "porous" for manifold environmental influences that affect them, but that they may affect in turn: when the child moves, the sun and the moon they see in the sky move with them, and when the child stops, so do they (Piaget 2007, p. 215). Correspondingly, the archaic person is not helplessly at the mercy of multiple threats from the environment, but can defend themselves against them: witches may conjure a thunderstorm to destroy a crop, but the farmer in turn may shoot skyward with his slingshot to hit the demons, or he may ally with the gods or God against them.

In summary, it can be said that magic as an expression of epistemological egocentrism is an essential component in all traditional cultures known to us (see Müller 1987, 2010) and used to cope with life in a practical way and to ward off existential threats. Since every society needs specialists to contact in case of an emergency, it should not come as a surprise that, in archaic systems, these occupations were closely linked to magical ideas. While Western medicine specializes in the treatment of isolated symptoms, traditional cultures do not focus "just on the content of the disease, but also on its context" (Selin and Shapiro 2003, p. XIX), in accordance with the rather egocentric notion that the human being is an open system in intimate interaction with the environment and its influences. One of the prototypes of this approach is shamanism, which we will now address.

2.2 The Precursor of Psychotherapy in Folk Culture

2.2.1 Shamanism and Archaic Medicine

2.2.1.1 The Shaman

What exactly makes a shaman (the following see Rieken 2011b, pp. 4–9) is widely discussed among researchers, but the majority defines the term as a person "who attained altered states of consciousness in order to mediate between human beings and the supernatural world" (Price 2001, p. I). This is tied to a dualistic attitude that distinguishes this world as a dwelling of mortal plants, animals, and people from a beyond, or otherworld, where powerful immortal spirits reside alongside the souls of the departed. These dictate "ultimately all that happens on earth" (Müller 2006, p. 38) and may therefore also be responsible for sickness.

This becomes much clearer when one considers that, in the archaic understanding, the human body consists of three elements: (1) the ephemeral body, (2) the less ephemeral vital soul which maintains the organic functions and provides the body's life force, and (3) the autonomous and immortal free soul (Müller 2006, p. 11). The "corresponding peer entities" (Müller 2006, p. 114) of the immortal spirits on Earth are the souls, especially the free souls, and it is one of the main tasks of the shaman to take care of the same in critical situations, such as in the case of sickness, and to contact the otherworldly powers.

To meet these therapeutic challenges, one needs specific skills and special training, the aim of which is a fundamental transformation. This typically includes: (1) vocation by the otherworld in the form of sickness, visions, and dreams but also one's own accord, that is, as a result of social exclusion; (2) apprenticeship with another shaman in order to get to know the structures of the invisible world, learn to diagnose sickness, and take therapeutic measures; (3) the ability to fall into a trance, control it deliberately, and withdraw from it voluntarily; (4) a public test to demonstrate the acquired skills; and (5) a vow to use them for the public good (Müller-Ebeling 2002, p. 19).

This rather prosaic listing already indicates that not everyone was called to be a shaman and that it required specific personality traits and biographical characteristics that show some similarities with those of psychotherapists. Thus, from an early age, shamans often appeared "unbalanced and nervous [...] and by nature reserved, serious, thoughtful or even brooding, not playful and happy as other children" (Müller 2006, p. 51). The vocation usually occurred during and after puberty, usually between the ages of 15–30, and it was accompanied by crises, especially since the training and future career brought about hardship, toil, and torment (Müller 2006, p. 51, 54). The initiation required isolation from the environment and often a profound change of the candidate that was induced by going on spirit journeys and killing his old self to make room for the new one which, transformed from the ground up, corresponded with his changed profession (see Kraft 1995, pp. 20–33; Müller 2006, pp. 54–61). The parallels to psychotherapeutic training are obvious, because that, too, requires isolation from the environment due to years of psychotherapeutic self-awareness and plenty of time needed to process in between the therapy sessions. The candidate also takes a journey that—while it does not lead to the spirit world—carries them to the *undiscovered country of the soul* where they meet mysterious powers and experience a transformation that enables them to deal with themselves and with their clientele and their "demons" better than before (see Zwiebel 2007).

As a psychotherapist, like the shaman, they assume a special position; although they transformed their emotional wounds productively by using them for the benefit of the community as a therapist, they often remain marked to some degree because the emotional distress caused by their own life history can never be completely healed. In addition, it is also a part of therapeutic work to absorb the patient's suffering at least partially, so in principle therapists remain at risk and must remain at risk (see Jung 1966, p. 171; Sedgwick 1994). It was similar for shamans, and possibly their profession was an even greater burden because

> "the burden of their function and the responsibility they carried for their own clearly weighed them down. Gaunt and emaciated, often tired and exhausted by the constant physical and mental overexertion, they moved slowly, sometimes downright sluggishly, did not joke and did not laugh, appeared introspective, thoughtful, serious, even dark, kept away from others in everyday life" (Müller 2006, p. 99).

This and the fact that ecstatic states occur in trances that reportedly include, among other things, dismemberment and rebirth processes and flight experiences prompted past research to reduce shamanism to a slew of psychopathological phenomena that were even given names, such as "arctic hysteria "(see Znamenski 2007, pp. 79–107). This was based on the evolutionism of the late nineteenth and early twentieth century that classified indigenous cultures with their belief in spirits as a "primitive" stage of development, while the European and North American industrial societies were considered highly developed and able to explain the "true" correlations in nature by using modern science. One of the last well-known representatives of this line of thinking was ethno-psychoanalyst Georges Devereux, who around 1970 still in all seriousness held the opinion that the acquisition of shamanistic powers was "ultimately, nothing more than an authentic 'clinical' disorder" (Devereux 1974, p. 54) and the shaman himself "a fundamentally neurotic person" (Devereux 1957, p. 1044; see Devereux 1961). His judgment of the shamans' professional work and its benefits to the community was similarly harsh and aggressive: "His immediate clinical counterpart is the psychotic child that, in a family that suffers from a latent neurosis, takes on the role of the 'acting lunatic'" (Devereux 1974, p. 56).

No one today who is in any way proficient in ethnology holds such a view, for shamans are considered to be individuals quite capable of coping with life and superior to most people in terms of physical stamina and self-control. The "illness" overtakes them only during the vocation and initiation, "then, during all later séances, they controlled the 'symptoms', used them when their function demanded it, then shook them off again. The spirits that they called, they could always get rid of" (Müller 2006, p. 108).

This means that, in contrast to psychotics, shamans can control their altered states of consciousness, and they also do not cause disturbances in social interaction as they, quite the contrary, pursue the aim of overcoming the same. Accordingly, the indigenous people do not consider them insane but someone who is able to reduce emotional suffering (see Kraft 1995, pp. 34–40; Müller 2006, p. 108; Scharfetter 1983; Silverman 1967).

In summary, it should be noted that shamans share certain similarities with psychotherapists in terms of their biography and professional work and thus may be considered their precursors. As a kind of footnote, I would like to add that there are parallels between their initiation and the life of Jesus. These are especially striking in the episode where Jesus is led into the desert by the Holy Spirit and fasts there for 40 days and nights. Not only is he totally isolated, but he must also resist the temptations of the devil. Only following that is he willing to accept his predetermined fate (Matthew 4:1–11; Mark 1:12–13; Luke 4:1–13; see Kraft 1995, pp. 96–107). Isolation, tests, and the willingness to take on the suffering of the people are clear parallels to the initiation of the shaman and psychotherapist.

2.2.1.2 Archaic Explanations for Sickness

The analogies between shamanic and psychotherapeutic work also exist in terms of archaic explanations for sickness, because they do share similarities with present views on the etiology of mental disorders. Listed below are the most important ones: they are widely used and can be found in different parts of the world and also in Western traditional folk beliefs and traditional folk medicine.

2.2.1.2.1 Losing One's Soul

That the "soul," as an irreplaceable substance needed to sustain the body's life force, can leave the body on its own accord is a view known to many peoples on Earth (Bacalzo 1996; Ellenberger 1970, pp. 6–9; Elmendorf 1952; Haller 1996; Honko 1959, pp. 27–29; Vogel 1990, pp. 19–20). For example, it may be lost when someone is scared to death, when they sneeze, or when they sleep, but it can also be stolen by evil spirits. The task of the healer is then to recover the soul and return it to the sick person. A famous tool is the "soul catchers" of the aboriginal peoples along the Canadian Pacific Coast. These are carved and richly decorated bones supposed to lure in the lost soul with their attractive design (Haller 1996, p. 304).

A typical example of losing one's soul is a sickness called *susto* in Central and South America. *Susto* means "strong fright" (Ellenberger 1970, pp. 7–9; Rubel et al. 1991). It can be caused by natural forces such as thunder and lightning or a strong storm, but also by black magic. A treatment example: the Zapotecs of the Mexican state of Oaxaca first ask the sick person where the *susto* was triggered and what caused it. Subsequently, a cleansing ceremony is performed during which an egg is passed along the body of the patient to dissipate mental and physical pressure. In the further course of treatment, the patient must return to the place where they received the *susto*. There they deliver offerings to ensure "that the soul held by a foreign power will return to the sick person and restore the mental balance so that the body will be healthy again" (Hartmann 1997, p. 80).

There are several similarities between this and psychotherapeutic treatment: the cleansing ceremony, which is performed using the egg to provide mental and physical relief, has its parallel in the liberating function of talking about the problems weighing on the soul. Moreover, it is the connection with the cause in particular that poses a parallel to psychotherapeutic treatment: the patient must return to the place of horror to be able to recover. In behavioral therapy, this corresponds with the confrontation with the anxiety-inducing object, while in psychoanalysis it is the traumas that are traced back to their origins in order to alleviate their negative effects. The return to the place of the terror's origin as practiced in archaic treatments and the delivery of offerings thus correspond to Sigmund Freud's "remembering, repeating, and working-through" ("Erinnern, Wiederholen und Durcharbeiten") (Freud 1914).

A general parallel to losing one's soul is that psychotherapy often talks about self-alienation, meaning that the patient lacks something or lost something by losing touch with themselves, something they need to rediscover in therapy. Should not, asks Ellenberger, the psychotherapist who treats severely afflicted patients and tries "to establish a contact with the remaining healthy parts of the personality and to reconstruct the ego be considered the modern successor of those shamans who set out to follow the tracks of a lost soul, trace it into the world of spirits, and fight against the malignant demons detaining it, and bring it back to the world of the living?" (Ellenberger 1970, p. 9)

2.2.1.2.2 Spirit Possession

The realm of imagination of most peoples is inhabited by a variety of spirits, some of which are given good and others bad attributes. Malevolent beings, when they enter the body of a person, take control of them, which is called "possession" (Bourguignon 2004; Ellenberger 1970, pp. 13–22; Lewis 2003; Oesterreich 1930). Oesterreich (1930) considers its most striking feature, "that the patient's organism appears to be invaded by a new personality; it is governed by a strange soul" (p. 17). This changes physiognomy and voice, the latter not speaking in a way usually associated with its owner but in terms of a new individuality: "Its ego is the latter's, and is opposed to the character of the normal individual" (Oesterreich 1930, p. 21).

It is now the task of the healer to drive out the demon, using spells, commands, curses, and the like, the Christian version of which, as is well known, is called exorcism and still practiced today by the Catholic Church (see Sect. 2.3.1.3). A common treatment method is the transference of the sickness, i.e., by casting the spirit into an animal, a well-known example of which is the Biblical healing of the possessed from the Gerasenes region by Jesus. "No one," it is said in Scripture, "was strong enough to subdue him. Night and day among the tombs and in the hills he would cry out and cut himself with stones" (NIV Bible 2011, Mark 5, 4–5). Jesus then drives out the "impure spirits" and allows them to jump into a herd of pigs. "The herd, about 2000 in number, rushed down the steep bank into the lake and were drowned" (NIV Bible 2011, Mark 5:13).

Another option is that the healer absorbs the demon and then drives it out. Another example:

> "Among the Yakuts, the sorcerer—after a long period and many phases of shamanistic rites—touches the patient with his mouth, seeming to swallow the sickness-demon, then, writhing and yelling incantations, spits the demon on the floor in order to kick and beat it out of the yurt" (Honko 1959, p. 31).

While possession is viewed as something entirely negative in societies that have been influenced by Christianity and its related belief in the devil, there are certainly examples from other regions of the world with a much more differentiated view of the phenomenon. Possession is very common in the folk form of Indian Hinduism, for example, which differentiates between possession by gods and possession by spirits. While the former is desirable because it is considered a communion with transcendent powers, the latter represents a danger because it causes sickness (Dattenberg-Holper 2002, pp. 355–356). According to Hindu belief, spirits are the dead who for some reason cannot soon be reborn. These reasons include premature death, violent death, and immoral behavior. In the period between their death and rebirth, they seek to enter living people in order to satisfy their basic drives, namely, sexuality, power, and hunger. This is why the spirits of these dead are viewed as dangerous and/or unhappy creatures dominated by evil or irrepressible desires (Dattenberg-Holper 2002, p. 356). From a psychological point of view, one would interpret them as split personality traits, which Freud already pointed out in his essay *A Seventeenth-Century Demonological Neurosis*:

> "In our eyes, the demons are bad and reprehensible wishes, derivatives of instinctual impulses that have been repudiated and repressed. We merely eliminate the projection of these mental entities into the external world which the middle ages carried out; instead, we regard them as having arisen in the patient's internal life, where they have their abode" (Freud 1923, p. 72).

In this sense, there are also parallels to psychotherapy when it comes to spirit possession as a cause of sickness in archaic medicine, especially with severe symptoms such as personality disorders or psychoses. These patients often feel haunted by strange, sinister, and destructive forces, sometimes they behave as if they were "possessed" or had "taken leave of their senses," and yet they hope for "deliverance" from their suffering. This puts great demands on the therapist as they have to deal with destructive actions and withstand massive forms of projective identification. The actually indigestible is "transferred" to them; they must, as Honko says, "swallow the sickness-demon" to later, "writhing and yelling incantations [. . .] kick and beat it out of the yurt" or drive it out into a "herd of swine."

2.2.1.2.3 Taboo Crimes

It is a widespread notion that a transgression of rules of conduct or a breach of convention, morals, and the law calls higher powers on the plan who provide physical or mental infirmity as punishment. Healing is only possible after interrogation and confession, and in addition various reconciliation or cleansing rituals may be imposed (Dein 2003; Ellenberger 1970, pp. 22–25; Honko 1959, pp. 23–27; Schmid GB 2008, Schmid JC 2008; Schmid 2010). This was, writes Ellenberger, "not a, 'disease theory', but an actual fact, confirmed by many reliable eyewitnesses" (Ellenberger 1970, p. 22). Ellenberger is absolutely right; there is a wealth of relevant reports from past and present times. This perception of sickness was particularly pronounced in the Inca culture, for example, which in addition to conventional crimes such as murder, theft, or fornication also considered disobedience to the state leaders and even the mere thought of such acts a taboo crime (Honko 1959, p. 24). This evokes associations with modern surveillance states, but also with the religious domain where such ideas are still in vogue, if one keeps in mind that, for example, according to Catholic doctrine one must not sin in thoughts, deeds, or words. Some examples may illustrate what has been said, the first one from the ethnological field (New Zealand):

> "On another occasion, while my informant resided on the same spot, passing a tapued place one day he saw some fine peaches and kumaras, which he could not resist the temptation of appropriating. On his return home, a native woman, the wife of a Sawyer, requested some of the fruit, which he gave to her, informing her, after she had eaten it, where he had obtained it. Suddenly, the basket which she carried dropped from her hands, and she exclaimed, in agony, that the attua of the chief whose sanctuary had been thus profaned would kill her. This occurred in the afternoon, and next day, by twelve o' clock, she was dead." (Brown 1845, p. 76)

The second example mentioned, however, comes from the medical field: when a 42-year-old patient with left-sided upper lobe pneumonia threatens to die in the hospital, she tells the doctor on duty that she is now receiving her just rewards. The doctor responds confidently: "Well, then you will *not* die. We will see to it that you pay the penalty above the earth and not below" (Ellenberger 1970, p. 25). She tells him then that she contracted the pneumonia in the very spot where she had cheated on her husband. Immediately thereafter, the symptoms lessen and the patient rapidly recovers (Ellenberger 1970, p. 25).

These examples will probably make the reader draw immediate connections to psychopathology and psychotherapy, since a variety of mental disorders deal with feelings of guilt or conflict. This applies primarily to the field of depression, which is one of the most common mental disorders. The relationship between guilt and infirmity is a ubiquitous pattern of interpretation, but especially common in the predominantly Christian Western world because of the close relationship between "sin" and punishment. The Bible refers to this connection as early as in Genesis, in the context of the flood narrative (Gen 6–9), and from then on—in some cases up to the present day (Rieken 2005, pp. 296–301, pp. 343–362)—it became the most prominent explanation for disasters: these are always a punishment from God for the "sinful" behavior of the people (Rieken 2013). This was illustrated, to use an example from the recent past, by the comments of strictly religious groups of people in connection with the flooding of New Orleans as a result of hurricane Katrina in 2005 (Rieken 2007).

2.2.1.2.4 Projectile

Sickness can be caused by harmful substances that penetrated a person's body in the form of a projectile. This is one of the oldest and most widespread ideas, as Finnish anthropologist Lauri Honko proved in his award-winning dissertation (Honko 1959; see Chaumeil 2004; Ellenberger 1970, pp. 9–12; Somé 2004). Even today, German phrases use comparisons such as something or an affliction having been "driven into someone" ("in jemanden gefahren") or "flown at" ("angeflogen") them. An echo of such ideas can be found in the common term "Hexenschuss" (literal translation: "witch's shot") for lumbago, for example. Martin Luther's view, according to which the sudden lower back or lumbar pain is caused by projectiles originating from witches (Grabner 1997, p. 127), is well known.

The task of the healer is to suck the projectile from the body of the afflicted person, in order to then destroy it or return it to the sender. Interesting from our perspective is the question of the reality of the projectile, because healers often already have an item at hand before the procedure starts that they present as the harmful substance afterward. This has led to Western accusations that healers were scammers, but that is not what this is about, because it is actually a part of the traditional ritual and the item must be presented in the right way at the right moment. Some people, such as the Dakota tribes, repeatedly present one and the same object and put it on public display when not in use. You could also say it has symbolic functions and serves to illustrate, similar to the Christian communion wafer (Honko 1959, pp. 204–207; p. 229). Honko thus aptly refers to the projectile explanation as a "psychotherapeutic means of illustration" (Honko 1959, p. 204).

Such ideas may seem strange or absurd, but if, for example, a patient has been relieved of a foreign object that caused them acute pain and the doctor presents it to them, this will likely trigger a relief similar to what suffering people feel in archaic societies when they see the sickness-inducing projectile. The same applies to psychotherapy when troublesome, formerly repressed experiences are examined thoroughly and the patient experiences a feeling of liberation from something that, until then, distressed or "poisoned" them. In the process, the psychotherapist must take the pathogenic patterns into themselves and then expel them—like the shaman does with the projectile. The therapist may not "suck" on the patient, but it is their task to draw out the disease. Often, this leads to a transference neurosis, which, as the therapist works through it, can be "shown" to the patient like the projectile is shown to the shaman's client (Ellenberger 1970, p. 12). Thus, in this case, the shamanic and psychotherapeutic works have in common that a "foreign object" has penetrated the patient and must be "extracted." In the case of psychotherapy, these are, among other things, problematic internalizations, for example, "introjected objects" which, when they are primarily aggressive, are construed as "bad" introjections and thus show phenomenological similarities with the projectiles of shamanism. The etymology of the noun "introjection" hints at this context, as it derives from the Latin "intro" = "inside" and "iacere" = "to throw" or "to fling."

2.2.1.3 The Professional Socialization of the Shaman and the Psychotherapist: A Comparison

In connection with the projectile explanation, an autobiographical account of the professional socialization of a shaman emerged, recorded by Franz Boas. It is about a member of the Kwakiutl Indians called Giving-Potlatches-in-the-World, who as a sorcerer was called Qā'selīd (Boas 1930, pp. 1–41; see Ellenberger 1970, pp. 9–12; Frank and Frank 1993, pp. 95–96; Znamenski 2007, pp. 117–120). Qā'selīd "desired to learn about the shaman, whether it is true or whether it is made up and (whether) they pretend to be shamans" (Boas 1930, p. 1). To find out, he takes part in a shamanic treatment in which the healer begins to suck on a spot on the patient's body where he suspects the seat of the disease and then pulls a tuft of bloody feathers from his mouth. This, he placed therein beforehand, but now explains that he sucked out the disease. Qā'selīd, though irritated, declares himself willing to undergo shamanic training. Soon he starts to do practical work, and since he is successful and the people consider him a great healer, he proceeds to dutifully conduct the shamanistic rites, defends his method of the bloody feather against other practices, and is proud of his achievements. He abandons his original goal of unmasking the shamans as frauds entirely. This is even more astonishing since, as Harry Whitehead found out, Qā'selīd was by no means a typical, indigenous tribesman, but had his roots in Western culture. His real name was George Hunt. Although his mother was a member of the Tlingit people in Alaska, his father was an Englishman who worked as a trader for the Hudson's Bay Company and brought him into contact with the achievements of European civilization (Whitehead 2000, 2009).

In his essay "The Sorcerer and his Magic" (Lévi-Strauss 1963, pp. 167–186), Lévi-Strauss explains Qā'selīd's conversion from skeptic to practicing shaman with healer, patient, and group being embedded in a common system where socially accepted symbols—in that case, among other things, the tuft of feathers as a manifestation of the disease—would emotionally affect even people who do not necessarily believe. Consequently, Lévi-Strauss writes that Qā'selīd did not become a great shaman because he cured his patients. Rather, the reason why he was so successful with his therapies was that he was considered a great shaman by the group and the sick people (Lévi-Strauss 1963, p. 180). This view certainly has its place, but it favors a linear line of argument ("if-then"), instead of assuming a set of interdependent conditions, especially since he did achieve demonstrable results at the beginning of his healing activities—as the text proclaims—only due to which the people started to consider Qā'selīd a great shaman in the first place.

Another aspect of Lévi-Strauss' ideas may be equally as one sided as the previous one as it also argues linearly, but is no less interesting. He postulates a substantial likeness between psychoanalysis and shamanism, which means he outright reverses the pathologization of shamanism conducted by senior scientists. The only difference between the two treatment methods consisted in the fact "that in the shamanistic cure the sorcerer speaks and abreacts for the silent patient, while in psychoanalysis it is the patient who talks and abreacts against the listening therapist" (Lévi-Strauss 1963, p. 183). Although this is a somewhat outdated notion of psychoanalysis, because it neglects the interdependent complexity of transference-countertransference events—viz., it ignores the fact that the therapeutic setting produces an interactional field—the indication that the healing process in both cases is connected with abreaction or emotional release is plausible (for a critical look at Lévi-Strauss, see Enderwitz 1977; Schmidbauer 1969; for similarities and differences between shamanism and psychotherapy, see Knoll 2012).

However, it is—thus following Lévi-Strauss and contradicting him at the same time—the interactional aspect in particular that helps explain structural similarities between shamanism and psychotherapy. For candidates in psychotherapeutic training programs often respond in a similar way as Qā'selīd, who initially was a skeptic and then became a practitioner, when they see for themselves only in the course of training therapy or training analysis that not everything is about interesting theories but also about the effectiveness of therapeutic methods that they are now experiencing firsthand. This is not only by virtue of individual experience but is also due to the interactional events between the teaching therapist, who generally believes in what she/he is doing, and their candidates. This mutual experience is at the same time highly charged emotionally and cannot be adequately understood in a cognitive way. From the perspective of *natural* science, this is a problem, because traditional science seeks to gain insight into the subject matter through a distanced, "objective" stance, but that is not possible in this case, because in order to understand the process, one has to "relationally engage" with it as a subject.

A typical example of this problem is the field research of Favret-Saada about witchcraft in the Bocage, a rural area in Normandy (France). The book carries the suggestive title *Deadly Words: Witchcraft in the Bocage* (Favret-Saada 1980), because the locals are of the opinion that even words are a dangerous weapon, which is why you cannot simply talk about magic since that would already mean to perform magic. Inevitably, this means one must give up the distanced perspective of the researcher and engage in the ethnographic "field": "When I was in the field, I had no choice but to accept being affected by witchcraft" (Favret-Saada 1990, p. 189).

Apparently, emotionally highly charged phenomena such as psychotherapy, shamanism, and sorcery, as well as some scientific approaches for their study, require an intersubjective methodology that relies on empathy in the sense of the German term *Einfühlung*: "In German philosophy, *Einfühlung* refers to an understanding so intimate that the feelings, thoughts, and motives of one person are readily comprehended by another" (Mossière 2007, p. 8).

However, it is necessary to make a distinction regarding the *Einfühlung*: while it is possible for the researcher to experience this only temporarily, because at some point they can leave the "field" or the research, with shamans or psychotherapists, it may result in a long-term or even lifelong identification. Michael Balint has drawn attention to the similarities between psychotherapy training and archaic initiation rites as early as in the 1940s by pointing out, "that the general aim of all initiation rites is to force the candidate to identify himself with his initiator, to introject the initiator and his ideals, and to build up from these identifications a strong superego which will influence him all his life" (Balint 1965, p. 261). He wrote this with (self-) critical intent, since he accuses the training institutions of "secretiveness about our esoteric knowledge, dogmatic announcements of our demands and the use of authoritative techniques" (ibid). This criticism has still not abated (see, i.e., Kernberg 2000, 2006, 2007; in German-speaking countries, i.e., Rieken 2003; Streeck 2008), and it reveals the Janus-faced nature of psychotherapy, which is profession and science at the same time and therefore is a field of study that is located between "faith" and science (Rieken 2011a). While it was relatively normal for the shaman and his patients—at least as long as they could be helped—to consider a worldview and the remedies derived from it as "true," today's psychotherapists are faced with a myriad of pluralistic treatment methods that all claim the right to exist (see Chap. 15). This does not necessarily lead to uncertainty within the narrower context of their own profession, but when one enters the field of academic research, some problems may arise. This includes, among other things, the allegation of a lack of intersubjective verifiability of case vignettes, which conflict with the standards of contemporary research, but it also includes the allegation of an inability to develop sufficient distance from one's own school of therapy in order to give unprejudiced consideration to and appreciate psychotherapy research, which at least raises the theoretical claim to consider all schools of psychotherapy equal, "objectively." On the other hand, the craft of psychotherapeutic work cannot simply be regarded as applied science, since it has a lot to do with life experience, intuition, *Einfühlung*, etc. And because the therapist-client experience is a shared phenomenon, treatment success is also dependent on how much the psychotherapist is convinced of the "rightness" of their method (for a discussion and empirical evidence, see Leykin and DeRubeis 2009; Wampold 2001). This tense relationship between natural science and profession, between objectivity and subjectivity, and between distance and "faith" cannot be resolved entirely (e.g., by revolving to the methods of human science) but must be endured to some degree. In this respect, the psychotherapist has at least one foot in a tradition which originated in archaic treatment methods, especially in shamanism: the belief in one's own actions and one's own method as the fruit of "archaic" initiation rites.

This applies, because the therapist-client experience is also reciprocated by the patient and his belief in the success of the therapy. The placebo effect, undisputedly effective not only with regard to drugs but also surgery, eloquently attests to that (see Wampold 2001 for a discussion). A well-known example is the study by Moseley et al., where 180 patients with osteoarthritis of the knee were randomly assigned to receive arthroscopic débridement, arthroscopic lavage, or placebo surgery. The latter only received two small incisions that were stitched up afterward, though these patients were shown images of a real surgery on a monitor to remove any doubt as to the performance of the same. Regarding the treatment success, there was no difference between the groups; 2 years later, the patients who received the placebo treatment were as satisfied as those with arthroscopic lavage or arthroscopic débridements (Moseley et al. 2002).

2.2.2 Folk Medicine in Europe and North America

This section cannot offer more than preliminary observations, because so far, the field of folk medicine in Europe and North America since the Middle Ages has not or not explicitly been examined from the research perspective of to what extent it holds precursors of psychotherapy. This is due to the fact that recorded histories barely differentiate between the healing arts of traditional indigenous peoples (see Sect. 2.2.1) and the healing arts of broad segments of the medieval and modern population of Western countries. This is why often enough examples are drawn from the field of European and North American folk medicine when archaic-shamanic healing methods are discussed (Ellenberger 1970; Frank and Frank 1993). One might assume that another reason for the difficulties in representing psychotherapeutic treatment methods used in folk medicine is that the distinction between physical and mental suffering is still new and was hardly of great importance in folk medicine. While this is true, it also applies to the field of archaic medicine or shamanism which, as we saw, definitely does share analogies with the psychotherapeutic experience, so this argument is invalid.

Nevertheless, there is heuristic value in distinguishing between folk remedies of archaic societies and those of Western premodern or modern societies. The healer of European and North American societies takes up a different position than the shaman or medicine man, because the latter is usually responsible not only for the health of the individual but also for the well-being of the group by taking over religious duties, preserving traditional mythology, or trying to influence the weather. They take up a special, exalted position, while the folk healers of Western societies are usually less isolated, as they are often people who practice without any formal training or in addition to their regular job, because they believe that they are "more capable than others" in certain areas – a somewhat cryptic description of people who are in any way considered knowledgeable about magic. In contrast to the exclusive character of the shaman, one should not underestimate the size of this group of people, because magical knowledge and magical thinking were widespread in the (European) Middle Ages and the modern period (Kieckhefer 2003, pp. 56–57). The existing source material is misleading, since medical works were written primarily by scholarly authors in the religious or medical profession, whereas folk knowledge was written down only rarely and, when dealing with magical practices, also can be problematic to collect empirically in the present. This is due to the fear of losing one's healing abilities if one reveals information about them, but legal reasons or fear of ridicule plays a role, too (Simon 2003, pp. 159–163). However, this problem can be somewhat mitigated by applying careful methods of field research and employing confidence-building measures, which were already discussed in see Sect. 2.2.1.3 in relation with Favret-Saada's research and in connection with the German term *Einfühlung*. And as for the widespread of magical thinking in the Middle Ages and the (early) modern period, this can be accessed indirectly, firstly by ecclesiastical sources and also by texts of authors in the Enlightenment tradition, because both groups—as much as they may differ in their beliefs—pay considerable attention to the fight against "superstition" and often present the contents of the same in detail.

In addition to the differing functions of the healer, there is another reason why it makes sense to differentiate between archaic and (early) modern folk medicine, and that is the dominant role of Christianity. This shows, among other things, in the widespread use of spiritual healing (faith healing), which assumes that sickness can be neutralized by divine power, such as prayers, blessings, and the like. Existing evidence ranges from the beginning of Christianity, such as Jesus healing the possessed man from the region of the Gerasenes (see Sect. 2.2.1.2.2 about spirit possession), to the present (Calestro 1972; Ehrenwald 1991, pp. 81–151; Ernst 2011; Olbrecht 1999, 2000; Schoepflin 1988). The connection with psychotherapy lies in the healing power of words, the emotions tied to them, as well as the shared worldview of the clients and their healers (see Frank and Frank 1993).

Though the Church, as already mentioned, has always tried to combat magical practices, it failed again and again, because the majority of the population saw no conflict between religious and magical practices but used both of them in perfect *syncretism*. The Church's repeated declarations of the dichotomy between religion and magic did not and do not address the reality of a broad segment of the population, because "in popular religiosity within the high religions, almost all forms of magic, from animism and magical imagery to elements of sympathetic, contagious, and imitative magic, are common" (Petzoldt 1999, p. 9). Therefore, in summary, not only the person of the healer is diverse, but folk medicine, too, is an inextricable conglomerate of empirical, magical, and religious beliefs (Hand 1980; Kieckhefer 2003, pp. 56–94; Kirkland et al. 1992; Ruff 2003; Thomas 2003; Wiegelmann 1987).

With regard to the perception of sickness, one might assume that the field of folk medicine is similar to shamanism, meaning that it includes the loss of the soul, possession, taboo crimes, and the projectile explanation (see Sect. 2.2.1.2). According to my experiences in this field though, this is only partially true, namely, with regard to possession, taboo crimes, and the projectile explanation. Because of the large number of cases that involve possession that were reported in modern period sources, possession is a frequently occurring phenomenon (see Sect. 2.3.1.3), as is the projectile explanation, because it was a widespread practice in the field of black magic in the form of the evil eye, curses, and the like. Taboo crimes also happened a lot, mainly because of the potential for conflict between Christian norms and actual behavior, which was often decried a "sin" by the Church leaders. In contrast, the loss of the soul appears to have been too archaic an explanation for sickness to have spread widely in the folk medicine of the early modern period. Stories about it exist primarily in the context of popular belief, the most common version being that the souls of witches could leave their sleeping body and cause harm (Frenschkowski 2007, p. 484; Meier 1852, p. 184). This is because Christian thinking tended to project all evil onto marginalized people, and it need not surprise that not only did "pagan" and Christian thought go hand in hand but also, as mentioned above, magical and religious elements meshed into an inextricable tangle in folk medical practices. The following example from the sixteenth century shows this clearly:

> "A young woman from Lyon was ailing because a witch put a hate spell on her at the request of her jealous mother-in-law. She could not bear the sight of her husband and his presence. A famous sorcerer examined the woman, put her in chains and rubbed her down with tree bark. Then he filled a cup with herbs, ensorceled it with incantations, and bit the young woman in the arm" (Ruff 2003, p. 80). Gradually, she recovered, but was plagued by severe pain caused by a needle that had migrated from her heart. The sorcerer pulled it out with another bite to the forearm (Ruff 2003, p. 80). "Meanwhile, an abbot, who had been sent for, arrived. A lay brother now pulled the remaining needles effortlessly from the body. They were kept as evidence for years. 'The Abbot touched the wound amid prayers and swore by the virtue of his faith that no more iron or steel would come out. And so it happened, alas the substance changed: small oak or ash wood chips and thicker blackthorns, sixteen pieces in a day.' After prayers, absolution, and the holding of a mass, the last in a series of wood chips appeared. It was shown publicly in the chapel. After that, the patient was healed and appreciated her husband again" (Ruff 2003, p. 80).

In this example, magical folk medicine and Christian treatment methods go hand in hand: a "famous sorcerer" examines the patient; makes a diagnosis (hate spell), probably with her help; and takes therapeutic measures that may be part empirical (herbs), part magical (incantations). While he is successful, the patient then suffers from severe pain, the cause of which, however, he recognizes (needle in the body) and fixes in accordance with the projectile explanation (bite to the forearm). But then the clergymen come along—why, we do not know, maybe the sorcerer was overwhelmed, maybe news of the woman's sickness had already spread and called the Church representatives on the plan, because the expulsion of items was considered a sure sign that someone had been hexed in the early modern period (Ruff 2003, p. 79). This also explains why the objects were shown publicly in the chapel after the medical procedure: they were meant to demonstrate the superiority of the Church over demonic powers and at the same time exhort people to live a God-fearing life.

In addition to the projectile explanation, taboo crimes also seem to play a role, because in the Christian understanding hating your spouse is a sin. From a psychotherapeutic perspective, it is interesting that the source of the curse is the negative or perceived negative attitude of the mother-in-law towards the patient, as is the violent aggression the patient developed towards her husband. In this context, the swallowing of objects also has meaning, be it real as harmful behavior towards one's own person or imagined as a hysterical mode, but both probably in the context of self-punishment mechanisms due to a guilty conscience.

That apparently the objects contained in the patient's body reached the surface through magical-religious procedures may seem as strange to us as the curse as an expression of black magic, but in the context of an early modern attitude towards life, which was shaped by magical thinking, these are appropriate therapeutic measures. After all, as we are assured by the source, they did lead to the desired results, especially since magical measures were and are an expression of practical life aid, as anthropologist Margaret Ruff aptly explained in her thesis (Ruff 2003). In this respect, the folk medical-magical procedures of the early modern period are indeed quite important for the history of psychotherapy.

The second example does not lead us into the past, but takes place in the present and my own psychoanalytic-therapeutic practice (Rieken 2012). It leads us to magical mental structures as they are still alive today in Eastern Europe, in this case in Serbia. One day, an about 35-year-old woman came to me requiring therapy for a panic disorder that had started after her husband was first diagnosed with liver carcinoma and then, on top of that, suffered a stroke shortly after the surgery. In the course of the anamnesis, it turned out that the patient's relationship with her husband was characterized by vehemently repressed feelings of hatred that resulted in an unconscious death wish against him. This was fulfilled in some way by the liver carcinoma and the stroke, which is why she responded with extreme feelings of anxiety, especially since she had been suffering from massive abandonment issues since early childhood. A psychoanalyst could henceforth simply have treated the unconscious conflict, but the problem went deeper than it seems. When the patient talked about her fear of the dark in one of the subsequent therapy sessions, I asked her if she was afraid of demons—and she answered this question in the affirmative. In her village, she explained, there were two old women who as witches dealt in black magic. Her husband's house was also tainted, because in their parents' generation, one of the children died early for a neighbor did some harm to them with the evil eye. Also, something had been off with her oldest daughter, because when she had been a child, she had cried constantly. Only when a wise woman from her village had advised her to turn her daughter's clothes inside out had she quieted down. This measure is a common form of defensive magic in traditional societies: confuse the malicious spirits—which are not necessarily considered particularly smart beings—and thus render them harmless.

In addition, she reported that her husband had been cursed several times, among others, by a neighbor of his first wife as well as by the patient's sister-in-law, who she said dealt in a particularly effective form of black magic, because she had help from a priest of another religion—a common belief in countries where Catholic, Orthodox, and Muslim clerics are of equal importance. This shows that in the popular belief not only is the perceived or real contradiction of religion and magic difficult to comprehend, but that, on the contrary, clergymen who are not members of one's own church may under certain circumstances be considered capable of particularly nasty abilities in the field of black magic.

After the patient gave an account of manifold curses, I asked her whether she herself may have once cursed her husband: after some hesitation, she answered "yes." This makes the panic attacks as a result of her husband's illness even more understandable: this is not simply about unconscious wish fulfillment in the psychoanalytic sense and being frightened by it but also about wish fulfillment and being frightened by it in the context of magical thinking.

In this case, it would be a mistake to assume a severe psychopathology, such as from the areas of paranoid schizophrenia, paranoia, or schizotypal disorder, because delusion is characterized primarily as a private reality through which the patient is removed from their relationship with others and their environment. But the world in which the patient lives is shaped both by normal social contact and the fact that she shares her magical ideas with a great number of people from her home village and also with some people in Vienna, her current home, who are important to her (Rieken 2012, pp. 102–104).

This is interesting for several reasons. For one, it is important for the diagnosis of mental illness with regard to immigrants from countries where magical thinking is more prevalent than in Western societies. With them, one needs to be careful with hasty pathologizing because it neglects the cultural context (see Gelo et al. in press for a discussion), in abovementioned case, the widespread acceptance of magical thinking in Eastern Europe. Viewed in this light, the history of psychotherapy also affects its present. The premodern period, as already mentioned, is heavily influenced by a worldview that perceives people not so much as defined individuals but rather as open systems, that is, as someone in a reciprocal relationship with multiple external influences (see Sect. 2.1).

The fact that a mental illness of the person concerned is put in a magical context also demands a "division of labor" type of therapeutic process. I can explain to the patient, for example, that the psychotherapist, in this case my person, is responsible for the psychological treatment of the panic disorder, something with which I have made some considerable progress (Rieken 2012, pp. 109–112), but with regard to the curse she is under, I do not have the means to help her. Thus she knows to maintain her contact with people knowledgeable about magic in order to neutralize the dreaded consequences of the curse, in addition to the psychotherapy sessions. Under no circumstances would I advise to try to rid the patient of their "superstition" in such cases where there is no doubt about the existence of black magic, because that would only alienate the patient from psychotherapy and/or the therapist. Driven by the impetus to "enlighten," one would achieve the opposite of what one wanted to achieve, especially considering how much is already gained if the patient placed so much trust in the psychotherapist as a representative of "enlightened" Western medicine that they admitted to being rooted in magical thinking.

The two case vignettes presented here are intended to illustrate not only the close relationship between Christian and magical thinking but also draw attention to a possible link between magic and psychotherapy. Both examples feature a curse the clients are diagnosed with, which is traced back to family dynamics and treated in a "division of labor" type of process by several healers, in the first case sorcerer and priests and in the second case people knowledgeable about magic and a psychoanalyst. Although the examples are taken from different eras, namely, the early modern period and the present, they do show structural similarities. They illustrate that magical thinking is an expression of Piaget's epistemological egocentrism and that people are perceived as open systems in intimate interaction with the supernatural influences that affect them, but which they are capable of affecting in turn. These are deep-seated structures that have not become completely obsolete even in modern societies and thus count among the *vulgus in populo*, the "folk in the population," to use a term from older European ethnology (Hoffmann-Krayer 1946, p. 2). In other words, they tell of the "simultaneity of the nonsimultaneous" as a mark of the modern period.

2.3 Precursors of Psychotherapy in Advanced Civilizations

2.3.1 Religion and the Church

2.3.1.1 Sickness as a Result of Sin and as an Expression of the Divine Plan of Salvation

As mentioned earlier (see Sect. 2.2.1.2.3 about taboo crime), sickness was often considered a punishment from higher powers for a violation of rules or commandments. In the primarily Christian world, this was a common interpretation pattern that, in its specific form, is relevant for the history of psychotherapy, which is why it is mentioned here: while the idea of sin as a cause of sickness is ubiquitous in traditional societies, the notion that, on top of this, sickness and evil are to be considered in the context of a divine plan is characteristic for Christian civilization. Medical historian Rothschuh called this concept *iatrotheology* (Rothschuh 1978, pp. 47–72), a term that is now enshrined in German-speaking medical history (Gerabek et al. 2005, pp. 657–658). In the Old Testament, mental and physical sickness or disasters such as famines, floods, and locust plagues are often considered divine punishment. The following passage from the Book of Deuteronomy is a typical example that explains what happens when people do not obey God:

> "The LORD will plague you with diseases until he has destroyed you from the land you are entering to possess. The LORD will strike you with wasting disease, with fever and inflammation, with scorching heat and drought, with blight and mildew, which will plague you until you perish" (Deut. 28, 21–22). And a few lines later it says: "The LORD will afflict you with madness, blindness and confusion of mind" (Deut. 28, 28).

In the course of Church history, the belief that illness and misfortune were a tool for the perfection of man in God's plan of salvation became equally important as the view that they were punishments for sinful behavior. For example, it says in the *Lorscher Arzneibuch* (*Lorscher Pharmacopoeia*), an eighth-century medical compendium: "Very beneficial is indeed a sickness that shatters the hardness of the spirit, yet very pernicious is health that leads man into disobedience" [Stoll 1992, p. 55; original text: "Valde enim salubris est infirmitas, quae mentem a durutia frangit, sed valde perniciosa sanitas, quae ad inoboedientiam hominem ducit" (Stoll 1992, p. 54)]. Thus, from an iatrotheological perspective, sickness may signify many things: it delivers people from sin and is a means for the purpose of internal refinement, trial, or purification, a sign of God's omnipotence through auspicious healing, or the healing itself may be an act of grace for a soul God loves especially [Gerabek et al. 2005, pp. 657–658 (with further references), p. 803; Rothschuh 1978, pp. 47–72; Vollmer 2011]. Given the importance of the iatrotheological concept of sickness, the claim of a well-known psychotherapy textbook that "a somatogenic (humoral) and demonological understanding of mental illness" prevailed in historical times can hardly be maintained (Hautzinger 2007, p. 10; see Jütte 1996, p. 67).

The interesting thing about the iatrotheological model is that health and sickness are relativized before the backdrop of the Christian doctrine of salvation and thus lose their unambiguousness. Someone who is bursting with health my go astray when they forget about God, while someone else may come to their senses only due to illness and thus choose the right path. Similarly to the psychotherapy of the present, this is about nothing less than the question of the "right" life. Nowadays, someone may be professionally very successful, but the driving force behind it may be narcissistic deficits, so the outward bustle is supposed to conceal an inner emptiness. Conversely, someone who leads an outwardly diminished life in comparison to others due to a depressive disposition may actually be a thoughtful person inside with a wide knowledge of philosophy and draw from this to give meaning to their life. The questions one asks about life that provide information about the value of the same are therefore similar in the context of the Christian worldview of the past and a contemporary psychotherapeutic framework. Only the answers differ, because they conform to the respective historical background.

The similarities between the worldviews become even more apparent when considered in the context of Aristotelian causality. A fundamental aspect of this is the distinction between the efficient cause and the final cause (Aristotle 1992, 194b–195b), which in the scholastic reception of Thomas Aquinas are referred to as *causa efficiens* and *causa finalis* (Thomas of Aquin 2011, lib. 1 l. 4 n. 2; see Chap. 4). The *causa efficiens* is the classic cause of modern understanding, because it asks "whence" and "why." For Aristotle, however, the final cause was more important, because it focuses on the self-concept of people whose actions usually can only be sufficiently understood when one knows the goal—aim, intention, purpose, and meaning—linked to it. However, this is not an attempt to pit the *causa efficiens* and the *causa finalis* against each other, but to discuss them as equals, because they complement each other. While the *causa efficiens* directs our attention to the past by asking "whence," the *causa finalis* draws attention to the future by focusing on the "where to" and "why." This covers essential areas when someone is striving not only to understand problems or setbacks but also to overcome them.

Both causes are essential for iatrotheology as well as psychotherapy. From an efficient-causal perspective, God punishes people because they have sinned in the past. But the action is also final causal insofar as that he is trying to bring them to their senses so they will lead a life in accord with the Christian order in the future. He endeavors to protect them from further temptations and to lead them into a more conscious life. The situation is similar in the psychological field: current problems that prompt a person to seek therapeutic treatment generally originate in the past. Someone who cheats on his wife, for example, may have a shared history with her that has not been very satisfactory for some time (*causa efficiens*). He may want to improve his life by cheating and unconsciously even give his own marriage fresh impetus, provided he has the hope that his wife, when she learns the truth, will not separate from him but put more effort into their relationship (*causa finalis*). If the man is now having erection problems when having sex with another woman or is starting to suffer from a guilty conscience that causes a depressive state, then this is, from an efficient-causal perspective, an inner conflict between base instincts and morality, while from a final-causal point of view, the unconscious goal is to refrain from the undesirable behavior.

Thus, there are some analogies to the Christian context, which would speak of sin, guilt, and catharsis with reference to the above example, whereas in the psychotherapeutic context, the descriptions used would be more along the line of *feelings* of guilt and problem handling or similar terms. The difference between the two fields is therefore mainly the fact that a psychotherapist does not act as a judgmental but as an understanding and accompanying instance that does not lay down rules of conduct but primarily listens, so that the patient can *talk* about the problems that distress them. This, however, provides another similarity that will be the focus of the following chapter.

2.3.1.2 Confession

A fundamental connection between psychotherapy and religion is confession, which is an institution inherent in Christianity. The commonality between the two lies in the fact that they both offer patterns of self-thematization to the individual so they may talk about themselves and their shortcomings (see Scheule 2001, p. 227). To express something burdensome often has a cathartic function; this applies to psychotherapy, which was called the "talking cure" by Sigmund Freud's and Josef Breuer's famous patient Anna O. (Freud and Breuer 1895, p. 30), as well as to confession. The etymology of the English term is narrower than that of the German word ("Beichte"). While the former is reduced to the semantic content of an "admission" and furthermore denotes the religious avowal, the latter traces back to the Old High German noun "bigiht" ("promise," "confession") (Schützeichel 1974, p. 15) which in turn derives from the Old High German verb "jehan," which in addition to the rather specific "confess" also includes the less specific meanings "speak" and "say" (Schützeichel 1974, p. 93f.). Thus, an etymological connection exists between speech and admission or confession that provides mental relief, which demonstrates that *homo narrans* is a fundamental anthropological category of our species, because talking contributes to self-assurance and problem relief to a decisive extent. It is primarily about things that have not been talked about, a secret that burdened the individual and alienated them from other people. Both, however, are essential for psychotherapy as well as for confession, which was already pointed out by C.G. (Jung 1933, p. 31; see Kidder 2010, pp. 230–232).

One big difference between psychotherapy and confession, however, is that the former is focused on the major difference between sickness and health, whereas the latter concentrates on grace and sin. As already indicated at the end of the last chapter, this is connected with another difference, namely, the difference between *feelings* of guilt and guilt or sin, meaning between subjective self-attribution in relation to alleged or actual norm violations and "objective" violations of the religious or moral order. Regarding this, the psychotherapist is not an attorney of a "higher power" who sits in judgment over right and wrong, good and evil, but primarily a companion who is supposed to understand the patient. If Christian authors of today find that the loss of importance of confession in present times had to do with the growing importance of psychotherapy (Kidder 2010, pp. 230–242), then this is due to exactly this circumstance, namely, that—unlike the priest—the therapist does not consider themselves an attorney of an "objective" higher power, but primarily refers to the subjectivity of the patient. This is an appropriate attitude towards the plurality of lifestyles in the postmodern societies of the present, which have difficulties with "objective" engagement. The individualization processes of modern times that implemented this development require emotional healing in a context where two individuals meet and learn to trust each other. This takes time, which is why the relationship between therapist and patient is much more intimate than the one between priest and penitent.

Conversely, one might speculate whether traditional societies with their more hierarchical structure facilitated mental relief and behavioral changes by means of confession to a greater extent than today. That is to say, individualization, as already explained in Sect. X.1, also means an increase in complexity, and as individuality and self-identity played a lesser role in times past and collective orientation patterns dominated instead, this may have made changes easier than today.

In this context, it is perhaps logical—albeit, from a different perspective, also amazing—that the European Church throughout its history has not created any kind of treatment method from the three elements sin, confession, and repentance, although similarities exist in particular with regard to taboo crimes (see Sect. 2.2.1.2.3 about taboo crimes). "All elements," writes Lauri Honko, "for this are, *each on its own*, available: sin, the divine punishment for which is sickness, and the confession of sin that frees man from sin and its consequences" (Honko 1959, p. 25). One may speculate about the reasons; maybe it seemed sufficient to give moral and educational instruction—and maybe that was enough in the context of traditional societies. Regardless, the Church will have feared a "contamination" with elements from the field of folk medicine, since secular healers, as discussed in the last chapter, usually worked "syncretically" by blending Christian with magical healing rituals and did not consider this inappropriate at all.

Let's leave it at that. Apart from the fact that an overview cannot delve into the issue in depth, these are questions that—explicitly in the context of a psychotherapy historiography—are yet largely unexplored. Though it would be particularly interesting to see how effectual the options for relieving mental distress as provided in times past were in the context of the mental background of the respective era and insofar comparable with current psychotherapy, which, given the complexity of the modern individual, is linked with high expectations. One way to reduce this academic void, for example, might be to use sources like autobiographical reports from the past that focus on personal processes of change, but also empirical-qualitative research that does the same for traditional societies of the present. Even though one must always be aware of the effects of the industrialized modern period on the latter, some analogous conclusions should certainly be possible.

2.3.1.3 Possession and Exorcism

While confession is rather similar to a therapy session that is carried out in a relatively calm way, possession is an extraordinary phenomenon that matches most closely with certain phases of very severe mental illnesses, such as psychosis or some personality disorders. The demons invoked in exorcism thus correspond with destructive split personality traits, which was already pointed out in Sect. X.2.1.2 about spirit possession, with reference, among other things, to Freud's essay *A Seventeenth-Century Demonological Neurosis* (Freud 1923).

It is interesting that, in the course of history, possession phenomena were not only observed with individuals but also entire collectives. Well-known examples are the Salem (Massachusetts) witch trials in the late seventeenth century (Boyer and Nissenbaum 2002; Caporael 1976) or the Annaberg witch hunts in the Erzgebirge (Ore Mountains) in the early eighteenth century (Rychlak 2001, 2009). Depending on the scientific perspective, the assumed causes are social conflicts and psychological influences such as mass hysteria, but also physiological components, ergotism (ergot poisoning), in the case of Salem and Annaberg. Poisoning as a cause has been proved, at least for an incident in the recent past that has gone down in history under the name of "l'affaire du pain maudit" ("The Case of the Cursed Bread"). This occurred in 1951 in the southern French town of Pont-Saint-Esprit where contaminated bread caused symptoms of a mass psychosis (see Kaplan 2008). I mention this because a recent publication argues that the CIA wanted to test the effects of LSD and for this purpose exposed the population of Pont-Saint-Esprit to the drug (Albarelli 2008, pp. 270–279). The legitimate and extensive research of historian Steven Kaplan (Kaplan 2008) proves that this is hardly possible, but it shows that even in the secular society of the present, substitutes for the devil and other demons may be found, in this case the CIA, which some people believe capable of every conceivable evil.

It would take up too much space to go into detail about collective possession here. It makes more sense instead to focus on a single historical event in order to illustrate the similarities with certain phases of the psychotherapeutic process when it comes to serious mental illness. The one about to be presented here is well documented and was also made available to an English-speaking readership by Ellenberger's monograph (Ellenberger 1970, pp. 18–22). It is the case of a 28-year-old woman named Gottliebin Dittus, who was possessed by demons and was successfully treated by the evangelical pastor Johann Christoph Blumhardt. The story takes place in Möttlingen, a town in the Black Forest, in the years from 1842 to 1843 and is documented in the clergyman's records (Blumhardt 1979; see Ising 2002, pp. 148–169); there are also depth-psychological interpretations of the case, among which the work of psychiatrist and psychosis specialist Gaetano Benedetti (Benedetti 1960; further literature in Ellenberger 1970, pp. 21–22) should be noted in particular.

Since 1840, Gottliebin Dittus lived in poverty with her siblings in the downstairs apartment of a haunted house. "What you heard was a recurrent banging and slurping in the chamber, living room, and kitchen that sometimes lasted all night, which often frightened the poor siblings very much, also worried the people living upstairs, as much as they were shy of letting this be known" (Blumhardt 1979, vol. 1, p. 34). When the banging increased until it was also heard by the neighbors and all the attention of the village focused on the haunted house, Blumhardt as the local pastor was forced to act. Following his advice, Gottliebin moved in with a cousin; while the haunting of the old dwelling stopped, though, it continued at the new location. On top of that, Gottliebin was shaken by convulsions and foaming at the mouth. A few days later, Blumhardt heard her speaking in a strange voice. When he talked to her, he learned that it was the spirit of a deceased woman who had murdered her two children and could not find peace. Then Gottliebin told him of many other demons that were around and inside her, though at first his intervention caused her condition to worsen: "She beat her chest, plucked out her hair, writhed like a worm, and seemed to be a completely lost person" (Blumhardt 1979, vol. 1, p. 44). Still the pastor stayed loyal to her, and gradually she started to trust him, especially when painful bleedings she had suffered and which the doctor who had been called had not been able to stop "ended the day I first began to seriously attend to her" (Blumhardt 1979, vol. 1, p. 45). He then also took up the fight against the demons who felt more and more pressured: "No one in the world," they said to him, "would have cast us out; only you, with your eternal praying and holding on, prevailed" (Blumhardt 1979, vol. 1, p. 48). Another demon, though, showed remorse and wanted to come into the church. Initially frightened, Blumhardt then answered: "If you promise me that you won't bother anyone and will never become visible, on the condition that Jesus gives you his permission, I do not mind" (Blumhardt 1979, vol. 1, p. 53). Only Gottliebin then saw the demon in the far corner of the church building, but after some time it disappeared. In the end, she was completely healed and her strength was coming back. She was much obliged to Blumhardt, and after some time she was accepted into his home, where she became not only "my wife's truest and wisest aide in matters of the household and child rearing" (Blumhardt 1979, vol. 1, p. 77) but also "virtually indispensable for the treatment of mentally ill people, because they soon place the most unreasonable trust in her, so that my dealing with them requires little time" (Blumhardt 1979, vol. 1, pp. 77–78).

Benedetti stresses that in the "attempt to interpret the known medical history of Gottliebin Dittus, which was written down by Pastor Blumhardt in 1848, [...] the similarity between his experiences and those of our medical procedure" catches the eye (Benedetti 1960, p. 474). This opinion is justified, because the notable characteristic in the pastor's report is that he did not really carry out an exorcism—thus violently using force against force—but first of all was merely there for Gottliebin by giving her pastoral care and supporting her and her demons, and he did this, as he points out frequently, through prayer and fasting. Only after she came to trust him did he become more active and dealt with the numinous figures. This at first led to a worsening of her condition, as is often the case in psychotherapy when changes are imminent, but he held out against all the hostility. He was able to do this because of his worldview, namely, that good may defeat evil at the end if one makes an effort, which connected him with his identity and offered him stability much like the therapist should be convinced of the effectiveness of their actions. Not only did he remain steadfast, but, as any experienced therapist, he was also flexible in the event of unusual questions in that, for example, he allowed a particular demon to retreat into the church building, provided Jesus gave permission.

Other similarities with a professional psychotherapeutic attitude are that Blumhardt did not condemn Gottliebin, who cast the worst aspersions on him, but held out against them and tried to understand her: it was the demons that spoke through her, not she herself. Thus he saw, without judging her, her ambivalence: "She felt tied down with a certain force on one side, the Satanic; and at her core she was searching for the other side, the divine" (Blumhardt 1979, vol. 1, p. 72). In addition, Blumhardt had a sense for the importance of childhood influences on later life, for he writes that the origins of her behavior were to be found in this period, as sorcerers had tried to get a hold of Gottliebin from a young age, by snatching her from her mother: her mother "often told her that she'd had the child next to her in bed, and in her sleep suddenly became anxious about the child [...]. Something fell to the ground by the chamber door, and it was the child" (Blumhardt 1979, vol. 1, p. 68). Looking at the symbolism and transferring the results to a therapeutic framework, one might speculate that the spatial separation between mother and child at night, the child falling to the floor, and the fears of the mother caused traumatic effects.

Also interesting is the happy ending of the story. A mutually trusting relationship develops, which is so stable that Blumhardt and his wife not only assign Gottliebin educational responsibilities for their children, but Blumhardt also allows her to attend to "mentally ill people, because they soon place the most unreasonable trust in her" (Blumhardt 1979, vol. 1, p. 78). Apparently she was able, like it is often the case with psychotherapists, to transform her afflictions and traumas into something productive—and it was a very severe affliction, perhaps comparable with the well-known case history of psychoanalyst Marguerite Sechehaye, in which she describes how her patient Renée was cured of psychosis (Sechehaye 1956)—the same Renée who she adopted later and who then became a psychoanalyst herself under the name Louisa Sechehaye-Duess (Cifali 2005).

The three elements of pastoral care and of dealing with problems in life described in this chapter—sickness as a result of sin and as an expression of the divine plan of salvation, confession, and the expulsion of demons—demonstrate that there are remarkable analogies to psychotherapy. It is possible that this is an adequate response to emotional problems in a thoroughly Christian-oriented world that has not yet been caught up in processes of individualization and where people identify themselves primarily through groups and collective orientation patterns. Under these conditions, people are more willing to submit to authority than in a society defined by the idea of self-realization. In this respect, it seems to be not only the directive element characteristic for traditional societies that makes it easier to influence the psyche than is the case in modern Western societies, but also dichotomous worldviews that may lack differentiating nuances but make a clear distinction between good and evil.

2.3.2 Philosophy

While the Christian religion is steered and controlled by intellectual elites but claims to serve broad segments of society, philosophy is to a large extent a concern of cultural elites for cultural elites without direct impact on the majority of the population. Still it is relevant in the context of a history of psychotherapy, because the two fields share some common ground.

The term "philosophy" comes from ancient Greek and means "love of wisdom." The latter is described as a basic human mind-set, which is based on life experience and the understanding of life in terms of its origin and its meaning and also addresses so-called essential questions (see Speer 2004). Similar to religion, the focus is also and in particular the problem of the "right" life, though while religion attaches great importance to faith, philosophy advocates rational activity. From today's perspective, which increasingly draws attention to psychological factors, these perceptions are too one sided, because they underestimated or underestimate the role of emotions and affects. A classic example for this is the philosophy of the Enlightenment, the first great practical application of which in politics, namely, the French Revolution, ended in a bloodbath and the subsequent reinstitutionalization of monarchy. Nevertheless, in the long run, the Enlightenment contributed to the humanization of society, in that, for example, the Fundamental Rights have been incorporated in the constitutions of Western democracies, which had a broad impact on the distribution of the ideas of equality and self-realization of man, among other things, which is also important for psychotherapy (see Rieken 2011b, pp. 13–21).

However, these are processes that went on for centuries and effectively changed the lives of individuals only in homeopathic doses. Therefore, it is not a surprise that at the end of the twentieth century, which historian Eli Zaretsky dubbed "Freuds Jahrhundert" (according to the German translation of Zaretsky 2004; the English translation is "Freud's Century") and which is marked to an increasing extent by a "culture of self-help" (Illouz 2008), philosophy, too, delves into the issue of how more rapid processes of individual change might be facilitated. The discipline that focuses on this was established in the German-speaking countries in the early 1980s and calls itself "Philosophische Praxis" ("Philosophical Practice") (Achenbach 1984; Ruschmann 1999; Staude 2010), while the English-language counterpart is called "Philosophical Counseling" (Marinoff 2002; Raabe 2001) and was established in the United States in the early 1990s. It is a form of life coaching, its relationship to psychotherapy controversial (see Achenbach and Macho 1985; Achenbach 2010a, b; Brandt 2010; Schuster 1999), but the lowest common denominator being the "clarification and orientation through independent, critical thinking" (Staude 2010, p. 7), with the addendum that "the critical reflection of oneself, of one's own development and contingencies [remains] a central challenge of human growth as a person and a sustainable development of society" (Staude 2010, p. 7).

An important theoretical basis of philosophical practice—to circle back to the history of psychotherapy now—is maieutic, called the art of midwifery, which is attributed to Socrates (see Lütchen 2013; Ruschmann 1999; Schuster 1999; see also Overholser 1993a, b, 1994, 1995, 1996, 1999; Maranhão 1986). It was passed down to us through Plato's dialogue *Theaetetus*, where he puts the following words in Socrates' mouth:

> "All that is true of their art of midwifery is true also of mine, but mine differs from theirs in being practised upon men, not women, and in tending their souls in labor, not their bodies. But the greatest thing about my art is this, that it can test in every way whether the mind of the young man is bringing forth a mere image, an imposture, or a real and genuine offspring. For I have this in common with the midwives: I am sterile in point of wisdom, and the reproach which has often been brought against me, that I question others but make no reply myself about anything, because I have no wisdom in me, is a true reproach" (Plato 2006, 150b, c).

If he says at the beginning of the quote, "all that is true of their art of midwifery is true also of mine," then this refers to a spiritual midwifery, which explains the paradox in the following sentence that this referred to men and not to women and also not to the body but to the soul. Because this was the patriarchal world of ancient Greece, where philosophy was reserved for men. The biggest similarity between the real and the philosophical art of midwifery, according to Socrates, is that one does not give birth oneself, but only assists in the birth process.

In other words, by asking the appropriate questions, one can help someone else gain greater awareness by making them track down the facts in question independently and thus "give birth" to insight. At this point, there are similarities to the psychotherapeutic process, provided it is designed to be nondirective and allows the patient to approach knowledge they already have through appropriate questions. Another aspect, however, when transferred to psychotherapy, only works in part, namely, that maieutic claims to be able to verify whether the mind of the young man "is bringing forth a mere image, an imposture, or a real and genuine offspring." Because every psychotherapist knows errors and wrong turns in the process and more than a few therapies end with only conditional success or even cancelation. On the other hand, when everything goes well, patients are taught to pay better attention to their own needs, and they gain autonomy, so that they then are able, to some degree, to verify themselves whether they are dealing with "a mere image, an imposture, or a real and genuine offspring."

The obvious question for psychoanalysts, whether the "birthing" of knowledge that someone was not previously aware of constitutes "unconscious knowledge," will only be touched upon briefly here. Gottfried Fischer, who has made great contributions to the philosophical foundations of psychotherapy as an independent science see Chap. 4, answered this question with a resounding "yes" (Fischer 2008, p. 106; Fischer 2011, p. 20). We, however, are a little more skeptical about this approach, because one must keep in mind that the concept of the unconscious was completely alien in ancient times and it could also only have been applied to the soul if the authors of that time had made distinctions between different parts that allowed at least analogies to the unconscious, preconscious, and consciousness, or the id, ego, and superego. But that is not the case, as although there is a tripartite division of the soul in Plato as there is in Freud, it is designed in analogy to the structure of the State and its estates as he created them in his republic. Plato distinguishes the "appetitive" (epithymētikón), the "spirited/passionate" (*thymós*), and the "logical" (*logistikón*) ability (Plato 2000, 439d; 441e) and links the logical ability to the wisdom of the rulers and the spirited/passionate ability to the bravery of the warriors, while the appetitive ability corresponds to the third class, the common people, and the craftsmen. Regardless, one should remember that maieutic is not less focused on emotional processes as on the gaining of knowledge. In contrast to this, psychotherapy is much more than a philosophical conversation because, although new knowledge is generated, it is also concerned with new relationship experiences and the satisfaction of emotional needs or deficits. Nevertheless, Fischer is right about one thing: the common ground between maieutic and psychotherapy is that both aspire to shine a light on knowledge that somebody possesses in potentiality but not yet in reality in their "logical ability," but which can be teased out by clever questions. Insofar, philosophy with its specific technique of maieutic has in fact earned a worthy place in the history of psychotherapy.

Conclusion

The history of psychotherapy is a short one, because it barely reaches back to the nineteenth century, but the prehistory of psychotherapy can be traced back all the way to illiterate cultures. However, if one was to measure the practices of the archaic and the premodern period by today's standards, then the methods, particularly in the fields of shamanism and folk medicine, would inevitably appear strange, archaic, or abstruse, especially since in the perception of human or written sources, they are often associated with so-called superstitious and supernatural phenomena. But when one considers the traditional treatment methods in the context of their time, it becomes clear that a large number of them is used "by modern psychotherapy, even though in a different form" (Ellenberger 1970, p. 3). If you consider that, you can recognize them as sincere efforts to deliver people from physical, emotional, and mental distress. They also demonstrate that, due to the similarities between traditional and contemporary psychotherapeutic treatment methods, it seems that there is a limited repertoire of treatment methods in terms of structure that has proven effective throughout the epochs (see Frank and Frank 1993; see also Chap. 4). Thus, people could learn from the past, the patient, as well as the professional or scientist.

In addition, the historical perspective teaches us two things: first, that in ancient societies, healing usually went hand in hand with meeting spiritual needs and, second, that no difference was made between physical and mental suffering. The former may not be transferable without modification to the secularized societies of the Western modern period, but what is still worth considering is the question of the meaning of life, which arises again and again in the case of severe mental shocks, as demonstrated by the high suicide rate in certain mental disorders, among other things. The other aspect—the unity of body, soul, and spirit—is connected with this, because it clearly shows that previous eras favored a holistic approach of looking at people, which is obviously a basic human need. It is important to consider, though, whether the contemporary mainstream of psychotherapy research is suited to fully understand phenomena such as wholeness and meaning, because the ideal of objectivity in association with the model of functional dependencies that aims to identify causal relationships as precisely as possible is not generally concerned with these phenomena. To answer the question why the mainstream does not concern itself with this, another look back in history might be in order, in this case the history of science, because this shows that in the course of the development of modern science since about 1500, important strands for the understanding of the *conditio humana*, the human condition, have been lost. This is what the next chapter is all about.

References

Achenbach GB (1984) Philosophische Praxis. Verlag für Philosophie Dinter, Köln

Achenbach GB (2010a) Philosophie, Philosophische Praxis und Psychotherapie. In: Achenbach GB (ed) Zur Einführung der Philosophischen Praxis. Vorträge, Aufsätze, Gespräche und Essays, mit denen sich die Philosophische Praxis in den Jahren 1981 bis 2009 vorstellte. Eine Dokumentation. Verlag für Philosophie Dinter, Köln, pp 289–303

Achenbach GB (2010b) Philosophische Praxis als Alternative zu Psychotherapie und Seelsorge. In: Achenbach GB (ed) Zur Einführung der Philosophischen Praxis. Vorträge, Aufsätze, Gespräche und Essays, mit denen sich die Philosophische Praxis in den Jahren 1981 bis 2009 vorstellte. Eine Dokumentation. Verlag für Philosophie Dinter, Köln, pp 305–315

Achenbach GB, Macho TH (1985) Das Prinzip Heilung: Medizin, Psychoanalyse, philosophische Praxis. Verlag für Philosophie Dinter, Köln

Albarelli HP (2008) A terrible mistake: The murder of frank Olson and the CIA's secret cold war experiments. Independent Publishers Group, Chicago

Aristotle (1992) Physics, books I and II. Translated by W Charlton. Oxford University Press, New York

Bacalzo D (1996) Erschreckte Kinderseelen auf den Philippinen. In: Keller FB (ed) Krank warum? Vorstellungen der Völker, Heiler, Mediziner, 2nd edn. Cantz, Stuttgart, pp 298–305

Balint M (1965) On the psycho-analytic training system. In: Balint M (ed) Primary love and psychoanalytic technique, 2nd edn. Tavistock Publications, London, pp 253–274

Beck U, Beck-Gernsheim E (2010) Individualization. Institutionalized individualism and its social and political consequences. Sage, London

Benedetti G (1960) Blumhardts Seelsorge in der Sicht heutiger psychotherapeutischer Kenntnis. Reformatio Zeitschrift für evangelische Kultur und Politik: 474–487:531–539

NIV Bible (2011) The new international version (NIV) bible, http://www.biblica.com/niv/ (15.02.2013)

Blumhardt JC (1979) Der Kampf in Möttlingen. Gesammelte Werke, Reihe 1, vol. 1 (Texte) and 2 (Anmerkungen). Vandenhoeck & Ruprecht, Göttingen

Boas F (1930) The religion of the kwakiutl indians. Part II—translations. Columbia University Press, New York

Borscheid P (2004) Das Tempo-Virus. Eine Kulturgeschichte der Beschleunigung. Campus, Frankfurt am Main, New York

Bourguignon E (2004) Possession and trance. In: Ember CR, Ember M (eds) Encyclopedia of medical anthropology. Health and illness in the world's cultures. Kluwer, New York, pp 137–145

Boyer P, Nissenbaum S (2002) Salem possessed: the social origins of witchcraft, 25th edn. Harvard University Press, Cambridge, MA

Brandt D (2010) Philosophische Praxis. Ihr Begriff und ihre Stellung zu den Psychotherapien. Alber, Freiburg München

Brown W (1845) New Zealand and its aborigines. Smith, Elder, and Co., London

Burckhardt J (1990) The civilization of the renaissance in Italy. Translated by S.G.C. Middlemore. Penguin, London

Calestro K (1972) Psychotherapy, faith healing, and suggestion. Int J Psychiatr 10(2):83–113

Caporael LR (1976) Ergotism: the Satan loosed in Salem? Science, New Series, Vol. 192, No. 4234 (Apr. 2, 1976): 21–26

Chaumeil JP (2004) Magic darts as viruses. In: Narby J, Huxley F (eds) Shamans through time. 500 years on the path to knowledge. Jeremy P. Tarcher/Penguin, New York, pp 272–279

Cifali M (2005) Sechehaye, Marguerite (1887-1964). In: Mijolla A de (ed.) International dictionary of psychoanalysis. Thomson Gale, Detroit http://www.enotes.com/psychoanalysis-encyclopedia/sechehaye-marguerite (10.08.2013)

Dattenberg-Holper T (2002) Spirit obsession and exorcism in India in traditional and western terms. In: Gottschalk-Batschkus CE, Green JC (eds) Handbuch der Ethnotherapien/handbook of ethnotherapies. ETHNOMED—Institut für Ethnomedizin e.V. München, pp 355–360

Dein S (2003) Psychogenic death: Individual effects of sorcery and taboo violation. Ment Health Relig Cult 6:195–202

Devereux G (1957) Dream learning and individual ritual differences in Mohave shamanism. Am Anthropol 59:1036–1045

Devereux G (1961) Shamans as neurotics. Am Anthropol 63:1088–1090

Devereux G (1974) Normal und Anormal. In: Normal und Anormal. Aufsätze zur allgemeinen Ethnopsychiatrie. Suhrkamp, Frankfurt am Main, pp 19–130 [engl. edn.: Devereux G (1980) Normal and abnormal. In: Basic problems of ethnopsychiatry. University of Chicago Press, Chicago, pp 3–71].

Düsing W (2007) Tragisch. In: Müller JD (ed) Reallexikon der deutschen Literaturwissenschaft, vol III. De Gruyter, Berlin, NY, pp 666–669

Ehrenwald J (ed) (1991) The history of psychotherapy. Jason Aronson, Northvale, NJ

Ellenberger HF (1970) The discovery of the unconscious. The history and evolution of dynamic psychiatry. Basic Books, New York

Elmendorf WW (1952) Soul loss illness in Western North America. In: Tax S (ed) Indian tribes of aboriginal america. University of Chicago Press, Chicago, pp 104–114

Emrich W (1981) Deutsche Literatur der Barockzeit. Athenäum, Königstein/Ts

Enderwitz U (1977) Schamanismus und Psychoanalyse. Zum Problem mythologischer Rationalität in der strukturalen Anthropologie von Claude Lévi-Strauss. Heymann, Wiesbaden

Ernst W (2011) Beschwörungen und Segen. Angewandte Psychotherapie im Mittelalter. Böhlau, Köln Weimar, Berlin

Favret-Saada J (1980) Deadly words: Witchcraft in the Bocage. Cambridge University Press, Cambridge

Favret-Saada J (1990) About participation. Cult Med Psychiatry 14:189–199

Fischer G (2008) Logik der Psychotherapie. Philosophische Grundlagen der Psychotherapiewissenschaft. Asanger, Kröning

Fischer G (2011) Psychotherapiewissenschaft. Einführung in eine neue humanwissenschaftliche Disziplin. Psychosozial Verlag, Gießen

Frank JD, Frank JB (1993) Persuasion and healing. A comparative study of psychotherapy (3rd edn). The John Hopkins University Press. Baltimore, London

Frenschkowski M (2007) Seele. In: Brednich RW (ed) Enzyklopädie des Märchens. Handwörterbuch zur historischen und vergleichenden Erzählforschung, vol 12. De Gruyter, Berlin, pp 476–489

Freud S (1914) Remembering, repeating and working-through. The standard edition of the complete psychological works of Sigmund Freud, vol. XII. The Hogarth Press and the Institute of Psycho-Analysis, London, pp 145–156

Freud S (1923) A seventeenth-century demonological neurosis. The standard edition of the complete psychological works of Sigmund Freud, vol. XIX. The Hogarth Press and the Institute of Psycho-Analysis, London, pp 67–108

Freud S, Breuer J (1895) Studies on hysteria. The standard edition of the complete psychological works of Sigmund Freud, vol II. The Hogarth Press and The Institute of Psycho-Analysis, London

Gelo OCG, Vilei A, Maddux JE, Gennaro A (in press) Psychopathology as social construction: the case of anorexia nervosa. J Constr Psychol

Genelot D (1992) Manager dans la complexité. Réflexions à l'usage des dirigeants. INSEP éd, Paris

Gerabek WE, Haage BD, Keil G, Wegner W (eds) (2005) Enzyklopädie Medizingeschichte. De Gruyter, Berlin

Gergen KJ (1991) The saturated self: dilemmas of identity in contemporary life. Basic Books, New York

Giedion S (2009) Mechanization takes command: a contribution to anonymous history. New York Review Books, New York

Grabner E (1997) Krankheit und Heilen. Eine Kulturgeschichte der Volksmedizin in den Ostalpen (2nd edn). Verlag der Österreichischen Akademie der Wissenschaften, Wien

Gryphius A (1972) Ermordete Majestät. Oder Carolus Stuardus König von Groß Britanien. Trauer-Spil. Reclam, Stuttgart

Gryphius A (1981) Catharina von Georgien. Oder Bewehrete Beständigkeit. Trauer-Spiel. Reclam, Stuttgart

Haller T (1996) Raub der "Seelenschatten" in Nord-Kamerun. In: Keller FB (ed) Krank warum? Vorstellungen der Völker, Heiler, Mediziner, 2nd edn. Cantz, Stuttgart, pp 302–305

Hand WD (ed) (1980) American folk medicine. A symposium. University of California Press, Berkeley

Hartmann M (1997) Gegenwart und Zukunft der "traditionellen Medizin" in Mexiko, vorgestellt am Beispiel des Bundesstaates Oaxaca. In: Ambatielos D, Neuland-Kitzerow D, Noack K (eds) Medizin im kulturellen Vergleich: die Kulturen der Medizin. Waxmann, Münster, pp 69–84

Hautzinger M (2007) Entwicklung und Geschichte der Psychotherapie. In: Reimer C, Eckert J, Hautzinger M, Wilke E (eds) Psychotherapie, 3rd edn. Springer, Berlin, pp 9–16

Hernegger R (1978) Der Mensch auf der Suche nach Identität. Kulturanthropologische Studien über Totemismus, Mythos, Religion. Habelt, Bonn

Hernegger R (1982) Psychologische Anthropologie. Von der Vorprogrammierung zur Selbststeuerung. Beltz, Weinheim

Hoffmann-Krayer E (1946) Die Volkskunde als Wissenschaft (1902). In: Geiger P (ed) Kleinere Schriften zur Volkskunde. Krebs, Basel, pp 1–23

Honko L (1959) Krankheitsprojektile. Untersuchung über eine urtümliche Krankheitserklärung. Academia Scientiarum Fennica, Helsinki

Illouz E (2008) Saving the modern soul. Therapy, emotions, and the culture of self-help. University of California Press, Berkeley

Ising D (2002) Johann Christoph Blumhardt. Leben und Werk. Vandenhoeck & Ruprecht, Göttingen

Jaspers K (1947) Von der Wahrheit. Piper, München

Jung CG (1933) Modern man in search of a soul. Harcourt Brace, New York

Jung CG (1966) The practice of psychotherapy: essays on the psychology of the transference and other subjects (The collected works of CG Jung, vol 16). Routledge, London

Jütte R (1996) Geschichte der Alternativen Medizin. Von der Volksmedizin zu den unkonventionellen Therapien von heute. Beck, München

Kaplan SL (2008) Le pain maudit; retour sur la France des années oubliées, 1945-1958. Fayard, Paris

Kernberg OF (2000) A concerned critique of psychoanalytic education. Int J Psychoanal 81:97–120

Kernberg OF (2006) The coming changes in psychoanalytical education: part I. Int J Psychoanal 87:1649–1673

Kernberg OF (2007) The coming changes in psychoanalytical education: part II. Int J Psychoanal 88:183–202

Kidder AS (2010) Making confession, hearing confession: a history of the cure of souls. Liturgical Press, Collegeville, MN

Kieckhefer R (2003) Magic in the middle ages. Cambridge University Press, Cambridge

Kirkland J, Mathews HF, Sullivan CW III, Baldwin K (eds) (1992) Herbal and magical medicine: traditional healing. Duke University Press, Durham

Knoll A (2012) Resonanzmomente. Beziehungsphänomene in Schamanismus und Psychotherapie. Monsenstein und Vannerdat, Münster

Köller W (2004) Perspektivität und Sprache. Zur Struktur von Objektivierungsformen in Bildern, im Denken und in der Sprache. de Gruyter, Berlin

Kraft H (1995) Über innere Grenzen. Initiation in Schamanismus, Kunst, Religion und Psychoanalyse. Diederichs, München

Le Goff J (ed) (1996) Der Mensch des Mittelalters. Magnus, Essen

Lévi-Strauss C (1963) Structural anthropology. Basic Books, New York

Lewis IM (2003) Ecstatic religion. A study of shamanism and spirit possession (3rd edn). Routledge, London

Leykin Y, DeRubeis RJ (2009) Allegiance in psychotherapy outcome research: separating association from bias. Clin Psychol Sci Pract 16(1):54–65

Lütchen J (2013) Das Bildungswegmodell zur Rehabilitation der sokratischen Mäeutik—Pädagogische und therapeutische Transformationsarbeit. Kovač, Hamburg

Maasen S, Elberfeld J, Eitler P, Tändler M (eds) (2011) Das beratene Selbst. Zur Genealogie der Therapeutisierung in den “langen” Siebzigern. Transcript, Bielefeld

Maranhão T (1986) Therapeutic discourse and Socratic dialogue. University of Wisconsin Press, Madison, WI

Marinoff L (2002) Philosophical Practice. Academic, San Diego, CA

Meier E (1852) Deutsche Sagen, Sitten und Gebräuche aus Schwaben, vol 1. Metzler, Stuttgart

Moseley JB, O’Malley K, Petersen NJ, Menke TJ, Brody BA, Kuykendall DH, Hollingsworth JC, Ashton CM, Wray NP (2002) A controlled trial of arthroscopic surgery for osteoarthritis of the knee. N Engl J Med 11:81–88

Mossière G (2007) Sharing in ritual effervescence: emotions and empathy in fieldwork. Anthropology Matters 9: 1. http://anthropologymatters.com/index.php?journal=anth_matters&page=article&op=view&path[]=59&path[]=114 (03.02.2013)

Müller KE (1987) Das magische Universum der Identität. Elementarformen sozialen Verhaltens. Ein ethnologischer Grundriss. Campus, Frankfurt New York

Müller KE (2006) Schamanismus. Heiler, Geister, Rituale (3rd edn). Beck, München

Müller KE (2010) Die Siedlungsgemeinschaft. Grundriss der essentialistischen Ethnologie. V&R Unipress, Göttingen

Müller-Ebeling C (2002) Not all healers are shamans—a survey about the variety of healing methods. In: Gottschalk-Batschkus CE, Green JC (eds) Handbuch der Ethnotherapien/handbook of ethnotherapies. ETHNOMED—Institut für Ethnomedizin e.V. München, pp 17–20

Oesterreich TK (1930) Possession, demoniacal and other, among primitive races, in antiquity, the middle ages, and modern times. R.R. Smith, New York

Olbrecht AJ (1999) Die Welt der Geistheiler. Die Renaissance magischer Weltbilder. Böhlau, Wien, Köln, Weimar

Olbrecht AJ (2000) Die Klienten der Geistheiler. Vom anderen Umgang mit Krankheit, Krise, Schmerz und Tod. Böhlau, Wien, Köln, Weimar

Overholser JC (1993a) Elements of the Socratic method: I. Systematic questioning. Psychother Theory Res Pract Train 30(1):67–74

Overholser JC (1993b) Elements of the Socratic method: II. Inductive reasoning. Psychother Theory Res Pract Train 30(1):75–85

Overholser JC (1994) Elements of the Socratic method: III. Universal definitions. Psychother Theory Res Pract Train 31(2):286–293

Overholser JC (1995) Elements of the Socratic method: IV. Disavowal of knowledge. Psychother Theory Res Pract Train 32(2):283–292

Overholser JC (1996) Elements of the Socratic method: V. Self-improvement. Psychother Theory Res Pract Train 33(4):549–559

Overholser JC (1999) Elements of the Socratic method: VI. Promoting virtue in everyday life. Psychother Theory Res Pract Train 36(2):137–145

Petzoldt L (1999) Magie. In: Brednich RW (ed.) Enzyklopädie des Märchens. Handwörterbuch zur historischen und vergleichenden Erzählforschung, vol 9. De Gruyter, Berlin, pp 2–13

Piaget J (2007) The child’s conception of the world. Rowman & Littlefield, Lanham

Piaget J, Inhelder B (1956) The child’s conception of space. Routledge, London

Plato (2000) The republic. Ed by Ferrari GRF. Cambridge University Press, Cambridge

Plato (2006) Plato in twelve volumes, vol 7: Theaetetus, Sophist. Harvard University Press, Cambridge, MA

Price NS (ed) (2001) The archaeology of shamanism. Routledge, London

Raabe PB (2001) Philosophical counseling: theory and practice. Praeger, Westport, CT

Rieken B (2003) Gegenübertragungsprobleme. Beziehungsanalyse und Selbstenthüllung im Schatten der Therapieausbildung Fallbeispiele und Überlegungen aus individualpsychologischer Sicht. Zeitschrift für Individualpsychologie 28:332–353

Rieken B (2005) “Nordsee ist Mordsee”. Sturmfluten und ihre Bedeutung für die Mentalitätsgeschichte der Friesen. Waxmann, Münster

Rieken B (2007) Vom Nutzen volkskundlich-historischer Zugänge für die Katastrophenforschung: New Orleans 2005. In: Hartmann A, Meyer S, Mohrmann RE (eds) Historizität. Vom Umgang mit Geschichte. Waxmann, Münster, pp 149–162

Rieken B (2011a) Psychotherapiewissenschaft, Hermeneutik und das Unbewusste. In: Rieken B (ed) Alfred Adler heute. Zur Aktualität der Individualpsychologie. Waxmann, Münster, pp 41–59

Rieken B (2011b) Zur Vorgeschichte der Psychotherapie. In: Rieken B, Sindelar B, Stephenson T (eds) Psychoanalytische Individualpsychologie in Theorie und Praxis. Psychotherapie, Pädagogik, Gesellschaft. Springer, Wien, pp 1–21

Rieken B (2012) Schwarze Magie in der therapeutischen Praxis. Psychoanalytisch-ethnologische Zugänge anhand eines Fallbeispiels. In: Wahl P, Lehmkuhl U (eds) Die Magie des Bösen. Vandenhoeck & Ruprecht, Göttingen, pp 97–116

Rieken B (2013) Learning from disasters in an unsafe world: considerations from a psychoanalytical-ethnological perspective. In: Egner H, Schorch M, Voss M (eds) Learning and calamities. Practices, interpretation, patterns. Routledge, London

Rothschuh KE (1978) Konzepte der Medizin in Vergangenheit und Gegenwart. Hippokrates, Stuttgart

Rubel AJ, O'Nell CW, Collado-Ardón R (1991) Susto, a folk illness. University of California Press, Berkeley, LA

Ruff M (2003) Zauberpraktiken als Lebenshilfe. Magie im Alltag vom Mittelalter bis heute. Campus, Frankfurt am Main New York

Ruschmann E (1999) Philosophische Beratung. Kohlhammer, Stuttgart

Rychlak G (2001) Die Annaberger Hexenkrankheit. In: Simon M (ed) Auf der Suche nach Heil und Heilung. Religiöse Aspekte der medikalen Alltagskultur. Thelem bei w.e.b.-Universitätsverlag, pp 101–117

Rychlak G (2009) Hexenfieber im Erzgebirge. Die Annaberger Krankheit 1712-1720, Diss. phil. Johannes-Gutenberg-Universität Mainz, http://ubm.opus.hbz-nrw.de/volltexte/2009/2159/pdf/diss.pdf (07.08.2013)

Scharfetter C (1983) Der Schamane—Das Urbild des Therapeuten. Praxis der Psychotherapie und der Psychosomatik 28:81–89

Scheule RM (ed) (2001) Beichten. Autobiographische Zeugnisse zur katholischen Bußpraxis im 20. Jahrhundert, Böhlau, Wien

Schmid GB (2008) Consciousness medicine: what can we learn about mind-body healing from psychogenic death phenomena? In: De Luca BN (ed) Mind-body and relaxation research focus. Nova Biomedical Books, New York, pp 93–138

Schmid JC (2008) Instabilität in Natur und Wissenschaft. Eine Wissenschaftsphilosophie der nachmodernen Physik. de Gruyter, Berlin

Schmid GB (2010) Tod durch Vorstellungskraft. Das Geheimnis psychogener Todesfälle, 2nd edn. Springer, Wien

Schmidbauer W (1969) Schamanismus und Psychotherapie. Psychol Rundsch 20:29–47

Schoepflin RB (1988) Christian science healing in America. In: Gevitz N (ed) Other Healers. Unorthodox medicine in America. Johns Hopkins University Press, Baltimore, pp 192–214

Schulze G (2005) Die Erlebnisgesellschaft. Kultursoziologie der Gegenwart (2nd edn). Campus, Frankfurt am Main New York

Schuster SC (1999) Philosophy practice: an alternative to counseling and psychotherapy. Praeger, Westport

Schützeichel R (1974) Althochdeutsches Wörterbuch, 2nd edn. Niemeyer, Tübingen

Sechehaye MA (1956) A new psychotherapy in schizophrenia: relief of frustrations by symbolic realization. Grune and Stratton, New York

Sedgwick D (1994) The wounded healer. Countertransference from a Jungian perspective. Routledge, London

Selin H, Shapiro H (eds) (2003) Medicine across cultures. History and practice of medicine in non-western cultures. Kluwer, Dordrecht

Silverman J (1967) Shamans and acute schizophrenia. Am Anthropol 69:21–31

Simon M (2003) "Volksmedizin" im frühen 20. Jahrhundert. Zum Quellenwert des Atlas der deutschen Volkskunde. Gesellschaft für Volkskunde in Rheinland-Pfalz e.V., Mainz

Somé MP (2004) Invisible projectiles in Africa. In: Narby J, Huxley F (eds) Shamans through time. 500 years on the path to knowledge. Jeremy P. Tarcher/Penguin, New York, pp 238–242

Speer A (2004) Weisheit. In: Ritter J, Gründer K, Gabriel G (eds) Historisches wörterbuch der philosophie, vol 12. Wissenschaftliche Buchgesellschaft, Darmstadt, pp 371–397

Staude D (ed) (2010) Methoden philosophischer Praxis. Ein Handbuch. Transcript, Bielefeld

Stoll U (1992) Das "Lorscher Arzneibuch": ein medizinisches Kompendium des 8. Jahrhunderts (Codex Bambergensis medicinalis 1): Text, Übersetzung und Fachglossar. Steiner, Stuttgart

Streeck U (2008) Lehranalyse. In: Mertens W, Waldvogel B (eds) Handbuch psychoanalytischer Grundbegriffe, 3rd edn. Kohlhammer, Stuttgart, pp 431–434

Thomas K (2003) Religion and the decline of magic. Penguin, London

Thomas of Aquin (2011) Sancti Thomae de Aquino Sententia libri Metaphysicae. Textum Taurini 1950 editum ac automato translatum a Roberto Busa SJ in taenias magneticas denuo recognovit Enrique Alarcón atque instruxit, http://www.corpusthomisticum.org/cmp0104.html (07.08.2013)

Tucholsky K (1926) Interessieren Sie sich für Kunst? In: Zürcher Student 2, 1. Mai 1926: 64

Vogel VJ (1990) American Indian medicine. University of Oklahoma Press, Norman

Vollmer M (2011) Sünde—Krankheit—"väterliche Züchtigung". Sünden als Ursache von Krankheiten vom Mittelalter bis in die Frühe Neuzeit. In: Classen A (ed) Religion und Gesundheit. Der heilkundliche Diskurs im 16. Jahrhundert. De Gruyter, Berlin, pp 261–286

Wampold BE (2001) The great psychotherapy debate: Models, methods and findings. Mahwah, NJ: Lawrence Erlbaum

Whitehead H (2000) The hunt for Quesalid: Tracking Lévi-Strauss' Shaman. Anthropology and Medicine: 7:149–168

Whitehead H (2009) Quest for Quesalid: myth-making and rationality in the initiation of a Shaman. In: Georganta K, Collingnon F, Millim AM (eds) The apothecary's chest: magic, art and medication. Cambridge Scholars Press, Newcastle upon Tyne, pp 129–144

Wiegelmann G (ed) (1987) Volksmedizin heute. Coppenrath, Münster

Zaretsky E (2004) Secrets of the soul: a social and cultural history of psychoanalysis. Knopf, New York (deutsch: Zaretsky E [2006] Freuds Jahrhundert. Die Geschichte der Psychoanalyse. Wissenschaftliche Buchgesellschaft, Darmstadt)

Znamenski AA (2007) The beauty of the primitive: shamanism and western imagination. Oxford University Press, New York

Zwiebel R (2007) Von der Angst. Psychoanalytiker zu sein. Das Durcharbeiten der phobischen Position. Klett-Cotta, Stuttgart

Historical Paths in Psychotherapy Research

3

Diana Braakmann

Contents

Abstract

The history of psychotherapy research can be viewed on the basis of four phases that differ in general streamings, aims, achievements, and protagonists, respectively. In the first phase (1920–1954), phenomena of private practices became objects of scientific investigation and basic outcome research was "invented." The first systematic sound recordings by Carl Rogers and his team represented the roots of process and process-outcome research. In the second phase (1955–1969), pre-post-follow-up designs were developed. Process research was intensively advanced and questions were posed in a more complex way. The refinement of research questions and further development of methods—especially meta-analytic strategies that allowed summarizing a large body of information across outcome studies—were major achievements of phase III (1970–1983). The fourth phase (1984 to now) is characterized by an intensive deepening of process and process-outcome research and by the emergence of mixed-method approaches, the investigation of unsuccessful cases, intercultural issues, as well as client and therapist factors and their interaction. Commensurate with the enormously quick increase of the importance of the Internet in everyday life, settings of online psychotherapy became a matter of interest. With respect to the enormous influence the idea of common therapy

D. Braakmann (✉)
Department of Psychotherapy Science, Sigmund Freud University, Freudplatz 1, 1020 Vienna, Austria
e-mail: diana.braakmann@sfu.ac.at

O.C.G. Gelo et al. (eds.), *Psychotherapy Research*,
DOI 10.1007/978-3-7091-1382-0_3, © Springer-Verlag Wien 2015

factors that can be observed across all therapeutic school settings has won in psychotherapy research, a second chapter is dedicated to a detailed view on the "birth" and further research developments in this field. The concluding paragraph offers a short glance on possible future perspectives.

3.1 Introduction

The historical traces of psychotherapy research are an essential and necessary context for the understanding and further development of psychotherapy research today. Therefore a chapter in a handbook on psychotherapy research needs its introduction from a historical perspective. The history of psychotherapy research has been described by several authors (e.g., Lambert et al. 2004; Muran et al. 2010; Orlinsky and Russel 1994; Strupp and Howard 1992). The present chapter aims at providing the reader with information on the historical phases of psychotherapy research, as they have been already differentiated by Orlinsky and Russel (1994). As to the very early roots, the chapter widens the view and goes beyond the beginning in 1920. Streamings and paradigms will be described as well as the role of key persons who affected the development and whose achievements still radiate today on the field of psychotherapy research and its dynamics. The birth and advancement of the idea of common factors is dealt with in detail with respect to its timeliness.

3.2 The Phases of Psychotherapy Research

This chapter is structured by the idea of four phases of the history of psychotherapy research, being proposed by Orlinsky and Russel (1994). Although the division states an oversimplification of the history, it provides boundaries that facilitate the description and understanding as well as distinguishing between streams and aims, which differ between the phases. In general, there have been two major traditions in psychotherapy research that have caused a lot of friction and are still controversial today, namely, the one being characterized by logical positivism and operationalism and the other by structuralism, phenomenology, and hermeneutics (see Ponterotto 2005 and Chap. 4; see also Gelo 2012). The two traditions especially differ in their epistemological pre-assumptions and have been challenged frequently during the last decades. Today there are increasingly more attempts to combine the approaches, to aim at synergetic effects, and to take a position of methodological plurality (Muran et al. 2010).

3.2.1 Phase I (1920 to the Birth of Psychotherapy Research in 1954) and Some Events Much Earlier

In general, the main concern of the first phase was "to demonstrate the feasibility and necessity of applying scientific methods to the study of psychotherapy" (Orlinsky and Russel 1994, p. 191). The beginning of the first phase is mainly described from the 1920s on, but there are even some earlier roots we should not forget.

3.2.1.1 Nearly Forgotten Roots and Famous Ones

Hardly anyone would expect the very first publications of systematic reflections on psychotherapeutic methods to be even enrooted in the eighteenth century. Indeed, it was more than 100 years before Hippolyte Bernheim (1840–1919) introduced the term "psychotherapy" (Bernheim, 1892), see when Karl Philipp Moritz (1756–1793), a philosopher, writer, and teacher, founded the Journal *Erfahrungsseelenkunde* or *Journal of Psychology from Experience*. The periodical was created as a reader for scholars and non-scholars and was published up to 1792. It provided the possibility to everyone who was interested to publish knowledgeable observations and thoughts on issues of mental disorders and the respective treatment options of that time.

Many contributions focused on questions of how to understand mental disorders more deeply but also how affected authors cured themselves (Fiedler 2010).

The better-known origins of psychotherapy research are the *Studies on Hysteria* by Breuer and Freud (1895). They contained a number of case studies reflected from a neurophysiological and psychological point of view. As it appears during the early stages of clinical sciences, the very first research steps were done in the form of single-case studies that provided the first evidence for theories and practice of psychotherapies. Freud's analytical hypotheses were mainly supported by clinical case studies, which are especially applicable to deeply exploring the therapeutic process and generating new hypotheses to be investigated more systematically (Hersen et al. 1984). To date, it is still difficult to understand why it was not until the 1990s (e.g., Faller and Frommer 1994) that case studies *really* had their renaissance in the field of psychotherapy research, except for the maintenance of more anecdotal case studies in the meantime.[1]

3.2.1.2 The Early Beginning from the 1920s to the 1950s

Between 1920 and 1940 there was a slow but steady rate of publications, with a discontinuation during the war (Orlinsky and Russel 1994). In the 1930s, institutions started outcome research activities by documenting treatment results. The studies were mostly comprised of simple tallies of therapist-perceived improvement. After the war research activities reoccurred in the beginning of the 1950s, aiming at investigating the many facets of psychotherapy. The Menninger Psychotherapy Project (see also Sect. 3.2.2.6) started in the mid-1950s and can be viewed as a major milestone of the reentry into outcome as well as process research interests after the war (Strupp and Howard 1992). In general, central concerns of psychotherapy research in the 1950s included patient and therapist characteristics, process of psychotherapy, and common treatment factors but also possible limitations of psychotherapy that were increasingly perceived and observed.

3.2.1.3 The Catalyst Effect: Eysenck

The proliferation of uncontrolled and also anecdotal clinical case studies at the beginning of the 1950s became increasingly criticized in favor of more systematic clinical surveys with increasing sample sizes and also experimental investigations due to historical trends and important events (Hersen et al. 1984)—one of them undoubtedly being H.J. Eysenck's attack on the effects of psychotherapy in general. He provocatively asserted that empirical research did not support the claim that psychotherapeutic approaches were more efficacious than neutral (control) conditions and that recovery of psychopathology was just reflecting *spontaneous remission* rates (Eysenck 1952). One early rejoinder was Lester Luborsky's rebuttal (Luborsky 1954) that stressed flaws in Eysenck's control group and in the assessment of outcome. Eysenck's provocation evoked a challenging starting point of the career of young Luborsky (Crits-Christoph et al. 2010). In the same year Rosenzweig (1954), in his reply to Eysenck, criticized the different standards of severity of illness and standards of recovery in his empirical data. He evaluated Eysenck's comparison to be of little validity and his generalizations to be highly questionable because of low resemblance in the named standards for the experimental and control group. Nevertheless, Eysenck's attack had an immense catalyst effect on the further development of psychotherapy research in general, especially aiming at refuting his assertions, and therefore justifying the discipline, as will be described later in this chapter.

[1] Obviously, the reason is that the development of psychotherapy research in the beginning happened in accordance with the imperatives of logical positivism that considers single-case research as marginal and consequently excludes it.

3.2.1.4 The Roots of Outcome Research

3.2.1.4.1 Counting and Statistics

Thirty years after the *Studies on Hysteria*, the first statistics-based outcome studies were published in the late 1920s (Fenichel 1930, cited in Bergin 1971; Huddleson 1927; Matz 1929). A very early British work by Neustatter (1935) was even published in the *Lancet*, which has continued to be one of the most influential journals in the field of medical research until today. This is astonishing, since still today, having a psychotherapy research study accepted by the evaluators of this journal is a difficult and demanding task. Until 1940 the efforts focused on very elementary outcome research aimed at a status of scientific legitimacy. Most of the studies dealt with therapist-perceived improvement, diagnoses were vague, and samples were heterogeneous and small (Bergin 1971). Therefore, they did not allow for deep interpretations or broad generalizations. The efforts were intensified after Eysenck's provocative attack on the efficacy of psychotherapy, as mentioned above (Eysenck 1952). Psychometric scaling was used as a means of quantifying phenomena, after Thorndike (1918) had formulated much earlier, "Whatever exists at all, exists in some amount. To know it thoroughly involves its quantity as well as its quality" (p. 16). He thereby took an acerbic position of positivism, which was heavily criticized in later stages of the development of the field of psychotherapy research.

3.2.1.5 The Roots of Process and Process-Outcome Research

3.2.1.5.1 The Revolution: Sound Recordings and Sequential Process Research

The striving for scientific legitimacy of psychotherapeutic treatments was consistent with an inherent characteristic of psychotherapy and its representatives, viewing psychotherapy as corresponding to applications of science of the mind. This means at the same time a theoretical allegiance to the ideal of natural science, following the logical positivism paradigm (i.e., objectivity, replicability, etc.) (Orlinsky and Russel 1994). As a revolution in psychotherapy research of the 1950s, for the very first time, sound recordings of therapy sessions were applied as a means of a scientific approach to psychotherapy. The beginning of systematic phonographic recordings of sessions can be viewed as the root of process research, invented and inspired by Carl Rogers and his team at the Ohio State University (Rogers 1942b). "The Case of Herbert Bryan" was the first fully transparent (through transcriptions) psychotherapeutic case ever published (Rogers 1942a). With this innovation, Rogers and his team tried to find an approach to illuminate the arcane characteristics of therapeutic sessions (Rogers 1942a). Classifications of therapist responses (e.g., questions, giving information, interpreting) or categorizations of "directive" vs. "nondirective" therapist behavior were made in the beginning. The very first sequential process research study was accomplished by Snyder (1945) under the supervision of Rogers. Both client and therapist responses were rated, and which therapist behavior prompted which client reaction was traced. Among other results, Snyder found that simple acceptance and clarification of feelings led to a higher degree of client insight than questions and interpretations by the therapist (Elliott and Farber 2010).

Given the pioneer status, Rogers' significant contributions were a strong emphasis on the importance of research in psychotherapy as well as the attempt to investigate the factors that constitute an effective therapeutic treatment. In this way, Rogers and his team (Gordon et al. 1954) invented a new genre of research—the process-outcome research—with its main characteristic being the sampling of key therapy process variables used to predict post-therapy outcome (Elliott and Farber 2010).

3.2.1.6 Major Developments and Achievements

As a main achievement the protagonists of the first phase showed that phenomena in private practice became objects of scientific investigation. Outcome research that was very basic in the beginning was especially refined after Eysenck's attack. Studies of this kind still strongly relied on a (post)positivistic model of science and empirical investigation. Moreover, the introduction of sound recordings meant the first sparks to the later and still current fireworks of process and process-outcome research, lighting the darkness of the therapeutic session.

3.2.2 Phase II (1955–1969): The Second Attack and the Advancement of Process Research

Immense growth in the field of psychotherapy research could be observed from the middle of the 1950s. The major task of this period can be described as fulfilling the promise of building a scientific field of the study of psychotherapy (Orlinsky and Russel 1994). A second attack conducted by Eysenck (see Sect. 3.2.2.1) again had a catalytic impact on the field and stimulated many of new investigations. This impetus was also accompanied by a general, greater concern with efficacy of psychotherapy by researchers (Hersen et al. 1984). It shaped in a way the pursuit of mostly outcome ideas, because general justification was demanded to help psychotherapy to gain an acknowledged position in the scientific field and society in general. The second phase was therefore very much characterized by the aim of justifying the psychotherapeutic profession through research. Moreover, this phase was characterized by a proliferation of process studies, especially by client-centered researchers, aiming at the validation of Rogers' necessary and sufficient factors for therapeutic change (Rogers 1957).

3.2.2.1 Eysenck's Second Attack

In the 1960s psychotherapy researchers were again facing a difficult situation, when Eysenck repeated his provocative thesis, with a second attack referring to (seemingly) more supportive data than in 1952 (Eysenck 1960). Although the body of knowledge in psychotherapy research had already grown significantly and especially research questions and associated methods had reached a much more elaborate and sophisticated state than ten years before, there was still not enough solid evidence concerning the general efficacy of psychotherapy to clearly refute Eysenck's assertions. A key event was Bergin's (1963) review and scrutiny of data that Eysenck leaned upon heavily in support of his pessimistic position expressed in the first and second attack. From today's perspective it can be viewed as a turning point in the altercation. The surprising part of Bergin's results was the observation that therapists could be divided into two groups: one producing positive and another producing negative results. Therefore, the calculated mean of the effects had produced a parameter that seemingly supported the assertion that psychotherapy was uniformly not effective. The publication of this reanalysis in the *Journal of Counseling Psychology* stated a milestone for refuting Eysenck's attack (Hersen et al. 1984). A flood of research activities on therapist variables was triggered, which, among other topics, also investigated the performance of lay persons (e.g., Rioch et al. 1965) and paraprofessionals (e.g., nurses; Tharp and Wetzel 1969), being trained, for example, for behavior modification.

3.2.2.2 Justification Informed by Logical Positivism

The prevailing philosophy of science at the beginning of this period was still logical positivism with the focus on overt behaviors (referring to observable aspects of behavior like aggression or anxious avoidance). Subjective states in this context were mainly considered as objectively unverifiable, and the role of observers was understood as scientifically trustworthy (Anchin 2008), which from a current point of view, of course, has to be heavily criticized and viewed as insufficient to achieve deep knowledge about changes in experience and behavior. Since a main concern in the second phase was justification, nomothetic group designs and respective statistical analyses were major elements of the predominant methodology approaches in process and outcome research, although they did not necessarily reflect the researchers' personal convictions and interests.

3.2.2.3 Initial Conferences and Reorganization of the Field

3.2.2.3.1 Initial Conferences

Three initial conferences in 1958, 1962, and 1966 caused significant interest in psychotherapy practice and research all over the world. The venues were Washington, D.C.; Chapel Hill; and Chicago, respectively. They were organized by the *American Psychological Association* (APA) and financed by the *National Institute of Mental Health* (NIMH). The major aims of the very initial conference were a) the evaluation of the state of the art of psychotherapy research and b) the stimulation of research. Significant participants like Lester Luborsky, Jerome Frank, Joseph Matarazzo, Morris Parloff, Carl Rogers, and Hans Strupp exchanged their ideas with colleagues, and the proceedings were published by Rubenstein and Parloff (1959).

The two following conferences hosted the full range of representatives of the psychotherapeutic schools. Clinicians discussed theory and concepts as well as methodology, aiming at elaborating and refining psychotherapy research (Strupp and Luborsky 1962; Shlien et al. 1968). The results were significant for the community for many years, also supporting independent researchers by providing them with a significant amount of knowledge and proceedings as well as inspiration for research ideas.

3.2.2.3.2 Reorganization of the Field

Another major development influenced the field of psychotherapy research in the 1960s: the upcoming behavior therapy. The yearly chapters of *The Annual Review of Psychology* on psychotherapy reveal that at the latest 1965 behavior therapy was viewed as a new force in the field (Hersen et al. 1984). Unfortunately, at that time integration of these two existing psychotherapy research fields seemed to be nearly impossible because of differing clinical theories and their consequences for research approaches, although it might have had a very fruitful effect on the general development of research activities. Hence, during the following years the development of the two research branches seemed to be still quite distant from another.

The growth of the field revealed the need for new organizational structures that resulted in two split branches: On the one hand, the provisions of Kenneth Howard and David Orlinsky found their culmination point in the first meeting of the *Society of Psychotherapy Research* (SPR) in 1970 in Chicago (Muran et al. 2010). On the other hand, ten behavioral therapists (John Paul Brady, Joseph Cautela, Edward Dengrove, Cyril Franks, Martin Gittelman, Leonard Krasner, Arnold Lazarus, Andrew Salter, Dorothy Susskind, and Joseph Wolpe) founded the *Association for the Advancement of Behavior Therapy* (AABT) in 1966 in Washington, D.C. (Franks 1987, 1997). According to the development of behavior therapy and its discourses during the following decades, the AABT was renamed twice, which resulted in the current name the *Association for Behavioral and Cognitive Therapies* (ABCT).

The parallel development of the two branches symbolized a splitting of the field of psychotherapy research, mostly due to differing clinical theories and their effect on research models. Although the gap was maintained over decades and can sometimes still be sensed today, both "sides" show their commitment to bridge the gap, aiming at synergies and fruitful cooperation for the further development of the psychotherapy research field in general.

3.2.2.4 Outcome Research in Phase II

3.2.2.4.1 Controlled Experiments, Tests, and Interview Techniques

The activities of outcome research in this phase were closely linked to the necessity of producing convincing rejoinders to Eysenck's provocative statements. Although some behaviorally oriented researchers used single-case experimental designs to support the influences of their treatment methods (e.g., Baer et al. 1968), a major portion of research activities focused on the refinement and application of controlled experiments, aiming at proving the efficacy of psychotherapeutic interventions compared to control conditions. Major developmental steps were therefore a consequence of the context of justification. Quasi-experimental pre-post-follow-up designs (without randomized assignment to clinical groups) were the predominant design, comprising assessments of personality and psychopathology as outcome variables (Orlinsky and Russel 1994). For this purpose, tests and interview techniques had to be elaborated, modified, or newly developed.

Analogue research designs were quite prominent, which means that researchers became interested in contrived or simulated therapy situations. For example, patient samples with mild clinical problems (i.e., snake phobia) were treated by trained graduate students (Lang and Lazovik 1963). On the one hand, the application of these studies fostered the shift from survey research to quasi-experimental controlled designs (i.e., because of design economy and avoidance of ethical constraints), and on the other hand, it was heavily criticized for removing studies too far from the clinical situations (Hersen et al. 1984) to allow any meaningful conclusions for the psychotherapeutic practice. With respect to the complexity of the therapeutic process from today's point of view, single-controlled experiments are not appropriate to demonstrate the efficacy of psychotherapeutic treatment approaches. Nevertheless, the merits of researchers of that time remain unquestionable, taking into account their dependency on the state-of-the-art methods on the one hand and being confronted with major pressure to justify the field of psychotherapy in general on the other hand.

3.2.2.5 Process Research in Phase II

3.2.2.5.1 Sound Recordings and Nonparticipant-Observational Measures

The development of formerly so-called objective measures for the analysis of sound recordings made important progress for process research, which was still conducted quantitatively. For instance, the counting of self-references in the verbal behavior, thought units, and chronological periods were analyzed in the sense of process variables. In addition, Rogers traced clients' thematic patterns across sessions and change in clients' sense of self as matters of interest (Elliott and Farber 2010). The collection of immense amounts of recorded sessions led to the necessary development of approaches toward time sampling (e.g., a proportion of the beginning, middle, and end of the process). The calculation of averages served as estimation for specific aspects of the process. Unfortunately, process indices often seemed to be far from clinical experiences and the underlying theoretical pre-assumptions, but nevertheless stated an important approach, which provided a basis for the development that followed (Orlinsky and Russel 1994).

The 1960s were dominated by client-centered researchers. They primarily tried to validate Rogers' necessary and sufficient conditions for therapeutic personality change (Rogers 1957). A paradox could be observed in this context: While emphasizing the importance of the clients' experience, he made use of nonparticipant-observational measures (at least partly based upon the bias of positivism). These measures were mostly therapist ratings of client behavior in the sense of, for example, greater integration, fewer internal conflicts, or changes toward more mature behavior. Independent from this critique, the work of Rogers and his team stressed the relevance of the therapeutic relationship factors and made a great effort to investigate them in a comprehensive and detailed way. Later, from the middle of the 1970s, a decrease of this specific kind of work could be observed.

3.2.2.6 Process-Outcome Research in Phase II

3.2.2.6.1 The Menninger Project

As to the field of psychoanalysis, in the mid-1950s Karl Menninger, an American psychiatrist and founder of the Menninger Clinic, initiated an impressive 30-year longitudinal process-outcome study to investigate the psychoanalytic treatment of 42 patients, supported by talented investigators like Robert Wallerstein, Otto Kernberg, Lester Luborsky, and others. The definite closure of this huge project was marked by the publication of *Forty-Two Lives in Treatment: A Study of Psychoanalysis and Psychotherapy* (Wallerstein 1986). Mainly, two questions were addressed during the research process: What changes take place in psychotherapy, and how do those changes come about? The investigation was realized by taking three major cross-sectional perspectives ("initial, termination, and follow-up study"). In addition, the patients' personality organization and life situation (in the sense of outcome variables) as well as the therapeutic process were taken into account. Various additional publications arose from the Menninger Project, dealing with facets of the study like psychological testing (Appelbaum 1977), the role of situational variables, factor-analytic aspects (Kernberg et al. 1972), and individual prediction of therapeutic success (Horwitz 1974).

3.2.2.6.2 More Ingredients of the Process

Besides relating client and therapist variables to outcome of psychotherapy (see Sect. 3.2.2.7), there was an intense interest in analyzing alternative elements that might characterize the psychotherapeutic process. Some studies focused on ideas of verbal reinforcement, referring to the idea—derived from learning theory—that therapists (not necessarily consciously) could shape their clients' behavior through selective reinforcement of behavior patterns or the choice of topics being dealt with in sessions. In this context, transcripts of sessions conducted by Rogers were also analyzed by Truax (cited in Truax and Mitchell 1971, Hersen et al. 1984). They revealed, for example, that the selective use of empathy and warmth as reaction to a client's reports and behavior seemed to follow such a shaping behavior. In this context, also psychoanalytic interpretations were shown to reinforce client responses independent from their accuracy (Noblin et al. 1963). This finding is generally related to the current evidence-based assumption that a rationale itself is understood as a common factor within the complex psychotherapeutic process because it offers a plausible explanation for psychological problems and a prognosis for how to change it (Frank and Frank 1991; Wampold 2001). Therefore, the usage of a rationale is accompanied by hope and positive expectancies in clients, independent from the theory it is based upon. Nevertheless, the former and the current results differ in their ideas about the respective mechanisms of change: The explanation of research results in the 1960s was rooted in learning theories, whereas the current understanding of the role of the rationale is based upon more general psychological mechanisms (e.g., Nelson and Borkovec 1989).

3.2.2.7 Client and Therapist Factors: More Questions

The crossing from phase I to II was characterized by interests in the role of client characteristics. The great variety of dimensions of interest included age, sex, race, education levels, religious affiliation, motivation, insight or defensiveness, and many more. In addition, differences between clients with regard to their developmental experiences, personality organization, social skills, and resources were taken into account (Hersen et al. 1984). The potential mediating or moderating effects of the socioeconomic status on the efficacy of psychotherapy were investigated and became a leading idea of more complex outcome studies (Rosenthal and Frank 1958). On the whole in this period's results remained contradictory, and numerous new questions were raised.

Difficulties in identifying significant client predictors influenced a growing interest in the relation between therapist characteristics and outcome. For instance, therapist psychopathology was found to inhibit efficacy of psychotherapeutic outcome (Bandura et al. 1960; Holt and Luborsky 1958). The 1950s resulted in posing questions rather than giving comprehensive empirical answers. One main conclusion from single studies was that more complex models were needed that entailed interaction and combination of client and therapist characteristics, leading to a great variety and amount of process-outcome research efforts in the following decades.

3.2.2.8 Differences and Common Ground

These examples mentioned above were challenging peaks of the phase, which somehow separated researchers from another, differing in their beliefs about which elements influence the psychotherapeutic process and outcome and to what extent. These beliefs were (and still are) closely linked to the respective metatheories of psychotherapy. There was a huge amount of research activities taking place on a more common ground for the community. Their main commonality was the enterprise to understand and improve psychotherapy through the identification of key elements like the therapeutic relationship, client and therapist variables, as well as their match and interaction and relating them to outcome variables (Butler 1952; Strupp 1957; Truax and Carkhuff 1965; Truax 1968; Hagebak and Parker 1969). These ideas were ancestors of what we consider today "common factors." The consistent labeling as such in the community started with the formulation of the first explicit common factor model by Frank (1961).

3.2.2.9 Major Developments and Achievements

3.2.2.9.1 Goodbye Simplicity: Complex Relationships Between Process and Outcome

Retrospectively, one might complain about the naivety of merely considering quantitative variations in treatment in that time, but studies had pilot status, in the sense that they stated initial steps that resulted in more refined and systematic research.

The results suggested a complex relationship between process and outcome instead of simple linear relations that had been assumed before, and therefore stated a call to further investigate this complexity in the future.

One achievement was the development of pre-post-follow-up designs, conducted by means of elaborate measures, interview techniques, and tests. These steps can be viewed as (forced) appropriate answers and rejoinders to Eysenck's criticism. Subsequently, it is not by chance that a list of "landmark volumes in psychotherapy research" being reviewed and compiled by Orlinsky and Russel (1994, pp. 187–190) contains titles with terms like "evaluation," "effective psychotherapy," or "outcome."

At the end of the 1950s, questions began to be posed in a growing, elaborate, and complex way, and also methods and techniques got more sophisticated. Simple case studies paled in favor of (many analogues) experimental controlled studies using elaborate techniques for assessing the communication of therapists and clients (Saslow and Matarazzo 1962). Moreover, process research was advanced in a very energetic and fruitful way (Orlinsky and Russel 1994). This means that the promise of building up a scientific field was fulfilled with success, independent of the fact that still major developments and changes were expected and were self-evidently viewed as eligible.

3.2.3 Phase III (1970–1983): Refinement and Challenge of the Mainstream

The tasks of the third period were the expansion and refinement within the methodological mainstream of process and outcome research. The experimental mainstream was elaborated and further developed (Orlinsky and Russel 1994). The main achievement was the convincing answer to Eysenck's criticism that clearly said: Psychotherapy works! Meta-analyses as a new statistical technique provided the researchers with the possibility to ascertain the general value and utility of psychotherapy (Smith et al. 1980, see Sect. 3.2.3.3). Process and process-outcome studies were designed in a renewed way, including new concepts and methods (e.g., Gomes-Schwartz and Schwartz 1978; O'Malley et al. 1983; Mintz and Luborsky 1971).

The publication of the first *Handbook of Psychotherapy and Behavior Change* (Bergin and Garfield 1971) amazingly summarized the new variety of actions and streams in the community. The significance of this *opus* for communicating progress and development in psychotherapy research is outstanding and unquestionable, readily integrating new streams into the body of knowledge. The current version is already in its 5th edition (Lambert 2004).

Generally, researchers felt freed from the necessity of exclusively justifying and offered much more variations of research questions. The emphasis on the psychotherapeutic process as well as on issues like "psychotherapy in the ghetto" (Richter 1974), "the lives of psychotherapists" (Henry et al. 1974), and the "therapeutic discourse" (Glaser 1977; Gross 1978) revealed a more playful and creative approach to the choice of issues, instead of being forced to work solely on justification.

3.2.3.1 Negative Effects and Accountability

In the 1970s researchers became concerned with the possible negative effects of psychotherapeutic treatments (Bergin 1971; Goth et al. 1980; Strupp and Hadley 1977). Bergin (1971) can be viewed as a pioneer who dealt with this topic by reanalyzing cases with minor changes in treatment outcome studies. The main reasoning was that if psychotherapy possesses the potential to effectuate positive change, the same potential should be present in a negative direction, subsequently a deteriorating impact (Strupp et al. 1976). The explicit identification and naming of negative effects of psychotherapy would perhaps have caused difficulties in earlier justification stages of psychotherapy research, although of course there already had been awareness in the community for the importance of respective topics. The issue can therefore be seen as a sign of more freedom in designing the research field. This might also have been associated with an increase of topics chosen because of personal epistemological interests of clinicians and researchers, but this has to be viewed as hypothesis.

The associated issue of accountability also became a key consideration for psychotherapists and researchers in the 1970s, most probably with the greatest impetus toward issues associated with governmental agencies and insurance carriers. Under deteriorating economic conditions, third-party payers got more concerned with the efficacy of psychotherapeutic treatments offered to patients (Hersen et al. 1984).

3.2.3.2 The Scope of the Community

As already mentioned, this phase was very important for the scope of the community in a concrete sense, because the collegial communication was outstandingly supported by the creation of the *Society for Psychotherapy Research* (SPR) in 1970 and the *Advancement of Behaviour Therapy* (AABT) in 1966, which highly met the needs of the research community. The aims of the SPR were (and are still today), among others, (a) to encourage the development of scientific research on psychotherapy; (b) to foster the communication, understanding, and use of research results; and (c) to enhance the social value and the efficacy of psychotherapy.

The community's pursuit of an increasing methodological rigor had its impact on viewing process and outcome research as two separate fields, a kind of dichotomization, although there already have been critical voices against this artificial separation (Orlinsky and Russel 1994).

3.2.3.3 Outcome Research in Phase III

Once it was shown that psychotherapy works, the next idea was to find out if some therapeutic approaches are potentially more effective than others. Moreover, the proliferation of different therapeutic models taking place in the third phase prompted the increasing accomplishment of comparative outcome studies. In particular, ambitions for the design of randomized controlled trials (RCTs) emerged. In general, outcome research by that time was characterized by keeping up the ideal of controlled conditions and a growing interest in the use and investigation of manualized treatments.

From the 1970s onward, psychotherapy research adopted RCT design from pharmacological research as the new ideal of psychotherapy research (Desmet 2013). The main differentiating characteristics of RCTs (also referred to as efficacy studies) compared to quasi-experimental designs are the randomized assignment of participants to experimental and control groups and the accomplishment of the trials under extremely controlled conditions. The critique from today's point of view focuses on ethical troubles as well as a tremendous gap between research and practice being caused by RCTs. Instead, naturalistic effectiveness studies in the form of quasi-experimental design are fostered as an alternative.

3.2.3.3.1 The Treatment of Depression Collaborative Research Program

The launch of the *Treatment of Depression Collaborative Research Program* (TDCRP) (e.g., Elkin 1994; Elkin et al. 1989), coordinated by Irene Elkin, represents a very meaningful methodological advancement in outcome research in psychotherapy. The uniqueness of the study for psychotherapy research was realized by a collaborative, multisite, controlled, comparative trial design, investigating a large sample size. The effects of two manualized psychotherapeutic treatments for depression, namely, cognitive therapy (Beck et al. 1979) and interpersonal psychotherapy (Klerman et al. 1984), were precisely investigated in an outpatient setting and compared to the psychopharmacological effects. Besides the comparative investigation, the TDCRP aimed at advancing psychotherapy research methods in a general way by determining the feasibility of the multisite (collaborative) clinical trial design for the field of psychotherapy. This design had been widely used in psychopharmacological research before. Elkin tried to equilibrate the rigors of research methods and the preservation of the complex human qualities of psychotherapy by creating the opportunity to investigate many key theoretical and practice-relevant questions about mechanisms of change to be investigated via precisely collected and archived TDCRP data beyond efficacy issues, which is an outstanding and admirable characteristic of her achievements (Moras and Shea 2010).

3.2.3.3.2 Meta-Analytic Strategies

Another major milestone in the field of outcome research was the development of meta-analytic strategies. These new statistical methods allowed the aggregation of the results of single investigations, aiming at proving the effects of psychotherapy in thereby summarized research fields. The prior means of evaluating the effects of psychotherapy had been the calculation of box scores. This means simply counting outcomes for and against the (positive) effects of psychotherapy. Rather than relying on simply adding results, meta-analyses calculate effect sizes. They are combined in a formula aiming at increasing the probability that different evaluators will come to the same conclusion. The first analysis of 475 studies (Smith et al. 1980) proved the superiority of psychotherapy to no treatment and treatment control conditions with effect sizes of up to .85. Although in a later reanalysis the effect size in the same data set had to be relativized to .60 (Shadish et al. 1997), the results showed that psychotherapy without a doubt works. This meta-analytic study and many other reviews came to the same conclusion then drawn by Luborsky et al. (1975), suggesting the equivalence paradox (Dodo Bird Verdict, 3.3.1) that states that all psychotherapies, regardless of their specific components, produce equivalent outcomes (Lambert and Ogles 2004).

The flourishing activities of the former phases (especially phase II) were strengthened in their function as a rejoinder to Eysenck by their summary by means of statistical procedures. This new period of outcome research provided the community with new research interests, e.g., in the effects of components of specific treatments[2] and comparisons of alternative treatments for specific disorders. However, meta-analytic strategies have been criticized by authorities of the field (Garfield 1981; Wilson and Rachman 1983), particularly with respect to the possible biases and arbitrariness of the method, problems of clinical vs. statistical significance (see also Sect. 3.2.4.3), and shortcomings in the selection of studies.

3.2.3.3.3 Outcome Measures and Single-Case Experimental Approaches

A lot of attempts were made aiming at enriching and professionalizing the field of outcome measures. Waskow and Parloff (1975) organized a panel on outcome measures for the NIMH and

[2] This interest mainly implies an adherence to a medical model of psychotherapy, which has to be differentiated from a contextual model (Wampold 2010) (see Sect. 2.1.1), which presumes that a "surgical" subdivision of a treatment approach into its single elements is not possible because of the interaction and transaction of involved variables.

published a comprehensive outcome measure collection, comprised of variables rated by patients, therapists, and significant others as well as independent clinical evaluator variables. Besides the measures themselves, they tried to heighten the precision of the process of choosing the clinically appropriate outcome measures.

Single-case experimental approaches were conducted in the field of behavior therapy in a more refined way than before (see Sect. 3.2.2.4), providing a better control of confounding factors in comparative studies and permitting an analysis of the vicissitudes of the treatment by the use of repeated measures during baseline and treatment (Hersen and Barlow 1976). A critical altercation with the methodological and interpretive problems evolved at the same time, focusing on problems like decisions on when to alter conditions in experiments, definition of evaluation criteria for treatments, and the clinical significance of effects (Kazdin 1978).

3.2.3.4 Process and Process-Outcome Research in Phase III

3.2.3.4.1 The Working Alliance

Although the beginning recognition of *process* research with focus on the complexity of phenomena in psychotherapy already started in the middle of the 1960s, this approach began to really flourish in the third phase of psychotherapy research. In the middle of the 1970s, Bordin (1979) offered a reformulation of the therapeutic relationship, and the term "working alliance" (see Chap. 16) emerged and would not be changed until today. The working alliance was conceptualized as a construct with distinguishable components; research activities intensively focused on this concept, including the construction and application of new instruments in process research.

The preparatory period for the emergence of *process-outcome* studies as a specific field in psychotherapy research had already begun in the 1950s (see Sect. 3.2.2.6). The flourishing of process-outcome research in this phase depended on the prior development of systematic outcome research and objective process research. Many researchers claimed that solely research activities connecting process with outcome variables can really answer the question about the value of psychotherapy. Process variables that showed to be quite robustly linked to therapeutic success were, for example, the working alliance (or group cohesion in group sessions), patient openness vs. defensiveness, patient expressiveness, or reciprocal affirmation (Orlinsky et al. 2004).

3.2.3.4.2 Kiesler's Influence: A Major Methodological Advancement

Kiesler assumed that the development and maintenance of individuals' patterns of behaving and experiencing are mainly influenced by interpersonal relationships through patterned interaction styles. His book *The Process of Psychotherapy: Empirical Foundations and Systems of Analysis* (1973) more generally communicated significant methodological advances and the refinement of measurements in the field of process research without being exclusively circumscribed to alliance issues. It can be viewed as the equivalent to the outcome measure collection by Waskow and Parloff (1975) (mentioned in Sect. 3.2.3.3) for the field of process research.

Kiesler (1973, 1982a) created a new conceptual and methodological basis for analyzing the therapeutic relationship by developing an observational system based upon his (nowadays more than well-known) circumplex model. His work on this topic can be viewed as a constitutive milestone for process research, in the form of offering a comprehensive, precise theoretical model, a circumplex providing an interpersonal circle taxonomy (Kiesler 1982), as well as major methodological advancements, namely, the development of the *Impact Message Inventory* (IMI) and *Checklist of Interpersonal Transactions* (CLOIT). The IMI measures impacts corresponding to the interpersonal circle categories and has been widely used in research on interpersonal elements of depression, personality disorders, and other psychopathologies (Kiesler 2001b), whereas studies using the CLOIT rather focused on interpersonal transactions in therapy like metacommunication, patient-therapist matching, countertransference, and therapeutic alliance (Kiesler 2001a).

Several years before, Kiesler (1966) had authored his famous article, "Some myths about psychotherapy research and the search for a paradigm." This publication summarized rejoinders to Eysenck and designed the type of research that was needed to refute Eysenck's provocations. By delineating (among others) the "patient uniformity myth" and the "therapist uniformity myth," he reasoned that the question "Does psychotherapy work?" should be turned into "What works for whom?" Based upon the idea that a minimal but general common paradigm in psychotherapy research should take into account current theoretical inadequacies and empirical learning, he suggested that subsamples of research groups should be grouped depending on patient and therapist variables (e.g., experience, attitudes, and personality variables). Opposing the uniformity myths mentioned above, he referred to the idea that patients compared to each other as well as therapists compared to each other are more different than alike:

> "Hence, my final point would be that before we can validly assess the outcome or therapy evaluation problem, it is vitally necessary that we attempt to isolate therapist dimensions that will accurately reflect heterogeneity of therapist performance." (Kiesler 1966, p. 113)

Many years later, the *Clinician's Research Digest* identified this publication as one of 12 significant articles in clinical psychology (Wagner and Safran 2010).

Another fundamental contribution of Kiesler was the refutation of the *spontaneous remission myth,* stating a direct counterreaction to Eysenck's claims (see Sect. 3.2.1.3). With great detail, Kiesler carves out that the base rate of two thirds of spontaneous remission in patients, stated by Eysenck based upon studies by Landis (1938) and Denker (1947), and at the same time being the core of his line of argumentation, is questionable and invalid for the following reasons: (1) The studies included problematic diagnostic groups, (2) the process of remission was not explained at all, and (3) there is no support from learning theory that could explain such a remarkably high spontaneous remission rate that implies a deep change of attitudes and habit systems without any intervention (Kiesler 1966).

One example for the currency of the impact of Kiesler's model on research and clinical practice is the *cognitive behavioral analysis system of psychotherapy* (CBASP), developed by James McCullough for patients suffering from chronic depression (McCullough 2005), which is based upon the theoretical basis of viewing, observing, and influencing the therapeutic relationship in the sense of Kiesler.

As an anecdotal digression, it is worth mentioning that Kiesler had quite painful experiences in his role as a leading team member of Rogers' innovative process research project on the efficacy of client-centered therapy for schizophrenia. He experienced emotionally escalating scenarios as a consequence of nontransparent communication when a major problem with the database occurred that heavily endangered the continuance of the project. Undoubtedly, these experiences fostered his interests in the impact of incongruent communication on interpersonal problems (Wagner and Safran 2010).

3.2.3.5 Major Developments and Achievements

The refinement of research questions and further development of methods in the sense of more concisely and detailed formulated issues can be viewed as one of the major achievements of phase III. The development of meta-analytic strategies allowed the summary of a large body of information across outcome studies inside specific research fields. It thereby contributed to the stability of evidence for the effects of psychotherapy. Being freed from reduction to justification, the researcher utilized the newly won degrees of freedom to challenge mainstream approaches, especially in the field of process and process-outcome research, and finally to ask more creative questions and conduct the further, associated developments of methods.

3.2.4 Phase IV (1984 to Now): Discovery and Micro-dynamics

3.2.4.1 From Verification to Discovery Informed by Constructivism-Interpretivism

The movement in the fourth phase until today can mainly be described as a shift from verification to the context of discovery which is, among other aspects, illustrated by the increasing use of qualitative research. Shapes of process-outcome relations in the sense of linear and nonlinear models of change represent a return of major interests to phenomena and exploration. Qualitative research may be generally framed within the constructivist-interpretivist paradigm, which developed as a consequence of the criticisms to the dominant (post)positivistic paradigm. Its main roots are, among others, philosophical hermeneutics, according to which meaning always emerges from a process of individual understanding and is, therefore, interpretative, and phenomenology, according to which investigation of subjective experiences is considered to be possible only to the extent to which we are able to assume the first-person perspective of the subjects being investigated (see Gelo 2012; see also Rennie 2012; see also Chap. 4).

Client variables, therapist variables, systematic treatment selection and placement, as well as bridging the chasm between research and clinical work are some topics that began to receive more attention in this phase. This development is highlighted by Orlinsky and Russel (1994), by summarizing the essence of several authors' acknowledgment in *Reassessing Psychotherapy Research* (1994) that "simplicity has seemed to have had its day" (p. 204). The role of context variables is viewed as absolutely crucial, and the ambiguity of the communication between therapist and patient is stressed. The necessity of overcoming an oversimplifying view of the methods needed to empirically investigate them has been focused and discussed (Elliott and Anderson 1994).

The major concern in the former three phases had been the task to demonstrate that psychotherapeutic interventions achieve significant positive effects compared to control conditions. After this was successfully achieved, a second exigent question gained increasing weight: *How* are the significant positive effects of psychotherapy achieved? This question was directly connected to issues to process and process-outcome activities because the community had realized solely that the connection of process and outcome variables would enable researchers to answer this question (see Sect. 3.2.3.4). Of course, the main question of how effects are achieved implies loads of sub-questions, which certainly will still be dealt with during the next decades. Moreover, critical discussions emerged on different philosophies of science and the associated methods as well as on issues of clinical significance and growth models. Therefore, this phase is also characterized by controversy and fundamental critique.

3.2.4.2 The Shift of Paradigms

In the fourth phase a relevant shift of paradigms that were viewed to be legitimately applied in psychotherapy research could be observed. The significant rise of qualitative psychotherapy research was confirmed by the publication of the special issues or sections on the subject in the *Journal of Counseling Psychology* (Hill 1994) and *Psychotherapy Research* (Elliot 1999). Qualitative research in general aims at a deep understanding of human behavior, which especially asks the question of *why* people behave in a certain manner. This means that instead of verification and generalization, discovery is a major aim. This implies (a) a critical view on traditional quantitative research designs and (b) the advancement of new research paradigms. Despite the permanent but slowly increasing relevance of qualitative paradigms in psychotherapy research, still a disbalance in favor of the quantitative approaches can be observed. But a major stream and continuous development aims at methodological pluralism in the sense of complementary approaches that in coexistence should make it more possible to meet the degree of complexity of phenomena that are dealt with Lambert (2013).

3.2.4.3 Outcome Research in Phase IV

3.2.4.3.1 Skepticism Toward RCTs

Researchers were faced with the problem that some treatments with evidence of efficacy gained under controlled conditions did not prove efficiency in naturalistic designs (Weisz et al. 1993). Findings like these nurtured the skepticism toward RCTs, and outcome research had to be specified in the sense that naturalistic settings of research had to be heightened. This means a turn from questions of *efficacy* to *effectiveness*. Efficacy refers to research designs under systematically controlled conditions with internal validity being paid most attention to. Effectiveness studies instead investigate the impact of treatments under "natural" conditions in the sense of clinical settings, with external validity and generalization being the most important quality marker (Lambert and Ogles 2004).

3.2.4.3.2 Statistical vs. Clinical Significance

One very closely associated topic is the debate about statistical vs. clinical significance. As an example, Nietzel et al. (1987) resumed in their meta-analytic study about the treatment of unipolar depression that "critical scholarship, clinical acumen, and thoughtful debate" (p. 160) should be utilized to define criteria for clinical significance in the respective research context. This suggestion clearly deviates from classical ways of dealing with outcome scores in an exclusively statistical sense and the according calculated differences. In this context, the establishment of a closer link between outcome and epidemiological research is also being discussed (Russell and Orlinsky 1996). The two most prominent approaches to measure clinical significance are the investigation (1) if clients show statistically reliable significant changes after treatment (Jacobsen et al. 1999) and (2) if clients can be empirically distinguished from "normal" control persons after treatment (Kendall et al. 1999). Another approach states the calculation of the *reliable change index* (RCI; Jacobsen et al. 1984; Jacobsen and Truax 1991). The RCI is calculated as a difference score (posttreatment minus pretreatment) divided by the standard error of measurement, based upon the reliability of the measure. The parameter has been widely used and can be a valuable assessment of clinical significance when used in conjunction with reliable measures and appropriate cutoff scores (Kendall et al. 2004). Primary studies as well as meta-analyses reveal that many clients achieve clinically meaningful changes, according to the two approaches. For example, a summary of 28 clinical trials by Hansen et al. (2002) yielded 58 % of the clients with clinical significant changes in outcome variables (Lambert and Ogles 2004).

3.2.4.4 Process and Process-Outcome Research in Phase IV

3.2.4.4.1 Psychological Processes Instead of Diagnoses

The major role of the assignment to diagnostic categories in research designs began to be criticized during phase IV. The single classification of individuals in the sense of mental disorders, including labeling them with diagnoses, states an oversimplification of case conceptualizations and omits relevant predictive variables and their complex interaction, being associated with psychotherapeutic process and outcome (Clarkin and Levy 2004). The extent of the problem of simply classifying clients due to standard diagnostic classification systems becomes even more apparent, facing the fact that definitions of diagnoses underlie changes due to regular revisions of the classification systems (WHO 1992; APA 2000). Therefore, the focus on psychological processes underlying the fulfillment of diagnostic criteria was and is increasingly viewed to lead to more significant findings (Persons 1986). Subsequently, rather psychological variables such as cognitive functions, emotional regulation, personality structure, and attachment history are discussed to interact relevantly with treatment than the nosological diagnoses in the sense of the ICD or DSM.

3.2.4.4.2 Elaborated Quantitative Analytical Methods

Quantitative process approaches have increasingly concentrated on characteristics within and across session patterns. Examples for elaborated analytical methods of quantitative process research applied to respective data bases are, for example, growth curve analysis (e.g., Goldman and Anderson 2007; Sauer et al. 2003; Tschacher and Ramseyer 2009), dynamic factor analyses, P-technique (Czogalik and Russell 1995), and multivariate time series analyses (e.g., Feiler et al. 2005; Pole et al. 2002). The techniques have in common the consideration of the development of variables over time. The flourishing of these approaches finally focused the refined longitudinal perspective which has to be taken if we want to deeply understand psychotherapy as a process that aims at changing emotions, cognitions, and behavior over time (Salvatore and Tschacher 2012). These kinds of quantitative process approaches help to overcome the problem that cross-sectional data on the process of psychotherapy disregard its temporal dimension (Tschacher and Ramseyer 2009).

3.2.4.4.3 The Qualitative Helpful Factor Design

The intensification of qualitative research also influenced the kind of process-outcome research being conducted. The qualitative helpful factor design was developed as an increasingly popular approach (Elliott 2010) that comprises two main alternative methods: (1) The application of a qualitative change interview, asking the patients at the end of therapy, or partway through, open-ended questions that focus on what clients experienced as helpful, important, or hindering during the process, including delayed effects that were not immediately apparent as well as to what they attribute changes that they have made during the psychotherapeutic process (Elliott et al. 2001); and (2) the application of the helpful aspects of therapy form (HAT, Llewelyn 1988), a post-session questionnaire prompting clients to describe the most helpful or important aspect of the session they just completed. By focusing on immediate effects of important change processes, the HAT allows for considerable insight in the texture of actual therapeutic change (Elliott 2010).

3.2.4.4.4 The Task-Analytic Approach

A major impulse that challenged the traditions of the mainstream was the emergence of the task-analytic approach (Rice and Greenberg 1984). Rice and Greenberg (1984) criticized the mainstream approach of investigating groups of participants, which pre-assumed that they react in a homogenous way to a specific treatment because of their similarity in certain variables. Stressing the complexity of human experience and behavior as well as the richness of the therapeutic process, they stated that this approach is not appropriate for gaining significant answers in psychotherapy research. Instead, they argued that change events within sessions have to be focused and that observable markers of clients' and therapists' behavior must be identified to investigate the process of change (Greenberg 1986). Subsequently, groups of *events* should be investigated, indicating that a client is experiencing a state or significant event at a specific point of time, rather than groups of *people* (Goldman et al. 2010). Through this work, Rice and Greenberg significantly influenced a paradigm shift in process-outcome research, assuming that groups of particular change events lead to a positive outcome.

3.2.4.5 Cost-Effectiveness and Sociopolitical Pressure

A generally heightened concern with cost-effectiveness and cost-benefit analyses reflects the growing sociopolitical pressure on psychotherapy research activities. Outcome of therapy has to be viewed as relative, and different perspectives and evaluation criteria of success cause problems in research on psychotherapeutic outcome. Moreover, it is stressed that solely professionals should be allowed to appraise therapeutic success. There is also a deficiency in taking long-term results as well as on research of negative effects (e.g., Caspar 2009) so that, especially in this field, there are numerous and concrete future tasks for the community. Cost-benefit analyses have to consider different aspects of costs (e.g., direct, indirect, and intangible costs), in case the economical effectivity—and therefore also its societal meaning – shall be ascertained (e.g., Lamprecht 2006). Future designs in psychotherapy research have to face these sociopolitical pressures and offer empirical answers to respective questions.

3.2.4.6 Major Developments and Achievements

The fourth phase is especially characterized by an intensive deepening of process and process-outcome research and by the emergence of qualitative and mixed-method approaches which leveraged psychotherapy research not only in justification but also in discovery. *The Psychotherapeutic Process: A Research Handbook* by Greenberg and Pinsof (1986) stresses the significance of this field of interest. Investigation and comparisons of successful and unsuccessful cases (e.g., Detert et al. 2006; Hersoug 2010), also with respect to client and therapist factors as well as their interaction (e.g., Macdonald et al. 2007; Schindler et al. 1989; Wiseman and Rice 1989), are utilized to depict and analyze the psychotherapeutic process, revealing that process research is increasingly connected to outcome variables, independent of whether it is dealt with qualitative, quantitative, or mixed-method approaches. The deepening of process and process-outcome research was accomplished by increasingly focusing on dynamics on a microlevel (e.g., in-session level). Examples for client-therapist interaction factors, which allow a differentiation between successful and unsuccessful cases, are mutual therapeutic engagement, therapeutic negotiation, undirected client reminiscence, and sustained therapist work (Czogalik and Russell 1995). Collectively, the most robust influence on therapeutic outcome, across single studies and meta-analyses, was found for the working alliance, especially from the clients' perspective (Orlinsky et al. 2004). The concept of adaptive prognoses entails the idea that process characteristics allow for more precise prognosis than comparable stable factors being measured at the beginning of therapy. Among others, the very promising impulses might stem from the field of monitoring the patients' outcome, such as by the consideration of recovery curves (Lambert et al. 2001) and the associated treatment optimization, enhancement of treatment effects, and avoidance of negative effects.

Commensurate with technical media developments including the enormously quick increase of the importance of the Internet in everyday life, studies also investigate process-outcome relationships in online psychotherapy (individual and group approaches) and, for example, e-mail follow-up care of inpatient psychotherapeutic treatment (Haug et al. 2008a, b).

3.3 The Birth and Development of Common Factors

After common factors were introduced under more general aspects above, the following part of the chapter offers a more detailed view of contributions to the development of the concept by significant persons as well as the shaping of the construct during decades of research (see Chap. 11 and 15 for a discussion).

3.3.1 The Origin: Saul Rosenzweig

It was Saul Rosenzweig (1907–2004), an American psychologist and therapist, who gave birth to the idea of common (pan-theoretical) factors in psychotherapy, assigning more importance to them than to school-specific therapeutic elements (Rosenzweig 1936). Rosenzweig suggested factors like catharsis, the "indefinable effect" of the personality of a good therapist, the "formal consistency" of the therapeutic doctrine as a basis for the clients' psychological reintegration as a sign for their recovery, as well as the alternative formulation of psychological events and the concept of interdependence of personality organization. He hypothesized the named aspects to be potent, implicit therapeutic factors in psychotherapy that by that time had not been explicitly formulated as curative factors. Moreover, he argued that the coexisting success of different treatment approaches (as to theory and techniques) means that the respective "therapeutic result is not a reliable guide to the validity of the theory" (p. 412). Given the interdependence of personality constituents, the particular (theoretical and technical) point from which change is approached should not be decisive for the therapeutic effect (Rosenzweig 1936). The background of Rosenzweig's work was a historical research on (also religious and supernatural) precursors of psychotherapy, resulting in his finding that they resemble each other with respect to ideas of healing (interview with Saul Rosenzweig in October 2000, Duncan 2010). His creativity and interest in literature led to the now-famous introduction of the metaphor of the race announced by the dodo bird in Lewis Carroll's *Alice's Adventures in Wonderland* (1865). By the use of this metaphor, he aimed at depicting the state of outcome research in psychotherapy. The race ended with the decision that "everybody has won, and all must have prizes," which from Rosenzweig's point of view stated a perfect illustration of the equivalence of efficacy of different psychotherapeutic treatments.

A few years later, Heine (1953) referred to Rosenzweig and agreed to the idea that theoretical approaches and specific interventions might be less important than, for example, the therapist. In addition, he argued that one single psychotherapy (an early idea of psychotherapy integration) should be developed, instead of keeping up and further developing various therapeutic schools.

3.3.2 The Medical Model vs. the Contextual Model

Two competing meta-models are referred to in the context of understanding and explaining the nature of psychotherapy (Wampold 2001). The idea that treatments can achieve different punched-out effects is mainly based upon the idea of a medical model of psychotherapy (e.g., Macklin 1973). This model assumes that there is a disorder or problem that can be psychologically explained and be related to a specific mechanism of change that corresponds to a theoretical explanation of the problem. Hence, from this perspective, particular therapeutic interventions should be used that are viewed as the cause of the later positive outcome of psychotherapy. The model is called "medical," because of its correspondence to the way of describing, explaining, and treating diseases in medicine, with the core characteristic that a particular disease can be cured by means of a particular substance or "ingredient." In the context of psychotherapy, this idea of particular effects of treatments is referred to as specificity (Wampold 2010). On the contrary, the contextual model is the "derivative of the common factors view" (Wampold 2001, p. 20). It was originally proposed by Jerome Frank (Frank and Frank 1991) and stresses contextual factors of psychotherapy like the relationship with a helping person, the healing setting, and the conceptual scheme or rationale that is provided as the causal influences on clinical change. These can be considered as common characteristics of all psychotherapies that, following the contextual model, can be attributed to the majority of the benefits of psychotherapy. Following Frank's model, specific techniques and ingredients are necessary to create a treatment setting that is reliable and conclusive for the client, as well as evoking hope, and at the same time a frame of action that the therapist is convinced of (Frank and Frank 1991).

3.3.3 The First Common Factor Model and a Gap of References

The contextual idea of therapeutic change was the basis of the very first conceptualization of a common factor model by Rosenzweig (1936). Accordingly, several common factor models were formulated, one of them being Frank's contextual model (Frank 1961; Marmor 1962; Garfield 1995). Jerome Frank (1961) was the first to publish a whole book on common factors across different forms of mental healing, including psychotherapeutic treatment approaches. He was also a key person in the *Johns Hopkins Psychotherapy Research Project*. Based upon a conclusion of preceding comparative study of psychotherapeutic approaches, it investigated the common healing factors of psychotherapy (Frank 1992).

In general, he added the idea of potential effects of expectation and of placebo to the existing conceptualization of the efficiency of psychotherapy. He described a search for similarities between different healing approaches and identified four features being an integral part of all effective therapies: (a) an emotional confiding relationship, (b) a healing setting, (c) a rationale that provides explanation and a curing procedure, and (d) rituals with active participation of client and therapist (Frank 1973).

Unfortunately, the development of models subsequent to Rosenzweig's considerations and conceptualizations entailed a gap of references to Rosenzweig during the following decades which led to a misconception of the creatorship of the first common factor model as well as the dodo bird metaphor. But both, the first model and the metaphor, have to be clearly accentuated as Rosenzweig's brainchild in 1936 (Luborsky et al. 1975; Duncan 2010). Being asked about his reaction to this gap of reference, Rosenzweig himself reacted in a very composed way:

> My passion lies in my current work. The joy is the moment of discovery [. . .] And maybe, somewhere down the line, someone will pick up on it—if they reference me fine, if not, that is the way it goes. I doubt if I'll notice when it is all said and done. (quoted from interview transcript, Duncan 2010, p. 20)

And indeed a lot of "someones" picked it up. The core similarity of all common factor models is the significance of the collaborative work of client and therapist to the disadvantage of specific ingredients or interventions in psychotherapy.

3.3.4 The Very First Panel on Common Factors: Fitness of Interpretations vs. Correctness

In 1940, a very early panel on—among others—ideas of common factors was organized by Goodwin Watson as part of a conference of the American Orthopsychiatric Society (Goldfried and Newman 1992). The evolving *Areas of Agreement in Psychotherapy* (Watson 1940) was published, with one main conclusion being the significance of the fitness of psychological interpretations (more than correctness) for a specific client.

Carl Rogers presented his ideas about working with children, while Rosenzweig depicted his concept of implicit factors. Although it remains unclear how much Rogers was influenced by Rosenzweig's thoughts on the qualities of a good therapist, Rogers no doubt kept referencing Rosenzweig and also invited him to speak to his colleagues in Chicago in 1945 (Duncan 2010). Although Carl Rogers is not even mentioned as a participant of the panel in 1940 in historical material (interview transcript from 2000, Duncan 2010), he referenced him in his book *Counseling and Psychotherapy*, published in 1942, and kept stressing his impact in later publications.

3.3.5 Evidence for Common Factor Models

The development of psychotherapy in many countries has been very closely linked to and intertwined with medicine. From this perspective, specific psychological treatment ingredients have been argued to cause specific changes in psychopathology. Following Wampold (2010), "the status of superiority of treatment method, above all else, may well indeed be a consequence of history rather of science" (p. 53).

On the basis of the current state of research, change in psychotherapy emerges from a core set of pan-theoretical factors that transcend different treatment approaches. An analysis by Wampold (2001) reveals a difference of specific treatment models accounting for just 1 % of the variance of psychotherapeutic outcome. This result reveals an even lower impact than in Lambert's early estimation of 15 % (Lambert 1992).

The current interpretation of common factors and their contextual embedment was aptly worded by Hubble et al. (2010): "Accepting the premise that therapeutic factors constitute the engine of change, then monitoring and feedback offers the means to deliver them" (p. 40).

The statement summarizes the changes that recently took place in the common factor research field: the orientation toward the contextualization of common factors. Although there have not been major changes in the type of common factors of interest, the context of the factors as well as their interactional relationship has been the main interest of recent approaches. Former studies estimated contributions of single factors (e.g., Lambert 1992). Despite the awareness of this illegitimate oversimplification of the psychotherapeutic process, the first comprehensive reviews of studies implied the notion of factors being invariant and proportionally fixed. Pie chart models were frequently used to illustrate estimated proportions (Hubble et al. 2010).

Instead of this linear idea of the effects of common factors, recent approaches clearly view therapy as a reciprocal process with the inseparable, interdependent, fluid, and dynamic contributions of common factors over the therapeutic course being the major catalyst of therapeutic outcome (Wampold 2010). The interdependent factors that are assigned major significance to can be grouped as follows.

3.3.5.1 Working Alliance

A positive alliance from the client's perspective states one of the most powerful predictors of therapeutic outcome (e.g., see Horvath et al. 2011 and Chap. 16). The alliance is perceived in a positive way in the context of therapy if it offers a promising notion in direction of achieving the client's goals in the given treatment frame. Especially the alliance formation in the initial stage (usually within the first three to four sessions) of therapy decrees a positive predictive power (Horvath and Bedi 2002).

3.3.5.2 Therapist Factors

There is a contradiction between the robustness of therapist factors as predictors for treatment outcome and their disregard in research up to recent times. Major findings support the delicate idea that some therapists are more successful than others. The recent state of evidence shows that better therapists seem to make better use (also of their knowledge) of the common factors to strive for good treatment outcomes (Hubble et al. 2010). Successful therapists seem to make greater (and more skillful) contributions to the formation and maintenance of the therapeutic alliance, taking dynamic and interactional facets of their contribution into account. Hence, a major part of the variability in therapists' efficacy can be explained by differences in building and maintaining the therapeutic bond (e.g., Baldwin et al. 2007). This contains also significant implications for training or research on training, because one important part could be improvement of abilities to form alliances while taking a dynamic perspective.

3.3.5.3 The Rationale

The rationale for the explanation of the client's problems and the treatment, also called the "myth" by Frank and Frank (1991), states an important common factor, in case it is convincingly communicated. It does not necessarily have to reflect "scientific truth," but has to be accepted by the client to enfold its impact in psychotherapy by leading to adaptive responses (Imel and Wampold 2008). This view is very similar to the early descriptions of Rosenzweig (1936), who stressed the importance of formal consistency (compared to "correctness"). From today's point of view, his very early statements can be viewed as crystal ball insight.

Due to their little differential efficacy, techniques can be viewed as general healing factors.

This means that they are not viewed as curative in a specific sense, but generally powerful in setting up a consistent treatment setting, enhancing hope, expectations of change, and problem resolution strategies in clients who have accepted the rationale as a treatment basis. It has been found that negative treatment outcome is related to a lack of focus and structure in the psychotherapeutic process (Lambert and Bergin 1994).

3.3.5.4 Client Factors

Hubble et al. (2010) stress that clients are the most neglected impact factor in psychotherapy research, including internal and external resources. Strengths and resources as well as readiness to change (McCarthy and Barber 2007), hope (Hubble et al. 1999; Larsen and Stege 2010), social support (Marziali 1987), and life events (Pilkonis et al. 1984) have, among others, been assigned significance as client characteristics. Independent of the therapeutic approach, therapy should therefore be specifically tailored to the respective client's needs and conditions. This idea is closely associated with the claim for the assessment of the quality, progress, and outcome of psychotherapy by clients.

3.3.6 Integrative Approaches

The development of integrative approaches for specific clinical problems can be viewed as a significant step, being closely associated with the movement of psychotherapy integration (Goldfried 2010, overview: Norcross and Goldfried 2005). Surprisingly, a very early ancestor can be traced back to the 1930s, when Thomas French was the first speaker in a meeting of the American Psychiatric Association who promoted an integrative idea of psychotherapeutic approaches (French 1933). More recent examples like cognitive analytic therapy (Rile 1995), mindfulness-based cognitive therapy (Segal et al. 2002), or dialectic behavior therapy for borderline personality disorder (Linehan 1993) should be labeled "integrative" rather than eclectic, because they combine certain strategies and techniques from different therapeutic schools under the roof of a new conceptualization of change, e.g., in the latter case from a philosophical dialectic perspective. This has to be differentiated from being merely eclectic in the sense that the treatment is based upon a whole new theoretical building. Despite the proven superiority of common factor impacts, in the area of very high symptom severity or severe personality disorders, the limits of common factors are to a certain degree tested and challenged. Therefore, especially for these aims, respective approaches and their refinement as well as their scrutiny for effectiveness are relevant also for future developments and high quality of clinical work and research.

3.4 Future Perspectives

With no doubt the further refinement of research methods is a topic of the history of psychotherapy research but also of the future. Quantitative methods should be enhanced in order to enable researchers to take the contextuality and time dependency of change processes more into account. The current intensive efforts to refine qualitative process-outcome methodologies, embracing the complexity of mechanisms of change, are and will with no doubt be maintained and intensified. This endeavor entails also the further consideration of qualitative outcome criteria. Mixed-method approaches have the potential to unify the strengths of both quantitative and qualitative and should as well be fostered in the upcoming years. A desirable aim is not just to strengthen the three branches in a parallel independent way, but to strive for a permanent interaction between the three approaches. This might impact the amelioration of especially common factor research in the future.

Moreover, although much is said and written about intercultural issues and their relevance for psychotherapy, the empirical basis for reasoning in this field is comparatively thin. Various questions arise in this field, not only giving attendance to the role of cultural characteristics as potential relevant client variables but also as therapist variables and the fit of characteristics in a therapeutic bond and their interaction. The same is true for the interaction of client and therapist variables in general, and respective research questions will most probably be investigated during the forthcoming years. There is a strong need associated with socio-political pressures to develop adequate evaluation designs for whole delivery systems with a focus on psychotherapy.

The strict adherence to traditionally dominant theories of change seems to fade in favor of micro-theoretical interests, with the central (more pragmatic) question being, "What works for whom or with this type of case?" (Lambert et al. 2004, p. 806).

Fortunately, there are so many creative minds out there all over the world, being ready and capable of facing these major challenges; being interconnected through societies, conferences, and modern media approaches; being full of spirit, who will reliably foster the development of psychotherapy research and will work on the ongoing insemination of research and practice.

References

American Psychiatric Association (APA) (2000) Diagnostic and statistical manual of mental disorders, fourth edition, text revision. American Psychiatric Association, Washington, DC

Anchin JC (2008) Contextualizing discourse on a philosophy of science for psychotherapy integration. J Psychother Integr 18(1):1–24. doi:10.1037/1053-0479.18.1.1

Appelbaum SA (1977) The anatomy of change: a Menninger foundation report on testing the effects of psychotherapy. Plenum, New York

Baer DM, Wolf M, Risley TR (1968) Some current dimensions of applied behavior analysis. J Appl Behav Anal 1:81–97

Baldwin SA, Wampold BE, Imel ZE (2007) Untangling the alliance-outcome correlation: exploring the relative importance of therapist and patient variability in the alliance. J Consult Clin Psychol 75:842–852. doi:10.1037/0022-006X.75.6.842

Bandura A, Lipsher DH, Miller PE (1960) Psychotherapists' approach-avoidance reactions to patients' expression of hostility. J Consult Psychol 24:1–8

Beck AT, Rush AJ, Shaw BF, Emery G (1979) Cognitive therapy of depression. Guilford, New York

Bergin AE (1963) The effects of psychotherapy: negative results revisited. J Couns Psychol 10:244–250

Bergin AE (1971) The evaluation of therapeutic outcomes. In: Bergin AE, Garfield SL (eds) Handbook of psychotherapy research and behavior change, 1st edn. Wiley, New York, pp 217–270

Bergin AE, Garfield SL (1971) Handbook of psychotherapy and behavior change, 1st edn. Wiley, New York

Bernheim H (1892) Hypnotisme, suggestion, psychothérapie. Études nouvelles. Doin, Paris

Bordin ES (1979) The generalizability of the psychoanalytic concept of working alliance. Psychotherapy 16:252–260. doi:10.1037/h0085885

Breuer J, Freud S (1893–1895/1955) The standard edition of the complete psychological works of Sigmund Freud: Vol. II. Studies on hysteria. Hogarth Press, London

Butler JM (1952) The interaction of client and therapist. J Abnorm Soc Psychol 47(2):366–378. doi:10.1037/h0063157

Caspar F (2009) Was genau ist "good for people"? Ein differenzierter Diskussionsbeitrag zur aktuellen Psychotherapieforschung. What does "good for people" mean? A contribution to current psychotherapy research. Psychoscope 30:8–11

Clarkin JF, Levy KN (2004) The influence of client variables in psychotherapy. In: Lambert M (ed) Bergin and Garfield's handbook of psychotherapy and behavior change, 5th edn. Wiley, New York, pp 805–821

Crits-Christoph PC, Barber JP, Grenyer BFS, Diguer L (2010) Lester Luborsky: a trailblazer in empirical research on psychoanalytic therapy. In: Castonguay LG, Muran JC, Angus L, Hayes JH, Ladany N, Anderson T (eds) Bringing psychotherapy research to life: Understanding change through the work of leading clinical researchers. American Psychological Association Press, Washington, DC, pp 39–49

Czogalik D, Russell RL (1995) Interactional structures of therapist and client participation in adult psychotherapy: P technique and chronography. J Consult Clin Psychol 63(1):28–36. doi:10.1037/0022-006X.63.1.28

Denker R (1947) Results of treatments of psychoneuroses by the general practitioner. A follow-up study of 500 cases. NY State J Med 46:2164–2166

Desmet M (2013) Experimental and naturalistic psychotherapy research: consequences for researchers, clinicians, policy makers and patients. Psychoanalytische Perspectieven 31(1):59–78

Detert NB, Llewelyn S, Hardy G, Barkham M, Stiles WB (2006) Assimilation in good- and poor-outcome cases of very brief psychotherapy for mild depression: an initial comparison. Psychother Res 16(4):393–407. doi:10.1080/10503300500294728

Duncan BL (2010) Prologue: Saul Rosenzweig: the founder of the common factors. In: Duncan BL, Miller SD, Wampold BE, Hubble MA (eds) The heart and soul of change. Delivering what works in therapy, 2nd edn. American Psychological Association, Washington, DC, pp 3–23

Elkin I (1994) The NIHM treatment of depression collaborative program: where we began and where we are. In: Bergin AE, Garfield SL (eds) Handbook of psychotherapy and behavior change, 4th edn. Wiley, New York, pp 114–139

Elkin I, Shea MT, Watkins JT, Imber SD et al (1989) The national institute of mental health treatment of depression collaborative program: general effectiveness of treatments. Arch Gen Psychiatry 46:971–982. doi:10.1001/archpsyc.1989.01810110013002

Elliot R (ed) (1999) Special issue: qualitative psychotherapy research. Psychother Res 9(3): 251–257

Elliott R (2010) Psychotherapy change process research: realizing the promise. Psychother Res 20(2):123–135. doi:10.1080/10503300903470743

Elliott R, Anderson C (1994) Simplicity and complexity in psychotherapy research. In: Russel RL (ed) Reassessing psychotherapy research. Guilford, New York, pp 185–214

Elliott R, Farber BA (2010) Carl Rogers: idealistic pragmatist and psychotherapy research pioneer. In: Castonguay LG, Muran JC, Angus L, Hayes JH, Ladany N, Anderson T (eds) Bringing psychotherapy research to life: Understanding change through the work of leading clinical researchers. American Psychological Association Press, Washington, DC, pp 17–27

Elliott R, Slatick E, Urman M (2001) Qualitative change process research in psychotherapy: alternative strategies. In: Frommer J, Rennie DL (eds) Qualitative psychotherapy research: methods and methodology. Pabst Science, Lengerich, pp 69–111

Eysenck HJ (1952) The effects of psychotherapy: an evaluation. J Consult Clin Psychol 16:319–324. doi:10.1037//0022-006X.60.5.659

Eysenck HJ (1960) Learning theory and behavior therapy. In: Eysenck HJ (ed) Behavior therapy and the neuroses. Pergamon, London

Faller H, Frommer J (1994) Qualitative Psychotherapieforschung. Grundlagen und Methoden. Asanger Verlag, Kröning

Feiler S, Muller KG, Muller A, Dahlhaus R, Eich W (2005) Using interaction graphs for analysing the therapy process. Psychother Psychosom 74(2):93–99. doi:10.1159/000083167

Fiedler P (2010) Verhaltenstherapie mon amour. Schattauer, Stuttgart

Frank JD (1961) Persuasion and healing. Johns Hopkins University Press, Baltimore

Frank JD (1973) Persuasion and healing, 2nd edn. Johns Hopkins University Press, Baltimore, MD

Frank JD, Frank JB (1991) Persuasion and healing: a comparative study of psychotherapy, 3rd edn. Johns Hopkins University Press, Baltimore

Frank JD (1992) The Johns Hopkins psychotherapy research project. In: Freedheim DK (ed) A history of psychotherapy: a century of change. American Psychological Association, Washington, DC, pp 392–396

Franks CM (1987) Behavior therapy and AABT: personal recollections, conceptions, and misconceptions. Behav Ther 10:171–174

Franks CM (1997) It was the best of times, it was the worst of times [special issue: thirty years of behavior therapy]. Behav Ther 28:389–396

French TM (1933) Interrelations between psychoanalysis and the experimental work of Pavlov. Am J Psychiatr 89:1165–1203

Garfield SL (1981) Evaluating the psychotherapies. Behav Ther 12:295–307. doi:10.1016/S0005-7894(81)80119-0

Garfield SL (1995) Psychotherapy: an eclectic-integrative approach, 2nd edn. Wiley, New York (originally published in 1980)

Gelo OCG (2012) On research methods and their philosophical assumptions: "raising the consciousness of researchers" again. Psychotherapie und Sozialwissenschaft 14(2):111–130

Glaser SR (1977) An analysis of the psychotherapeutic interview as a rhetorical process by applying the methods of rhetorical criticism to ongoing therapeutic discourse. Dissertation Abstracts International, vol 38 (2-A)

Goldfried MR (2010) The future of psychotherapy integration: closing the gap between research and practice. J Psychother Integr 20(4):386–396. doi:10.1037/a0022036

Goldfried MR, Newman CF (1992) A history of psychotherapy integration. In: Norcross JC, Goldfried MR (eds) Handbook of psychotherapy integration. Basic, New York, pp 46–93

Goldman GA, Anderson T (2007) Quality of object relations and security of attachment as predictors of early therapeutic alliance. J Couns Psychol 54: 111–117. doi:10.1037/0022-0167.54.2.111

Goldman RN, Angus L, Safran JD (2010) Leslie Greenberg: emotional change leads to positive outcome. In: Castonguay LG, Muran JC, Angus L, Hayes JA, Ladany N, Anderson T (eds) Bringing psychotherapy 1987 research into life. Understanding change through the work of leading clinical researchers. American Psychological Association, Washington, DC, pp 186–195

Gomes-Schwartz B, Schwartz JM (1978) Psychotherapy process variables distinguishing the inherently helpful person from the professional psychotherapist. J Consult Clin Psychol 46(1):196–197. doi:10.1037/0022-006X.46.1.196

Gordon T, Grummon DL, Rogers CR, Seeman J (1954) Developing a program of research in psychotherapy. In: Rogers CR, Dymond RF (eds) Psychotherapy and personality change. University of Chicago Press, Chicago, pp 12–34

Goth N, Goth J, Weigelin J (1980) Zum Problem der negativen Effekte in der Psychotherapie. Psychiatr Neurol Med Psychol 32(9):550–556

Greenberg L (1986) Change process research. J Consult Clin Psychol 54(1):4–9. doi:10.1037/0022-006X.54.1.4

Greenberg LS, Pinsof WM (eds) (1986) The psychotherapeutic process: a research handbook. Guilford, New York

Gross HS (1978) Therapeutic discourse: psychotherapy as a conversation. J Nerv Ment Dis 166(12):897–900. doi:10.1097/00005053-197812000-00014

Hagebak RW, Parker GVC (1969) Therapist directiveness, client dominance, and therapy resistance. J Consult Clin Psychol 33(5):536–540. doi:10.1037/h0028298

Hansen N, Lambert MJ, Forman EM (2002) The psychotherapy dose-response effect and its implication for treatment delivery services. Clin Psychol 9:329–343. doi:10.1093/clipsy.9.3.329

Haug S, Strauß B, Gallas C, Kordy H (2008a) New prospects for process research in group therapy: text-based process variables in psychotherapeutic Internet-chat groups. Psychother Res 18:88–96. doi:10.1080/10503300701368008

Haug S, Sedway J, Kordy H (2008b) Group processes and process evaluations in a new treatment setting: inpatient group psychotherapy followed by internet-chat aftercare. Int J Group Psychother 58(1):35–53. doi:10.1521/ijgp.2008.58.1.35

Heine RW (1953) A comparison of patients' reports on psychotherapeutic experience with psychoanalytic, nondirective and Adlerian therapists. Am J Psychother 7:16–23

Henry WE, Sims J, Spray SL (1974) The public and private lives of psychotherapists. Psychotherapy 11 (4):390–391

Hersen M, Barlow DH (1976) Single-case experimental design: strategies for studying behavior change. Plenum, New York

Hersen M, Michelson L, Bellack AS (1984) Historical overview. In: Bellack AS, Hersen M, Michelson I (eds) Issues in psychotherapy research. Plenum, New York, pp 3–33

Hersoug AG (2010) A closer look at good and poor outcome in psychodynamic, psychotherapy: a case comparison study. Clin Case Stud 9(2):135–153. doi:10.1177/1534650110364415

Hill CE (ed) (1994) Special section: qualitative research in counseling process and outcome. J Couns Psychol 41(4)

Holt RR, Luborsky L (1958) Personality patterns of psychiatrists. Vol. II. A study of methods for selecting residents. Basic Books, Oxford

Horvath AO, Bedi RP (2002) The alliance. In: Norcross JC (ed) Psychotherapy relationships that work. Therapist contributions and responsiveness to patients. University Press, Oxford, pp 37–69

Horvath AO, Del Re AC, Flückiger C, Symonds D (2011) Alliance in individual psychotherapy. Psychotherapy 48(1):9–16. doi:10.1037/a0022186

Horwitz L (1974) Clinical prediction in psychotherapy. Jason Aronson, New York

Hubble MA, Duncan BL, Miller SD (1999) Directing attention to what works. In: Hubble MA, Duncan BL, Miller SD (eds) The heart and soul of change: what works in therapy. American Psychological Association, Washington, DC, pp 407–448

Hubble MA, Duncan BL, Miller SD, Wampold BE (2010) Introduction. In: Duncan BL, Miller SD, Wampold BE, Hubble MA (eds) The heart and soul of change. Delivering what works in therapy, 2nd edn. American Psychological Association, Washington, DC, pp 23–46

Huddleson GH (1927) Psychotherapy in two hundred cases of psychoneurosis. Mil Surg 60:161–170

Imel Z, Wampold D (2008) The importance of treatment and the science of common factors in psychotherapy. In: Brown SD, Lent RW (eds) Handbook of counseling psychology. Wiley, New York, pp 249–262

Jacobsen NS, Truax P (1991) Clinical significance: a statistical approach to defining meaningful change in psychotherapy research. J Consult Clin Psychol 59: 12–19

Jacobsen NS, Follette WC, Revenstorf D (1984) Psychotherapy outcome research: methods for reporting variability and evaluating clinical significance. Behav Ther 13:336–352

Jacobsen NS, Roberts LJ, Berns SB, McGlinchey JB (1999) Methods for defining and determining the clinical significance of treatment effects: description, application, and alternatives. J Consult Clin Psychol 67:300–307. doi:10.1037//0022-006X.67.3.300

Kazdin AE (1978) Methodological and interpretive problems of single-case experimental designs. J Consult Clin Psychol 46:629–642. doi:10.1037//0022-006X.46.4.629

Kendall PC, Marrs-Garcia A, Nath SR, Sheldrick RC (1999) Normative comparisons for the evaluation of clinical significance. J Consult Clin Psychol 67(3): 285–299. doi:10.1037/0022-006X.67.3.285

Kendall PC, Holmbeck G, Verduin T (2004) Methodology, design, and evaluation in psychotherapy research. In: Lambert M (ed) Bergin and Garfield's handbook of psychotherapy and behavior change, 5th edn. Wiley, New York, pp 16–43

Kernberg OF, Berstein ED, Coyne L, Appelbaum A, Horwitz L, Voth H (1972) Psychotherapy and psychoanalysis: final report of the Meninnger foundation's psychotherapy research project. Bull Menninger Clin 36:1–375

Kiesler DJ (1966) Some myths of psychotherapy research and the search for a paradigm. Psychol Bull 65: 110–136. doi:10.1037/h0022911

Kiesler DJ (1973) The process of psychotherapy: empirical foundations and systems of analysis. Aldine, Chicago

Kiesler DJ (1982) Confronting the client-therapist relationship on psychotherapy. In: Anchin JC, Kiesler DJ (eds) Handbook of interpersonal psychotherapy. Pergamon, Elmsford, pp 274–295

Kiesler DJ (2001a) Empirical studies that used the checklist of interpersonal/psychotherapy transactions: an annotated bibliography. Retrieved from http://www.vcu.edu/sitar/cloit.pdf

Kiesler DJ (2001b) Empirical studies that used the impact message inventory: an annotated bibliography. Retrieved from http://www.vcu.edu/sitar/imi.pdf

Klerman GL, Weissman JM, Rounsaville BJ, Chevron ES (1984) Interpersonal psychotherapy for depression. Basic Books, New York

Lambert MJ (1992) Psychotherapy outcome research: implications for integrative and eclectical therapists. In: Norcross JC, Goldfried MR, Marvin R (eds) Handbook of psychotherapy integration. Basic Books, New York, pp 94–129

Lambert MJ, Bergin AE (1994) The effectiveness of psychotherapy. In: Lambert M (ed) Bergin and Garfield's handbook of psychotherapy and behavior change, 4th edn. Wiley, New York, pp 143–184

Lambert MJ (2004) Bergin and Garfield's handbook of psychotherapy and behavior change, 5th edn. Wiley, New York

Lambert MJ (2013) Bergin and Garfield's handbook of psychotherapy and behavior change, 6th edn. Wiley, New York

Lambert MJ, Ogles BM (2004) The efficacy and effectiveness of psychotherapy. In: Lambert M (ed) Bergin and Garfield's handbook of psychotherapy and behavior change, 5th edn. Wiley, New York, pp 139–193

Lambert MJ, Hansen NB, Finch AE (2001) Patient-focused research: using patient outcome to enhance treatment effects. J Consult Clin Psychol 69:159–172. doi:10.1037/0022-006X.69.2.159

Lambert MJ, Garfield SL, Bergin AE (2004) Overview, trends and future issues. In: Lambert M (ed) Bergin and Garfield's handbook of psychotherapy and behavior change, 5th edn. Wiley, New York, pp 805–821

Lamprecht F (2006) Kosten-Nutzen-Erwägungen in der Psychotherapie. Cost-benefit analyses in psychotherapy. In: Strauss B, Geyer M (eds) Grenzen psychotherapeutischen Handelns. Vandenhoeck & Ruprecht, Goettingen, pp 91–103

Landis C (1938) Statistical evaluation of pychotherapeutic methods. In: Hinsie SE (ed) Concepts and problems of psychotherapy. Heineman, London, pp 155–165

Lang PJ, Lazonik AD (1963) Experimental desensitization of phobia. J Abnorm Soc Psych 66(6):519–525. doi:10.1037/h0039828

Larsen DJ, Stege R (2010) Hope-focused practices during early psychotherapy sessions: Part I: implicit approaches. J Psychother Integr 20(3):272–292. doi:10.1037/a0020820

Linehan MM (1993) Dialectic behavior therapy for borderline personality disorder. Guilford, New York

Llewelyn S (1988) Psychological therapy as viewed by clients and therapists. Br J Clin Psychol 27:223–238. doi:10.1111/j.2044-8260.1988.tb00779.x

Luborsky L (1954) A note on Eysenck's article 'The effects of psychotherapy: an evaluation'. Br J Psychol 45(2):129–131

Luborsky L, Singer B, Luborsky L (1975) Comparative studies of psychotherapies: is it true that "everyone has one and all must have prizes"? Arch Gen Psychiatry 32:995–1008

Marmor J (1962) Psychoanalytic therapy as an educational process. In: Massernan JH (ed) Science and psychoanalysis. Grune and Stratton, New York, pp 286–299

Macdonald J, Cartwright A, Brown G (2007) A quantitative and qualitative exploration of client-therapist interaction and engagement in treatment in an alcohol service. Psychol Psychother 80(2):247–268. doi:10.1348/147608306X156553

Macklin R (1973) The medical model on psychoanalysis and psychotherapy. Compr Psychiatry 14(1):49–69. doi:10.1016/0010-440X(73)90055-2

Marziali E (1987) People in your life: development of a social support measure for predicting psychotherapy outcome. J Nerv Ment Dis 175(6):327–328

Matz PB (1929) Outcome of hospital treatment of ex-service patients with nervous and mental disease in the U.S. Veterans Bureau. Med Bull 5:829–842

McCarthy K, Barber JP (2007) Review of ambivalence in psychotherapy: facilitating readiness to change. Psychother Res 17(4):504–506

McCullough JP Jr (2005) Cognitive behavioral analysis system of psychotherapy: treatment for chronic depression. In: Norcross JC, Goldfried MR (eds) Handbook of psychotherapy integration, 2nd edn. Oxford University Press, London, pp 281–298

Mintz J, Luborsky L (1971) Segments vs. whole session. Which is the better unit for psychotherapy process research? J Abnorm Psychol 78(2):180–191

Moras K, Shea MT (2010) Irene Elkin: "the data are always friendly". In: Castonguay LG, Muran JC, Angus L, Hayes JH, Ladany N, Anderson T (eds) Bringing psychotherapy research to life: Understanding change through the work of leading clinical researchers. American Psychological Association Press, Washington, DC, pp 77–88

Muran JC, Castonguay LG, Strauss B (2010) A brief introduction to psychotherapy research. In: Castonguay LG, Muran JC, Angus L, Hayes JH, Ladany N, Anderson T (eds) Bringing psychotherapy research to life: understanding change through the work of leading clinical researchers. American Psychological Association Press, Washington, DC, pp 3–13

Nelson RA, Borkovec TD (1989) Relationship of client participation to psychotherapy. J Behav Ther Exp Psychiatry 20(2):155–162. doi:10.1016/0005-7916(89)90048-7

Neustatter WL (1935) The results of fifty cases treated by psychotherapy. Lancet 1:796–799

Nietzel MT, Russell RL, Hemmings KA, Gretter ML (1987) Clinical significance of psychotherapy for unipolar depression: a meta-analytic approach to social comparison. J Consult Clin Psychol 55(2):156–161. doi:10.1037//0022-006X.55.2.156

Noblin CD, Timmons EO, Reynard MC (1963) Psychoanalytic interpretations as verbal reinforcers: importance of interpretation content. J Clin Psychol 19: 479–481

Norcross JC, Goldfried MR (eds) (2005) Handbook of psychotherapy integration (2nd edn). Oxford University Press, New York

O'Malley S, Suh CS, Strupp HH (1983) The Vanderbilt psychotherapy process scale: a report on the scale-development and a process-outcome study. J Consult Clin Psychol 51(4):581–586. doi:10.1037/0022-006X.51.4.581

Orlinsky DE, Russel RL (1994) Tradition and change in psychotherapy research. Notes on the fourth generation. In: Russel RL (ed) Reassessing psychotherapy research. Guilford, New York, pp 185–214

Orlinsky DE, Rønnestad MH, Willutzki U (2004) Fifty years of psychotherapy process-outcome research: continuity and change. In: Lambert M (ed) Bergin and Garfield's handbook of psychotherapy and behavior change, 5th edn. Wiley, New York, pp 307–389

Persons JB (1986) The advantages of studying psychological phenomena rather than psychiatric diagnoses. Am Psychol 41(11):1252–1260. doi:10.1037//0003-066X.41.11.1252

Pilkonis P, Imber SD, Rubinsky P (1984) Influence of life events on outcome in psychotherapy. J Nerv Ment Dis 172(8):468–474. doi:10.1097/00005053-198408000-00005

Pole N, Ablon J, O'Connor L, Weiss J (2002) Ideal control mastery technique correlates with change in a single case. Psychother Theory Res Pract Train 39(1): 88–89. doi:10.1037//0033-3204.39.1.88

Ponterotto JG (2005) Qualitative research in counseling psychology. A primer on research paradigms and philosophy of science. J Couns Psychol 52(2):126–136. doi:10.1037/0022-0167.52.2.126

Rennie DL (2012) Qualitative research as methodical hermeneutics. Psychol Methods 17(3):385–398. doi:10.1037/a0029250

Rice LN, Greenberg LS (eds) (1984) Patterns of change: intensive analysis of psychotherapy practice. Guilford, New York

Richter HE (1974) Community development and psychotherapy in slum ghetto. Psychother Psychosom 24 (4–6):269–280

Rile A (1995) Cognitive analytic therapy: developments in theory and practice. Wiley, New York

Rioch MJ, Elkes C, Flint AA, Usdansky BS, Newman RG, Silber E (1965) Pilot project in training mental health counselors (U.S. Public Health Service Publication No. 125, 1965). US Government Printing Office, Washington, DC

Rogers C (1942a) Counseling and psychotherapy. Houghton Mifflin, Boston

Rogers C (1942b) The use of electrically recorded interviews in improving psychotherapeutic techniques. Am J Orthopsychiatry 12:429–434. doi:10.1111/j.1939-0025.1942.tb05930.x

Rogers C (1957) The necessary and sufficient conditions of therapeutic personality change. J Consult Psychol 21(2):95–103. doi:10.1037//0022-006X.60.6.827

Rosenthal D, Frank JD (1958) The fate of psychiatric clinic outpatients assigned to psychotherapy. J Nerv Ment Dis 127:330–343. doi:10.1097/00005053-195810000-00004

Rosenzweig S (1936) Some implicit common factors in diverse methods of psychotherapy. Am J Orthopsychiatry 6:412–415. doi:10.1111/j.1939-0025.1936.tb05248.x

Rosenzweig S (1954) A transvaluation of psychotherapy: a reply to Eysenck. J Abnorm Psychol 49:298–304. doi:10.1037/h0061172

Rubenstein EA, Parloff MB (1959) Research in psychotherapy, vol 1. American Psychological Association, Washington, DC

Russell RL, Orlinsky DE (1996) Psychotherapy research in historical perspective. Implications for Mental Health Care Policy. Arch Gen Psychiatry 53:708–714. doi:10.1001/archpsyc.1996.01830080060010

Salvatore S, Tschacher W (2012) Time dependency of psychotherapeutic exchanges: the contribution of the theory of dynamic systems in analyzing process. Front Psychol 3:253. doi:10.3389/fpsyg2012/00253

Saslow G, Matarazzo JD (1962) A technique for studying changes in interview behaviour. In: Rubenstein V, Parloff MB (eds) Research in psychotherapy, vol 3. American Psychological Association, Washington, DC

Sauer EM, Lopez FG, Gormley B (2003) Respective contributions of therapist and client adult attachment orientations to the development of the early working alliance: a preliminary growth modeling study. Psychother Res 13:371–382. doi:10.1093/ptr/kpg027

Schindler L, Hohenberger-Sieber E, Hahlweg K (1989) Observing client-therapist interaction in behaviour therapy: development and first application of an observational system. Br J Clin Psychol 28(3):213–226. doi:10.1111/j.2044-8260.1989.tb01371.x

Segal ZV, Williams JMG, Teasdale JD (2002) Mindfulness based cognitive therapy for depression. A new approach to preventing relapse. Guilford, New York

Shadish WR, Matt GE, Navarro AM, Siegle G, Crits-Christoph P, Hazelrigg MD, Jorm AF, Lyons LC, Nietzel MT, Prout HT, Robinson L, Smith ML, Svartberg M, Weiss B (1997) Evidence that therapy works in clinically representative conditions. J Consult Clin Psychol 62:992–1002

Shlien AM et al (eds) Research in psychotherapy: vol. III. American Psychological Association, Washington, DC

Smith ML, Glass GV, Miller TI (1980) The benefits of psychotherapy. John Hopkins University Press, Baltimore

Snyder WU (1945) An investigation of the nature of nondirective psychotherapy. J Gen Psychol 33: 193–223. doi:10.1037/10841-035

Strupp HH (1957) A multidimensional comparison of therapist activity in analytic and client-centered therapy. J Consult Psychol 21(4):301–308. doi:10.1037/h0045423

Strupp HH, Hadley SW (1977) A tripartite model of mental health and therapeutic outcomes. With special reference to negative effects in psychotherapy. Am Psychol 32(3):187–196. doi:10.1037//0003-066X.32.3.187

Strupp HH, Howard KI (1992) A brief history of psychotherapy research. In: Freeman DK, Freudenberger HJ, Kessler JW, Messer SB, Peterson DR, Strupp HH, Wachtel PL (eds) History of psychotherapy: a century of change. American Psychological Association, Washington, DC, pp 309–334

Strupp HH, Luborsky L (1962) Research in psychotherapy, vol 2. American Psychological Association, Washington, DC

Strupp HH, Hadley SW, Gomes B, Armstrong SH (1976) Negative effects in psychotherapy: a review of clinical and theoretical issues together with recommendations for a program of research. Report to the National Institute of Mental Health (Contract No. 278-75-003)

Tharp RG, Wetzel RJ (1969) Behaviour modification in the natural environment. Academic, New York

Thorndike EL (1918) The nature, purposes and general methods of measurements of educational products. In: Whipple GM (ed) National society for the study of educational products: seventeenth yearbook. Public School Publishing, Bloomington, pp 16–24

Truax CB (1968) Therapist interpersonal reinforcement of client self-exploration and therapeutic outcome in group therapy. J Consult Psychol 15(3):225–231

Truax CB, Carkhuff RR (1965) Client and therapist transparency in the psychotherapeutic encounter. J Couns Psychol 12(1):3–9

Truax CB, Mitchell KM (1971) Research on certain therapist interpersonal skills in relation to process and outcome. In: Bergin AE, Garfield SL (eds) Handbook of psychotherapy and behavior change, 1st edn. Wiley, New York, pp 299–344

Tschacher W, Ramseyer F (2009) Modeling psychotherapy process by time-series panel analysis (TSPA). Psychother Res 19(4–5):469–481. doi:10.1080/10503300802654496

Wagner CC, Safran JD (2010) Donald J. Kiesler: interpersonal manifesto. In: Castonguay LG, Muran JC, Angus L, Hayes JH, Ladany N, Anderson T (eds) Bringing psychotherapy research to life: Understanding change through the work of leading clinical researchers. American Psychological Association Press, Washington DC, pp 211–220

Wallerstein RS (1986) Forty-two lives in treatment: a study of psychoanalysis and psychotherapy. Guilford, New York

Wampold BE (2001) The great psychotherapy debate: models, methods, findings. Lawrence Erlbaum Associates, London

Wampold BE (2010) The research evidence for the common factor models: a historically situated perspective. In: Duncan BL, Miller SD, Wampold BE, Hubble MA (eds) The heart and soul of change. Delivering what works in therapy, 2nd edn. American Psychological Association, Washington, DC, pp 49–81

Waskow IE, Parloff MB (1975) Psychotherapy change measures: report of the clinical research branch outcome measures project. National Institute of Mental Health, Rockville

Watson G (1940) Areas of agreement in psychotherapy. Am J Orthopsychiatry 10:698–709

Weisz JR, Weiss B, Donenberg GR (1993) The lab vs. the clinic: effects of child and adolescent psychotherapy. Annual Progress in Child Psychiatry and Child Development: 47:441–458

Wilson GT, Rachman S (1983) Meta analysis and the evaluation of psychotherapy outcome: limitations and liabilities. J Consult Clin Psychol 51:54–64. doi:10.1037//0022-006X.51.1.54

Wiseman H, Rice LN (1989) Sequential analysis of therapist-client interaction during change events: a task-focused approach. J Consult Clin Psychol 57(2): 281–286. doi:10.1037//0022-006X.57.2.281

World Health Organization (1992) The ICD-10 classification of mental and behavioural disorders. Clinical descriptions and diagnostic guidelines. World Health Organization, Geneva

4 The Philosophy of Psychotherapy Science: Mainstream and Alternative Views

Bernd Rieken and Omar Carlo Gioacchino Gelo

Contents

Abstract

The aim of this chapter is to show that determinism, reductionism, and mechanism have dominated people's lives since the early modern period and, as a consequence, have been representing a monopoly in sciences in general and in psychotherapy science in particular ever since. In addition, it will raise the issue of what other approaches to understanding reality and human beings have unjustly been forgotten—unjustly, because they might contribute to a more comprehensive understanding and examination of human life and with it also of psychotherapy. These include, as we will attempt to demonstrate in the following, intentionality, wholeness, and the analogical thinking, which lay the groundwork for emerging alternative research approaches. Finally, the implications of the above for a pluralistic psychotherapy science will be presented.

B. Rieken (✉)
Department of Psychotherapy Science, Sigmund Freud University, Freudplatz 1, 1020 Vienna, Austria
e-mail: bernd.rieken@sfu.ac.at

O.C.G. Gelo
Department of History, Society and Human Studies, University of Salento, Via Stampacchia 45, 73100 Lecce, Italy

Department of Psychotherapy Science, Sigmund Freud University, Freudplatz 1, 1020 Vienna, Austria
e-mail: omar.gelo@unisalento.it; omar.gelo@sfu.ac.at

4.1 Introduction

In order to understand the behavior and experience of a person, it can be helpful to concern oneself with their life history as well as their implicit and explicit theoretical beliefs. This is similar with regard to science: what is natural for us has its own history which could have taken a different course and that is why scientific approaches that were once available to us are

O.C.G. Gelo et al. (eds.), *Psychotherapy Research*,
DOI 10.1007/978-3-7091-1382-0_4,

buried today. Moreover, scientists often tend not to reflect enough on the implicit presuppositions of their approaches, and so they pay little attention to alternatives to their own method(s) (Gelo 2012; Slife 1998).

This actually outlines the topic of this chapter: the tacit philosophical assumptions of science, including the aspects of their historical development, and how these ground our conception(s) of psychotherapy science. It makes sense to focus on this, because our specific understanding of psychotherapy science derives from our understanding of science in general. Usually people do not think about this, because it is assumed implicitly that science must be practiced the way it has always been done—and the way science is mostly practiced nowadays conforms to the principles of natural sciences. Only few authors, such as Gottfried Fischer in the German-speaking world (Fischer 2008, 2011; see also Rieken 2013) and Brent D. Slife in the English-speaking world (Slife 2004; Slife and Gantt 1999; Slife et al. 2005; see also Gelo 2012), have dealt with alternative approaches and tried to point out that our understanding of science in general and its implications for psychotherapy science depend on ideas, values, and beliefs that do not only exist "objectively" but are there because we believe in them.

In the present chapter, we first outline some of the implicit beliefs characterizing the mainstream in science and psychotherapy science in its historical development and highlight its strengths and weaknesses; thereafter, we draw attention to alternative views that are important for human sciences in general and psychotherapy science in particular.

4.2 Science in the Mainstream

4.2.1 *Homo Faber* and the Relationship Between Cause and Effect as *Causa Efficiens*

From the plethora of ascriptions that claim to capture the "essence" of man (see Wuketits 1985, pp. 262–263), the dominating idea since the science of the *modern* period has been that *Homo sapiens* is primarily a *Homo faber* (Frisch 1959) who is characterized by the ability to use or make tools. But this ability does not account for the exceptional position of humans in evolution, for they share it with other living beings such as birds, which build nests, or beavers, which construct dams. Still it pushes other concepts of the human being into the background, especially concepts from the field of the humanities—such as that of the *Homo symbolicus* (Cassirer 1953–1957), the *Homo ludens* (Huizinga 1980), or the *animal metaphysicum* (Schopenhauer 1958). However, the view that human beings are primarily characterized through their activities as *Homo faber* and the ability to manufacture or use tools still continues to shape science and the public opinion (see Mumford 1967–1970). When, for example, an article was published in the *Proceedings of the National Academy of Sciences of the United States of America* (PNAS) in 2013 that had found evidence that not only *Homo sapiens* but Neanderthals also used special tools made of bone, called lissoirs, to process leather (Soressia et al. 2013), this message went around the world and quickly spread in the popular media (about 25,000 results on Google by entering the keywords "Lissoirs Neanderthal" on 29/08/2013).

Why does the *Homo faber* shape humans' self-image so much even though alternative attributions are available that are also of significance for them? Obviously, there are fundamental experiences that reinforce this and always have: the primitive hunter who shoots an arrow at a deer and kills it notices *causality*, a connection between cause and effect, which is linked to *activity* and *movement*. Thus, the hunter can actively change the environment which, simultaneously, does not only lead to practical certainty, which is essential for life, but also an understanding of its processes.

Psychological ontogenesis works similarly in children, as they gradually learn to coordinate schemata of grasping and looking via the interplay of assimilation and accommodation, so that they can finally reach for an object in order to examine it more closely, or examine it in order to touch it more precisely (Piaget 1953). In this respect, the intimate connection between "grasping" ("grasp" in the sense of "to reach for something") and "grasping" ("grasp" in the sense of "to understand") is not only semantic but also real. The child's "grasping" is followed by an "understanding," similar to how the primitive hunter made the connection between the firing of the arrow and the killing of the deer. Ever since Aristotle, the philosophy of science has called this correlation the *causa efficiens*; however, while in Aristotle this is only one of several causes (see Sect. 4.3.1), in the early modern period it became the sole cause—the definition of philosopher David Hume is paradigmatic with this regard, describing cause "as an object, followed by another, and whose appearance always conveys the thought to that another" (Hume 2007, No. 76, p. 70). This way of conceptualizing causality is the hallmark of the modern *causal-analytical* thinking (see Sect. 4.3.3, for an antithetical view).

With regard to psychotherapy science, the textbook examples for this are the efficacy studies in outcome research in which the isolated and controlled treatment conditions represent the *causa efficiens* and the treatment outcome, systematically assessed through pre-post measures, is identified as effect (see Chap. 26 Lambert 2013). Actually, mainstream psychotherapy research seems not to be able to conceive any other form of causality legitimately grounding the scientific investigation of treatment outcomes (see Slife et al. 2005 for a discussion).

4.2.2 Empiricism, Reductionism, and Determinism: Observation and Experiment

The insight gained from everyday life about the connection between cause and effect is not yet scientific knowledge, but knowledge gained from experience. In order to turn it into scientific knowledge, it needs to be systematized in several ways. This includes the acknowledgment that direct perception can be deceptive, which is why it is necessary to take a step back, so to speak, to be able to observe what one wants to examine from a certain distance. In other words, a separation of subject and object is required (as discussed in more detail in Chap. 4), dealing with the fundamental changes of the self and self-perception in Renaissance culture. This separation also means relinquishing the magical-mythical view of nature, which is based on the notion of humans being a part of and in constant interaction with nature as a living organism. The objectification of nature, which goes hand in hand with the insistence on the human ability to "create distance," enhances the status of the intellectual at the expense of the emotional capacity. Philosophy henceforth calls the former "higher faculty" and the latter "lower faculty," thus contrasting reason and emotion in a hierarchical relationship (see Gloy 1996, pp. 7–8).

The mind may now, without having to rely on the "lower faculty," systematically *observe* its subject; this should be done repeatedly over time and by several people independently, so that the observation becomes *verifiable* and *repeatable*. Moreover, scientists should measure the phenomena under investigation in order to carry out *reliable* observations. It is also possible to intervene with the observed system in the form of an *experiment* and systematically alter specific influencing (independent) variables with instruments and devices in order to measure the resulting changes in other (dependent) variables. These are important differences that separate modern from ancient and medieval science: first, there was little interest in intersubjective verifiability and/or shareability in antiquity and the Middle Ages. This is partly due to an alternative conception of truth, which was based on the confirmation by authority and less on *empiricism*—according to which knowledge is derived from our sense experience. Also, the focus was not on things that change—movement and variables—but rather on things that remain static, because ultimately, movement served only to achieve a "natural" state of rest. Aristotle's famous statement that man begets man (Aristotle 1930, II, 2, 194b) makes it clear that what is reproduced is always the same, in this example an individual of the same species. A third point is that the aim of investigation was, in line with the primacy of the static, to observe the natural processes of the world without interruption, but not to change them. This is radically different in the modern period: the experiment has a special status in the empirical sciences of the modern era, because it systematically intervenes in nature and thus "each experiment [poses] [. . .] a question to nature," to quote the famous philosopher Schelling from the year 1799 (Schelling 2004, p. 33).

With the experiment, humans develop an active relationship with nature. They assume that the bewildering diversity of natural phenomena hides simple, eternal laws. In reality, however, these cannot be observed in direct form, though the movements of the planets come pretty close. Isaac Newton (1643–1727) used them to develop his three basic laws of motion in the *Philosophiae Naturalis Principia Mathematica*: the law of inertia, the law of force, and the law of interaction (Newton 1999). The movements of the planets may occur under conditions that largely correspond to the Newtonian laws, but the conditions on Earth are more complicated. Therefore, in an experiment, the appropriate conditions must first be created. All factors in the course of an event that do not correspond to the postulated law must be declared disruptive factors and eliminated, regardless of the role they play in the normal processes that do not take place under experimental conditions. The success of science thus came at the cost of a radical simplification of natural conditions. Only on this basis was it possible to attain reliable and generally applicable scientific data. This means that the inscrutable wealth of subjective impressions was replaced by a world of simpler and eternal laws. In this way, the processes that were studied could be traced back to the laws of motion and explained in a strictly deterministic way through the principle of cause and effect, which led to a mechanization of nature (Dijksterhuis 1961; Dupuy 2000; Giedion 1948; see Sect. 4.2.3).

What I have described above holds also and especially for the empirical sciences of today. They are characterized by *empiricism*, which derives substantiated, "objective" knowledge from what is gained through sense experience, specifically through measurement and experiment. A critical point, however, is that the decision about what makes experience is made beforehand and thus is not gained by experience itself. This is what Slife criticizes when he writes "that the formulation of any method must assume, before investigation, a certain type of world in which that method would be effective. Indeed, every occasion that a method is applied to a new population, place, or time—and is thus, in a sense, *re*formulated—it has to make pre-investigatory assumptions about the nature of that population, place, or time" (Slife 2004, p. 50). The sciences aligned with empiricism are further characterized by *reductionism*, because they simplify spheres of reality in their complexity based on the model of physics and the physical experiment, and they are *deterministic* in that any event is necessitated by an antecedent set of causally sufficient conditions.

Mainstream psychotherapy science has long adopted empiricism, reductionism, and determinism. This is evidenced by the fact that, for example, *nonempirical* issues (Kukla 1989) have been marginalized in conventional psychotherapy research, with philosophical or theoretical analysis seen as unnecessary speculation and "armchair philosophizing" (Barker et al. 2002, p. 10), at most, as an auxiliary support at the service of empirical investigation (Salvatore 2011; Slife 2004). This is related to the fact that the cornerstone of contemporary psychotherapy research is to provide *empirical evidence* to the efficacy and mechanisms of actions of psychotherapeutic interventions.[1] Methodologically, the

[1] It should be noted that, when talking about empirical evidence, the term "empirical" is most of the time understood sensu stricto as indicating the *standardized measurement* of a certain phenomenon; as a consequence, qualitative research is considered not at all, or at least less, empirical than quantitative research and is therefore disqualified as pseudoscientific or, in any case, as less scientific than the dominant quantitative approaches. On the contrary, we consider the term "empirical" as indicating the fact that some data about a phenomenon of interest are *systematically* gathered and analyzed (see also Barker et al. 2002); following this, both quantitative and qualitative researches may be considered empirical approaches, though different in their foundations and

"gold standard" to provide this empirical evidence is the randomized clinical trial (RCT; see Chap. 26) which, developed in analogy with biomedical research, requires the researcher to *manipulate* and *control* the research environment in order to increase the internal validity of the results (i.e., that the observed clinical outcome actually depends on the administered treatment): treatments need to be manualized, an experimental group and a control group are required, patients must be randomized to these two groups, the effects of the treatments have to be measured by means of standardized instruments, etc.

4.2.3 The Mechanization of Worldview and Science: Innovation and Consequences

The term "mechanization" in this context is not defined in the usual sense as the production or use of machines to assist people or to increase productivity, but as a term rooted in philosophy or the philosophy of science, derived from physics (Dijksterhuis 1961): mechanics is the branch of science that deals with the motion of objects and physical forces producing it, and, in this context, mechanization means to attribute natural processes and phenomena of the living to the laws of motion and to explain them strictly deterministically according to the principle of cause and movement in the sense of the *causa efficiens*. Firstly, mechanization—as already mentioned—introduced research methods that rely on measurement and experiment as their source of information and mathematical formulations as a means of description and explanation. Secondly, it promoted the development of technology and thus led to the industrialization of the world, on which the following will focus first.

Despite or because of its reductionism and determinism, mechanistic thinking was a huge success and changed the world to a degree that never before occurred in human evolution. This was because when nature is explained by determining the laws by which it operates, practical utilization is not long in coming: "Human knowledge and human power meet in one; for where the cause is not known the effect cannot be produced. Nature to be commanded must be obeyed" (Bacon 2000, Aphorism 3). This is a key phrase of the modern period, the more popular version of which is "knowledge is power" (German: "Wissen ist Macht"). This is a quote from Francis Bacon (1561–1618), one of the greatest pioneers of *natural* science. In the early modern period, it was mainly inventions such as the telescope, microscope, compass, and gunpowder that were used to explain the world and subdue it. Later, steam engine, internal combustion engine, electric motor, and the computer were added; they changed the world fundamentally by mechanizing, industrializing, and digitalizing it.

The success of classical physics and in particular of mechanics convinced and still convinces generations of scientists so much they also became the model for various human sciences that consider themselves "empirical," such as medicine, psychology, or sociology. If they explain the processes they examine deterministically and reductionistically, according to the principle of cause and effect of independent and dependent variables, this means they build on a mechanistic worldview or a machine model of man such as was developed as early as the European modern period based on Newton's *Principia*, René Descartes' (1596–1650) *Principia Philosophiae* (Descartes 1988), and La Mettrie's (1709–1751) infamous memoir *Man a Machine* (Mettrie 1994). Particularly interesting with regard to this is *Laplace's Demon*, an idea developed by the marquis de Laplace (1749–1827) of a higher intelligence that would one day be capable of accurately calculating all world affairs in terms of the mechanistic worldview:

> "We ought then to regard the present state of the universe as the effect of its anterior state and as the cause of the one which is to follow. Given for one instant an intelligence which could comprehend all the forces by which nature is animated and the

implementations (see Gelo, Braakmann, & Benetka 2008, 2009; Gelo 2012).

> respective situation of the beings who compose it—an intelligence sufficiently vast to submit these data to analysis—it would embrace in the same formula the movements of the greatest bodies of the universe and those of the lightest atom; for it, nothing would be uncertain and the future, as the past, would be present to its eyes" (Laplace 2007, p. 4).

Similar notions can also be found in standard scientific works of the present, for example, when a widely used psychology handbook claims "that the human soul is moved by the same laws as other natural objects [...]. A machine now is nothing more than an arrangement of causal laws," which is why "there is no avoiding a machine conception of the human soul [...]" (Dörner 2004, p. 35). This, however, blurs the principal difference between inorganic and organic matter. Living beings are characterized by the requirements of their metabolism; they exist through exchange and their structure is dynamic and dissipative, i.e., it must constantly be supplied with energy, because otherwise the structure would dissolve. While inorganic matter is characterized by "uniformity, rigidity, and stability," living things excel through "diversity, dynamic, and flexibility" (Bammé et al. 1983, p. 134). According to dynamic systems theory, this difference can be explained considering that living systems—together with other complex systems which change over time—are comprised of a set of mutually interacting elements giving rise to *emergent* systemic properties, that is, properties exhibited by the system as a whole and not by any of its individual components. To illustrate this with an analogy, the individual components of an automobile do not constitute a vehicle with which you can move. This is only possible if they are connected with each other in a specific way, because only then the car can be started (Wuketits 1985, pp. 96–97). Driving is therefore an emergent systemic property of the motor vehicle, just as thinking is an emergent systemic property of the brain, because the whole is more than the sum of its parts (see Sect. 4.3.2). However, this cannot be "seen" when only the individual parts are analyzed.

Another example, one of the best-known German methods handbooks for psychology says that "it [is] not a difference in principle but only in degree when new physical phenomena are 'explained' by (presumably) true physical laws, and new psychological phenomena by [...] psychological theories" (Bortz and Döring 2006, p. 17). The authors try to prove this assertion with two if-then relationships (see Rieken 2010a, pp. 21–22). From physics, they choose the theorem "if metal is heated, then it expands" (Bortz and Döring 2006, p. 16) and, from psychological aesthetics research, a phenomenon from the field of popular music, namely, that among the most popular hits are often songs with a particular sequence of harmonies, specifically those with a medium excitation level. From this they derive the following hypothesis: "If pop music follows a harmonic scheme of medium difficulty, then it is assessed positively" (Bortz and Döring 2006, p. 17). However, this need not be the case, because every metal expands when heated, but not every person takes delight in the most popular pop songs, because some people prefer folk music, others New Orleans jazz or classical music, etc. This means that it is, at best, only possible to make statements about a certain number of people, but not about humanity as a whole. And even the preferences of a single individual may change depending on their mood. Sometimes they might want to listen to the *Nocturnes* by Frédéric Chopin, then to Glenn Miller, and then yet another time to the *Rocky Horror Picture Show*. It may well be that a majority of people prefers a "harmonic scheme of medium difficulty," but such a statement should not be elevated to the status of a physical or physics-analogous law, because it is an exaggerated claim to want to establish laws with universal and eternal validity (see Salvatore and Valsiner 2010 for a discussion).

This claim in turn has to do with the historical context in which the experiment blossomed—the Age of Absolutism: "The experiment combines [...] the subjective arbitrariness of researchers with strict regularity, with methods that should allow a precise control and evaluation of reality. This structure shows in a specific way essential elements of absolutism. In absolutism, the reigning sovereign is the 'absolute master'; all government action should be centered toward the position of the ruler. This claim is expressed precisely by a saying of Louis XIV, the most prominent ruler of absolutism: '*L'etat, c'est moi*'—'I am the state'" (Vinnai 1993, p. 53). From a depth psychological perspective, exaggerated claims to power have to do with a defense against fears. In this respect, the practice-oriented natural sciences could be seen as gigantic companies that aim to reduce or even minimize fears—especially the fear of being dominated by nature, which is why one seeks to rule it as completely as possible. Hannah Arendt has pointed out with regard to the hitherto unsuspected power potential of mechanization that all manufacturing is violent, because humans interfere with the balance of nature by destroying living things, for example, such as felling a tree to gain wood or preventing slow natural processes from completing when they break iron or stone from "the womb of the earth" (Arendt 1998, p. 139). And Ludwig von Bertalanffy, one of the greatest biologists and systems theorists of the twentieth century, wrote—probably still affected by the Second World War in the early 1950s—the following: "The attitude that considers physical phenomena as the sole standard-measure of reality, has led to the mechanization of mankind and to the devaluation of higher values. The unregulated domination of physical technology finally ushered the world into the catastrophical crises of our time" (Bertalanffy 1950, p. 165). Sigfried Giedion expressed something similar in his monograph *Mechanization Takes Command* when at the end of the chapter on the mechanization of the meat industry he links the same with the allegorical image of the Dance of Death and states that the associated neutrality of killing was displayed on a large scale during the Second World War (Giedion 1948).

This is not an attempt to condemn mechanization lock, stock, and barrel with its belief in explaining natural and human processes with the laws of motion and deterministically in line with causality. Mechanization is like a tool that can be used for good or evil and can help or hinder the pursuit of knowledge. It presents a simplification of the world, which has advantages and disadvantages, namely, on the one hand the capacity for targeted and efficient change where mono-causal relationships dominate but on the other hand little success or failure where multiple causes and interactions exist. No one in the Western industrialized societies would want to give up the comforts it brought, such as speedy travel in a car or plane, central heating, or computers. But at the same time, it had a huge impact on nature, society, and the individual, through resource extraction, pollution, climate change, and, for example, reducing the individual to a cog in the system of the economy, when you think of Taylorism ("scientific management"). The inner feelings of the individual often fall to the wayside, because they are less easily measured than behavior that can be observed from the outside. Typical examples are the ideological foundations of parliamentary democracy and capitalism as formulated by Immanuel Kant or Adam Smith, because they are based on mechanistic considerations. Kant said that even a nation of devils could be governed, namely, in the following manner: "So order and organize a group of rational beings who require universal laws for their preservation—though each is secretly inclined to exempt himself from such laws—that, while their private attitudes conflict, these nonetheless so cancel one another that these beings behave publicly just as if they had no evil attitudes" (Kant 2003, p. 23). This was not about the moral improvement of the people but only about using the "*mechanism* of nature" (Kant 2003, pp. 23–24, emphasis added: B.R.), meaning the system of the separation of powers in particular: while everyone wants to accumulate power, others want the same, and thus they keep each other in check, push against each other mechanically as it were. The same applies to Adam Smith's theory of capitalism, according to which mass affluence can be generated through the principle of competition, but businesspeople are prevented from becoming too powerful because they end up pushing against other people's strivings for power. Although Smith speaks of the "invisible hand" (Smith 2007, p. 352) to prove this success, which sounds a bit mythological, he is actually referring to a mechanical process similar to Kant, which is comparable with colliding billiard balls. Now undoubtedly democracy and capitalism have cleared the way for liberties and prosperity—undisputed advantages of mechanization—but problems such as the formation of cartels, corruption, exploitation of natural resources in developing countries, or the dubious and mostly failed attempts of the USA to establish democratic institutions in developing countries show that the "mechanism of nature" alone is not enough to solve certain problems, because that also requires consideration of the inner workings of the individuals involved.

But back to the questions of science in the narrower sense, something should be noted: when contemporary human sciences play the keyboard of mechanization by following the example of classical physics, they use nineteenth-century standards. Anyway, in contemporary natural sciences, nobody believes anymore that "the laws of nature [are] the real essence of nature, but only a theoretical *model*: an idealized concept of nature that does not exist in reality" (Bammé et al. 1983, p. 128). Mechanics creates—and, at the same time, requires the reference to—an oversimplified world: mass in free fall, for example, is considered with a point source to make it possible to perform calculations, and interfering factors such as air resistance or wind conditions are neglected, though they are major factors with other phenomena, such as the free fall of a goose feather. Newer approaches such as quantum physics, fuzzy logic, systems theory, and chaos theory have, on the contrary, relativized the simple causal-analytical worldview of mechanics. Quantum physics, for example, has reintroduced the observer as an influencing variable, because on a microscale, the observed is changed by the observation (Heisenberg's uncertainty principle), while fuzzy logic is a theory that operates with truth values but when applied has proved to be on a par with the classic causal-analytical models. Systems theory relativizes the unilinear causality model in favor of interactions, and chaos theory, while as deterministic as classical physics, is based on initial conditions that are so complex they cannot be determined with existing measurement methods and instruments at present and probably not in the long term either, such as the proverbial "flap of a butterfly's wing," which may have unforeseen long-term consequences (see Sect. 4.3.2).

Mechanization is evident in mainstream psychotherapy research and in the prescriptions of its quantitative methodology (see Chap. 12 and 13): experimental designs should be ideally used to test models of antecedent causality through the control of confounding variables and the exclusion of possible alternative explanations for the observed behaviors; big samples should be employed in order to allow time- and context-free generalizations of the results; standardized measurement by means of questionnaires and/or rating scales should be used for data collection, with the consequence of the richness of the patient's subjective experience being pushed into the background in favor of reliable measures of what is supposed to change; and statistics should be employed to describe and analyze relationships among the investigated constructs, so that the general laws governing the observed behaviors may be adequately tested.

Such a dominant (quantitative) paradigm of psychotherapy research has developed coherently with an oversimplified model of the world borrowed from the physical sciences (mechanics) of the nineteenth century (see Danziger 1985, 1990 for a general discussion; see also Gelo 2012, Slife 1998) and is therefore based on simplistic assumptions and related models of inquiry (Elliott and Anderson 1994); in other words, mainstream psychotherapy researchers must make a series of simplifying assumptions on psychotherapy in order to be able to investigate it, with the negative consequence of increasing the gap between research and practice (see Kazdin 2008). An example is the *drug metaphor* model described by Stiles and Shapiro (1989, 1994), according to which researchers assume a direct and linear relationship between the different aspects of the therapeutic process (e.g., therapists' interventions, patients' verbal and nonverbal expressions, etc.) and the therapeutic outcome.

4.2.4 Critics of Naturalism in Psychotherapy Science

As mentioned in the previous section, there are fundamental differences between living and nonliving systems and between organic and inorganic matter. This distinction is blurred by reductionism, which aims to explain life through mechanical principles of movement and also uses physical standards that have been relativized by modern physics (quantum theory, fuzzy logic, etc.). The determinism resulting from this reductionism is also faced with the problem set of free will/determination: if you understand life mechanistically, all behavior is causally determined because for every action there must be a preceding cause which in turn can be traced back to other conditional causes. This concerns psychotherapy science in particular, because it is about patients freeing themselves from (causal-analytically) conditional pathological patterns or at least putting them into perspective. In other words, it is the goal ("outcome") of any psychotherapy to gain a degree of inner freedom by the end of it. Also, behind this lies a much more general problem still: without the postulate of free will, there would be no responsibility and thus no way, for example, to protect society from criminals. Thus the special element of the outcome in psychotherapy and the general element of the attribution of responsibility in criminal offenders are reasons not to deny the postulate of free will entirely, which poses a conflict with the reductionist determinism of classical science and the psychotherapy science derived from it.

Reductionism may also conflict with the empiricism that is a refinement of objectivism. The mechanistic view is based on physics, but nowadays physicists do not consider their theories to be a reflection of the world but rather a simplified model. As already stated, empiricism overlooks that experience is only possible under the condition of conditions that cannot be experienced. And these conditions are not objective but, as Immanuel Kant pointed out in his *Critique of Pure Reason*, subject to specific categories as well as forms of intuition, namely, space and time. Knowledge is therefore not possible without perspective (Kant 1998), which is a view also shared by some philosophers of language, according to which language shapes the way people think and therefore also shapes their perception of the world (Köller 2004).

Therefore, it should not surprise that mainstream psychotherapy science is not met solely with agreement, and there are well-known researchers who have examined its grounding tacit assumptions critically. Brent D. Slife, for example, in the fifth edition of *Bergin and Garfield's Handbook of Psychotherapy and Behavior Change*, addresses the constraints that arise from a kind of thinking he calls *naturalism* (Slife 2004) and that is closely related to mechanization (Slife 2004; see Slife 1998; Slife and Gantt 1999; Slife et al. 2005). Naturalism as he describes it is characterized by five attributes that are all compatible with what has been outlined here, namely, objectivism, universalism, materialism, hedonism, and atomism. The author's criticism regarding *objectivism* is focused on the supposed value freedom (German: Wertfreiheit) of the traditional scientific method, which overlooks the fact that a researcher's implicit presuppositions grounding the scientific method used often remain unquestioned and/or cannot be tested, but still affect his/her research—in other words, objectivity cannot be value-free because it is a value itself. A well-known example is the work of Grawe (Grawe et al. 2001; Grawe 2004), whose recommendation for behavioral therapy might be considered to be rooted in his preference for empirical-quantitative psychology; both these two systems are based on the same mechanistic foundation, so it is not surprising that one is confirmed by the other. Slife (2004) therefore advises researchers as well as therapists to be aware of their own preconceptions, a view that is pretty close to the ethno-psychoanalytic mandate to reflect on one's "countertransference" in the research process.

Universalism shares some common ground with objectivism, because if one thinks it possible to capture the natural world beyond our perspectival perception, it also seems to be within the realm of possibility to make universal statements and attain "diagnostic and treatment 'universals'" in the area of therapy (Slife 2004, p. 48). This disregards the fact that unforeseen events happen in the therapy process that are completely unique, in other words, the fact that psychotherapy is a "science of subjectivity" (Pritz and Teufelhart 1996).

The term *materialism* broaches the issue of the philosophical mind-body problem, which may appear to be "solved" from a mechanistic point of view by advocating for monism but from a long-term perspective—that of over 2000 years of history of Western thinking—requires differentiation (see, e.g., Rentsch 1980). Slife (2004) points out that while biological factors do constitute an important basis for research, human action and experience cannot be reduced to them. He exemplifies inter alia using the example of love, which may trigger biochemical processes without there being any empirical ways to determine "what type of relationship the biochemical substrate has to the phenomenon" (Slife 2004, p. 55).

Finally, Slife also criticizes *hedonism* and *atomism*: the former because it steered toward selfishness due to misunderstood desires for self-realization, the latter because it saw the individual irrespective of the context. As an alternative, he recommends the consideration of altruistic potential as it was laid out, for example, in Alfred Adler's individual psychology ("community feeling") (Adler 1927), as well as interpersonal and relational aspects in research and profession. This set of problems, too, bears relation to mechanization, as mechanization analyzes and isolates individual factors in order to treat them effectively, as happens exemplarily in conventional medicine, for example, which successfully treats specific diseased organs but may not be quite as helpful when dealing with multicausal diseases or functional disorders with no organic findings.

Gottfried Fischer's approach is similar to Slife's. His aim is to establish psychotherapy as an independent science instead of a subdomain of medicine or psychology (Fischer 2008, 2011). According to Fischer, an important element in the conceptualization of psychotherapy science is ecological thinking in the sense of an inner reference to the environment, which is tantamount to a rejection of atomism. From there it is only a small step to intentionality (see Sect. 4.3.1), which the author considers a central element in understanding human subjects. That also provides a major criterion for the demarcation from the neighboring disciplines of medicine and mainstream psychology, which determine suffering with regard to some general modalities of functioning rather than with regard to individual personal experience. However, this does not advocate for subjectivist constructivism, because the systematic study of subjectivity is performed ecologically, thus maintaining a reference to environmental conditions.

This has several consequences for research, because the scientific objectives in psychotherapy science are different than in medicine and psychology: it is not only about the identification of generally applicable laws—for example, "if someone constantly washes their hands, they suffer from an obsessive-compulsive disorder"—but also about the experiences and actions of people in specific situations as well as their change or development and the expansion of possible actions, which poses some contrast to the static nature of laws. This is why qualitative methods in addition to quantitative ones are important, and in addition to *explanation*—in the sense of a deterministic, reductionistic, and mechanistic identification of the *causa efficiens*—is *understanding*, which is a multidimensional phenomenon closely interwoven with the interpretative elements of intentionality, wholeness, and analogical thinking. The following sections will explain what these three terms mean and their importance for (psychotherapy) science.

4.3 Alternative Perspectives in Science

So far, this text has outlined a view of science that may be the dominant perspective in contemporary science but by no means the only one possible. In the following sections, we will dive into realms that have become meaningless in the natural sciences of the present and therefore do not receive much attention in psychotherapy science either. More specifically, we will focus on intentionality, wholeness, and analogical rationality type.

4.3.1 Aristotelian Causality and Intentionality

Intentionality has always played a central role in the human sciences and still does so today; one aim of this section is to make it clear that it should not be neglected in the study of the human psyche.

In the science of the nineteenth century, the modern conception of the term intentionality emerges for the first time in the works of Franz Brentano (1838–1917), who used it in his descriptive psychology. He used the term to determine psychic phenomena, because in contrast to physical phenomena, they were characterized by their reference relationship to a content or (mental) object (Brentano 1995). Another groundbreaking text in this context is Martin Heidegger's essay "Being and Time" (German: "Sein und Zeit"), which calls attention to the fact that the original approach to the world was a practical attitude that he described as "readiness-to-hand" (German: "Zuhandenheit"). He wrote that, in contrast, the theoretical understanding, the "presence-at-hand" (German: "Vorhandenheit"), was a derivative that isolated the things of the world and made them lose their referral to each other: the practical reference was lost, a hammer was only a hammer, a nail only a nail, because in isolated analysis no reference could be formed, such as that someone might use the hammer to pound nails into wood to build a house for people. This could only happen with "readiness-to-hand" (Heidegger 1988).

The reference to content or an object puts the concept of intentionality in opposition to mechanistic thinking with its analyzing-isolating approach ("atomism"). However, in order to avoid playing off one against the other instead of thinking about how both may contribute to the enrichment of understanding mental processes, it seems appropriate to look back to ancient Greece and take a look at Aristotelian causality; the core of which is still considered one of the established parts of standard knowledge in philosophy (see Tetens 2001). Aristotle distinguishes four different forms of causality that in the Latin translation of Thomas Aquinas (Thomas Aquinas 2000, lib. 1 l. 4 n. 2) are termed as follows: (1) *causa materialis* ("material cause"), (2) *causa formalis* ("formal cause"), (3) *causa efficiens* ("efficient cause"), and (4) *causa finalis* ("final cause") (Aristotle 1930, Book II, Chapters 2–3, 194b; see Gloy 1995, pp. 116–133; Tetens 2001, pp. 378–380). Here is an example: If I eventually buy a particular house, then I may do so (1) because of the material, as it is made of bricks that create a good room climate and unlike prefabricated houses are durable. I will buy it (2) because of formal reasons, as its appearance is pleasing. (3) The *causa efficiens* plays a role that is understood as the "initial impetus" according to Aristotle (Aristotle 1930, 194b): I want to live in a house again because I did so as a child and I felt very comfortable there, but I later moved to the city and suffer from the constriction of the housing conditions. Finally, (4) the *causa finalis* is of importance, because in order to increase the quality of my life and really recover from the exertions of my professional routine, I aim to live in a house again.

It is not necessary to discuss the hotly debated issues of Aristotle-centered research more closely at this point, such as whether the doctrine of the fourfold cause claims to be complete, whether it is a system of necessary real causes or more a collection of topoi as methodological tools, etc. (see Gloy 1995, pp. 116–117; Tetens 2001, pp. 378–380). In this context, it is essential that two of the four causes, namely, the *causa efficiens* and the *causa finalis*, were going to be of major importance in the further course of the history of science. The *causa efficiens* (see Sect. 4.2.1) is the cause that has become essential for the scientific notion of causality in modern times. It is the question of why and whence, which in the sense of the modern period was the only approved connection between cause and effect and was considered the link between independent and dependent variables in an experiment.

There were several reasons for neglecting the *causa finalis*. First, it was not limited to the human realm in ancient and medieval philosophy, but also applied to animate and inanimate nature. Thus, for example, Aristotle did not explain the free fall of a stone with the force of gravity, as we do today, but with the argument that it was the stone's goal to get to the center of the Earth as the "natural place" of rest. While the "light elements" strived for the edge of the lunar sphere, the "heavy elements" aimed for the center of the imagined geocentric cosmos (Aristotle 1930, VIII, 4, 255a–255b).

On the other hand, the scholastic view of science, especially in the reception of Thomas Aquinas, granted the *causa finalis* a far higher priority than the *causa efficiens*, namely in the context of the Christian religion, which understands the world as a creation of God and thus a realization of a wise plan, which is why it assumes that there is a hidden purpose behind everything. In the Catholic Church, this view has survived to this day, as demonstrated by a New York Times article by Cardinal Christoph Schönborn, Archbishop of Vienna, in which he speaks of the divine design and the higher, namely, the divine aim of evolution that is equated "with final cause, purpose, or design" (Schönborn 2005; see Rieken 2010b).

Thus it should not surprise that the *causa finalis* lost more and more of its influence with the beginning of the success story of modern science, namely since the early modern period. It was too attached to metaphysics to be taken seriously in science, and indeed it does not really make sense to ask for what purpose, for example, New Orleans was devastated by hurricane Katrina in August 2005 (*causa finalis*), as opposed to why this happened (*causa efficiens*). Only religious fundamentalists advocated the *causa finalis* by arguing that God caused the hurricane with the intent to punish the city, as it was a den of iniquity built on decadence, debauchery, and voodoo (Rieken 2007).

Things look different in the human, non-metaphysical realm, because there, intentionality is equivalent to the question of the meaning and purpose of certain events and actions, or even the meaning of life. It is primarily the *human* science that deals with these questions and within them philosophy and literary studies in particular; the latter look for the meaning of fictional texts that often are closely connected to life (Gerigk 2006; Schapp 2004; Searle 2004; Spaemann and Löw 1985). These disciplines in no way question the validity of the *causa finalis*, because it is "based on the model of human action. Man is capable of setting goals and acting in order to achieve these goals. His actions often can only be understood when one knows the goal linked to the desired final state of an action" (Schiemann 1998, p. 3). Therefore, these sciences consider the neglect of the *causa finalis* and the sole focus on the *causa efficiens* typical of the *natural* sciences such as psychology or medicine reductionist. And in fact, natural sciences by their own admission do have problems exploring "research ideas with philosophical content" such as the empirical investigation of the "meaning of life" (Bortz 1984, p. 16).

Crisis situations, such as mental illness or traumatic events, in particular raise the question of the meaning of what happened to someone. To put it in the words of anthropologist Lauri Honko, "Every even somewhat more serious illness is a harrowing event in a human life that challenges one's continued existence. All patients have in common that, from the first stages of their illness, they try to explain its nature and causes somehow. The establishment of some sort of theory almost seems to be a human need" (Honko 1959, p. 19). And this theory does not only include the question of how it came that something happened to oneself (*causa efficiens*) but also what the point is and what one may learn from it (*causa finalis*).

For example, in 2008, Rieken conducted a field research in Galtür, a mountain village in the Austrian province of Tyrol that was affected by a catastrophic avalanche in 1999, in order to ascertain whether and to what extent the inhabitants have processed the disastrous event. The informants also provided intentional content, such as that they now live a more conscious life; that solidarity—in the sense of a social network—has become more important; or that they have learned to talk about personal problems. They also variously assumed ecological connections, such as that the environmental impact on nature was too much and it sometimes needed to "discharge," which then sometimes hit the wrong people, in this case the people of Galtür. In addition, in this village that is entirely Catholic, Christian faith proved helpful as it offered solace or encouraged the view that the rapid reconstruction and extensive outside support indicated that God was helping. All these arguments were communicated to me during the interview process, and they not only testify to an intensive reflection of the disaster but also make it clear that intentional aspects are important for comprehensive processing (Rieken 2010a). It is not about the extent to which these views, such as the reference to ecological aspects or to God, are "objectively" correct, but only whether they provide support for the respective subject to process traumatic events in a *meaningful* way. This is confirmed by results of resilience research, as far as they refer to Antonovsky's concept of salutogenesis, who considers comprehensibility and meaningfulness essential factors for a sense of coherence. What this means is that events are structured meaningfully that their internal cohesion can be comprehended and that one's own life and actions have a purpose (Antonovsky 1987).

Still, this is not about playing *causa efficiens* and *causa finalis*, natural and human science, against each other, because both highlight fundamental approaches to the human condition. Humans cannot bear isolated facts, because if something is not understood or not interpreted, it is perceived as a threat. This is why people make every effort to classify the phenomena they encounter into tangible contexts (see Köller 2004, p. 837), and *causa efficiens* and *causa finalis* are equally suited for this, as it may be enlightening to ask not only where something came from but also where it leads, what one wants to achieve with it and what its purpose is. This is also demonstrated by different schools of psychotherapy with their various priorities. Psychoanalysis, for example, is primarily committed to the *causa efficiens*, because it perceives a close correlation between the determinants of childhood and later adult life. The same applies to behaviorism with its connection between stimulus and response. Conversely, however, there are also references to the *causa finalis* in schools of therapy that, like behavioral therapy, are firmly anchored in the here and now, as, for example, the term "reframing" plays an important role at least in systemic family therapy and neurolinguistic programming. This means putting specific conditions into a new framework, for example, by allowing that compulsiveness has the goal of trying to achieve order in life (Andreas and Andreas 1982; Bandler et al. 1983; Satir and Baldwin 1983). From the humanistic schools of therapy, it is Viktor Frankl's logotherapy in particular that focuses mainly on the *causa finalis* since it considers the question of the meaning of life paramount and since Frankl believed that being human had to do with "self-transcendence," the ability to relate to others (Frankl 1975, 2004). This is in contrast to the before-mentioned atomism and is also confirmed by resilience research, because the existence of a well-functioning social network is considered important for mental health or for the recovery thereof. Also important in this context is Alfred Adler's individual psychology, which draws attention to unconscious, not conscious, intentionality, unlike in Brentano's philosophy. Being both a student of Freud and a psychoanalyst specializing in-depth psychology, Adler did believe that the *causa efficiens* was essential, because he knew about the formative influence of childhood on the character and adult life, but at the same time he focused on the *causa finalis*, because from the child's sense of "inferiority" arises the desire for compensation, social equality, power, and prestige—in short, from the beginning, people aim to increase their self-esteem (Adler 1912). In principle, like in individual psychology, both causes are applied in Freud's psychoanalysis, because the libido as an effective causal driving force simultaneously pursues the goal of obtaining satisfaction. Still both authors use a different focus, Freud more on the *causa efficiens* and Adler more on the *causa finalis*, which is also taken into account in modern psychoanalysis textbooks. Thomä and Kächele, for example, write the following about dreams: "As necessary and important as the dreamer's history is with its biographical obstacles to development, their life takes place in the here and now *and is future-oriented*" (Thomä and Kächele 2006, p. 180, emphasis added: B.R.).

The difference between *causa efficiens* and *causa finalis* is clearly stated in Thomä and Kächele's text. However, things tend to be less clear in everyday language as, at first glance, it does not make much difference whether someone says they go to school *because* they want to learn something (*causa efficiens*) or *to* learn something (*causa finalis*). However, in case of the former, the focus is on the past; in case of the latter, it is directed to the future, much as is the case with Thomä and Kächele. This differentiation is of particular interest especially with regard to psychotherapy. For example, if someone is suffering from depression, the effective cause may be a conflict such as a man cheating on his wife even though he is a devout Catholic. At least from a psychoanalytic point of view, an unconscious conflict is a frequent trigger for depression. In this case, the attention is focused on the past, because the conflict must already exist in order to cause the condition. From the perspective of the *causa finalis*, on the other hand, one may ask what the person in question, looking at the future, wants to achieve with their depression. The answer could be that he/she wants to unconsciously avoid the confrontational behavior, because if he/she is depressed, he/she will have no desire to be unfaithful – true to the motto: "Who does nothing, does nothing wrong." Another example would be inner distance in personal relationships, "philobatism" in the tradition of Michael Balint (Balint 1959). Anyone who has a fear of too much personal closeness is likely to have suffered through painful experiences with their parents (*causa efficiens*) and is aiming to protect themselves from further injury by keeping the partner at a distance so that they will not see one's supposed shortcomings (*causa finalis*).

Maybe these explanations make it clear why it makes sense to consider both forms of causality, because the consideration of "whence" and "why" covers a broader spectrum than the consideration of only one aspect. However, the more unusual and surprising approach is that of the *causa finalis*, because thanks to the dominance of mechanistic thinking (see Sect. 4.2.3), we are primarily used to consider the *causa efficiens* when asking questions about causes. It is the same with patients: they suffer; why should their suffering have meaning, a purpose, and a goal? But if they have use for this question, this often means a lot has been gained, because they no longer see themselves only as a *passive* sufferer who had something happen to them but instead realize that they are also *actively* contributing something to their suffering and are possibly even actively holding on to it because they are afraid of change. Many therapists know from their practice that patients "also want to cry or attack, complain and blame, and sometimes very much 'need' their problems" (Buchholz 1999, p. 72)—the "need" again representing the intentional aspect. And when they have realized all of these, then they can *actively* distance themselves from it in the longer term. In other words, the consideration of intentionality can help gain a better understanding of mental illness and thus also contribute to recovery.

In the field of psychotherapy research, the application of *qualitative* methods (Frommer and Rennie 2001; McLeod 2013; see Chaps. 20 and 21) may make it possible to adequately take into account such issues as *causa finalis* and intentionality. Consider, for example, being interested in the outcome of a treatment: in quantitative outcome research, patients are usually asked to provide information on how they are doing "*at that moment*" (for exceptions see Elliott et al. 1999) before and after the therapy—with the change faced by the patient being reflected in the pre-post difference. In contrast, a possibility in qualitative outcome research is to explicitly ask the patients, before the beginning of the therapy, "*what they would change*" about themselves, thus calling into play the intentionality of the patients and allowing to identify the *causa finalis* of the treatment according to their perspective; in a second interview, conducted at the treatment termination, patients are then asked to critically reflect on the content of the first interview based on the changes effectively experienced during the treatment (see Chap. 27 for an overview on qualitative outcome research). Such an approach presents an example of how it is possible to investigate the outcome of psychotherapy by taking into account the in-depth analysis of the final cause of the therapeutic process. Other examples are provided by any qualitative research making use of *experiential* methods, that is, involving "the conceptualization of meanings of experiences" reported by patients and/or therapists (Rennie 2012, p. 385); in fact, we believe that any reconstructed experience of the participants is imbued with their intentionality, at least in Brentano's sense.

4.3.2 Wholeness

Intentionality is closely connected with another term that also has its origin in Greek antiquity and met the same fate, namely to be marginalized in the modern period in the course of the mechanization of science: holistic thinking. Although some representatives of this may be found in the natural philosophy of the Renaissance and it was later recognized by well-known authors such as Schelling and Goethe, it has been doomed to a shadowy existence ever since (Gloy 1996; Kaulbach and Beck 1974)—the causal-analytical influence on the world has become too powerful. The term "whole" or "holon" takes a prominent place in Plato, for in the *Timaeus* he speaks of the Creator God who wants to create a creature that is as perfect as possible, lacks nothing, and is thus labeled "whole" or "holon" (Plato 1929, 32d). Equally well known is the Aristotelian notion that there are things "which have a plurality of parts, and which are not a total aggregate but a whole of some sort distinct from the parts" (Aristotle 1933, book 8.6, 1045a)—a notion that prompted later generations to formulate the phrase "the whole is more than the sum of its parts." This formulation is, as hinted at in Sect. 4.2.3, also a key sentence of modern systems theory (Ropohl 2012, pp. 25–26): if a number of elements are combined in a specific way, new system properties may occur that the individual elements do not possess.

But what now is the connection between intentionality and wholeness? Hardly anybody has described this as vividly as the Austrian-American psychiatrist and individual psychologist Erwin Wexberg, whose words deserve an extensive quote:

> "Every organism forms a cohesive unit. This is precisely where it differs from inanimate matter. One can take away half the stones from a pile of stones, leaving a smaller pile, but its essence is still the same [...]. An organism, however, cannot be split, it is indivisible—in-dividual—and is no longer alive, no longer an organism but dead matter if separated [...]. Thus the concept of wholeness remains inextricably linked to the concept of living, coincides with it. Apparently, there are also inanimate things that carry the character of wholeness, for example a house [...]. For a completely impartial observer, such as a resident of an area where houses are unknown, a house really is inanimate matter, without meaning, without wholeness. For them, the building in ruins means nothing less and nothing other than the intact building. For us as house-dwellers though, the house has meaning, because we have given this pile of inanimate matter a purpose. Thus, for us the house has a kind of life, though naturally a life that we have breathed into it. And because it is organized in the sense of this borrowed animation, it appears to us as a whole." (Wexberg 1987, pp. 12–13)

While you can split inorganic matter without changing anything except for its size, this is not something that can be done with living organisms or with those phenomena people have breathed life into. In addition, the above quote also demonstrates that intentionality does not necessarily need to involve irrationality or metaphysics but that it counts as one of the vital needs of human beings, because it is them and not some otherworldly entity that are responsible for creating meaning.

When a person identifies with their house, this also means a certain lifting of the subject-object division characteristic for the mechanistic model. Related to this as a consequence of this "identification" is an attachment to the object and a consideration of emotion to an extent that is at least equal to the intellectual property. This also contrasts the mechanistic belief that emotions are among the "lower faculties" whereas the mind counts among the "higher faculties." And finally, wholeness means a relativization of the quantitative mode of cognition, which is about the isolation and analysis of the individual parts (see Gloy 1996, p. 7).

The desire for wholeness arises from a basic human need that is mainly addressed in gestalt therapy. The gestalt is considered "an indivisible, but transposable relationship structure, like a melody," then "a pattern of behavior (i.e., survival strategies through withdrawal, adaptation, or preemptive defense)," and finally "a self-image (the conciliator, the eternal loser, the one-eyed king, the gray eminence)" (Hartmann-Kotteck 2003, p. 183). Thus exist references to the concept of the character as used in psychoanalysis (König 2011), to the "lifestyle" of individual psychology (Adler 1933), and to the ego identity of psychoanalytic ego psychology (Erikson 1950).

What has already been formulated in the previous sections of this chapter applies here, too, namely, that this is not about playing one off against the other. It is one of the fundamental insights of hermeneutics (see Gadamer 1989) that the whole must be understood through the individual and the individual through the whole, a principle that is generally referred to as the hermeneutic circle (see Chap. 6; see also Chap. 20) but should more accurately be called "hermeneutic spiral" because it is about mutually reinforcing processes that lead to an increase of knowledge. The associated problem is impossible to solve logically, because in order to understand individual parts, one needs a prior understanding of the context, but in order to gain a preliminary understanding of the context, one must already have understood some of its parts (see Gadamer 1989). This means, however, that cognitive appropriation cannot be a purely rational act, because it is also about hunches, intuition, partial understanding, etc., from which emerges an increase of knowledge and significance in a spiral pattern. Aside from that, however, the hermeneutic circle suggests that analytic and holistic thinking do not have to remain in opposition, but can complement each other. A well-rounded picture is only created by looking at both the details and the whole. This is particularly important for patients in traumatic situations, because major life events are often perceived as a turning point, as a radical disruption of life, which is why therapies are concerned with mending the "common thread."

The important question behind this is, "who am I?" This is a fundamental and very early need, which—according to Lacan—emerges in a baby's life when they discover their mirror image. Their own form, which previously was only visible to them in individual parts, is now perceived as something whole. But at the same time, the picture they see evokes imperfection, because they cannot yet experience the body as such. Someone's outside appearance can be seen in the mirror where one is not, and one can feel what is inside of oneself as something not whole where one does not see (Lacan 2001). This causes an alienation that persists for the rest of the subject's life in the form of a longing for unity and should therefore be taken into account in psychotherapy as a profession and science. In fact, it can be taken into account by asking appropriate questions such as inquiring about formative episodes from the subject's life history and trying to learn why (*causa efficiens*) and for what purpose (*causa finalis*) they are of such great importance to the patient. Other lines of inquiry that serve to guide the focus to holistic aspects would be, for example, to ask about the "common thread" in life or typical character traits and then connect those to previously discussed details of the life history, very much in the spirit of the hermeneutic circle.

In at least the last two decades, there have been increasingly more calls for a methodological sophistication in psychotherapy research able to take into account the complex wholeness of clinical practice (e.g., Elliott and Anderson 1994; Greenberg 1986; Laurenceau et al. 2007). Traditional (quantitative) psychotherapy research is in fact considered to be simplistic by assuming a direct and linear causality between the phenomena under investigation and by "concentrating on the isolation of effects and on deriving universal laws, while the practice of psychotherapy is characterized by complex and highly individual interrelations between phenomena" (Smith and Grawe 2003, p. 275). The processes as well as the effects of psychotherapy should be conceived in terms of interacting patterns of reciprocal modifications instead of as an additive and cumulative collection of independent individual features (see Chap. 10). When dealing with reciprocal functional interactions, as is the case in psychotherapy, the attempt to isolate single variables has turned out to be problematic (Salvatore and Tschacher 2012; Schiepek et al 1992), hence the need to develop new research strategies which take into account the *patterned complexity* as well as the *contextuality*, *contingency*, *nonlinearity*, and *circularity* of the therapeutic process (Greenberg 1991; Stiles and Shapiro 1994). With regard to this, successful attempts have been made in the past years.

First is the increasing application of *qualitative* methods in psychotherapy research, which represents without doubt the elective approach in switching the focus from mechanistic causal models to holistic ones; in fact, qualitative research emphasizes the intentional and narrative structure of meaning through the depiction of multilayered, circular, and reciprocal interactions and relationships between dimensions of the human experience as it is reflected in language. An example of this is the *qualitative helpful factors design*, consisting of applying qualitative methods in order to identify what patients recognize as helpful factors of their treatment (Elliott 2010; see Chap. 20 for an overview of the qualitative methods in psychotherapy process research and Chap. 21 for an overview of its applications; see Chap. 27 for an overview of qualitative methods in psychotherapy outcome research and examples of its application).

Second is the refinement of existing *quantitative* methods and the development of new ones. An example is the *microanalytic sequential process design* characterized by the question "what patients processes are triggered by what therapist responses under what conditions?" (Elliott 2010, p. 128). It consists of the quantitative within-session investigation of the turn-to-turn interaction between patient and therapist, coded on rating scales and/or category systems, in order to test micro-theories of clinically productive processes. Another example is the application of *dynamic systems theory* (DST) to the study of psychotherapy (e.g., Pascual-Leone 2009; Salvatore and Tschacher 2012; Salvatore et al. 2010; see Chap. 10 for a general account of psychotherapy process from this perspective; see Tschacher, Gelo, Koch, & Salvatore (2014) for some empirical applications); DST describes clinical change in terms of nonlinear and discontinuous dynamics between stability and instability (i.e., self-organization), thus emphasizing the complex, multi-determinate nature of the therapeutic process. Both of these approaches—microanalytic sequential process design and DST—share the use of modern statistical procedures able to take into account the time-dependent nature of the investigated variables (e.g., sequential analysis, time-series analysis, growth curve analysis), thus representing "an important conceptual advance, from a temporally decontextualized synchronic representation of therapeutic process [. . .] to a truer representation of process as patterns of change or trajectories across sequential time points" (Orlinsky et al. 2004, p. 360; see Chap. 12 for an introduction of statistical data analysis in psychotherapy process research and Chap. 13 for an overview of quantitative approaches to the study of psychotherapy process and its relation to outcome; see also Chap. 26 for a discussion of quantitative methods in outcome research).

Third is the development of complex *mixed-method* designs combining both qualitative and quantitative approaches. An example is the *significant events approach*, which focuses on clinically relevant moments in therapy such as insight, resolution of therapeutic tasks, assimilation of problematic experiences, relational ruptures, etc. (Elliott 2010; see Chap. 21 for an overview of mixed-method applications to psychotherapy process research). This approach usually requires the researcher (1) to empirically identify clinically significant moments and the related patient's and/or therapist's behavior within the analyzed sessions in order to develop a qualitative model of in-session change which takes into account the step-by-step unfolding of the behavior considered (2) and to quantitatively connect these within-session processes with post-session and eventually posttreatment outcomes.

4.3.3 Analogical Thinking

In this section, we will describe *analogical thinking*, which suffered the same fate as the *causa finalis* and wholeness—it fell into oblivion due to the dominance of mechanization, which has definitely no coincidence as it shares certain similarities with holistic thinking.

Language is characterized, among other things, by the fact that it uses images and metaphors, which are based on *analogical similarities*. The analogical relation between a signifier and signified does not only apply to language but is also connected with the structure of thinking (see also Hofstadter and Sander 2013; Lakoff and Johnson 1999). For example, metaphors play a relevant role in the natural sciences for concept formation as, for example, in the case of "atomic nucleus" (German: "Atom*kern*") or "black hole" (German: "schwarzes Loch"); moreover, we know from psychotherapy research that metaphorical thinking plays a key role in the therapeutic process (e.g., Buchholz 2003; Gelo 2008; Gelo and Mergenthaler 2012; McMullen 2008). In modern cognitive science, analogical thinking (also called analogical information processing) is defined as the process of establishing an analogical correspondence between two different domains of experience and/or knowledge (Gentner 1983; Gentner et al. 2001). This kind of analogical correspondence results from *projecting* the relational structure (i.e., the set of relationships between the elements, independently of the properties of the elements themselves) of a *source* domain (usually more concrete and familiar) into a *target* domain (usually more abstract and unfamiliar). In this way, the target domain is enriched, restructured, or even generated anew based on the relational structure of the new one. As a result of this, the two domains will share the same relational structure and, as a consequence of this, will show analogical similarity.

According to Rieken (2010c), the most primal mode of acquiring the world is in reference to one's own person, or, in the language of Jean Piaget, the epistemological egocentrism as we find it in the thinking of the child (Piaget 2007) and also in the mundane imagination not only of the indigenous but also of modern societies, as established plausibly by anthropologist Klaus E. Müller (1987). This is because in order to get one's bearings, one's own lifeworld must make sense, and it does when it is connected to oneself, when the person in question focuses on themselves and discovers analogical similarities between themselves and the environment.

Applied sciences do the same thing, provided they operate with models, such as simulating actual flow conditions at a particular coastal strip in a pool of water, for example, or learning from a specific environmental process. One of the best-known examples is the work of French engineer Sir Marc Isambard Brunel (1769–1849), who was charged with, among other things, building a tunnel under the Thames in London. At first, this seemed to be an impossible task: how could one dig a tunnel into soft, permeable stone without water penetrating? He didn't find a solution until he started to pay attention to the behavior of the naval shipworm, Lat. *teredo navalis*: it digs through wood and secures the rear of the tunnel with endogenous calcareous secretions. The engineer translated this process from nature to technology and developed a construction method that he had patented in 1818: he called it shield tunneling, which is done by successively digging a tunnel and then immediately securing each newly dug section. Brunel was successful; the Thames Tunnel was completed in 1843 (Beamish 1862, pp. 202–225). Nowadays, it is traversed by subway trains.

Analogical thinking is even tentatively making an appearance in modern medicine, namely in the field of vaccination, which is the administration of antigenic material. This causes an infection without pronounced symptoms which in turn causes the immune system to produce antibodies that preclude the disease for a time; the principle of analogical similarity in this case is the limited pathogenicity of the infectious agents. Except for that this kind of thinking is only considered important in alternative medicine that is not compatible with the causal-analytical model, such as homeopathy or traditional Chinese medicine (TCM), both of which operate on the principle of analogical similarity rule.

However, the thing that has made analogical similarity thinking seem particularly suspect from the perspective of modern science is its close connection with magical ideas. Magic lives, as Klaus E. Müller phrased it, by "two antithetical principles of force," is the rule of similarities that was just mentioned above (*similia similibus*) and the rule of opposites (*contraria contrariis*) (Müller 1987, p. 202). According to the rule of opposites, in order to heal, one has to fight evil with good and cast out sickness demons with divine assistance, for example, as is the case with exorcisms. According to the simile rule, on the other hand, it is possible to cause a disease by replicating the target in the shape of a doll and stabbing a needle in it. The idea of healing according to the simile rule is widespread: measles is treated using agents that have a reddish tint, while liverwort with its three-lobed shape is evocative of the liver with its three lobes and used accordingly in liver disease.

It is a fact that analogical thinking cannot be understood by using conventional causal relationships as, for example, the behavior of the naval shipworm (cause) stands in no direct relation to the possibility of digging a tunnel under the Thames (effect). But the same problem also arises in experimental psychology. Strictly speaking, the Milgram experiment (Milgram 1974), for example, reveals nothing about the willingness to obey authority, only about the willingness to obey university psychologists in the laboratory. This is because the concept of theory that is used by empirical psychology "permits, in a strict sense, only laws that are accessible to experimental testing, it does not permit laws that give evidence about the ratio of experimental reality and true social reality" (Vinnai 1993, p. 43). Even a natural science-oriented psychologist such as Theo Herrmann admits this when he writes that for this "a theory of everyday reality [would be required] that does not exist, that in relation to scientific theories would be a superordinate 'super theory', but in its construction the everyday reality itself would be conceptualized and thus on the one hand reduced exemplarily and, on other hand, constituted theoretically, so that it would no longer be that which is simply experienced which is by what the theory in question should originally have been measured" (Herrmann 1979, p. 75). Although this dilemma could be avoided by creating analogical similarity between obedience in the laboratory and in everyday life, this would not be acceptable for academic psychology. Thus, following the considerations quoted above, Theo Herrmann warns explicitly against "calling the problem areas related to nomological theories empirical models," because that "proves to be a metaphor" (Herrmann 1979, p. 75), which he apparently does not consider scientific due to its similarity structures.

This, however, can be critically questioned. Thinking based on analogical similarity might be, to quote science historian and philosopher Karen Gloy, "not accepted as a form of rationality from the perspective of our current type of science, intent on specification and classification [...], because with the development and enforcement of our conception of science and reason it was no longer understood, fell into disrepute, and was finally suspended. However, since it is a formal method that can be schematized and uses generally understandable laws, which is universally applicable and intersubjectively communicable and, just like the classificatory model, follows the scientific criteria of comprehensibility, semantic clarity and precision, logical consistency—although a different one than specification or classification—operational handling, etc., it cannot be denied the status of its own type of rationality" (Gloy 2001, pp. 207–208; see Gloy and Bachmann 2000).

What is formulated theoretically here finds its application in everyday thinking but also in the construction of models in applied sciences, even though their understanding of rationality follows the mechanistic design. In addition, the *analogical rationality type*, as Karen Gloy calls it, plays a dominant role at least in psychodynamic therapeutic methods, notably with the elements of (1) transference, (2) projection, and (3) free association:

1. Transference is concerned with, for a start, a common human phenomenon, namely, the ability to enter into closer contact with other people. But in psychotherapy, "the common personal encounter becomes the special case of the analytic situation" (Herold and Weiß 2008, p. 799), during which, spontaneously or gradually, behavior and thinking patterns emerge that are similar to those used with significant attachment figures in the past.
2. Projection shares a certain kinship with transference, because both will assign something to someone else that does not exist in the presumed form; only in the case of projection the focus is not on early relationship patterns but on traits a person himself/herself possesses. The term is somewhat outdated, because nowadays it is mostly subsumed under the collective designation of externalization (Mentzos 2008, p. 189), but it does have heuristic value, because—similar to transference—it starts with a common human phenomenon that, as already mentioned, became the center of Jean Piaget's theory: the egocentric tendency to judge the things of this world and the people with whom one interacts by oneself in order to transform the unknown into the familiar.
3. In his novel *Klein and Wagner*, Hermann Hesse puts the following words in the mouth of his protagonist: "What you had to seek and learn was a different kind of thinking. Was it a form of thinking at all? It was a condition, an inner state, which could last only for moments and was spoiled by strenuous efforts to think. In this highly desirable state you had inspirations, memories, visions, fantasies, insights of a special kind" (Hesse 1970, p. 78). This is a poetic description of free association, which is of genuine analogical quality. This is because the question of what this dream or that event spontaneously inspires often calls forth memories of similar constellations from the past. Sometimes, this causes stressful or traumatic events to surface, and these must then be worked through, which means emotionally reliving the same ordeal in a weakened form. And that now is of genuine analogical quality, because things are the same and at the same time different: the trauma is experienced in a similar way as before, but the context is different, seeing as it is a non-damaging relationship in a therapeutic context.

In summary, it can be said that analogical thinking is of great importance not only in everyday life but also in sciences in the construction of models. It is also easily substantiated through scientific theory, as Karen Gloy has demonstrated, and while it does play a major role primarily in psychodynamic therapy, it is also a valuable factor in, for example, gestalt therapy and its perception exercise of the "empty chair," which acts as a transfer object and permits dialogue with people, parts of oneself, or with actual or imagined relationships (see O'Leary 2013, pp. 76–77). Since specific studies exist (Buchholz 2003; Gelo 2008; Gelo and Mergenthaler 2012) about special phenomena contiguous with the analogical rationality type, such as projection (Werner and Langenmayr 2005a, pp. 82–113) or the composition of metaphors and analogies (Werner and Langenmayr 2005b, pp. 14–56), the analogical rationality type can be employed in psychotherapy science.

The relevance of analogical thinking has long been neglected in mainstream psychotherapy research that, on the contrary, has heavily relied on causal-analytical thinking (see Sects. 4.2.1 and 4.2.3). This is especially evident in statistical *hypothesis testing* and the related *hypothetico-deductive* method that dominates contemporary research in psychotherapy: one or a few assertions are derived from a theory, stated in the form of one or a few hypotheses and compared with observations gathered from a large, representative sample in order to find out if the confidence in the statement(s) is significantly increased (i.e., not due to chance; $p < .05$).

Such an approach has several limitations. For example, researchers working within this framework tend to consider only one—typically, the favored—hypothesis and ignore alternative and/or other relevant ones (*confirmation bias*; Dunbar and Fugelsang 2005). Moreover, the assumptions which have to be satisfied in order to work within a quantitative hypothesis-testing framework are mostly unable to address the richness and context sensitivity of clinical theories (Greenberg 1991; Stiles 2009). In accordance with these observations, Mahrer (1988) stated that "hypothesis-testing research is essentially inadequate and unproductive for serious confirmation or disconfirmation of the propositions that make up theories of psychotherapy and also for contributing to a purportedly cumulative body of psychotherapeutic knowledge" (p. 701).

For these reasons, there has been an increasing call for *discovery-oriented* psychotherapy research in the past years (Mahrer 1988) which, contrary to hypothesis-testing research, emphasizes the intention to learn and the possibility to be surprised by means of adequately exploring the data with the aim of *hypothesis generation* and *theory building* (see the significant event approach described by Elliott 2010; see also Chaps. 3 and 8). Analogical thinking plays a significant role in this kind of research. "Scientists use analogies to form a bridge between what they already know and what they are trying to explain, understand, or discover. In fact, many scientists have claimed that the use of certain analogies was instrumental in their making a scientific discovery and almost all scientific autobiographies and biographies feature an important analogy that is discussed in depth" (Dunbar and Fugelsang 2005, p. 713). Analogical reasoning is useful for generating new hypotheses and to build explicative models of unexpected findings (Dunbar and Fugelsang 2005; Clement 2008); this is possible because analogy *projects* the relational structure of a *source* knowledge domain (i.e., what is already known) into a *target* knowledge domain (i.e., what can be discovered), so that new features of the latter may be highlighted and/or new sets of relations may emerge (Gentner 1983; Gentner et al. 2001). Moreover, analogy may activate *abduction* (Clement and Núñez Oviedo 2003), a form of inference which allows us to use (unexpected) observations to recursively and creatively modify and extend an existing theory or generate a new one (Haig 2008; see also Salvatore and Valsiner 2010; Stiles 2009; see Chap. 6).

Conclusion: Toward a Pluralistic Psychotherapy Science

The history of science shows that the individual scientific disciplines have branched out more and more since the early modern period. While at the beginning of the university development in medieval Europe there were only four faculties with few subjects (*artes liberales*, law, medicine, theology), over the past centuries and especially in the decades after the Second World War, it has been possible to observe an increasing specialization which gave rise to, among other things, an independent psychotherapy science, no longer considered merely a branch of psychiatry and clinical psychology (see Rieken 2012, 2013; see also Chap. 5). The main idea of this chapter is that psychotherapy science could be put on a broader foundation if it followed not only the scientific *mainstream* but also took into account the *alternative* frameworks of understanding outlined in this text.

In the course of the European modern period, the assumptions described at the beginning of this chapter produced—and, at the same time, were the expression of—a mathematical-scientific-technological image of nature and science (the so-called *received view of science*; Suppe 1977) that, with all its advantages and disadvantages, has changed the world as never before in the cultural evolution of man. Natural processes are attributed to mechanical laws and explained deterministically according to the principle of the *causa efficiens*. This also applies to many disciplines usually considered extremely relevant in the field of psychotherapy, such as biological psychiatry and experimental psychology, since they share the basic assumptions of the received view of science. This may have explanatory value, especially in those areas in which humans may be considered to behave "similar to machines" following deterministic laws, such as in low-level learning processes (see, e.g., the classic stimulus-response model) and related targeted interventions associated with restricted degrees of freedom (as it might be the case, e.g., in some purely behavioral interventions). The human psyche cannot be reduced to this, though, because the reference to universal regularities by means of reductionist and deterministic laws cannot fully take into account the context-bound development of individuality and subjectivity, which play such a fundamental role in psychotherapy.

Thus, we believe that the consideration of *causa finalis*, wholeness, analogical thinking alongside the *causa efficiens*, determinism, and mechanism might permit a more comprehensive and useful approach to the scientific investigation of humans, their mental problems, and the way to treat them than what the latter can offer on their own. All of these components could contribute to psychotherapy as a science developing a more embracing profile. From the perspective of the philosophy of science, mechanization, *causa efficiens*, and analytical thinking are one, and wholeness, *causa finalis*, and analogical thinking the other side of a coin and from the perspective of psychotherapy science only the combination of both these "angles" provides a more complete view of the human condition. Slife expressed this in a similar way when he spoke of a *methodological pluralism* (Slife and Gantt 1999; see also Elliott 2010), which means that science works with different methods based on different philosophies, the use of which depends on our interests, inclinations, and our particular research questions.

Such a kind of pluralism may allow us to avoid the absolutistic *monopoly* of any specific scientific approach without falling into relativism and "anything goes" positions. In fact, this pluralism underlines that the specific research method to be used (e.g., quantitative, qualitative, mixed methods) should be driven by the subject matter being investigated and the research questions being asked (e.g., "to explain a general phenomenon" vs. "to understand a subjective experience"; see Dillon 1984 for a review), and not by the abstract epistemologies comprising our ideologies (e.g., "reality can be objectively analyzed" vs. "reality is a sociocultural construct). In order to do this, researchers should, first of all, become aware that any specific research method they might apply is *conceivable* only on the basis of a set of metatheoretical (i.e., philosophical) assumptions, beliefs, and values (Gelo 2012; Slife 1998; Slife and Williams 1995); and, second, they should engage in constructive *dialogues* with the proponents of different approaches with the aim of increasing mutual sharing and understanding (Gelo and Gelo 2012; Smaling 2000). We hope that this chapter could make a contribution into this direction.

References

Adler A (1912) The neurotic character. Fundamentals of individual psychology and psychotherapy. In: Stein HT (ed) The collected clinical works of Alfred Adler, vol 1. Classical Adlerian Translation Project, Bellingham, WA

Adler A (1927) Understanding human nature. Garden City, New York

Adler A (1933) What life should mean to you: the psychology of personal development. Oneworld, Oxford

Andreas S, Andreas C (eds) (1982) Reframing: neuro-linguistic programming and the transformation of meaning. Real People Press, Moab

Antonovsky A (1987) Unraveling the mystery of health: how people manage stress and stay well. Jossey-Bass, San Francisco

Arendt H (1998) The human condition. University of Chicago Press, Chicago

Aristotle (1930) Physica. In: Ross WD (ed) The works of Aristotle, vol 2. Clarendon Press, Oxford

Aristotle (1933) Metaphysics. In: Aristotle in 23 Volumes, Vols.17, 18, Transl. by Hugh Tredennick. Harvard University Press, Cambridge MA, William Heinemann, London

Bacon F (2000) Novum organum. Cambridge University Press, Cambridge

Balint M (1959) Thrills and regressions. The Hogarth Press, London

Bammé A, Feuerstein G, Genth R, Holling E, Kahle R, Kempin P (1983) Maschinen-Menschen, Mensch-Maschinen. Grundrisse einer sozialen Beziehung. Rowohlt, Reinbek bei Hamburg

Bandler R, Grinder J, Andreas S, Andreas C (1983) Reframing: neuro-linguistic programming and the transformation of meaning. Real People Press, Moab

Barker C, Pistrang N, Elliott R (eds) (2002) Research methods in clinical psychology: an introduction for students and practitioners, 2nd edn. Wiley, Chichester

Beamish R (1862) Memoir of the life of Sir Marc Isambard Brunel. Longman, London

Bortz J (1984) Lehrbuch der empirischen Forschung. Springer, Heidelberg

Bortz J, Döring N (2006) Forschungsmethoden und Evaluation für Human- und Sozialwissen-schaftler, 4th edn. Springer, Heidelberg

Brentano F (1995) Psychology from an empirical standpoint. Routledge, London

Buchholz MB (1999) Psychotherapie als Profession. Psychosozial, Gießen

Buchholz MB (2003) Metaphern der "Kur". Eine qualitative Studie zum psychotherapeutischen Prozess. Psychosozial, Gießen

Cassirer E (1953–1957) The philosophy of symbolic forms, vol 3. Yale University Press, New Haven

Clement J (2008) Creative model construction in scientists and students: imagery, analogy, and mental simulation. Springer, Dordrecht

Clement J, Núñez Oviedo M (2003) Abduction and analogy in scientific model construction. Paper presented at the national association for research in science teaching conference, Philadelphia. Retrieved from http://people.umass.edu/~clement/pdf/clement_nunez_paper.pdf

Danziger K (1985) The methodological imperative in psychology. Philos Soc Sci 15(1):1–13. doi:10.1177/004839318501500101

Danziger K (1990) Constructing the subject: historical origins of psychological research. Cambridge University Press, New York

de La Mettrie JO (1994) Man a machine. Hacket, Indianapolis, Ind

Descartes R (1988) Principles of philosophy. Mellen, Lewiston

Dijksterhuis EJ (1961) The mechanization of the world picture. Clarendon, Oxford

Dillon JT (1984) The classification of research questions. Rev Educ Res 54(3):327–361

Dörner D (2004) Der Mensch als Maschine. In: Jüttemann G (ed) Psychologie als Human-wissenschaft. Ein Handbuch. Vandenhoeck & Ruprecht, Göttingen, pp 32–44

Dunbar K, Fugelsang J (2005) Scientific thinking and reasoning. In: Holyoak KJ, Morrison R (eds) Cambridge handbook of thinking. Cambridge University Press, Cambridge, pp 705–725

Dupuy JP (2000) The mechanization of the mind. Princeton University Press, Princeton

Elliott R (2010) Psychotherapy change process research: realizing the promise. Psychother Res 20(2):123–135. doi:10.1080/10503300903470743

Elliott R, Anderson C (1994) Simplicity and complexity in psychotherapy research. In: Russell RL (ed) Reassessing psychotherapy research. Guilford, New York, pp 65–113

Elliott R, Shapiro DA, Mack C (1999) Simplified personal questionnaire procedure manual. University of Toledo, Department of Psychology, Toledo

Erikson E (1950) Childhood and society. Norton, New York

Fischer G (2008) Logik der Psychotherapie. Philosophische Grundlagen der Psychotherapiewissenschaft. Asanger, Kröning

Fischer G (2011) Psychotherapiewissenschaft. Einführung in eine neue humanwissenschaftliche Disziplin. Psychosozial-Verlag, Gießen

Frankl VE (1975) Anthropologische Grundlagen der Psychotherapie. Huber, Bern

Frankl VE (2004) On the theory and therapy of mental disorders: an introduction to logotherapy and existential analysis. Brunner-Routledge, New York

Frisch M (1959) Homo faber. A report. Abelard-Schuman, London

Frommer J, Rennie DL (eds) (2001) Qualitative psychotherapy research: methods and methodology. Pabst Science Publishers, Lengerich

Gadamer HG (1989) Truth and method, 2nd edn. Sheed and Ward, London

Gelo OCG (2008) Metaphors and emotional-cognitive regulation in psychotherapy. Ulmer Textbank Verlag, Ulm

Gelo OCG (2012) On research methods and their philosophical assumptions: "raising the consciousness of researchers" again. Psychotherapie und Sozialwissenschaft 14(2):111–130

Gelo OCG, Gelo C (2012) Dialogical relationship among scientific paradigms in psychotherapy research. Paper presented at the 3rd Joint Meeting of the European and the United Kingdom Chapters of the Society for Psychotherapy Research, Porto, October 10–13

Gelo OCG, Mergenthaler E (2012) Unconventional metaphors and emotional-cognitive regulation in a metacognitive interpersonal therapy. Psychother Res 22:159–175. doi:10.1080/10503307.2011.629636

Gelo OCG, Braakmann D, Benetka G (2008) Quantitative and qualitative research: beyond the debate. Integr Psychol Behav Sci 42(3):266–290. doi:10.1007/s12124-008- 9078-3

Gelo OCG, Braakmann D, Benetka G (2009) Erratum to "Quantitative and qualitative research: beyond the debate". Integr Psychol Behav Sci 43(4):406–407. doi:10.1007/s12124-009-9107-x

Gentner D (1983) Structure-mapping: a theoretical framework for analogy. Cogn Sci 7:155–170. doi:10.1207/s15516709cog0702_3

Gentner D, Holyoak KJ, Kokinov BN (eds) (2001) The analogical mind: perspectives from cognitive science. MIT Press, Cambridge

Gerigk HJ (2006) Lesen und Interpretieren, 2nd edn. Vandenhoeck & Ruprecht, Göttingen

Giedion S (1948) Mechanization takes command: a contribution to anonymous history. Oxford University Press, New York

Gloy K (1995) Das Verständnis der Natur, vol. 1: Die Geschichte des wissenschaftlichen Denkens. Beck, München

Gloy K (1996) Das Verständnis der Natur, vol. 2: Die Geschichte des ganzheitlichen Denkens. Beck, München

Gloy K (2001) Vernunft und das Andere der Vernunft. Alber, Freiburg (Breisgau), München

Gloy K, Bachmann M (eds) (2000) Das Analogiedenken. Vorstöße in ein neues Gebiet der Rationalitätstheorie. Alber, Freiburg im Breisgau München

Grawe K (2004) Psychological therapy. Hogrefe & Huber, Cambridge

Grawe K, Donati R, Bernauer F (2001) Psychotherapie im Wandel: von der Konfession zur Profession, 5th edn. Hogrefe, Göttingen

Greenberg LS (1986) Change process research. J Consult Clin Psychol 54(1):4–9. doi:10.1037/0022-006X.54.1.4

Greenberg LS (1991) Research in the process of change. Psychother Res 1:3–16. doi:10.1080/10503309112331334011

Haig BD (2008) An abductive perspective on theory construction. J Theory Constr Test 12(1):7–10

Hartmann-Kotteck L (2003) Gestalttherapie. In: Reimer C, Rüger U (eds) Psychodynamische Psychotherapien. Lehrbuch der tiefenpsychologisch orientierten Psychotherapien, 2nd edn. Springer, Berlin, pp 178–233

Heidegger M (1988) Being and time. Harper and Row, New York

Herold R, Weiß H (2008) Übertragung. In: Mertens W, Waldvogel B (eds) Handbuch psychoanalytischer Grundbegriffe, 3rd edn. Kohlhammer, Stuttgart, pp 799–811

Herrmann T (1979) Psychologie als Problem. Herausforderungen der psychologischen Wissenschaft. Klett-Cotta, Stuttgart

Hesse H (1970) Klein and Wagner. In: Klingsor's last summer (trans: Winston R, Winston C). Farrar, Straus and Giroux, New York

Hofstadter R, Sander E (2013) Surfaces and essences: analogy as the fuel and fire of thinking. Basic Books, Perseus Book Group, New York

Honko L (1959) Krankheitsprojektile. Untersuchung über eine urtümliche Krankheitserklärung. Academia Scientiarum Fennica, Helsinki

Huizinga J (1980) Homo Ludens: a study of the play-element in culture. Routledge and Kegan Paul, London

Hume D (2007) An enquiry concerning human understanding: and other writings. Cambridge University Press, Cambridge

Kant I (1998) Critique of pure reason. Transl. and ed. by Guyer P, Wood AW. Cambridge University Press, Cambridge

Kant I (2003) To perpetual peace: a philosophical sketch. Hackett Publishing, Indianapolis, Ind

Kaulbach F, Beck H (1974) Ganzes/Teil. In: Ritter J (ed) Historisches Wörterbuch der Philosophie, vol 3. Wissenschaftliche Buchgesellschaft, Darmstadt, pp 3–20

Kazdin AE (2008) Evidence-based treatment and practice: new opportunities to bridge clinical research and practice, enhance the knowledge base, and improve patient care. Am Psychol 63(3):146–159. doi:10.1037/0003-066X.63.3.146

Köller W (2004) Perspektivität und Sprache. Zur Struktur von Objektivierungsformen in Bildern, im Denken und in der Sprache. de Gruyter, Berlin

König K (2011) Kleine psychoanalytische Charakterkunde, 10th edn. Vandenhoeck & Rup-recht, Göttingen

Kukla A (1989) Non-empirical issues in psychology. Am Psychol 44:785–794. doi:10.1037//0003-066X.44.5.785

Lacan J (2001) The mirror-stage as formative of the function of the I. In: Écrits: a selection (trans. Sheridan A). Routledge, London, pp 1–7

Lakoff G, Johnson M (1999) Philosophy in the flesh: the embodied mind and its challenge to western thought. Basic Books, New York

Lambert MJ (2013) The efficacy and effectiveness of psychotherapy. In: Lambert MJ (ed) Bergin and Garfield's handbook of psychotherapy and behavior change, 6th edn. Wiley, Hoboken, pp 169–218

Laurenceau JP, Hayes AM, Feldman GC (2007) Some methodological and statistical issues in the study of change processes in psychotherapy. Clin Psychol Rev 27(6):682–695. doi:10.1016/j.cpr.2007.01.007

Mahrer AR (1988) Discovery-oriented psychotherapy research: rationale, aims, and methods. Am Psychol 43(9):694–702. doi:10.1037/0003-066X.43.9.694

Marquis de Laplace PM (2007) A philosophical essay on probabilities. Cosimo, New York

McLeod J (2013) Qualitative research: methods and contributions. In: Lambert MJ (ed) Bergin and Garfield's handbook of psychotherapy and behavior change, 5th edn. Wiley, New York, pp 49–84

McMullen LM (2008) Putting it in context: metaphor and psychotherapy. In: Gibbs R (ed) The Cambridge handbook of metaphor and thought. Cambridge University Press, Cambridge, pp 397–411

Mentzos S (2008) Externalisierung. In: Mertens W, Waldvogel B (eds) Handbuch psycho-analytischer Grundbegriffe, 3rd edn. Kohlhammer, Stuttgart, pp 189–191

Milgram S (1974) Obedience to authority: an experimental view. Harper & Row, New York

Müller KE (1987) Das magische Universum der Identität. Elementarformen sozialen Verhaltens. Ein ethnologischer Grundriss. Campus, Frankfurt

Mumford L (1967–1970) The myth of the machine, vol 2. Harcourt, New York

Newton I (1999) The Principia: mathematical principles of natural philosophy. University of California Press, Berkeley

O'Leary E (2013) Techniques, experiments, and dreams. In: O'Leary E (ed) Gestalt therapy around the world. Wiley, New York, pp 61–91

Orlinsky D, Rønnestad M, Willutzki U (2004) Fifty years of psychotherapy process-outcome research: continuity and change. In: Lambert M (ed) Bergin and Garfield's handbook of psychotherapy and behavior change, 5th edn. Wiley, New York, pp 307–390

Pascual-Leone A (2009) Dynamic emotional processing in experiential therapy: two steps forward, one step back. J Consult Clin Psychol 77(1):113–126. doi:10.1037/a0014488

Piaget J (1953) The origin of intelligence in the child. Routledge & Kegan, London

Piaget J (2007) The child's conception of the world. Rowman & Littlefield, Lanham

Plato (1929) Timaeus. In: Plato in 12 Volumes, Vol. 9: Timaeus; Critias; Cleitophon; Menexenus; Epistles. Harvard University Press, London, pp 1–253

Pritz A, Teufelhart H (1996) Psychotherapie—Wissenschaft vom Subjektiven. In: Pritz A (ed) Psychotherapie—eine neue Wissenschaft vom Menschen. Springer, New York, pp 1–18

Rennie DL (2012) Qualitative methods as methodical hermeneutics. Psychol Methods 17(3):385–398. doi:10.1037/a0029250385

Rentsch T (1980) Leib-Seele-Verhältnis. In: Ritter J, Gründer K (eds) Historisches Wörterbuch der Philosophie, vol 5. Wissenschaftliche Buchgesellschaft, Darmstadt, pp 185–206

Rieken B (2007) Vom Nutzen volkskundlich-historischer Zugänge für die Katastrophenforschung: New Orleans 2005. In: Hartmann A, Silke M, Mohrmann RE (eds) Historizität. Vom Umgang mit Geschichte. Waxmann, Münster, pp 149–162

Rieken B (2010a) Schatten über Galtür? Gespräche mit Einheimischen über die Lawine von 1999. Ein Beitrag zur Katastrophenforschung. Waxmann, Münster

Rieken B (2010b) Wiederentdeckung des teleologischen Denkens? Der anthropogene Klimawandel aus ethnologisch-psychologischer und wissenschaftsgeschichtlicher Perspektive. In: Voss M (ed) Der Klimawandel. Sozialwissenschaftliche Perspektiven. VS Verlag für Sozial-wissenschaften, Wiesbaden, pp 301–312

Rieken B (2010c) Das Analogiedenken und seine Bedeutung für Medizin und Psychotherapie. Curare. Zeitschrift für Medizinethnologie 33:192–199

Rieken B (2012) Psychotherapie als Bildungsprozess am Beispiel der Sigmund-Freud-Privatuniversität Wien. Zeitschrift für Psychotraumatologie, Psychotherapiewissenschaft, Psychologische Medizin 10:95–102

Rieken B (2013) Überlegungen zur Akademisierung der Psychotherapie—am Beispiel der Sigmund-Freud-Privatuniversität Wien. Z Individ 38:285–302

Ropohl G (2012) Allgemeine Systemtheorie: Einführung in transdisziplinäres Denken. Edition Sigma, Berlin

Salvatore S (2011) Psychotherapy research needs theory. Outline for an epistemology of the clinical exchange. Integr Psychol Behav Sci 45:366–388. doi:10.1007/s12124-011-9180-9

Salvatore S, Tschacher W (2012) Time dependency of psychotherapeutic exchanges: the contribution of the theory of dynamic systems in analyzing process. Front Psychol 3:1–14. doi:10.3389/fpsyg.2012.00253

Salvatore S, Valsiner J (2010) Between the general and the unique: overcoming the nomothetic versus idiographic opposition. Theory Psychol 20(6):817–833. doi:10.1177/0959354310381156

Salvatore S, Gelo OCG, Gennaro A, Manzo S, Radaideh A (2010) Looking at the psychotherapy process as an intersubjective dynamic of meaning-making. A case study with the discourse flow analysis. J Constr Psychol 23(3):195–230. doi:10.1080/10720531003765981

Satir V, Baldwin M (1983) Satir step by step: a guide to creating change in families. Science and Behavior Books, Palo Alto

Schapp W (2004) In Geschichten verstrickt. Zum Sein von Mensch und Ding (4th edn). Klostermann, Frankfurt am Main//Empêtrés dans des histoires: l'être de l'homme et de la chose. Editions du Cerf, Paris 1992

Schelling FWJ (2004) Einleitung zu seinem Entwurf eines Systems der Naturphilosophie. In: Schriften (1799–1800). Historisch-kritische Ausgabe, Reihe 1, Vol. 8. Frommann-Holzboog, Stuttgart, pp 1–86

Schiemann G (1998) Ohne Telos und Substanz. Grenzen des naturwissenschaftlichen Kau-salitätsverständnisses. Vortrag am 20. Weltkongress für Philosophie, Boston (Massachusetts), 10.08.–15.08.1998. http://www.philosophie.uni-wupper-tal.de/fileadmin/philosophie/PDFs_allg/Schiemann/Aufs%C3%

A4tze_neu/18Ohne_Telos_und_Substanz_1.pdf (28.08.2013)

Schiepek G, Fricke B, Kaimer P (1992) Synergetics of psychotherapy. In: Tschacher W, Schiepek G, Brunner EJ (eds) Self-organization and clinical psychology. Springer, Berlin, pp 239–267

Schönborn C (2005) Finding design in nature. New York Times, 07.07.2005. http://www.nytimes.com/2005/07/07/opinion/07schonborn.html?_r=0 (02.09.2013)

Schopenhauer A (1958) On man's need for metaphysics. In: The world as will and representation, vol 2 The Falcon's Wing Press, Indian Hills, Colorado, pp 160–189

Searle JR (2004) Mind: a brief introduction. Oxford University Press, New York

Slife BD (1998) Raising the consciousness of researchers: hidden assumptions in the behavioral sciences. Adapt Phys Act Q 15(3):208–221

Slife BD (2004) Theoretical challenges to therapy practice and research: the constraint of naturalism. In: Lambert MJ (ed) Bergin and Garfield's handbook of psychotherapy and behavior change, 5th edn. Wiley, New York, pp 44–83

Slife BD, Gantt E (1999) Methodological pluralism: a framework for psychotherapy research. J Clin Psychol 55(12):1–13

Slife BD, Williams RN (1995) What's behind the research: discovering hidden assumptions in the behavioral sciences. Sage, Thousand Oaks

Slife BD, Wiggins BJ, Graham JT (2005) Avoiding an EST monopoly: toward a pluralism of philosophies and methods. J Contemp Psychother 35(1):83–97

Smaling A (2000) What kind of dialogue should paradigm-dialogues be? Qual Quant 34(1):51–63

Smith A (2007) Wealth of nations. Cosimo, New York

Smith EC, Grawe K (2003) What makes psychotherapy sessions productive? A new approach to bridging the gap between process research and practice. Clin Psychol Psychother 10(5):275–285. doi:10.1002/cpp.377

Soressia M, McPherronc SP, Lenoire M, Dogandžić T, Goldberg P, Jacobs Z, Maigrot Y, Martisius NL, Miller CE, Rendu W, Richards M, Skinner MM, Steele TE, Talamo S, Texier JP (2013) Neandertals made the first specialized bone tools in Europe. Proc Natl Acad Sci USA 110(35):14186–14190

Spaemann R, Löw R (1985) Die Frage Wozu? Geschichte und Wiederentdeckung des teleologischen Denkens, 2nd edn. Piper, München

Stiles WB (2009) Logical operations in theory-building case studies. Pragmatic Case Studies in Psychotherapy 5(3): Article 2, 9–22. http://hdl.rutgers.edu/1782.1/pcsp_journal

Stiles WB, Shapiro DA (1989) Abuse of the drug metaphor in psychotherapy process-outcome research. Clin Psychol Rev 9:521–543. doi:10.1016/0272-7358(89)90007-X

Stiles WB, Shapiro DA (1994) Disabuse of the drug metaphor: psychotherapy process-outcome correlations. J Consult Clin Psychol 62(5):942–948. doi:10.1037/0022-006X.62.5.942

Suppe F (1977) The structure of scientific theories, 2nd edn. Illini Books, Champaign-Urbana

Tetens H (2001) Ursache/Wirkung. In: Ritter J, Gründer K, Gabriel G (eds) Historisches Wörterbuch der Philosophie (vol 11). Wissenschaftliche Buchgesellschaft, Darmstadt, pp 377–412

Thomä H, Kächele H (2006) Psychoanalytische Therapie. Grundlagen, 3rd edn. Springer, Heidelberg

Thomas of Aquin (2000) Sancti Thomae de Aquino Sententia libri Metaphysicae. In: Corpus Thomisticum S. Thomae de Aquino Opera Omnia. Recognovit ac instruxit Enrique Alarcón electronico Pampilonae ad Universitatis Studiorum Navarrensis aedes A.D. MM. http://www.corpusthomisticum.org/cmp0104.html. Accessed on 28 Aug 2013

Tschacher W, Gelo OCG, Koch SC, & Salvatore S (2014) Dynamic systems theory and embodiment in psychotherapy research. A new look at process and outcome (Special issue). Front Psychol 5:1089. http://journal.frontiersin.org/ResearchTopic/1744#overview

Vinnai G (1993) Die Austreibung der Kritik aus der Wissenschaft: Psychologie im Universitätsbetrieb. Campus, Frankfurt am Main New York. http://psydok.sulb.uni-saarland.de/volltexte/2005/547/. Accessed on 31 Aug 2013

von Bertalanffy L (1950) An outline of general system theory. Br J Philos Sci 1(2):134–165

Werner C, Langenmayr A (2005a) Das Unbewusste und die Abwehrmechanismen. Vandenhoeck & Ruprecht, Göttingen

Werner C, Langenmayr A (2005b) Der Traum und die Fehlleistungen. Vandenhoeck & Ruprecht, Göttingen

Wexberg E (1987) Individualpsychologie. Eine systematische Darstellung, 3rd edn. Hirzel, Stuttgart

Wuketits F (1985) Zustand und Bewusstsein. Leben als biophilosophische Synthese. Hoffmann und Campe, Hamburg

Psychotherapia Academica Universitatis: A Philosophical Argument for the Academic Discipline of Psychotherapy

5

Kurt Greiner

Contents

K. Greiner (✉)
Department of Psychotherapy Science, Sigmund Freud University, Freudplatz 1, 1020 Vienna, Austria
e-mail: kurt.greiner@sfu.ac.at

Abstract

An academic psychotherapy (*psychotherapia academica universitatis*) can only be termed as such when the inhomogeneous movement-specific models, methods, and practices of psychotherapy (*psychotherapia*) enter into a systematic dialogue of reflection both with each other and with other cultural constructs so that an increasingly differentiated level of self-conception in terms of psychotherapeutic modes of thinking and acting may gradually emerge, which, not least, may render visible their limits of meaning and the commitment dimensions of various psychotherapeutic findings.

This chapter methodically provides arguments for this claim, which I endeavor with reference to arguments found in Friedrich G. Wallner's "constructive realism" (CR). CR is a cultural-constructivist approach to the philosophy of science which was conceived in the 1990s at the University of Vienna. In the course of a constructive-realist discussion, it becomes plausible that scientific activities in the academic sense are neither the representation, description, or explanation of a prefabricated world nor the unraveling, decoding, or deciphering of some structures of objective reality, but exclusively the production, application, and reflection of various contexts of argumentation and action ("microworlds"). A short introduction to constructive-realist methodology is followed by the philosophical

O.C.G. Gelo et al. (eds.), *Psychotherapy Research*,
DOI 10.1007/978-3-7091-1382-0_5,

argumentation for the *academic discipline of psychotherapy (psychotherapia academica universitatis)* and the application of terminological principles of CR to the *therapeutic practice of psychotherapy (psychotherapia)*. The chapter will demonstrate that, because of its pluralism of arguments, its linguistic diversity, and its methodological heterogeneity, contemporary psychotherapy has not only a vast head start in research theory but also enormous reflection-scientific advantages in comparison with a large number of other academic disciplines.

5.1 Introduction

Although the therapeutic practice of psychotherapy (*psychotherapia*) has been striving for academic recognition since Sigmund Freud's attempts at conceptualizing the first therapeutic-scientific treatment method, it was continually refused its long-awaited access to the circle of established disciplines in university research throughout the twentieth century. There are several reasons for this troubling situation, and all of them have very little to do with psychotherapy itself, but rather pertain to the culture and politics of science, which I shall not discuss here. The scientific phenotype of psychotherapy has the ideal preconditions to become an independent discipline in its own right—not least because the field of psychotherapeutic practice is split up into a large number of highly diverse and varied schools, approaches, systems, models, branches, and positions. From a science-philosophical point of view, we are dealing with various "microworlds" (F.G. Wallner) of psychotherapy, that is, *constructed, artificial realities of psychotherapeutic activity* which in no way can be ascribed to a common structural logic or a paradigmatic basic principle that all commit to. Each of these *psychotherapeutic microworlds* determines for itself how to understand the psychotherapeutic object of research, so that an efficient epistemic approach to it becomes possible, which subsequently answers questions specific to the object of research and eventually enables activities to solve the problem.

In order to be accepted as an academic discipline, psychotherapy first has to operate adequately within its different school contexts (*technical level*). If, however, psychotherapy does not claim more for itself than to operate adequately, it downgrades itself to a mere *technique of healing and convalescence* and thus remains on the level of psychotherapeutic practice (*psychotherapia*). If psychotherapy wants to position itself as an academic discipline in the occidental cultural sense (*psychotherapia academica universitatis*), it has to make an effort to *gain deep insights into the complex structures of its professional activities*. This means it is paramount for school-based psychotherapeutic microworlds to critically reflect their respective modes of operation in order for a differentiated self-comprehension of psychotherapeutic thought and practice to emerge (*level of insight into technical aspects*). Critical reflection of a psychotherapeutic microworld succeeds via dialogic encounters with other psychotherapeutic schools as well as artistic media and other constructions of meaning. In order to implement and carry out such dialogic encounters methodically and systematically, the approach of *transfermeneutic psychotherapy science/experimental hermeneutics* has developed special tools that are applied at the Sigmund Freud University in Vienna (SFU) in research projects about psychotherapy science (cf. Greiner et al. 2009; Greiner 2012, 2013a). The reflection methods are so-called experimental hermeneutic methods, i.e., innovative tools of meaning comprehension which help gain differentiated self-reflexive insights into the specific modes of psychotherapeutic operations (*insight into technical aspects*).

Consequently, we may already state the following in this introduction: From the point of view of contemporary scientific theory (cf. Wallner 1997b, 2002, 2005; Wallner et al. 2010; Lan et al. 2013), we can speak of an academic psychotherapy (*psychotherapia academica universitatis*) only when the inhomogeneous school-specific tenets, methods, and practices of psychotherapy (*psychotherapeutic microworlds*) enter a systematic dialogue of reflection both with each other and with other cultural constructs (*dialogue of psychotherapeutic microworlds*) so that gradually an increasingly differentiated level of self-comprehension in terms of psychotherapeutic modes of thinking and acting may emerge, which, not least, may render visible their boundaries of meaning and the commitment dimensions of various psychotherapeutic findings.

I attempt to incrementally substantiate this claim in this essay. The text is structured into two main parts. Part one, *The Two Levels of Academic Sciences* (see Sect. 5.2), introduces readers to the kind of basic concepts of science and research which characterize the so-called constructive realism (CR) according to Friedrich G. Wallner (cf. Wallner 1992a, 1994, 1997b, 2002; Slunecko 1997; Greiner 2005a; Jandl and Greiner 2005). CR is a cultural-constructivist approach to the philosophy of science (cf. Wallner 2009, 2011; Wallner et al. 2010), which was conceptualized in the 1990s at the University of Vienna to tie in with positions of the philosophy of language as well as postmodernism, particularly Ludwig Wittgenstein's (1966, 1968) and Paul Feyerabend's (1985). In the course of a constructive-realist discussion, it becomes plausible that *scientific activities in the academic sense* are neither the representation, description, or explanation of the prefabricated world nor the unraveling, decoding, or deciphering of some structures of objective environments, but exclusively the *production, application, and reflection of various "microworlds"* (cf. Wallner 2005; Wallner and Greiner 2006; Greiner and Wallner 2009).

Part two, *Academic Psychotherapy* (see Sect. 5.3), deals with a science-philosophical substantiation of the *academic discipline of psychotherapy* (*psychotherapia academica universitatis*) by way of a constructive-realist argumentation, i.e., by applying the terminological principles of *constructive realism* (CR) to the *therapeutic practice of psychotherapy* (*psychotherapia*). This shall demonstrate that because of its pluralism of arguments, its linguistic diversity, and its heterogeneity of methodologies, contemporary modern psychotherapy has not only a vast head start in research theory but also enormous reflection-scientific advantages in comparison with a large number of other academic disciplines.

5.2 The Two Levels of Academic Science: Arguments of a Contemporary Philosophy of Science

The philosophy of science of constructive realism (CR) in its current form states that scientific action and activity may never be associated with the *progress of epistemic approaches* about the methodological orientation toward the *object of observation comprehended as structurally prefabricated* (*objective environment*). Much rather, the subject of investigation—the studied, observed object—is *structurally anticipated*, i.e., the object of investigation is in a way *captured* and *included* and therefore does not encounter the researcher as an independent entity, a "thing-in-itself," so to speak, but is an *integral part* of the *active or creative research activity* from the outset. This special conception of science obviously requires explanation, which I shall attempt in the following pages.

5.2.1 Starting Point: Epistemological Logics in the Object-Method Circle

In contrast to *conventional realists*, for instance, who cling to the *existence of an objective environment independent of observers*, "constructive realists" factor in that, on principle, scientific acts in the context of experiences which can be argued rationally proceed in a circular, structured fashion. The specific relation that develops between the research object and the investigative method can be termed "circle of object and method" (Wallner 1992a) or as "object-method circle" (Greiner 2005a), which means that the scientific object and the scientific method are in reciprocal reference to each other, i.e., in an inextricable interdependence (cf. Wallner 1992a: 39).

Certain convictions about the quality of the suitable research method develop for the investigation of a given object structure based on the conviction and the idea one has about the structure of this research object. In other words, pertinent knowledge about the object of research already exists before the object's scientific analysis. Therefore, the scientist must know the object he wishes to study and analyze before his research activity begins in order to be able to carry it out judiciously. In this sense, Hans-Georg Gadamer (1989), for instance, also draws attention to the impossibility of being without prejudice ("prejudgment," "preopinion") in generating knowledge and insights. From this we may deduce that the structural specificity and quality of a science always depend on the prescientific acquaintance with the object. The unavoidable reciprocal problem of a scientific method is evident in the circumstance that, in order to choose the most rational approach, one must already be acquainted with the object of analysis, but in order to recognize it in the first place, one requires an adequate method of research (cf. Wallner 1992a: 39–41).

If we look at the basic principles of any form of science or field of research, we will encounter this circle. Every academic and scientific institution certainly is interested in "concealing" the object-method circle in two ways: They not only wish to conceal "that the chosen method do not represent legitimized," but instead "historically developed decisions" embedded in research-traditional correlations, but, moreover, also conceal that "nobody truly knows about" the object of research, because it is only in the context of the analysis process that it is "defined," i.e., constructed and structured (cf. Wallner 1992a: 41).

If we take the epistemologically central figure of the object-method circle seriously and into consideration, it becomes clear why the traditional objectivist motif of conventional realism—which may be conceptualized in the expression *striving for objective knowledge of observer-independent environment structures*—represents a philosophically untenable ideology. Therefore, the next logical step is to bid farewell to the traditional notion that scientific activity has anything to do with *representation*, *description*, or *discovery*, or with *unraveling*, *decoding*, or *deciphering environments*, the *world*, or *nature*, and to replace it with a *constructivist* notion of scientific and research-related activity.

Constructivist approaches of all provenances (i.e., not only constructive realists but also methodical culturalists, radical constructivists, social constructionist, etc.) indeed work under the assumption that scientists and researchers still "create knowledge," as the German word "Wissenschaft"—"Wissen schaffen"—insinuates (cf. Hartmann and Janich 1996; Glasersfeld 1998; Gelo et al. in press). Constructivists do not in any way question whether science works (*technical level*) but instead always already expect the professional qualifications of the "working scientist" and the professionalism of his specific actions and their results (cf. Wallner 1992a: 12, 1997a: 20). However, they suspend the *truth* of the produced results of a scientific activity (statements, theories) from the *correspondence-theoretical postulate* of the (in principle non-verifiable) correspondence with structures of an objectively present and observer-independent, prefabricated environment.

This obviously raises the following question: If we shift the basic philosophical understanding of science and reality, because science and research clearly do not provide knowledge of objective environments by representation, description, or explanation, do we not also automatically disband the typically European (Western) claim to gaining knowledge and insight? In the constructivist paradigm, is science not instrumentalistically reduced to its applicatory function and thus downgraded to the *purely technical level*?

Of course not! In constructive realism, for instance, the concept of "knowledge" and "insight" gets reoperationalized via the *tactics of the about-turn of the object*. Because of the insurmountable basic epistemological problem (object-method circle), knowledge and insight are no longer able to refer to the objects of an (ostensibly) objective environment that needs to be represented, described, or deciphered.

Knowledge and insight can, however, be directed at the *actual activities* scientists and researchers carry out professionally when they *create knowledge*. In constructive realism, knowledge and insight refer exclusively to gaining deeper insights into the complex structures of scientific action and activity, while scientists themselves need to put a critical-reflexive focus on that which happens in science on the *technical level* in order for differentiated self-awareness and self-comprehension of scientific thought, research, and activity to be successful. If scientists become active in research in a critical, self-reflexive manner, they move away from the *technical level* and toward a *level of insight into technical aspects*. Only by combining these two levels of knowledge can the status of academic matters be characterized in the occidental cultural sense (cf. Wallner 1992a: 60–66; cf. Slunecko 1996b: 146).

The epistemological logic within the object-method circle and the science-philosophical consequences we can deduce from it and have briefly mentioned above are the starting points for further, advanced arguments in constructive realism. Everything centers on the two basic levels of a *science in the academic sense*: 1. the *technical level* and 2. the *level of insight into technical aspects*.

5.2.2 The Technical Level: Science Must Work

The *technical level* is about the actual scientific activity of *creating knowledge*. This is not about the question of *how questions or problems can be answered or solved in a scientific-systematic way*. On this scientific level, *functional knowledge* is developed and used with regard to the solution-oriented ways of dealing with a given object or field.

5.2.2.1 Science Invents Artificial Realities: "Microworlds"

As we have argued in our *starting point*, science and research do not unravel, decode, or decipher the purported environment; they are in no way able to describe, explain, or represent the world (ostensibly objectively present) and environment structures (seen as prefabricated). By way of methodical-systematic and intersubjectively understandable scientific activity, however, scientists and researchers manage to produce *artificial realities*, i.e., *artificial worlds*, which need to function meaningfully insofar as they have to fulfill certain tasks related to given applications. In the course of their professional activity within specific scientific communities, scientists thereby structure and construct specific *manners of environment* and do not *discover* the *world* with them but rather *invent different worlds* (cf. Wallner 1993: 24, 1997a: 21, 2002: 211 f.). These invented environment structures which are developed in scientific activity in the context of specific object-method circles can be termed "microworlds" (cf. Wallner 1993, 1997a, 2002; Greiner 2005a; in Greiner 2007, they are termed "scientific microrealities"). We find similar considerations in Thomas Kuhn (1970) and Nelson Goodman (1978).

A concrete microworld thus represents *a certain scientific context of argumentation and action* which is "coherently and logically congruent" and where "scientific experience" is seen as "true" (cf. Wallner 2002: 204 and 211). Usually, such microworlds are conceptualized and applied in institutionalized structures of special academic disciplines within the organizational framework of colleges and universities. Thus, one may find different microworlds of psychiatric thought and action in the *academic discipline* of medicine (e.g., the mighty pharmacological microworld and various microworlds of psychoanalysis and depth psychology) and microworlds of developmental psychology, social psychology, differential psychology, and others in the *academic discipline* of psychology. We will discuss the microworlds of psychotherapy below (see Sect. 5.3.1).

The larger the number of different microworlds within an academic discipline, the more varied are the modes of operation of this discipline—i.e., the more differentiated is the level of *functional knowledge* in terms of solution-oriented ways of examining a given object or field. Of course, we need to beware of the misconception that what is perceived as *scientific progress in a technical sense* has nothing to do with an *increasingly exact approach toward objective knowledge of prestructured environments*. The actual advantage of the science-philosophical term *microworlds* is rather more in the framework of comparing scientific conceptualizations (methodologies, theories, paradigms) far beyond the problematic concept of science in conventional realism. It is only through such comparisons and reciprocal encounters and dialogic confrontations that the necessary provision of an overview and the creation of order and rules in scientific language in relation to scientific practices become possible (cf. Wallner 2002: 204). Not least this helps maintain boundaries of meaning and commitment of scientific contexts of argumentation and action (microworlds). The latter consideration already focuses our attention on the second basic level of academic science. However, it is only possible to explore this *level of insight into technical aspects* in Sect. 5.2.3 of our science-philosophical discussion.

5.2.2.2 The Dependency of Scientific Knowledge on Culture

The circle problem of the object-method relation as an integral part of scientific action—which I have already mentioned above—is illustrated in the circumstance that one needs to know the object of scientific research in some way beforehand in order to be able to investigate it in the first place. How, then, can this become actualized? To what extent can we know an object that is to be studied before the investigation? Here prerequisites and conditions come into play that we usually do not normally consider or only barely think about. In every scientific context of argumentation and action (microworld), a certain conception of the structural constitution of the object of research initially exists, in which these specific ideas and forms of prescientific knowledge of the object are based on *various traditions of comprehension and approach*, which were enabled to develop in disciplinary and subdisciplinary fields (cf. Wallner 1992a: 39–41). In this context we might also speak of *object perspectives dependent on the respective research tradition, which,* via *the more or less divergent certainties, examine how a concrete object of research can, in fact, rationally only be viewed in advance*.

We might then infer from these considerations that the qualitative structure of scientific action is always dependent on the prior, prescientific knowledge of reality. With this essential thought we address the central topic of the *basic cultural dependency of scientific activity*, because the *object perspectives dependent on the respective research tradition*, which I have just mentioned, obviously did not "appear out of nowhere" but are embedded in the superordinate overall context of a specific cultural development (cf. Wallner 2002: 197). *Culture-specific potentials of dealing with the world* have emerged in the course of history in sociocultural overall contexts (world cultures). The analytic-reductionist approach with its rigorous focus on the dominating somatic modern medicine is a typical example of a *specific potential of dealing with the world*, which was able to emerge in the framework of the occidental, Western culture. Conversely, in the context of Chinese culture, a *specific potential of dealing with the world* becomes distinct only in the system-oriented holistic approach, taking into consideration the body-mind relation which characterizes traditional Chinese medicine (TCM) (see Rieken, Chap. 2). Although both medical systems have different prerequisites and operate with completely divergent instruments, they are—each in its own specific way—successful (cf. Lan et al. 2013). The corresponding *matrix of thought, action, and behavior in occidental, Western culture* represents the basis on which institutionalized activities of systematic research were able to gradually develop, which may be summarized in the term *academic science*. That the scope of disciplinary production performances (microworlds) of academic science is limited by the basic conditions of the overall context of Western culture is a fundamental insight, and its significance cannot be overestimated (cf. Wallner 2002: 197).

In order to keep the terminology manageable, I will summarize the specific relationship of the concepts introduced above: The significant cultural sector of *academic science*, which is characterized by a multitude of *academic disciplines*, within which a diversity of *microworlds* has been able to develop, has emerged in the overall sociocultural context of *Western culture*. Since scientific performances are in principle *culture-specific performances*, no culturally independent—i.e., objective—scientific knowledge that is absolutely, universally binding can therefore exist and can at best only be "feigned" (cf. Wallner 1992a: 33 ff.).

If we take into consideration the fact of science's culture relativity or, more precisely, culture *relationality*, it becomes more understandable that scientific action on the basis of Western culture must feature other structural qualities than scientific endeavors in other sociocultural contexts, because of this very difference in the prerequisite knowledge of reality (cf. Wallner 1992a: 39), i.e., based on the dissimilitude with regard to the generated *culture-specific potentials of dealing with the world.* At this point I should indicate that the intellectual value of divergent culture-specific research activities cannot be determined with the question of which culture comes closer to the "objective truth" with its special efforts to gain knowledge. Much rather, concepts such as Karl Popper's "idea of approximation," i.e., the philosophical conviction of a gradual approach to truth (cf. Popper 1963), should be seen as situated in their own cultural foothold. On the other hand, the divergent structuring measures of scientific methods obviously impinge on the technical usability of their products, which is why—seen exclusively from the standpoint of this instrumental level—culturally determined differences in the quality of *creating knowledge* can and must be assessed.

The character of (prescientific) *knowledge of reality*—which in some measure represents the basis of the structuring quality of scientific activities as an anticipation of *what* and *how* reality (environment, world, or nature) *is*—is, in the end, always dependent on the overall sociocultural context. Of course, we need to add: the more differentiated the manner in which a culture has developed, the more layers the prescientific knowledge of reality has and the more diverse the disciplinary structuring measures are.

We occidental people—conditioned by culture and milieu—take for granted a culture-specific way of *Western life*, i.e., of Western thought, action, and behavior, to such an extent that what is *specific to this culture* often goes unnoticed. Here one must always consider that the coexistence of non-Western overall sociocultural contexts (world cultures) cannot be denied (cf. Wallner 1997a: 23, 2002: 207 f.). In this sense, the term "culture" refers to generated and established systems of convictions and rules that prove meaningful and useful because they have proven functionally valuable over more or less extensive periods of time (visibility factor). In this instrumental regard, *cultural regulating systems* guide a multitude of everyday conducts and behaviors, thus minimizing the pressure to make decisions in everyday situations and, not least, determining the—more or less nuanced—culture-relational *knowledge of reality*, which eventually also affects microworldly preconvictions of the only rationally imaginable structure of a certain object of research (cf. Wallner 2002: 208 f.).

In summary, a reflection of the combination of academic science with Western culture makes evident that certain sciences always belong to certain cultures—or, to put it differently: "that different cultures generate different sciences" (cf. Wallner 2002: 197). Since there can be no science beyond or outside a specific sociocultural framework, the following always applies in principle: science and research are culture dependent.

5.2.2.3 From the Technical Level to the Level of Insight into Technical Aspects

I have already stated that scientific syntactic systems do not describe or explain an object of "objective environment" but rather are mere action regulations which indicate what to do in order to reach a concrete goal (technical aspects). Specific syntactic systems within certain microworlds represent tested and approved rules, instructions, and guidelines which show how to adequately handle information or phenomena and areas where such phenomena occur. This way, structuring rules are produced within the professional framework of microworlds which reveal nothing about the condition of the things of the world, or the environment's objects, but rather how they are to be *managed*. Whoever possesses such a system that works and leads to a successful technical manageability of the world does not gain a "structural representation of the world" but rather, and exclusively, an instrumental-technical knowledge without the function of insight (cf. Wallner 2002: 200, 211 ff., 215 u. 219 f.). The "instrumentalist" concept of science that Wallner proposes is, of course, nothing new. One of the more prominent historical positions of instrumentalism is "American pragmatism" (cf. James 2014), but we also find considerations of this nature in Kant scholar Hans Vaihinger's work (1924).

The instrumental manageability of the world and the *technical level* are without doubt important and fascinating but on their own do not amount to an *academic* science. Many of the present-day scientists and researchers who, in fact, abandon any claim to scientific insight and knowledge because to them it seems irredeemable apparently do not understand that they ruin the Western cultural phenomenon of *academic science* at large. After all, the pragmatic withdrawal into pure instrumentalism (technical level) signifies nothing other than the definitive disintegration and destruction of the conventional occidental idea of science. In this manner, science would be replaced by "pure technique" (cf. Wallner 2002: 193 f., 214–220).

Of course, we might ask: What would be the harm in all this? After all, it should suffice if science manages to provide successful basic services for the development of functioning technologies. Is it not perfectly enough if science and research prove useful and suitable in instrumental terms (technical level) for the improvement of our living conditions? Why do we still need "knowledge" or "insight" into the functional level of science (reflection on technical aspects)?

A substantial number of contemporary research theoreticians and science scholars locate the "actual crisis of science" (Wallner 2002: 199) we lament today in the very circumstance of losing this dimension of reflection and knowledge. Since there are no insights in the critical-reflexive sense to be gained on the technical level, we place purely instrumentalistically oriented science far below the intellectual level of sophistication that academic science has claimed for itself for more than two millennia. By foregoing the culturally significant aspect of insight, science and technique de facto coincide in instrumentalistic thought. What separates the analytical and interpretive moment from science, however, not only promotes the "total instrumentalization of the world" but also at the same time arrests or restricts those critically reflexive references and discussions within one's own microworld, which represent the very preconditions that are necessary for creative innovations, fruitful developmental encounters, and successful possibilities of change (cf. Wallner 2002: 213 f.).

Furthermore, we need to consider the following: If one abandons the occidental concept of science oriented toward insight and knowledge, one will have to expect unpleasant sociocultural consequences sooner or later, especially when taking into consideration the enormous "human need for knowledge." With the disappearance of the *epistemological science* and its substitution with a *technical* science, the phenomena of "knowledge" and "insight" would slip into the sphere of influence of dubious ideologies, shady cults, and other totalitarian entities (cf. Wallner 2002: 194).

5.2.3 The Level of Insight into Technical Aspects: Science Must Critically Reflect Its Modes of Operation

The *level of insight into technical aspects* is motivated by a *self-referential interest in knowledge*. Here everything revolves around the question: *How can the specific practices of thought and action on the technical level be understood (or conceive of themselves) in a differentiated manner?* On this level of science, functioning microworlds are analyzed and interpreted, i.e., critically reflected.

5.2.3.1 Gaining Critical-Reflexive Insight into the Factual Mechanisms of Science

There are obviously good reasons why a critical reflection and interpretation level should never be unhitched from scientific action. At the same time, we need to bluntly remind ourselves again that endeavors toward knowledge and insight can no longer be applied in the traditional "objectivist sense" of conventional realism. From a contemporary science-philosophical perspective, the naïve-realistic program of *representing and describing objective environments* must in any event be viewed as a failure. Interpretation and critical reflection can only refer to the instrumental functional level of science, i.e., the *technical level*. In this sense, "insight" is clearly no longer about an *explanation of the world* but rather about how to structure *artificial worlds (microworlds)*, i.e., we are specifically concerned with *gaining critical-reflexive insight into the factual mechanisms of science* (cf. Wallner 1992a: 63 ff., 2002: 209; cf. also Gelo 2012; Slife 1998).

In contrast to the metaphysical fiction of a prefabricated, objective environment, constructed microworlds are epistemologically relevant, as they represent epistemic objects as fabricated, self-produced artifacts. Giambattista Vico already called attention to the fundamental connection between recognizability of self-created things (1725, *Scienza Nuova Prima*), when he claimed that man cannot recognize nature in the actual sense and instead only recognizes what he himself brings forth, i.e., only phenomena created by man himself (*verum et factum convertuntur*) (cf. Pompa 1990). To this extent, the basic interest at the core of scientific endeavors toward insight must be explicitly geared toward the special construction methods and structuring activities within concrete microworlds. Therefore, we need to pose the question of which specific actions are necessary to be able to develop specific statement systems. The motif of critical-reflexive insight must be carried by the intent to explore which structure of preconditions is necessarily prerequisite in order for a meaningful special argumentation context to be created and subsequently applied (cf. Wallner 1992a: 40, 2002: 216).

Only by incrementally answering and gradually clarifying these questions are we able to gain insight and an overview of the concrete commitment areas of a microworldly syntactic system. It is, in turn, this very commitment-related manner of gaining knowledge that is essential and significant for the question of the position and *ranking* of certain scientific activities in relation to alternatives to such activities. That is to say, the more one is able to find out about the complex and, in many cases, unarticulated basic structures of special scientific manners of construction, the more obvious a certain manner of argumentation's commitment dimensions and boundaries of meaning will be. We can therefore also comprehend that, although microworlds are "purely fictional," they are, at the same time, equally "binding"—in a *methodical sense* (cf. Wallner 1992a: 33–36, 2002: 218).

In comparison with an action-reflexively oriented epistemological science, pure instrumentalism and pure technique have no functions of insight, because they exist as exclusively application-related and always within the boundaries of their own systems. In contrast, gaining critically reflexive knowledge always presupposes a transgression of the system, because only those get to glimpse into its field of action who manage first to distance themselves from conventional, methodically correct, and functional activities. Therefore, the converse also holds: Whoever does not dare exit their acquired activity territory will not understand it in a differentiated manner and cannot gain any critical-reflexive knowledge. Gaining insight and knowledge in the critical-reflexive sense always involves questioning, and not describing, the "given," and therefore it is necessary to place this "given" into a "foreign environment" in order to actually be able to create new knowledge about the "structure of the given" (cf. Wallner 1992a: 60–65, 2002: 220 f.). In this context, in the philosophy of science of constructive realism (CR), we speak of "knowledge by strangification" and of "insight by change of context" (cf. Wallner 1992a, b, c, 1997a, 2002; Slunecko 1994, 1996a, b; Parfy 1996; Greiner 2005a, b, 2006; Greiner et al. 2006).

5.2.4 Summary: The Two Fundamental Levels of Academic Science

Thus far, we have placed at the center of our science-philosophical argumentation the consideration that science in the academic sense is marked by a combination of the following two fundamental levels: Specific microworlds are developed and applied on the *technical level*, on which *science must operate*. The *level of insight into technical aspects*, where *science must critically reflect its modes of operation*, is concerned with gaining differentiated insights into the complex structural relations of functioning microworlds. These two levels—*technical* and *reflection on technical aspects*—characterize the Western cultural phenomenon of *academic science* and therefore offer a distinguishing criterion in comparison with others (e.g., technical-instrumental, lifeworldly, religious, spiritual-magical, esoteric, hetero-cultural) forms of knowledge (cf. Wallner 2002: 214 u. 220).

In this regard, constructive realists give explicit warning about disregarding the *level of insight into technical aspects*. If this knowledge level is ignored, the occidental invention of academic science degenerates and intellectually atrophies to become radical instrumentalism and eventually disintegrates completely on the purely technical level (cf. Wallner 2002). Essentially, every scientist needs to fight this sign of deterioration, since it bears unfathomable dangers—in both scientific and political respects.

Interestingly enough, it is the therapeutic practice of psychotherapy (*psychotherapia*), of all areas, which has great reflexive potential on its own turf, which has to do with its singular methodological phenotype. In comparison, psychotherapy, with its radically pluralistic approaches, polymorphic concepts and heterogeneity in its methods, differs distinctly from all other academic disciplines and therefore enjoys a *special research-structural position*. This structural attribute characteristic of psychotherapy will be the focus of our science-philosophical discussion below, which shall use terminological principles of constructive realism to argue for *psychotherapy as a new academic discipline (psychotherapia academica universitatis)*.

5.3 Academic Psychotherapy: The Microworlds of Psychotherapy in a Critical-Reflexive Dialogue

Judging from a contemporary perspective of a philosophy of science, *academic science* is composed of two basic levels. Only when the *technical level* is combined with the *level of insight into technical aspects* can we speak of a *science in the academic sense*. To put it differently: Since *technique* without *reflection on technical aspects* does not yet represent a *genuine science in the academic sense*, we can argue that academic science not only *must work*, but also must *critically reflect on its modes of operation* at all times.

Against the background of this constructive-realist understanding of science, the therapeutic practice of psychotherapy (*psychotherapia*), of all fields, emerges as a field of research that veritably *embraces reflection* and *evokes self-knowledge*. This is a claim which obviously warrants discussion. In the course of my discussion, I shall develop science-philosophical arguments specifically for *psychotherapy as an independent academic discipline (psychotherapia academica universitatis)*.

5.3.1 Technical Level: Psychotherapy Works in a Multitude of Microworlds

In our constructive-realist discussion in the first main part (Sect. 5.2), we were able to gain the following basic insight in terms of a philosophy of science: If scientists learn to understand, by way of critical-reflexive insight (reflection on technical aspects) into their respective practices of thought and action (technique), that scientific activity has to nothing to do with a decoding of environment structures, but rather, and more importantly, with the production and application of functional microworlds, they will gradually increase their ability to state in a differentiated manner *what* they actually do when they *create knowledge*. Thus, they will have achieved the highest state of freedom in the scientific context of activity. By developing adequate competences for self-reflection in regard to their scientific activity, scientists will automatically increase their creative scope in their own field of thought and research and will overcome the irrational and counterproductive fear of an intradisciplinary pluralism of arguments and the related methodological heterogeneity.

5.3.1.1 Innovation, Development Impulses, and Academic Disciplines

With regard to the question of concrete possibilities of implementing reflexive competences with far-reaching consequences and looking at independent academic disciplines and the evaluation of their specific manifestations, we could speak of *milieus with a tendency to promote development* and *milieus with a tendency to inhibit development*. It is rather easy to determine that some academic disciplines are, methodologically speaking, relatively "open" for pluralistic developmental impulses, and that others in comparison are rather "sensitive" toward change of this kind and may even "reject" it. The degree of structural-scientific elasticity and the methodological flexibility of an academic discipline are, of course, also measures of its ability for discourse and thus also hint at the long-term prospects of survival within the territory of institutionalized science. The question of how accessible a discipline is to methodological transformations and tentative expansion is directed at future opportunities and possibilities of the continued existence of a scientific domain.

Primarily, branches of study unshakably rooted in objectivism, fixed in rigorous discipline, and featuring metaphysical claims to commitment are said to tend to *inhibit development* in this sense. We might mention the "hard sciences" as an example, exact biosciences, as well as all empirical fields of research which strictly follow the "scientistic" (disciplinary) method-monism of the world of natural sciences. Of course there are also other disciplinary fields in the universe of academic science with an *atmosphere that promotes development*. One field of thought and research which offers a particularly welcoming general framework and veritably ideal discipline-related preconditions for critical-reflexive scientific ambitions is the therapeutic practice of psychotherapy in its current status quo. Due to its science-structural peculiarity and methodological extraordinariness, contemporary psychotherapy stands in stark contrast to all other established academic disciplines.

5.3.1.2 The Microworlds of Psychotherapeutic Practice

Both the usual introductory literature and most psychotherapy textbooks today present an image of its practice that features a pluralism of paradigms, polymorphous concepts, and heterogeneity in its methods. It presents its various psychotherapeutic methods in the contextual framework of their systems of creation and origin and assigns them to basic superordinate paradigmatic positions. Among the most important psychotherapeutic paradigms are, for instance, the psychodynamic (depth-psychological), the behavioristic, the humanistic, the systemic, and the existential position. Among the best-known schools of psychotherapy are the psychoanalytical, cognitive behavioral, person-centered, gestalt, and logotherapy approaches. These few examples shall suffice to serve as an illustrative list, although, of course, we must note that by now there is an almost unmanageable number of different psychotherapeutic approaches and systems, and that psychotherapy itself is therefore continually diversifying (cf. Stumm and Wirth 1994: 5 f.; Slunecko 1996b: 128). When we look at the development of psychoanalysis in the twentieth century alone and are here confronted with the internal differentiation of psychoanalysis into countless sub-schools, orientations, positions, and doctrines (cf. Young-Bruehl and Dunbar 2009), we gain at least a sense of the claimed unmanageability in regard to psychotherapy as a whole.

Evidently, the practice of psychotherapy, with its genuine pluralism of theories and methods, has successfully managed to develop a scientific self-conception beyond the reach of the ideological straitjacket of the objectivity craze of conventional realism (cf. Heinz von Foerster 1981). At least many representatives of individual psychotherapeutic schools have in their concepts long been accounting for the grave epistemological faux pas of the disciplinary program and generally reject "the belief in the possibility of a universal theory of human relations independent of space, time, observer, and methods" (Wagner 1996: 243). From the viewpoint of a contemporary understanding of science, the medical specialist and psychotherapist Elisabeth Wagner, for instance, already indicates that "ontological reasons" are insupportable and observes that

> *the models and theories of various schools of therapy help to organize the one's impressions from a therapeutic situation, and thus allow the therapist to act rationally and consistently. In their own right, they do not lay claim to an ultimate knowledge, but represent instructions (for action) to structure therapeutic phenomena in an individually corresponding manner.* (Wagner 1996: 243)

One might still establish a widespread tendency in psychotherapeutic correlations of thought and action toward self-conception aiming for the definition of a "consciously multi-paradigmatic science" (Wagner 1996: 245) and thus amounting to a specialized self-conception far beyond the old objectivity-dogmatic fixation of conventional realism. There are increasingly clear signs in psychotherapy of a "perspectival understanding of science and research," which is "a position of knowledge particularly suitable for the psychotherapeutic situation," which "leaves the paradigm of truth and objectivity behind and deals with the construction and deconstruction of different views of reality" (Wagner 1996: 243).

By bringing forth and developing an almost inexhaustible science-structural diversity, psychotherapy has attained an incomparable methodological status on the technical level, which today tends to determine its scientific self-conception and self-awareness. In their entirety and from a constructive-realist point of view, the various and nonuniform systems, approaches, doctrines, and procedures of psychotherapy represent the *microworlds of psychotherapy*. In this regard, we may speak of, for instance, the *psychoanalytic microworld according to Sigmund Freud*, the *psychoanalytic microworld according to Jacques Lacan*, the *individual psychological microworld according to Alfred Adler*, the *analytical-psychological microworld according to Carl Gustav Jung*, the *daseinsanalytical microworld according to Ludwig Binswanger*, the *self-psychological microworld according to Heinz Kohut*, the *gestalt-therapeutic microworld according to Friedrich Perls*, the *cognitive-mediational therapeutic microworld according to Richard Lazarus*, the *cognitive behavioral therapeutic microworld according to Aaron Beck*, the *holotropic therapeutic microworld according to Stanislav and Christina Grof*, the *systemic-therapeutic microworld according to Paul Watzlawick*, the *systemic-therapeutic microworld according to Steve de Shazer*, etc.

The reason for allowing the diverse, nonuniform microworlds of psychotherapy to exist equally side by side is that there is no immanent, disciplinary compulsion for uniformity. As long as no branch lays claim to power within psychotherapy's territory of thought and practice, theoretical and methodical heterogeneity is guaranteed, which means nothing else than the wealth of psychotherapeutic *science cultures*, i.e., of diverse forms and languages of therapy (microworlds), will continue to flourish in these conditions.

No comparable field of study currently exists in the entire Western cultural phenomenon of academic science with as highly a differentiated methodological structure as psychotherapy. It is exactly because this polymorphism in the structure of psychotherapy (pluralism of arguments and heterogeneity of methods) has increased invariably, i.e., has steadily increased in density, that it seems ever more pressing to answer the question of how much claim each specific epistemic achievement from the individual psychotherapeutic microworlds may lay to scientific commitment.

5.3.1.3 Does Commitment Disintegrate in the Territory of Heterogeneous Theories and Pluralistic Methods?

Ultimately, we will, without doubt, attain completely different results in the course of examining one particular case within the context of argumentation and action of psychotherapeutic microworld A (e.g., bioenergetic analysis according to Alexander Lowen) than within the context of argumentation and action of psychotherapeutic microworld B (e.g., transactional analysis according to Eric Berne). Results one attains in psychotherapeutic microworld C (e.g., psychosynthesis according to Roberto Assagioli) may even potentially contradict the results one may develop in psychotherapeutic microworld D (e.g., guided affective imagery according to Hanscarl Leuner) with regard to the exact same object of analysis and research context. One may fear that, at worst, the scientific claim to commitment in the psychotherapeutic territory of pluralistic methods and polymorphic concepts may disintegrate entirely due to the mutual foreignness of the forms of therapy.

Here I must once again reference the epistemological figure of the object-method circle and remind readers that each microworld has its own way of conceptualizing, specifying, and structuring the object of research, which immediately renders mention of "the exact same object of analysis" obsolete. This also lets the demand for a commitment related to research and science lose relevance in an absolute and objective sense, because we can no longer assume that such a thing as a knowledge-related approach (as in, e.g., Karl Popper's "asymptotic approximation") to "objective truth" is even possible in principle. From a contemporary, science-philosophical point of view, no single discipline may legitimately claim for itself a commitment of the metaphysical or absolute kind in terms of its results and gained knowledge (cf. Wallner 1992a: 33 ff.)—neither in physics nor in biology and, of course, also not in psychotherapy.

Yet, the idea of commitment and the claim to commitment in microworldly contexts of action remain meaningful and even necessary, although they must not be applied in a metaphysical manner but should rather be understood in a *relativistic sense*. To speak of commitment in scientific contexts is only sensible if one looks, with a reflective intent to know, at the complex structure of methodical presuppositions, which *must be presupposed* for an instrumental and technical argument to be *added thereafter* in a meaningful (professional) fashion. Commitment in the context of science and research can rationally only refer to a commitment *in the methodical sense*. By self-reflexively clarifying the rational and methodical commitment of a microworldly procedure, we gain insight into the legitimate scope of its obtained results and outcomes, which means nothing other than that a matter has to be successfully defendable, communicable, discussible, and criticizable with regard to the phenomenon of *relative/methodical commitment*, if science and research are not to be ruined by the use of undifferentiated, absolute and objective—i.e., metaphysical—claims to commitment (cf. Wallner 1992a: 33–36, 1997a: 24 ff.).

Accordingly, all instrumental and technical outcomes, results, and knowledge gained in the specific context of individual psychotherapeutic microworlds are always binding in relation to the methodical process of gaining them. Simultaneously, they are based on constructed, self-determined, and fabricated preconditions and prerequisites and thus exist on a purely fictional *culture-relational* basis. In this sense, we may also claim that psychotherapeutic knowledge—and also every other scientific knowledge—is always "binding and chosen freely at the same time" (cf. Wallner 1992a: 77 ff., 2002: 218). On the basis of this contemporary scientific perspective, the following *constructive-realistic definition of psychotherapeutic activity* takes shape:

> *In compliance with its specialist orientation* (relational to therapeutic schools) *psychotherapists re-/produce microworldly ways of therapeutic thought and action that are specific to each orientation* (theoretical aspect) *and thereby create forms of professional understanding and solution-oriented practice that are typical for each therapeutic system* (practical aspect) *for complex problems of individual lifeworlds* (treating culturally specific "suffering").

5.3.2 Level of Insight into Technical Aspects: Psychotherapy Reflects Its Modes of Operation in Dialogue with Psychotherapeutic Microworlds

One can get more or less comprehensive information about the explicit or manifested axioms, assumptions, and premises of individual psychotherapeutic systems, branches, and procedures (microworlds) in introductory literature and psychotherapy textbooks. In addition, however, or rather, *beneath* all these, there are the implicit, unarticulated, unreflected, and even latent preconditions and prerequisites, the unspoken, *unaddressed*, and therefore also undetected basic structures of a scientific context of argument and action that turn out to be more interesting and, most importantly, much more effective in terms of the methodological characteristics or the identity of a special psychotherapeutic microworld. These fundamental background (or rather, underground) principles ultimately determine the blind spots in the researcher's own approach to research and practice and may often seduce researchers to consider their thoughts and actions "objectively binding," i.e., to metaphysically exaggerate them and thus to misunderstand them. Therefore, a critique in terms of a philosophy of science and, subsequently, a reflective science have to address this issue and to attempt to render these unseen, undetected, and uncomprehended structures visible, detectible, and comprehensible with text- and theory-analysis tools (cf. Wallner 1992b: 84–89, 1997a: 26 f.).

5.3.2.1 Quest for Critical-Reflexive Insight into Implicit Structural Relations of Psychotherapeutic Microworlds

In keeping with this structure, there is the epistemic motif on the self-reflexive level of an autonomous academic discipline characterized by the *quest for critical-reflexive insights into the specific basic structures of created microworlds.* To remind readers, we cannot automatically assume that scientific syntactic systems are *critically reflexively* understood in a differentiated manner only by correctly applying and adequately using scientific syntactic systems in microworldly semantic contexts. Whoever uses disciplinary modes of thought and action successfully so that a scientific system is said to work satisfactorily appears to have learned the derivation rules, sign uses, and application principles correctly and also to have correct command of them—but this does not yet give any information about the extent of the *self-reflexive knowledge of action.* Scientific syntactic systems are known to be structuring rules first and foremost, offering directions and instructions about how to master and change phenomena and fields of phenomena (cf. Wallner 2002: 215). In this respect the various syntactic systems of psychotherapeutic microworlds initially only offer application-specific know-how, i.e., instrumental and technical knowledge about how to meaningfully deal with a subject matter with therapeutic intent.

In order to gain adequate insight into the complex basic structures of its theoretical steps, its abstract thought processes, and the resulting technical maneuvers and strategies as well as the—related—necessary manageability of the rational/methodical commitment of its different microworldly epistemic achievements, it is imperative for academic science—as I have pointed out repeatedly—to develop a critical-reflexive level of knowledge, a successful form of differentiated self-comprehension (level of insight into technical aspects). If it fails to do so, it will not be able to continue to exist as a *science in the occidental, Western sense*, because it will intellectually reduce itself to absurdity by the obvious danger of unreflected fixation on the instrumental-technical level (technical level).

The necessary preconditions and prerequisites that generally need to be created in order for scholars to be able to strive for *critical-reflexive insights into the implicit structural relations of microworlds* are already automatically on hand in the therapeutic practice of psychotherapy. Due to its special science-structural characteristics revealed in its incomparable wealth of microworlds, i.e., in its diversity of forms of therapy and its foreignness to theoretical language or its "consciously multi-paradigmatic" status (E. Wagner), opportunities and possibilities of reflection-scientific epistemic approaches through "strangification" and "contextual changes" present themselves almost automatically (cf. Slunecko 1994; Parfy 1996; Greiner 2006). An axiom from the logotherapeutic microworld according to Victor Frankl may be transferred or "strangified," by way of trial, into the psychodramatic microworld according to Jacob Moreno, or a theory from the individual psychological microworld according to Alfred Adler, into the person-centered microworld according to Carl Rogers, or a principle from the analytical-psychological microworld according to Carl Gustav Jung, into the character-analytical microworld according to Wilhelm Reich, or a formula from the holotropic microworld according to Stanislav Grof, into the systemic-therapeutic microworld according to Paul Watzlawick, etc.

This scientific idea has, in fact, already been implemented in research practice. In the past 5 years, a fundamental research program in psychotherapy has been established at the Sigmund Freud University (SFU) under the banner of such a dialogue of psychotherapeutic microworlds. Of course this is not an actual dialogue but a fictitious one, i.e., it is about intermedial contacts by way of pseudo-dialogues initiated by the representative of a certain school of therapy and directed at the theoretical basis of another school of therapy or a structural logic or formal principles of cultural constructs with the goal of attaining critical-reflexive knowledge. The so-called transfermeneutic psychotherapy science (or *experimental hermeneutics*) is a theory-analytical approach to research in the sense that it uses innovative tools of understanding meaning (*experimental hermeneutic approaches*) which are all founded on the basic constructive-realist idea of strangification (cf. Greiner 2012, 2013a; Greiner and Jandl 2012; Greiner et al. 2013).[1]

[1]The individual methods of analysis of transfermeneutic (=transfer-hermeneutical) psychotherapy science can be allocated to the two largest process groups: (a) *experimental hermeneutic processes for dialogue between psychotherapeutic microworlds* and (b) *experimental hermeneutic processes for dialogue with artistic media*. The following list represents instruments of the process group (a): *Experimental Trans-Contextualization* in *Therapy Schools Dialogue (ExTC/TSD)*, the *Intertherapeutic Text Puzzle (ITTP)*, the *Intertherapeutic Picture Process (ITPP)*, and *Intertherapeutic Media Games (ITMG)* in its three intertherapeutic process modes of *Psycho Mimicry Analysis (PmiA)*, *Psycho Music Analysis (PmuA)*, and *Psycho Dance Analysis (PDA)* (cf. Greiner 2012, 2013a). Analysis tools of process group (b) are the *Psycho Text Puzzle (PTP)*, the *Psycho Picture Process (PPP)*, and *Psycho Media Games (PMG)*, also conceptualized in three versions, analogous to the ITMG (cf. Greiner 2013b, c). While the intertherapeutic (=therapy-school-interdisciplinary) analysis process of Experimental Trans-Contextualization (ExTC), which characterizes the field of research of the so-called Therapy Schools Dialogue (TSD), has already proven effective in several research projects at Sigmund Freud University (cf. Greiner et al. 2009; Greiner and Jandl 2010; Greiner 2011, 2012, 2013a), the practical scientific suitability of the more recent experimental hermeneutic methods and techniques has only been tested in a handful of paradigmatic

This theoretical representation should be followed by at least one concrete example from experimental hermeneutic research practice, which shows in an exemplary fashion how Experimental Trans-Contextualization (ExTC) in Therapy Schools Dialogue (TSD) works. Since we use special technical terms in TSD, this practical example should be preceded by an explanation of terms and the process-related structural pattern of ExTC, in order to prevent terminological ambiguities and misunderstandings in the course of the paper.

The *origin context (OC)* is the (same) therapy system in which the TSD user has been socialized in terms of practical science. In contrast to this, the *strangification context (SC)* refers to the heteromorphic therapy system in whose structure an ExTC is to take place. The *discourse field (DF)* refers to the thematic or theoretical basis of the OC from which a "transpose" (T) is extracted (e.g., basic assumptions and views in anthropology, the philosophy of science, the theory of socialization, ethics, the theory of sexuality, the theory of personality, psychopathology, therapeutics, etc.). The *transpose (T)* is the sort of typical concept or characteristic statement in the OC which is to be *experimentally trans-contextualized* (i.e., is transferred by way of trial, provisionally translated) in the chosen SC. Each T must contain in principle two different *Transpose Aspects (TA)*. An *ostensibly integration-friendly Transpose Aspect (aifTA)* is a TA which promises a high heterocontextual possibility of integration and a high aptitude for transference in relation to the SC, whereas an *integration-resistant Transpose Aspect (irTA)* refers to a TA where the heterocontextual possibility of integration is highly questionable and the aptitude for transference in relation to the SC is called into question.

After *determining* the OC, SC, and DF, one will start the actual analysis process (ExTC), which is called *dialogue operation* and consists of five *dialogue-operative phases* and a *dialogue summary*. The first dialogue-operative phase (*1. Transpose Selection and Identification*) conceptualizes the T, its aifTA, and its irTA. The second dialogue-operative phase (*2. Brief Explanation of the Ostensibly integration-friendly Transpose Aspect in its Original Structural Context*) gives an overview of the actual context of use and application of the aifTA in the OC. The third dialogue-operative phase (*3. Translation and Installment*) has three substages. The first substage of the third dialogue-operative phase (*3.1 Location and Conceptualization of a Heterocontextual Coupling for the aifTA*) seeks the heterocontextual coupling, which is to be presented subsequently. This is a possibility of integration and a corresponding opportunity for the aifTA to connect and link in the OC. The second substage of the third phase (*3.2 Brief Explanation of the Heterocontextual Coupling in its Original Structural Context*) gives an overview of the actual context of use and application of the found heterocontextual coupling in the SC. The third substage of the third phase (*3.3 Demonstrating the Intersections in the Discourse Field*) illustrates the detected number of elements of conviction, opinion, and comprehension both dialogue partners or therapy systems (OC and SC) have in common in the discourse field (DF). Much as the third phase, the fourth dialogue-operative phase (*4. Critical Testing of Heterocontextual Integration Attempts*) also has three substages. The first substage of the fourth phase (*4.1 Focus on the Integration-Resistant Aspect of the Transpose*) directs the attention to the irTA in the context of its original structural context. In the second substage of the fourth phase (*4.2 Review of the Heterocontextual Aptitude for Transference with Regard to the irTA*), critical testing must encounter a contradiction at a certain point. This is then the "site of contradiction," the point of absurdity in the SC where the translation attempt definitely fails. Under the title, *Presentation of the Extracted Contradiction*, the point of absurdity (site of contradiction) is ultimately identified. The third substage of the fourth phase again (*4.3 Heterocontextual*

procedural examples (cf. Greiner 2013a, b, c). Fortunately, most of these processes obtain their first concrete opportunities for application within the context of several current qualification studies at SFU.

Transference Breach with the Contradiction), and for reasons of plausibility and better comprehensibility, briefly discusses the failure to integrate in a summarizing argument. In the fifth, and final, dialogue-operative phase (*5. Reflection Profits*), the serious and thorough examination of the contradiction which caused the failure of the attempt at heterocontextual integration ultimately offers possibilities of insight into the implicit structure of preconditions and commitment, i.e., in unarticulated structures of prerequisites which must be at the core of the T in the OC (context-specific logic), so that absurdities and contradictions do not arise there—as opposed to the SC. Reflexive findings of this kind have inspiring effects and are conducive to creativity; they may thus stimulate theoretical, methodological, and process-related modifications in a researcher's own therapy system (OC).

The phase of dialogue summary (summary of dialogue results) must recapitulate findings in three individual stages: *results of the dialogic confrontation between therapy system A (OC) and therapy system B (SC) in the discourse field (DF) 1 with transpose (T) x according to the used data base*. The first summary stage is entitled *Transpose-Relative Intersection in Discourse Field (DF) 1 Based on Data Used*; the second stage is entitled *Transpose-Relative Difference in Discourse Field (DF) 1 Based on Data Used*; the third stage is entitled *Transpose-Relative Reflection Profit for Therapy System A (OC)*.

5.3.2.2 Experimental Hermeneutics Practical Example: Trans-Contextual Dialogue Operation between Analytical Psychology (C.G. Jung) and Structural Psychoanalysis (J. Lacan)

Within the context of this dialogue-operative illustrative example, we can develop the process of an Experimental Trans-Contextualization (ExTC) which confronts the *Analytical Psychology according to Carl Gustav Jung* with the *Structural Psychoanalysis according to Jacques Lacan*. Psychotherapeutic thought and action according to Jung is tied to the following subject-theoretical perspective: "[The self] is strange to us and yet so near, wholly ourselves and yet unknowable, a virtual centre of [...] mysterious [...] constitution" (Jung 1966: 237). For exemplary purposes, we shall trans-contextualize this central notion, which can be viewed as a characteristic structural element of Jungian Analytic Psychoanalysis, into the thought and action system of Lacanian Structural Psychoanalysis (2001) by way of trial.

Definitions *Origin Context (OC)*: The following example will view Jungian Analytical Psychology as the "original" therapy system.

Strangification Context (SC): Lacanian Structural Psychoanalysis will serve as the heteromorphic therapy system in the structure of which an ExTC shall take place.

Discourse Field (DF): A *transpose* (=a theoretical statement to be transferred) shall be extracted from the basic area of *subject theory* in the origin context.

1. *Selection and Determination*
   Transpose (T): "[The self] is strange to us and yet so near, wholly ourselves and yet unknowable, a virtual centre of [...] mysterious [...] constitution" (Jung 1966: 237).
   Ostensibly integration-friendly Transpose Aspect (aifTA): "[The self] is strange to us and yet so near, wholly ourselves and yet unknowable."
   Integration-resistant Transpose Aspect (irTA): "[The self] is [...] a virtual centre of [...] mysterious [...] constitution."
2. *Brief Explanation of the aifTA in Its Original Structural Context*
   "[The self] is strange to us and yet so near, wholly ourselves and yet unknowable"—with this aifTA, Jung informs us that we cannot say much about the contents of the "self." In fact, according to Jung, we can only "experience" this "self" and cannot rationally grasp it, which is why each attempt at closer definition invariably reaches the "limits of our cognitive faculty"—exactly because we are dealing with something we are able to individually

experience and at the same time unable to conceptually define (cf. Jacobi 1993: 131), the Jungian "self" is a typical "transcendental postulate," which, "although justified psychologically, does not allow of scientific proof" (Jung 1966: 240). Jung speaks of a "paradox [which] is inescapable, as always, when we try to define something that lies beyond the bourn of our understanding" (ibid: 238). Ultimately, Jung sees in the "self an indication of a primal psychic source par excellence, which is not justifiable. It is the ultimate thing in and of the psyche that one is able to experience" (Jacobi 1993: 132).

3. *Translation and Installment*

3.1 *Location and Conceptualization of a Heterocontextual Coupling for the aifTA*

As is generally known, "self" is "other" for Jacques Lacan (2001), who sees the subject as neither the autonomous center of itself nor the initiator of its conscience-based relationship to the world. Lacan's notion of I ("je"), which is not me ("moi"), makes the subjectivity-centrism of the Cartesian tradition of self-certitude lose its footing (cf. Pagel 1991: 14 and 24) and, as a provocative understanding of "subject," offers a possible connecting factor for the aifTA from the Jungian theory of the self. The idea that the self "is strange to us and yet so near, wholly ourselves and yet unknowable" seems to be rather capable of connecting to the special subject perspective, which Lacan's I-formulas—"the I (je) is not the me (moi)" and "self is other"—offer.

Heterocontextual Coupling for the aifTA: "the I (je) is not the me (moi)" and "self is other" (Jacques Lacan).

3.2 *Brief Explanation of Heterocontextual Coupling in Its Original Structural Context*

This consequential "je-moi difference" or I-me distinction according to Lacan (2001) has its earliest roots in infantile experiences during the "mirror stage" (at 6–18 months of age). Pagel (1991: 33 f.) summarizes the essence of Lacan's mirror theory in three points: (1) The producing-the-self of the "me" is characterized by an imaginary feature; it strives toward an illusory unit of what is produced and producing, which Lacan characterizes as the difference between "moi" ("me") and "je" ("I") as the true subject. (2) In Lacan, the moi appears as the imaginary site of recognition and false recognition; the movement of development is caught by a mirrorlike "wholeness." The "moi" aspires to autonomy but is thrown back to the state of alienation due to its imaginariness and its having been produced. (3) "The mirror stage represents the matrix of all identification processes" (ibid). The mirror is meant as a metaphor and generally constitutes the description of an imaginary intersubjectivity, with which it illustrates the narcissistic character of finding the self—the pursuit of a unity of moi and je that is as necessary as it is futile.

3.3 *Demonstrating the Intersections in the Discourse Field (Df)*

According to Lacan, this fictional me (moi), with its form of intersubjectivity governed by self-love, is only responsible for the distance separating the subject from its "actual (unreflexive) I." Lacan calls this "true I" the "je" or "sujet de l'inconscient," which as the "subject of the unconscious" is never directly present (cf. Pagel 1991: 40 f. and 51). Lacanian psychotherapists therefore have to clearly differentiate between the unfolding speech of the imaginary "moi" and the concealed "other speech" of the unconscious hidden behind it, in order to perceive this "it speaks" in the first place, where the "true" subject of the "je" articulates itself (cf. Pagel 1991: 118). After all, it is the aim of the Lacanian analyst "to lead the subject to its actual being or to his 'missed being' in speech in order to let truth step forward from behind the fake objectivism" (Pagel 1991: 122 f.). Apparently, it is unproblematic to integrate the aifTA from Jungian self-perspective into Lacan's representation of the "true subject" ("je"/I): *The self* ("je"/I) *is strange to us* ("other speech," "it speaks") *and yet so near* ("actual I," "actual being"), *wholly ourselves* ("true subject") *and yet unknowable* ("unreflexive I," "subject of the unconscious," "never directly present").

4. *Critical Testing of the Heterocontextual Integration Attempt*
   4.1 *Focus on the Integration-Resistant Transpose Aspect (irTA)*
   The *irTA* is: "The self is a virtual centre of mysterious constitution." In fact, the "concentric self-positioning" (*a virtual center*) and the "suggested self-ontologization" (*of mysterious constitution*), which Jung also carries out in his attempt at a definition (transpose), seem to cause significant transference difficulties.
   4.2 *Review of the Heterocontextual Aptitude for Transference with Regard to the irTA*
   A main qualitative characteristic of Lacanian Structural Psychoanalysis is, of course, the radical transcendence of the traditional Occidental fixation on "centrism" (critique of logocentrism and egocentrism). Such a psychoanalytical standpoint at least seems incompatible with a therapeutic enterprise aiming to make the self the new gravity center of the individual (cf. Jung 1970: 40), because it claims to recognize that "the beginnings of our whole psychic life seem to be inextricably rooted in this point and all our highest and ultimate purposes seem to be striving towards it" (Jung 1966: 238). The concentric and the ontological aspect of the Jungian "self" can in no way be reconciled with the Lacanian understanding of "je"/"I." When asked about the essence of the "true subject," "Lacan allocates it eccentricity's, or rather *ex-sistence*'s way of being. As such, however, we cannot attribute it a proper essence. Because no matter how we call it, we miss its center, its being" (Pagel 1991: 40 f.
   Extracted contradiction: Jacques Lacan allocates the essence of the "true subject" ("je"/"I") "eccentricity's, or rather *ex-sistence*'s way of being. As such, however, we cannot attribute it a proper essence. Because no matter how we call it, we miss its center, its being" (Pagel 1991: 40 f.).
   4.3 *Transference Breach with the Contradiction*
   The *aifTA*, i.e., the ambivalent structure in the Jungian figure of the self, which reveals itself in the strangeness and simultaneous closeness of the ultimately unrecognizable being self, seems to be capable of being integrated into the Lacanian thought horizon. Translating Jung's concentric-ontological self-definition into Lacan's psychotherapeutic domain fails, however. The transference of this irTA seems to break due to a different notion of "being" and "essence" of the "true subject" (contradiction). Lacanian analytical work does not aim at an illusory act of centering but rather focuses on the "other speech," the dimension of the "it speaks," "which we have to reveal and develop, in order for the subject can understand and experience itself as a being and saying subject based on this eccentricity" (Pagel 1991: 41 f.).

5. *Reflection Profit*
   It is the very fact of heterocontexual failure, however, which puts some—more or less implicit—basic prerequisites in psychotherapeutic thought and action according to Carl Gustav Jung more clearly into the foreground, which renders them more accessible to a reflexive examination. Categories such as, e.g., "centering" and "positioning" or

"tangibility," "essentiality" and "gestalt," which seem to play a certain role in Jung's self-theoretical context, are definitely dismissed in Lacan's structural-psychoanalytic approach. Yet the concept of the subject may still find a theoretically meaningful and practical use in this therapeutic realm. This realization may now be used by Jungian psychotherapists as a potential incentive to develop by way of trial an alternative "understanding of self" beyond the ontic and concentric dimension. Obviously, a therapist would have to assess whether such an innovation actually proves advantageous or more useful in his or her own practice. It is only the Jungian psychotherapist himself or herself, of course, who can make judgments about this.

Summary of Dialogue Results We shall now examine the results of the dialogic confrontation between the therapy system *Analytic Psychology according to Carl Gustav Jung* (OC) and *Structural Psychoanalysis according to Jacques Lacan* (SC) in the discourse field (DF) *subject theory* based on the transpose (T) of *The self is strange to us and yet so near, wholly ourselves and yet unknowable, a virtual centre of mysterious constitution* (Jung 1966: 237) and based on the used database:

Transpose-Relative Intersection in the Discourse Field (DF) of Subject Theory Based on Used Data The transpose-related similarity in subject-theoretical thought between Analytic Psychology according to Carl Gustav Jung and Structural Psychoanalysis according to Jacques Lacan can be discerned in the specific subject-structural ambivalence which shows itself in the phenomenon of strangeness and simultaneous closeness of the ultimately unrecognizable. What Lacan alleges for the "true subject" of the "je" or "I" in a similar way also applies to Jung's figure of the "self": *The self* ("je"/I) *is strange to us* ("other speech," "it speaks") *and yet so near* ("actual I," "actual being"), *wholly ourselves* ("true subject") *and yet unknowable* ("unreflexive I," "subject of the unconscious," "never directly present").

Transpose-Relative Difference in the Discourse Field (DF) of Subject Theory Based on the Used Data The transpose-related difference in subject-theoretical thought between Analytic Psychology according to Carl Gustav Jung and Structural Psychoanalysis according to Jacques Lacan is represented in the dialogue at hand as follows: While the analytic-psychological therapy system according to Jung views the "self" as a "virtual centre of mysterious constitution" (*irTA*), the "true subject" of the "je"/"I" in the structural-psychoanalytic therapy system according to Lacan is merely a phenomenon of eccentricity that cannot be further defined. If Jung at least hints at something like "positioning," "essentiality," and "tangibility" in connection with the question of the "self," in Lacan the "actual I" radically eludes any kind of closer assignation, so that, even if one wished to define it, one will never reach the "true subject."

Transpose-Relative Reflection Profit for the Therapy System Analytical Psychology According to Carl Gustav Jung (OC) Gaining transpose-related knowledge in the therapy system of Analytical Psychology according to Carl Gustav Jung can be summarized as follows: Both the ontic and the concentric dimensions, which in Jung's therapeutic approach have quite an essential subject-theoretical significance, are deliberately dropped in Lacan's therapeutic approach. Nevertheless, even the Lacanian analyst can find meaningful and productive use for subject-theoretical terms in the psychotherapeutic context. An increase in insight of this kind can potentially inspire methodological steps toward innovation, which may also contribute to working out and developing alternative—and perhaps even useful—"ways of understanding self."

This illustration from experimental hermeneutics should demonstrate in what methodical way the postulate in a philosophy of science *of gaining critical-reflexive insight in implicit structural relationships of psychotherapeutic microworlds* can be transferred into psychotherapeutic practice at the Sigmund Freud University in Vienna. Subsequent, more detailed illustrations of experimental hermeneutics would go beyond the scope of this science-philosophical explanatory argumentation, which leads me to no other option than to suggest to the inclined reader wishing to delve into the matter, to sample the books listed in the bibliography at the end of this chapter.

5.3.3 Summary: The Two Basic Levels of Academic Psychotherapy

A science that is no longer interested in the prevalent fiction of a *knowledge-related approximation* ("asymptotic approximation") to the true structure of *objective environments* is also no longer pressured or forced to advance to the *only true statement about reality*. In contrast to the conventional-realistic scientific action of unraveling, decoding, and deciphering, which is tied to the correspondence-theoretical truth dogmatic of a *compulsory correspondence of scientific theory with objective environment*, a contemporary research goal with an understanding of science based in cultural constructivism in no way intends to "reduce a given matter to a few sentences" or "trace a given matter back to a few characteristics" (cf. Wallner 1996: 355) but instead strives for a pluralism of arguments and a heterogeneity of methods.

It is exactly this science-structural pair of features—*pluralism of arguments and heterogeneity of methods*—which has been characterizing the therapeutic practice of psychotherapy from the outset. From the first successful methodological steps of separation and movements toward a detachment from Sigmund Freud's psychoanalytic therapy monopoly (Alfred Adler, Carl Gustav Jung), psychotherapy represents a genuinely multi-conceptual form of thought and practice. Compared to established disciplines, the polymorphism that is typical for psychotherapy renders it unique in two ways: *1. with regard to the level of psychotherapeutic functions (technical aspects)* and 2. *with regard to the level of insight into psychotherapeutic functions (reflection on technical aspects).*

5.3.3.1 Academic Psychotherapy and Its Technical Level

The technological polymorphism of an academic discipline has the advantage of including many differently conceptualized research objects in many different microworlds, which allows for greater manageability and transparency in a given field of study and phenomena (*polymorphic microworldification*) than with a voluntary limitation to the application of a monoperspective (*scientistic discipline ideal*). Through the very path of generation, differentiation, and application of diverse microworlds (*heterogeneous therapy languages*), psychotherapy manages to produce varied and different knowledge-related achievements (cf. also Wallner 1996: 355 ff.).

Only with the help of heterogeneous forms of argumentation can a larger diversity of knowledge be achieved. It allows for more insights in terms of different views and approaches in connection with a given field of subjects and phenomena. With this in mind, we may also argue that we can consequently differentiate and—due to repeated "views"—are better able to "see" the research object (cf. Wallner 1996: 357). Without doubt all fields of research and academic disciplines of the twenty-first century can learn from a methodological orientation of this kind and a contemporary scientific culture such as what we find in psychotherapy.

5.3.3.2 Academic Psychotherapy and Its Level of Insight into Technical Aspects

Due to its specific structure of research and practice, psychotherapy has a reflection-methodological competitive advantage in principle and may therefore also serve as a role model where *reflection on technical aspects* is concerned. Critical reflections on technical aspects in psychotherapy may be undertaken in its own scientific domain, because it is structured multi-conceptually and pluralistic in terms of methods as well as heterogeneous in terms of theories and thus potentially offers ideal possibilities for "strangification" and "context changes," which in many established academic disciplines are not automatically given.

These factors of a structure which is so intrascientifically complex and strange that it seems impossible for all the established academic disciplines (yet) to implement to the extent that is specific to psychotherapy are not only a fundamental methodological criterion of distinction from other fields of research but actually also render the characteristic structure of psychotherapy comprehensible as an exemplary condition for science-reflexive endeavors. In fact, no other academic discipline has as high a level of study-related reflection provocation as psychotherapy. This quality feature alone encourages critical-reflexive epistemic acts which have been systematically carried out at Sigmund Freud University, Vienna, for years within the context of the basic-analytical research approach of *transfermeneutic psychotherapy science/experimental hermeneutics*, with which psychotherapy also makes its academic status of a genuine university subject (*psychotherapia academica universitatis*) plausible.

References

Feyerabend PK (1985) Realism, rationalism and scientific method. Philosophical papers, vol 1. Cambridge UP, Cambridge

Gadamer H-G (1989) Truth and method, 2nd edn. Sheed and Ward, London

Gelo OCG (2012) On research methods and their philosophical assumptions: 'raising the consciousness of researchers' again. Psychother Sozialwiss 14(2): 109–128

Gelo OCG, et al (in press) Psychopathology as social construction: the case of Anorexia Nervosa. J Constructivist Psychol

Goodman N (1978) Ways of worldmaking. Hackett, Indianapolis

Greiner K (2005a) Therapie der Wissenschaft. Eine Einführung in die Methodik des Konstruktiven Realismus. Peter Lang, Frankfurt am Main

Greiner K (2005b) Knowledge of life world by functional strangification of high-tech equipment: instruction for a thought experiment. In: Jandl MJ, Greiner K (eds) Science, medicine and culture. Festschrift for Fritz G. Wallner. Peter Lang, Frankfurt am Main, pp 339–343

Greiner K (2006) The epistemological method of strangification in constructive realism: two examples of application. In: Bayat A (ed) Proceedings of the 1st international conference on research methodologies in science, engineering and technology, May 30–31 2006. ICRMSET, Tehran, pp 23–28

Greiner K (2007) Psychoanalytik als Wissenschaft des 21. Jahrhunderts. Ein konstruktivistischer Blick auf Struktur und Reflexionspotential einer polymorphen Kontextualisations-Technik. Peter Lang, Frankfurt am Main

Greiner K (2011) Integrationsprogramm Therapieschulendialog (TSD). Entwicklung einer textanalytischen Grundlagenforschung in der Psychotherapiewissenschaft. Peter Lang, Frankfurt am Main

Greiner K (2012) Standardisierter Therapieschulendialog (TSD). Therapieschulen-interdisziplinäre Grundlagenforschung an der Sigmund-Freud-Privatuniversität Wien/Paris (SFU). Sigmund-Freud-Privatuniversitäts-Verlag, Vienna

Greiner K (2013a) Methodenfahrplan Inter-Therapeutik (ITK). Transfermeneutische Psychotherapiewissenschaft an der SFU Wien. Sigmund-Freud-Privatuniversitäts-Verlag, Vienna

Greiner K (2013b) Psycho-Text-Puzzle: Theoriendiskursives Spielverfahren für die Psychotherapiewissenschaft. In: Lan F, Wallner FG, Schulz A (eds) Concepts of a culturally guided philosophy of science. Contributions from philosophy, medicine and science of psychotherapy. Peter Lang, Frankfurt am Main, pp 85–107

Greiner K (2013c) Psycho-Bild-Prozess (PBP): Imaginationsförderndes Reflexionsinstrumentarium für die Psychotherapiewissenschaft. In: Lan F, Wallner FG, Schulz A (eds) Concepts of a culturally guided philosophy of science. Contributions from philosophy, medicine and science of psychotherapy. Peter Lang, Frankfurt am Main, pp 109–126

Greiner K, Jandl MJ (2010) Novum Therapieschulendialog (TSD). Methodologische Prinzipien einer theorien-integrativen Psychotherapiewissenschaft. In: Greiner K, Jandl MJ, Wallner FG (eds) Aus dem Umfeld des Konstruktiven Realismus. Studien zu Psychotherapiewissenschaft, Neurokritik und Philosophie. Issue 14 in the series Culture and Knowledge. Edited by Friedrich G. Wallner. Peter Lang, Frankfurt am Main, pp 15–41

Greiner K, Jandl MJ (2012) Das Psycho-Text-Puzzle und andere Beiträge zu Psychotherapiewissenschaft und Philosophie. Sigmund-Freud-Privatuniversitäts-Verlag, Vienna

Greiner K, Wallner FG (2009) Innovative ontology and methodology: an introduction into constructive realism (CR). In: Wallner FG (ed) Five lectures on the foundations of Chinese medicine. Peter Lang, Frankfurt am Main, pp 17–24

Greiner K, Wallner FG, Gostentschnig M (eds) (2006) Verfremdung—Strangification. Multidisziplinäre Beispiele der Anwendung und Fruchtbarkeit einer epistemologischen Methode. Peter Lang, Frankfurt am Main

Greiner K, Jandl MJ, Paschinger O (eds) (2009) Programmatik und Praxis im Therapieschulendialog (TSD). Erste Beiträge zur dialogexperimentellen Theorien-Integration in der Psychotherapiewissenschaft. Sigmund Freud Privatuniversitäts-Verlag, Vienna

Greiner K, Jandl MJ, Burda G (2013) Der Psycho-Bild-Prozess und andere Beiträge zu Psychotherapiewissenschaft und Philosophie. Sigmund-Freud-Privatuniversitäts-Verlag, Vienna

Hartmann D, Janich P (eds) (1996) Methodischer Kulturalismus. Zwischen Naturalismus und Postmoderne. Suhrkamp, Frankfurt am Main

Jacobi J (1993) Die Psychologie von C. G. Jung. Eine Einführung in das Gesamtwerk. Fischer, Frankfurt am Main

James W (2014) Pragmatism: a new name for some old ways of thinking [1907]. Cambridge UP, Cambridge

Jandl MJ, Greiner K (eds) (2005) Science. Medicine and culture. Festschrift for Fritz G. Wallner. Peter Lang, Frankfurt am Main

Jung CG (1966) "The relations between the ego and the unconscious." Two essays in analytical psychology [1953]. The collected works of Jung CG, vol 7, 2nd revised edn. Edited and translated by Gerhard Adler and Richard Francis Carrington Hull. Princeton/Bollingen, Princeton, pp 123–244

Jung CG (1970) "Commentary on 'The Secret of the Golden Flower.'" Alchemical Studies [1967]. The Collected Works of C.G. Jung, vol 13, 2nd printing. Edited and translated by Gerhard Adler and Richard Francis Carrington Hull. Princeton/Bollingen, Princeton, pp 1–56

Kuhn T (1970) The structure of scientific revolutions, 2nd revised edn. Chicago UP, Chicago

Lacan J (2001) The mirror-stage as formative of the function of the I. In: Écrits: A Selection. Translated by Bruce Fink. Routledge, London, pp 1–7

Lan F, Wallner FG, Schulz A (eds) (2013) Concepts of a culturally guided philosophy of science. Contributions from philosophy. Medicine and science of psychotherapy. Peter Lang, Frankfurt am Main

Pagel G (1991) Lacan zur Einführung. Junius, Hamburg

Parfy E (1996) Die Integration von psychotherapeutischen Theorien unterschiedlicher Schulen. In: Psychotherapie Forum. 1996/4. Springer, Vienna, pp 84–99

Pompa L (1990) Vico. A study of the new science, 2nd edn. Cambridge UP, Cambridge

Popper KR (1963) Conjectures and refutations. The growth of scientific knowledge. Routledge & Kegan, London

Slife BD (1998) Raising the consciousness of researchers: hidden assumptions in the behavioral sciences. Adapt Phys Act Q 15(3):208–221

Slunecko T (1994) Plädoyer für einen Grundlagendiskurs in der Psychotherapieforschung. In: Psychotherapie Forum, 1994/2. Springer, Vienna, pp 128–136

Slunecko T (1996a) Einfalt oder Vielfalt in der Psychotherapie. In: Pritz A (ed) Psychotherapie—eine neue Wissenschaft vom Menschen. Springer, Vienna, pp 293–321

Slunecko T (1996b) Wissenschaftstheorie und Psychotherapie. Ein konstruktiv-realistischer Dialog. WUV UP, Vienna

Slunecko T (ed) (1997) The movement of constructive realism. Braumüller, Vienna

Stumm G, Wirth B (eds) (1994) Psychotherapie—Schulen und Methoden. Eine Orientierungshilfe für Theorie und Praxis. Falter, Vienna

Vaihinger H (1924) The philosophy of "As If". A system of the theoretical, practical and religious fictions of mankind. Kegan, London

von Foerster H (1981) Observing systems. Seaside, California

von Glasersfeld E (1998) Radikaler Konstruktivismus. Ideen, Ergebnisse, Probleme. Suhrkamp, Frankfurt am Main

Wagner E (1996) Psychotherapie als Wissenschaft in Abgrenzung von der Medizin. In: Pritz A (ed) Psychotherapie—eine neue Wissenschaft vom Menschen. Springer, Vienna, pp 219–247

Wallner FG (1992a) Acht Vorlesungen über den Konstruktiven Realismus. WUV UP, Vienna

Wallner FG (1992b) Wissenschaft in Reflexion. Braumüller, Vienna

Wallner FG (1992c) Konstruktion der Realität. Von Wittgenstein zum Konstruktiven Realismus. WUV UP, Vienna

Wallner FG (1993) Der Konstruktive Realismus. Theorie eines neuen Paradigmas? In: Wallner FG, Schimmer J, Costazza M (eds) Grenzziehungen zum Konstruktiven Realismus. WUV UP, Vienna, pp 11–23

Wallner FG (1994) Constructive realism. Aspects of a new epistemological movement. Braumüller, Vienna

Wallner FG (1996) Eine neue Ontologie für Psychotherapien. In: Pritz A (ed) Psychotherapie—eine neue Wissenschaft vom Menschen. Springer, Vienna, pp 341–357

Wallner FG (1997a) Aspekte eines Kulturwandels. Der Bedarf nach einem neuen Begriff des Wissens. In: Wallner FG, Agnese B (eds) Von der Einheit des Wissens zur Vielfalt der Wissensformen. Erkenntnis in Philosophie, Wissenschaft und Kunst. Braumüller, Wien, pp 11–27

Wallner FG (1997b) How to deal with science if you care for other cultures. Constructive realism in the intercultural world. Braumüller, Vienna

Wallner FG (2002) Die Verwandlung der Wissenschaft. Vorlesungen zur Jahrtausendwende. Kovac, Hamburg

Wallner FG (2005) Structure and relativity. Peter Lang, Frankfurt am Main

Wallner FG (2009) Five lectures on the foundations of Chinese medicine. Edited by Florian Schmidsberger. Peter Lang, Frankfurt am Main

Wallner FG, Greiner K (2006) Theoretical frameworks for research methodology. The new approach to science. In: Bayat A (ed) Proceedings of the 1st international conference on research methodologies in science, engineering and technology, May 30–31, 2006. ICRMSET, Tehran, pp 1–13

Wallner FG, Schmidsberger F, Wimmer FM (eds) (2010) Intercultural philosophy. New aspects and methods. Peter Lang, Frankfurt am Main

Wallner FG, Lan F, Jandl MJ (eds) (2011) Chinese medicine and intercultural philosophy. Theory, methodology and structure of Chinese medicine. Peter Lang, Frankfurt am Main

Wittgenstein L (1966) Tractatus Logico-Philosophicus [1921], 3rd edn. Routledge & Kegan Paul, London

Wittgenstein L (1968) Philosophical investigations [1953], 3rd edn. Blackwell, Oxford

Young-Bruehl E, Dunbar C (2009) One hundred years of psychoanalysis. A timeline: 1900–2000. Caversham, Toronto

Kurt Greiner, Univ.-Doz. DDr. phil., teaches philosophy of psychotherapy science and methodology of therapy schools research at Sigmund Freud University Vienna (SFU Vienna/Paris/Berlin) and invented the analysis program of experimental hermeneutics.

6 Interpretation as a Cognitive Instrument: Psychotherapy Science as an Attempt to Pool Paradigm-Based Systems of Interpretation

Thomas Stephenson

Contents

T. Stephenson (✉)
Department of Psychotherapy Science, Sigmund Freud University, Freudplatz 1, 1020 Vienna, Austria
e-mail: thomas.stephenson@sfu.ac.at

Abstract

Interpretation (German: "Deutung") is generally regarded as an exclusive instrument used by an elitist psychoanalysis. In this study we will broaden this perspective and reconstruct the cognitive process that is immanent to interpretations. This will be done against the backdrop of the discourse of abduction. We will first present several clarifications of the concept of abduction with reference to various forms of deduction and induction and introduce four basic forms of the knowledge-finding process in the production of "new" insights. We will then proceed to juxtapose Charles Sanders Peirce's ideas on abduction with Thomas Samuel Kuhn's theories on "Scientific Revolutions" and his concept of the paradigm. Explanations regarding the empirico-hermeneutic circle of scientific research will constitute the third part of the background against which the abductive paradigm shift will be explored microanalytically as exemplified in the interpretative patterns of Jean Michel Charcot and Sigmund Freud.

Finally, we will develop a concept of interpretation that can serve as a means for gaining knowledge in psychotherapy science by

O.C.G. Gelo et al. (eds.), *Psychotherapy Research*,
DOI 10.1007/978-3-7091-1382-0_6, © Springer-Verlag Wien 2015

networking six possible definitions in a categorical systematic account. This concept of interpretation will assume its legitimate place in psychotherapy science understood as a group of different paradigm-based systems of interpretation.

6.1 Introduction

> To put it simply, the idea of science is research, that of philosophy interpretation. (Adorno 1973, 334)

In the title of this study, "Deutung" (interpretation) is defined as a cognitive instrument of scientific research. The above quote, taken from Adorno, seems to rob this definition of its underpinnings. Even if we can assume that the author was not specifically thinking of this technical term of psychoanalysis, his statement does in fact point directly to a thorn in the side of psychoanalysis in particular and in psychotherapy science in general. What happens when both psychoanalysis and psychotherapy science use "interpretation" as a *cognitive instrument*? Are they engaging in a *serious* type of science? It is an instrument that is actually "only" used in the intimate working alliance between analyst and client, that is "with the exclusion of the public," to mitigate "private" states of suffering. What is more, doesn't it refer to something that *per definitionem* cannot be observed directly and thus ultimately eludes empirical verification? And this thorn does not become any less irritating by viewing human beings as an "interpretative system" (Straub 2009), that is, as a being that always has to have first "translated" the stimuli that it processes into its meaning-constructing inner systems to be able to explore what these stimuli signify. The German word "Deutung" cannot be identified with "interpretation"[1] (even if this commonly done in the psychoanalytic literature of the English-speaking world), as will become clear in the following. In this study I would like to show the following:

1. "Deutung," understood both in its specific psychoanalytic sense and in the more general scientific sense, contains the essence of all psychotherapy science thought.
2. The essence of all psychotherapy science-related thought in the sense of scientific research consists of specific characteristics in the sequence of abductive, inductive, and deductive thought which is typical of the thought process of interpretation.
3. This sequence becomes evident when one juxtaposes Charles Sanders Peirce's with those of Thomas Samuel Kuhn and uses this link as an interpretative pattern for the birth of psychotherapy.
4. If one traces the development of psychotherapy from this perspective, then one can note a certain constellation of characteristic traits in this "process of emergence" with respect to the inferential reasoning that can be observed both as a basic pattern inherent in the process of psychotherapy and a basic pattern in the diversification of psychotherapy in various schools.
5. This basic pattern has also shaped the research of psychotherapy science itself, independent of its research methodological orientation.
6. The study of this basic pattern is thus the main task of the theory of psychotherapy science.

In order to substantiate the above claims, I will proceed as follows. I will first present a number of "puzzle pieces" taken from various discourses of psychotherapy science (see Sect. 6.2) in a seemingly random way so as to ask the question what "in the innermost sense" holds these seemingly unrelated facts together. This will serve to stimulate discussion and to focus on the issues at hand. I will then examine more closely three implications of certain puzzle pieces (see Sect. 6.3) and concentrate on (a) the discourse of abduction (see Sect. 6.3.1), (b) the

[1] The problem lies in the fact that in German, there are two different terms: "Deutung" and "interpretation," while in English there is only "interpretation." In German the word "interpretation" has a very wide field of meaning. For referring to the specifically "psychoanalytical" form of interpretation, German-speaking analysts always use the term "Deutung."

discourse of paradigm (see Sect. 6.3.2), and, finally, (c) the development of Freud's ideas at the beginning of psychoanalysis (see Sect. 6.3.4). Against the backdrop of the findings of these reflections, I will then turn to Freud's theory of there being a "link between research and healing" and examine it from a new perspective, defining it as a cognitive instrument of psychotherapy science (see Sect. 6.4). In closing, we will attempt to answer some questions arising from the pieces of the puzzle we have examined and to take a look at the future of the activities of psychotherapy science in a theory of science and/or self-reflexive context.

6.2 Pieces of a Puzzle Taken from Discourses of Psychotherapy Science

First Puzzle Piece "Deutung" (interpretation) is often highlighted as a central instrument of psychoanalysis. Here there seems to something like a variation on the Cartesian existential creed that goes like this: "I interpret, I am thus a psychoanalyst!" The role of the psychoanalyst is classically regarded as that of one who uncovers unconscious contents, memories, connections, motivations, etc. Interpretation in this sense ("Deutung") is a statement that is used precisely for this process of unearthing, revealing unconscious contents. In interpretation something is directly and explicitly addressed, which not even the client was able to recognize—or to put it in more exact terms, what the client was not allowed to recognize. In this sense interpretation is clearly and unmistakably defined as an instrument that is supposed to lead to "private insights." What is realized is a part of the individual's psychic structure, the individual's unique life story, the individual's unique movements of thought and feeling, that is to say the "private logic."

Second Puzzle Piece Sigmund Freud, the "founding father" of psychoanalysis, the first version of modern psychotherapy (and thus ultimately the first pioneer of psychotherapy science), is also the "inventor" of (psychoanalytic) interpretation. He made a claim that is essential for the question of the scientific status of psychoanalysis—to the extent that (scientific research and teaching) psychoanalysis is part of psychotherapy science. He claims that in psychoanalysis, there is a "link between healing and research": When a psychoanalyst studies the "depths" of a client's psyche, he is also promoting his client's healing. And, inversely, when he wants to heal his clients, he has to study them. Freud himself made the following momentous statement: "*This prospect of scientific gain was the most dignified, most pleasant feature of analytical work*" (Freud 1927, p. 293). Here, however, he not only postulates a "scientific gain" of his procedure, he also exaggerates it with the assertion: "Our analytical approach is the only one, in which this valuable convergence is maintained" (ibid., italicized by TS).

Third Puzzle Piece In the almost 120 years of the history of the development of psychoanalysis, one can observe a change in perspective that is often described as a paradigm shift over the various preliminary stages and interim phases. In the "classical" interpretation of the analytical situation, a person who is suffering and does not know himself sufficiently and seeking help meets with a highly qualified expert who thanks to his competence and ingeniousness is able to offer this person in need of help insight into the causes of his suffering—according to the principle: "I know, thus I heal!" In the "relational" version of psychoanalysis (e.g., Mitchell 1988, 1998), by contrast, which has influenced ever-greater circles, the psychoanalyst sees himself as a specific part of the "therapist-client" team which works together, even if "with separate roles," to keep deepening the understanding of the client's development (and thus also his symptoms). Here both partners of this intersubjective process try to achieve an ever more complete and multilayered "reconstruction" of the client's biography. An integrative part of this "reconstructive work" is the reflection of what is taking place between the two "authors of the narrative," of what becomes tangible and can be experienced in the relationship during this work or what might be initially excluded from this feeling and experiencing and thus repressed. The motto here is: "Let us re-tell your story!"

Fourth Puzzle Piece A new discipline has established itself in the distinguished scientific landscape of this planet.[2] After the eventful history leading up to psychotherapy becoming a subject of academic study (Orlinsky 2004a, b; Wallerstein 2009), in 2005, the SFU, the Sigmund Freud Private University, was founded in Vienna. It was the first university worldwide to have made "psychotherapy science" as a separate (and central) faculty an integrative and autonomous part of university study and research (Rieken 2013; Stephenson 2011). A number of vehement scientific, epistemological, and methodological discussions were triggered not just in Austria but here in particular. These discussions are now in full swing both within this "psychotherapy science university" and in the rest of the scientific landscape. And it does not appear as if there will be any time soon a broad consensus on the scientific status of psychotherapy in general and psychoanalysis in particular.

Fifth Puzzle Piece Psychotherapy science, academically structured and established as part of a university, is in a sense paradigmatic within a field governed by very old but also very new discourses. These all relate to the question as to the relation of scientific status and whether a science can be attributed to certain "camps" within the great struggle for the "right science." These "camps" usually engage in certain polarizations, as are marked by conceptual dichotomies such as "nomothetic vs. idiographic," "sciences vs. humanities," "quantitative vs. qualitative," and "empirical vs. hermeneutical" (regarding these polarization discourses, see, e.g., Gelo et al. 2008, 2009; Salvatore and Valsiner 2010; Gelo 2012). To put it bluntly, there are two opposing camps facing each other when the predicates of science are being assigned to psychotherapy science. One subscribes to the combination "nomological-natural scientific-empirical-quantitative," while the other prides itself in being "ideographic-humanities-hermeneutic-qualitative."

Sixth Puzzle Piece A different type of troubleshooter has become an indispensable basic element of almost all textbooks in the realm of "qualitative research": abduction. Originally stemming from ancient times and taken up again in the nineteenth century by Charles Sanders Peirce as the only form of inference, within which something "new" can emerge: "Abduction is the process of forming explanatory hypotheses. It is the only logical operation which introduces any new idea" (Peirce CP 5.172). Peirce reformulated and expanded this notion, which pushes itself into the ambivalent link between the two great sacred columns of logic: deduction and induction. Abduction first claims to be an autonomous third form of logical inference, banking on those (scientific) thinking processes in which something "new" is created. Given the power of the possibilities of argumentation introduced to the discourse on truth and reality, abduction has, however, from the beginning the worst position. While deductions allow for crystal-clear insights by means of necessarily true statements, inductions can only claim to produce plausible possibilities of true statements. Abductions, by contrast, only evoke the hope (according to Peirce himself) that one has found something true or correct. Nonetheless, precisely the scientists of the "qualitative research program" adopt abduction as the "*via regia*" to pertinent research results with their "idiographic-humanities-hermeneutic-qualitative" approach and even postulate abduction as the scientific approach that is capable of offsetting the drawbacks and weaknesses of the "nomological-scientific-empirical-quantitative program." At the same time, both camps always claim to have hegemony and interpretative power in the social sciences and humanities.

Seventh Puzzle Piece The "humanities" had to swallow one of the great insults from one man who with just two terms rose to prominence in both scientific and nonscientific circles: since Thomas Samuel Kuhn (1962) introduced them, the expressions "scientific revolutions" and the

[2] Why the author is referring to the "planet" will become clear in Sect. 6.3.1.

word "paradigm" are quoted on every fitting and not-so-fitting occasion. And even (rather paradoxically!) in the social science circles... in spite of the fact that Kuhn discredited the social sciences in one extremely important respect. As this great historian of science stated, unlike the natural sciences, the social sciences had failed to reach the status of a "mature science" even in the twentieth century. According to the man who coined these terms, they had not succeeded in agreeing on a paradigm. The latter has the feature of being able to organize the concept of science and to bundle the forces contained in it so that the "normal science" that is thus established is able to intensively pursue its state of knowledge and to expand it. And if though there is no sign that this state of affairs could change in the twenty-first century, precisely the social sciences make use of the paradigm concept to underline the scientific status of their results.

6.2.1 Zooming in on the Subject Matter

As different as the phenomena described here appear to be, against this backdrop of this subject of this article, some questions arise:

1. To what extent is "interpretation" (in the sense of Deutung) an "elitist" instrument that is only accessible to a (controversial) subgroup within psychotherapy science and one that can only be used within psychoanalysis?
2. If it is more than just that which status can it assume within the repertory of research activities of psychotherapy science?
3. For what kind of knowledge can "interpretation" pertain to?
4. Does its (questionable) usability as "cognitive instrument" in psychoanalysis mean that "interpretation" cannot be used for "research from the outside" or precisely can be used?
5. What implications would there be if "interpretation" would not be a cognitive instrument that could "also" be used in psychotherapy science research but would even be regarded as a paradigm and core instrument of all psychotherapy science activity (and how could such a claim be legitimized)?
6. What meaning for this whole complex of questions does the fact have that "interpretation" in its meaning as psychoanalytic cognitive instrument is directed at something that *per definitionem* cannot be observed directly but only in its effects, namely, the effects on the "unconscious"?
7. To which "research-programmatic camps" can "interpretation" be attributed? Does it allow nomological or idiographical insights, ones that are natural scientific or humanities oriented, quantitative, or qualitative?
8. Can it be incorporated in "unifying" methodological concepts such as that of "triangulation" and "mixed methods"?
9. In what way does it relate to induction, deduction, and abduction?
10. Is it *part of a paradigm* or is it itself a paradigm?

I will try to base my elaborations on these questions so that the results provide answers to as many of these questions as possible.

6.3 Paradigms of Knowledge and the Abductive Birth of Psychotherapy Science

The ten questions that emerged from our preoccupation with the "puzzle pieces" open up a wide field. In this context, the search for answers is limited to the triad of knowledge-abduction-psychotherapy science. In the following, we will thus only focus on certain aspects of this puzzle pieces. Here it seems especially important to clarify the terms "abduction" (see Sect. 6.3.1) and "paradigm" (see Sect. 6.3.2) in their relation to "knowledge" (see Sect. 6.3.2.4) and their interconnections (see Sect. 6.3.3). It is also important to address the "microanalytical" reference to abductive and paradigmatic phenomena at the (historical) beginning of psychotherapy science (Sect. 6.3.4).

6.3.1 The Discourse of Abduction

For some considerable time, the concept of abduction has been assuming an increasingly prominent place in textbooks from the large field of "qualitative methods of research" (see, e.g., Kelle 1994, 2003, 2007; Strübing 2004; Reichertz 2004, 2010; Bohnsack et al. 2011; Keller 2013). Similar to the way "interpretation" (Deutung) was described as a defining feature of psychoanalysts in connection with puzzle piece 1, we could meanwhile say very simply: "I use abduction, I am thus a qualitative researcher!" As always, when a complex term mutates into a trendy word, which is used programmatically, its differentiating and clarifying potential is in danger of degenerating. It is the achievement of critical thinkers such as Jo Reichertz for having systematically reviewed the concept that Charles Sanders Peirce developed and changed numerous times in the course of his life as a researcher and having subject it to a clarifying reconstruction (see also Deutscher 2002). In this connection I refer the reader to publications (in particular Reichertz 2011, 2013) for a differentiated reception of this systematization, and I will also proceed from these results to develop my own ideas on this subject.

The following elucidation of the abduction discourse is based on a few basic clarifications. The idea of abduction will be limited to the meaning that can be found in Peirce's late writings and will be juxtaposed to the concepts of "induction" and "deduction." To offer both a rich diversity of perspectives and to provide clear explanation, we will use a descriptive model in which a fictive "alien example" is developed. This will allow for a short discussion of the basic forms of scientific thought (inferential, argumentative, discursive) and a differentiation of abductive thought along several lines of scientific action.[3]

6.3.1.1 Induction, Deduction, and Abduction in the Context of the Four Sections of Scientific Thought

6.3.1.1.1 Induction and Deduction

As all of us learned in school, Socrates is mortal even though he paradoxically became immortal for precisely this reason. When we then were supposed to learn what deduction and what induction is and how these two can be represented in a syllogism, we had to juggle with these sentences: Socrates is a human being. All humans are mortal. Socrates is mortal.

We then had to give various names to these three sentences: "premise 1," "premise 2," "conclusion" or also "top proposition," "bottom proposition," and "conclusion."

The names mark positions in a scheme and depending on what names and thus what position we give which of the three sentences, another logical pattern of thought emerges, in each case a different process of inference.

If the fact that all humans are mortal received the name "premise 1" and the even more trivial insight that Socrates was human was given the name "premise 2," then the designation "conclusion" remained for the sentence "Socrates is mortal"—and the whole thing was then called "deduction." If you let this all spin a bit further in a kind of merry-go-round, induction appeared: "If Socrates is mortal and if Socrates is human, then all human beings are mortal!"

This way we not only realized that in scientific thought logic relates to "thinking about the world" in the same way as a house built of Lego blocks does to a castle in Versailles. We also realized straight away that one procedure produced no doubt the right results, while the other one almost provoked doubts.

[3] For colleagues who are already taking issue with the seeming abstruseness of citing an "alien" in this text, this is less to make science more entertaining (which, I might add, is certainly underestimated) but more in response to the need to create a being for this fictive journey through various "scientific settings"—a being that can think of "newness" in terms of abduction and can be used to illustrate a lot of things that are "state of the art" for us, *essentially* new and sometimes at least in part not *contextual*. It couldn't be a child because this being had to be in full possession of the "mental structures" of an adult. What remained here was a scientist from a completely different star!

Why should one believe the assumption that all humans are mortal results from the fact that we know that Socrates is mortal and a human? It is also not correct that all people have white beards even though Socrates is human and had a white beard. Now it was also clear that both induction and deduction had to be linked if one wanted to obtain the "right" results. It is entirely possible that an alien (let's simply call him "Allen") who we put into a time machine that takes him back to 399 BC and then gets outs at the Acropolis in Athens is the first person in the world to see Socrates (who has just emptied the cup of hemlock). He finds out from us that Socrates is a human and then thinks to himself: well, if he has a white beard, then all people might very well have beards.

With this inductively found theory, he would then have to search for proofs, that is, he would have to do deductive empirical research. If the theory, "all people have a white beard" is to be true, then also the prediction "The next person that I bump into must have a white beard!" must also be correct. As long as Allen meets on or the other colleague of Socrates who also has a white beard, his theory remains valid. But one Allen actually enters Socrates' house, the theory would become falsified: Xanthippe could perhaps have a sharp tongue, but she would certainly not have a white beard—yet she would still be human! In order to not have to ditch his entire theory, Allen can now try to differentiate his theory. One part of humans have a white beard, the other part doesn't. The rest is then a matter of verification. Since Allen has other things to do, he comes up with a shortcut. If I take a certain number from all humans and look if they each have a white beard or not, then I can, to a certain degree, infer for all people—statistics is born! When we then think—Well, that might be good for an alien, but this is something we could have told him without all the research, we might hear our old philosophy professor admonishing us: "Yes, but only because you have already learned this thing with the *conditio humana*, while Allen hasn't!" This way we learn that in order to think scientifically, more is needed than just inferential thought in and for itself—namely, argumentation!

Then we cannot simply say in a cocky way to the alien as a scientist: "Tough luck, that's something we've known for a long time!" Instead we should make it clear to him that we can't for that reason believe that all people have to have a white beard only because Socrates had a white beard, because there can be other people who don't have a white beard and are still people. But, and this we can assure the alien, we can certainly believe that Socrates is mortal, simply because we know that he is a human, because "mortality" is part of the *conditio humana*, that is, to basic human disposition or "nature," and consequently is a necessary (if not sufficient) trait of the type "human being"—while "white beard" is not a necessary one!

We can thus say: Dear Allen, you can, if you now also see that the white-bearded Socrates (who, as already said, drank from the cup of hemlock and of whom we know that he is human) dies before your very eyes, inductively conclude with a clear conscience that "humans" are mortal. Now you can say that the feature of "mortality" by necessity belongs to him from the definition of the type "human" (theoretical argument), and we have yet to find one single species of this type that does not show this feature (empirical argument). We have thus provided him with an empirical argument why he should believe in the result of our induction that we learned in school and, inversely, must relativize the result of his induction. "Our induction is tenable (albeit not logically "provable") because we can show the empirical result that all of Socrates' contemporaries have died. Your induction is not tenable, because we are able to present an (empirical) counterargument. "See, Socrates' wife is also human, but she has no beard!"

And if we are lucky enough to have a scientifically far-developed alien before us, then he can show us that our approach is not the final word of all science. After going to church he asked us: "Was Jesus human?" We answer—a bit hesitantly, as we already sense doom—"Yes, he, too!" But now the alien has caught us, "Why could he then arise from the dead?" Now the inferential thinking that we unfolded in a dialogue has obtained the following form: "Since all humans are mortal, Socrates is mortal, because he is human, even though Jesus rose from the dead and was also human!" And how we have already received the higher honors of thinking and have entered the ranks of scientifically thinking individuals (one of which was Socrates), namely, the art of discursive though. Now we have to begin a discussion with the alien: "Your argumentation, that "mortality" is not an element of *conditio humana*, is unfortunately untenable, since Jesus was both man and the son of God. He died as a man, but he rose again as God's son. Now what do you say?" And if Allen is not smart enough to get back into his space ship and to fly back to his home planet where he can enjoy his immortal life (since that is part of the *conditio aliena*), then we would still be sitting there today since there is no natural end for a scientific discourse, only an end brought on by time constraints or desperation.

6.3.1.1.2 Abduction

What we can expect of an alien is not something we can expect of us adult human beings: namely, induction. The induction "all humans are mortal!" is nothing new, original. Yet for an immortal alien without a beard, the first impression of a dying, white-bearded person can be surprising, and his thought "Perhaps all humans are mortal and white-bearded!" could then be an abduction in the sense of Charles Sanders Peirce! Why?

Because the decisive difference between induction and abduction for Peirce only lies in the fact that in abduction a new rule, a new type is created in the theory system of the thinker!

From the moment that Allen has performed this first step in abduction (finding a new rule or a new type with defined characteristics whose "token" is the interesting phenomenon) and—maintaining the claim to the status of science—continues research to test his new theory, he returns to the eternal cycle of induction and deduction. From this moment on his statement: "All mortals are mortal and have white beards!" is also no longer new for him! From this moment, also all of his inductions are only "qualitative inductions": the next living being which crosses his path is identified as "human" because of certain characteristics (which each time means carrying out a "qualitative" (since it is oriented to certain traits) induction) and is now deductively examined for the existence of his mortality and beardedness.

6.3.1.1.3 Types of Abduction in Various Parts of Scientific Action

Our Allen example allows us to recognize a further differentiation. Let's suppose he would like to find out why all people have to die but also even the male old humans do not all have a white beard, even if many do. For him, it is a hypothetical explanation that goes: "Old male humans let a beard grow because that way they can document their social status as 'wise old men'"—a rather new idea which helps Allen explain his surprising experience (and thanks to which he will next time he sees an old wise man with a beard will no longer find this surprising but simply something worth investigating).

His next (scientific) goal, after having, by means of abduction, reached his mortality and beardedness hypothesis, will be to find out whether the "predictions" ("prognostic" claims) will really take place in an empirically observable way. And since he knows no other research method than to study all exemplars of the type "man," he soon faces a "surprising" aporia: Not only that in spite of his own immortality he would simply need too much time to witness the death of all of Socrates' contemporaries,[4] since he knows that he had not landed on earth at a time when already all humans have proved their mortality by their death (and "man" in this sense was extinct.) Since it became clear to him that for reasons of definition, he could never test never *ALL*[5] humans for their mortality, since the

[4] For this, we will simply assume that on his home planet "economical" has also gained currency as a criterion of scientificity.

[5] Strictly speaking, this means: "All humans who ever lived + all human who are alive at this moment + all humans who will be alive until humanity becomes extinct once and for all (otherwise until the end of all time)." And since this verification has to be carried out by a human being (if it is to be valid for human science, that is, excluding our fictive alien), it could not even determine the last live exemplar of humanity, since it would then still be living as a human being. At the moment this last human being also dies, it cannot make any more statements. Thus this universal statement is *in principle and non-verifiable a priori* (except by a nonhuman being with the capacity to make rational statements and to verify them both empirically and logically!) We have been

time machine in which we put him is unfortunately only able to travel into the past and not into the future. His method thus does not really lead him to the goal he is aspiring to: namely, the confirmation or refutation of his hypotheses. If he now does not simply blow off the entire project and instead desperately looks for ways out of his dilemma—and in so doing "invents" the inferential statistics, takes a sample, and is able to calculate statistical parameters for determining the probability of his hypothesis—then he has actually succeeded in performing an abduction of a cognitive instrument,[6] as opposed to his previous "typology abduction" (and the "explanation abduction" cited above!). As with deductions and inductions, we can thus distinguish at least four types of abductions: (1) abductions in the realm of scientific descriptive knowledge ("typologies" as category systems of phenomena), (2) abductions in the realm of scientific explanatory knowledge, (3) abduction in the realm of scientific cognition goals, and (4) abduction in the realm of scientific cognitive instruments (methods of study).

The fact that in our example we had to use Allen as the only exemplar of a separate "species" of scientists in order to see in Socrates' syllogism not just an induction but also an abduction and we as students (i.e., as "private persons") were able to speak with our old philosophy teacher (i.e., a person who pursues a profession) and in the process kept featuring science and research, two further dimensions have emerged which can be used to differentiate our "typology of abductions."

1. Private/professional/scientific abductions (deductions/inductions)
2. Individual/collective abductions (deductions/inductions)

In the deployment of Peirce's ideas presented here, several possibilities emerge that allow us to differentiate both the concept of abduction and that of induction and deduction as three forms of scientific inference and to distinguish them from other forms (professional, private[7])[8] (Fig. 6.1).

These three dimensions taken from the model of the empirical circle (EC) are those of the "positions" (private, professional, scientific), the "fields" (description, explanation, goals, means), and the "spaces" (individual, community) (see Stephenson 2003, pp. 113–133).

This systematic differentiation also seems necessary because Peirce usually deals with "new types" and "new explanations" in the scientific thought of one thinking individual, while the process of (human inferential) thought in general and that of inventing/finding the new in science in particular encompasses much more. It is thus not clear why abduction should only refer to one aspect of scientific action. The intellectual *ductus* of abduction lies, as said, in the core of the "late" Peircean concept only in the sequence:

"Surprising outcome" → "new rule"

Whether this rule only implies the construction of a new "type" by means of which a "strange exemplar" (="surprising even") can be incorporated now as a "token of a (new) type" (and thus is no longer surprising) or whether an

waiting for a long time to find such living beings like our alien. But until we actually do find one such example simply remains thought experiments.

[6] "An abduction of a **new** cognitive instrument" would thus be a pleonasm on the basis of the definition presented here.

[7] That all three positions can and must also be viewed from the perspective of logical argumentation is state of the art for qualitative researchers and/or social scientists. Qualitative research uses "common-sense constructions" as its point of departure (Przyborski and Wohlrab-Sahr 2008, 26ff).

[8] If, for example, Allen himself (as a "human" based on the observation of Socrates' death and his previous identity) were to infer the "mortality of man," then this would first be a *private individual* abduction in the realm of *categories* or *types*. Since he only "learns" from the philosophers on earth, he is only adopting a scientific model of deduction ("humans" are mortal, when the next being can be identified as human, it automatically follows (without it being necessary to verify this empirically) that it is mortal.) If, however, Allen as a *scientific emissary of his planet* comes up with the idea that the surprising fact that no all old men have white beards can be *explained* by the fact that the white beard is a sign of social status, as "old sage" and not all old men have to or want to bear such a sign, he created a *scientific individual* abduction in the realm of *explanatory models*.

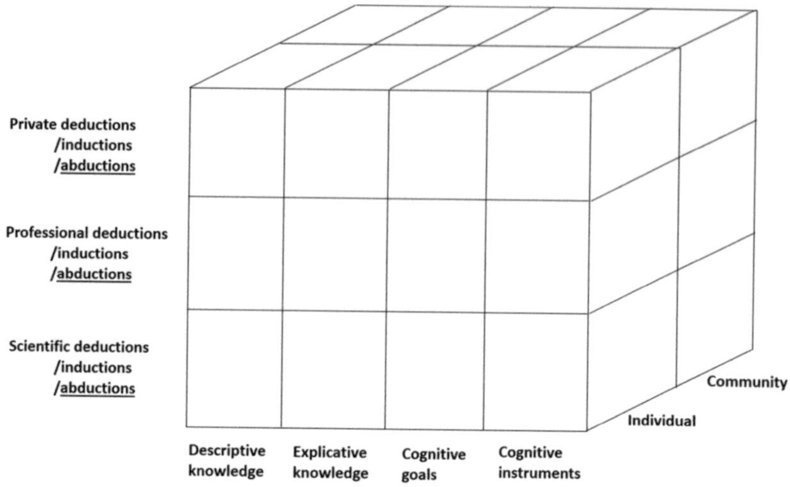

Fig. 6.1 A first systematic description of cognitive forms in deductive, inductive, and abductive thought on the basis of the three dimensions of the empirical circle (Stephenson 2003)

entire explanatory model is "invented," which furnishes us with the missing explanation for the emergence of a surprising phenomenon, does not change anything on the basic figure cited above ("surprising outcome" → "new rule"). And this basic figure remains valid, even when we define as "surprising event" as the moment at which we (enduringly, following many failed attempts) must note that the aspired result of our research with the existing means that we have learned to apply in "such cases" cannot be attained—and we thus have to invent a new method. The history of science is replete with achievements, which represents something new in the area of methodology. Each time such a new method is found or invented, in any case constructed, abduction is—if we follow Peirce—at work.[9] The demands and test criteria for new cognitive instruments (or new goals of cognition) are however different than those that apply in the introduction of a new phenomenon category for scientific forms of action of "describing phenomena" or "explaining phenomena"!

Up until now we know that what is characteristic of abduction is that it creates a new rule for a surprising result and that the act of thought taking place in it can be represented at least in its basic outlines or up to a certain degree in the form of a syllogism. But we have no idea what kind of new thing will emerge and to which elements of inferential thinking this new something must refer to.

6.3.1.2 Four Basic Forms of Gaining Knowledge in the Production of the "Novel"

Before we change sites and let Allen return to his home planet for the time being and then witness his flight from this planet back to earth, where he will land with his time machine first in 1969 and then in 1895, we must elaborate on several elements that will play a role in the following: (a) Peirce's use of the expressions "result," "case," and "rule," (b) a differentiation of the "new" and "surprising" in a scientific research concept, and (c) the steps in a scientific process of gaining knowledge in connection with the aspects of induction-deduction-abduction.

6.3.1.2.1 New "Conclusion" and New ""Result": "Final Elements" of Different Interpretations of the "New" in a Process of Gaining Knowledge

We used the familiar Socrates example to illustrate forms of scientific thought or argumentation. In the following, we will stick to this

[9] In the next stage of Allen's journey, we will also cite an example for abductions in the section on "cognitive goals."

example, because the other often used examples using a ball or beans can easily lead to confusion.

Let's revisit the three statements with which the differentiation of "deduction," "induction," and "abduction" juggles with and categories of "rule," "case," and "result":

- "All humans are mortal." (→ "rule")
- "Socrates is human." (→ "case")
- "Socrates is mortal." (→ "result")

"Result" here should not be confused with "conclusion." The above classification of the statements according to the Peircean categories of "rule," "case," and "result" always remains the same, while the three sentences change their status as "premise" or "conclusion." The quality of "newness" in one or more of these sentences can, however, be interpreted differently. The result of inference should in any case not be called a "new insight" from the outset, even though it actually is such in any case. When I "have" two or three elements, that is, the two premises are "familiar" and thus the "old elements," then the third element, which I use as a documentation of my insight automatically, becomes the "new" one. The decisive difference here is to be found in the fact whether the contents of my conclusion in my thinking existed before the conclusion already in my background knowledge. In this sense "insight" is represented in inferential reasoning either as a "rediscovery" or as a "new invention." In order to illustrate this, we need a colleague of Allen's, who comes from a planet of an even more remote galaxy, where the scientists do not even know that earth beings exist—those who Allen knows as "humans" (even if he does not know they are mortal.) Let's call this second "even more ignorant" alien "Tim."

Tim knows nothing about humans. Allen knows them, but does not know from his own conclusions that they are mortal. Both do not know Socrates before beginning their inferential act of thought.

For Tim, the statement "Socrates is 'human'!" is something completely new as conclusion, that is the final product of his inferential reasoning—(=new in both knowledge-relevant elements "Socrates" and "human"). It is thus also the result of the introduction of an unprecedented category (this is the criterion for inductive thought)—namely, "human"! For Allen, this conclusion is only a "new" designation for a new criterion, namely, "qualitative induction")! Thus for Tim a conclusion at the end of which "Socrates is mortal" stands, a multistep process of thinking in which all partial steps actually contain something new for Tim. At the end a real abduction takes place because both the premise "Socrates is human" and the premise "humans are mortal" were not part of his background knowledge before.

For Allen, by contrast, "all humans are mortal" is a "simple induction" [i.e., the creation of a "rule" that did not yet exist in the background knowledge because of a given case and an observation that was just made (as a "result") following a previous qualitative induction in which he identifies Socrates as an exemplar of the category "human" (which he was already familiar with)].

For us educated people of the twenty-first century, only a simple deduction can be carried out in that we show that Socrates who was known to us as an exemplar of our familiar category man who is, as we know, mortal, must also by necessity be mortal, but this does not really represent any "real" new element of our thinking."[10]

Figure 6.2 shows the marking points in the abduction discourse—points that have been identified in this chapter.

According to this table, deductive thought works without a new thought element, qualitative induction as "incorporating" with one "ampliative" induction (as the "classical" case of induction) with two and abduction as "generating induction" with three new elements. This is accompanied by an ever-greater degree of "insecurity"—with the conclusions becoming ever less logically cogent.

In the table, "P" (=premises) and "C" (=conclusion) also always designate the foundations (i.e., the premises) of our conclusions and the product (i.e., the conclusion as inferred knowledge or a goal and final result of

[10] Deduction, in its most stringent form, does not expand or even reform our knowledge—it only shows all *what is implicit in it*.

	Deduction (deductive)		Induction (incorporative =„qualitative I.")		Induction (ampliative)		Abduction (generative)	
Regel	P given theoretical rule	P given empirical rule	P given theoretical rule	P given empirical rule	C expanded theoretical rule	C expanded empirical rule	C new theoretical rule	C new empirical rule
Fall	P given theoretical case	P given empirical case	C given theoretical case	C given empirical case	P partially given theoretical case	P partially given empirical case	P new theoretical case	P new empirical case
Ergebnis	C given theoretical result	C given empirical result	P new theoretical result	P new Empirical result	P new theoretical result	P new empirical result	P new theoretical result	P new empirical result

Fig. 6.2 A second systematic representation of forms of knowledge as deriving, classifying, expanding, and generating thought (*C* conclusion, *P* premise), and conclusions are the final results of each inferential act of thought in the given cell, highlighted by being *circled* in

a given act of thought) of the given form of logical reasoning, with the product of knowledge being highlighted with a circle.

The category of the "new" assumes several differentiations in the table. A distinction is make between products of thought (individual statements and systems of statements) that are either present prior to the process of thinking, that is "given" or "new," that is during the process of thinking either (a) completely created new, found, and invented or (b) only "modified," that is, "expanded" (that is to say, are then "partly new").

6.3.1.2.2 The Sequence of Steps in the Scientific Process of Finding Knowledge and the Frequency of Abductions

How scientists pursue their research in a precise way, which steps they first take, which next steps they take, and where they end is, fortunately, not something that can be defined exactly. And we certainly have no desire to introduce such fixed rules.

For the line of thought that we have developed here, we simply have to take a closer look at this special procedure called abduction—in its contextualization in the entire research process.

The process of abduction on which we are focusing here, which is part of the research process, proves, on closer scrutiny, to be a more complex process, even if we try to simplify and reduce it. From the many variants, let's take a closer look at an "ideal type":

1. Initial state of research: the existence of a "surprising event"
2. Attempt, by means of (qualitative) induction to eliminate the surprise ("IA" = induction attempt)
3. Lasting failure of this attempt
4. Attempt, by means of abduction, to construct a new set of ideas which could serve as a candidate for analyzing and explaining the surprising event ("AA" = abduction attempt)
5. Successful attempt to eliminate the surprise
6. An attempt, by means of deduction, to apply the "completely" new "type" or the "completely" new rule in order to let previously "surprising" events become "not surprising" ones ("DA" = deduction attempt)
7. Successful use of the new "type" ("DS" = deduction success)
8. Use of the new type in all further results of the previously surprising kind—until the next surprising event occurs.

A crucial aspect is now the successful or failed attempts to proceed by means of induction or deduction. Abductions are not used at the beginning and in every case of a research process. On the contrary, in purely quantitative terms, they are "inferior" to the other forms of reasoning. In my estimate the average proportion between derivative, classificatory, expansive, and generative (that is to say, abductive in the narrowest sense) acts of thinking is 25:50:24:1. And this is true for science of all camps—be it "nomothetical," "ideographical," "quantitative," "qualitative," "empirical," or "theoretical" research! The crux lies in the course of point 3; in the vast majority of instances of scientific research, one or the other variant of elements already existing in background knowledge can be successfully used to determine goal, selection of means, the analysis, and explanation of the object of study. Abduction takes place—but extremely rarely. Yet in order to understand the prerequisites and implications of this claim to the full, we still need the empirical and theoretical results of two revolutionary projects of the last century. So let us once again follow Allen's tracks.

6.3.1.2.3 Allen's Journey Continues

Equipped with the new insight that humans on earth are mortal, Allen now returns to his planet. Here he will share this revolutionary discovery with his science colleagues in a lecture that has been eagerly awaited. He makes his story more interesting by predicting that with this new insight about the earth beings several to date unexplained phenomena can be explained in a very simple way. Science on Allen's planet has some optical data of the planet earth which allowed for it to be concluded, for instance, that there is life on this planet, also thinking beings with social structures that have a certain resemblance to those existing on Allen's planet. Allen's colleagues had, however, initially assumed that these beings were immortal just like on their planet. "Mortality" is not known as a concept in this community where there are only the most different forms of "change." Allen's report is, however, not met with a wave of enthusiasm as he had expected; he did not receive praise and awards. Rather he was horrified to see that many of his colleagues showed doubt regarding the truth of this discovery and some were even angry and directed hateful accusations at him. Those who were less furious and even disturbed and apprehensive voiced the concern that humanity might have been overcome by a virus, which had brought on this strange quality of mortality and were now worried that Allen may have imported this virus to their planet. Only a few of them came up to him after his lecture and congratulated him on this revolutionary discovery and asked him to tell them more. Unlike the others, these colleagues were also thrilled by the fact that certain phenomena on earth, which until then had only been explained by rather obscure ideas, could now be interpreted in a very simple way against the backdrop of this new image. Allen's science colleagues had for the longest time been mulling over data according to which humans had places where individual exemplars of their species were locked away in boxes and buried under the ground. Many scientists believed the theory that this practice was a special kind of torture and punishment, while others suspected that they were extreme forms of self-discovery attempts or even spiritual exercises of an especially strict order. In any case most scientists regarded this phenomenon as something marginal and not worth being pursued, while others were haunted by these strange phenomena. In any case they were unable to find any reasonable explanation that seemed to be compatible with all the available data.

Allen first tried to convince those scientists who were trying with all their might to discriminate and marginalize him for his scientific views, but he soon came to realized that these attempts would remain fruitless because his enraged opponents could hardly be reached by rational arguments and used all legitimate and non-legitimate means in discussions to maintain their own view.

Allen was so upset about this development and the same time so hell-bent to explain it that he spent a long time trying to find similar cases in the history of science of his own planet. He actually succeeded in discovering some and now tried to reveal the similarities between these cases.

He succeeded in identifying a number of such common features. One thing in particular caught his attention. On Allen's planet, there had on numerous occasions been discourses triggered by new theories. These were most frequent when the issue was concepts that pertained to a given object in the core of its definition, and this object was the central part of the self-definition of an entire discipline. There had, for instance, once been a controversy over a radically new theory, which was related to the planet earth. This, however, was the opposite of his case. A scientist had claimed, before the venerable Gaian society for biology, that life on its planet originated on the planet earth and that millions of years ago people had landed on Gaia to sough the seeds that had ultimately led to the present state of living being o that planet. Like his now, this theory had met with fierce opposition, and the scientist who had proposed this theory withdrew to a lonely island and had never again been heard from. Allen subsequently elaborated his theory of "scientific revolutions," the "scientific paragon," and the "transdisciplinary nucleodicts," but he refrained from presenting them to the science council of the Gaians—once bitten twice shy—our alien now avoided all discourse!

After having been admonished by his fans again and again to pursue his research on the earth beings based on his transdisciplinary[11] nucleodict "Man is mortal," Allen decided on day to board his time machine spaceship and return to earth. He arrived there in the year 1969, where he mingled with the audience of a lecture being held by an inhabitant of the planet earth known by the name of "Tom the Bold" before a community of earth scientists. The longer Allen listened to Tom, the more restless he became. This human being was speaking precisely about those things that he had discovered with such great effort on the planet Gaia. Tom the Bold called his "scientific upheavals" "scientific revolutions," his "scientific paragon" became "exemplar" and what Allen called "transdisciplinary nucleodict," Tom the bold called "paradigm." But it was entirely clear that they were both speaking of the exact thing. And in the audience, there were intense discussion going on, but no one seemed to be terribly excited about Tom's insights!

Feeling rather frustrated, Allen boarded his time-space machine and turned at the buttons. Finally he likes the number 1895, and since he always wanted to see Paris and visit an opera, he selects this city as his destination. His meanwhile rather overstrained time machine dropped him off about 5 km too far from the Paris opera, and so he landed in a place called "Salpetrière." He was a bit puzzled about this "surprising outcome" since he now found himself, for the third time, in a lecture being given by a man who clearly looks like a scientist to an elegantly dressed audience. Allen continues to be amazed: here the subject of the lecture is those patients who on Allen's home planet are known as "chameleon patients" suffering from an illness that has been known for centuries and is meanwhile curable. By means of joint travels into the supraconsciousness of the "chameleon," this illness can be quickly healed—a procedure which however has to first be approved by the ethics council since it always deals with very intimate, delicate issues and the healers are very much aware of their responsibility in this delicate interplay with the patient. Yet here this scientist was presenting the chameleon patients as if it were at a fairground attraction; yes he even tugs at their tongue and pinched the testicles of some of the male patients! And there was no mention of the supraconscious!

Disgusted by all of this, Allen gets the hell out of there. His next stop is Vienna where he lands right in the study of an older gentleman with a beard (he immediately recognizes that it is not

[11] The expression "transdisciplinary" also refers to something over-arching on Allen's planet which is valid for all disciplines of a group of sciences (social sciences, natural sciences, etc.).

Socrates). This gentleman is just in the process of filling page after a page with notes, in a visibly agitated state. As Allen reads while looking over his shoulder, he grins. The scientist is obviously just inventing the first transdisciplinary nucleo-dict, which every kid on Gaia already learns about in primary school. A bit reassured by the insight that he Allen and his Gaian community of scientists have long built up knowledge that is just beginning to emerge on earth, he collects his holographic notes and heads back to his home planet where he wants to share his latest insights on the specific characteristics of the earth beings with his small but growing group of followers.

6.3.2 Thomas Samuel Kuhn's "Scientific Revolutions" and "Paradigms" as Special Cases of the Cognitive Process

Thomas Samuel Kuhn (1922–1996) revolutionized thinking about science in the second half of the last century. He studied physics on his own and then became more and more interested in the general emergence of knowledge in the world of science. Contrary to popular opinion, Kuhn did not just deal with "natural sciences," he also described his experience with social sciences and claimed that this experience: "in a community composed predominantly confronted me with unanticipated questions about the differences between such communities and those of natural scientists among whom I had been trained. Particularly, I was struck by the number and extent of overt disagreements between social scientists about the nature of legitimate scientific problems and methods" (Kuhn 1962, ix–x).

We have already encountered these "differences" in several of the puzzle pieces at the beginning of this text. Kuhn took them as an occasion for further remarks on the essence of science and knowledge in scientific communities. The perception of special problems in the humanities prompted him to assume, as we already mentioned above, that this group of scientists apparently does not yet have access to the basic ideas of order, orientation, and consensus. With regard to the "overt differences in opinion" related to the "essence of the meaningful scientific problems and correct methods," he notes: "Both history and my own experience led me to doubt that natural scientists have more solid or lasting answers to such questions than their colleagues in the humanities" (loc.cit, 10). Yet he also underlines "somehow, the practice of astronomy, physics, chemistry or biology normally fails to evoke the controversies over fundamentals that today often seem endemic among, say, psychologists or sociologists" (loc.cit.).

He then develops his basic concept on the basis of this difference: "Attempting to discover the source of that difference led me to recognize the role in scientific research of what I have since called 'paradigms'" (loc.cit.). He does not further pursue the possible applications of his notion of paradigm in the various different scientific themes of the humanities but rather develops it against the backdrop of physics, chemistry, and astronomy.

Since Kuhn's most widely read book *The Structure of Scientific Revolutions* appeared in 1962, a vast number of people have made use of this word "paradigm" in private, professional, and scientific contexts of all kinds. The only thing that actually links everyone using this concept that we can acknowledge here is the blurred aspect of paradigm: it appears to be something important and significant which is present in every scientific (discipline) but is different in each case. With this vague and vacuous "smallest common denominator," the value of this concept degenerated to the point of becoming a kind of jolly joker in the scientific world, a word that, like in the "Emperors' New Clothes" only appeared to represent the illusion of authority in argumentative discourse. It assumed this role only after Kuhn and was now in danger of losing its original value.

This prompted me in 2003, as part of a large-scale study, to systematically reconstruct the paradigm concept (Stephenson 2003).

To illustrate the puzzle pieces described at the beginning of this text and show that interpretation ("Deutung") can serve as a legitimate "cognitive instrument" for psychotherapy science (and not just of it!), I will present the most relevant results for our lines of thought (see Stephenson 2003 for an in-depth construction of the results of the cited study). A link is to be established between the results we have obtained and the "abduction discourse."

6.3.2.1 "Exemplars," "Paradigms," and Kuhn's View of the "New" in Science

We must first distinguish between "exemplar" and "paradigm." "Exemplar" is a special, particular phenomenon (that is to say an especially prominent part of "casuistic (that is empirical) archives" of a scientific community), while a "paradigm" is a set of basic assumptions regarding the central subject matter of a discipline (i.e., part of a discipline's system of theories).

In essence, a "paradigm" has three characteristic features:

1. Creates new elements (in the sense of one's not present in the "old" paradigm)
2. In the definition found on the highest level of abstractions
3. Of the central object of study of the discipline

For the arguments developed here, it suffices to illustrate this central meaning of "paradigm" on the basis of the historical example of the essence of light, which Kuhn himself addressed so prominently. All of the studies in physical optics ("light" being the central object of study in this discipline) had been carried out on the assumption that "light" consists of "particles" ("material corpuscles," eighteenth century), while "today's physics textbooks tell the student that light consists is photons, i.e., quantum-mechanical entities that exhibit some characteristics of waves and some of particles" (Kuhn 1969, 11f).

The crucial point here is the "*Deutung*" (interpretation) of the phenomena related to "light," the central object of study: first, "light as particle," then "light as wave," and finally "light as photons," with "photons" showing characteristics of waves and of particles—but in any case conceived as an "autonomous" and thus as a really new entity.

Why "Deutung" and not just simply "interpretation"? The reason is that "Deutung" also essentially operates with the non-observable in the observable! (19)

This phenomenon of human thinking, to operate with the non-observable in the observable, can be found in all realms of human thought, in scientific thought but also in the natural sciences and in the so-called humanities. "Gravity," just like "the unconscious," cannot be directly observed, but the effects of both certainly can be!

In both cases, we are observing certain phenomena in which we can note certain common features, and so we postulate something that is "responsible" for these phenomena and for the common features between them as "something not observable in the observable" ("gravity," "unconscious"). In the following, this something will be the central characteristic of "thought based on 'Deutung' within inferential reasoning."

With this argument, I do not wish to claim that physics and psychoanalysis do not have many and also crucial differences in the way they obtain their insights. I would only like to underscore this essential fact which they both cannot elude: at certain points of both theoretical and empirical thought assumptions must be made which relate to something that can help us order the diversity of phenomena. These mental categories are however not directly observable. Whether we then assume that this "something" (be it a "thing," "process," or "holon") is "part of reality" that can be directly grasped or "part of a construction" that we produce follows a science theoretical paradigm, which is the basic assumptions regarding our cognitive activity. Yet neither "matter" nor "the construction" nor "reality" can be directly observed. Rather, what we observe directly is interpreted "as" that what the paradigm presents it to be.[12] And this is exactly what Kuhn is referring to when he says:

[12] In "interpretation 1" (German: *Deutung*) we create the referential categories for our observations; in "interpretation 2" (German: *Interpretation*), we incorporate what we have observed in the referential categories. This distinction will prove significant in the following!

"That which knows" first creates a foundation of knowledge by means of certain fundamental assumptions so as then, on the basis of these assumptions, to "see" everything "as" the fundamental assumptions claim. The entire mental work that we perform, be it privately, professionally, scientifically, or theoretically, functions according to this principle: the observable only becomes observable by defining and identifying the "non-observable in the observable."

6.3.2.2 Individual-Community Paradigm

Kuhn did not claim his understanding of paradigm to be "absolute" but rather intended it explicitly to be "relative to what knows." A paradigm shift means a change in the basic assumptions of the central object—but in the sense of "center of the background knowledge used in a particular case"! And this background knowledge can be that of an individual but also that of an entire community (or one of their subgroups)!

This distinction opens up the actual field of scientific revolutions. An individual ("the discoverer") uses his work on a specific phenomenon as an opportunity to change his background knowledge (which he shares with a specific group, i.e., the scientific community) in its central aspects. When this happens, a scientific revolution has taken place. Then the really exciting part begins: how will the community react to this? Kuhn claims: by being divided! The larger part of the community will react the way Allen experienced on his return to his home planet: with irritation, anger, resistance, devaluation, ignorance.... Another part will celebrate the discoverer as a messiah and become enthusiastic followers.

All these phenomena only appear in the interaction between individual and community when the very foundations are shaken, that is, when knowledge with a high paradigm value[13] is at stake! Only the context of the given community decides whether these are actually at stake. Physicists rather stoically took note of the paradigm shift implied by the interpretation of light "as photons" and reacted neither with defensive irritation nor fanatic enthusiasm. Optical physics was, by contrast, the epicenter of the revolution, and so this "new" discovery had far-reaching consequences here. All of its research work was based on a new foundation in the sense that its central object of study—"light"—was now interpreted in a new way. Thus also its empirical store, the "casuistry archives" of optical physics, was "purged" and filed with a new type of cases without this having immediate consequences on the casuistic archives and theoretical constructions of other subdisciplines of physics (at least not on all of them.)

The history of psychotherapy is marked by a long series of new communities being established—communities that emerged by precisely such divisions where the "inventors of new interpretations" of what psychotherapy essentially consists of, attracted followers or dissidents. How much this was actually a paradigm shift and scientific revolution will be analyzed in Sect. 6.3.2.

The "place" that can be seen as the "birthplace" of a paradigm is abductions. That is to say, each introduction of a new paradigm constitutes abduction. However, not ever abduction is a paradigm shift in Kuhn's sense. What he refers to as "micro-revolutions" assume a special position. These are ultimately synonymous with the concept of induction—and also with the concept of abduction. Each new insight changes—even if only minimally—both the empirical and theoretical background system. This phenomenon results from the "spiral characteristic" of two scientific circle processes: the "hermeneutic" and the "empirical" circles, which can be regarded as the two basic, interwoven aspects of all scientific thought. We need them to be able to grasp more precisely the thought patterns that have led to the birth of psychoanalysis and continue to decisively influence them to this very day.

[13] This "paradigm value" is higher, the closer the basic elements of the statement come to the core of the definition of the essential aspects of a central object in a given discipline.

6.3.2.3 The Empirico-hermeneutical Circle (Stephenson 2003) and the Four Segments of Scientific Thought

For two centuries, the concept of hermeneutical circle has kept haunting the scientific landscape (Ast 1808, Bohnsack et al. 2011). Without being able to delve into this far-reaching, ramified discourse, I would like to remind the reader of Wolfgang Stegmüller's view of the hermeneutic circle (Stegmüller 1974). Stegmüller showed that this cognitive process should actually be called "hermeneutic spiral" (given the fact that "preliminary knowledge" and "case knowledge" mutually expand each other) while also undermining the dichotomization of natural sciences and humanities by describing the interpretation processes that take place in the hermeneutic spiral as ones that all scientific thought is based on.

The four dimensions of scientific thought (cognitive goals, cognitive instruments, descriptive knowledge, explicative knowledge) described in Fig. 6.3 and to be found in the model of the "empirico-hermeneutical circle"[14] (EHC) also stand in a circular relationship of reference. Which goals do we pursue and which cognitive instruments do we use has a direct effect on which data we can "wrestle" from the phenomena. And which data we are able to collect in observation marks the framework within which we are able to construct our explanatory models of observation.

The connection between both circular processes of cognition is represented in the following figure (Fig. 6.3):

In all four dimensions, "theory" furnishes the "background knowledge" which serves as a "model" on the basis of which we make case-related decisions, that is, which concrete goals we will focus on, which concrete methods referring to the case we will use in our study, which concrete contents from the observation of the given case we will insert in the theoretically given categories of observation, and finally according to which familiar models of explanation we will explain the present case.

And the realization of both takes place through reciprocal enrichment and concentration but more in the sense of a spiral than a circle (see Stegmüller 1974).

With the understanding of each case, my background knowledge also becomes more differentiated, and with greater background knowledge, I am able to approach each new case with a more differentiated perception.

With the understanding of each detail, my understanding of the entire case grows; with increased knowledge about the entire case, my perception of the next detail becomes more differentiated.

If a symptom becomes an object of study, then all three components of observation in the hermeneutical circle are activated. The researcher approaches the "text"[15] of the symptom with "background knowledge," and his background knowledge increases after successfully tackling the "symptom text." At the same time, the understanding of the current symptoms grows with knowledge about its development. And while the dialogue between "subject of knowledge" and "object of knowledge" aims at understanding the symptoms, mutual understanding grows.

Up to this point, the issue was always general principles of scientific thought and inference. And even though, implicitly, all of the principles named thus far were also conceived as binding for psychotherapy science, we will now turn our attention explicitly (and until the end) to this link with psychotherapy science. Precisely this last level is of decisive importance for the phenomena of psychotherapies. Here the two protagonists of psychotherapeutic processes are subject and

[14] This connection of empiricism and hermeneutics is not just based on the "mainstream," where these two often irreconcilable opposites are often addressed. For an inference and argumentation of this "new" conceptuality, see Stephenson (2003).

[15] "Text" here is used in the broadest sense. The Latin word "textum" is the "tissue" that also "covers" what it "marks" (and "protects") as the "tissue"—"tego" meaning "to cover." In this sense everything that humans use in communication (words, gestures, sounds, images, etc.) is "text," i.e., both "indicating and covering." The sense and meaning of a "textum" must also be first grasped. This is something that all scientists processing their "raw data" with natural scientific, nomothetical, empirical means—this data must first be interpreted before insights can be inferred from them!

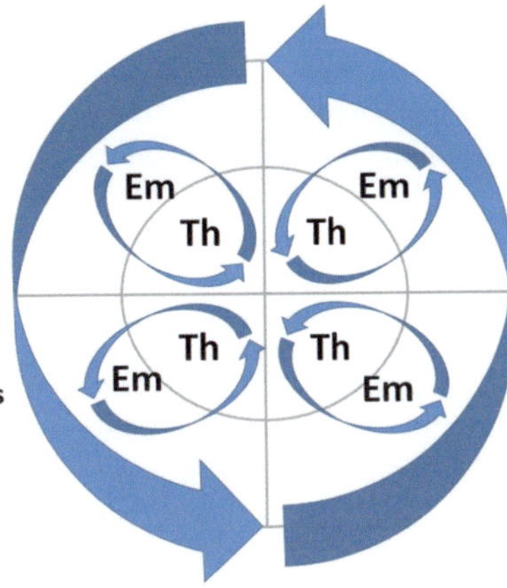

Fig. 6.3 The empirico-hermeneutic circle (*Th* theory, *Em* empiricism)

object at the same time and in a dual sense. The therapist has to see the client both as (his) "object of knowledge" and as a (autonomous) "subject of knowledge." And the client as a *subject of knowledge* also has himself as an *object of knowledge*. Both are implicated in all of the dimensions of the hermeneutic circle described above. What implications this has for psychotherapy science and "interpretation as a cognitive instrument of psychotherapy" will be addressed in Sect. 6.4.

6.3.2.4 Knowledge and Change

The reference just made to the psychotherapeutic situation directs our gaze to a "bifurcation" in the empirical circle with regard to the "goals and means" (i.e., the "left half of the circle" of the empirical circle) in the special case of the psychotherapeutic situation. Diagnosis and therapy are two processes here, both of which are based on descriptions and explanations. However, they are very different in terms of goals and means. The "diagnostic circle" remains within the realm of knowledge. Goals here can only be "cognitive goals"—a "clarification" of the diagnosis will only be guided by the goal of trying to reach an understanding of the client's situation with greater precision or also with confirmation. "Therapy" by contrast turns to the *goals of change* following description and explanation of symptoms. If a situation has been sufficiently grasped and can be explained satisfactorily, then there is the question how it can be changed to the client's benefit. The same is true for the "instruments" of diagnosis and therapy: diagnostic instruments are *cognitive instruments*; therapeutic instruments ("interventions") are "*instruments of change*." We need this distinction in the following when we would like to try, at least tentatively, how, by focusing on "interpretation," it is possible to systematize inferential thinking in psychotherapy science.

6.3.3 Abductions with Varying Paradigm Value in the Empirico-hermeneutical Circle

Before we turn to the situation in which Allen first observes the scientist "fiddling with his testicles"[16] on the stage and then looks over the shoulder of the "bearded scientist" writing a text that is to leave its mark on the world of psychotherapy, we should sum up the categories and distinctions that we have discussed as the foundation of defining "interpretation" (*Deutung*) as a "cognitive instrument."

In inferential thinking, both the descriptive and explicative knowledge and the goals and instruments of knowledge and change are realized as derivative (→*deduction*),

[16] From the original text of the lecture where Charcot actually did this before an audience of men and women: "You remember that (...) on March 15, the continuing pressure on the hysterogenous zone next to the pen... led to a completely classical hysteroepileptic attack happened" (Charcot 1886, p. 269).

incorporative (→*qualitative* "*induction*"), *ampliative* (→*induction*), and *generative* (→"*abduction*") mental acts (and thus as different variants and combinations of *deductive* and *inductive* thought).

The "*newness value*" in the elements of these mental acts *increases* from deductive to generative, while the *frequency* of these mental acts *drops* dramatically from deductive to generative.

In the process, coordination and adaptation take place *within* and *between* the levels of concrete phenomena ("*empiricism*") and the level of generalizations ("*theory*").

In the course of these empirical and theoretical inferences, various types of "*newness*" emerge. From "*expected newness*" in deduction, "*newly refound*" in "qualitative induction" to "*newly created categories in old systems of categories*," newness culminates in abduction by "*new category (systems) with types of cases*," which can also have "the character of revolutionizing science" in a *few* cases.

The range of the effects that this "novelty" then has on all previous and future inferences determines its "paradigm value" which is basically to be found in *the degree of abstraction in the determination of an object*.

To what extent which type of "novelty" is to be found in a given insight (as a product of inferential thinking) depends o the personal context. For two individuals or for an *individual* and his *community*, one and the same insight can be "new" or "old." For a *group*, a new category can show relatively *low* paradigm value, even though a *high* paradigm value exists for a *subgroup*.

All these determinations and distinctions can be used for "private" (psychotherapy clients), "professional" (psychotherapists), and "scientific" (psychotherapy scientists) insights.

6.3.4 The Abductive Paradigm Shift in the Interpretation Patterns of Charcot and Freud

In 1885 when Allen was able to observe him at the Salpetriere giving his lectures, Jean Martin Charcot was a neurologist who was famous and recognized far beyond the circle of specialists. His area of expertise was "neuroses" and here, more specifically, "hysterias." When Allen entered the auditorium, Charcot was just presenting one of his "favorite" group of patients, the "hysterical paralyses." What Allen could not know at this moment is that the man who is sitting next to him and assiduously taking notes is the scientist with the beard whom he will a bit later be looking over his shoulders at Berggasse 19: Sigmund Freud who translated Charcot's lectures from French into German and subsequently was to do a very different type of "translation work."

6.3.4.1 The Failure of Charcot's Abductive Attempts at Interpretation

Charcot had ". . . turned away from the study of nervous disorders that are based on organic changes . . . so as to devote himself exclusively to the study of neuroses, in particular hysteria. . ." (Freud 1886, p. 3). However, he took with him all of the interpretative patterns of his neurological perspective. And his cognitive goals and cognitive instruments were influenced by all of the empirical and theoretical underpinnings of deduction of this particular community. This meant that only a certain group of descriptive insights and only certain types of explanatory insights were possible for him. Precisely with these, he constantly encountered in these cases, which he studied that which Kuhn called "anomalies." The "hysterical" paralyses showed characteristics that let qualitative-inductive classifications under the "nervous disorders based on organic changes" fail. For instance, these disorders could be made to disappear or reappear through by hypnosis. This is a sign of "anomaly" to the extent that such phenomena do not, in certain central elements, correspond to the "normal" combination of neurological paralyses—a "surprising outcome" in Peirce's sense! An element that in inferential reasoning could lead to abductions! If we trace exactly how first Charcot and then Freud reacted to these anomalies, we are able to recognize the different character of abductions with low paradigm value and abductions with high paradigm value—and to thus pave the way for a further epistemological and theory of science definition of interpretation ("*Deutung*").

The decisive passage in Charcot's conclusions reads as follows:

> The monoplegia in question can, however, be explained by a lesion in the cortex which mainly affects the cortical position of the arm, but it is not a serious, material lesion but only a "dynamic" one, a lesion "sine material", in short one that as we are used to assuming, to explain the development and the continuation of the various permanent symptoms of hysteria (loc.cit., 234).

In this way, Charcot is performing an induction in the sense of an expansive introduction of a new category, whose abduction character in the sense of Peirce and whose paradigm value in Kuhn's sense can be verified.

Abductive is the conclusion on the basis of our considerations up until now, to the extent that a "surprising event" (paralysis that can be triggered and reversed by means of hypnosis) which strongly resists all attempts to be incorporated in terms of given qualitative-inductive categories. For him, this had the result that he introduces a "new category" ("dynamical/functional lesion sine material") in the "old system of categories" (=the neurological category system of paralyses) and at the same time specifies the patient as a case of this new category.[17]

The paradigm value of this abduction is however rather low. The degree of generalization is high, but the new category is merely a "stop-gap, it is added as a "complement" to the basic category "organic lesion" ("lesion sine material" which in the organic medical-neurological conceptual system leads to a paradoxical, "non-organic organic lesion"). This is a typical "categorical neutralization" of anomalies: All phenomena whose imprecise match we were unable to explain or change with regard to the previous categories of comprehension were classified under "miscellaneous."

Thus Charcot's conclusion is also not a "Deutung" in the following sense—something we had defined above as its specific characteristic:

"Interpretation" (*Deutung*) also operates in essence with "non-observable in the observable"!

The "non-observability" is to be found in the fact that represents a typical sign of a further "emergency measure" given an imminent paradigm shift. Before the paradigm shift takes place, the basic categories of the old paradigms are expanded and distorted inadmissibly. That he had carried out such an inadmissible inference is something that even Charcot recognizes—and then he tries a further "trick":

> He can only consider those lesions that elude our present-day anatomical methods of study and for which one has agreed to use the designation "dynamical" or functional lesions for lack of a better expression (Charcot 1886, p. 260).

The "lesion" can thus not be observed because the investigative instruments of neurology are not developed far enough for one to be able to make the "material" of the "lesion" visible. The paradigm tries to salvage itself.

We thus have to withdraw the title of "Deutung" from Charcot's statement (and to put it down as an inadmissible abduction-deduction trick) and will not be able to introduce it before Freud who introduced something *per definitionem* non-observable, but something that can be grasped as a category as an always inclusive element of all his conclusions: the unconscious!

6.3.4.2 Freud's Abductive Attempts at Interpretation Reach the Necessary Paradigm Value

The element which in the microanalytical study of the difference between Charcot's and Freud's abductions is the most effective in providing knowledge is the concept of the "voluntary motoric actions" of the patients.

Charcot's and Freud's patients were not capable of performing certain motoric acts even though they wanted to! This fact fulfilled a criterion for "paralysis." If a group of muscles or part of the body cannot be moved, then it is "paralyzed." The anomaly only became visible

[17] For Kuhn this would be an *exemplar* used *to preserve the old paradigm*.

in the neurological examination, and the anomaly grew with the intensive, meticulous application of neurological instruments that were available at the time. These could not recognize any physiological or anatomic obstacles for carrying out the desired movements. When, however, a functional muscle which could be tensed by the deliberate will of the individual on the basis of his physiological disposition and then in spite of deliberate will could not be tensed, then abduction will by necessity have to be directed at something fundamentally different than physiology, if no permanent physiological causes for the "paralysis" can be noted.

And this is something that Freud did: he did not direct his attention to the nerve cells but to the will! And his abduction has the highest value as a paradigm: in addition to deliberate will, there is a different type of will in us, and this resides I the unconscious!

Thus he interprets the neurological conceptual system "neurosis-hysteria"—"hysterical paralyses"—in such a radically new way that he not only departed from the field of "medicine-neurology"; he also created a separate new discipline: psychoanalysis as the first version of psychotherapy science! Here, from the beginning, what is *per definitionem* non-observable in the observable, which can still be grasped in category and thus be studied systematically, is an all-inclusive element of all inferences: the unconscious! And this basic figure of interpretative thinking does not depend on the selection of the name "unconscious" but from the non-observables that can be grasped on categories on the basis of inferential thought that can be "seen" in what can be observed. These "interpretations in the broadest sense" characterize all versions of PT and psychotherapy science to this very day![18]

[18] I know that this is a bold claim. And it is clear to me that meanwhile even the psychotherapeutic system of behavioral therapy works with a variation of the concept, simply because it is impossible otherwise to explain certain phenomena. This in itself is an interesting phenomenon.

Proceeding from this paradigmatic first step of founding a specific way of thinking Freud constructs the first foundations of a new discipline. When Allen looks over his shoulder, Freud is just writing the following passage in one of his examples which he uses to create and expand his paradigm, the case history of Miss Elisabeth v.R. The analysis had reached a point where a memory that had been repressed up until now surfaced in the patient's consciousness and Freud rejoices:

> Now of course everything was clear. The analyst's efforts were being richly rewarded. The ideas of "defense" of an unbearable idea, the emergence of hysterical symptoms through conversion of psychic excitation into the physical, the formation of a separate psychic group through the act of volition, which leads to defense—all of this became so clear, so tangible to (...) This is the way things happened and no other way. This girl had given her brother-in-law a tender gesture... She had succeeded in sparing herself of the painful certainty that she loved her sister's husband by creating physical pains for this, and in moments in which this certainty sought to impose itself (on strolls with him, during a morning reverie, while bathing, before her sister's bed), those pains emerged through successful conversion into the somatic. (Freud 1895, p. 222)

For us, the joy Freud found in such abductive creation of categories of defense, conversion, etc., is not so interesting as the fact that Freud here already begins to differentiate his conceptual system, which congruently follows the first paradigm created. He has already completed the greatest paradigm shift! For this is a paradigm shift in the purest sense: located in the highest generalization of the object "man," it regulates the relations of the worlds which "man" partakes of; mind and matter, the so-called psychophysical relation comes into play.

Petra Stoerig's elaborations on the "psychophysical problem" illustrate especially well how specifications (and thus also abductions) on this level show the highest value as paradigm and how this can be demonstrated in relation to the example taken up by both Freud and Charcot: "hysterical paralyses."

> The special sciences show which structures are needed to smoothly execute an arbitrary

> movement, in which areas process of the central nervous system take place, when the activity in the movement of the muscle groups involved is coordinated... and where and when which patterns of excitation accompany the deliberate decision of a motoric act. They thus answer the question as to the physical foundation of the possibility of voluntary movements... They thus expand our knowledge of the body and these results can be integrated specifically in psychophysical solutions attempts. (Stoerig 1985, 108f, italicized by T.S.)

> Can the necessary conditions defined by the special sciences ... be seen as sufficient for the execution of an voluntary movement?... The answer depends on the *psychophysical view* that one holds (...) A parallelist, an epiphenomenalist, an identity theoreticians, will see the conditions as sufficient, whereas a mentalist, an interaction dualist, an interaction emergentist will regard the *mental act of deciding* as the one *actually* triggering the action. (...) The active creation of holistic neuronal patterns in the motoric association cortex can be identified with the decision, can be understood as parallel action or as something that was mentally triggered, but it can also be interpreted as the cause of the epiphenomenal (...) decision. (loc. cit., italics by T.S.)

Freud in a certain sense changed Charcot's interpretation of phenomena "neurosis," "hysteria," and "hysteric paralyses," which gave his abductions maximum value in the sense of creating a paradigm. Charcot posits one world in which all phenomena are material and that which he calls "psychical" is then merely a "epiphenomenon," that is, a sort of "appendix" in a world in which everything is in essence matter and thus all illnesses are physical or organic. Thus, the appendix "dynamic or functional" lesions, whose "material" had already been found or had to be found. What Freud did in this respect was actually the shift of the paradigm of the highest order, which influenced all of the "subordinate" parts of the paradigm. Freud juxtaposed a "theory of interaction" to Charcot's epiphenomenalism and decided to focus of the world of the "psyche," the "mind" (or whatever other name one might give this highest concept), and to make it the primary object of study. In this "world of the psyche" which in all explanatory models of (not only) "neurosis," "hysteria," and "hysterical paralysis" are seen as the "prima causa," he then separated, in a second act of creation, "lightness" from "darkness." In the world of the psyche, the "conscious" is now juxtaposed with the "unconscious," and they, too, mutually influence each other just as psyche and soma also stood in a reciprocal relation on equal footing.

In summary, we can state the following in the "language of inferences":

"Interpretation" in the Freudian sense is every inference that identifies an "outcome" that can be observed in the physical or psychical realm as a "case" of the effect of the unconscious ("rule") as the "non-observable in the observable."

6.3.4.3 The Traces of the "Basic Interpretative Pattern" in the History of the Diversification of Psychotherapy

The claim made at the beginning of this study is that in the development of psychotherapy, it is possible to detect a characteristic basic pattern of both the psychotherapy process and the diversification of psychotherapy schools. Here, however, we can only give a cursory overview of the basic trait with a few examples.

The "highest paradigm" ("psyche as *causa prima*") retains its effect in all "dissident" cases of the history of the psychotherapy,[19] which could at the same be described as paradigm shift. In the structure of the large areas of the therapeutic process (interpersonal aspects in the therapist and client and the relationship between the two, etc.), the later founders of their own schools again and again posited paradigm-like abductions of an interpretative nature. Adler, for instance, undermined Freud's "monism of drives" and postulating, next to the sexual drive, an aggression drive, which resulted not only on all "subordinate levels" dramatic changes with implications for personality theory and practical treatment. Because of the high par-

[19] And it gives the entire discipline its name: psychotherapy science as the science that studies the "treatment" of the *psyche*!

adigm value of his abductions, it also led to Adler being banished from the Wednesday Society associated with the Freud paradigm. Jung postulated, by abduction, his own paradigmatic realm of the unconscious, which was also formative for his entire "analytical psychology": the collective unconscious. Rogers initiated a paradigm shift on the level of the relational structure between therapist and patient, postulating an existential equivalence of the two persons involved in the process. He thus undermined the old "rift between doctor and patient," lending humanist psychology its typical characteristic.

In all of these cases and in many others, we can find the "characteristic of interpretation" postulated here—the aggression drive, the collective unconscious, and in Carl Roger's "organismic valuing" all represent something *per definitionem* non-observable in the observable, which can still be grasped in categories and studied systematically and is treated as an element that must always be included in all inferences. This process reflects a certain sequence of abductive, inductive, and deductive thinking. In the beginnings of the schools of systemic therapy, one finds the new paradigm of the "third beings," the personal system that emerges when at least two people come together, and this is more than just the "addition of these two individuals." As the "third being," it is invisible but at the same time it can be grasped in categories as a basic constant and can thus be differentiated as a foundation for all theories and interventions. Even in behavioral therapy, one can note such a characteristic from the beginning to the present. The "black box" of the Stone Age of behavioral therapy is even the most extreme hard-core example of this. In the observable aspects of the stimuli-reaction process, there is something non-observable *per definitionem*—namely, the black box. We cannot see into this box, and thus nothing more is said on what numerous fundamental changes took place in the course of the development of the behavioral therapy schools. This not only changed nothing about the previous introduction of the black box as "something lying between the stimuli and reaction," it also became an extreme expression of non-observability.

To what extent the "characteristic of interpretation" and the aspect of paradigm shift can be applied to the "basic pattern of the process of psychotherapy" will be examined in Sect. 6.4.

6.4 "Interpretation" as a Means of Gaining Knowledge in Psychotherapy Science

At the end of our journey, we can now take a look at the various discoveries we have made against the backdrop of our "puzzle pieces" and the different aspects of "interpretation." This will allow us to give a systematic summary. But before we do that, let's look over the shoulders of Tim and Allen and let them have the final word.

6.4.1 Interpretations in General Science, Psychotherapy Science, and Psychoanalysis

In general science, every inference that uses what is non-observable (in the sense that it can only be indirectly observed through its effects) in the observable as part of its premise-conclusion structure can be seen as a general scientific interpretation (Deutung GS), that is, an interpretation in the widest sense. From this perspective, the use of the term "gravity" in physics is an interpretation.

A psychotherapeutic interpretation (interpretation PTS) as an inferential interpretation in a wider sense can be found in a premise-conclusion statement structure, when an inference is made from an observable surface structure of human behavior to non-observable deep structure and the surface structure is interpreted on the basis of its effect. Here speaking of the unconscious in this sense as speaking of social systems of the black box placed between stimulus and reaction and the "organismic valuing" can be seen as interpretation in a further sense since in each case it is a construction that cannot be directly observed.

And those inferences that refer to a psychoanalytical deep structure (interpretation PA) can be seen as interpretation in the narrowest sense. An explanation of certain behavioral modes within the therapeutic relationship as the effect of unconscious components such as transference and countertransference would be such an interpretation.

To what extent psychotherapy science research can identify interpretations in the widest, wider, or narrowest sense is an issue for self-reflection in psychotherapy science. In any case we can note a differentiation as is presented in Fig. 6.1, elaborated on in the chapter on "Types of Abductions" (see Sect. 6.3.1) and summarized in the following in Sect. 6.4.6.

6.4.2 Interpretation in the Context of Inferential Thinking

Interpretations in the broadest, broader, and most restricted sense, that is to say interpretations in general science, psychotherapy science, and psychoanalysis, are based on a sequence of various types of inferences. This mental pattern refers to the combination of inductive, deductive, and abductive thought. Here the specific nature of interpretation only represents the non-observable deep structure of the object of study—a structure that is then an integrative part of the deductive, inductive, and abductive thought. Figure 6.4 depicts all "stations" from 1 to 10 or steps of interpretation.

1. When what we perceive on the surface structure of behavior can no longer be grasped and explained without recourse to the non-observable, we first use deductive, that is, derivative interpretations. Here everything we already know about the given deep structure is used.
2. When a deduction fails, we first
3. try to carry out other interpretive classifications, i.e., to interpret on the basis of qualitative induction.
4. If this succeeds, then everything begins again with 1.
5. If these attempts fail, then we look for a solution in ampliative, i.e., inductive thinking.
6. If existing categories can be expanded by means of subcategories, then everything begins again with 1.
7. If the deductive experiment also fails with the expanding results of induction (permanently)
8. Then we begin trying abductive interpretations (at first with low paradigm value).
9. If this is successful, then everything begins again with 1.
10. If attempts at abductive interpretation with low paradigm value do not prove successful,

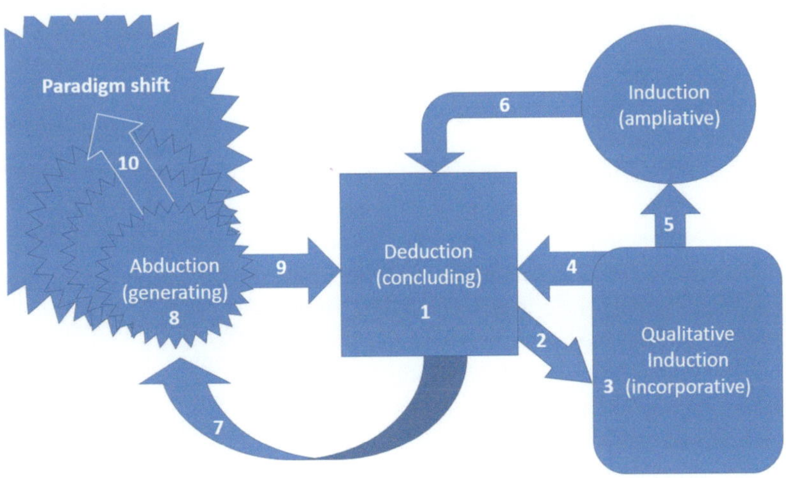

Fig. 6.4 Interpretation in the context of inferential thinking

the paradigm value of the next abductive interpretation is increased until a paradigm change takes place.

11. From this point on, there is a for the most part new referential system for the interpretation steps described in 1–9 in which the steps 1–9 can be carried out over a very long period of time.

What is activated here is a kind of backup system which allows for paradigm change only as a very last resort and lets such events become extremely rare.

The specific aspect of interpretation as a means for gaining knowledge is to be found in the fact that interpretation, proceeding from grasping an observable surface structure of human behavior, infers a non-observable deep structure the effect of which is interpreted as the surface structure.

"Interpretation" provides "translation" of everyday descriptions in (special) scientific "interpretation"—(a) already infers and (b) using non-observable elements in the premises and/or conclusions.

6.4.3 Interpretation as Derivative, Classifying, Expanding, and Generating Means of Gaining Knowledge

In the above description of the steps in inferential-interpretative thought, we postulated that there are deductive, qualitative-inductive, inductive, and abductive interpretations—all with various value as paradigms. These categories correspond to what we have called derivative, classifying, expanding, and generating thought. How can we see this in connection with interpretation?

Examples of interpretations in the most restricted sense, i.e., psychoanalytical interpretations, are most illustrative here. Simply put, deductive-derivative interpretations proceed from already familiar unconscious structural aspects and contents of a client so as to interpret "in the usual fashion" surprising current reaction modes (or also dreams). They sometimes appear as "predictions," i.e., as hypotheses on how the client will react in an imminent situation in keeping with his familiar transference trends.

Qualitative-inductive interpretation attempts are activated when the client, for instance, reports in such a situation that he reacted differently than expected. Interpretations of this can be "incorporative" and thus qualitative-inductive in the sense that others are used from the "pool" of the client's already known unconscious structures and contents so as to be able to interpret and incorporate the "surprising reaction."

If this does not succeed definitively, the process has reached a point where "new" aspects of the unconscious deep structure have to be studied and grasped. A new category of unconscious conflicts can then be the result of such "inductively expanding interpretation."

If one encounters a completely new category of behavioral modes, abductive interpretation is called for. This can have a "revolutionary" effect in varying degrees. If it leads to the creation of an entirely new "section" of unconscious deep structure, the paradigm value of the corresponding interpretations increases. An example of this would be "coming out" experiences that take place in the course of an analysis. Here a person's total sexual orientation and/or the entire gender self-definition become called into question, as is the case in transsexuality, undergoing a radical change. The crux for "interpretation" is that before the "new" orientation had been one that was only *unconscious*.

6.4.4 Interpretation as an Idiographic and Nomothetic Instrument for Gaining Knowledge on Psychotherapy Processes

Using the above example of reorientation, we can also illustrate the distinction between "idiographic" and "nomothetic" interpretations. "Idiographic" interpretations are in certain sense "situation-bound" interpretations, that is, "individualized" interpretations geared to "individual instances" of concrete situations. The concrete "empirical" scenes that constitute the client's biography, lined up like pearls on a string, are directly interpreted in relation to the unique situation—taking into account the unconscious categories appearing here, unconscious explanations, unconscious goals, and unconsciously used "instruments."

In the process there are always possibilities of generalization—common aspects that exist between scenes or certain reactions and behavioral modes allow us to conclude that we are dealing here with a general principle in the client's perception or behavior (or even of the therapist as "private person"), a "private law" or a "private theory" on which the client's individual perceptions and acts are oriented. To determine these by means of interpretation is the task of "nomothetic" interpretations.

Such nomothetic interpretations in particular (but not only) are often the basis for further deductive interpretations that are oriented on the found "private unconscious laws"—interpretations of further or newer situations and of the client's reactions that can be observed here. Here Fig. 6.4 comes to mind where we saw that deduction is the point of departure for every process of interpretation—no matter how diverse it might be. "Nomothetic interpretations" thus exist—just like all other types of interpretations—in both an inductive and abductive version. Out of the generalization of idiographic interpretations (i.e., ones oriented to an individual situation to be interpreted) nomothetic interpretations (i.e., interpretations oriented to a common structure that is superordinate to this and similar situations) could be generated by means of generalization.

6.4.5 Interpretation as an Instrument for Gaining Knowledge on the Process of Psychotherapy from Various Positions

Not just the distinction between deductive, inductive, and abductive thought but also, even more importantly, the reference to explanations, descriptions, goals, and instruments and to

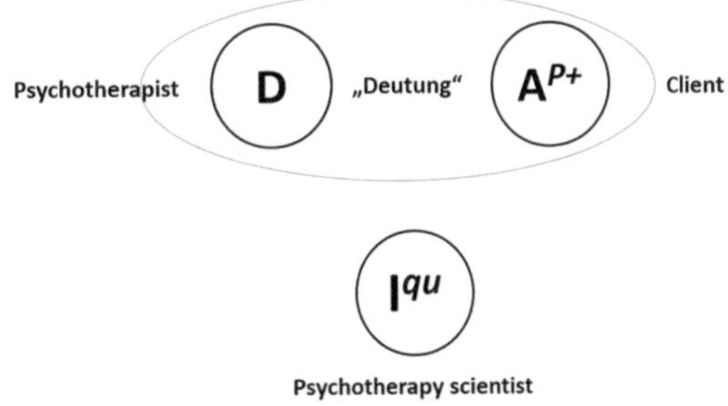

Fig. 6.5 Three positions (*D* deduction, A^{P+} abduction with high paradigm value, I^{qu} qualitative induction)

"idiographic" and "nomothetic" thought require that three positions be distinguished in the process of psychotherapy: that of the client, the therapist, and the scientist. In one and the same situation in the psychotherapeutic process, various types, forms, and contents of interpretations can become visible in the three positions. This is to be illustrated with an example (see Fig. 6.5).

For the client (see Fig. 6.5 where the psychotherapist and the client are marked with an oval as elements of an interactive "therapeutic team"), a certain interpretation can be an element of an abduction with high paradigm value (abduction), while for the psychotherapist it is a product of his deductive thinking (deduction). For the psychotherapy scientist, it can, in turn, be a premise which leads to a conclusion of qualitative-inductive, that is, integrative thinking (induction) when he assigns the interpretation that took place in the process of psychotherapy to one of his categories of interpretation types.

In each of these cases, "interpretative thinking" means something different in the various positions. Most importantly, interpretative thinking does not have to be given in all three positions at the same time. The psychotherapy scientist can, for instance, keep track of and compare "not interpreting" the number of "interpretations in the more restricted sense" as opposed to two certain time periods in the process of the psychotherapy he is observing. In doing so, he remains completely on the surface structure of the object of study he has selected (thus inferring in an interpretive sense, but not "interpreting"!), while in the "professional" position and the "private" position, interpretative thinking and thus an understanding of an unobserved deep structure is taking place.

For us, the decisive conclusion of this line of thought where we move from the level of psychotherapy science to the level of psychoanalysis is to be found in the following thesis: specific psychoanalytic phenomena such as interpretations (in the most restricted sense) as realization of psychoanalytic knowledge of change can be interpreted in the sense of psychotherapy science or research without interpretation! They have both a surface structure and a deep structure—and I can study both empirically provided they are part of a categorical system and can be realized in time and space as concrete singular phenomena.

6.4.5.1 Interpretation as an Instrument for Gaining Knowledge (for the Psychotherapy Client)

In psychoanalysis the client explores his own deep structures from a self-reflexive position (just as the psychotherapist does this from his professional position and the psychotherapy scientist does from the position of his discipline[20]). This requires the client sharing the therapist's paradigm, being convinced in one or the other way that the "unconscious exists." Many analyses have an initial phase in which the client has to be convinced of the purpose of introducing categories of one's own unconscious perceptions, unconscious systems of convictions, how the world and life is to be explained, unconscious (neurotic and non-neurotic) goals of the use of certain means to reach one's own unconscious goals—before analysis "gets going." If this succeeds, then this ultimately means that the client has partaken of the "top paradigm shift".[21] For most clients this is initially a bit like entering a new world in which almost all insights have abductive value, many even resemble paradigm shifts in what is taken for granted. Idiographic and nomothetic hear also refer to one's own "empirical" and "theoretical" background.

6.4.5.2 Interpretation as an Instrument for Gaining Knowledge for the Psychotherapist

For the psychotherapist, each client means a new realm of experience. The "empirical and theoretical knowledge" of the therapist regarding the laws and specificities of both conscious surface structures and unconscious deep structures is incomparably greater than that of the client. And this knowledge refers to what he has learned in training and what he has learned from experience. His goals and instruments for gaining knowledge and bringing about change, the possibilities and limits thereof, are "professional" and are derived or created anew for each therapeutic process. They refer to the work with the client (and to the reactions that might appear in the therapist during the therapeutic process) and not to one's own life (as in the case of the client).

At the same time, he shares "community knowledge" with other colleagues who have received training for the same school of therapy. This knowledge develops further in the course of one's own professional experience. The psychotherapists who work "in the solitude" of their own practice, those who do not engage in any exchange with colleagues, develop a rather "individual-professional" background knowledge. A comparison of interpretations and their backgrounds between psychotherapists of the same school can yield very different results. For the therapist, "nomothetic" inferences mean inductions on the basis of the cases available to him. It can be assumed that a rather large

[20] Here we once again have the perspective of a "double hermeneutics," as, for instance, is highlighted by Smith (2004). He refers to "double hermeneutics: The participant is trying to make sense of their personal and social world; the researcher is trying to make sense of the participant trying to make sense of their personal and social world" (p. 40).

[21] Practical insights to the effect that clients undergoing Freudian analysis increasingly dream more "Freudian" (or dream more "Adlerian" or more "Jungian" when undergoing Adlerian or Jungian analysis) are proof of even more far-reaching "co-optations."

percentage of "solitary" psychotherapists have already created abductive products of thought with a high paradigm value and proceed on the basis of these by deductive means. Who knows how many "new schools" Allen was able to see from his space ship—schools that never saw the light of day in the world of professional communities.

6.4.5.3 Interpretation as a Means of Gaining Knowledge for the Psychotherapy Scientist

In addition to his observations and generalizations, the work of the psychotherapy scientist is enriched by yet another dimension, especially since the scientific principle compels him to engage in exchanges with his community and he is able to benefit from ongoing discussions.

He is interested in integrating the processes taking place between individual therapists and clients in general models of psychotherapy or expanding these models and restructuring them on the basis of new insights. He grasps, interprets, and "reads" interpretations (which results in a sort of "dual hermeneutics"; see Giddens 1984, p. 200). Within the psychotherapeutic processes that he observes or the information he gets from therapists or patients, he reads these interpretations as a text.

In addition to the "working conditions" to be found in all sciences, psychotherapy science offers a unique case in that it is a special "synthesis/pool of paradigmatic patterns of interpretation." Most psychotherapy scientists are psychotherapists (not absolutely necessary but usually the case). Thus the community ("psychotherapy scientists") is essentially a constellation of subgroups ("psychotherapy scientists with psychoanalytic paradigms," "psychotherapy scientists with behavior theory paradigms," etc.) As we saw above, any psychotherapeutic process that is governed by the paradigms of a certain school of psychotherapy can, in principle, be studied by any psychotherapy scientist (our "non-interpreting" scientist who counted the "interpretations" does not by necessity have to be a psychoanalyst). But for a number of reasons, the right "expertise" of each school can have advantages in researching a certain object of study. Assuming that "critical reflection of the boundaries of meaning and validity of the schools and disciplines of thought and action in psychotherapy" (Greiner 2013, p. 91) can, and should, be regarded as a special achievement of psychotherapy science as a timely research platform, then one could come to believe "that precisely for its pluralism of arguments, its diversity of languages and its heterogeneous methodology contemporary psychotherapy not only has an edge in theoretical research but also advantages in terms of scientific reflection as compared to all other academic movements in science" (Greiner in this volume, Chap. 5).

6.4.6 Interpretation and the Fundamental Issue of Psychotherapy Science

The phenomenon in the psychotherapeutic situation that has been addressed here for illustrative purposes, namely, the psychotherapeutic outcome (see parts II and III of this volume), is the primary issue of psychotherapy science but certainly not the only one. The study of culture-specific and social "surrounding conditions" of this psychotherapeutic phenomenon (e.g., Orlinsky 2004a, b) is just as legitimate objects of psychotherapeutic study and the historical developments of various schools of psychotherapy (Frank and Frank 1993), theoretical and philosophical approaches (see Chaps. XXX Rieken and XXX Greiner; Slife 2004), and much more. Psychotherapy scientists should have "a model (i.e., a simplified version) of psychotherapy which has a heuristic (orienting, describing) function" (Gelo 2013) which can be taken from current discussions.

In such models basic categories and the fundamental of the therapeutic process are described. David Orlinsky, for instance, describes in his "generic model" six such basic categories: the therapeutic pact, the techniques used to implement the pact, the therapeutic alliance, the self-references of those involved in the interaction, the repercussions of the given session, and the temporal sequence of events within and following the sessions (Cf. Orlinsky 2004a, b, p. 88).

There are pre-structured "surrounding conditions" that can be used to study the therapeutic process. Here one also finds the different types of categories in which social, economic, cultural, religious,[22] and other parameters are networked with the structural elements of the psychotherapeutic process (see above). Here descriptive and explicative knowledge and the "interpretive patterns" of inferential thought come to bear in psychotherapy science. These, too, are pre-structured just as the respective goals of research and the cognitive instruments that are used.

In all of the different "models of interpretation" that one can find in the pertinent literature of psychotherapy science, one is able to note the typical traits of "interpretative patterns." We will hear a little bit more about this from Tim and Allen, our "alien companions."

6.5 Outlook

Tim and Allen are getting back into their time-space machine. They have peeked over our shoulders, and each has experienced in his own way the ideas that we presented here as a "surprising outcome." Other results that might strike us as "surprising" are our "old ALTER HUT" for them. In any case, they found it really interesting to watch people think on this planet. They took back a lot of data for their own research back home. And they will apply for funding from their ministry of research and provide us, in turn, with a certain kind of knowledge that cannot even be sketched in the mental processes described here. The knowledge regarding the "black box" in which the unobserved processes, what lies between the lines of our explicit knowledge, constitutes the greatest part of our thoughts and acts, resides here. When they give us this knowledge, the storm of paradigm shifts will be unprecedented not just in psychotherapy science.

[22] Just by virtue of the very use of this name such a categorization is taking place!

There is one thing that Allen already learned when he completed his studies on the old mortal scientist with the white beard. Socrates was, in reality, also an alien in connection with Allen's and Tim's knowledge. Their translation of his most famous statement "ouda ouk eidos" (which is usually falsely translated as: "I know that I know nothing!") "ouda ouk eidos," in the inversion, contains a significant reference to this "black box." When Socrates exclaimed: "I, a knower, do not know!" and thus identified the uncertainty of all our knowledge as a certainty, he was also expressing the opposite "We non-knowers know": Allen and Tim already studied the foundations of the non-observable in the observable aspects of thought. This refers to what we call "implicit knowledge" or "intuition"—that which we only know plays a really crucial role in psychotherapies and about which we still have only questions but hardly any answers. We are thus anxiously waiting for the time-space machine that will bring us this knowledge for the psychotherapy science of the future.

References

Adorno TW (1973) Philosophische Frühschriften (Band 1 der gesammelten Schriften). Suhrkamp, Frankfurt am Main

Ast F (1808) Grundlinien der Grammatik, Hermeneutik und Kritik. Thomann, Landshut

Bohnsack R, Marotzki W, Meuser M (2011) Hauptbegriffe Qualitativer Sozialforschung. Verlag Barbara Budrich, Opladen

Charcot JM (1886) Neue Vorlesungen über die Krankheiten des Nervensystems, insbesondere über Hysterie. Toeplitz & Deuticke, Leipzig

Deutscher G (2002) On the misuse of the notion of 'abduction' in linguistics. J Linguis 38:469–485

Frank JD, Frank JB (1993) Persuasion & healing. A comparative study of psychotherapy, John Hopkins Paperback Editions. Johns Hopkins University Press, Baltimore, MD

Freud S (1886) Vorwort des Übersetzers. In: Charcot JM (ed) Neue Vorlesungen über die Krankheiten des Nervensystems, insbesondere über Hysterie. Toeplitz & Deuticke, Leipzig, pp III–IV

Freud S (1895) Studien über Hysterie. GW I, 81-251. Frankfurt am Main: Fischer (1999)

Freud S (1927) Nachwort zur Frage der Laienanalyse. Erstveröff.: Zeitschrift für Psychoanalyse, XIII.Jg, Heft 2 und 3, GW XIV, 207–296

Gelo OCG (2012) On research methods and their philosophical assumptions: "raising the consciousness of researchers" again. Psychotherapie Sozialwissenschaft 14(2):111–130

Gelo OCG (2013) Perspektiven der Psychotherapiewissenschaft. Vorlesungsmanuskript. SFU, Burnaby, BC

Gelo OCG, Braakmann D, Benetka G (2008) Quantitative and qualitative research: beyond the debate. Integr Psychol Behav Sci 42(3):266–290. doi:10.1007/s12124-008-9078-3

Gelo OCG, Braakmann D, Benetka G (2009) Erratum to "Quantitative and qualitative research: beyond the debate". Integr Psychol Behav Sci 43(4):406–407. doi:10.1007/s12124-009-9107-x

Giddens A (1984) The constitution of society, outline of the theory of structuration. Polity Press, Cambridge

Greiner K (2013) Was ist Psychoanalytische Forschung? Eine zeitgemäße Antwort wissenschaftstheoretischer Art. In: Fengli; Wallner u. Schulz, pp 127–136

Kelle U (1994) Empirisch begründete Theoriebildung. Zur Logik und Methodologie interpretativer Sozialforschung. Deutscher Studienverlag, München

Kelle U (2003) Abduktion und Interpretation. Die Bedeutung einer 'Logik der Entdeckung' für die hermeneutische Sozialforschung. In: Ziebertz H-G, St. Heil, Prokopf A (Hrgs) Abduktive Korrelation. LitVerlag, Münster, S.109–S.124

Kelle U (2007) Die Integration qualitativer und quantitativer Methoden in der empirischen Forschung. VS Verlag, Wiesbaden

Keller R (2013) Doing discourse research. Sage, London

Kuhn TS (1962) The structure of scientific revolutions. University of Chicago Press, Chicago

Mitchell S (1988) Relational concepts in psychoanalysis. An integration. Harvard University Press, Harvard

Mitchell S (1998) Relationality: from attachment to intersubjectivity. Analytic Press, Hillsdale, NJ (2003)

Orlinsky D (2004a) Der menschliche Kontext von Psychotherapien. Eine handlungstheoretische Systemanalyse von Einflüssen auf therapeutische Kontexte von Psychotherapien. Teil 1: Der soziale und kulturelle Kontext von Psychotherapie. Psychotherapeut 49:88–100

Orlinsky D (2004b) Der menschliche Kontext von Psychotherapien. Eine handlungstheoretische Systemanalyse von Einflüssen auf therapeutische Kontexte von Psychotherapien. Teil 2: Die individuellen Kontexte von Psychotherapie. Psychotherapeut 49: 167–181

Przyborski A, Wohlrab-Sahr M (2008) Qualitative Sozialforschung. Ein Arbeitsbuch. Oldenbourg Verlag, München

Reichertz J (2004) Abduction, deduction an induction in qualitative research. In: Flick U et al (eds) Companion to qualitative research. Sage, London, pp S.159–S.165

Reichertz J (2010) Abduction: the logic of discovery of grounded theory. In: Bryant A, Charmaz K (eds) The Sage handbook of grounded theory. Sage, London, pp S.214–S.229

Reichertz J (2011) Abduktion. In: Bohnsack u.a. pp 11–14

Reichertz J (2013) Die Abduktion in der qualitativen Sozialforschung: Über die Entdeckung des Neuen. Springer Fachmedien, Wiesbaden (2003, 2013)

Rieken B (2013) Überlegungen zur Akademisierung der Psychotherapie – am Beispiel der Sigmund-Freud-Privatuniversität Wien. Ztschr. F. Individualpsychologie 2013, Jg. 38 Heft 03, 285–302

Salvatore S, Valsiner J (2010) Between the general and the unique. Overcoming the nomothetic versus idiographic. Theory Psychol 20(6):817–833

Slife BD (2004) Theoretical challenges to therapy practice and research: the constraint of naturalism. In: Lambert MJ (ed) Bergin and Garfield's handbook of psychotherapy and behavior change, 5th edn. Wiley, New York, pp 44–83

Smith JA (2004) Reflecting on the development of Interpretative phenomenological analysis and its contribution to qualitative research in psychology. Qual Res Psychol 1:39–54

Stegmüller W (1974) Das Problem der Induktion: Humes Herausforderung und moderne Antworten./Der sogenannte Zirkel des Verstehens. Wissenschaftliche Buchgesellschaft, Darmstadt

Stephenson T (2003) Paradigma und Pädagogik. Wissenschaftsanalytische Untersuchungen im Spannungsfeld zwischen Pädagogik, Therapie und Wissenschaft. Empirie Verlag, Wien

Stephenson T (2011) SFU-IP –Erste Konturen einer sich neu bildenden Community. In: Rieken B (Hg) Alfred Adler heute. Zur Aktualität der Individualpsychologie. Waxmann, Münster, pp S.9–S.39

Stoerig P (1985) Leib und Psyche. Eine interdisziplinäre Erörterung des psychophysischen Problems. Fink, München

Straub HR (2009) Das interpretierende System: Wortverständnis und Begriffsrepräsentation in Mensch und Maschine: Mit einem Beispiel zur Diagnose-Codierung. ZIM-Verlag, Wolfertswil

Strübing J (2004) Grounded theory. VS für Sozialwissenschaften, Wiesbaden

Wallerstein RS (2009) Psychoanalysis in the university: a full-time vision. Int J Psychoanal 90:1107–1121

Institutional Parameters of Psychotherapy Education as a Prerequisite for Systematic Psychotherapy Research 7

Alfred Pritz

Contents

Abstract
Admission requirements for psychotherapy training have been defined historically and are different across countries. In European certificates, which have a synoptic regulation with modern content and include different psychotherapy degrees, general basic requirements for comparative, empirical psychotherapy research are missing or rudimentary. There is a need to create a better description of the basic premises in research projects.

A. Pritz (✉)
Department of Psychotherapy Science, Sigmund Freud University, Freudplatz 1, 1020 Vienna, Austria
e-mail: alfred.pritz@sfu.ac.at

7.1 Introduction

Psychotherapy research, which, generally speaking, measures its worth by results, needs a mandatory introductory amount of basic data and a certain homogeneity of the group under investigation. This chapter aims to show that the basic data and the homogeneity of the researched group—namely, psychotherapy as it is practiced by psychotherapists in several countries—are sparse due to different historical and institutional developments (Pritz 2002a). It is thus necessary to communicate the historical facts and institutional frames in the training of psychotherapy to foster a comprehensive understanding for any particular research enterprise on psychotherapy. Psychotherapy as a human science of subjectivity (Pritz 1996, 2008) needs to describe its content as well as its borders.

7.2 On the Regulation of Psychotherapy Training

Sigmund Freud established regulated psychotherapy education in the 1920s. Three elements were implemented: the training analysis, the analysis that a psychoanalytic candidate undergoes, and the theoretical training and the supervision of psychotherapy performed by the candidate. This training triad is found today in most psychotherapy curricula (Pritz 2002a).

O.C.G. Gelo et al. (eds.), *Psychotherapy Research*,
DOI 10.1007/978-3-7091-1382-0_7, © Springer-Verlag Wien 2015

Only in recent decades has the need for a regulated training for psychotherapists developed, mainly due to the intensified focus on the legalization of psychotherapy as a profession. Nine European countries have professional regulation for psychotherapists; this first began in Sweden in 1985. As of 2014, Finland, Sweden, Italy, Germany, Austria, Switzerland, France, Netherlands, and Malta have these regulations. A legal, partially regulated division (sphere/area/domain) for the practice of psychotherapy exists in other countries such as Hungary and Bulgaria. All these countries have legal regulations for admission to and requirements of the training and predetermined conditions for completion. The juristic regulations are different in many ways, but one commonality is noticeable. Countries outside the European Union have regulations for psychotherapy training, but they are part of the regulations of an occupational group. There is, for example, a regulation for psychiatrists who want to practice psychotherapy in Russia and similar regulations for clinical psychologists in Chile, Canada, and many states in the USA (see more different regulations in Pritz 2002b).

None of the juristic regulations for psychotherapists developed in recent decades are intended for a medical doctor monopoly, meaning doctors' exclusive access to psychotherapy training and the authorization to practice. This is remarkable inasmuch as the struggle for autonomy for psychotherapy has been going on for approximately 100 years (Pritz 2011). The first hurdle was the emancipation from the exclusive doctor yoke. Sigmund Freud cherished this notion in his near-prophetic publication "Zur Frage der Laienanalyse," in which he said that a doctor is an amateur of psychoanalysis if he or she has not learned it, equal to everyone else (Freud 1926). This publication came about after Otto Rank was supposed to take over the administration of the psychoanalytic outpatient clinic at the Vienna General Hospital (which was then, as it is now, the largest hospital in Austria).

The Austrian Medical Chamber denounced him in court because as a psychologist he had no authorization to treat patients. After Freud's publication, Rank immigrated to Berlin, and the trial ceased. It became clear that independence from the medical profession would need to be fought for because it put the monopoly doctors had on the treatment of all illnesses into question. This was not achieved in Austria until a federal law was passed in 1990. However, a threefold claim was made that included required training, the requirement to treat psychological disorders independently from medical practitioners, and independence from other professions, such as medicine. The last aspect naturally reflects the situation of psychoanalysis in the decade after the First World War, when more and more psychologists and graduates from other professions were accepted to psychoanalytic training.

This conflict would continue in countries like Germany, the USA, England (which to this day has no legal psychotherapy regulation), Italy, France, and numerous other countries, although a certain tolerance is maintained in countries without legal regulations, as long as the demand to treat patients is not raised (like in Great Britain and Spain).

Another commonality is admission to the training from different caring professions, and the differences lie in which lobbies were able to push their interest during the creation of the law. Only in the Netherlands, Italy, and Switzerland were psychologists privileged to be the second group besides medical doctors admitted into psychotherapy training, whereas various professional groups were allowed in other countries. Furthermore, a commonality lies in the specification of training standards, which are also very different in their details. With the exception of France, where only professions such as doctors, psychologists, and, notably, psychoanalysts (all three professional groups without a proof of education) are legitimized, laws across all other countries require proof of education. The title of medical doctor is provided after the completion of training and the permission to practice as a psychotherapist. Another similarity is the training for different psychotherapy modalities, whereby psychoanalysis is legally licensed in all countries and other psychotherapy schools vary in licensure.

Table 7.1 Psychotherapy education of licensed professional groups in 21 EU countries

Professional group	*N*
Psychologists	21
Medical doctors	21
Social workers	15
Pedagogues	11
Nurses	12
Social pedagogues	5
Teachers	3
Theologians	3
Other professions	10

N number of EU countries

Public forms of payment for psychotherapeutic treatment exist, to a certain extent, in countries with a psychotherapy law (exceptions: Italy and France), and payment is usually regulated by health insurance.

As previously noted, there are considerable differences in legal regulations between countries; these differences are illustrated through the features of the admission to training and the current regulated training. Strauss (Strauss, B. cit. in Pritz 2011) researched completed education prior to psychotherapy training in Europe (see Table 7.1).

As seen, psychologists and medical doctors are the two professional groups most admitted to psychotherapy training in the 21 EU countries considered, followed by social workers and pedagogues. Based on these differences, one can understand the difficult battle between the different professional groups; the differences show who was successful in this battle and who was defeated. These battles were admittedly waged with arguments, but from a distant perspective, the divide is not really an argument for the main debate.

For example, how is it that in Switzerland only psychologists and doctors are admitted to psychotherapy training, whereas in neighboring Austria, theologists, communication researchers, nurses, medical-technical professionals, and pedagogues, among others, are also permitted? How does this situation influence psychotherapy research? There are currently no comparative data on this topic.

The differences in the training parameters are also considerably noticeable. For example, Germany requires a 3- to 4-year postgraduate training for psychologists and social pedagogues, whereas non-medical practitioners who have permission to practice psychotherapy need a training of only approximately a half year (minimum). There are also considerable differences for doctors in Germany. If a doctor aspires to complete additional training, he must complete several hundred hours to become a specialist for psychosomatic medicine and psychotherapy to complete a psychoanalytic or behavioral therapy training. In regard to legally defined training parameters, Germany simultaneously has the highest and lowest requirements for psychotherapy training.

The differences are also particularly obvious in the recognition of professional training in individual psychotherapeutic methods: it ranges from two psychotherapeutic methods in Germany to 22 in Austria. There are 20 modalities in Italy. It is important to recognize that psychotherapy training is offered for different methods in every country, many of which do not fall under national laws and therefore, in the admission of training candidates, have significant competitive disadvantages and less access to research funds.

The situation in the nonregulated countries is more heterogeneous: the training is in the hands of private training facilities. These are often societies but are also private institutions that usually represent a specific school of psychotherapy. The training programs are organized differently; some programs have a few courses, and some last many years. The schools of psychotherapy are various. The quality requirements are very different depending on the training establishment.

In the USA, psychotherapy is essentially integrated as a part of the professional group of psychiatrists, psychologists, and social workers. Training in a psychotherapeutic method is often offered as part of a PhD program. Furthermore, there are numerous additional developments to the integrated training structure as well as a myriad of training and further education opportunities for all people with or without the necessary qualifications; these people are not included in the statistics of the psychotherapy profession. School specificity is also not regulated in the USA. Thus, the specificity of psychotherapy is only structurally recognized according to internal rules of professional conduct. Accordingly, the American Psychological Association differentiates between 59 "divisions," i.e., topic-centered areas of responsibilities of psychologists. One of them, Division 29, is titled "Psychotherapy." However, there are other divisions that could be assigned to psychotherapy; therefore, there is a separate division for "psychoanalysis" and "trauma therapy." The difficulty with regard to the qualifications of psychotherapy training in the USA is that one cannot initially identify whether a person has completed psychotherapy training and what level of qualification they have, due to the overlapping job titles of psychiatrist, psychologist, and social worker.

Meanwhile, there is a new structure of university-based admission parameters. Since 2005, Sigmund Freud University, Vienna, allows 18-year-olds who qualify for admission to university to begin a bachelor's degree in psychotherapy science after they have completed the admission procedure. The admission procedure consists of two personal interviews and attendance at a self-experience group. The bachelor's plus master's program includes more than just theoretical psychotherapy content; psychotherapy training is fully integrated into the curriculum and is scientifically based. Students graduate with a BA and an MA and are fully trained psychotherapists (see Rieken 2012, 2013). Since 2013, the Karl Landsteiner Private University in Krems, near Vienna, has offered a bachelor's in psychotherapy science. The criteria for admission are not yet known but will be provided.

7.3 The Strasbourg Declaration on Psychotherapy and the European Certificate for Psychotherapy

The European Association for Psychotherapy (EAP), which was established in 1992, merges approximately 140 psychotherapeutic organizations in Europe. The World Council for Psychotherapy (WCP), founded in 1995, has chapters on all continents. Both the EAP and the WCP have established certifications that lead to the conferral of a diploma, and both have based their training content on the Strasbourg Declaration on Psychotherapy, which is also taught in psychotherapy training. The idea was to develop a training framework that is applicable across different schools and countries and enables students, professionals, and researchers to have a common structure for trained psychotherapists (European Association for Psychotherapy 1990).

Strasbourg Declaration on Psychotherapy (European Association for Psychotherapy 1990, p. 1)

In accordance with the aims of the World Health Organization (WHO), the non-discrimination accord valid within the framework of the European Union (EU) and intended for the European Economic Area (EEA), and the principle of freedom of movement of persons and services, the undersigned agree on the following points:

1. Psychotherapy is an independent scientific discipline, the practice of which represents an independent and free profession.
2. Training in psychotherapy takes place at an advanced, qualified and scientific level.
3. The multiplicity of psychotherapeutic methods is assured and guaranteed.
4. A full psychotherapeutic training covers theory, self-experience, and practice under supervision. Adequate knowledge of various psychotherapeutic processes is acquired.
5. Access to training is through various preliminary qualifications, in particular human and social sciences.

The goal of the efforts of these two organizations is to define the standards for psychotherapy education in Europe and worldwide. In both cases, it is clear that the criteria are to be kept general enough to include all types of psychotherapy training under one roof. Therefore, these trainings described are based on content and are less formal. Admission criteria are defined only insofar as the Strasbourg Declaration's (see above) statement that human and social sciences are seen as a qualification for psychotherapy training.

When discussing admission criteria in psychotherapy training, some considerations can be made. It should be noted that as of 2014, there is no legal training in psychotherapy provided in most countries worldwide. Nevertheless, there are formalized psychotherapy training establishments in most countries: in all states of North and South America, in almost all European countries, in some countries in Asia, in Australia, and also in some African countries. Psychotherapy training is in a globalization trend. We have taken a closer look at the countries that have legal regulations for psychotherapy as an independent profession because they represent a certain indicator function for future development (Pritz 2011).

The admission criteria for psychotherapy training have come a long way in the last 100 years: they have developed from doctors' privilege—whereby "laypeople," i.e., not doctors, were barely tolerated and often prohibited from the full practice of the profession—to today's regulations, which accept many qualifying professions, to the latest development of an independent, scientific study with specific entrance requirements (Rieken 2012, 2013).

To understand the different admission requirements for training in psychotherapy, one must review the recent history of modern psychotherapy, around the turn of the twentieth century. In 1900, a group of interested people formed around Sigmund Freud and dedicated themselves to different educational and ideological formations of psychoanalysis and, later, other schools of psychotherapy. These groups generated great interest in the media, but they remained small groups that initially did not have any specific professional perspective. Only since the 1950s has there been a worldwide movement that has led to the development of a psychotherapeutic practice profession.

Within this development, certain professional groups demanded that psychotherapy be a part of only their profession and be excluded from other professional groups. In 1926, this medical hubris opposed Sigmund Freud on the question of lay analysis. The next professional group that wanted to dominate the field of psychotherapy was psychologists. This often successful struggle is reflected in the legal regulations created in the 1990s. For example, as of 2014, there is still no law in Germany that regulates the authorization for psychologists to practice in various professional fields, but there has been such a law for "psychological psychotherapists" since 1990. However, other professional groups, such as social workers, educators, theologians, nurses, and others, are fighting to get a "piece of the cake." As previously mentioned, admission to psychotherapy training according to pre-psychotherapeutic principles has been allowed.

In addition to the interest in wielding power, the lack of authorization is also about substantive issues, questions of ethics and identity and the professional self-image, not to mention research interests and access to research funds. For example, doctors argued once that a complete understanding of the functions of the human body enables holistic psychotherapy. Psychologists argued that a diversity of psychological knowledge should be known before one can even begin to learn psychotherapy. A particularly popular argument was the issue of the "maturity" of the personality, which would be addressed in psychotherapy training. This debate especially played a role in the academization of psychotherapy: on the one hand, people argued that 18-year-olds were too young, possessed too little life experience, and therefore should only enter psychotherapy training only after having a previous profession. On the other hand, proponents for the academization of psychotherapy thought that the same requirements might as well be applied to future physicians, psychologists, nurses, educators, etc., which are highly specialized and stressful human professions for which no one has suggested allowing admission to the actual career choice only after completing vocational training. Rather, the formation of identity is more moldable if the training begins early, and the practice of the profession is more effective after the training. Fiegl (2014) was able to show that these arguments were based on traditional patterns and that younger therapists achieved equally effective results as older therapists. Specifically, representatives of "source professions" argue that their specific trade provides the best conditions for subsequent psychotherapy training.

For the patient/client in the process of looking for support and help, it comes down to truth and guidance. The dilemma that arises in this context is the often many years of futile searching for the right treatment. If another professional group masks as psychotherapy, the search process often takes a long time or the patient may encounter false treatment. In this scenario, the power of better public relations reigns.

Some legal requirements are relatively specific in the list of seminars, supervision, and theoretical training (Austrian psychotherapy law, German law for psychological psychotherapists), whereas others are more general (Swedish Psychotherapy Act, Dutch Psychotherapy Act, Italian Psychotherapy Act), and some mostly just define admission (French psychotherapy law, Finnish psychotherapy law). Each psychotherapeutic method provides a more concrete description of the amount of supervision, theoretical seminars, and teaching therapy.

The training requirements include current training courses that have been developed by psychotherapy associations throughout past decades and then transformed into law. Since 1996, the European Certificate of Psychotherapy (ECP) has attempted to subsume the various types of training to enable registration of psychotherapists from every European country:

4. Length and Content of Psychotherapy Training (Excerpt from the ECP; European Association for Psychotherapy 2012, p. 4)

4.1. The total duration of the training will not be less than 3,200 h, spread over a minimum of 7 years, with the first 3 years being the equivalent of a university degree. The later 4 years of which must be in a training specific to psychotherapy. The EAP will, in collaboration with NAOs and EWAOs, determine the proportion of the training elements that need to be completed prior to the ECP being awarded.

4.2. The training meets the EAP's criteria for basic professional training, and includes the following elements:

4.2.1. Personal Psychotherapeutic Experience, or equivalent: This should be taken to include training analysis, self-experience, and other methods involving elements of self-reflection, therapy, and personal experience (not less than 250 h). No single term is agreed by all psychotherapeutic methods. Any training shall include arrangements to ensure that the trainees can identify and appropriately manage their involvement in and contributions to the processes of the psychotherapies that they practice in accordance with their specific methods.

4.2.2. Theoretical Study: There will be a general part of university or professional training and a part which is specific to psychotherapy. University or professional courses leading to a first University degree or its equivalent professional qualification in subjects relevant to psychotherapy may be allowed as a part of, or the whole of, the general part of psychotherapy theory, but cannot contribute towards the 4 years of specific psychotherapy training. Theoretical study during the 4 years of training specific to

(continued)

psychotherapy should include the following elements:
- Theories of human development throughout the life-cycle
- An understanding of other psychotherapeutic approaches
- A theory of change
- An understanding of social and cultural issues in relation to psychotherapy
- Theories of psychopathology
- Theories of assessment and intervention

4.2.3. Practical Training: This will include sufficient practice under continuous supervision appropriate to the psychotherapeutic modality and will be at least 2 years in duration.

4.2.4. Placement in a mental health setting, or equivalent professional experience: The placement must provide adequate experience of psycho-social crisis and of collaboration with other specialists in the mental health field.

4.3. Supervision, training and, where applicable, personal psychotherapy should be provided by practitioners whose training meets the criteria of the ECP. Advanced trainings for trainers and supervisors are not covered by these criteria, but will be required.

Compared to the attention that has been focused on the laws of admission criteria, the content of training steps has been discussed in less detail. Rather, the law lays out the training requirements with respect to authorized training organizations that are required to have the necessary authorization from the state education authority. Training organizations that do not have this education authority—because, for example, they teach a method that is not recognized by the law—can operate their training, but their graduates have significant disadvantages in the regulated market for psychotherapy; they might not even able to practice. The question of method is slightly influenced by research results, but it is strongly determined by the influence of lobbying interests of both health insurance and course representatives of each method. What one could expect would be a set of "basic skills." These would not be defined in the content of the laws if not structurally required, for example, in Austrian law, in regard to an overview of the psychotherapeutic methods (Kierein et al. 1991). However, what concrete training for basic skills looks like is again left to the training institutions.

In some countries, psychotherapeutic methods are recognized that have very little scientific basis but have practical competence. However, a comparison of method-specific training presents a fundamental obstacle, similar to the different requirements for admission criteria. The idea of a synoptic view on psychotherapy is widespread and must be recognized in the evaluation of research findings (Pritz 1996, 2005, 2008).

In matters of psychotherapy law in Europe, product safety for the consumer, or patient, is often argued. A clear designation would help the consumers of psychotherapeutic services to separate the wheat from the chaff. Therefore, the laws in various countries mandate the use of a title. The violation of this is punishable: if someone who is not authorized uses the psychotherapist title, they can be punished. However, the title designation law says that the person concerned is only authorized to use the title of psychotherapist—and therefore offer public psychotherapy services—in their own country. The mandatory use of a title transnationally within or even outside the European Union does not yet exist.

There is, however, the recognition of the duty of each registrant who wants to emigrate from one country to another and practice in the host country. The host country is obligated (EU Directive 2005) to accept the registration of another country's state-approved psychotherapeutic training. Thus, a European matrix of mutual interstate recognition is slowly being created. However, this is still in its infancy and involves many bureaucratic hurdles. This regulation does not apply to countries where no psychotherapy law exists, i.e., most countries in the EU. Psychotherapists who emigrate from non-EU countries in Europe, the USA, South America, and Russia often have considerable bureaucratic recognition problems due to the differences in psychotherapeutic training in their countries of origin. But the first step has been made.

7.4 Implications for Empirical Psychotherapy Research

The dynamics in the development of the psychotherapeutic profession are taken into account in psychotherapy research insofar as the studies are becoming more refined and adapted to the psychotherapeutic reality (see also Chap. 3). However, from the perspective of the different admission requirements and the different training curricula, as well as the different statutory and non-statutory regulations, the question must be raised as to what extent modern psychotherapy research should take these developments more strongly in to account.

Thus, in the future, the following factors should be given more attention in research design:

1. Both admission criteria and training aspects, as well as the completion situation of the psychotherapist taking part in the study, must be explicit. Currently, typically only the psychotherapeutic method for which the participating psychotherapist completed training is taken into account in research studies. Additionally, the level of experience is usually not evaluated. In addition, the contextual conditions in which the study was developed should be described. Comparative psychotherapy research is needed that crosses national borders (see Orlinsky et al. 1994).
2. The evaluation of psychotherapeutic competence of the participating psychotherapists is a prerequisite for the qualitative evaluation of a study.
3. A synopsis of the psychotherapeutic structural dimension of the participating psychotherapists, along with a description of the method and the selection of the study participants, is further prerequisite to accurately evaluate the results of a research study. For example, studies in which the head researcher and the participating psychotherapist are the same person have less validity than a study with many participating psychotherapists who have a similar age and experience and are independent from the investigator.
4. In any case, the aspect of institutional requirements in the selection of psychotherapists should be assessed appropriately and in detail in both process studies and outcome studies.

References

European Association for Psychotherapy (1990) Strasbourg declaration on psychotherapy. http://www.europsyche.org/download/cms/100510/EAPLogo-Strassburg-Dekl-e. pdf. Accessed 19 July 2013

European Association for Psychotherapy (2012) The European certificate for psychotherapy (ECP). ECP official document, version 5. http://www.europsyche.org/download/cms/100510/ECP-document_version-5-0-voted-AGM-Valencia-July-2012.pdf. Accessed 21 July 2013

EU Directive (2005) http://ec.europa.eu/internal_market/qualifications/policy_developments/legislation/index_en.htm

Fiegl J (2014) Direct academic psychotherapy training. In: Poster presentation at the conference Practice Oriented Psychotherapy Research, Vienna, Austria, 7–8 Nov 2014

Freud S (1926) Zur Frage der Laienanalyse. Internationaler Psychoanalytischer Verlag, Leipzig Wien Zürich

Kierein M, Pritz A, Sonneck G (1991) Psychologengesetz, Psychotherapiegesetz. Orac, Wien

Orlinsky DE, Grawe K, Parks BK (1994) Process and outcome in psychotherapy – noch einmal. In: Bergin AE, Garfield SL (eds) Handbook of psychotherapy and behavior change, 4th edn. Wiley, New York, NY, pp 270–376

Pritz A (ed) (1996) Psychotherapie – eine neue Wissenschaft vom Menschen. Springer, Wien

Pritz A (ed) (2002a) Wörterbuch der Psychotherapie. Springer, Wien

Pritz A (ed) (2002b) Globalized psychotherapy. Facultas, Wien

Pritz A (ed) (2005) Personenlexikon der Psychotherapie. Springer, Wien

Pritz A (ed) (2008) Einhundert Meisterwerke der Psychotherapie. Springer, Wien

Pritz A (2011) The struggle for legal recognition of the education of psychotherapy and an autonomous psychotherapy profession in Europe. Eur Psychother 10:5–20

Rieken B (2012) Psychotherapie als Bildungsprozess am Beispiel der Sigmund-Freud-Privatuniversität Wien. Zeitschrift für Psychotraumatologie, Psychotherapiewissenschaft, Psychologische Medizin 10: 95–102

Rieken B (2013) Überlegungen zur Akademisierung der Psychotherapie – am Beispiel der Sigmund-Freud-Privatuniversität Wien. Zeitschrift für Individualpsychologie 38:285–302

Theory Building, Enriching, and Fact Gathering: Alternative Purposes of Psychotherapy Research

8

William B. Stiles

Contents

W.B. Stiles (✉)
Department of Psychology, Miami University, Oxford OH 45056, USA

Department of Psychology, Appalachian State University, Boone NC 28608, USA
e-mail: stileswb@miamioh.edu

O.C.G. Gelo et al. (eds.), *Psychotherapy Research*,
DOI 10.1007/978-3-7091-1382-0_8, © Springer-Verlag Wien 2015

Abstract

In this chapter, I draw distinctions among three classes of research purposes: theory building, enriching, and fact gathering. Theory-building research seeks to test, improve, and extend a particular theory. Enriching research seeks to deepen and enrich people's appreciation or understanding of a phenomenon. Fact-gathering research seeks to discover facts without explicitly focusing on a unified theory or systematically unpacking the meanings in a phenomenon. Insofar as the distinction concerns the *purposes* of research, not the methods, any method may be used to advance any of the purposes.

8.1 Introduction

In this chapter, I draw distinctions among three classes of research purposes in psychotherapy research. I call them theory building, enriching, and fact gathering. Table 8.1 summarizes the comparison that this chapter elaborates.

Briefly, theory-building research seeks to test, improve, and extend a particular theory by comparing it and reconciling it with observations, working toward a unified best account within the domain of the theory. Enriching research seeks to deepen and enrich people's appreciation or understanding of a phenomenon by considering it in alternative perspectives and unpacking the explicit and implicit meanings involved. Note that enriching *people* rather than enriching theories is a key feature. Whereas theory building focuses on a particular theory, enriching research may consider many theories as alternative, potentially useful viewpoints. Theory-building and enriching purposes might be described as scientific and hermeneutic, respectively. However, the terms *science* and *hermeneutics* carry powerful connotations of value and status, and they are understood in widely varied ways by different people, so I have chosen the terms *theory building* and *enriching* in an effort to remain relatively neutral, descriptive, and stable.

For this chapter, I added a third category, fact gathering, to an originally dichotomous distinction (Stiles 2006) to encompass the many studies in psychotherapy research (probably a majority) that seem aimed neither at building a specific theory nor at systematically unpacking the meanings in a phenomenon. As our field develops, I would expect increasingly more of the research to advance either theory-building or enriching purposes.

My distinction concerns the *purposes* of research, not the methods. In principle, each of the purposes may be addressed with any method. Thus, although theory-building purposes have been more often addressed with quantitative and nomothetic methods, whereas enriching purposes have been more often addressed with qualitative and idiographic methods, at least in psychotherapy research, these previous affinities are not necessary or fixed. I have argued elsewhere that qualitative and idiographic methods may be particularly appropriate for theory-building research on psychotherapy (Stiles 2009) and that numbers can be enriching (Stiles 2006). Thus, importantly, the theory building versus enriching distinction is not parallel to quantitative versus qualitative research. Both

Table 8.1 Comparison of theory-building, enriching, and fact-gathering research

Section heading	Theory-building research	Enriching research	Fact-gathering research
Goals	Work toward a unified account	Work toward enriching and deepening	Build an evidence base
Recent examples	Petrowski et al. (2013)	Oddli and Rønnestad (2012)	Lutz et al. (2013)
	Caro Gabalda and Stiles (2013)	Harris et al. (2012)	Flückiger et al. (2013)
Strategies	Hypothesis testing and qualitative theory building	Unpacking historicity	Draws on both theory-building and enriching strategies
Generality	Scope of theory	Transferability	Analogy
Meaning of terms	Stable meanings of terms (within theory)	Rich, evocative expression	Vulnerable to inconsistent meanings
Common versus diverse understanding	Common understanding	Diverse understandings	–
Coherence versus balance	Logically coherent	Multiple perspectives, balance, fairness	–
Locus of the benefit	Benefit is improved theory	Benefit is enriched people	–
Written reports	Orthodox research reports	Conventional and innovative formats (e.g., performance texts)	–
Investigator values	Open-minded, dispassionate	Fairness, balance, social benefit	–
Investigators' relationship to theory	Own the theory (able to change it)	Understand the theory (how to apply it)	–
Purposes viewed from each other's perspectives	May view enriching research as scattered and off-topic, fact gathering as haphazard	May view theory-building research as narrow and tedious, fact gathering as pointless or unexamined	May view theory building as premature, enriching as speculative

qualitative and quantitative methods may be used to advance any of the three purposes (see also Rennie 2012).

In academia, theory-building purposes and enriching purposes are associated with mature sciences and humanities, respectively. The distinction overlaps with Guba and Lincoln's (1994; see also Gelo 2012) categories of positivism/postpositivism versus constructivism-interpretivism/critical-ideological, but without the implication that each entails distinct methods. It overlaps to some degree with the distinction between realism and relativism (see, e.g., Rennie 2000, 2012), though without the ontological basis. It is an attempt to draw the distinction between what many have seen as different realms of research purposes.

Following Kuhn (1970), I understand fact-gathering research as representing an early stage of scientific development characterized by the lack of a *paradigm*, which can be understood as an agreed theory together with a body of cardinal examples, practices, and problems to be addressed. In the absence of a paradigm, scientists focus on finding facts rather than interpreting them within a larger framework. Arguably, psychotherapy research could be considered as pre-paradigmatic in Kuhn's terms. As Kuhn put it, "It remains an open question what parts of social science have yet acquired such paradigms" (p. 15). Kuhn's theory thus suggests that a good deal of psychotherapy research may be fact gathering, and my informal observations confirm this expectation. In a historical sense, Kuhn described fact gathering as preliminary to theory building (Kuhn did not address enriching research). In practice, however, fact gathering, enriching, and theory building are distinct purposes. Investigators do not expect to start with one and then move on to another; each is considered (by investigators who have that purpose) to be complete in itself.

Is it possible for research to have more than one of these purposes? Perhaps. But the differences between purposes are more profound than they may seem at first, and researchers used to advancing one may not appreciate how different the others are (at least this was my personal experience). Among other things, I think that readers and reviewers tend to approach research reports tacitly expecting just one of these purposes to be advanced. If the authors' purpose does not match readers' expectations, readers are likely to find the product confusing, unsatisfying, or wrongheaded, as addressed later. I comment on combinations of purposes in the final discussion.

After an introductory explanation of what I mean by the term *theory*, this chapter is organized around a series of distinguishing characteristics: goals, strategies, generality, meaning of terms, common versus diverse understanding, coherence versus balance, locus of the benefit, written reports, investigator values, investigators' relationship to theory, and purposes viewed from each other's perspectives (see Table 8.1). In each section, I have tried to compare and contrast theory-building and enriching—and sometimes fact-gathering—purposes with respect to that characteristic. Fact-gathering research seems less differentiated, and I have omitted it under about half of the headings. I believe that particular instances of fact-gathering research may be oriented toward theory building or enriching, but in an unarticulated way, so that this dimension of the purpose is not clear in the research report.

8.2 What Is a Theory?

The concept of *theory* is central to the distinction between theory building and enriching, but theories play very different roles in advancing these two purposes. Theory-building research has improving a theory as its product. Enriching research uses alternative theories as a way of appreciating a phenomenon. Fact-gathering research may aspire to either or to being atheoretical. I use the term *theory* extensively in this chapter, so I begin by trying to say what I mean.

As I use the term (e.g., Stiles 2009), theories are explanations of aspects of the world, such as how psychotherapy works, stated in words or numbers or diagrams or other *signs*. Signs, as I use the term (Stiles 2009, 2011), are tangible and observable—marks on a page or a screen or vibrations in the air. However, the meanings of signs are in people's private experience. Theories must be distinguished from the epistemologically private ideas the theories express or convey. Insofar as the theories are made of signs—words, numbers, diagrams, and so forth—they are public and observable, unlike their meanings.

Meaning, as I use the term, is a subjective process that accompanies hearing, seeing, writing, or speaking a sign. That is, meanings cannot be directly observed by others. Insofar as people never understand each other perfectly, sign meanings are generally different for the sign's *author* and *addressee* (e.g., speaker and hearer, author and reader). They are different or for different authors or addressees (people say, write, hear, and read things differently). And they are different at different times for the same author or addressee (understandings grow and change).

In this chapter, I am concerned mainly with *explanatory theories* (cf. Miller 2004; Held 2007), as distinct from *treatment theories*, which are meant to guide clinicians in conducting therapy. Explanatory theories express people's ideas and understandings, for example, about how psychotherapy works. They describe things and events in the world and relations among them. They suggest how observation of one event may indicate that other events have taken place or will take place. Treatment theories may be far simpler than explanatory theories. "All you need is love" is psychotherapeutic treatment theory that might plausibly have some efficacy, but it is a woefully imprecise explanatory theory. Explanatory theories may be judged by how general, precise, and realistic they are (Levins 1968). Treatment theories may be judged by how well they work, or more technically, how efficacious and effective they are (see Sussman et al. 2006). These two types of theories are often confused in psychotherapy research, I think, because some of our most familiar treatment theories (e.g., psychoanalytic theory, cognitive theory) aspire to be both. In what follows, when I use the term *theory* unmodified, I mean explanatory theory.

Although the discipline of psychotherapy is, arguably, pre-paradigmatic, the alternative explanatory theories of psychotherapy may be considered as candidate paradigms. That is, theory-building research can be conducted within them. The theories can also be used for enriching purposes; the array of alternatives available (see any textbook of theories or personality or psychotherapy) offers a diversity of perspectives that can enrich people's knowledge and appreciation of the phenomenon.

A theory (i.e., an explanatory theory) is a good one if people observe what the theory leads them to expect, that is, if the theoretical descriptions match the descriptions of the observations, or still more technically, if people's experiences of the theoretical descriptions (i.e., the meanings of the descriptions) correspond with their experiences of observing the things and events in the world that the theory describes. I have elsewhere called this the *experiential correspondence* theory of truth (Stiles 1981, 2006). That is, truth is a property of statements, including theoretical statements, as understood by people. It is a correspondence of people's understanding of theoretical statements with their understanding of their observations or their understanding of others' descriptions of observations.

Living theories are never finished. They are always subject to modification by further observations, which may strengthen or weaken confidence in them or illuminate aspects that might be elaborated or extended. This chapter is meant as theory building; the typology attempts an account of research purposes. It is not a finished product and is subject to evaluation and change.

8.3 Alternative Goals

8.3.1 Theory-Building Research Seeks a Unified Account

Theory-building research aims to construct an internally consistent, explicit explanation. It need not presume that there is a positivistically true or crystalline account, but it does seek a unified and logically coherent account.

Explanatory theories arise and are elaborated and extended, I think, when people describe their observations of the world and then revise the descriptions in light of further observations. Theory-building research provides quality control on theories by gathering observations and comparing them with what the theory leads them to expect (experiential correspondence). The observations may confirm or disconfirm or strengthen or weaken the theory, leading to increased or reduced confidence in aspects of the theory.

In principle, a theory that fails to account for even one observation could be rejected (Popper 1959), but this is rare (Lakatos 1978; Meehl 1990). More often, investigators seek methodological explanations for divergent observations.

Observations that persistently or convincingly diverge from theoretical expectations may suggest modifications or extensions to the theory. Modifications or new tenets may be incorporated through a process of *abduction* (Rennie 2000, 2012; Salvatore and Valsiner 2010; Stiles 2009; see also Chap. 6); investigators reason that if the modified tenet were part of the theory, then the otherwise divergent observation would be expected. This justifies tentatively retaining the modification and making further observations. Through this process, the theory changes to fit new observations.

Most scientific theory-building research aims to assess and improve existing theories rather than to construct new theories.[1] As Kuhn (1970) explained, in sciences with an established paradigm, new theories arise only when the existing paradigm falters. Even in pre-paradigmatic areas like psychotherapy research, constructing a completely new theory forgoes the benefits of cumulative improvements. Far fewer readers or researchers are likely to care about a new theory constructed ad hoc than about extending a familiar theory to encompass new observations.

The purpose that I call theory building encompasses all stages of the work of constructing explanatory accounts—exploration, testing, validating or invalidating, modifying, elaborating, extending, and so forth. That is, it encompasses both the context of discovery and the context of justification. Both quantitative and qualitative methods can be used for theory building. Importantly, enriching research is not another name for the early, exploratory stages in the development of a science but rather a separate purpose.

From a theory-building perspective, theories are important because they knit observations together. Through adjustments in light of accumulating observations across many studies, theories come, in effect, to compactly share the accumulated experience of many researchers with readers who have not personally had all those experiences. Theories can mediate the effect of research on practice by distilling observations into theoretical principles and conveying them in a way that they can be used.

8.3.2 Enriching Research Seeks a Richer, Deeper, Broader, More Profound Appreciation of the Object of Study

It aims to enrich the experience of readers, investigators, and research participants. Observation and interpretation are designed to illuminate phenomena and perspectives in new, constructive, or satisfying ways. Enriching research uses multiple and varied methods, qualitative (e.g., Madill and Gough 2008) and quantitative (e.g., Westerman 2006; Yanchar 2006), to advance the goal of advancing people's deeper and richer appreciation of the phenomenon.

Enriching research considers multiple perspectives and alternative ways of understanding a phenomenon without necessarily seeking to resolve them into a unitary account. Enriching research has also been described as *interpretive* (e.g., Kral 2008; Westerman 2006). It makes distinctions to open possibilities for alternative interpretations. In the search for alternative interpretations, the research may draw on a wide range of scholarly traditions, such as ethics, aesthetics, political praxis, and epistemology, as well as pragmatic, cultural, and historical perspectives. It often uses an evocative descriptive language and explores varied meanings of terms within the same project. In striving for greater depth, it may give particular attention to less-heard views, and for this reason it may give relative emphasis to oppressed or marginalized perspectives.

Importantly, enriching research is *not* a preliminary step in theory building but rather an altogether different project—an activity that has a different purpose. I emphasize this because, as someone whose orientation has long been toward theory building, I spent many years being

[1] Despite its name, grounded theory research (Glaser and Strauss 1967; Levitt 2015) seldom seems to be theory building in the sense I'm using the term. This point is addressed in Sect. 8.3.2.

exposed to enriching research in psychotherapy and related areas of psychology, often feeling critical or befuddled about it, without appreciating that its practitioners had a fundamentally different purpose from mine. Enriching is the point of the project; it is the end in itself rather than leading toward a statistical test of alternatives or other empirical assessment of the validity of the interpretation.

In my use of the term *enriching research*, it is *people*—readers, investigators, participants, and perhaps others—rather than theories, whose enrichment I am referring to. That is, the primary product of enriching research is in the private understanding of people who encounter the research. This contrasts with theory-building research, where the primary product is in the theory (a semiotic construction) and the understanding of the theory by people is derivative.

Both theory-building and enriching research seek understanding, but *understanding* has different meanings in the two contexts. Theory-based understanding is a cognitive map of the world, a grasp of how things work (including, potentially, people and psychotherapy); Gelo (2012), following Dilthey (1977), distinguished this sort of understanding as *explaining*. Enriching-based understanding is an aesthetic, empathic, historical appreciation of phenomena (including people and psychotherapy). Both sorts of understanding seem valuable and desirable (to me at least), but they are different and attained differently.

As I noted earlier, enriching research might also be called hermeneutic research, albeit risking misunderstandings. Many major investigators have used the umbrella term *qualitative research* to describe the wide variety of approaches sharing the purpose that I am calling enriching research (e.g., Denzin and Lincoln 2005; Gelo 2012; Guba and Lincoln 1994; Morrow 2007). In my view, this use of *qualitative research* conflates purpose with method, overlooking the important theory-building possibilities of qualitative methods (e.g., Stiles 2009) and the enriching possibilities of quantitative methods (e.g., Westerman 2006).

Enriching research informs therapeutic practice by giving therapists a deeper sense of people and processes. In psychotherapy, a rich appreciation of the client's experience and context of action facilitates appropriately responsive interventions. One colleague suggested using the term *pragmatic* to describe the enriching purpose in psychotherapy research.

In contrast to theory-building research's focus on assessing and elaborating a particular theory, enriching research often considers multiple theories and alternative interpretations as well as the historical and potential meanings of texts and events. In this respect, enriching research resembles the work often done by clinicians to understand a case: applying multiple theories, not with the goal of improving the theories or even deciding which theory is the right one for the case, but rather with the goal of building a richer and more rounded view of the case.

Enriching research may develop new interpretations along with exposing, exploring, and criticizing old ones. It may evaluate alternative interpretations, rejecting some as inferior or inadequate, while advocating others. However, it does not presume that any one interpretation is the only, best, or final account. On the contrary, part of the point of enriching research is to uncover, understand, and appreciate multiple accounts. Rather than starting with one theory and seeking to test or extend it (using either qualitative or quantitative methods), enriching research starts with a text, a topic, a person, or a phenomenon and seeks to deepen understanding of it.

Ironically, most grounded theory research (see Glaser and Strauss 1967; Levitt 2015; Mörtl and Gelo 2015; Rennie 2000) seems to be enriching rather than theory building. Although its nominal purpose is building a theory, this theory is not meant as the one best account of a domain, to be incrementally improved in subsequent studies. Rather, it is meant as a novel interpretation, an enriching perspective that grows out of intimate contact with the focal topic. As Levitt (2015) has put it, "a core premise of grounded theory is that many different valid understandings can emerge from different perspectives on the same data" (p. 473). This contrasts with the theory-building project of working toward a unified best account that is as general, precise, and realistic as possible.

The difference between grounded theory and theory building is not so much semantic as strategic. The word *theory* has roughly the same meaning in both contexts, but grounded theory usually seeks a new and enriching perspective, whereas theory building seeks to confirm or improve a unified best account.

When I have previously presented the distinction between theory-building and enriching research purposes, some qualitative researchers have seemed uncomfortable, insisting that their research purposes encompass both. Of course, to fully consider this claim, one would have to examine particular studies. But I think the research they do usually turns out to be enriching. Enriching research may develop new interpretations or comment on various theories as a way of enriching the readers, but it does not aim toward a unifying theory. Combining theory building with enriching is a characterization of enriching purposes.

8.3.3 Fact-Gathering Research Aims to Build an Evidence Base

Its goal is making and reporting observations that might contribute to a future understanding or that might be pragmatically useful. It seeks to establish facts with sufficient reliability and rigor that they can be viewed as trustworthy.

A *fact*, I think, is an observational statement about which there is social consensus. That is, observational statements that are socially shared and endorsed are considered as facts. This understanding of facts seems roughly compatible with the legal conception, in which facts are decided by agreement among members of a jury. However, in research, the facts can be changed by further observation. If someone observes something different and so disagrees—or, at least, if enough people or the right people observe something different and disagree—then the statement is no longer a fact.

In Kuhn's (1970) account, fact gathering is understood as historically preliminary to theory building. Fact-gathering researchers sometimes seem to expect that when enough facts have accumulated, a comprehensive theory will emerge or be synthesized. Fact gathering may also be preliminary to enriching; the observations might be intended for readers' own idiosyncratic use. For example, many studies seem to offer findings not to confirm, disconfirm, or extend a theory but rather simply to inform the reader of facts that may be used as they see fit. Such studies could be said to be preliminary to enriching purposes, particularly if their discussion sections offer alternative interpretations.

The anticipation of future use is sometimes explicit; for example, Fishman (2005) proposed systematic collection of case studies as a data bank for future theoretical synthesis. Often, however, I find it unclear whether fact-gathering researchers understand their work as leading toward an eventual unifying synthesis (theory building) or toward varied understandings and applications by different readers (enriching) or perhaps toward both or neither. I take the unclarity to be diagnostic of fact-gathering research, that is, as showing that the interpretation of the findings is unfinished and preliminary.

An important subcategory of fact-gathering research can be called *product-testing research*. In psychotherapy research, products include treatment packages and assessment procedures. Clinical trials seek to evaluate treatment packages; reliability and validity studies seek to evaluate psychological tests. Such product-testing research aims to evaluate packages rather than to build an understanding. Clinical trials may aim to evaluate the efficacy or effectiveness of treatment theories, but they do not primarily seek to build explanatory theories.

In calling fact gathering an embryonic or preliminary purpose, I do not mean to imply that it is necessarily unsophisticated. On the contrary, fact-gathering studies can be methodologically sophisticated and conceptually thoughtful, often more so than theory-building or enriching studies in psychotherapy research. In Kuhn's scheme, fact gathering is an appropriate purpose for research conducted in the absence of a paradigm.

8.4 Illustrative Recent Examples

To illustrate these purposes using current research on psychotherapy, I selected articles from issues of the journals *Psychotherapy Research* and *Psychology and Psychotherapy: Theory, Research and Practice* that had been published recently at the time of my revising this chapter (January 2013).

8.4.1 Theory-Building Studies

Working within attachment theory, Petrowski et al. (2013) examined the relation between the therapist's own attachment representation and the patient's attachment relationship to the therapist. Comparisons of 22 therapists' Adult Attachment Interviews with 468 patients' scores on the Client Attachment to the Therapist Scale showed that therapists' preoccupied attachment status was associated with patients' preoccupied-merger attachment to the therapist, while therapists' dismissing attachment status was associated with patients' avoidant-fearful attachment to the therapist. That is, specific types of therapist insecurity were associated with particular patient's attachment-related experience. This work was interpreted as evidence supporting a modification and elaboration of an attachment theory account as it applies to psychotherapy.

Caro Gabalda and Stiles (2013) addressed the contradiction between the assimilation model's suggestion that progress in psychotherapy follows a regular eight-stage developmental sequence and the common clinical observation that therapeutic advances alternate with setbacks. Examination of 466 setbacks in the therapy transcripts of two clients suggested that most of what appeared to be setbacks involved switches to a related but less advanced strand of a problem. Thus, rather than contradicting the theory, this study's results yielded an elaboration of it.

8.4.2 Enriching Studies

Oddli and Rønnestad (2012) examined how therapists introduce the technical aspects of therapy within the working alliance in a naturalistic study of the practices of nine experienced therapists. They focused on the concept of agency, distinguishing eight therapist action descriptions, which they categorized as either (1) supporting the client's agency or (2) expressing agency themselves. They described their method as a variant of grounded theory analysis. But their purpose, clearly demonstrated in their discussion, was not constructing a unified, general theory of agency but rather exploring varied understandings of therapist power, negotiation, consensus, and collaboration.

Harris et al. (2012) applied Interpretative Phenomenological Analysis (Smith and Osborne 2003) to transcribed interviews with eight service users about their experiences of being in contact with an early intervention for psychosis program. They distinguished five major themes: stigma, relationships, understanding the experiences, sense of agency, and impact, and they examined possible meanings of these themes from professional perspectives (clinicians, care coordinators) as well as the service users themselves. Their purpose appeared not to be specifying a theory but rather promoting an enriched and empathic understanding of the experiences of the people in such health-care systems.

8.4.3 Fact-Gathering Studies

As expected, a substantial majority of the articles in these journal issues were fact-gathering studies. The first two fact-gathering studies in the first 2013 issue of *Psychotherapy Research*—by Lutz et al. (2013) and Flückiger et al. (2013)—were both sophisticated analyses of longitudinal (session-level) data using structural equation modeling techniques. Lutz et al. (2013) examined sequences of session reports, identified clients who experienced sudden gains and sudden losses in treatment, and linked these respective patterns to the degree of treatment success. Flückiger et al. (2013) examined the relation of early session experiences to prediction of psychotherapy outcome while controlling statistically for intake distress and early response; results suggested that these factors were robust predictors of treatment effectiveness. These studies cited and reviewed conceptual as well as empirical literature; for example, Flückiger et al. focused on "dual models" of psychotherapy, which stress the balance between interpersonal and task aspects of the process. In both studies, however, the principal conclusions were cast in neutral and pragmatic terms rather than in terms of building a particular unified theory.

8.5 Alternative Strategies

8.5.1 Two Theory-Building Strategies

Both quantitative and qualitative methods can be used to provide quality control on theory. To illustrate, in this section, I contrast statistical hypothesis testing with qualitative case study. Both can be effective, but they use very different strategies (Stiles 2003, 2005, 2007, 2009, 2010).

The familiar (to psychologists) statistical hypothesis-testing strategy uses the hypothetico-deductive method. Investigators derive one statement or a few statements from a theory and compare the statement with many observations. If the observations tend to match the statement, then confidence in the statement is substantially increased (e.g., not due to chance, $p < 0.05$). This confidence in one statement yields a small increment of confidence in the theory from which the statement was deduced. For example, empirical support for a hypothesized association between therapist attachment representation and patient attachment relationship to the therapist yields a small increment of confidence in attachment theory more broadly.

Qualitative theory-building research, such as a theory-building case study (Stiles 2009), addresses many theoretical issues in the same study rather than only one or a few. It does this by comparing many theoretically based statements with qualitative observations in the same case, assessing how well the theory accounts for the details (see Campbell 1979). Because only one or a few observations bear on each statement, the change in confidence in any one statement may be small. Because many statements are examined, however, the number of empirical observations, and hence the gain (or loss) in confidence in the full theory, may be as large as from a statistical hypothesis-testing study.

Observations that fail to correspond to the theory—failed hypotheses or unexpected qualitative observations—can stimulate improvements in the theory. New research results can thus permeate the theory in the form of tenets that are added or elaborated or modified to accommodate new observations (abduction). However, earlier thinking and results are retained. For example, based on his observations and interpretations in the case of Dora, Freud (1905) began incorporating the concept of transference into his developing psychoanalytic theory. Thus, through changes in confidence and abduction, observations accumulate in theories.

Qualitative theory-building research has some advantages for psychotherapy research. Theories of psychotherapy aim to account for distinctive details of clinical cases that may not be shared with other cases. As Rosenwald (1988) argued, social phenomena are manifested differently in each case, so it is essential to understand the distinctive features. Qualitative theory-building research does not require large number of similar cases to make observations scientifically useful, as illustrated in a study by Brinegar et al. (2006) described at the end of the following Sect. 8.5.2.

8.5.2 Unpacking Historicity as an Enriching Strategy

One major strategy of enriching research can be understood as unpacking the *historicity* of texts, objects, and events. Historicity refers to the meaning that words and other signs accumulate through use (Bakhtin 1981, 1986; Stiles 2011; Voloshinov 1986). When you understand my words, you share some of my experience. That is, the meaning of my words to you is your experience of my experience. When you repeat my words to others, then your audience shares some of your experience but also some of my experience, which is carried in the words. For example, if you now tell someone about the concept of historicity, your audience will share not just your experience but also a bit of my experience. They will also share a bit of the experience of Leiman (1992, 2011; Leiman and Stiles 2002), who taught me about Bakhtinian semiotics, and the experience of Bakhtin (1981, 1986) and Voloshinov (1986), who wrote about this property of words. To say this another way, each use of a word (or any sign) changes its meaning by adding something of the experience of its author and addressee. In a sense, each word or phrase or story or image or icon (or number; think of the unlucky number 13 or the magical number 7 plus or minus 2) carries echoes of the experience of all who have used it previously. Even artifacts and natural objects carry meanings, which trace to the experience of previous speakers and authors (e.g., through previous authors, a fence can be a metaphor for limits; a flower can be a metaphor for love). In this view, essentially everything has semiotic properties and carries meaning derived from people's previous experience of it. Insofar as words and other signs have been accumulating these meanings though used by people for many generations, the meanings have enormous depth. As Bakhtin (1986) put it, "the word . . . is bottomless" (p. 127).

Unpacking historicity thus involves explicating the meanings of signs. In psychotherapy, the signs of particular interest are clients' expressions of their experiences (unpacking therapists' expressions can be interesting too). The concept of historicity suggests that people cannot be fully aware of their own meanings (there are far too many), so that therapists and, secondarily, researchers can usually unpack more than the client knew.

As an example of this enriching strategy, McLeod and Lynch (2000) conducted a qualitative enriching study of the case of Margaret, a 58-year-old woman who was seen for 17 sessions in a clinical trial of process-experiential treatment for depression (Greenberg and Watson 1998). McLeod and Lynch aimed at a broad and deep understanding, drawing on alternative accounts to show how "a sense of what is 'good' in life, an implicit notion of the 'good life', both underpins and guides everyday action" (McLeod and Lynch 2000, p. 389). Their aims were advanced by presenting multiple perspectives, including Margaret's own story using her own words, the therapist's story, the authors' summary account of the case as a whole, and their interpretation in terms of narrative processes, drawing particularly on the ideas of Polanyi (1985) regarding the practice of storytelling and Taylor (1989) regarding the concept of strong evaluation.

As a contrast, Brinegar et al. (2006) conducted a qualitative theory-building study based on the same case material. Margaret's case provided a particularly clear example of therapeutic work between stages 3 (problem statement) and 4 (understanding) in the developmental sequence posited by the assimilation model. This case study (like many others; see Stiles 2001, in press) provided empirical support for the assimilation model by making many observations on varied aspects of the cases, as described in the preceding section (see Campbell 1979; Stiles 2009). The work also led to proposing a series of four substages between stages 3 and 4. That is, whereas Brinegar et al. (2006) used the case of Margaret to elaborate a particular theory, McLeod and Lynch (2000) used it for unpacking the meaning of the good life as it emerged in Margaret's therapy.

8.5.3 Fact-Gathering Strategies Draw on Theory-Building and Enriching Strategies

Perhaps the commonest examples of quantitative fact-gathering psychotherapy research are hypothesis-testing studies whose hypotheses are not explicitly derived from theory but rather come from clinical intuition or lore or intuition

(Rosenwald 1986, called this *pre-theoretical knowledge*) or by analogy from previous research.

If the hypotheses were not derived from a theory, there is no theory to be strengthened, weakened, modified, or extended. Instead, the results may be offered as speaking to several theories, as illustrated by the fact-gathering studies reviewed in Sect. 8.4.2. A supported hypothesis from fact-gathering research seems to be advanced as a free-standing finding (e.g., justified as resembling previous results) rather than a test or extension of a general theory. Similarly, qualitative studies whose results are not unpacked or specifically brought to bear a unified theory may also be considered as fact gathering. For example, Grant et al. (2012) interviewed 16 expert supervisors about how they managed difficulty in supervision and distilled 4 major approaches that encompassed most of the responses and discussed these in terms of their clinical and practical usefulness. The treatment packages or assessment procedures studied in product-testing psychotherapy research may be based on treatment theories, but the research evaluates efficacy or usefulness rather than examining theoretical tenets.

Fact-gathering studies frequently discuss multiple interpretations of their results, for example, comparing their results with those of other studies. Sometimes it is difficult to distinguish such discussions from the sort of unpacking used in enriching studies. However, whereas enriching studies characteristically offer the multiple interpretations to foster broader understanding or deeper appreciation, fact-gathering studies characteristically offer these as alternative candidate accounts to be tested in future work.

8.6 Alternative Understandings of Generality

8.6.1 In Theory-Building Research, the Theory Bears the Burden of Generalization

In principle, each quantitatively or qualitatively assessed statement is embedded in the theory and depends on the theory for its meaning. The theory specifies its own degree of generality—its range of convenience, the circumstances or topics to which it is applicable. Evidence addressing any statement bears on the whole theory to the extent that the statement is logically linked to the rest of the theory. If the theory is general and logically coherent, support for any assessed tenet strengthens confidence in its specified generality.

Each study concerns only a part of a theory, typically a very small part. Its impact is not on the generality of the theory but rather on confidence in the whole theory. If the hypothesis is confirmed, the whole theory is strengthened; if the hypothesis is disconfirmed, the whole theory is weakened. For example, psychoanalytic theory describes the situations to which it is applicable. Empirical findings for or against some small part of psychoanalytic theory, whether they are statistical hypothesis tests or qualitative clinical observations, strengthen or weaken the theory. Sometimes they may suggest ways to broaden (or narrow) the scope of the theory. That is, they may suggest abductions that could make the theory more general. But in theory-building research, the generality—the range of application—is a property of the theory rather than the finding. In this respect, theory-building research contrasts with fact-gathering research, where concern focuses on the generality of the finding ("external validity").

8.6.2 The Enriching Research Analogue of Generality Is Described as Transferability (E.g., Lincoln and Guba 1990; Morrow 2005)

Transferability refers to whether those involved in the research as researchers, participants, or consumers can *transfer* the observations to their own lived experiences and contexts. It is a form of usefulness that relies on the users' own integration of the understanding rather than their application of a general theory.

Whereas generality refers to the truth of a particular statement or theory across contexts, transferability refers to the usefulness and applicability of personal understandings gained from the research. Rather than strengthening a theory, enriching research deepens and broadens the practical, empathic, aesthetic, historical understanding of those who read or hear about the research or participate in it. It is successful to the extent that it can be applied or extended to the reader's own sphere, that is, to the extent that the reader can see implications in their own lives (e.g., their practice of psychotherapy). Transferability, then, describes how much the research affects the world through the activities of the people who learn about the research.

What is transferred may vary from person to person. Whereas a theory specifies its own range of generality, the nature and range of application of enriching research depends on the needs and capacities of the people who are influenced by it. Different people may understand the work differently and may apply it in different, even contradictory, ways.

8.6.3 In Fact-Gathering Research, Generalization Is Mainly by Analogy

Fact-gathering findings are generalized to circumstances that seem intuitively similar. Generality is cast at the level of particular statements, rather than at the level of a general theory.

I think the concept of generality of *findings* (including qualitative observations) draws on the concept of statistical generalization. A statistical hypothesis supported in a sample drawn randomly from some specified population can be generalized to that population (with specified confidence). In a technical statistical sense, there is no basis for generalization of hypothesis tests beyond the population from which the sample was drawn. And very few psychotherapy studies draw samples randomly from the population of interest, for practical and ethical reasons. As a result, the generalization of most fact-gathering research is technically unwarranted. On the other hand, the findings may have some transferability; that is, they may have generality in the sense used in enriching research.

In fact-gathering research, findings are formulated in words. Although the statistical generalization of a finding can be only to the population from which participants were randomly sampled, the verbal formulation of the finding may be transferred approximately to other settings. For example, a tested statement about one group may be presumed to apply to a population that seems similar.

In fact-gathering research, this form of generality is sometimes called *external validity*, which can be understood as the strength of the analogy between the study and the broader clinical situation of interest. This may be a useful strategy in clinical trials, for example, but the logic is sharply distinct from generality in theory-building studies, where generality concerns the range of application of the theory.

8.7 Meanings of Terms

8.7.1 Theory Building Requires Stable Meanings of Terms

Stable meanings of terms are essential for the logical interconnection that allows empirical observations on one tenet of a theory to affect confidence in other tenets (Stiles 2009). Requiring that terms have fixed meanings is major restriction, frequently violated in practice, as words change meaning continually in natural language (Stiles 2009, 2011).

If signs change meaning, logic fails. As I have pointed out elsewhere (Stiles 2009, p. 12), the classic syllogism seems unassailably valid on first reading:

All men are mortal.
Socrates is a man.
Therefore, Socrates is mortal.

Yet any educated person knows that Socrates is immortal, alive, and influential throughout Western scholarship through two and a half millennia.

The verbal paradox arises because the meaning of *Socrates* and *mortal* changes from the flesh-and-blood man who drank a cup of poison hemlock and died to his enduring shared memory and his cultural impact. In the same way, the logically (mathematically) derived relationship, $E = mc^2$, is not true for all E, m, and c. We cannot decide that E now stands for empathy or extraversion and expect the formula to remain valid.

The need for stable meanings makes quantification attractive. Numbers have the remarkable property of meaning more or less the same thing to everyone, across the time and context (Stiles 2006). In the human sciences, where people's experience is a central topic and the most direct access is via verbal report, data are often not easily quantified, and the precision achieved by quantification is balanced by an unacceptable loss of realism or generality.

Meanings of such terms as transference, alliance, conflict, stimulus, automatic thoughts, emotion, self-disclosure, and empathy shift continually in informal psychological discussions, so getting them to hold still within a theory is challenging, and failures to do so may be overlooked. Analogous shifts in mathematics or chemistry would be noticed much more quickly.

Although numbers are attractive, they are not necessary for theory building, nor are they unassailable. No terms, not even numbers, have exactly the same meaning to everyone or at all times. And in psychotherapy research, many of the most interesting and important phenomena are not easily quantified. Qualitative methods may be necessary to address such phenomena. And we must accept a degree of imprecision in communication in our field.

8.7.2 Enriching Research Favors Rich, Evocative Expression

In enriching research, words can retain their natural language meaning or assume the different meanings they have in different theories. The meanings need not be the same throughout a research report; indeed, an important part of the work is exploring the alternative meanings that words or statistics may have (historicity). Enriching research affords the use of images, visual and verbal. Thus, enriching research not only acknowledges the difficulty of achieving stable terms (particularly in psychological domains) but may take the diversity of meaning as a strength and a focus.

Enriching research does not require standard meanings for terms because internal consistency is not essential. Even numbers are bottomless, and their use in a context can be unpacked (e.g., they may connote precision, symmetry, luck, similarities to quantities of other things). Using and appreciating the diversity of meanings of signs can be profoundly enriching. For example, in the Oddli and Rønnestad (2012) study reviewed in Sect. 8.4.2, unpacking the meanings of power, negotiation, consensus, and collaboration was a central contribution.

8.7.3 Fact-Gathering Research Seems Vulnerable to Inconsistent Meanings

Fact-gathering research often seems to presume that natural language terms have fixed, shared meanings, as do technical terms in paradigmatic sciences. Findings in chemistry or physics seem expressed in terms with common definitions because the definitions offered by the underlying theory are generally accepted. This is not the case in pre-paradigmatic fields like psychotherapy research.

Implicitly assuming that natural language meanings are universal may tempt researchers to move freely between theories or attempt direct comparisons of theoretical explanations. However, terms rarely if ever have common meanings across theories, and the assumption that they do can be problematic in studies considered as preliminary to theory building (Leiman and Stiles 2002). Operational definitions and standard measures can provide consistent meanings within a particular study, but the meanings lose precision beyond the study if they are not anchored by an internally consistent theory. For example, defining depression as score on the Beck Depression Inventory offers standardization within a line of research, but theoretical uses of the term *depression* seldom have precisely that meaning (Leiman 2010). Maintaining consistent meanings for treatment package names in clinical trials of psychotherapy is even more problematic (Stiles 2013).

If a fact-gathering study is considered as preliminary to enriching research, the inconsistency of term meanings across people and contexts is less serious, though of course it may still interfere with addressees' understanding of authors' meanings.

8.8 Common Versus Diverse Understanding

I have not included characterizations of fact-gathering research under this or the subsequent five major headings because I could not distinguish distinctive features in these areas. Insofar as fact gathering may be considered as a preliminary stage, it may share some characteristics with either theory building or enriching.

8.8.1 Theory Building Aims for a Common Understanding

A good theory says the same thing to everybody and offers a framework for a common understanding of observations. As noted, theory-building researchers (quantitative or qualitative) aspire to maintain consistent meanings for terms throughout the theory and to convey the same meaning to all users of the theory. There is an underlying presumption that the world is consistent and an intent to construct the best possible account of it. If a theory says different things to different people, yet the world is consistent, then at least some people will be misled (Stiles 2006, 2009).

8.8.2 Enriching Research Permits and Encourages Diverse Understandings

Insofar as enriching research seeks transferability rather than generalization, different readers may understand and appreciate its results (quantitative or qualitative) in different ways. The potential meanings of any text or observation far exceed any one person's grasp, so it is understood that different readers will focus on different aspects and find different value in them. There is no presumption that there is a best way to understand the world—or at least not the aspect of the world under investigation—so there is no point in seeking uniformity.

8.9 Coherence Versus Balance

8.9.1 Theory Building Seeks Logical Coherence

Theories aim to be internally consistent, in the sense of not including direct contradictions. Its tenets should also be expressed in a common set of terms, with logical relations among tenets. Theory-building research requires that observations on one part of a theory—or logical derivations from the theory—bear on the trustworthiness of the theory as a whole. The observation that starlight bends around the sun (Dyson et al. 1920) made all of Einstein's general relativity theory more trustworthy because this derivation was a logical derivation from the theory. If the theory's parts were not internally consistent and interrelated, observations on one aspect of a theory would not bear on other aspects. To say this another way, without a logical link between the theory and the observation, finding empirical support for a hypothesis would not affect confidence in the rest of the theory. This link is essential in both statistical hypothesis-testing and qualitative theory-building strategies.

In particular, then, new empirical observations must be described in the terms of the theory and assessed for logical consistency with the theory. If observations are not consistent with theory in this sense, then either there is some fault in the observation or the theory requires modification. (In Popper's (1959) classical account, the theory is rejected, though in fact, complete rejection is rare.) Observations that are not inconsistent but also not logically linked to the theory may point to abductions—ways of elaborating or extending the theory.

8.9.2 Enriching Research Seeks Multiple Perspectives and Balanced Representation

Whereas theory-building research seeks logical consistency, enriching research seeks fairness. For example, insofar as each topic of study embodies the experience of many people (because of its historicity), a responsible unpacking must represent multiple and varied perspectives. This may take the form of presenting alternative interpretations or competing theoretical accounts, perspectives of different communities or cultures or roles or statuses (e.g., client, therapist, observer). The goal is not necessarily to reach a conclusion or a resolution (though authors often express their opinions and preferences) but rather to ensure that the alternatives are exposed. The goal of balance applies to both qualitative and quantitative studies; it would apply, for example, both to enriching studies of interviews with clients' parents and to enriching studies of distributions of personality factors in different groups.

The goal of balance and fairness entails special efforts to represent a diversity of perspectives including those of people less privileged on such social dimensions as ethnicity, gender, residence, age, and class. This is a powerful entailment, insofar as most published scientific literature, and indeed most literature of all kinds, is written from the perspective of individuals who are respected within society, powerful, and relatively wealthy. Relative to most other genres, then, enriching research differentially incorporates and represents the perspectives of those who are otherwise underrepresented, particularly including the oppressed, the weak, and the impoverished.

8.10 Locus of the Benefit

8.10.1 The Benefit of Theory-Building Research Is in an Improved Theory

As explained earlier, theories are composed of signs—words, formulas, diagrams, and so forth—all of which are external and observable, as distinct from people's private understanding of the theory. Thus, the product of theory-building research is an improved semiotic construction, an observable thing.

8.10.2 The Benefit of Enriching Research Is in People's Experience

The product of enriching research is not a unified theory but a richer or deeper appreciation of the object of study by people, including readers, researchers, and, sometimes, participants. Whereas the product of theory-building research is external, represented in words or other signs, the product of enriching research is internal, lodged within the experience of the people who read the research reports and the reverberations of the ways they change as a result. From their encounter with the research (e.g., reading a research report), people find their own meanings and uses. Arguably, it also extends to others who are subsequently affected by those who have read or learned about the research.

8.11 Written Reports

8.11.1 Theory-Building Studies Characteristically Use Orthodox Research Reports

They generally follow the introduction-method-results-discussion outline. The goal of common understanding tends to favor a common, familiar format. Even reports of qualitative theory-building studies are constrained for this reason, though they may require a broader explication of the theory and different quality control criteria (Elliott et al. 1999; Stiles 1993, 2003).

8.11.2 Enriching Studies More Often Use Different and Innovative Formats

Authors of enriching research reports are not restricted to the conventional forms but can draw on a wide range of expressive techniques to convey their observations and interpretations. Thus, enriching research reports may use narrative, poetry, varieties of performance texts, and other nontraditional forms (e.g., Glesne 1997; Lincoln 1997; Richardson 2002). Such formats may not normally be accepted in many psychotherapy research journals, but they are common in journals devoted to qualitative research, such as *Qualitative Inquiry*.

8.12 Investigator Values

8.12.1 Theory-Building Research Values Open-Mindedness, Dispassionate Observation

Theory-building research entails a commitment to a particular theory. This is not an unquestioning belief in the theory's current tenets. On the contrary, the research enterprise demands open-minded attention to new observations that put the theory at risk or that may extend the theory's scope. Instead, it values a motivation to check and improve the theory's generality, precision, and realism.

8.12.2 Enriching Research Values Fairness, Relationships, and Social Benefit

The goal of exposing diversity of meaning tends to position enriching research in opposition to forces that would restrict diverse understanding or dictate meanings. This easily becomes a political position, insofar as interpretive orthodoxies tend to go hand in hand with concentrations of power. Diverse understandings are likely to challenge authority, including scientific authority.

Whereas theory-building research requires recognition of inconsistent observations, enriching research requires openness to alternative interpretations. Enriching research demands choices and evaluations and invokes researchers' values and personal positions. As multiple perspectives and interpretations are exposed, researchers' positions proceed not from consistency with a particular theory but from attitudes around issues of value and power.

As striving for balance tends to expose socially suppressed experiences and meanings, enriching researchers may find that their work places them actively in opposition to social injustices and oppression. Social action may be incorporated into the research (for one illustrative line of work, see Kidd and Kral 2005; Kral 2008; Kral and Idlout 2009).

8.13 Investigators' Relationship to Theories

8.13.1 Theory-Building Researchers Must Feel They Own the Theory They Are Building

Insofar as theory-building research may lead modifications of the theory, researchers must feel entitled to make such changes. If they feel that the theory is the best available account of the phenomenon under study, then failures of the theory to account for their observations represent problem in their conception of the world, which demands a solution. If researchers regard the theory as belonging exclusively to someone else (e.g., Sigmund Freud, Carl Rogers, Aaron Beck), then they can comment on it or try it or use it, but they are likely to feel they lack the standing to improve it.

Such ownership grows from intimate knowledge of the theory. Theory-building research requires sufficient familiarity with the theory to recognize when the theory fails to account for an observation (qualitative or quantitative). Ownership also involves the courage to propose changes in response to observations that can modify or extend the theory.

8.13.2 Enriching Researchers Must Understand the Theories They Apply

Whereas theory-building investigators must take responsibility for the theory they address in order to change it, enriching researchers must understand and convey others' theories and perspectives to achieve balance. Thus, breadth and depth of scholarship are central values along with the breadth and depth of exploration of the perspectives of people whose lives are observed and reported.

In enriching research, then, theories are treated as the views of their authors, to be grasped and unpacked. Enriching researchers do not take ownership but rather respect the ownership of whoever produced them. Alternative concepts are presented and compared. Often, critical reflection on alternative views and theories is central to an enriching contribution.

8.14 Purposes Viewed from Each Other's Perspectives

I think the differences among theory-building, enriching, and fact-gathering purposes are a source of significant misunderstanding. The purposes are not opposed to each other, but they lead to very different expectations about what will be accomplished and reported. Readers, particularly other researchers, who encounter even high-quality research with one purpose when they expected another are likely to be uncomprehending or disappointed and may be disparaging or even contemptuous.

8.14.1 Readers Expecting Theory-Building Research

Readers expecting theory-building research who encounter enriching research may view it as undisciplined or off-topic, perhaps exploring interesting possibilities but failing to identify or resolve contradictions to advance a theory, and therefore pointless. They may strongly object the intrusion of subjectivity, or bias (Madill and Gough 2008). If they encounter fact-gathering research, they may find it interesting to the extent that they can find a place for the facts in their own theory building, but otherwise it is likely to seem unguided and haphazard, and therefore uninteresting, describing findings without showing their scientific purpose.

8.14.2 Readers Expecting Enriching Research

Readers expecting enriching research who encounter theory-building research are likely to view it as narrow, overly selective, or rigid, arbitrarily focusing on one perspective while ignoring other equally important perspectives. The expectation that there could be a unified theory may seem restrictive or even arrogant. Both theory-building and fact-gathering research may seem narrow and tedious. The findings may occasionally be of interest but picky and interpreted in unnecessarily conventional ways. It may appear as part of an established scientific hegemony and shaped to preserve existing power structures. Enriching researchers may oppose the notion that important psychological phenomena are susceptible of being explained within one unified theory. Similarly, fact-gathering research may seem narrow, partial, and incomplete.

8.14.3 Readers Expecting Fact-Gathering Research

Readers expecting fact-gathering research may view theory-building research as premature. Presumably if they were proponents of the theory being built, they would not be expecting fact-gathering research. They may view enriching research as speculative and insufficiently rigorous.

8.15 Discussion: Mixed Purposes

Many of the key terms I have used in this chapter, including *theory building* and *enriching*, can have multiple meanings in colloquial use. I have tried to make clear the specific meanings I intend, but I may not have succeeded, and to the extent I have failed, the chapter is likely to be confusing. If it still seems to you that the purposes overlap or are difficult to distinguish, such a failure of communication about the meaning of terms may be responsible.

Of course, research with one purpose can serve other purposes than those the researcher intended. For example, theory-building researchers may see enriching research (or fact-gathering research) as exploratory, as research in the context of discovery, and thus as a possible source of hypotheses to be tested. The deeper appreciation or new perspective that comes from enriching research can inform theory building. Thus, theory builders may understand an enriching study as preliminary to a confirmatory study.

Conversely, good theories and established facts can yield valuable alternative perspectives, and in this sense, a theoretical analysis can contribute to the enriching project. Enriching researchers may make use of the product of theory building or fact gathering as a perspective to be included and respected in their own work. Considering only one theoretical view would be considered as foolishly narrow in an enriching study, however.

Fact-gathering researchers may view their own work as preliminary to theory building, though the eventual synthesis may be understood as far away (e.g., Fishman 2005). Or they may consider their work as preliminary to enriching, leaving the interpretive elaboration to readers.

Acknowledgment I thank Mehdi Farshbaf, Claudia Meystre, Katerine Osatuke, David Rennie, and the Qualitative Research Group at Miami University for comments on drafts of this chapter.

References

Bakhtin MM (1981) Discourse in the novel. In: Holquist M (ed) The dialogic imagination. Four essays by M. M. Bakhtin. University of Texas Press, Austin, TX, pp 259–422

Bakhtin MM (1986) Speech genres and other late essays. University of Texas Press, Austin, TX

Brinegar MG, Salvi LM, Stiles WB, Greenberg LS (2006) Building a meaning bridge: therapeutic progress from problem formulation to understanding. J Couns Psychol 53:165–180. doi:10.1037/0022-0167.53.2.165

Campbell DT (1979) “Degrees of freedom” and the case study. In: Cook TD, Reichardt CS (eds) Qualitative and quantitative methods in evaluation research. Sage, Beverley Hills, CA, pp 49–67

Caro Gabalda I, Stiles WB (2013) Irregular assimilation progress: reasons for setbacks in the context of linguistic therapy of evaluation. Psychother Res 23: 35–53. doi:10.1080/10503307.2012.721938

Denzin NK, Lincoln YS (2005) Introduction. In: Denzin NK, Lincoln YS (eds) The Sage handbook of qualitative research, 3rd edn. Sage, Thousand Oaks, CA, pp 1–32

Dilthey W (1977) Descriptive psychology and historical understanding. Nijhoff, The Hague. doi:10.1007/978-94-009-9658-8

Dyson FW, Eddington AS, Davidson C (1920) A determination of the deflection of light by the Sun’s gravitational field, from observations made at the total eclipse of 29 May 1919. Phil Trans R Soc Lond 220A:291–333. doi:10.1098/rsta.1920.0009

Elliott R, Fischer C, Rennie D (1999) Evolving guidelines for publication of qualitative research studies in psychology and related fields. Br J Clin Psychol 38:215–229. doi:10.1348/014466599162782

Fishman DB (2005) Editor’s introduction to PCSP: from single case to database. Pragmatic Case Studies in Psychotherapy 1(1):1–50, http://pcsp.libraries.rutgers.edu

Flückiger C, Grosse-Holtforth M, Znoj HJ, Caspar F, Wampold BE (2013) Is the relation between early post-session reports and treatment outcome an epiphenomenon of intake distress and early response? A multi-predictor analysis in outpatient psychotherapy. Psychother Res 23:1–13. doi:10.1080/10503307.2012.693773

Freud S (1905) Bruchstück einer Hysterie-Analyse. Mschr Psychiat Neurol XVIII:285–310, 408–467; G. W., V, p 161–286; Fragment of an analysis of a case of hysteria. Standard Edition 7:1–122

Gelo OCG (2012) On research methods and their philosophical assumptions: “raising the consciousness of researchers” again. Psychotherapie & Sozialwissenschaft 14:109–128

Glaser BG, Strauss AL (1967) The discovery of grounded theory: strategies for qualitative research. Aldine, Chicago, IL

Glesne C (1997) That rare feeling: re-presenting research through poetic transcription. Qual Inq 3:1–13. doi:10.1177/107780049700300204

Grant J, Schofield MJ, Crawford S (2012) Managing difficulties in supervision: supervisors' perspectives. J Couns Psychol 59:528–541. doi:10.1037/a0030000

Greenberg LS, Watson J (1998) Experiential therapy of depression: differential effects of client centered relationship conditions and active experiential interventions. Psychother Res 8:210–224. doi:10.1093/ptr/8.2.210

Guba EG, Lincoln YS (1994) Competing paradigms in qualitative research. In: Denzin NK, Lincoln YS (eds) Handbook of qualitative research. Sage, Thousand Oaks, CA, pp 105–117

Harris K, Collinson C, das Nair R (2012) Service-users' experiences of an early intervention in psychosis service: an interpretative phenomenological analysis. Psychol Psychother Theory Res Pract 85:456–469. doi:10.1111/j.2044-8341.2011.02043.x

Held BS (2007) Psychology's interpretive turn: the search for truth and agency in theoretical and philosophical psychology. American Psychological Association, Washington, DC. doi:10.1037/11588-000

Kidd SA, Kral MJ (2005) Practicing participatory research. J Couns Psychol 52:187–195. doi:10.1037/0022-0167.52.2.187

Kral MJ (2008) Psychology and anthropology: intersubjectivity and epistemology in an interpretive cultural science. J Theor Philos Psychol 27:257–275. doi:10.1037/h0091296

Kral MJ, Idlout L (2009) Community wellness and social action in the Canadian Arctic: collective agency as subjective well-being. In: Kirmayer LJ, Valaskakis G (eds) Healing traditions: the mental health of aboriginal peoples in Canada. University of British Columbia Press, Vancouver, BC, pp 315–334

Kuhn TS (1970) The structure of scientific revolutions. University of Chicago Press, Chicago, IL

Lakatos I (1978) The methodology of scientific research programs. Cambridge University Press, Cambridge

Leiman M (1992) The concept of sign in the work of Vygotsky, Winnicott and Bakhtin: further integration of object relations theory and activity theory. Br J Med Psychol 65:209–221. doi:10.1111/j.2044-8341.1992.tb01701.x

Leiman M (2010) Mitä Beckin depressioasteikko mittaa (What does the Beck Depression Inventory measure?). Psykologia 45:22–30

Leiman M (2011) Mikhail Bakhtin's contribution to psychotherapy research. Cult Psychol 17:441–461. doi:10.1177/1354067X11418543

Leiman M, Stiles WB (2002) Integration of theory: methodological issues. In: Säfvestad-Nolan I, Nolan P (eds) Object relations and integrative psychotherapy: tradition and innovation in theory and practice. Whurr Publishers, London, pp 68–79

Levins R (1968) Evolution in changing environments: some theoretical explorations. Princeton University Press, Princeton, NJ

Levitt HM (2015) Study-driven guidelines for designing and evaluating grounded theory research: a constructivist-social justice approach. In: Gelo OCG, Pritz A, Rieken B (eds) Psychotherapy research: foundations, process, and outcome. Springer, New York, NY

Lincoln YS (1997) Self, subject, audience, text: living at the edge, writing in the margins. In: Tierney WG, Lincoln YS (eds) Representation and the text: reframing the narrative voice. State University of New York Press, Albany, NY

Lincoln YS, Guba EG (1990) Judging the quality of case study reports. Qual Stud Educ 3:53–59. doi:10.1080/0951839900030105

Lutz W, Ehrlich T, Rubel J, Hallwachs N, Röttger M-A, Jorasz C, Mocanu S, Vocks S, Schulte D, Tschitsaz-Stucki A (2013) The ups and downs of psychotherapy: sudden gains and sudden losses identified with session reports. Psychother Res 23:14–24. doi:10.1080/10503307.2012.693837

Madill A, Gough B (2008) Qualitative research and its place in psychological science. Psychol Methods 13:254–271. doi:10.1037/a0013220

McLeod J, Lynch G (2000) "This is our life": strong evaluation in psychotherapy narrative. Eur J Psychother Couns Health 3:389–406. doi:10.1080/13642530010012039

Meehl PE (1990) Appraising and amending theories: the strategy of Lakatosian defense and two principles that warrant it. Psychol Inq 1:108–141. doi:10.1207/s15327965pli0102_1

Miller RB (2004) Facing human suffering: psychology and psychotherapy as moral engagement. American Psychological Association, Washington, DC. doi:10.1037/10691-000

Morrow SL (2005) Quality and trustworthiness in qualitative research in counseling psychology. J Couns Psychol 52:250–260. doi:10.1037/0022-0167.52.2.250

Morrow SL (2007) Qualitative research in counseling psychology: conceptual foundations. Couns Psychol 35:209–235. doi:10.1177/0011000006286990

Mörtl K, Gelo OCG (2015) Qualitative methods in psychotherapy process research. In: Gelo OCG, Pritz A, Rieken B (eds) Psychotherapy research: foundations, process, and outcome. Springer, New York, NY

Oddli HW, Rønnestad MH (2012) How experienced therapists introduce the technical aspects in the initial alliance formation: powerful decision makers supporting clients' agency. Psychother Res 22:176–193. doi:10.1080/10503307.2011.633280

Petrowski K, Pokorny D, Nowacki K, Buchheim A (2013) The therapist's attachment representation and the patient's attachment to the therapist. Psychother Res 23:25–34. doi:10.1080/10503307.2012.717307

Polanyi L (1985) Telling the American story: a structural and cultural analysis of conversational storytelling. Praeger, New York, NY

Popper K (1959) The logic of scientific discovery. Basic Books, New York, NY, Original work published 1934

Rennie DL (2000) Grounded theory methodology as methodological hermeneutics: reconciling realism and relativism. Theory Psychol 10:481–502. doi:10.1177/0959354300104003

Rennie DL (2012) Qualitative research as methodical hermeneutics. Psychol Methods 17:385–398. doi:10.1037/a0029250

Richardson L (2002) Poetic representation of interviews. In: Gubrium JF, Holstein JA (eds) Handbook of interview research: context and method. Sage, Thousand Oaks, CA. doi:10.4135/9781412973588.d50

Rosenwald GC (1986) Why operationism doesn't go away: extrascientific incentives of social-psychological research. Philos Soc Sci 16:303–330. doi:10.1177/004839318601600302

Rosenwald GC (1988) A theory of multiple case research. J Pers 56:239–264. doi:10.1111/j.1467-6494.1988.tb00468.x

Salvatore S, Valsiner J (2010) Between the general and the unique: overcoming the nomothetic versus idiographic opposition. Theory Psychol 20:817–833. doi:10.1177/0959354310381156

Smith JA, Osborne M (2003) Interpretative phenomenological analysis. In: Smith JA (ed) Qualitative psychology: a practical guide to methods. Sage, London, pp 51–80

Stiles WB (1981) Science, experience, and truth: a conversation with myself. Teach Psychol 8:227–230. doi:10.1207/s15328023top0804_11

Stiles WB (1993) Quality control in qualitative research. Clin Psychol Rev 13:593–618. doi:10.1016/0272-7358(93)90048-Q

Stiles WB (2001) Assimilation of problematic experiences. Psychotherapy 38:462–465. doi:10.1037//0033-3204.38.4.462

Stiles WB (2003) Qualitative research: evaluating the process and the product. In: Llewelyn SP, Kennedy P (eds) Handbook of clinical health psychology. Wiley, London, pp 477–499. doi:10.1002/0470013389.ch24

Stiles WB (2005) Case studies. In: Norcross JC, Beutler LE, Levant RF (eds) Evidence-based practices in mental health: debate and dialogue on the fundamental questions. American Psychological Association, Washington, DC, pp 57–64

Stiles WB (2006) Numbers can be enriching. New Ideas Psychol 24:252–262. doi:10.1016/j.newideapsych.2006.10.003

Stiles WB (2007) Theory-building case studies of counselling and psychotherapy. Couns Psychother Res 7:122–127. doi:10.1080/14733140701356742

Stiles WB (2009) Logical operations in theory-building case studies. Pragmatic Case Studies in Psychotherapy 5(3):9–22, http://jrul.libraries.rutgers.edu/index.php/pcsp/article/view/973/2384

Stiles WB (2010) Theory-building case studies as practice-based evidence. In: Barkham M, Hardy G, Mellor-Clark J (eds) Developing and delivering practice-based evidence: a guide for the psychological therapies. Wiley-Blackwell, Chichester, pp 91–108. doi:10.1002/9780470687994.ch4

Stiles WB (2011) Coming to terms. Psychother Res 21:367–384. doi:10.1080/10503307.2011.582186

Stiles WB (2013) The variables problem and progress in psychotherapy research. Psychotherapy 50:33–41. doi:10.1037/a0030569

Stiles WB (in press) Signs and voices fifteen years on. In: Strauss B, Barber J, Castonguay LG (eds) Visions in psychotherapy research and practice: reflections from the presidents of the society for psychotherapy research. Routledge, London

Sussman S, Valente TW, Rohrbach LA, Skara S, Pentz MA (2006) Translation in the health professions: converting science into action. Eval Health Prof 29:7–32. doi:10.1177/0163278705284441

Taylor C (1989) Sources of the self: the making of modern identity. Cambridge University Press, Cambridge

Voloshinov VN (1986) Marxism and the philosophy of language. Harvard University Press, Cambridge, MA

Westerman MA (2006) Quantitative research as an interpretive enterprise: the mostly unacknowledged role of interpretation in research efforts and suggestions for explicitly interpretive quantitative investigations. New Ideas Psychol 24:189–211. doi:10.1016/j.newideapsych.2006.09.004

Yanchar SC (2006) On the possibility of contextual-quantitative inquiry. New Ideas Psychol 24:212–228. doi:10.1016/j.newideapsych.2006.09.005

Part II

Psychotherapy Process Research

Introduction to Psychotherapy Process Research 9

Gillian E. Hardy and Sue Llewelyn

Contents

Abstract

In this chapter we unpack what is meant by psychotherapy process research and what are the overarching aims of such research. We then look at types of process research and some of the methodologies that have been used in pursuit of these aims. The limitations of these methodologies are then discussed and some emerging methods are presented.

9.1 What Is Process Research?

Although we have made great advances in psychotherapy research, so that we can now say with confidence that many psychological treatments lead to significant therapeutic change, there are still many questions to which we do not know the answer. Perhaps the most important of these questions is, 'What is it that happens in the psychotherapy session that is helpful?' or, put another way, 'How does psychotherapy work?' Of course this question is inextricably linked to the question 'Does it work?' But it is the focus that is different, the focus of what it is that happens within the system—that of the client, therapist and their interactions—that somehow enables change to occur. This is the focus of process research.

There is a range of definitions of process research such as that from Greenberg and Pinsoff (1986) who describe it as the study of the interaction between patient and therapist systems,

G.E. Hardy (✉)
Clinical Psychology Unit, Department of Psychology, University of Sheffield, Sheffield S10 2TN, UK
e-mail: g.hardy@sheffield.ac.uk

S. Llewelyn
Isis Education Centre, Warneford Hospital, University of Oxford, Headington, Oxford, UK

O.C.G. Gelo et al. (eds.), *Psychotherapy Research*,
DOI 10.1007/978-3-7091-1382-0_9, © Springer-Verlag Wien 2015

with the goal of identification of change processes as these systems interact. Other definitions include the following: 'addresses what happens in psychotherapy sessions, examining variables such as therapist behaviours, client behaviours, and interactions between therapists and clients during treatment' (Lambert and Hill 1994, p. 72); and our own definition includes 'the content of psychological therapy sessions and the mechanisms through which client change is achieved, both in single sessions and across time' (Llewelyn and Hardy 2001, p. 2). All of these definitions point to the central focus of the research being on what it is that underlies, enables or drives therapeutic change.

At their core, psychotherapy processes include client change processes and how these may result from therapy interventions and interactions. These dynamics are not always straightforward, however, nor are they easy to observe. Client change processes may or may not occur within the therapy session; they may or may not be amenable to verbal description, and events that occur in the therapy session may be helpful, unhelpful or neutral with regard to their impact on client change. As in all areas of research, it is therefore important to provide both theoretical and empirical evidence for the way in which therapy processes or activities are linked to client change processes. Further, research must involve identifying and understanding both client and therapy processes so that, as Kazdin (2009) states, we can develop 'evidence-based explanations' of why a treatment works and how changes come about.

In 1991, a central researcher in psychotherapy process work, Robert Elliott, introduced a five-dimensional model of therapy process. This model is useful to help researchers and practitioners think about what process they are interested in exploring. Elliott's five dimensions are (1) perspective of observation, (2) person/focus, (3) aspect of the process, (4) unit level and (5) sequential phase. In conducting process research, Elliott suggests that the researcher first asks the questions 'Who observes?'—which might be the client, therapist, supervisor or observer—then 'Who is being studied?' and then 'What aspect of the process is being studied?' such as, for example, client or therapist behaviours, intentions, style or the content or quality of the dialogue. Next they should clarify the unit level, which refers to the boundaries of analysis, such as is the level of focus a single word, speaking turn event, whole session or the whole of therapy? Finally, the sequential phase is determined by whether the focus is on active processes that are part of temporal or causal sequences. So, for example, one might look at clients' views (perspective) of their therapists' (person/focus) skilfulness (aspect) in answering personal questions (unit level) on the quality of the therapeutic alliance (sequential phase). Elliott's model is a good starting point for any process researcher in considering how their own area of interest fits in to other works in the field and what its particular reference points should be. We will return to this model later in this chapter.

9.2 Aims of Process Research

There are four primary aims of process research. The first is perhaps the core aim, which is to understand the mechanisms of treatment processes and client change processes in psychotherapy. While outcome is the key question for funding bodies, who want to provide effective treatments, as it is of course for both clients in distress and for therapists who want to alleviate that distress, nevertheless, it is unsatisfactory for many reasons not to know *why* something works, even if it does work. The question of what exactly are the specific ingredients of change has intrigued psychotherapy researchers for many years, although this issue has not attracted the level of funding that has been provided for outcome research. Consequently there has been relatively little research concerning process issues compared with the number of studies concerning questions about psychotherapy outcome. Although psychodynamic therapy researchers, and other therapies such as Gestalt, person-centred and psychodynamic-interpersonal, have had a long and distinguished history of interest in process work, until relatively recently very few cognitive-behavioural researchers in particular have addressed this issue (Lambert et al. 2004). Furthermore, it seems that this question is considerably less easy to answer than outcome work, in that the number of clear-cut and robust research findings about mechanisms is surprisingly small (Orlinsky et al. 2004). Nevertheless, most therapists at some time or another have asked themselves what it is about their work with clients that has had the most (or least) impact, and the question of mechanism remains an intriguing area of debate.

The second aim of process research is to improve the quality of therapy, by understanding which aspects of treatment are the most important in effecting change, and therefore to emphasise or develop those aspects, rather than aspects which are less critical. For example, Scholing and Emmelkemp (1996) showed that exposure is as effective as a more complex cognitive-behavioural treatment in treating social phobia, suggesting that the quality of the therapeutic intervention would be boosted by placing relatively more emphasis on this element. Likewise, process studies of the therapeutic relationship, and how it is best developed, can improve quality; for example, Hill and Knox (2002) have shown how and when therapist self-disclosure can best contribute to the formation of the therapeutic alliance. Importantly, process studies have also been able to show that some aspects of therapy in fact have relatively little effect on the quality of the experience of clients, for example, gender (Beutler et al. 2006), age or ethnicity (Beutler et al. 2004). This is also clearly highly relevant for service delivery.

The third aim is to contribute to the development of theories, which provide the underpinning rationale and consequently offer a sound structure to the work of therapy. Therapeutic work that is not based securely on theory is likely to have a limited impact and to risk losing focus. Theoretically based work can also build on what has been shown to be effective in the past and can suggest strategies for future interventions which are likely to be effective. Close examination of a process can reveal features of the therapeutic interaction which may not be observed in outcome studies and which can thereby support or refute theoretical postulates. Process work on mechanisms of change, for example, can provide insight into exactly which features of therapeutic intervention lead to what outcome, which will allow the confirmation or disconfirmation of the theory which proposes that it should be effective. Hence, the relative importance of some aspects of theory can be strengthened, while other parts can be modified or even discarded. An example is the role of transference interpretations: a series of studies by Piper and colleagues (e.g. Piper et al. 1991) examined the number and type of interpretations in relation to therapeutic outcome, leading Orlinsky et al. (2004), amongst others, to conclude that evidence does not support the use of transference interpretations in brief psychotherapies, which arguably does raise questions about some aspects of the underlying theory. A related but key issue here has been the recognition of the importance of the therapeutic relationship itself and the so-called non-specific factors in contributing to change [see, e.g. the review by Cooper (2008)]. Indeed, there has been research on the process of therapy which has demonstrated unequivocally that although therapists from different theoretical orientations do behave differently from each other, nonetheless, therapeutic efficacy across a variety of theoretical approaches is broadly equivalent (see, e.g. Ablon and Jones 1999; Stiles et al. 1998).

Finally, process work aims to assist in the development of effective training, by closely linking with the other three aims noted above. Hence, process work aims to enable therapists to learn to deliver forms of intervention that are most likely to result in effective outcomes, to improve quality and to ensure that the theories that underpin the approaches studied are supported by evidence. Observation of what has the most impact clearly has implications for what should be taught to novice therapists. Likewise supervision: many therapists routinely listen to audiotapes of psychotherapy sessions; this practice of review shares many of the features of process research in that attention is paid to features of the session which may be difficult to pick up in real-time practice, or which are characteristics of the client, therapist or setting, and which can reveal aspects of what is taking place. This can then lead to effective learning by the therapist. For example, comprehensive process analysis (CPA) was designed to provide a methodology for an intensive investigation of some chosen aspect of the therapeutic encounter, for example, how a client attains insight within a particular therapeutic model (for an application, see Elliott et al. 1994). But while CPA is a research tool, it also has educative functions. Engagement particularly in qualitative research such as this can itself act as a forum for learning, which allows the researcher to gain personal clinical understandings about what is helpful, as well as providing data for wider publication through completion of the formal research project or paper.

For example, in Leeds, UK, a research clinic was set up in partnership with local clinical psychologists. Therapy training and supervision were offered to the therapists along with an invitation to take part in research projects. A therapist led one such study and looked at what clients found helpful in therapy. Post-therapy interviews were conducted and analysed using qualitative methodology (Clarke et al. 2004).

9.3 Types of Process Research

There are many ways in which the broad topic of process research can be approached so that a study can be focussed on a specific area of concern. For example, the influential series of texts concerning empirical evidence and psychotherapy, originally edited by Bergin and Garfield (1994) and more recently edited by Lambert (2004), chose to divide the investigation of the ingredients of therapeutic efficacy to a number of domains including therapist and patient variables, comparison and causality factors and common factors. Cooper (2008) also divided his succinct and accessible examination of the field into therapeutic orientation, client factors, therapist factors, relationship factors and technique factors.

In our own work (Llewelyn and Hardy 2001), we have used a Kuhnian model of scientific inquiry to structure and map out the field of process research. In doing so we outlined three broad types of process study: descriptive, hypothesis testing and theory building. That is, we proposed that a helpful way to structure the field was to move from observation through hypotheses building and testing and finally to theory construction with particular emphasis on different ways of accounting for change. Although the Khunian heuristic has anomalies, it does allow an understanding of the precise nature of the underlying question posed by the research. Thus we can ask: is the study trying to understand what is happening in a complex encounter or process by carefully observing at least some of its components without having a specific model in mind (observation), or is it trying to examine certain variables or elements which given theories or models indicate are likely to be important (hypothesis or theory testing), or is the study examining links between specific underlying general processes and therapeutic change (theory construction)? The research methods used by each of these three types also vary, and each approach can include quantitative and qualitative work, as well as an intensive and mixed method approach that integrates the two.

These broad types will now be explained in more detail.

Descriptive studies are typically those which aim to provide a clear account of behaviours and processes which can be observed to occur during therapy, or in the accounts, beliefs, feelings and behaviours of participants, and which do not yet have a theoretical base. Focussing on observation is a crucial stage of inquiry, where the phenomena of therapeutic interaction or thought can be examined and key patterns detected. This approach can make use of the clinical skills and expertise of therapists who may have developed a rich understanding of what is happening and want to start to systematise their perceptions.

Examples of descriptive studies include the work of Rennie (1994) who showed by detailed examination of therapeutic transcripts how clients find subtle methods of influencing their therapists, of which therapists may be unaware. Another example is the study by Macran and Shapiro (1998) on how helpful therapists consider their own therapy has been and how they considered it as beneficial. Such studies do not propose causality, but suggest that a full understanding of process needs to be mindful of its complexity.

Hypothesis testing studies normally attempt to predict outcome from a number of variables, which are assumed to be critical in determining whether or not therapy is effective. The vast majority of published process studies can be subsumed under this heading, whereby numerous researchers have attempted to provide evidence for various aspects of the therapeutic encounter that are assumed to be crucial. What is striking about this approach is that despite many thousands of studies, few variables have been found to consistently predict outcome across most therapies. The most robust finding has been the contribution of the quality of the therapeutic relationship and the quality of client participation (Castonguay and Beutler 2006; Lambert 2004), although methodological difficulties complicate the picture, for example, it has been suggested that measures of therapeutic relationship, which consistently predict outcome, in fact constitute an early measure of outcome, thus conflating the measure of process with outcome, thereby arguably rendering the reported link theoretically uninformative.

Despite this, there are four main hypothesis testing approaches which can be distinguished: studies that examine the impact of specific techniques, those examining selected patient or therapist characteristics, those that consider the timing and context of therapeutic interventions and those that consider poor outcome and ineffective therapy. The first category is essentially theory driven and may use a variety of research methods to examine the effectiveness of a theoretically important technique. For example, working within a cognitive perspective, Tang and DeRubeis (1999) reported that significant changes in client reporting of symptoms were preceded by large in-session cognitive changes, as might be predicted from a cognitive model of change. A similar result was reported in psychodynamic therapy by Andrusyna et al. (2006) who showed that significant change followed sessions in which there were a greater number of accurate interpretations and an improved therapeutic relationship, again both theoretically indicated variables.

The second category consists of studies looking at characteristics of therapy participants which clinical experience, theory or other empirical studies suggest are likely to affect outcome. For example, Benjamin and Karpiak (2002) describe a series of studies on client variables that show how having the diagnosis of personality disorder impacts on therapy, such that those with borderline or dependent personalities appear to have particularly poor outcomes. As an example of research concerning therapist variables, Cooper (2008) summarises a series of studies showing that therapist ethnicity, age and gender do not have a major impact on outcome, although there is a link to the frequency of premature termination and dropout. Looking at variables concerning both participants, Hilliard et al. (2000) examined therapists' and patients' developmental history and linked both these to indices of process and outcome.

The third category of hypothesis testing study concerns timing and context. For example, studies by Silberschatz et al. (1986) showed that the impact of interpretations may vary depending on when they are given, and studies by Meyer and Pilkonis (2002) showed that clients with dismissive attachment styles develop their ability to relate to the therapist after initial wariness, suggesting that the approach of therapists may need to adapt over time.

Finally, within the fourth category, some process studies have focussed on what happens when aspects of therapy are harmful or ineffective. For example, Safran and Muran (2002) have suggested that repair of ruptures may hold a key to effective therapy, although many therapists struggle to respond to alliance-threatening events with appropriate skill and attention. Safran and Muran indicate that therapeutic work that specifically targets the repair of ruptures results in significant improvement and reduces dropout from treatment, irrespective of other interventions in the treatment.

Theory building. The last of the three broad types of process research, included in our 2001 Khunian model, examines the links between psychotherapeutic processes and theories of change. Many of these studies concern concepts or models that are still at the stage of theory development. Investigations in this category aim to examine how psychological change itself occurs, often from a multi-theoretical perspective. Examples here include the assimilation model (Stiles et al. 1990) and Prochaska's (1999) model of change. A key component of many of these models is that they do not assume that there is only one route to change, but instead that change is multidimensional, being influenced by internal and external events. Another key assumption is that in many respects psychological change is understood to be technically chaotic, that is, that it is difficult to predict reliable causal chains and that some key factors may interact with each other in unique, relatively unpredictable ways. Noting that a high proportion of other process studies rely on correlational analyses, these models by contrast assume that the frequency of a technique or variable does not necessarily imply its value. Indeed, as noted in our earlier paper, these models assume that 'key components of therapy may have their effect only occasionally, when conditions are right, while at other times these same components are functionally inert. Alternatively, these key components may set up processes in action that then have their potent impact at some later point...' (Llewelyn and Hardy 2001, p. 11).

Related to this work has been the contribution of writers such as Hubble et al. (1999) who point out that psychotherapy researchers have systematically attended to therapist-driven features of the therapeutic encounter, whereas it is in fact essentially the 'heroic' client who does the changing. Possibly understandably, researchers have examined those aspects of the process over which they have the most control, namely, themselves and the techniques that they use, while ignoring the far more significant client who inhabits an ever changing and influential world outside therapy and actually does the changing themselves.

9.4 Research Methodology

There is no single, widely accepted or aspirational standard for process research methods. The randomised control trial (RCT) design, a gold standard for outcome research, does not seek to answer process research-type questions, and no equivalent research method has reached pre-eminence within psychotherapy process research. However, the development of electronic methods to record therapy sessions is probably the most important event that has encouraged the scientific study of therapy processes. Early process researchers only had therapists' notes to indicate what happened in therapy sessions, and this did not of course lend itself to rigorous methods of study.

Audiotapes and then videotapes have therefore provided researchers with rich observable data that can be measured, examined and assessed using many methods such as coding schemes, rating scales, descriptive analyses and quantitative, qualitative and exploratory analyses. These have been effectively summarised in reviews by Kiesler (1973), Bergin and Garfield (1994), Orlinsky et al. (2004) and Cooper (2008). These types of data, in comparison to self-reported data, however, do not necessarily tell us what is happening inside the therapist and client—what their intentions, thoughts, feeling and their experiences of the therapy events are. The wish to gain greater access to such 'invisible' data has led to the development of a range of alternative measures to obtain participants' perceptions and reactions to therapy. Examples of these include the therapist session intentions measure and the session evaluation questionnaire (Stiles et al. 1994, 1996, respectively). Such measures ask the therapist, client or both participants to rate their private thoughts and feelings about the psychotherapy session that they have experienced. As with more observable data, the particular perspective, focus, aspect, unit and time point will vary from measure to measure. Indeed, this has led to a complex matrix of approaches to process research, summarised in Elliott's dimensional model of psychotherapy process, described at the beginning of this chapter.

As with all research, the type of process research methods used depends on the questions being asked, and process researchers have employed both qualitative and quantitative research methods. What matters most in selecting the methodology is that it is capable of answering the question, and both qualitative and quantitative approaches have a role to play. Details of these methods will be discussed in later chapters of this book. Here, we will take the three broad types of process research questions that we outlined above and will give examples of the range of research methods available to the researcher to answer these questions. We will then briefly review the limitations of the methods used in the literature and conclude with a section describing some promising new research methods.

Before doing so, a cautionary note must be sounded. There are now a huge range of established measures that purport to assess specific aspects of psychotherapy processes. Hill and Lambert (2004) have detailed some of the most common process measures that have been used to assess constructs focussing on the therapist, for example, social influence, facilitative conditions, techniques, intentions, helpfulness of interventions and verbal and nonverbal behaviours. They have also listed measures focussing on the client, for example, experiencing behaviour, verbal and nonverbal behaviour, intentions and reactions, as well as measures focussing on both the therapist and client, for example, control, dominance, values and alliance. Hill and Lambert's chapter includes measures with good and clearly demonstrated validity and reliability. However, it is evident from the wider literature that many researchers have developed measures and scales for their own particular study, where few validity and reliability data are available. These measures tend to be used only in a few studies and therefore make it difficult to compare findings across studies. The process researcher is well advised to pay particular attention to issues of reliability and validity when seeking to evaluate any measures included in a study or when they themselves conduct process research. Hill and Lambert (2004) also discuss a number of additional issues that need to be considered during data collection. These include practical factors that could impact on the quality of data collected, such as participant burden, missing data and the effects of the research on the therapy itself. Questions about sampling and uses of judges (number, level of expertise, training, bias and drift) are also important to consider.

9.4.1 Examples of Research Questions

Descriptive questions are usually answered using quantitative methods. For example, researchers might want to know how often therapists use questions and how many of these are 'closed' questions. This could be done by coding the therapist's speech, perhaps using a verbal response mode system (e.g. Hill et al. 1979). One of the response modes might be 'closed' questions, for example, and by coding a session, estimates of the frequency of such an event can be measured. Such studies could inform the researcher about the typical profile of a therapist using a particular type of therapy or with a specified client group. Qualitative methods can also be used for descriptive studies, such as the work by Rennie (1994).

Examples of the second type of research, that is hypothesis testing studies, tend to take the form of quantitative, within-study comparisons, or correlational studies looking at the frequency of behaviour in relation to outcome or at which aspects of therapy vary together. Here, for example, the study might test the hypothesis that cognitive therapists are more collaborative than psychodynamic therapists, by counting how many collaborative questions are used within a specific time frame. The limitations of such methods have been well described by Hill (1982), Stiles (1988) and others. The biggest problem is that recording the frequency or relative proportion of a specific behaviour within a given time frame does not give any indication of the quality or appropriateness of that behaviour nor, as noted above, of its clinical or therapeutic significance.

Designs employing experimental and quasi-experimental designs have been less frequently utilised but can be used to look at the impact of therapy techniques on outcome. In such studies clients are randomly assigned to receive a type of therapy that contains or does not contain the therapist behaviours of interest. For example, Hoglend et al. (2007) randomly assigned patients to receive brief dynamic therapy in which transference interventions were either prescribed or proscribed. Such studies are often designed to follow the randomised control model, although such approaches are fraught with difficulty, given the very considerable problems in controlling all the salient variables. Other problems also beset this type of work, not least of which are issues of client acceptability and ethical concerns.

Finally, theory development research often utilises qualitative methodology. This includes research that is definitional and asks questions such as 'What is the nature of this particular therapeutic phenomenon?' or 'What defines it?' Such studies may employ phenomenological research or grounded theory methods. Methods where interpretation of events is the focus include comprehensive process analysis (Elliott 1989) (noted above), task analysis (Greenberg 1984; Bennett et al. 2006) and narrative case study (Grafanaki and Mcleod 1999; Polkinghorne 1988).

What this brief summary of research methods used by process researchers shows is the huge variety of data collection methods, ranging from interviews, questionnaires and therapy review procedures such as interpersonal process recall (Elliott 1986, 1989) and brief structured recall (Elliott and Shapiro 1988) to data derived from observation or ratings of therapy session audio or video recordings. Similarly, designs and methods of analysis are numerous. The types of questions one can ask include definitional, descriptive, quantificational, interpretive, critical, comparative, relational or deconstructive, while analyses can cover all aspects of qualitative and quantitative methods.

9.4.2 Limitations of Process Research Methodology

As noted above, the range and diversity of measures used and the varied basis for selecting units and categories, as well as the repeated use of new, potentially unreliable content analysis or categorisation systems for analysis, are highly problematic for the field. These features of many existing process studies have limited the comparison we can make across studies, impede the accumulation of knowledge and may be some of the factors that lead to the lack of consistency in findings in this area.

Other methodological problems include the use of small unrepresentative samples, the use of differing definitions of the same construct and an over-reliance on correlational data. Researchers have also neglected to use control or comparative groups and have often not specified the theoretical assumptions underpinning their research. There have been concerns about the limited ecological validity of some research, the limited attention to the interpersonal context and an emphasis on therapist actions.

9.5 Historical Developments in Process Research

It is, of course, somewhat arbitrary to separate the achievements of process and outcome research. To most observers, the term 'psychotherapy research' is generally thought of in terms of whether a particular treatment works, that is, the evidence base to support the use of a particular treatment with specific client groups. This research has largely been driven by the requirement to find out if psychotherapy is effective, by users and commissioners of services, and has been structured by available outcome research methods. However, though important and necessary, such outcome studies do not address the questions of how an intervention works or of what particular intervention is most appropriate with this client at this particular time that process research seeks to address. Such questions are important to practitioners, and in fact process research has the potential for bridging the researcher-therapist divide by seeking answers that are highly relevant to practitioner decision-making. This is indeed another good reason to support process research, as the gap between the concerns of practitioners and researchers does not have positive consequence for either grouping.

In this final section, we briefly overview the focus of process research over the last 60 years (see also Chap. 3). The first generation of research has been described by Orlinsky et al. (2004) as 'justification' (1950s and 1960s) and was concerned primarily with describing and measuring therapy processes: What happens in therapy and can we measure it? As noted, the use of audiotapes of therapy sessions enabled researchers to conduct fine-grained analyses of the activity of the therapist and client. This included the development of measures such as the verbal content and vocal expression of therapist and client speech, for example, examination of the verbal content of sessions in psychodynamic therapy by Brody et al. (1951) and on facilitative conditions in counselling by Rogers (1957).

This focus on therapy content was subsequently replaced by a focus on the links between the processes happening within sessions and therapy outcome. This second generation of research has been called 'specificity' and includes publications from the 1970s to the 1980s. Working in this tradition, Greenberg and Pinsoff (1986) called explicitly for more research that aimed to explain exactly how therapy produces change. The most obvious example of this type of research is looking at the working or therapeutic alliance and outcome, such as the studies by Horvarth and Greenberg (1989), or empathy (Barrett-Lennard 1986).

Between the late 1980s and the present, psychotherapy researchers have tended to seek to identify specific elements in therapy and change processes within clients that would improve the quality of psychotherapies, including questions such as 'How does change occur?' Such research has highlighted markers that impacted on client outcomes and ways to intervene in those markers. The seminal rupture and repair work of Safran and colleagues exemplifies this type of work (Safran and Muran 2002; Safran et al. 2002).

9.6 Emerging Process Research Methodologies

Panchankis and Goldfried (2007) have recently described how advances in statistics have now made it possible to track much more realistically client change over time at an individual and group level, providing 'individual trajectories over time, discontinuities and transition points and dynamic systems of change'. These methods include growth curve modelling and multilevel modelling. Such analyses require clients to complete assessments more frequently and hence allow researchers who are using these assessments to identify points of change (either improvement or deterioration). Such methods therefore enable researchers to address the limitations of earlier research by considering outcomes within a specific context and having greater ecological validity and offer an improved opportunity to address the concerns of clinicians as well as researchers.

Developments in qualitative research methods have also taken place. These include refinements of existing methods, but a variety of new approaches have also been introduced, such as those described by Elliott et al. (2009) and Schielke et al. (2009). Elliott and colleagues advocate the use of mixed methods, borrowing from the legal adversarial system, to weigh up evidence in a hermeneutic single-case design. In this method 'evidence' from many sources of a clients' progress including questionnaire data, interview transcripts, process notes, etc. are presented to and discussed by two groups of analysts—those in support of successful change and those who do not support change. Schielke and colleagues, borrowing from architecture, describe a method of building consensus between different interpretations of qualitative data. They call this the Ward method, where researchers cycle between working individually and then in a group, all the time seeking to come to a common, agreed understanding. During the meetings individuals aim to understand the perspectives of other group members and not challenge or disagree but to use the information to inform the next iteration of their own individual interpretation of the data. This process continues until consensus is reached.

Conclusion

All of the above approaches offer researchers further opportunities for answering the key questions in process research, by building on earlier investigations that used simpler research methodology. It is hoped that these more sophisticated approaches will start to reveal more consistent findings, so that progress can be made in meeting the four main aims of process research, that is, the development of understanding, the enhancement of quality, the development of theory and the provision of improved opportunities for training and clinical supervision. This will then also allow process research to contribute even more significantly to the work of outcome researchers, in improving the overall effectiveness of psychotherapy services for clients.

References

Ablon JS, Jones EE (1999) Psychotherapy process in the national institute of mental health treatment of depression collaborative research program. J Consult Clin Psychol 67:64–75

Andrusyna DO, Luborsky L, Pham T, Tang TZ (2006) The mechanisms of sudden change in supportive-expressive therapy for depression. Psychother Res 16:526–535

Barrett-Lennard GT (1986) The relationship inventory now: issues and advances in theory, method and use. In: Greenberg LS, Pinsoff WM (eds) The psychotherapeutic process. Guilford, New York, NY, pp 439–476

Benjamin LS, Karpiak CP (2002) Personality disorders. In: Norcross JC (ed) Psychotherapy relationships that work. Oxford University Press, New York, NY, pp 423–438

Bennett D, Parry G, Ryle A (2006) Resolving threats to the therapeutic alliance in cognitive analytic therapy. Psychol Psychother 79:395–418

Bergin AE, Garfield SL (eds) (1994) Handbook of psychotherapy and behavior change, 4th edn. Wiley, New York, NY

Beutler LE, Malik M, Alimohamed S, Harwood MT, Talebi H, Noble S et al (2004) Therapist variables. In: Lambert MJ (ed) Bergin and Garfield's handbook of psychotherapy and behavior change, 5th edn. Wiley, Chicago, IL, pp 227–306

Beutler L, Blatt SJ, Alimohamed S, Levy KN, Angtuaco L (2006) Participant factors in treating dysphoric disorders. In: Castonguay LS, Beutler LE (eds) Principles of therapeutic change that work. Oxford University Press, New York, NY, pp 13–63

Brody EB, Newman R, Redlich FC (1951) Sound recording: the problem of evidence in psychiatry. Science 113:379–380

Castonguay LG, Beutler L (2006) Principles of therapeutic change that work. Oxford University Press, New York, NY

Clarke H, Rees A, Hardy GE (2004) The big idea: clients views of cognitive therapy. Psychol Psychother 51:81–92

Cooper M (2008) Essential research findings in counselling and psychotherapy. Sage/BABCP, London

Elliott R (1986) Interpersonal process recall (IPR) as a psychotherapy process research method. In: Greenberg LS, Pinsoff WM (eds) The psychotherapeutic process. Guilford, New York, NY, pp 503–527

Elliott R (1989) Comprehensive process analysis: understanding the change process in significant events. In: Packer M, Addison RB (eds) Entering the circle: hermeneutic investigation in psychology. SUNY Press, Albany, NY, pp 165–184

Elliott R, Shapiro DA (1988) Brief structured recall: a more efficient method for identifying and describing significant therapy events. Br J Med Psychol 61: 141–153

Elliott R, Shapiro DA, Firth-Cozens J, Stiles WB, Hardy GE, Llewelyn S, Margison F (1994) Insight in interpersonal-dynamic therapy: a comprehensive process analysis. J Couns Psychol 41:449–463

Elliott R, Partyka R, Wagner J, Alperin R, Dobrenski R, Messer SB, Watson JC, Castonguay LG (2009) An adjudicated hermeneutic single-case efficacy design of experiential therapy for panic/phobia. Psychother Res 19:543–557

Grafanaki S, Mcleod J (1999) Narrative Processes in the construction of helpful and hindering events in experiential psychotherapy. Psychother Res 9: 289–303

Greenberg LS (1984) Task analysis: the general approach. In: Rice L, Greenberg LS (eds) Patterns of change. Guilford, New York, NY, pp 124–148

Greenberg LS, Pinsoff WM (1986) The psychotherapeutic process: a research handbook. Guilford, New York, NY

Hill CE (1982) Counselling process research. Philosophical and methodological dilemmas. Counsel Psychol 10:7–19

Hill CE, Knox S (2002) Self-disclosure. In: Norcross JC (ed) Psychotherapy relationships that work. Oxford University Press, New York, NY, pp 255–265

Hill CE, Lambert MJ (2004) Methodological issues in studying psychotherapy processes and outcomes. In: Lambert MJ (ed) Bergin and Garfield's handbook of psychotherapy and behavior change, 5th edn. Wiley, Chicago, IL, pp 84–135

Hill CE, Thames TB, Rardin DK (1979) Comparison of Rogers, Perls, and Ellis on the hill counselor verbal response category system. J Couns Psychol 26: 198–208

Hilliard RB, Henry WP, Strupp HH (2000) An interpersonal model of psychotherapy: linking patient and therapist developmental history, therapeutic process and types of outcome. J Consult Clin Psychol 68: 125–133

Hoglend P, Johansonn P, Marble A, Bogwald KP, Almo S (2007) Moderators of the effects of transference interpretations in brief psychotherapy. Psychother Res 17:162–174

Horvarth AO, Greenberg LS (1989) Development and validation of the working alliance inventory. J Couns Psychol 36:223–233

Hubble M, Duncan BL, Miller SD (eds) (1999) The heart and soul of change: what works in therapy. American Psychological Association, Washington, DC

Kazdin AE (2009) Understanding how and why psychotherapy leads to change. Psychother Res 19:418–428

Kiesler DJ (ed) (1973) The process of psychotherapy: empirical foundations and systems of analysis. Aldine, Chicago, IL

Lambert MJ (ed) (2004) Bergin and Garfield's handbook of psychotherapy and behavior change, 5th edn. Wiley, Chicago, IL

Lambert MJ, Hill CE (1994) Assessing psychotherapy outcomes and processes. In: Lambert MJ (ed) Bergin and Garfield's handbook of psychotherapy and behavior change, 4th edn. Wiley, Chicago, IL, pp 72–113

Lambert M, Bergin G, Garfield SL (2004) Introduction and historical overview. In: Lambert M (ed) Bergin and Garfield's handbook of psychotherapy and behavior change, 5th edn. Wiley, New York, NY, pp 139–193

Llewelyn S, Hardy GE (2001) Process research in understanding and applying psychological therapies. Br J Clin Psychol 40:1–21

Macran S, Shapiro DA (1998) How does personal therapy affect therapists' practice. J Couns Psychol 71:13–25

Meyer B, Pilkonis PA (2002) Attachment style. In: Norcross JC (ed) Psychotherapy relationships that work. Oxford University Press, New York, NY, pp 367–389

Orlinsky DE, Ronnestad MH, Willutzki U (2004) Fifty years of psychotherapy process-outcome research: continuity and change. In: Lambert MJ (ed) Bergin and Garfield's handbook of psychotherapy and behavior change, 5th edn. Wiley, Chicago, IL, pp 307–389

Panchankis JE, Goldfried MR (2007) On the next generation of process research. Clin Psychol Rev 27:760–768

Piper WE, Azim HFA, Joyce AS, McCallum M (1991) Transference interpretations, therapeutic alliance, and outcome in short-term individual psychotherapy. Arch Gen Psychiatry 48:946–953

Polkinghorne DE (1988) Narrative knowing and the human sciences. SUNY, Albany, NY

Prochaska JO (1999) How do people change and how can we change to help many more people? In: Hubble M, Duncan BL, Miller SD (eds) The heart and soul of change: what works in therapy. American Psychological Association, Washington, DC, pp 227–255

Rennie DL (1994) Client deference in psychotherapy. J Couns Psychol 41:427–437

Rogers CR (1957) The necessary and sufficient conditions of therapeutic personality change. J Consult Psychol 21:95–103

Safran JD, Muran JC (2002) Negotiating the therapeutic alliance: a relational treatment guide. Guilford, New York, NY

Safran JD, Murran JC, Samstag LW, Stevens LC (2002) Repairing alliance ruptures. In: Norcross JC (ed) Psychotherapy relationships that work. Oxford University Press, New York, NY, pp 235–254

Schielke HJ, Fishman JL, Osatuke K, Stiles WB (2009) Creating consensus on interpretations of qualitative data: the ward method. Psychother Res 19:558–565

Scholing A, Emmelkemp PMG (1996) Treatment of generalised social phobia: results at long-term follow-up. Behav Res Ther 34:447–452

Silberschatz G, Fetter PB, Curtis JT (1986) How do interpretations influence the process of therapy? J Consult Clin Psychol 54:646–652

Stile WB (1988) Psychotherapy process-outcome correlations may be misleading. Psychotherapy 25:27–35

Stiles WB, Elliott R, Llewelyn S, Firth-Cozens J, Margison F, Shapiro DA, Hardy GE (1990) Assimilation of problematic experiences by clients in psychotherapy. Psychotherapy 27:411–420

Stiles WB, Reynolds S, Hardy GE, Rees A, Barkham M, Shapiro DA (1994) Evaluation and description of psychotherapy sessions by clients using the session evaluation questionnaire and the session impacts scale. J Couns Psychol 41:175–185

Stiles WB, Startup MS, Hardy GE, Barkham M, Rees A, Shapiro DA, Reynolds S (1996) Therapist intentions in cognitive-behavioral and psychodynamic-interpersonal psychotherapy. J Couns Psychol 43:402–414

Stiles WB, Barkham M, Twigg E, Mellor-Clark J, Cooper M (1998) Effectiveness of behavioural, person-centred, and psychodynamic therapies in UK primary-care routine practice: replication in a larger sample. Psychol Med 38:677–688

Tang TZ, DeRubeis RJ (1999) Sudden gains and critical sessions in cognitive-behavioral therapy for depression. J Consult Clin Psychol 67:894–904

Outlines of a General Theory of the Psychotherapy Process. The Clinical Exchange as Communicational Field: Theoretical Considerations and Methodological Implications

10

Sergio Salvatore and Alessandro Gennaro

Contents

Abstract

Psychotherapy process research nowadays is facing the need to make research evidence from different clinical approaches reciprocally commensurable. This seems possible through the design of general metatheoretical models of the clinical process that can both describe the clinical process and its working and pinpoint the dynamics regulating this process as well as the conditions that favour its functioning. This chapter outlines a semiotic and dynamic perspective in which the clinical process is conceived in terms of communicational dynamic field focusing on the ontological status of psychotherapy and the modelling of its basic modality of functioning. Finally, some methodological implications are outlined in terms of psychotherapy process modelling as a field phenomenon and strategies of knowledge building.

10.1 Research *In* and *On* the Process

In recent years *process research* has produced a huge amount of empirical data as a result of different approaches (single case studies, intensive qualitative and/or quantitative analysis, naturalistic studies and so on) and different data analysis strategies (use of standardised methods, hermeneutic approaches, discourse analyses and so on), and this trend still is ongoing

S. Salvatore (✉) • A. Gennaro
Department of History, Society and Human Studies, University of Salento, Via Stampacchia 45, 73100 Lecce, Italy
e-mail: sergio.salvatore@unisalento.it

O.C.G. Gelo et al. (eds.), *Psychotherapy Research*,
DOI 10.1007/978-3-7091-1382-0_10, © Springer-Verlag Wien 2015

(e.g. Lambert 2004; Elliott et al. 2009; Matos et al. 2009; Pascual-Leone et al. 2009), in the attempt to recognise the role played by components/variables in promoting clinical change (such as therapeutic alliance, therapist interventions, defence mechanisms, etc.; for a systematic review of the factors/components of psychotherapy, see Orlinsky et al. 2004).

However, in recent years some researchers have pointed out that such progress, despite its desirability, is still not satisfying: the dynamic sustaining change in the therapeutic process has to be explained too, namely, those mechanisms that allow a specific component of the clinical process to produce an effect on the patient's psychological state (Salvatore 2011). This underlines the need to develop a *general theory of the therapeutic process* (Mergenthaler 1996; Salvatore and Valsiner 2010a, b) that can show not only *what* works in regulating the clinical process but also *why* and under *which conditions* this happens.

In this perspective, it is possible to identify and distinguish two different focuses in the study of the course of psychotherapy: research *in* the process versus research *on* the process (Manzo 2010; Salvatore and Valsiner 2010a, b). The former focuses on those dimension-specific constructs acknowledged as being significant from a clinical viewpoint (i.e. therapeutic alliance, therapist interventions, defence mechanisms, metacognitive functioning). This approach considers the clinical process as a container in which such variables are displayed—thus, the process as such does not represent the target of this kind of research; rather it is the context within which it operates. The second perspective, research on the process, reflects a different and broader aim: the development of a theory of the clinical process, conceiving the process as a phenomenon existing per se, which has to be described and modelled as a whole (Salvatore et al. 2007b). This research focus deals with questions like: what does the psychotherapy process consist of? How does it work? What is clinical change? What is the dynamics of its functioning? What are the vectors and regulators of such dynamics?

Actually, few researchers have addressed the task of establishing a general theory of the process capable of addressing such questions (e.g. Mergenthaler 1996; Bucci 1997; Gonçalves et al. 2009; Salvatore et al. 2010a, b). This could be comprehensible: due to the plurality of psychotherapeutic approaches, *research on the process* is rather complex, since it is strictly connected to the elaboration of general models that are both quite abstract and able to grasp the specificity of the clinical intervention. Nowadays the definition of a general theory of the clinical exchange (here and henceforth this term is used as an equivalent of the psychotherapy process) is a priority for process research, which needs to look for a metatheoretical framework that is transversal to the clinical approaches (i.e. psychoanalysis, cognitivism, etc.) and thus capable of orienting analyses focused on specific aspects of the clinical exchange and to make them reciprocally commensurable.

The present work addresses this need. It proposes a semiotic and dynamic view of the psychotherapy process as a communicational dynamic field and discusses theoretical and methodological implications that can be drawn from it. It is divided into three parts. The first section outlines the semiotic model of the psychotherapy process as communicational field. The second section examines in greater depth some theoretical aspects associated with such a view—specifically, two aspects will be focused upon: the ontological status of psychotherapy and the modelling of its basic modality of functioning. The third section discusses some methodological implications of the model—namely, what modelling the psychotherapeutic process as a field phenomenon means and which strategies of knowledge building can be used to do it.

10.2 Section I: A Semiotic and Dynamic Look at the Psychotherapy Process

10.2.1 Clinical Exchange as a Communicational Field

The psychotherapy process is a communicative exchange. From a semiotic perspective (Salvatore and Gennaro 2012), communicative exchange represents the very substance of the clinical process. However, even those who do not share this theoretical framework should have no difficulty acknowledging that communicative exchange is the main vector of clinical factors, namely, that which allows psychotherapy to carry out its clinical function. The therapist operates in terms of acts (not only linguistic acts) which have an impact on the patient according to the way the latter interprets them in their role as communicative events (Austin 1962), and vice versa.

In brief, the conceptualisation of the communicative exchange in terms of field consists of the basic idea that the experience of the clinical relationship works as a regulator of participants' mind processes (Salvatore and Tschacher 2012). Such a view gives central importance to the conceptual issue of how meaning is intended and how it works. As the conception of meaning changes, the view of communication changes as well, along with the mode of conceiving and studying the clinical exchange. This conceptual task has to be considered as a general, foundational operation that crosses a plurality of research domains (clinical research, but also the general modelling of the mind, the psychosocial analysis of economic behaviours, the analysis of educational, organisational and socio-institutional settings; see Salvatore et al. 2009b, 2003, 2006/2009; Salvatore and Freda 2011; Salvatore and Zittoun 2011). It has led to a shift towards a semiotic view conceiving of human communication in terms of sensemaking, namely, as a dynamics of exchange of signs. According to this view, psychological processes are sustained and shaped by persons, who interpret the experience through the mediation of signs (e.g. words, meanings, images, beliefs, acts; cf. Salvatore and Zittoun 2011; Valsiner 2007). Communication and the person's mental activity associated with it are recursive chains of interpretations, namely, signs performed in interpreting the previous signs, in their turn performed in order to interpret the previous signs and so forth in an endless forward-backward process of semiosis (Salvatore 2011). Thus, to conceive of communication as a semiotic dynamic means addressing it as an ongoing activity of sensemaking. A central aspect of the semiotic view (in particular in Peirce's [1897/1932] version adopted here) is that meaning is not a fixed entity held in signs. Rather, it emerges within and through the way signs combine with each other in the semiotic chain. Thus, meaning is continuously shaped and reshaped by the interpretative activity comprising communication (Peirce 1897/1932; Wittgenstein 1958). This basic tenet has as an important corollary—the displacement of the theoretical and analytic focus from the content of signs to their structure and dynamics. Understanding sensemaking, therefore, means modelling the dynamic relationships among signs (Valsiner 2001) or the action they perform with each other. The way the experience is shaped and interpreted—namely, what people think, feel and enact—reflects this structural and dynamic relationship among signs.

The model of meaning and communication outlined above is quite removed from the commonsensical standpoint and also from most models in clinical psychology, which take meanings to be static and invariant entities, predefined and discrete properties to be applied to objects. On the other hand, a plurality of developments of contemporary psychology, in particular from what is broadly speaking the socio-constructivist framework (cf. inter alia Bruner 1990; Cole 1996; Gergen 1999; Edwards and Potter 1992; Valsiner and Rosa 2007), has highlighted the need to focus psychological analysis on actors' interpretative activity, intended as the process allowing the meaning to be co-constructed, rather than merely applied.

Socio-constructivism rejects the idea of meanings as fixed entities in the symbolic universe and maintains that meanings are not pre-existent to social and communicative exchange; rather they are built and redefined continuously by the communicative exchange itself. Meanings are contingent to intersubjective negotiations, and such negotiations, rather than being the results of abstract rules, are themselves social acts, oriented and organised by pragmatic and rhetorical instances of social regulation.

Some characteristics of what meaning is are outlined below, together with the relevant implications for clinical practice that can be drawn from them (Forges et al. 2008; Salvatore et al. 2009c).

Pragmaticity Thinking is not a neutral operation; rather, it is always a social act, sourced and fed by any form of intentionality (whether it be communicative, expressive or the like). In other words, the way actors interpret experience is one of the basic devices through which they are able to hold and promote their perspectives, world views, systems of interest and—in the final analysis—their identity. This means that people's thoughts and interactions are not limited to the aseptic application of computational rules, driven by criteria of truth, blind to their consequences. On the contrary, they organise thoughts, use rhetorical strategies, assume discursive positions and make use of communicational strategies in order to affirm/sustain a specific viewpoint, thus regulating the social exchange in which they are involved. In this sense thinking and communicating are social acts. This perspective entails a basic heuristic and methodological implication: the need to take into account the pragmatic dimension of meaning. While this aspect may seem obvious, it is not always taken into account within the field of psychotherapy process research, where often the focus is confined to the semantic and/or syntactic components of language (Manzo 2010).

Contextuality Sensemaking is not the product of an operative function located inside the mind but an inherently social process displayed through communicative exchange. Semantic structures (frames, schemata, scripts) regulating the mind's functioning must not be conceived in Kantian terms—like a priori forms constituting the human mind. Rather, they are to be seen as historical products: symbolic artefacts that the culture of a certain social group makes available to its own members (Cole 1996). From a clinical viewpoint, this means that what happens in the clinical process has to be considered in the light of the socio-symbolic context of which it is part, rather than as the immanent expression of an isolated mind.

Situativeness Meanings do not lie in a ubiquitous universe, from which they regulate people's thoughts and discourses. In fact, after Wittgenstein (1958), we are aware that meanings are defined through the way people make use of signs—thus, through the way they act (Harrè and Gillett 1994). This means that meanings have to be considered as circularly connected to the circumstances of communication and action. Meanings, on the one hand, allow actors to communicate and act; on the other hand, they are systematically and recursively redefined by these circumstances of communication and action. We speak of situativeness of meanings to discourses, in order to highlight that meaning is not pre-existent to communication and action but emerges from such processes (Salvatore et al. 2006/2009d; Salvatore and Freda 2011), as a result of the situated modalities of social exchange (Gergen 1999; Salvatore et al. 2005). The acknowledgment of the situativeness of meanings has a significant consequence for clinical research. The super-ordered frames of meaning regulating thinking are defined locally, within and through the micro-social dynamics in which they are used. Consequently, in order to understand the sense of what happens inside the clinical process one cannot limit oneself to considering discrete communicational units, as if they were meaningful entities in themselves; one also has to take into account the here and now of the intersubjective micro-dynamics sustaining the clinical exchange (Stern 2004). The last statement clarifies the meaning of the methodological tenet of communicative exchange indexicality (Salvatore et al. 2007a). This claims that any act —in our case the acts produced inside the clinical process—assumes different meanings according to the intersubjective context in which it is performed, for instance, the same utterance can work as an insult, nonsense and a compliment, depending on the discursive circumstances in which it is uttered.

10.2.2 Communication as Nonlinear Dynamic Field

The semiotic dynamic view of the psychotherapeutic process can be synthesised in the definition of the clinical exchange as a *nonlinear field dynamics of communication* (henceforth, only communicative field) (as to psychotherapy as nonlinear, see Barkham et al. 1993; Greenberg 1991; Hayes et al. 2007). The psychotherapy process is characterised by a huge number of elements, far more than the ones that psychotherapy research could ever take into consideration (Bickhard 2009). Moreover, what has to be taken into account is the interaction between elements rather than the elements themselves, namely, their working as part of a whole (Salvatore and Valsiner 2010a, b). Consequently, no elements can be considered as having an invariant clinical value. Rather, the impact of one factor on the whole therapeutic process is mediated by the field, in the sense of the set of dynamically interrelated co-occurring elements (Salvatore et al. 2009c).

We claim that the view of clinical exchange as communicative field is a promising framework in order to seek a general theory of the therapeutic process. It represents the convergence of different theoretical and clinical approaches. The psychoanalytic theory has developed the notion of therapeutic field as the capacity of the clinical relationship to be experienced as a salient psychological object, as such able to affect the mind processes of those who participate in the exchange (Odgen 2004; Storolow et al. 1994). Semiotic cultural psychology has elaborated this idea in terms of generalised and polysemic meanings (field signs; Valsiner 2007), embodied in sensemaking (Salvatore and Freda 2011), working as assumptions regulating the self and the interpretation of experience (Zittoun 2011). In the psychotherapy process research field, the acknowledgment of the field nature of the clinical exchange has led some authors to adopt concepts and methods developed in dynamic system theory (Salvatore and Tschacher 2012).

As intended here, the communicative field is the context of meaning emerging as the interaction of the structural (i.e. participant characteristics, treatment conditions, duration) and dynamic elements (i.e. therapeutic interventions, states of mind, elaborative styles, defence mechanisms, transference and counter-transference dynamics, narratives adopted, thematic contents, discursive forms) characterising the *hic et nunc*—the *present moment* (Stern 2004) of the clinical exchange.

The communicative field is constantly fed, reproduced and modelled over time by the same communicative acts (and corresponding intrapsychic configurations) sustaining clinical exchange. At the same time, the communicative field works as the semiotic environment in and through which the dynamics of clinical exchange unfolds. In other words, the communicative field defines those conditions and constraints in terms of which the elements of the therapeutic process interact and in so doing produce their clinical effects.

It is worth noting that the construct of communicative field does not add elements to the array of factors recognised as relevant by process research. Rather, the construct of communicative field is intended as the ground of a general explicative model of the clinical exchange; in other words a basic theory aimed at highlighting why and under which conditions therapeutic factors are able to produce change. This kind of theory does not replace specific clinical models, focused on the role played by particular factors in the therapeutic process but works as an explicative framework of such models, for it offers them an understanding of basic mechanisms mediating the salience of the factors studied. To express this with an image, the relationship between the general theory and specific models is analogous to that between molecular biology (i.e. the general theory modelling the basic mechanisms) and pharmacology (i.e. the discipline that studies the clinical effects of a certain drug).

10.3 Section II: Theoretical Considerations

10.3.1 The Ontological Status of the Psychotherapy Process

The view of the clinical process in terms of communicative field brings the issue of the ontological status of the psychotherapy process to the foreground. We devote this section to dealing with this very basic aspect, with the aim of helping to broaden the debate in psychotherapy research, still too weakly committed to the theoretical grounds underpinning empirical investigation (for significant exceptions, Slifes 2004; Gelo 2012).

To start with, take the following imaginary situation. Two people are playing roulette on different tables in a casino. The first person has come to the casino to have a relaxing night after a boring psychotherapy research meeting. The other one is a professional gambler, who lives thanks to his casino wins. It is easy to see that the two players have different aims in their gambling and this will be reflected in the way they play (betting organisation, reactions to results, attention to other players' wins and so on). Yet, the functioning of the roulette does not change—it remains constant, regardless of the difference in the gamblers' goals.

The same seems not be at stake if one considers psychotherapy instead of gambling. As a matter of fact, often clinical researchers tend implicitly to consider the therapeutic process as a specific object with its own functioning, differing from other human relationships. This assumption corresponds to believing that a specific human relationship (i.e. between therapist and patient) acquires a specific way of functioning due to its aim (i.e. psychotherapy).

We have already discussed the epistemological and theoretical issues raised by this implicit belief (Salvatore 2011; Salvatore and Valsiner 2006, 2010a, b; Salvatore et al. 2009a, 2010b, c). Here we will simply highlight the main point in terms of a paradox: if the socially defined aims driving a certain human relationship were able to configure the basic functioning of this relationship, then a research domain would have to be defined for each socially defined practice. For instance, it would be necessary to define specific theories dealing with having a pizza, visiting a museum, engaging in a romantic relationship, playing golf, going to a football match and so on. Of course someone might object that not all those process are important enough to justify a research domain, but this objection will make the situation even more complicated: without denying the model-specific characteristics of the phenomenon, it would mean that what is worth considering of scientific interest is established by socially defined hierarchies of values and interests.

The thesis of the ontological non-specificity of the psychotherapeutic process—as claimed here—empowers the heuristic possibilities of process research. Accordingly, the clinical process lends itself to be viewed as a local manifestation of general sensemaking dynamics, taken as the fundamental object of psychological inquiry. This perspective entails a distinction between the *dynamics* of the object and the *process* instantiating it (Salvatore and Valsiner 2010a, b; Salvatore 2011). The dynamics is the constitutive form of the phenomenon, its basic modality of coming to be. The dynamics is invariant and atemporal; consequently, it could be modelled in terms of universal rules. On the other hand, sensemaking is realised within and through specific sociocultural contexts, qualifying the aims, and therefore the conditions and constraints of happiness of the communicative exchange. Thus, the same dynamics can sustain different processes according to the field parameters (i.e. the characteristics defining the dynamic organisation of the field) defining the modalities of its instantiation (Salvatore 2011).

Consider physics. It deals with generalised phenomena, abstracted from their contingent empirical content—bodies, rather than stones, shoes, dishes and the like. Even if the dynamics is invariant, it brings about widely differing processes, due to the variety of field parameters involved. The trajectory of a bullet, the falling of stones, the orbit of a planet and so forth are covered by the same fundamental dynamics, but are different processes due to the field parameters associated with their functioning. Thus, processes have to be studied locally. This is what disciplines like ballistics, astronomy and hydraulics do, as domains of knowledge addressing specific phenomenic fields. Yet, the shape/way of functioning of these phenomenic fields (in the terminology adopted here: the process) always reflects the basic dynamics concerning the general class of phenomena of which such fields are local instantiations. Thus, for example, the trajectory of a bullet at a level of observation follows specific rules, different from the ones followed, say, by the trajectory of a planet or a stone or a tennis ball; yet at a more general level, it follows the same dynamics as other bodies. What makes such processes specific are the field parameters mediating the instantiation of their common dynamics. Consequently, to understand the trajectory of the bullet, one has to study the bullet but also to refer it to the general dynamics. In other words, the modelisation (i.e. the conceptualisation of the phenomenon in terms of abstract constructs) of the dynamics is the grounds of the analysis of local processes.

The analogy with physics allows us to highlight the distinction process/dynamics, thus to better understand how the psychotherapy process lends itself to be considered a specific form of communication created by particular field parameters—namely, cultural and institutional (e.g. the social representation of psychotherapy function, the organisational forms in terms of which the psychotherapy is performed), interpersonal (i.e. quality of the relationship), biopsychological (states of mind, personality, psychopathology and so forth) as well as technical (setting parameter) conditions. Such conditions make psychotherapy a unique form of human communication, compared with an infinite number of other versions of the same general phenomenon—i.e. human communication—such as romantic engagement, participating in a work meeting, giving a present, selling a car and so forth.

The distinction of dynamic/process and the idea of the non-autonomy of psychotherapy are not a mere philosophical discussion. On the contrary, it is immediately relevant to research, due to its conceptual and methodological implications. Insofar as aspects affecting the clinical process—be they specific or not—work on the grounds of basic mechanisms, the same identifiable in other forms of communicative exchange, and therefore understanding the psychotherapy process require three complementary lines of investigation:

(a) Modelling the clinical exchange's ways of working.
(b) Interpreting them as specific modalities of functioning of the basic dynamics of communication (and more in general of mental functioning) (see the next section).
(c) Identifying the conditions (field parameters) that constrain/allow such modalities to operate and produce clinical effects.

In the final analysis, this means reinterpreting the distinction between specific and nonspecific therapeutic factors in terms of the specific-general dichotomy (see Chap. 15).

10.3.2 A Dynamic and Semiotic Model of the Psychotherapy Process

In what follows a model of the psychotherapy process is presented: the Two-Stage Semiotic Model (TSSM, Salvatore et al. 2010a, b, c). The TSSM is a specific interpretation of the conceptual framework discussed in the first section, namely, the view of the psychotherapy process as a communicational field. It is based on a basic tenet and three assumptions derived from the tenet.

Basic Tenet: Psychotherapy as Sensemaking Dynamics Clinical exchange is an intersubjective dynamics of sensemaking aimed at modifying patients' affective and cognitive modalities of interpreting experience. Patients arrive at psychotherapy with a more or less rigid system of declarative and procedural assumptions (conception of self and others, affective schemata, metacognitive modalities, relational strategies, unconscious plans and so on) working as super-ordered meanings—in other words, premises of sense regulating the way of understanding their own experience (Valsiner 2007). Such assumptions represent both the source of the problem leading the patient to look for a psychological intervention and the ground and the constraints of sensemaking. Symptoms, intrapsychic and relational conflicts could be conceived of as the consequence as well as a form of expression of such super-ordered meanings. This leads us to conclude that the super-ordered meanings are the motive, the object and the aim as well as the mediator of the psychotherapeutic intervention.

Assumption 1: *The two-stage articulation*. In the initial moments of treatment, the clinical dialogue exposes the patient to the encounter with a different system of assumptions, which is part of and expressed by the clinical setting (therapist attitude, rules, modalities of relating). This difference works as a constraint on patient's system of assumptions. If it were not so, the patient could not but generalise her/his way of interpreting experience to the relationship with the therapist and in so doing fully reproduce within the clinical setting those critical elements (i.e. way of thinking, feelings, behaviours and attitude) that the clinical setting has been designed to address. For instance, a paranoid patient who considers everyone as wanting to attack and destroy him will have little chance of benefitting from psychotherapy if he assimilates the setting to his paranoid schema and thus feels that the therapist aims to hurt him. This first stage is therefore fundamentally a deconstructive process, in which the therapeutic dialogue works as an external constraint on the regulative activity of the patient's problematic super-ordered meanings (Salvatore and Valsiner 2006). The weakening of patient's critical super-ordered meaning paves the way for the second stage of psychotherapy characterised by patient elaboration of new assumptions. Thus, in the second stage, patient-therapist dialogue is supposed to implement new super-ordered meanings, replacing the previous system of assumptions regulating the patient's sensemaking experience.

Obviously, the two stages are not totally distinct and mutually exclusive. In any case, the two-stage assumption asserts that, at the macro-analytical level, in a clinically efficacious psychotherapy process it is possible to discriminate between one phase where deconstructive sensemaking is prevalent and another where clinical activity works in support of the patient's activity of exploring and creating new super-ordered meanings.

Assumption 2: *Nonlinearity of the psychotherapy process* The two-stage articulation of psychotherapy described by the first assumption implies that the clinical exchange performs different functions in the two stages: a deconstructive and a constructive function, respectively. Consequently, despite the traditional way of viewing the psychotherapy process, sensemaking does not follow a linear way of functioning over the course of the psychotherapy: sensemaking works in terms of change of patterns of functioning rather than as a summative modification of independent elements (on the nonlinear nature of the clinical process, see Russell 1994).

Assumption 3: *The quasiperiodic mechanism of sensemaking*. This third assumption concerns the micro-semiotic mechanism underlying sensemaking. In accordance with the nonlinearity of the clinical process (Lauro–Grotto et al. 2009), the TSSM assumes a quasiperiodic mechanism as the basis of the communicative exchange. This mechanism is characterised by a "fits and starts" trajectory, similar to a heartbeat trend, where moments of "basic" sensemaking are interrupted by circumscribed outbreaks of semiotic variability, or in other words of recombination between meanings.

10.3.2.1 Empirical Evidences About TSSM

A method of psychotherapy process analysis coherent with TSSM has been developed: the Discourse Flow Analyzer (DFA, Salvatore and Valsiner 2010a, b). The DFA has been applied to a sequence of psychotherapy cases (Gennaro et al. 2009, 2011; Nitti et al. 2010), in accordance with the logic of abductive generalisation (see the next section). A presentation of the method is provided in Sect. III; in what follows we simply report the main results, in order to provide some evidence of the TSSM construct validity:

(a) In each case analysed, the trend of super-ordered nodes follows a U shape. This trajectory is consistent with the initial deconstructive phase envisaged by the TSSM, where the clinical dialogue works in order to reduce patient super-ordered meanings, followed by a second constructive phase where the clinical process is characterised by the development of new meanings.
(b) Case analyses have highlighted how the two stages foreseen by TSSM are characterised by different patterns of functioning. For instance, correlations between relevant variables change—both in terms of their entity and in terms of their direction—from the first to the second stage.
(c) Analyses have highlighted a fits and starts trend of the sensemaking micro-dynamics. This trend is consistent with the third TSSM assumption, which claims that the course of sensemaking is characterised by circumscribed moments of semiotic variability breaking into the basic functioning.

10.4 Section III: Methodological Implications

10.4.1 Studying the Psychotherapy Process as a Communicative Field

The view of the psychotherapy process as a communicative field, with the ontological and theoretical implications highlighted above, leads us to conceive of the study of the clinical exchange in terms of two main complementary aims (Salvatore 2011): on the one hand, the identification of field parameters marking the dynamics of clinical exchange (in other words, the understanding of the mechanisms that allows the clinical exchange to work and make it specific, unlike other ways of human communication, as a communicative modality) and on the other hand, the understanding of the way such mechanisms mediate the interaction between elements of the clinical field (setting conditions, patient's and therapist's characteristics, therapeutic orientation, therapist's interventions, transference and counter-transference dynamics, therapeutic alliance, etc.) and their clinical impact. In sum, conceiving the clinical process in terms of communicative field implies the integration of two complementary investigative aims: on the one hand, the building of a model dealing with its emergence in the clinical process (and its reproduction over time) as a global property of the clinical exchange, able to characterise it as different from other human communicative forms (*upward causality*), and on the other hand, the modelling of the way the communicative field acts on the clinical exchange itself and on its ability to produce change (*downward causality*).

The above general aims can be broken down into the following complementary goals:

1. To highlight the action in the clinical exchange carried out by a higher-order context of meaning, which lends itself to be interpreted as communicative field.
2. To identify the specificity of such communicative field as compared to other forms of human communication.
3. To describe the dynamics that sustains the communicative field—that is, its emergence and its display over time.
4. To analyse the influence of the communicative field, both on the behaviour of the elements of the communicative exchange, their interaction, and on the global qualities of the process. In so doing one can expect to obtain a typology of field dynamics that can explain the different process-outcome trajectories (good outcome,

drop out, non-good outcome, therapeutic stalemate).

5. To detect the conditions and modalities allowing therapeutic interventions—and in a wider perspective: what happens in the clinical exchange—to affect the communicative field dynamics.

It is worth noticing that goals 1–5 reflect a set of working assumptions on the basic mechanisms sustaining the therapeutic process, taken from the current clinical literature and from general psychological models dealing with human communication. These are:

(a) Each therapeutic treatment is characterised by its own higher-order contextual meaning (Salvatore et al. 2012a, b).
(b) In the light of some characteristics (dynamicity, emergence), such meaningful context can be interpreted in terms of the communicative field (Salvatore et al. 2006/2009d; Schiepek et al. 1997).
(c) Independently from its contents, which are case-specific, the dynamics and the structure of the communicative field tend to show prototypical characteristics, which make psychotherapy a unique form of human communication. Specifically, the communicative field of the clinical exchange is characterised by an alternation of phases of opening and closing of the sensemaking dynamics, corresponding respectively to moments focusing on the production of innovative meaning and moments in which already consolidated meanings are used (Mergenthaler 1996; Bucci 1997; Gennaro et al. 2009).
(d) The communicative field emerges at the beginning of the clinical exchange between the first therapist–patient interactions, and it follows a nonlinear dynamics (Salvatore et al. 2006/2009d).
(e) The behaviour of salient elements of the psychotherapeutic process and their interaction is contingent to the communicative field. In other words, the trend of variables (and their combination) cannot be mapped as a stationary trajectory (i.e. a trend which can be described by a single model). Instead, it depends on the field conditions: it changes its way of working over time (i.e. two variables could correlate positively in a specific phase of the treatment and could correlate negatively in a following phase, once field conditions have changed) (Hayes et al. 2007).
(f) Following the above hypotheses, the communicative field is taken as a main factor on which the whole clinical quality of the therapeutic process and outcome depends. Consequently, one has to expect to find that the quality and efficacy of the clinical process are a function of the (dynamic and structural) model of the communicative field (Kraemer et al. 2007; Tschacher et al. 1998).
(g) Within the therapeutic process, a dynamics of upward causality is also in operation: what happens in the clinical exchange (acts, meanings, feelings, . . .) is not only influenced by the field but also influences it. The modalities and the conditions activated by such upward causality are—at least at a certain level of abstraction—similar among cases and therefore can be generalised.

Before concluding this section, an implication directly linked to the considerations made above needs to be highlighted. It is the idea that psychotherapy process analysis could benefit from different scientific disciplines and approaches, which developed models for the analysis and interpretation of human communication phenomena (i.e. ethnomethodology; conversational analysis; discourse analysis; cultural psychology; communication philosophy; neuroscience, infant research). The multidisciplinary dialogue offers the scientific space useful in understanding which aspects of the therapeutic process work (producing effects) as a reflection of more general modalities of communicative speech and which work as a result of specific dynamics of this peculiar form of communication.

10.4.2 The New Methodological Approach

In recent years the acknowledgment of the field, dynamic and nonlinear nature of the clinical exchange has led researchers to develop innovative strategies of analysis. For example, Ribeiro et al. (2012) analysed the semiotic and dialogic mechanism which, under specific conditions, sustains the reproduction of regressive and progressive components of patient narratives, while—under different condition—it favours the transition from one to the other. Tschacher and Ramseyer (2009) analysed the patient-therapist micro-dynamics of attunement, showing that an increase in the synchronisation of nonverbal behaviours of the therapeutic dyad is connected significantly to the quality of outcome. Salvatore et al. (2006/2009d) adopting an analysis method based on the dimensionality of the clinical exchange's phase space described the emergence and the maintenance of a shared frame of meaning in the clinical exchange, interpreted as evidence of a discursive attunement between patient and therapist.

In parallel with such methodological innovations, new procedures of data analysis have begun to be used in the field of psychotherapy research—e.g. pattern analysis (Santos et al. 2009), transition pattern analysis (Salvatore et al. 2012a, b) and network analysis (Nitti et al. 2010; Tschacher et al. 1998). In most of the cases, such procedures have been developed in other consolidated scientific domains (i.e. mathematic theory of dynamic systems; cf. Schiepek et al. 1997; Tschacher et al. 1992), where the dynamic nature of analysed objects is a consolidated acquisition. These innovative strategies of analysis, whether they may be different in focus and aims, share two basic methodological principles:

(a) The choice of micro units as observational data (e.g. utterances, or words of the clinical exchange; body micro movements); that is, observational units whose "resolution" is higher than the phenomenological experience.
(b) Data analysis is carried out in terms of analysis of dynamic transitions, based on the main idea that psychotherapy is a field phenomenon, defined by the interactions of its microcomponents over time (Lauro-Grotto et al. 2009; Tschacher and Grawe 1996).

10.4.2.1 The Logic of Investigation of the Psychotherapy Process as Field Dynamics

The communicative field represents a higher-order level of functioning. This high-order level has to be interpreted in epistemological rather than ontological terms. In other words, the communicative field must not be considered a separate reality but an observational level, which allows a structure of order to be recognised in the behaviour of specific components of the clinical exchange as well as in their interaction.

This brings into the foreground the methodological issue of how to model this structure of order. In what follows we present a logical architecture informed by the theory of dynamic systems and designed to address this issue. It integrates idiographic and nomothetic perspectives, in a two-step strategy.

Step 1: Intensive Analysis of a Set of Cases

Each case has to be analysed in parallel following the logical phases below:

1. Local analysis of a set of major components of the clinical exchange (e.g. therapeutic alliance; defence mechanisms; characteristics of setting, narratives; level/model of patient mentalisation) and their interaction (e.g. mentalisation/narratives). This means modelling the behaviour of such elements over time, in order to identify markers of field effects (auto-regression, nonlinearity, bifurcations, attractors, dissipative dynamics). The results of this phase will allow the elaboration of hypotheses about the global dynamics depicting the clinical exchange (e.g. in terms of periodic trajectories, nonlinear dynamics, self-organisation), which can guide the subsequent choice of a

mathematical model to adopt for the mapping of the communicative field.
2. Individual case analysis in terms of patterns of functioning. The analysis is organised in the following substages: (a) multidimensional breakdown of the molar characteristics of the therapeutic process and (b) their bottom-up reaggregation in terms of stable patterns identified in the multidimensional space (phase space) obtained from the previous breakdown.
3. Description of the identified pattern trajectories through time (in terms of emergence phenomena, stability, bifurcations, peaks, meta-trends). This operation involves the qualitative-quantitative description and the formal modelling of the trajectories that patterns display in the phase space.
4. Interpretation of the role played by the patterns identified. Patterns have to be considered as second-order latent constructs, working as mediator/moderator in the relationship between relevant clinical aspects of the process and their clinical effect.
5. Analysis of clinical exchange conditions determining pattern evolution—control parameters, in terms of the dynamic system theory. This operation calls for the identification of clinical exchange's local states associated with relevant variation points in the field dynamics (i.e. the characteristics of therapist intervention just preceding a peak in the trajectory of the communicative field).

The output of this idiographic level of analysis results in the mapping of each case, thus in the definition of a pool of explicative models of the dynamics of clinical change (in the hypotheses that there will not be a single dynamics explaining change, but a limited set of trajectories, each one associated to specific major characteristics of the clinical exchange).

Step 2: Generalisation of the Explicative Models

To this end, explicative models can be validated by evaluating their abilities to work as models that can explain change in new cases (estimation of the goodness of fit).

10.4.3 Modalities of Knowledge Building: The Problem of Generalisation

The peculiarity of the two-step strategy presented above lies in the fact that the aggregation of the information about cases needed for the generalisation process is developed at the level of those models, which map the whole dynamics of the same cases, rather than at the level of the specific elements (i.e. a specific narrative content, a specific therapist intervention).

This strategy comes from the recognition of the fact that, in field phenomena (as assumed for the therapeutic process), specific elements do not have one single meaning; rather, their meaning is contingent to the field; consequently, elements cannot be directly aggregated among cases (Salvatore and Valsiner 2010a, b).

10.4.3.1 Field Phenomena Have to Be Investigated in Idiographic Terms

The clinical process is a single event, implying two (or more) persons for a more or less long time period. On the other hand, scientific research requires the knowledge concerning single events to go beyond the boundaries of the single and thus become generalisable.

This clash between uniqueness and generalisability needs to be discussed in terms of a critical reading of the classical nomothetic-idiographic contrast (Salvatore and Valsiner 2009; Salvatore et al. 2009a, b, c, d, 2010a, b; Molenaar and Valsiner 2009). Following the lesson of Windelband (1904/1998; see also Lamiell 2003), the terms form a complementary relationship, rather than an opposition. Due to their dynamic (time dependent) and contextual nature, psychological phenomena are unique, in the sense that their way of working is mediated by the contingence of field conditions. Consequently, scientific psychology cannot but be intrinsically idiographic, in the sense that it cannot but take into account phenomena which are unique and irreversible (on this topic see also Toomela 2009). At the same time the aim of any scientific knowledge is intrinsically nomothetic, that is, devoted to building general knowledge, beyond the phenomenical field that serves as its source. Hence, the problem of psychology, therefore of psychotherapy process research, is the identification of a logical model of generalisation that is coherent with the idiographic nature of the object in analysis.

In some recent works (Salvatore and Valsiner 2009, 2010a, b), abduction has been suggested as the basic form of psychological knowledge. According to the argument put forward in these works, the uniqueness of psychological objects disproves the possibility of making a generalisation through induction, namely, as accumulation of empirical occurrences, each of which come from an individual observation. Peirce (1897) talks about induction in terms of acquisition of a habit: if an event occurs *n* times, then we could induce that it has a regularity that gets one accustomed to considering valid for the future too. The conceptual inconsistency of induction derives from the recognition that individual cases, insofar they are unique, cannot be compared with each other; consequently, it has to be concluded that it is impossible to liken observation coming from different cases. This principle has been described from a psychometrical perspective by Molenaar in terms of the violation of the ergodic assumption characterising psychological processes (Molenaar 2004; Molenaar and Valsiner 2009).

Abductive generalisation represents an alternative to inductive generalisation (Di Nuovo 2010). Like induction, the abductive generalisation starts from data but is oriented to the construction of a theoretical local model, namely, a model that can depict and interpret the phenomenical occurrences of the single case (to encompass the totality of predicates, to recall Pierce's image). On the other hand, the theoretical local model is produced on the ground and within the constraints of the general theory underlying the inquiry. Thus, it is the relationship between local theory and general theory that is generalised, rather than the redundancy/regularities of data, as in inductive generalisation. This is the same as saying that abductive generalisation concerns the construction of an intermediate model that is between the general and the local model, namely, a model that can be grounded and reflect the general theory's assumption and at the same time abstract enough (i.e. expressed in independent terms from the empirical content of the single case[1]) to be able to interpret the plurality of cases.

Let us consider the series C of cases (1,2,3,. . ..,*n*) and the set of occurrences O_c of which any single case *c* consists. The inductive generalisation defines the superset (S_I) of the sets of occurrences O_c. S_I cumulates all the occurrences, which are (in accordance to the observer's standards) *descriptively* similar among them, regardless which cases they belong to. On this basis, the general rule mapping the behaviour of the S_I set is assumed to be valid for all *c* cases too. In contrast, in the case of abductive generalisation, it is the O_1 set (namely, the occurrences concerning case 1) which is modelled as a single and unrepeatable phenomenon, as such not encompassing the occurrences concerning other cases. This operation generates the local model L_1, which is developed on the

[1] For instance, take into account the case characterised by the occurrences: a, b, b, a, b, b, b, a, b, b, b, b, a. The empirical content of such a process is unique; thus it could not be generalised if such content were taken as the object of analysis. In contrast, the pattern characterising the relationship a-b could be analysed beyond (but not independently from) its empirical content—i.e. in terms of the tendency of the second element of the dyad (b) to increase its incidence through time. Now, this model represents an abstract map of the case, a representation of it devoid of empirical content. On the other hand, "giving up" the reference to the empirical makes it possible to develop a generalisation among different cases through abstraction—for instance, it could be argued that a case highlighting the pattern m, n, n, m, n, n, n, m, n, n, n, n, m, in spite of the different empirical content, follows the same model as the former case.

ground and within the constraints of the general theory (T_C) framing the investigation. Once developed, L_1 is used to interpret O_2, namely, the occurrences comprising case 2. In this interpretative process, L_1 undergoes abstraction in order to include the local specificity of case 2. Thus L_1 is transformed into a more generalised model $L_{(1,2)}$. $L_{(1,2)}$ is able to keep the ability of working as a map of both O_1 and O_2. Insofar as $L_{(1,2)}$ proves to be consistent with T_C, then $L_{(1,2)}$ is considered a generalisation of $L_{(1)}$ within the frame of the general theory. The recursive application of such abductive procedure to the succession of cases C will produce the model $L_{(1,\ 2,\ldots,n)}$ which constitutes the *generalised local model*, endowed with the abstractive level needed to interpret the specificity of each single case of C.[2]

In short, the fundamental difference between induction and abduction is that the former is aimed at detecting what is common among cases, while the latter strives to strengthen the theory, through its accommodation in coping with the variability of cases. An example might be useful to highlight this difference. Take two researchers, *Induct* and *Abduct*, interested in studying the relationship between therapist's interventions and symptomatology. Induct makes use of the inductive approach. Thus she takes into consideration a single case verifying, say, the frequencies of certain therapist's interventions in each session and patient's symptomatology at the end of each session. Imagine that *Induct* finds that the symptomatology level is lower at the end of a session characterised by a higher number of therapist interventions. Now *Induct* analyses several different cases discovering that in most circumstances (or in all circumstances, the difference is irrelevant here) the results are similar. On this basis, she concludes: "In the cases analyzed, I observed systematically that a higher frequency of therapist intervention produces a decrease in patient symptoms". Having at her disposal a huge number of cases supporting this relationship, *Induct* is legitimated (is inducted) to conclude that the relationship between the frequency of therapist interventions and the reduction of symptomatology is a universal rule, valid for all cases. Thus *Induct* has operated an inductive generalisation. To use the terminology adopted above, she has collected the set of descriptively similar O_c occurrences (symptomatology and intervention frequencies) from each case of the series C, in so doing creating the generalised class S_I, where the map of S_I—i.e. symptomatology (S) is a function of the frequency of therapist intervention (*int*); in other words, $S = f(Int)$—has been invested with the rule valid for all the cases.

From what has been observed above, one can conclude that inductive generalisation is an *extensional* modality of building knowledge, consisting of the possibility of increasing the number of cases for which the law—originally referred to a restricted number of cases—can be considered valid.

Abduct decides to follow a different strategy—abductive generalisation. To this end, she takes as reference a general theory (T_C), preceding (and driving) the empirical inquiry. Let's say *Abduct* adopts the intersubjectivist standpoint claiming the contingency of the patient's mind to the clinical relationship; on this basis, she grounds the inquiry on the general theory (T_C), namely, on the model, $S = f(R)$; the symptomatology level S is a function of the patient-therapist relationship (R). As one can see, *Abduct*'s starting point—the general theory—coincides with *Induct*'s conclusion. According to T_C, *Abduct* starts the analysis of case 1. T_C guides and constraints Abduct both in the selection of the relevant occurrences—i.e. symptomatology and markers of the clinical relationship—and in modelling their linkage. Thus T_C enables *Abduct* to develop an interpretative model (L_1) of the case 1: $S = f(Int)$. It is worth underlining that even if it is not different from *Induct*'s, this model is strictly local and therefore, unlike *Induct*'s, its validity is circumscribed to case 1—it is a kind of idiographic knowledge. *Abduct* goes on with her inquiry and examines case 2, interpreting it in terms of the local model as previously defined

[2] An example of a research method following such logic is task analysis (cf. Pascual-Leone et al. 2009).

(L_1). But in case 2, *Abduct* identifies a pattern which cannot be likened to L_1: in a limited number of sessions the higher frequency of intervention is associated to an increase rather than a decrease in patient symptoms. If *Abduct* took into account the global set of occurrences observed, this would only be a marginal aspect, an exception that could be put aside. Yet this is precisely the pattern that *Abduct* focuses on, forcing her to accommodate L_1 in order to make it able to encompass the divergent pattern too. In so doing, *Abduct* comes to define a new local model $L_{(1,2)}$, more general than $L_{(1)}$, that can both interpret case 2 and provide a reinterpretation of case 1. The model, for instance, could be $S = F(Int_{rel})$: "the level of symptomatology depends on the proportion of therapist intervention as compared to linguistic acts produced by the patient (Int_{rel})". It can be observed that $L_{(1,2)}$ belongs to a more abstract level than $L_{(1)}$ in the sense that: (a) it concerns a pattern more distant from contingent empirical data (i.e. the same value of *Int* could refer to two different values of Int_{rel} and vice versa) and (b) it focuses on a more specific and circumscribed aspect, as a result of a more powerful operation of selection of the pertinent elements (about the idea of abstraction as pertinentisation, see also Salvatore and Valsiner 2009). *Abduct*, then, analyses case 3, producing $L_{(1,2,3)}$ and so forth, continuing in her operation of accommodating the local model due to divergent patterns retrieved from the other cases. This process of generalisation through abstractive accommodation goes on until the generalised local model is able to work as an interpretative theory of subsequent cases without any need for further accommodation. On the other hand, in parallel, the generalisation of the local model through abstractive accommodation generates a "tension" on the general theory T_C. Thus, the development of the generalised local model works as a dialectic factor for the validation and/or the redefinition of the general theory—in accordance to T_C's ability to bear the pressure of the generalisation of the local model. Otherwise it needs to be developed in order to allow the latter's abstractive accommodation.

One can thus conclude that if inductive generalisation is an extensional way of building knowledge, abductive generalisation follows an *intensional logic*: a model of knowledge consisting of the progressive development (articulation/abstraction) of theory through the dialectics among levels of modelisation (local vs. general).

Before concluding this section, it is worth highlighting some implications that make the discussion on abduction of immediate interest for clinical research. Firstly, abductive logic gives primacy back to theory. Abductive generalisation is driven by theory. Knowledge is developed as a recursive process of theory development, resulting from the systematic attempt to produce local interpretations of phenomena in the light of generalised assumptions. This means that in the abductive logic the primacy of theory does not mean denying the role played by empirical investigation. Rather, empirical research is valorised, not as a substitute for theory, but it works as the dialectic lever of the theoretical development.

Secondly, abductive logic activates a peculiar logic (and culture) of research, which is different from the one on which induction is based. The abductive development of theory is committed to the heuristic valence of theory; the choice of the phenomena to be studied aims for marginal and divergent events, namely, data disconfirming previously acquired interpretations, therefore able to force the researcher to accommodate (re-modulate, re-elaborate) the theory. In sum, marginal cases, which are regarded by mainstream inductive methodology as noise preventing the identification of regularities, are conceived of as source of knowledge in the logic of abduction.

Finally, abductive logic provides evidence of the utility in psychology (and therefore in clinical psychology) of developing formalised languages to carry out case modelling. Insofar as generalisation is performed through progressive abstraction, then formalised languages are useful tools for the development of clinical theory.

Conclusions

In this work we have tried to highlight the need for a general theory of the psychotherapy process and to take some steps towards developing one. Psychotherapy research calls for a theory of such kind, because it may not limit itself to recognise the role played by this or that element in promoting clinical change—the empowerment of clinical interventions, both in terms of effectiveness and efficiency, requires that research being able to explain why and under which conditions the clinical process succeeds in promoting change, too.

In our view, in order to address such a conceptual task, psychotherapy research has to rediscover conceptual analysis. Needless to say, as used here, conceptual analysis is not a substitute for empirical investigation but its complement: the awareness of the epistemological, theoretical and methodological assumptions on which empirical investigation is grounded is a way of strengthening the latter, making it more consistent both with actual clinical practice and psychological scientific models.

Acknowledgments We want to thank Paolo Allegrini, Enrico Ciavolino, Antonello Colli, Claudio Gentili, Angelo Gimignani, Margherita Lang, Flavia Lecciso, Vittorio Lingiardi, Gianluca Lo Coco, Laura Parolin, Diego Rocco, Claudia Venuleo and Alessandro Zennaro who read parts of the manuscript, providing us with insightful comments.

References

Austin J (1962) How to do things with words. Oxford University Press, Oxford

Barkham M, Stiles WB, Shapiro DA (1993) The shape of change in psychotherapy: Longitudinal assessment of personal problems. J Consult Clin Psychol 61:667–677. doi:10.1037/0022-006X.61.4.667

Bickhard MH (2009) Interactivism: a manifesto. New Ideas Psychol 27:85–9. doi:10.1016/j.newideapsych.2008.05.001

Bruner J (1990) Acts of meaning. Harvard University Press, Cambridge

Bucci W (1997) Psychoanalysis and cognitive science. Guilford, New York

Cole M (1996) Cultural psychology. A once and future discipline. Harvard University Press, Cambridge

Di Nuovo S (2010) Back to phenomenology: An (old) new way for psychotherapy research. In: Salvatore S, Valsiner J, Gennaro A, Traves J (eds) Yearbook of idiographic science, vol 2. Firera Publishing Group, Roma

Edwards D, Potter J (1992) Discursive psychology. Sage, London

Elliott R, Partyka R, Alperin R, Dobrenski R et al (2009) An adjudicated hermeneutic single-case efficacy design study of experiential therapy for panic/phobia. Psychother Res 19(4–5):543–57. doi:10.1080/10503300902905947

Forges Davanzati G, Potì S, Salvatore S (2008) L'economia irregolare come fenomeno culturale. Note per una interpretazione psicosociale.[Irregular economy as cultural phenomenon. Highlights for a psychosocial interpretation] Il pensiero economico moderno XXVIII (4): 63–88

Gelo OCG (2012) On research methods and their philosophical assumptions: "Raising the consciousness of researchers" again. Psychotherapie und Sozialwissenschaft 2:111–130

Gennaro A, Al-Radaideh A, Gelo OCG, Manzo S, Nitti M, Auletta AF, Salvatore S (2009) Modelling the psychotherapy process as a sensemaking dynamics. The Two Stage Semiotic Model (TSSM) and the Discourse Flow Analyzer (DFA). In: Salvatore S, Valsiner J, Traves Simon JB, Gennaro A (eds) YIS: Yearbook of idiographic science, vol 2. Firera Publishing Group, Roma, pp 131–170

Gennaro A, Gonçalves M, Mendes I, Ribeiro A, Salvatore S (2011) Dynamics of sensemaking and development of the narrative in the clinical exchange. Res Psychother Psychopathol Process Outcome 14(1): 90–120

Gergen K (1999) An invitation to social construction. Sage, London

Gonçalves M, Matos M, Santos A (2009) Narrative therapy and the nature of "innovative moments" in the construction of change. J Constr Psychol 22:1–23. doi:10.1080/10720530802500748

Greenberg LS (1991) Research on the process of change. Psychother Res 1:3–16. doi:10.1080/10503309112331334011

Harrè R, Gillett G (1994) The discursive mind. Sage, London

Hayes AM, Laurenceau JP, Feldman G, Strauss JL, Cardaciotto L (2007) Change is not always linear: The study of nonlinear and discontinuous patterns of change in psychotherapy. Clin Psychol Rev 27:715–723. doi:10.1037/a0014488

Kraemer S, Lihl M, Mergenthaler E (2007) Schlüsselstunden im Verlauf kognitiver

Verhaltenstherapie von schizophrenen Patienten: Ein Beitrag zur Prozessforschung. Verhaltenstherapie 17:90–99. doi:10.1159/000101472

Lambert MJ (2004) Bergin and Garfield's handbook of psychotherapy and behavior change, 5th edn. Wiley, New York

Lamiell JT (2003) Beyond individual and group differences. Sage, Thousand Oaks

Lauro–Grotto R, Salvatore S, Gennaro A, Gelo OCG (2009) The unbearable dynamicity of psychological processes: highlights of the psychodynamics theories. In: Valsiner J, Molenaar PCM, Lyra M, Chaudhary N (eds) Dynamics process methodology in the social and developmental sciences. Springer, New York, pp 1–30

Manzo S (2010) La ricerca di processo nel decennio 1998–2007 [Process research in the 1998–2007 decade]. Ricerca in psicoterapia/Res Psychother Psychopathol Process Outcome 13(1):92–119

Matos M, Santos A, Gonçalves M, Martins C (2009) Innovative moments and change in narrative therapy. Psychother Res 19(1):68–80. doi:10.1080/10503300802430657

Mergenthaler E (1996) Emotion abstraction patterns in verbatim protocols: a new way of describing therapeutic processes. J Consult Clin Psychol 64:1306–1315. doi:10.1037/0022-006X.64.6.1306

Molenaar PCM (2004) A manifesto on psychology as idiographic science: bringing the person back into scientific psychology, this time forever. Measurement 2:201–218. doi:10.1207/s15366359mea0204

Molenaar PCM, Valsiner J (2009) How generalization works through the single case: A simple idiographic process analysis of an individual psychotherapy. In: Salvatore S, Valsiner J, Strout S, Clegg J (eds) YIS: Yearbook of idiographic science, vol 1. Firera Publishing Group, Rome, pp 23–38

Nitti M, Ciavolino E, Salvatore S, Gennaro A (2010) Analyzing psychotherapy process as intersubjective sensemaking. An approach based on discourse analysis and neural networks. Psychother Res 20 (5):546–563. doi:10.1080/10503301003641886

Odgen TH (2004) The analytic third. Implications for psychoanalytic theory and technique. Psychoanal Quart 73(1):167–194. doi:10.1002/j.2167-4086.2004.tb00156.x

Orlinsky DE, Ronnestad MH, Willutzki U (2004) Fifty years of psychotherapy process-outcome research: continuity and change. In: Lambert MJ (ed) Bergin and Garfield's handbook of psychotherapy and behaviour change, 5th edn. Wiley, New York, pp 307–389

Pascual-Leone A, Greenberg LS, Pascual-Leone L (2009) Developments in task analysis: new methods to study change. Psychother Res 19(4):527–542. doi:10.1080/10503300902897797

Peirce CS (1897/1932) In Hartshorne C, Weiss P (eds) Collected papers of Charles Sanders Peirce, vol 2. Harvard University Press, Cambridge

Ribeiro PA, Gonçalves MM, Santos A (2012) Innovative moments in psychotherapy: From the narrative outputs to the semiotic-dialogical processes. In: Salvatore S, Gennaro A, Valsiner J (eds) Yearbook of idiographic science, vol 4. Information Age Publishing, Charlotte, NC, pp 149–175

Russell RL (1994) Reassessing psychotherapy research. Guilford Press, New York

Salvatore S (2011) Psychotherapy Research Needs Theory. Outline for an Epistemology of the Clinical Exchange. Integr Psychol Behav Sci 45:366–388. doi:10.1007/s12124-011-9180-9

Salvatore S, Freda MF (2011) The role of the unconscious in communication. Outlines for a comprehensive model of sensemaking. New Ideas Psychol 29(1):119–135. doi:10.1016/j.newideapsych.2010.06.001

Salvatore S, Gennaro A (2012) The inherent dialogicality of the clinical exchange. Int J Dial Sci 1:1–14

Salvatore S, Tschacher W (2012) Time dependency of psychotherapeutic exchanges: the contribution of the theory of dynamic systems in analyzing process. Front Psychol 3:253. doi:10.3389/FPSYG.2012.00253

Salvatore S, Valsiner J (2006) 'Am I really a psychologist?' Making sense of a super–human social role. Eur J School Psychol 4:5–30

Salvatore S, Valsiner J (2009) Idiographic science on its way: Towards making sense of psychology. In: Salvatore S, Valsiner J, Strout-Yagodzynski S, Clegg J (eds) Yearbook of idiographic science, vol 1. Firera & Liuzzo Group, Rome, pp 9–19

Salvatore S, Valsiner J (2010a) Idiographic Science as a non-existing object: The importance of the reality of the dynamic system. In: Salvatore S, Valsiner J, Gennaro A, Traves Simon JB (eds) Yearbook of idiographic science, vol 3. Firera & Liuzzo Group, Rome, pp 7–26

Salvatore S, Valsiner J (2010b) Between the general and the unique: overcoming the nomothetic versus idiographic opposition. Theory Psychol 20(6):817–833. doi:10.1177/0959354310381156

Salvatore S, Zittoun T (eds) (2011) Cultural psychology and psychoanalysis in dialogue. Issues for constructive theoretical and methodological synergies. Information Age Publishing, Charlotte

Salvatore S, Freda MF, Ligorio B, Iannaccone A, Rubino F, Scotto di Carlo M, Bastianoni P, Gentile M (2003) Socioconstructivism and theory of the unconscious. A gaze over a research horizon. Eur J School Psychol 1(1):9–36

Salvatore S, Ligorio MB, De Franchis C (2005) Does psychoanalytic theory have anything to say on learning? Eur J School Psychol 3(1):101–126

Salvatore S, Gennaro A, Grassi R, Manzo S, Melgiovanni S, Mossi P, Olive C, Serio V (2007a) Lo studio del processo terapeutico in termini di analisi della dinamica discorsiva. Applicazione del DFA (Discourse Flow Analyzer) al caso Katja [Therapeuthic process research in terms of discorsive analysis. DFA (Discourse Flow Analyzer) application to Katja case]. In: Salvatore S, Nicolò G, Salvatore S, Nicolò G (eds) La ricerca sulla psicoterapia. Prospettive e materiali di studio dal contesto italiano [Psychotherapy research. Research perspective from the italian context]. Edizioni Carlo Amore, Rome

Salvatore S, Mossi P, Gennaro A (2007b) Il discorso sulla psicoterapia, tra dinamiche istituzionali, concezioni della mente, modelli di intervento, pratiche di ricerca. [Engl. Tr. Approaching psychotherapy between institutional dynamics, mind conception, model of intervention, research practices]. In: Salvatore S, Nicolò G (eds) La ricerca sulla psicoterapia. Prospettive e materiali di studio dal contesto italiano [Psychotherapy research. Research perspective from the italian context]. Edizioni Carlo Amore, Rome, pp 43–66

Salvatore S, Valsiner J, Strout-Yagodzynski S, Clegg J (2009a) Yearbook of idiographic science. Firera & Liuzzo Group, Rome

Salvatore S, Forges Davanzati G, Potì S, Ruggeri R (2009b) Mainstream economics and sense-making. Integr Psychol Behav Sci 43(2):158–177. doi:10.1007/s12124-008-9084-5

Salvatore S, Lauro-grotto R, Gennaro A, Gelo OCG (2009c) Grasping the dynamic nature of intersubjectivity. In: Valsiner J, Moolenar PCM, Lyra MCDP, Chaudhary N (eds) Dynamic process methodology in the social and developmental sciences. Springer, New York, pp 171–190

Salvatore S, Tebaldi C, Poti S (2009) The discursive dynamic of sensemaking. In Salvatore S, Valsiner J, Strout S, Clegg J (eds) YIS: Yearbook of idiographic science 2008, vol 1. Firera Publishing, Rome, pp. 39–72. First published 2006, in International Journal of Idiographic Science [On Line Journal], Article 3.

Salvatore S, Gelo OCG, Gennaro A, Manzo S, Al-Radaideh A (2010a) Looking at the psychotherapy process as an intersubjective dynamic of sensemaking. A case study with discourse flow analysis. J Construct Psychol 23(3):195–230. doi:10.1080/10720531003765981

Salvatore S, Valsiner J, Travers–Simon J, Gennaro A (2010b) YIS: Yearbook of idiographic science, vol 2. Firera Publishing Group, Rome

Salvatore S, Valsiner J, Travers–Simon J, Gennaro A (2010c) YIS: Yearbook of idiographic science, vol 3. Firera Publishing Group, Rome

Salvatore S, Gennaro A, Auletta A, Tonti M, Nitti M (2012a) Automated method for content analysis. A device for psychotherapy process. Psychother Res 22 (3):256–273

Salvatore S, Gennaro A, Auletta A, Grassi R, Rocco D (2012b) Dynamic Mapping of the Structures of Content in Clinical Setting (DMSC). A new coding system for analyzing the patient's narratives. Psychother Theory Res Pract 85(4):391–423. doi:10.1111/j.2044-8341.2011.02038.x

Santos A, Goncalves MM, Matos M, Salvatore S (2009) Innovative moments and change pathways. A good outcome case of narrative therapy. Psychol Psychother Theory Res Pract 82:449–466. doi:10.1348/147608309X462442

Schiepek G, Kowalik ZJ, Schiitz A, Kohler M, Richter K, Strunk G, Miihlnickel W, Elbert T (1997) Psychotherapy as a chaotic process I: coding the client-therapist interaction by means of a sequential plan and the search for chaos: a stationary approach. Psychother Res 7(2):173–194

Slifes BD (2004) Theoretical challenges to therapy practice and research: The constraint of naturalism. In: Lambert MJ (ed) Bergin and Garfield's handbook of psychotherapy and behavior change, 5th edn. Wiley, New York, pp 44–83

Stern D (2004) The present moment in psychotherapy and everyday life. Norton, New York

Storolow RD, Atwood GE, Brandchaft B (1994) The intersubjective perspective. Jason Aronson, Hillsdale, NJ

Toomela A (2009) How methodology became a toolbox – and how it escapes from that toolbox. In: Valsiner J, Moolenar PCM, Lyra MCDP, Chauldary N (eds) Dynamic methodology in the social and developmental science. Springer, New York

Tschacher W, Grawe K (1996) Selbstorganisation in Therapieprozessen—Die Hypothese und empirische Prufung der "Reduktion von Freiheitsgraden" bei der Entstehung von Therapiesystemen. Z Klin Psychol 25:55–60

Tschacher W, Ramseyer F (2009) Modelling psychotherapy process by time-series panel analysis (TSPA). Psychother Res 19(4–5):469–81. doi:10.1080/10503300802654496

Tschacher W, Schiepek G, Brummer EJ (eds) (1992) Self-organization and clinical psychology. Empirical approaches to synergetics in psychology. Springer, Berlin

Tschacher W, Scheier C, Grawe K (1998) Order and pattern formation in psychotherapy. Nonlin Dynam Psychol Life Sci 2:195–215

Valsiner J (2001) Culture and human development. Sage, London

Valsiner J (2007) Culture in minds and societies. Foundations of cultural psychology. Sage, New Delhi

Valsiner J, Rosa A (2007) The Cambridge handbook of sociocultural psychology. Cambridge University Press, New York

Windelband W (1998) History and natural science. Theory Psychol 8: 5–22. Original version published in 1904. doi: 10.1177/0959354398081001

Wittgenstein L (1958) Philosophical investigations. Basic Blackwell, Oxford

Zittoun T (2011) Meaning and change in psychotherapy. Integr Psychol Behav Sci 45:325–334. doi:10.1007/s12124-011-9166

11 The Relationship: How It Works

Stephanie L. Budge and Bruce E. Wampold

Contents

Abstract

As tension continues to exist between those who endorse contextual versus medical explanations for the efficacy of psychotherapy, it remains undetermined *how* psychotherapy works. One of the primary purposes of this chapter is to provide a rationale on evolved social and relational characteristics for the efficacy of psychotherapy. In conjunction with an evolutionary explanation for why psychotherapy is effective, we provide compelling evidence that there is a neurological and social context for three separate pathways—which we call the tripartite model of the relationship. The first path includes the real relationship between the patient and the therapist. The second path is comprised of expectations that are maintained and generated via cogent rationales and treatments. The third path consists of the benefits of healthy actions and how specific ingredients contribute to these behaviors.

S.L. Budge (✉)
University of Wisconsin-Madison, Louisville, KY, USA
e-mail: budge@wisc.edu

B.E. Wampold
University of Wisconsin-Madison, Madison, WI, USA

Forskningsinstituttet, Modum Bad Psychiatric Center, Vikersund, Norway

11.1 Introduction

One of the primary points of contention among researchers over the last several decades regards what makes psychotherapy work. The focus of this research has varied, from studying

O.C.G. Gelo et al. (eds.), *Psychotherapy Research*,
DOI 10.1007/978-3-7091-1382-0_11, © Springer-Verlag Wien 2015

techniques (e.g., specific ingredients of therapy such as exposure or systematic desensitization), common factors (e.g., variables found in most therapies apart from theoretical orientation, such as empathy, alliance, acceptance), expectancy (e.g., placebo effects, client and therapist belief in treatment), and extratherapeutic factors (e.g., social support, spontaneous remission) (Lambert and Barley 2002) (see Chap. 15). As psychotherapy research has continued to evolve in studying these factors, the focus of research recently, it seems, is on identifying specific treatments for specific disorders. Within the empirically supportive treatment (EST) movement, specific guidelines have been set as to how researchers can correctly and competently run a psychotherapy research trial in order to determine if a treatment is effective, such as having a tightly controlled randomized trial with treatment manuals (see Task Force on Promotion and Dissemination of Psychological Procedures 1995). Norcross (2011) indicated that there are three main pieces that are missing from this type of research: (a) the person of the therapist, (b) the therapy relationship, and c) the patient's nondiagnostic characteristics. The purpose of this chapter is to present a model that integrates the common factors (e.g., a core group of therapeutic factors shared by all treatments that contribute to change) and specific ingredients, and this integrated model shows why psychotherapy works. This model is based on evolved human traits, and it is our contention that psychotherapy is effective because humans have evolved to respond to psychotherapy.

11.1.1 Can Common and Specific Factors Coexist?

In this chapter, we propose a model that integrates the specific factors and the common factors at a level of abstraction that does not give primacy to one over the other or that proposes that one is necessary but not sufficient (see also Chap. 15). We make the claim that neither the common factor nor the specific ingredient models capture the essence of *why* psychotherapy is truly effective. Indeed, we wish to move beyond the language of common factors and specific ingredients to talk about the factors that make psychotherapy therapeutic.

Generally speaking, researchers fall into two camps: those who believe that treatment ingredients are the core of effective therapy and those who believe that common factors, patient factors, and interactions are important. There is a partial, although unsatisfying, resolution of these two positions, by recognizing that the common factors are in a sense necessary to deliver particular treatments for particular disorders, but the specific ingredients "do the heavy lifting." But clearly, there remains a divide, well expressed by David Barlow, who makes a distinction between psychological treatments and generic psychotherapy. Psychological treatments contain important "specific psychological procedures targeted at the psychopathology at hand" which is differentiated from psychotherapy that is built on the common factors found in a variety of treatments, including "the therapeutic alliance, the induction of positive expectancy of change, and remoralization" (Barlow 2004, p. 873).

11.1.2 Lack of Treatment Differences in Psychotherapy

As psychotherapy research has attempted to attain scientific rigor, a medical model of treatment efficacy has been adopted. It is clear within medicine that some treatments are more effective than others in that specific ingredients address the basic illness processes. As psychotherapy research has modeled itself, to a great extent, after the medical field, there has been a focus on searching for treatment differences—treatments with ingredients that address deficits of various psychopathologies should be more effective than treatments without these ingredients (Barlow 2004). Indeed, Eysenck (1952, 1961, 1966) argued that psychotherapy as a whole may actually be harmful, but that specific treatments could be designed to pinpoint symptoms in order to increase positive outcomes. Although Eysenck discussed this point nearly

60 years ago, proponents of specific treatments continue to indicate that therapy will not be effective unless there are specific treatments for specific presenting concerns (Barlow 2010).

Although the debate between common factors and specific factors remains heated, there is an overwhelming amount of evidence to indicate that there are more similarities in efficacy among treatments than there are differences. In their seminal study regarding treatment efficacy of psychotherapy, Smith and Glass (1977) reported two major findings: (a) psychotherapy is effective, and (b) when controlling for confounding variables, there were no significant differences among treatments. One particular example of this is illustrated in a study conducted by Jacobsen et al. (1996), where three treatments were compared: behavioral activation (BA), activation and modification of dysfunctional thoughts (AT), and cognitive therapy (CT). Post-treatment, 6-month, and 24-month follow-up all indicated that the treatments were equally effective and that no specific component of the treatments contributed to the changes. The authors indicate some surprise by the results, as theory for behavioral and cognitive treatments should support differing outcomes.

The majority of treatments in psychotherapy trials are being tested to prove that one of the treatments is more effective than another treatment. As noted by the APA Task Force on Promotion and Dissemination of Psychological Procedures (1995), one of the methods of proving that a treatment is an evidence-based treatment (EBT) is to compare one treatment to an additional bona fide treatment. Bona fide treatments are provided by trained therapists—usually at the master's level—and are based upon fundamental psychological assumptions and operable treatments offered in the community or contain specified elements (Wampold et al. 1997). Shadish and Sweeney (1991) indicate that the studies that incorporate a direct comparison between two treatments provide the best evidence about treatment superiority because they control for confounds. In order to address this concern, Wampold et al. (1997) conducted a meta-analysis of direct comparisons to determine the differences among treatments. The results from this meta-analysis indicated that the treatments were all approximately equally effective. Since that time, meta-analyses have shown similar findings when focused on specific disorders, for example, post-traumatic stress disorder (Benish et al 2008), alcohol-use disorders (Imel et al. 2008), depression (Cuijpers et al. 2005), and childhood disorders (Spielmans et al. 2010; Miller et al. 2008).

11.1.3 Common Factors

As the discussion continues to unfold regarding specific versus common factors that contribute to the benefits of psychotherapy, so too continues a discussion of what the nonspecific factors really are. In 1936, Rosenzweig coined the term "implicit common factors" to explain how psychotherapy treatment works. Rosenzweig discussed four common factors: (a) the therapist's personality being perceived as motivating or encouraging, (b) using a therapeutic theory to apply to the client's personality, (c) providing a space for catharsis, and (d) reinventing psychological events.

Although these four factors contributed tremendously to the understanding of the components that contribute to psychotherapy effectiveness, the most notable model regarding the common factors was first presented by Jerome Frank (1961, 1973) and extended in 1991 by Frank and Frank. The common factors outlined in this model include the following: (a) a helping relationship that allows therapeutic space to emote and confide in the therapist, (b) a rationale rooted in the therapeutic context that is accepted by both the therapist and the patient, and (c) the provision of a ritual that ensures both the patient and therapist are participating in the process—and that this participation must be believed as helpful and viable. There are a myriad of rituals that can exist within the psychotherapeutic context—Frank and Frank outline six elements that will be common to beneficial rituals. The first is to attend to the patient's experiences of demoralization and continue to maintain and develop a relationship throughout this emotional process. The second is the importance of the therapist instilling hope and expectation that therapy will be helpful. Next, the therapist assists the patient by establishing a new way of understanding presenting issues through self-discovery, guidance, and illustration. The fourth and fifth relate to rituals that involve emotional arousal and that enhance patient self-efficacy. Last, the therapeutic context exists as a forum to practice newfound skills regarding self-discovery and affective processes.

As the conversation continues to grow in regards to common factors, the number of factors has also risen. Prior to Frank and Frank (1991) publishing their most recent model of common factors, a content review found that almost 90 common factors had been outlined in the psychotherapy literature (Grencavage and Norcross 1990). This content review paired down the 90 common factors by overlapping themes, which resulted in five separate domains that included client factors, therapist factors, therapeutic processes, structure of therapy, and relationship factors. As a result of this abundance of common factors, authors have attempted to reign in the theory to collapse the fundamentals of common factors (e.g., Tracey et al. 2003).

There is strong research evidence in support of common factors. Although the research evidence supporting common factors is primarily correlational, the amount of evidence is difficult to dispute. There are several examples of the evidence for common factors—especially when the outcome for common factors was unexpected (e.g., Jacobson et al. 1996). Beyond overall treatment effectiveness, studies have shown that it is not the specific ingredients that make changes at posttreatment, but that clients show changes throughout different phases of the therapeutic process—which is attributable to common factors. For example, early responders to a supportive therapy control group specifically focused on the relationship had higher rates of remission than patients in the experimental conditions (Renaud et al. 1998). Indeed, this lends to empirical evidence supporting that patients improve in phases, rather than solely responding to techniques to improve symptoms. For example, the phase model of change has been empirically supported to indicate that common factors improve well-being, symptom reduction, and life functioning (Kopta et al. 1994). Common factors have been shown to be especially essential within separate phases, such as positive expectancies, role preparation, and collaborative goal formation being particularly important within the early process of psychotherapy (see Defife and Hilsenroth 2011).

In addition to overall treatment and phase outcomes, there is a large basis of support for specific common factors. For example, the alliance has been shown to have an overall effect size of 0.28 on treatment outcome (Horvath et al. 2011), 0.22 in child and adolescent populations (Shirk et al. 2011), and 0.26 in couple and family therapy (Friedlander et al. 2011). In addition to the alliance contributing a moderate effect to positive treatment outcomes, several other common factors indicate similar effects, such as empathy ($r = 0.31$; Elliott et al. 2011), positive regard ($r = 0.27$; Farber and Doolin 2011), and genuineness ($r = 0.24$; Kolden et al. 2011) (see also Chap. 15). While these effect sizes are indicators of moderate effects on treatment outcomes, they all account for a portion of the variance related to the effectiveness of psychotherapy. The effect sizes presented in the meta-analyses also provide an undeniable contribution of the common factors to how patients respond to psychotherapy.

11.1.4 Healing

One method for bridging the gap that exists between the two separate schools of thought for the level of specificity of treatments is to examine the origins of healing. We contend throughout this chapter that psychotherapy is effective because there is an evolutionary basis to the responsiveness to psychotherapy. Essentially, the main reason why psychotherapy emerged was because it employs the human characteristics that enable healing. We contend throughout this chapter that, as a field, we have forgotten one of the fundamental components of why psychotherapy research exists in the first place—we want to know if and how it works. Thus, bridging the gap between common factors and specific ingredients is not proving which one works, but coming to a consensus that both work because humans are hardwired to respond to psychotherapy.

Although healing occurs in many forms across species, faith healing is uniquely human. There is an evolutionary significance related to human characteristics. Although humans and animals have evolved in similar ways, there are human practices that have occurred cross-culturally from the beginning of humankind that are universally and distinctively human—and do not exist in infrahuman species (Wilson 1978). One of these practices is, interestingly, faith healing. Jerome Frank (Frank and Frank 1991) discussed the similarities of faith healing and psychotherapy:

> Methods of supernatural healing highlight the close interplay between assumptive systems and emotional states and the intimate relation of both to health and illness. Healing rituals also bring out the parallels between inner disorganization and disturbed relationships with one's group, and illustrate the healing power of patterned interactions of patient, healer, and group within the framework...certain properties of healing rituals in the nonindustrialized societies resemble naturalistic methods of psychotherapy in ways that may serve to increase our understanding in both (p. 87–88).

Academic discussions regarding faith healing and mental healing appear to have begun as early as 1913. Painter (1913) provided the historical connection between faith and mental healing where he describes healing practices that were recorded prior to 1500 B.C., such as healing by magic at the hands of physicians and priests. He proceeds to describe a rich cross-cultural history, spanning from Jews, Babylonians, Egyptians, Chaldeans, Hindus, Chinese, and early Greeks who were told by healers to appeal to their imagination, even when drugs were administered. Shapiro and Shapiro (1997) and Fabrega (1997) similarly provide a historic account of sickness and healing. As an extension of healing by the hands of priests, faith healing and psychotherapy have been described as similar healing practices (Dow 1986).

11.2 Humanistic Characteristics

While there are a myriad of ways in which faith healing and psychotherapy are interconnected, this chapter will focus on three core evolutionary hypotheses that explain how humans have evolved to gain positive outcomes from psychotherapy: (a) belongingness and social relatedness, (b) empathy, and (c) expectations.

11.2.1 Belongingness and Social Relatedness

According to Bowlby (1969, 1973, 1980), belongingness and social relatedness are characteristic of humans and are indeed necessary for survival and fitness. For example, to ensure survival, infants must have a caregiver who is responsive to the emotional and physical needs of the child. Even when infants are provided with the necessary means for physical survival (i.e., food, shelter), they may not survive due to the lack of emotional connection. One of the primary examples of this was demonstrated from an experiment conducted by Harry Harlow in the 1960s when he showed that rhesus monkeys will choose a surrogate "mother" made of cloth over a wire "mother" providing milk—indicating the importance of social comfort and contact. Provision of food (viz., the milk) was insufficient as these monkeys failed to thrive, displaying abnormal sexual and social behaviors in adulthood and lacking the necessary provision of care to their own infants.

In addition to attachment being a necessary component for survival, belongingness is a basic evolved human need (Baumeister 2005). One of the evolutionary reasons that belongingness is ultimately such a great need for humans is that it promotes reproduction by bringing potential mates into contact with one another. In addition, belongingness also stimulates social relations by ensuring that groups of individuals will share resources and care for one another in times of need (e.g., fighting off enemies and defending resources against predators).

The evolutionary evidence of belongingness is strong—unattached individuals are more likely to develop cancer, tuberculosis, and heart disease than those in romantic relationships (Baumeister 2005). As an extension of his argument, Baumeister provides additional evidence that social connectedness is a stronger predictor of happiness than any other factor and that mental illness is from 3 to 20 times higher among divorced than married people. Simple acts, such as being present with a significant other or holding the hand of a loved one, can increase the toleration of pain, with the expected concomitant neural processes (Benedetti 2011). Benedetti indicates that these specific types of relationships "benefit from greater regulatory effects on the neural system involved in negative emotions, e.g., the affective components of pain" (p. 149).

The evidence indicating that community can be created through faith healing is compelling. The concept of integrating outsiders into community based on faith healing is important; if belongingness existed only for those who were already connected, there would be a complete loss of hope for those who were displaced or those who needed to change community to gain a different healing perspective. Bringing in outsiders to establish belongingness has been at the forefront of how psychotherapy works—a stranger is meant to provide a supportive environment for one who needs healing. An example of this phenomenon is best illustrated by the importance of traditional healers and mental health professionals within indigenous communities (Kirmayer 2004). Both types of faith healing were seen as being an important aspect of creating belongingness within the community but also fostered the integration of those who were not already a part of the community.

As mentioned earlier in this chapter, social connectedness has an evolutionary basis, where attachments are innate connections that form the moment humans are born (Bowlby 1969) and that there is a fundamental need to belong that has been adaptive to help humans survive and reproduce (Leary et al. 1995). The concept of social contagion also has interesting implications for an evolutionary understanding of emotional reactions and social connectedness. Social contagion has been defined as "the spread of affect, attitude, or behavior from Person A (the "initiator") to Person B (the "recipient"), where the recipient does not perceive an intentional influence attempt on the part of the initiator (Levy and Nail 1993, p. 266)." According to Levy and Nail, the theory of social contagion has been around for over 100 years; however, recent analyses of social influence are beginning to shed light on the impact of social networks and emotions. For example, Fowler and Christakis (2008) conducted a study with data from the Framingham Heart Study, indicating that happiness was correlated with individuals who were connected within a social network. These data indicate that those associated with individuals who were happy also reported more happiness—thus concluding that happiness can be conceived as a form of "social infection."

To support the data and theories presented by Fowler and Christakis (2008), Hill et al. (2010) present the susceptible-infected-susceptible (SISa) disease model, connecting positive and negative affect to the number of connections that an individual has over periods of time. There is evidence of the contagiousness of certain moods, such as depression. In a meta-analysis with over 4,900 participants, depressive mood and symptoms were shown to be highly contagious, especially in studies with confederates and actual friends and acquaintances (Joiner and Katz 1999). Regarding positive mood, Hill et al. report data from the Framingham Heart Study, indicating that each content contact with another individual increases the probability of an individual becoming more content by 11 %; conversely, each discontent contact increased the likelihood of becoming discontented by 100 % per year. The authors determined that, after controlling for factors such as age, sex, or education, the results remained the same.

11.2.2 Empathy

Empathy is an additional mechanism that underlies the effectiveness of psychotherapy—and has evolved mainly to ensure that humans care for one another. Empathy is very complex and has many purposes. Beings can share the emotions of others, evaluate the causes for others' affective states, and identify with the other being by adopting his or her perspective. Empathy is necessary for the regulation of cooperation, goal sharing, and social interactions and allows beings to rapidly and automatically understand the emotional states of other beings (de Waal 2008). Frans de Waal has spent his career researching primates and emotional expression in separate species—eventually to provide evidence that indicates there is evolutionary pressure to have rapid emotional connectedness. The origin of empathy likely began with parental care, where a signaling infant in distress would urge the caregiver into action. This empathetic reaction led to more global empathetic aptitude in humans, transformed from raising children into broader social relationships, allowing for communities to band together, distribute resources, and survive (de Waal 2008).

Although the explanation for the evolutionary basis for empathy is fairly straightforward, the actual biological and social processes of empathy are more complex. The perception-action model (PAM) (Preston and de Waal 2002) describes the mechanisms of empathy:

> At the core of the empathetic capacity lies a mechanism that provides the observer [the subject] with access to the subjective state of another [the object] through the subject's own neural and bodily representations. When the subject attends to the object's state, the subject's neural representations of similar states are automatically and unconsciously activated. The more similar and socially close two individuals are, the easier the subject's identification with the object, which enhances the subject's matching motor and autonomic responses. This lets the subject get "under the skin" of the object, bodily sharing its emotions and needs, which in turn may foster sympathy and helping (de Waal 2008, p. 286).

PAM is especially important to understand when looking at the several different layers of empathy. De Waal (2008) describes these layers in the metaphor of the Russian doll. The innermost doll level is represented by PAM, which represents the unconscious, strictly biological mechanisms of empathy—a level at which motor mimicry (imitation) and emotional contagion (empathy) are engaged. The middle doll is exemplified by coordination, shared goals (imitation), sympathetic concern, and consolation (empathy). The outermost doll includes true imitation, emulation (imitation), perspective-taking, and targeted helping (empathy).

At its most basic, emotional contagion is demonstrated by feeling alarmed by the distress of others or a mother's distress provoked by her offspring's own distress. Motor mimicry, a form of empathy, represents automatically emulating another's posture, voice, or facial expressions—this occurs immediately and microscopically and often goes unnoticed by the perceiver. On the other hand, there is much top-down processing of the information about the internal states of others, particularly their goals, desires, motivations, and beliefs (Boyer and Barrett 2005; Hutto 2004; Stich and Ravenscroft 1994; Thomas 2001). This processing, which is typically referred to as theory of the mind (although some theorists refer to it interestingly as folk psychology—one's lay theories of behavior), has been defined as a person's own "description and explanation of mental function" (Thomas 2001, p. 3). A theory of mind is arguably uniquely human. These descriptions allow humans to understand others, to discriminate between those who will assist and those who will be a threat, and to create social groups. According to Boyer and Barrett (2005), a theory of mind leads to "coalitional alliance, based on a computation of other agents' commitments to a particular purpose.. . .as well as the development of friendship as an insurance policy against variance in resources" (p. 109). Not unexpectedly, there are cultural differences in such top-down processing (Thomas 2001).

Empathy is most often produced through facial expression of affect and other nonverbal cues, especially at the innermost perception-action level. We contend that empathy is an underlying evolutionary mechanism that contributes to the effectiveness of psychotherapy—when a patient expresses affect through vocal intonation, gestures, or facial expression, this will elicit the support from the therapist (Williams 2002). Thus, humans are predisposed to obtain assistance from designated caregivers and to depend on social support in times of need.

11.2.3 Expectations

The human brain is designed for the past and future as well as the present. That is, humans can recall the past, in vivid imagery, as well as anticipate the future. The expectations created thereby have powerful effects not only in the mind but on the body. The power of expectations becomes evident from examining the effects of placebos on humans.

Robust placebo effects have been demonstrated in many areas of medicine. The expectation that an inert substance (i.e., a placebo) will be analgesic not only affects patients' reports of pain reduction but demonstrably has been shown to result in the release of endogenous opioids, a substance with known analgesic effects (Amanzio et al. 2001; Levine et al. 1978). In addition, placebo medications given to patients with Parkinson's disease result in visible motoric activity but also result in an increase of endogenous dopamine (Benedetti 2011). A particularly informative meta-analysis examined the effects of adherence to medication regimens on mortality rates of several trials of effective and harmful drugs (Simpson et al. 2006). Not surprisingly, patients who adhered to the regimen of effective drugs had lower mortality rates than did patients who did not adhere. However, patients who adhered to the placebo regimens in these same trials also had lower mortality rates than those who did not adhere to the placebo regimen, suggesting that those who believed that the medication was effective and used it (ingested the placebo as instructed) benefited. Although there are other explanations (e.g., those who take medication also have healthier habits generally), another result of this meta-analysis supports the belief-expectation hypothesis. Not surprisingly, those patients who took harmful drugs (i.e., those that were less effective than the placebo) had poorer outcomes than those who did not take the harmful drugs. What is surprising is that those who took the placebo still had lower mortality rates than those who did not take the placebo, even for a condition in which it turned out the drug was harmful.

There is accumulating evidence that expectations created in the medical context are critical to the effectiveness of many medical procedures. In a series of studies, Benedetti and colleagues delivered analgesics to hospital patients in two conditions: (a) patients were aware that they were receiving the medication, as it was administered by a physician who told them that the medication was a powerful analgesic, and (b) patients were given the medication surreptitiously (i.e., were unaware that they received the analgesic). Patients in the former condition reported less pain and needed less additional medication to control pain than the patients in the former condition. Benedetti (2011) estimates that telling a patient that they will receive a powerful analgesic and getting a placebo is equivalent to 6 to 9 mg. of morphine. Kirsch and colleagues (see Kirsch 2009) estimate that more than 90 % of the effects of antidepressants are due to expectation effects.

There is evidence, as well, that the attributions made about the treatment, particularly about one's own ability to control internal states and external events, are critical for the benefits of treatments (Kirsch 1990). In an ingenious experiment in the 1970s, Jerome Frank and colleagues (Liberman 1978) designed an essentially bogus treatment for outpatient neurotics, which consisted of various laboratory tasks. Patients were told that performance on these tasks would lead them to be better able "to handle" their problems in real life, and they were given feedback that they would be gradually improving at performing the tasks, even if they were not. Surprising to some perhaps, the patients experienced significant symptom reduction and improved well-being. Patients in this treatment were randomly assigned to two conditions, designed to show the power of expectations. In one condition, patients were told that their performance on the laboratory tasks was due to their hard work—these patients generally maintained their treatment gains after treatment. Patients in the other condition had been given a placebo before treatment and after treatment were told that their increasingly successful performance on the laboratory tasks was due to the medication—these patients relapsed (relative to the other condition), presumably because they had been induced to attribute their success to the medication rather than to their ability to master issues in their lives (Liberman 1978; Wampold and Weinberger in press). Interestingly, this study was replicated (unknowingly) by Powers and Emmelkamp (2008) in a study that gave an herb to patients before they completed an in vivo exposure treatment for claustrophobia. Those patients who were told after the treatment that the herb was a sedative relapsed to a greater extent than patients who were told that the herb was a stimulant or that the herb was inert. Clearly, the attributions that one makes about one's efforts and the expectation that they can control or master their difficulties have an effect on symptoms (see Kirsch 1990).

There are instances in which placebo effects can be induced unconsciously through a conditioning paradigm, but such conditioning effects are relatively rare and it is difficult to rule out cognitive mediation of such effects (Benedetti 2011). Generally, there is evidence that the healing setting, the manner in which the healer explains the treatment and its effects, and the healing ritual exert particularly powerful effects through expectations. Indeed, there is much neuroscientific evidence for expectancy effect in the healing context (see Benedetti 2011).

There is some speculation that responses to placebos by way of expectancy are an evolved characteristic, although the evidence here is not conclusive. Evans (2004) contends that the psychological triggers that elicit a web of chemical messengers involved in the placebo response have been the result of millions of years of evolution. He states that one evolutionary argument for this expectation response is that placebo effects allowed earlier humans to survive and reproduce more successfully. For example, scientists indicate that many different types of mammals (e.g., rats, dogs, guinea pigs, etc.) are susceptible to a phenomenon known as immune conditioning, which is similar to the placebo response. However, Wall (1999) argues that the mechanisms involved in placebos and human pain are much more complex. He states that pain can sometimes be terminated by social events, such as care and attention from others and having the expectation that pain would decrease from these social events would be evolutionarily beneficial. The effects of expectancy seems to be a ubiquitous human characteristic, which is related to the rise of healing practices as the healer creates the expectations through the rituals of the practice and the cultural acceptance of the practice.

11.3 A Tripartite Model of the Relationship in Psychotherapy

We provide the following tripartite model in order to elucidate how evolutionary processes have contributed to the importance of the therapeutic relationship. This model was first presented in Wampold and Budge (2012) and is expanded upon in this chapter. The three relationship pathways contribute to mechanisms of change via separate but complementary paths. We first describe the real relationship between the patient and the therapist (Gelso 2009). Next, we describe how expectations are maintained and generated via cogent rationales and treatments

(Wampold 2007). Last, we describe the benefits of healthy actions and how specific ingredients contribute to these behaviors. Prior to describing the pathways, we provide a discussion of the therapeutic bond and its influence on the real relationship, the creation of expectations, and participation in healthy actions.

11.3.1 The Initial Therapeutic Bond

As the initial therapeutic work in psychotherapy begins, the therapeutic bond is formed—which then leads to an agreement of tasks and goals (Bordin 1979). The complex process of the working alliance includes both bottom-up and top-down processing that contributes to the patient's trust toward the therapist. This is an almost instantaneous determination. Humans are evolved to make very rapid determinations of whether someone is a friend or foe. A series of experiments have shown that individuals make explicit trait judgments based on photographic presentation of faces. Within 100 milliseconds of seeing a face, judgments are made; when exposure time increased to 500 ms, conclusions became more confident and negative (Willis and Todorov 2006). Benedetti (2011) suggests that these judgments indicate that exploring the face is not necessary given the speed at which the judgments are made. Although trust may be enhanced through several different mechanisms within the therapeutic relationship, it is important to note that patients likely make initial judgments about whether or not they can trust their therapist within milliseconds.

This initial judgment may impact therapy to some extent—however, patients' previous predisposition to healing also impacts the therapeutic relationship. As healing practices are ubiquitous across cultures, a positive orientation toward the healer and the healing setting is enhanced when the practice is unconditionally accepted by the predominant culture (Wampold 2001). In addition to a positive predisposition, patient motivation for change can impact the patient's engagement while in therapy, whether the client stays in therapy, and how positively the therapy can impact the patient (Prochaska and Norcross 2001; Ryan et al. 2011). Further characteristics that may impact the therapeutic bond include the patient's perception of the therapist's expertness (Frank 1961, 1964; Heppner and Claiborn 1989; Orne and Wender 1968) and similarity of group identification (Cabral and Smith 2011).

It would be impossible for patients to engage in a therapeutic relationship without having feelings, perceptions, and reactions toward their therapist—these judgments will most likely be based on previous or concurrent interpersonal relationships. According to psychodynamic schools of thought, this concept is considered to be transference. Patients arrive to therapy with predisposed schemas that will be influenced by the relationship with the therapist; countertransference will also contribute to the bond and how judgment is formulated within the dyad.

11.3.2 The Real Relationship

In the psychotherapy context, the real relationship is a connection based on realistic perceptions and genuineness (Gelso 2009). Realistic observations are perceptions that exclude transferential distortions, and genuineness is the ability to be transparent, honest, and authentic (Gelso and Carter 1994). Gelso and Carter explain:

> In general, as the participants work together, and as their working bond strengthens, they will come to experience more positive reactions toward one another. Tied to the manner in which the participants have worked together (and thus their working alliance), the client, for example, may come to see the qualities in the therapist (e.g., loyalty or a sense of humor) that the client realistically admires and likes. (p. 299)

One of the primary effective components within the therapeutic relationship involves the patient's ability to disclose difficult—often shameful—information and in return has the assurance of a continuing relationship with a therapist who is trained and expected to be empathic. Of course, patients who have had difficulty with attachment (e.g., anxious or avoidant) may particularly benefit from a therapist who understands these difficulties and replies deeply, authentically, and empathically to this patient (see Elliott et al. 2011; Farber and Doolin 2011). The therapeutic benefits of this relationship should not be underestimated.

The real relationship appears to be widely accepted as a concept; however there is a lack of understanding as to *how* it is therapeutic. We assert that the main way positive outcomes are achieved through the real relationship is through the salutary effects of being connected to another human being, particularly one who is invested in the other's well-being. Earlier, we discussed the evolutionary bases for belongingness and the importance of social connectedness for psychological well-being. We presented research evidence indicating that there are deleterious effects when individuals feel disconnected (Baumeister 2005) and that social connectedness acts as a buffer for mental health (Benedetti 2011; Hill et al. 2010). Many patients present with problems with attachment, social relationships, or insufficient social support—all prognostic indicators of psychopathology. Simply said, the real relationship is therapeutic because it is a real relationship with an important and significant other.

One of the primary benefits of the real relationship is that the general well-being of the patient is the focus of therapy—not symptom reduction. It is predictable that the effects of the real relationship would increase with each therapeutic "dose" of connectedness. Subsequently, the outcome of the real relationship is that psychological well-being will increase incrementally over the course of therapy. Academic scholarship has shown support that receiving "doses" of connectedness based on experiencing the real relationship *does* improve psychological well-being. The therapist's perception of the real relationship has been shown to predict the reduction of patient posttreatment symptoms, indicating that the real relationship can provide positive outcomes within psychotherapy (Marmarosh et al. 2009). In addition, patient-rated genuineness of the real relationship and therapeutic bond were related to improved outcomes in a brief therapy intervention (Lo Coco et al. 2011).

11.3.3 Creation of Expectations

We discussed previously that healing practices characterize all societies, past and present, and that much of the effect of healing practices involve expectation. The second pathway for the relationship is through the creation of expectations.

The provision of hope (e.g., "remoralization") as a positive expectation is a key factor in client improvement in the therapeutic process (Frank 1973). This concept is practically one in the same with the concept of expectations. Greenberg et al. (2006) provide illustrations of instilling hope, such as a therapist saying "It makes sense that you sought this type of help for your difficulties" or "depressions do respond to treatment and the prognosis is quite good" (p. 671)—which will contribute to positive psychotherapy outcomes. Before a relationship is even created, remoralization can occur from the moment the appointment is made to the minute the patient walks in the door for the first time (Frank and Frank 1991; Wampold 2001). In essence, it is therapeutic to simply seek services and expect that the services will be effective.

More broadly, this pathway is focused on specific coping expectations and procedures for solving specific problems. We contend that these expectations are generated via the relationship with the therapist. Patients typically present with "folk" psychology beliefs about their problems and do not allow for explanations that will solve these concerns (Wampold 2001, 2007; Wampold et al. 2007), For example, "I am lonely because I am physically unattractive and cannot therefore make friends." Of course, this is somewhat circular because if the patient's explanation were adaptive, the patient would enact the solutions. A primary therapeutic activity of the therapist is to provide an adaptive explanation. For example, the patient is lonely because she does not have social skills necessary to make friends. The patient's acceptance of an adaptive explanation creates the expectation that therapy will assist in enacting a solution (i.e., "something can be done to help me"). This explanation is powerful to the patient because it makes sense (i.e., is rational from the patient's perspective) but importantly because it is provided by a trusted therapist.

After the patient accepts the explanation, the patient participates in therapeutic rituals that the patient believes will be helpful. These rituals may not make sense necessarily to psychologists, as was clearly the case in Lieberman and Frank's (Liberman 1978) laboratory tasks discussed earlier in this chapter—the important aspect here is that the patient believes that the tasks will be helpful in coping with his or her problems, which then further creates the expectation that the patient has "control" over their problems. This "control" has been discussed in various ways, including mastery (Frank and Frank 1991; Liberman 1978), self-efficacy (Bandura 1986), or response expectancies (Kirsch 1990). Recent treatments created to contain no active ingredients, when provided by therapists who believe in them and they are acceptable to patients, perform as well as treatments containing "scientifically" derived ingredients. One particular example of this is present-centered therapy for PTSD, which contained neither of the ingredients specific to the experimental treatment, but was found to be as effective (McDonagh et al. 2005, see also Wampold et al. 2010).

The alliance literature provides the primary evidence indicating that both agreement to an adaptive explanation and participation in a therapeutic ritual are beneficial. Establishing goals and providing tasks of therapy are two major components that contribute to the alliance. Hundreds of studies show that early therapeutic alliance is related to outcome (Horvath et al. 2011). This evidence also indicates that there are no differences among treatments regarding the effectiveness of the alliance—that is, some tasks (e.g., CBT) are not more advantageous than agreement about other tasks that may be considered "less scientific" (see Flückiger et al. 2012; Horvath et al. 2011). There has been specific evidence in the literature that agreement on goals and engaging in tasks are related to both the therapeutic alliance and to positive psychotherapy outcomes, as evidenced by effect sizes of 0.34 and 0.27 respectively (Tyron and Winograd 2011). Allocation of tasks has also exhibited an impact on positive therapy outcomes. Psychotherapeutic tasks are outlined in a myriad of ways (e.g., homework, common factors, therapeutic actions). Homework has displayed a moderate relationship ($r = 0.36$) with therapy outcomes (Kazantzis et al. 2000).

It is critical that our main point is emphasized—expectations *rely on a coherent explanation and simultaneous therapeutic tasks.* Generating these expectations by merely connecting to the patient (keeping in mind that the real relationship is imperative) is not enough—specific ingredients, a term many use, are absolutely necessary to create the appropriate expectations.

11.3.4 Participation in Healthy Actions

We conclude our presentation of the tripartite model by explaining the third pathway—the patients' engagement in healthy behaviors. Thus far we have described the process of the relationship being used to incite participation within the therapeutic environment. Yet, participation in these activities is therapeutic for an important reason above and beyond the creation of expectations. All of these activities induce the patient to do something helpful—substitute adaptive attributions for maladaptive ones, address emotional issues with significant others, act assertively, develop friendships, express repressed emotions, and so forth. The particular activities differ dramatically among therapeutic orientations. Successful treatments induce the patient to act in ways that are healthy and contribute to increased functioning and more integration into their community.

As tension still exists between those who endorse contextual versus medical explanations for the efficacy of psychotherapy, it remains undetermined whether the benefits of participating in healthy behaviors are because of specific factors. Each of the actions may speak to a certain patient shortfall or generate a specific coping skill. Thus, the notion of specificity is on point in suggesting that the particular ingredient of treatment is therapeutic. However, the helpful aspects of the therapy possibly accumulate simply because the patient is engaging in healthy actions in and of themselves, regardless of what those actions are—a myriad of healthy actions for numerous mental disorders are established as therapeutic (Wampold 2007).

Conclusion

One of the primary purposes of this chapter was to provide a rationale for the evolutionary relational bases for the efficacy of psychotherapy. We believe that the heart of psychotherapy has been lost in the debate of specific versus nonspecific factors; in the end, we know that psychotherapy is effective, yet there continues to be a lack of understanding for the mechanisms of change within the process. Instead of debating these processes, we argue that humans are evolutionarily designed to respond to psychotherapy.

One possible solution in moving away from specific versus common factors is to acknowledge that faith healing is ubiquitous across cultures and that humans are primed to respond to psychotherapy as a healing practice. In this chapter, we provided compelling evidence that there is a neurological and social context for three separate pathways—which we call the tripartite model of the relationship. This model explicates a holistic process that may help the field to move forward. Energy and resources should be propelled into understanding more about *why* psychotherapy works, instead of primarily relying on efficacy studies that indicate one treatment might work better than another. Process-oriented research will most likely dominate the next phase of psychotherapy research. Researchers should focus more on ways to test how the components of the tripartite model are linked to one another—for example, how empathy and expectations present and are felt within therapy to contribute to the relationship and thus how these are combined with discussions of tasks and goals to lend to both global outcomes and symptom-specific outcomes. Researchers must embrace multiple methods in order to test the concentration of processes that occur within therapy—using fMRI technology to understand biological processes of empathy, using qualitative methods to understand a more nuanced look at the relationship, and developing quantitative measures to test how the processes are related to multiple types of outcomes. We believe that embracing the unique characteristics that allow us to respond to healing will move the field into a direction of having a richer understanding and appreciation of the process and outcome of psychotherapy.

References

Amanzio M, Pollo A, Maggi G, Benedetti F (2001) Response variability to analgesics: a role for non-specific activation of endogenous opioids. Pain 90:205–215. doi:10.1016/S0304-3959(00)00486-3

American Psychological Association, Task Force on Promotion and Dissemination of Psychological Procedures (1995) Training in and dissemination of empirically-validated psychosocial treatments: Report and recommendations. Clin Psychol 48:3–23

Bandura A (1986) The explanatory and predictive scope of self-efficacy theory. J Soc Clin Psychol 4:359–373. doi:10.1521/jscp.1986.4.3.359

Barlow DH (2004) Psychological treatments. Am Psychol 59:869–878

Barlow DH (2010) Negative effects from psychological treatments: a perspective. Am Psychol 65:13–20. doi:10.1037/a0015643

Baumeister RF (2005) The cultural animal: human nature, meaning, and social life. Oxford University Press, New York

Benedetti F (2011) The patient's brain: the neuroscience behind the doctor-patient relationship. Oxford University Press, New York

Benish SG, Imel ZE, Wampold BE (2008) The relative efficacy of bona fide psychotherapies for treating posttraumatic stress disorder: A meta-analysis of direct comparisons. Clin Psychol Rev 28:746–758. doi:10.1016/j.cpr.2007.10.005

Bordin ES (1979) The generalizability of the psychoanalytic concept of the working alliance. Psychother Theory Res Pract 16:252–260. doi:10.1037/h0085885

Bowlby J (1969) Attachment and loss. Vol. 1: Attachment. Basic Books, New York

Bowlby J (1973) Attachment and loss, Vol. 2: Separation-anxiety and anger. Basic Books, New York

Bowlby J (1980) Attachment and loss, Vol 3: Loss-sadness and depression. Basic Books, New York

Boyer P, Barrett HC (2005) Domain specificity and intuitive ontologies. In: Buss DM (ed) The handbook of evolutionary psychology. Wiley, Hoboken, NJ, pp 96–118

Cabral RR, Smith TB (2011) Racial/ethnic matching of clients and therapists in mental health services: A meta-analytic review of preferences, perceptions, and outcomes. J Couns Psychol 58:537–554. doi:10.1037/a0025266

Cuijpers P, van Lier PAC, van Straten A, Donker M (2005) Examining differential effects of psychological treatment of depressive disorder: An application of trajectory analyses. J Affect Disord 89:137–146. doi:10.1016/j.jad.2005.09.001

DeFife JA, Hilsenroth MJ (2011) Starting off on the right foot: common factor elements in early psychotherapy process. J Psychother Integr 21(2):172

de Waal FBM (2008) Putting the altruism back into altruism: the evolution of empathy. Annu Rev Psychol 59:279–300. doi:10.1146/annurev.psych.59.103006.093625

Dow J (1986) Universal aspects of symbolic healing: a theoretical synthesis. Am Anthropol 88:56–69. doi:10.1525/aa.1986.88.1.02a00040

Elliott R, Bohart AC, Watson JC, Greenberg LS (2011) Empathy. Psychotherapy 48:43–49. doi:10.1037/a0022187

Evans D (2004) Placebo: mind over matter in modern medicine. Harper Collins, London

Eysenck HJ (1952) The effects of psychotherapy: an evaluation. J Consult Psychol 16:319–324. doi:10.1037/h0063633

Eysenck HJ (1961) Handbook of abnormal psychology: an experimental approach. Basic Books, Oxford, England

Eysenck HJ (1966) The effects of psychotherapy. International Science Press, New York

Fabrega H (1997) Evolution of sickness and healing. University of California Press, Berkeley

Farber BA, Doolin EM (2011) Positive regard. Psychotherapy 48:58–64. doi:10.1037//0033-3204.38.4.390

Flückiger C, Del Re AC, Wampold BE, Symonds D, Horvath AO (2012) How central is the alliance in psychotherapy? – A multilevel longitudinal meta-analysis. J Couns Psychol 59(1):10–7

Fowler JH, Christakis NA (2008) Dynamic spread of happiness in a large social network: longitudinal analysis over 20 years in the Framingham Heart Study. Br Med J 337

Frank JD (1961) Persuasion and healing: a comparative study of psychotherapy. Johns Hopkins University Press, Baltimore

Frank JD (1964) Group psychology and the elimination of war. Int J Group Psychother 14:41–48

Frank JD (1973) Persuasion and healing, 2nd edn. Johns Hopkins University Press, Baltimore

Frank JD, Frank JB (1991) Persuasion and healing: a comparative study of psychotherapy, 3rd edn. Johns Hopkins University Press, Baltimore

Gelso CJ (2009) The time has come: the real relationship in psychotherapy research. Psychother Res 19 (3):278–282. doi:10.1080/10503300902777155

Gelso CJ, Carter JA (1994) Components of the psychotherapy relationship: their interaction and unfolding during treatment. J Couns Psychol 41:296–306. doi:10.1037/0022-0167.41.3.296

Greenberg RP, Constantino MJ, Bruce N (2006) Are patient expectations still relevant for psychotherapy process and outcome? Clin Psychol Rev 26:657–678. doi:10.1016/j.cpr.2005.03.002

Grencavage LM, Norcross JC (1990) Where are the commonalities among the therapeutic common factors? Profes Psychol Res Pract 21:372–378. doi:10.1037/0735-7028.21.5.372

Heppner PP, Claiborn CD (1989) Social influence research in counseling: a review and critique. J Couns Psychol 36:365–387. doi:10.1016/j.cpr.2005.03.002

Hill AL, Rand DG, Nowak MA, Christakis NA (2010) Emotions as infectious diseases in a large social network: the SISa model. Proc R Soc B 277:3827–3835. doi:10.1098/rspb.2010.1217

Horvath A, Del Re AC, Flu¨ckiger C, Symonds D (2011) The alliance in adult psychotherapy. Psychother Theory Res Pract Train 48:9–16. doi:10.1037/a0022186

Hutto DH (2004) The limits of spectatorial folk psychology. Mind Lang 19:548–573

Imel ZE, Wampold BE, Miller SD, Fleming RR (2008) Distinctions without a difference: Direct comparisons of psychotherapies for alcohol use disorders. Psychol Addict Behav 22:533–543. doi:10.1037/a0013171

Jacobson NS, Dobson KS, Truax PA, Addis ME, Koerner K, Gollan JK, et al (1996) A component analysis of cognitive-behavioral treatment for depression. J Consult Clin Psychol 64(2):295

Joiner TE, Katz J (1999) Contagion of depressive symptoms and mood: meta-analytic review and explanations from cognitive, behavioral, and interpersonal viewpoints. Clin Psychol Sci Pract 6:149–164. doi:10.1093/clipsy.6.2.149

Kazantzis N, Deane FP, Ronan KR (2000) Homework assignments in cognitive and behavioral therapy: a meta-analysis. Clin Psychol Sci Pract 7:189–202. doi:10.1093/clipsy.7.2.189

Kirmayer LJ (2004) The cultural diversity of healing: meaning, metaphor and mechanism. Br Med Bull 69:33–48. doi:10.1093/bmb/ldh006

Kirsch I (1990) Changing expectations: a key to effective psychotherapy. Brooks/Cole, Pacific Grove, CA

Kirsch I (2009) The Emperor's new drugs: exploding the antidepressant Myth. Random House, London

Kopta SM, Howard KI, Lowry JL, Beutler LE (1994) Patterns of symptomatic recovery in psychotherapy. J Consult Clin Psychol 62:1009–1016. doi:10.1037/0022-006X.62.5.1009

Lambert MJ, Barley DE (2002) Research summary on the therapeutic relationship and psychotherapy outcome. Psychother Theory Res Pract Train 38:357–361. doi:10.1037//0033-3204.38.4.357

Leary MR, Tambor ES, Terdal SJ, Downs DL (1995) Self-esteem as an interpersonal monitor. The sociometer hypothesis. J Pers Soc Psychol 68:518–530. doi:10.1037//0022-3514.68.3.518

Levine JD, Gordon NC, Fields HL (1978) The mechanism of placebo analgesia. Lancet 2:654–657. doi:10.1016/S0140-6736(78)92762-9

Levy DA, Nail PR (1993) Contagion: a theoretical and empirical review and reconceptualization. Genet Soc Gen Psychol Monogr 119:235–285

Liberman BL (1978) The role of mastery in psychotherapy: Maintenance of improvement and prescriptive change. In: Frank JD, Hoehn-Saric R, Imber SD, Liberman BL, Stone AR (eds) Effective ingredients of successful psychotherapy. Johns Hopkins University Press, Baltimore, pp 35–72

Lo Coco G, Gullo S, Prestano C, Gelso CJ (2011) Relation of the real relationship and the working alliance to the outcome of brief psychotherapy. Psychotherapy 48:1–9. doi:10.1037/a0022426

Marmarosh CL, Gelso CJ, Markin RD, Mallery C, Choi J, Majors R (2009) The real relationship in psychotherapy: relationships to adult attachments, working alliance, transference, and therapy outcome. J Couns Psychol 56:337–350. doi:10.1037/a0015169

McDonagh A, Friedman M, McHugo G, Ford J, Sengupta A, Mueser K (2005) Randomized trial of cognitive-behavioral therapy for chronic posttraumatic stress disorder in adult female survivors of childhood sexual abuse. J Consult Clin Psychol 73:515–524. doi:10.1037/0022-006X.73.3.515

Miller S, Wampold B, Varhely K (2008) Direct comparisons of treatment modalities for youth disorders: A meta-analysis. Psychother Res 1:5–14. doi:10.1080/10503300701472131

Norcross JC (ed) (2011) Psychotherapy relationships that work: evidence-based responsiveness. Oxford University Press, New York, NY

Orne MT, Wender PH (1968) Anticipatory socialization for psychotherapy: method and rationale. Am J Psychiatr 124:1202–1212

Painter CF (1913) The evolution of mental healing. Boston Med Surg J 169:605–611. doi:10.1056/NEJM191310231691703

Powers MB, Emmelkamp PMG (2008) Virtual reality exposure therapy for anxiety disorders: A meta-analysis. J Anxiety Disord 22(3):561–569. doi:10.1016/j.janxdis.2007.04.006

Preston SD, de Waal FBM (2002) Empathy: its ultimate and proximate bases. Behav Brain Sci 25:1–72. doi:10.1017/S0140525X02000018

Prochaska JO, Norcross JC (2001) Stages of change. Psychother Theory Res Pract Train 38:443–448. doi:10.1037//0033-3204.38.4.443

Renaud J, Brent DA, Baugher M, Birmaher B, Kolko DJ, Bridge J (1998) Rapid response to psychosocial treatment for adolescent depression: a two-year follow-up. J Am Acad Child Adolesc Psychiatry 37 (11):1184–1190

Rosenzweig S (1936) Some implicit common factors in diverse methods of psychotherapy. Am J Orthopsychiatry 6:412–415. doi:10.1111/j.1939-0025.1936.tb05248.x

Ryan R, Lynch M, Vansteenkiste M, Deci E (2011) Motivation and autonomy in counseling, psychotherapy, and behavior change: A look at theory and practice. Couns Psychol 39:193–260. doi:10.1177/0011000009359313

Shadish WR, Sweeney RB (1991) Mediators and moderators in meta-analysis: There's a reason we don't let dodo birds tell us which psychotherapies should have prizes. J Consult Clin Psychol 59:883–893. doi:10.1037/0022-006X.59.6.883

Shapiro AK, Shapiro E (1997) The placebo: Is it much ado about nothing? In: Harrington A (ed) The placebo effect: an interdisciplinary exploration. Harvard University Press, Cambridge, MA, pp 12–36

Simpson SH, Eurich DT, Majumdar SR, Padwal RS, Tsuyuki ST, Varney J et al (2006) A metaanalysis of the association between adherence to drug therapy and mortality. Br Med J 333:15. doi:10.1136/bmj.38875.675486.55

Smith ML, Glass GV (1977) Meta-analysis of psychotherapy outcome studies. Am Psychol 32:752–760. doi:10.1037/0003-066X.32.9.752

Spielmans G, Gatlin E, McFall J (2010) The efficacy of evidence-based psychotherapies versus usual care for youths: Controlling confounds in a meta-reanalysis. Psychother Res 20(2):234–246. doi:10.1080/10503300903311293

Stich S, Ravenscroft I (1994) What is folk psychology? Cognition 50:447–468

Task Force on Promotion and Dissemination of Psychological Procedures (1995) Training in and dissemination of empirically-validated psychological treatment: Report and recommendations. Clin Psychol 48:2–23

Thomas RM (2001) Folk psychologies across cultures. Sage, Thousand Oaks, CA

Tracey TJG, Lichtenberg JW, Goodyear RK, Claiborn C, Wampold BE (2003) Concept mapping of therapeutic common factors. Psychother Res 13:401–413. doi:10.1093/ptr/kpg041

Tyron G, Winograd G (2011) Goal consensus and collaboration. In: Norcross JC (ed) Psychotherapy relationships that work: evidence-based responsiveness. Oxford University Press, New York, NY

Wall PD (1999) The placebo and the placebo response. In: Wall PD, Melzack R (eds) Textbook of pain, 4th edn. Churchill Livingstone, New York

Wampold BE (2001) The great psychotherapy debate: model, methods, and findings. Lawrence Erlbaum Associates, Mahwah, NJ

Wampold BE (2007) Psychotherapy: *the* humanistic (and effective) treatment. Am Psychol 62:857–873. doi:10.1037/0003-066X.62.8.857

Wampold BE, Budge SL (2012) The relationship—and it's relationship to the common and specific factors of psychotherapy. Counsel Psychol 40:601–623

Wampold BE, Weinberger J (in press) Critical thinking in the design of psychotherapy research. In: Alarcón RD, Frank JB (eds) To persuade and to heal: a tribute to Jerome D. Frank. Johns Hopkins Press, Baltimore

Wampold BE, Mondin GW, Moody M, Stich F, Benson K, Ahn H (1997) A meta-analysis of outcome studies comparing bona fide psychotherapies: Empirically, "all must have prizes". Psychol Bull 122:203–215. doi:10.1037//0033-2909.122.3.203

Wampold B, Imel Z, Bhati K, Johnson-Jennings M (2007) Insight as a common factor. In: Castonguay L, Hill C (eds) Insight in psychotherapy. American Psychological Association, Washington, DC, pp 119–139

Wampold BE, Benish SG, Imel ZE, Miller SD, Laska K, Del Re AC, Baardseth TP, Budge SL (2010) What works in the treatment of PTSD? A response to Ehlers et al. Clin Psychol Rev 30:269–276. doi:10.1016/j.cpr.2010.06.005

Williams AC (2002) Facial expression of pain: an evolutionary account. Behav Brain Sci 25:439–488. doi:10.1017/S0140525X02000080

Willis J, Todorov A (2006) First impressions: making up your mind after a 100-ms exposure to a face. Psychol Sci 17:592–598. doi:10.1111/j.1467-9280.2006.01750.x

Wilson EO (1978) On human nature. Harvard University Press, Cambridge, MA

Quantitative Data Analysis in Psychotherapy Process Research: Structures and Procedures

12

Dan Pokorny

Contents

D. Pokorny (✉)
Department of Psychosomatic Medicine and Psychotherapy, Ulm University, Ulm, Germany
e-mail: dan.pokorny@uni-ulm.de

Abstract

This chapter outlines and discusses the structures and procedures of quantitative data analysis in psychotherapy process research. These aspects will be described in two main steps: (a) exploring the complex psychotherapy process and usefully constructing the data structures to simplify a targeted reality and (b) statistically analyzing the data and testing the results in the original material. Psychotherapy research is understood as a process that is substantially influenced by researchers' personal perspectives and attitudes. Finally, the statistical consultation within this creative process is discussed as interpersonal activity that relies on the working alliance of collaborating colleagues.

12.1 Psychotherapy Process in the Mirror Statistical Data Analysis

12.1.1 What Is the Psychotherapy Process?

The most open and, therefore, most eloquent definition describes the psychotherapy process as "any event occurring during psychotherapy" (Orlinsky et al. 2004). Consider the following example of such events:

The patient is sitting in the waiting room with the questionnaires the therapist asked her to

O.C.G. Gelo et al. (eds.), *Psychotherapy Research*,
DOI 10.1007/978-3-7091-1382-0_12, © Springer-Verlag Wien 2015

complete. (Let us presume first that the patient is a she and the therapist is a he; please reread this paragraph once more, later switching the gender roles.) She is reading the questions and crossing some answers rapidly and hesitating and biting the pencil during other ones. The therapist invites her to his room, and they are speaking with each other as they do each Friday from 3:00 to 3:50 pm. The voice recorder is recording their voices. They hear the speech melody and the pitch of the voice and the pauses; they understand the meaning of the words and try to understand the messages hidden behind the words. He observes the rhythm of her breath. Some neurons in her brain are extremely activated, and his mirror neurons take note of it. He does not consciously perceive the smells coming out of her skin. The therapist's dog sitting under the table can do this 500 times better. It licks the hand of the patient. The patient smiles. The therapist smiles, too. None of these lastly mentioned events—the breaking point of the therapy—was recorded by the high-tech machine.

In this chapter, we will try to describe the steps on the *way there*, from the complex nature of a real psychotherapy process to data structures that are quantitatively analyzable by statistical procedures, for one or many patients, as well as a very short outline of the *way back*, linking the statistical results with phenomena observed with an origin in the therapy sessions.

In our fictitious first example, we will call the patient *Alice* and the therapist *Bob*. These model names were introduced in cryptography research; Alice is sending the encrypted message to Bob, and Bob is trying to decrypt it. This is surely one of the aspects of communication in the therapeutic setting.

12.1.2 Psychotherapy Process Data

Daniel Stern (2004) has shown in his experiments that even during very simple activities, such as eating breakfast, humans reveal themselves as very complex. Following his empirical approach, we could fill this book whole with the description of the Friday session. Nevertheless, we would never be able to fully capture what the real psychotherapy process is. Following Stern's approach again, let us observe the activity of the psychotherapy researcher. The researcher radically reduces the scope of the empirical observation and gains the *data*. The data have the structure of one or more *data matrices*; their rows represent the *cases*, i.e., observations, and the columns represent the observed *variables*, i.e., their properties. This radical reduction of uncountable process events to a simple data structure can be inadequate, misleading, appropriate, clever, smart, creative, or—in a lucky case—even ingenious and leading to new discoveries, such as Luborsky and Crits-Christoph (1998), or opening new branches of psychotherapy research, such as Orlinsky and Howard (1967). Multiple different appropriate formalizations of the same reality are possible in most research situations. The search for correspondences between the complex world and simplified and useful formal structures is a basic challenge for data analysis, statistics, and mathematics in general.

Before we start the often nearly infinite process of data collection, as discussed below (Sect. 12.2.6), we have to consider the nature of collected data as variables and their organization into data structures. Variables differ according to the range of their possible values:

- *Dichotomous* variables have two possible mutually exclusive values, such as gender or secure/insecure attachment.
- *Nominal* variables have a finite range of unordered categorical values, for example, the classification of attachment representation into secure, dismissing, preoccupied, and unresolved trauma.
- *Ordinal* variables have a finite range of linearly ordered categories; a typical representative is the Likert scale with five ordered categories, such as "never," "rarely," "often," "mostly," and "always."
- *Interval*-scaled variables have a subset of real numbers as the range, such as the body temperature of a human being.

These basic variable types (see also Chap. 13 and Hill and Lambert 2004) are sufficient for most research situations and for most psychotherapy process researchers. Nevertheless, there are numerous other variable types, such as *circularly* scaled variables, where values are ordered in a cycle without a natural beginning or end, such as 7 days in the week. Circularly scaled variables are necessary for analyzing cyclic processes—for example, seasonal effects or disorder onsets—that repeat within a day, week, or year. These are also helpful during analyses of the circumplex structures introduced by Leary.

Another complexly organized situation—*hierarchically* ordered structure—arises in the classifications issued by diagnostic systems, such as *the International Classification of Diseases* ICD-10 (WHO 2010) or *the Diagnostic and Statistical Manual of Mental Disorders* DSM-V (APA 2013). Hot discussions on the DSM-V demonstrate the role of subjective opinions and personal or group interests in any formalization of real-life issues. A process research example of this structure is the system *Core Conflictual Relationship Theme—Leipzig-Ulm, CCRT-LU* (Albani et al. 2008, www.ccrt-lu.org)—which has five hierarchical levels with 2–120 relationship categories.

The scaling is chosen by the researcher rather than by observed objects per se. Our young psychotherapist Bob might tend to classify patients' problems into different categories, or he could prefer a model with more clear-cut ordinal dimensions. A transsexual researcher would likely distinguish four gender categories rather than two; a biologist could even consider gender a continuum. The choice of variable scaling could be freely associated to individuals' preferred *categorical* or *continuous* perspective of the world.

A statistical investigation of real-world events reflected in the data has two substantial consecutive phases:

- Design and creation of the data matrix (or matrices) for the data to be collected
- Statistical data analysis (or analyses)

We advocate strongly, during the planning of a study, the consideration of these two phases in this sequence. We discuss these two topics, data structures in Sect. 12.2, and data analysis in Sect. 12.3.

12.2 The Invention of a Data Matrix

12.2.1 History and Philosophy of the Data Matrix

In the pioneer times of statistics, mathematicians computed using paper, pencils, and their brain. The emphasis was on finding sophisticated mathematical formulas suitable for manual computations. In the pioneer times of computers, numerous programs were written for a great variety of statistical problems. Data structures differed from program to program; thus, it was necessary to prepare the data from the same study in multiple different ways to accommodate different programs. Over time, it became clear that data analyses could be more comfortable and efficient when all evaluation procedures operated with the same data structure.

This led to the development of statistical packages that used the same philosophy of data representation for all included procedures. These packages were developed step-by-step from samples of similarly designed programs into integrated systems based on a common executing engine in the core. Main contributors during this era were the statisticians at universities frustrated by user-unfriendly and inefficient software landscapes. Statistical program packages that substantially influenced the world of the data analysis in this period were "Biomedical Programs" (BMD, later BMDP), "Statistical Programs for Social Sciences" (SPSS), "Statistical Analysis System" (SAS), and numerous others.

The basic data structure of these systems is composed of the rectangular *data matrix* and the describing meta-information. The horizontal rows of the data matrix correspond to the *cases* from the investigated sample (like patients, sessions, or words) and its columns correspond to the observed *variables* (like gender, age, scores on psychometric instruments, and nearly

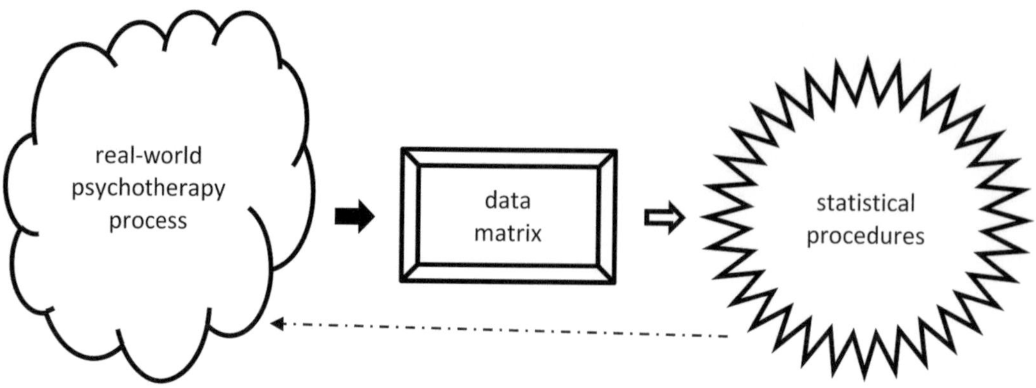

Fig. 12.1 The data matrix as a bridge between the real world and data analysis

anything else). The values in cells of the data matrix can be numbers or alphanumerical strings.

Within the descriptive meta-information, properties of the variables are captured using a concise *variable name* ("gender"), a sufficiently longer *variable label* ("gender of the patient"), and—particularly for categorical variables—the *value labels* (w = "woman," m = "man"). Hence, the system file contains a self-describing data structure, making the documentation tasks considerably more convenient.

The system currently most widespread—but not exclusively used—in the field of psychology and psychotherapy science is likely SPSS. (See www.spss.com and the links therein.) The data matrix is the basic file type of the system; there are also other file types where computational procedures (data manipulations, statistical computations) or results (tables, graphs) can be stored. SPSS is not the only system in the field; however, its system file is a de facto standard for data documentation and sharing between collaborating researchers and laboratories.

SPSS and similar systems were developed as program packages of tools and contain a very broad spectrum of data analysis procedures; even a very advanced specialist does not use them all. On the other side, the algorithms outside of this portfolio are not realizable in the rule. For this reason, these systems have been called "program cans"—you can select the food, you can warm it up quickly, but you cannot cook your own. The current system version offers advanced possibilities for data input and transformation, step result presentation, etc.; you can at least modify the canned food.

An alternative approach is offered by the *R Project for Statistical Computing* (www.r-project.org), a high-level programming language oriented to statistical applications that allows a do-it-yourself development of any statistical procedure. The project is a de facto standard for the publication or sharing of statistical algorithms. The system can be acquired as a free add-on of the SPSS system.

The data matrix is an interface between the psychotherapy process in the real world and quantitatively oriented statistical reasoning (see Fig. 12.1). The key to meaningful and innovative data analysis lies in finding and designing a suitable representation of the psychotherapy process using the data matrix. This representation (the black arrow in Fig. 12.1) requires focusing on selected aspects of the psychotherapy process and their radical simplification. And, clearly, there is no unique solution to this task. Once this part is managed, the next step, i.e., the selection of appropriate statistical procedures (the white arrow), will be comparably easy. Designing the data matrix can be a very complex, challenging, and creative process for some situations and relatively simple and nearly standard for others. The meaning of the dashed line will be explained later (see Sect. 12.3.4).

Table 12.1 Simple data matrix

Person	Nickname	Gender	Age	WAI
001	Alice	w	18	1.0
002	Carlos	m	27	6.5
003	Dolores	w	22	3.8
004	Eleonor	w	19	4.2
005	Franciscus	m	25	7.0

Table 12.2 Simple data matrix with two groups

Person	Group	Nickname	Gender	Age	WAI
101	p	Alice	w	18	1.0
102	p	Carlos	m	27	6.5
103	p	Dolores	w	22	3.8
104	p	Eleonor	w	19	4.2
105	p	Franciscus	m	25	7.0
201	t	Gina	w	24	6.3
202	t	Hubert	m	21	6.9
203	t	Ivana	w	18	6.2
204	t	Jana	w	19	6.9
205	t	Karl	m	22	6.0

12.2.2 Organization of a Data Matrix

Let us assume that Bob documented his patients' basic information. He designed a simple data matrix (Table 12.1) where gender, age, and working alliance are recorded. The Working Alliance Inventory (see Horvath and Greenberg 1989) is a 36-item instrument that assesses the working alliance attitude. Bob prefers its short version (Horvath 1981) that consists of 12 items, such as "My counselor and I trust one another," which are answered on a 7-level ordinal scale. The resulting score for each client is computed as the mean of the 12 items; the value 1.0 corresponds to the minimum and the value 7.0 indicates the maximum effectiveness of the working alliance. These data will help Bob monitor the distribution of his clients' gender and age and their experience of the therapeutic relationship.

We have thus simplified Bob's job. As discussed below, he stores (and hence documents) all 12 original items and lets the program compute the overall score.

Bob is a therapy trainer and is also interested in the working alliances of his trainees. Bob does not create two separate matrices for his patients and trainees; rather, he stores the data of both groups in one common data matrix and distinguishes the groups by a dichotomously scaled variable "group" (Table 12.2). Therefore, he will immediately be able to compare working alliances in the groups using an appropriate statistical test. Moreover, he has the flexibility to analyze different subsamples by selecting a variable or variables for grouping the data.

After Bob's patients and trainees finish therapy, Bob is interested in evaluating the change that occurred during the process. He asks clients to answer the WAI questionnaire again. Bob hesitates, wondering if he should add the new measurements to the bottom of the matrix as new cases after the rows for persons A, C, . . ., K or to the right as new variables.

His statistical advisor Dr. L strongly recommends the second option (Table 12.3). The reason is that data collected at the beginning and end of therapy are linked by the investigated client; both measurements of Alice and the other clients are in the same line, and the same is true for Carlos and other persons. This enables the application of powerful tests designed for pairwise observation.

Representing one person as two cases—i.e., as two rows in Table 12.3—would muddle the important fact that the two cases are related to the same person. Moreover, this representation would be statistically incorrect; it would reflect a sample of 20 persons instead of the actual 10 persons.

The variable WAI-t2 has *missing values* for Jana because she was absent for the last session. The occurrence of missing values in a data matrix is a rule rather than an exception in psychotherapy science. Using different alternative strategies, statistical procedures can address incomplete data pretty well.

The last column was added later using the transformation function in the program system. This variable contains the difference between the second and the first measurement, WAI_{t2} – WAI_{t2}. Alice's working alliance improved at +5.9 points, Hubert's alliance decreased by 0.1 point, and Franciscus' maximum score remained

Table 12.3 Data matrix with two groups and two repeated measurements

Person	Group	Nickname	Gender	Age	WAI t1	WAI t2	W2 − W1
101	p	Alice	w	18	1.0	6.9	+5.9
102	p	Carlos	m	27	6.5	6.8	+0.3
103	p	Dolores	w	22	3.8	4.7	+0.9
104	p	Eleonor	w	19	4.2	5.6	+1.4
105	p	Franciscus	m	25	7.0	7.0	0.0
201	c	Gina	w	24	6.3	6.6	+0.3
202	c	Hubert	m	21	6.9	6.8	−0.1
203	c	Ivana	w	18	6.2	6.5	+0.3
204	c	Jana	w	19	6.9	X	X
205	c	Karl	m	22	6.0	6.8	+0.8

unchanged. This once again clarifies the reason for storing repeated measurements within one case: It should be possible to create a new variable containing their difference.

Repeated measurements need not concern only time repetitions. Bob could ask a patient to estimate his relationship quality with other people close to him. In a sample of married couples, the answers of both partners can build one case that represents a pair of mutually linked people. (Note: When presenting the change results, be sure that mean differences, t-statistics, and effect sizes are described with a positive sign to indicate an increase and a negative sign to indicate a decrease.)

Investigation at two (or three or four) time points during, before, or after therapy is a central approach of *outcome research* (see Chap. 26); the task is to *quantify* and *prove* therapeutic change in large patient groups. On the contrary, *process research* is interested in when and how change happens; it aims to *understand* what goes on during the treatment and, particularly, the *dynamics* of the personal and therapeutic relationships (see Chap. 16; see also Chap. 11).

12.2.3 The Case of the Single Case

Bob, interested in investigating the course of Alice's therapy, asks her to complete his instruments immediately after each therapy session.

The philosophy of the data matrix and data organization is completely different from previously discussed cross-sectional designs. The row of the matrix still represents a case in a statistical sense. However, the case is one therapy session now, and we address the sample of one patient's sessions. Alice is our "universe of discourse" here.

Table 12.4 Simple single case analysis, the "Alice case"

Person	Session	Date	Day	WAI
1	1	Oct 03	0	1.0
1	2	Oct 10	7	7.0
1	3	Oct 17	14	3.2
1	4	Oct 24	21	3.7
1	5	Oct 31	28	4.5
1	6	Nov 07	35	4.6
1	7	Nov 14	42	4.0
1	8	Nov 21	49	5.3
1	9	Nov 28	56	5.7
1	10	Dec 05	63	6.4
1	11	Dec 12	70	7.0
1	12	Dec 19	77	6.9

This type of study is called a *single case study* in the fields of medical or psychotherapy sciences (see Chap. 20); this is sometimes expressed by "$N = 1$," meaning that only one person is in the spotlight. From a mathematical perspective, this metaphor is rather misleading. In the Alice case, 12 sessions constitute the sample, and the sessions are 12 cases from this sample.

Bob organizes the data into a data matrix shown in Table 12.4.; the matrix rows contain the information from one of Alice's sessions. The variables *date*, or alternatively *day*, are technically important for the therapy to maintain the time structure. Using these data, Bob can examine the nature of the development and determine whether he can see and statistically prove apparent increasing or decreasing trends.

Bob would likely wish that scores improve smoothly and steadily. This is usually not the case in real process research studies; typically, we see curves that show numerous leaps and bounds. In our fictitious example, after the first session, Alice answered all items extremely negatively as an expression of her resistance to the therapy. After the second session, she answered all items extremely positively for similar resisting reasons. After the third session, she started to collaborate and answer the question with honest self-reflection. It was the key session of the therapy when the dog was licking her hand.

Encouraged by the successful analysis of Alice's case, Bob started to collect session-by-session data from all of his patients and clients. The structure of his database is considerably more complex than the single case design in Table 12.4 (one patient with many sessions) or a cross-sectional design with two repetitions, such as in Table 12.3 (many patients with two sessions). Even the design with a fixed number or repeated measures would be a statistically easy case (for instance, many patients, each with exactly four measurements). Bob's challenge is that the number of therapy sessions with his patients differs from case to case. Nevertheless, within the frame of variance analysis (and elsewhere), there is a design for handling this difference. Bob will ask Dr. L for details.

12.2.4 More Complex Data Organizations

Until now, we have seen basic examples of how categorical or continuous data can be organized into a data matrix suitable for statistical analysis. Sometimes, the data organization in real-life research can be considerably more complicated: More matrices can be necessary for a useful representation of the situation at hand. For instance, when investigating the dynamic of the group therapy, the feelings of the therapist can be documented in one matrix, the patients' feelings can be documented in the second matrix, and the mutual evaluation of patients can be documented in the third. Current statistical software systems can handle these complex situations.

Statistical data analysis proceeds collected categorical or continuous data mostly in a quantitative way: The information in data matrices is elaborated to be described in terms of means, standard deviations, frequencies, correlations, effect sizes, statistics, or significance. The statistical considerations and consultations concerning the structure of the data matrix or matrices should take place *before* the study starts and focus on the organization of data structures first.

12.2.5 Coding the Events Inside the Therapy Session

The fictitious single case study of Alice addresses one aspect of the dynamics of the psychotherapy process, the self-estimation of the patient, which was performed immediately *after* the sessions but not *during* the sessions; observation of the process during the therapy sessions is much more challenging. The variety of channels and perspectives is potentially infinite and so is the variety of possible organizations of the data matrix. Let us mention, or at least imagine, some of them.

In the 1970s, psychotherapy researchers started to work very intensively with verbatim session protocols, and many research methods considered transcripts the basic data source for investigations. After a period of typewriting documents, text analysis assisted by computers played an increasing role (see Chap. 19 and Kächele and Mergenthaler 1983). Numerous computer programs that enabled or facilitated text analysis were developed, whereas statistical software systems were designed nearly exclusively to solve quantitative statistical tasks. During recent decades, statistical systems "learned" to work with textual information and sophisticated functions that manage text strings completed the traditional numerical functionality (cf. www.spss.com). Using these new system abilities, it is possible to analyze the transcribed session records step-by-step in the statistical system.

Using some simple tricks, the transcribed text can be transformed to the data matrix, corresponding to the first four columns of Fig. 12.2. The first three variables are the session number, the token word within the session, and the speaker's role (patient or therapist). The next variable, a *string* variable, contains the words in the sequence of how they were recorded. The current non-fictitious example presents a small part of a therapy session that was conducted using Guided Affective Imagery (cf. Stigler and Pokorny 2001).

This structure makes it possible to evaluate the occurrence frequencies of different words (types) in the whole therapy or differentiated by session and/or speaker. The vocabulary used by the patient and therapist can be analyzed by means of computer-assisted content analysis. Here, the Affective Dictionary Ulm ADU (Dahl et al. 1992), which classifies emotional words into 8 content categories, was applied. Using the functions of the SPSS system, the emotion categories could be added as a nominally scaled variable; see the fifth column in Fig. 12.2.

During the following technical steps, the nominally scaled variable ADU was expanded to the vectors of 8 categorical dichotomous variables that express the occurrence (yes or no) of particular emotion categories. The ADU category number 4 in the example is *joy*, and category number 8 is *anxiety*. The file containing this data matrix was huge; each token word from the transcript occupied one row in the matrix. The next step was an operation of *aggregation*; a new matrix with 25 lines corresponding to therapy units was created. Each line contained the occurrence frequencies of ADU categories. After transforming the absolute frequencies into relative ones, the sample could finally be analyzed by standard statistical methods for correlations and group comparisons. Hence, starting with pure text data, it was possible to continue until the classical quantitative methods were used, within the same system (here SPSS) and "under one roof."

This study has shown remarkable differences between the 6 imagery sessions and the remaining standard sessions (Stigler and Pokorny 2001). The *positivity index* (relative frequency of positive emotion words compared to all emotional words) was considerably higher in the imagery sessions than in standard sessions. This was the case for 5 out of 6 sessions. One imagery session contained negative emotional words in the category of anxiety, which was one of the patient's problems. The imagery session allowed patients to speak freely about their problems, and this session was identified as a key session of the therapy.

Context-free vocabulary analysis that counts the word occurrences is, by nature, not very sensitive to the semantic word meaning with respect to the given context. Additionally, the computer can hardly distinguish between a serious and sarcastic tone of voice. Hence, while the computer-assisted analysis is considerably quick, computer misunderstandings are to be expected. In contrast, ratings issued by human experts are much more sensitive—and immensely time-consuming, too.

One such approach is the method of the Central Relationship Conflict Theme (CCRT) founded in the 1970s by Lester Luborsky (Luborsky and Crits-Christoph 1998) with the innovated category system CCRT-LU (Albani et al. 2008). The procedure—analogous to previously mentioned ones—starts with qualitative decisions about the type of relationship elements, as described in Chaps. 19 and 20. The cases in the data matrix consist of sentences or clauses, the smallest meaningful sentence part other than individual words. These text parts are rated by humans, who produce a huge data matrix over several months; this matrix is then aggregated to relatively tiny matrices.

In the sake of controlling the subjective factors in the rating process, a study of *interrater reliability* is necessary: Two or more judges rate the same portion independently, and their ratings are then compared.

session	token	speaker	word	ADU
...	...	...	...	...
18	500	T	hmm	0
18	501	P	well	0
18	502	P	I	0
18	503	P	feel	0
18	504	P	the	0
18	505	P	wind	0
18	506	P	and	0
18	507	P	the	0
18	508	P	air	0
18	509	P	that	0
18	510	P	I	0
18	511	P	can	0
18	512	P	breathe	0
18	513	P	that	0
18	514	P	**fresh**	4
18	515	P	air	0
18	516	P	and	0
18	517	P	feel	0
18	518	P	such	0
18	519	P	a	0
18	520	P	feeling	0
18	521	P	of	0
18	522	P	**freedom**	4
18	523	P	but	0
18	524	P	if	0
18	525	P	I'd	0
18	526	P	come	0
18	527	P	too	0
18	528	P	close	0
18	529	P	I'd	0
18	530	P	have	0
18	531	P	such	0
18	532	P	a	0
18	533	P	feeling	0
18	534	P	in	0
18	535	P	my	0
18	536	P	stomach,	0
18	537	P	well,	0
18	538	P	like	0
18	539	P	**anxiety**	8
...	...	...	...	...

T = therapist, P = patient

ADU: Affect Dictionary Ulm, 0 = no emotional word (white), 1-8 affect categories (grey).

Fig. 12.2 Simple single case analysis, the "Alice case". *T* therapist, *P* patient, *ADU* Affect Dictionary Ulm, 0 = no emotional word (*white*), 1–8 affect categories (*gray*)

Similar to astronomers using instruments for different types of electromagnetic waves, psychotherapy researchers investigate the process from different research perspectives and personal positions. The proceedings of the Society of Psychotherapy Research in Copenhagen (SPR 2014) and previous regular meetings include reports on these channels:

- Relationship patterns in transcripts
- Attachment representation in projective or narrative text
- Affective dictionary
- Affective content coded second-by-second during the whole course of therapy
- Primary process markers
- Ruptures and their repairment
- Crying during the therapy session
- Laughing during the therapy session
- Stress measured by physiological parameters
- Tone of speech
- Mimic signals

  . . . and many other phenomena until . . .
- The commonly shared silence

12.2.6 Data Acquisition and Documentation

Bob tried to document the data as close to their original form as possible. He followed the advice of statistical consultant Dr. L not to lose the information through premature data reduction. For instance, he documented the age in years by the patient's last birthday like "24", rather than in decades like "until 20," "21–30," "31–40," etc. Anyway, Bob can categorize data from years to decades later should that be necessary. Furthermore, there is a spectrum of statistical procedures that can better manage original data in this case.

Bob stores all 12 items of each WAI questionnaire in a similar way and for similar reasons. It is a good principle to develop the schemes, or so-called masks, for the data input as closely as possible to the original sources gained by the process observation. For instance, many psychometric instruments work with a mixture of items formulated positively or negatively with respect to the intended scale concept in the background. A good strategy is to type the items' values into the matrix or mask in their original form. This makes the task easier for the documenting person; thus, the input process is more reliable and error-free.

The data can be transformed to the form necessary for computation by procedures that are saved and documented in a separate file. The procedures can then reverse the items, summarize them to scale, and do everything else that is necessary. In this discipline of data transformation, the computer is better than a human.

The strategy of dividing the phase of data documentation into two subphases has more advantages: (a) Bob can compare the original information with stored data easily and check its correctness; (b) corrections of mistyped data can be easily solved; (c) procedures for data manipulation—like building the scales from items or aggregating the time-dependent data—are transparent and can be checked again anytime; and (d) corrected data can be easily reanalyzed.

The correctness of stored data is one of the fundamental issues within the quality management of data analysis. In the early times of computer-based technology, research data were checked by inputting them manually twice, preferably by two different people. The alternative option was to read and control all data without typing twice. This has been called "optical control" and has been considered a quick-and-dirty procedure. Currently, this procedure is proudly called "100 % check." The data can be inputted considerably more quickly and easily nowadays; however, their reliability is lower.

These considerations concern mostly the smaller projects where manual paper-and-pencil data input is often still the most effective option. Anyway, a completely new field of data acquisition was created by modern computer technologies, which enabled direct data inputting through electronic systems, like online measurements of physiological parameters, clients answering questionnaires using a tablet, and Internet surveys. The reliability with respect to possible local minor mistakes is very high and satisfactory; the dangers lie instead in possible occurrences of global systematic errors. A carefully prepared Internet survey can be spoiled by one hacker unless the researcher prevents it.

Nevertheless, these electronic techniques are the data-acquisition highways of the future that have already started being paved. Further developments are still needed. For example, Bob successfully dictates his case reports into his voice recorder, which is equipped with the newest speech-recognition program. However, the program is still *not* able to transcribe reliably the patient's speech in the audio recordings of Bob's psychotherapy sessions.

12.3 The Landscape of Data Analysis

Try to imagine the learning of basic statistical methods as a holiday trip. Within the scope of this chapter, there are not enough places to organize this journey. Instead, we will try to present the map of the landscape of data analysis. We will refer to literature and software as if we were referring to travel bureaus organizing the expedition.

12.3.1 Basic Bivariate Methods

In the meantime, Bob conducted more extensive process research studies, and he would like to analyze his data. However, he is scared of thick textbooks full of mathematical symbols within the most important explanations. Fortunately, passing through the entrance gates to the landscape of data analysis is not as difficult as it seems. The prerequisite is to understand the basic principles of data organization discussed above and to clearly distinguish the basic variable scales: *dichotomous*, *nominal*, *ordinal*, and *interval*.

Most methods for the interval-scaled variables demand, moreover, a *normal* distribution, the well-known bell curve introduced mathematically by Gauss and demonstrated experimentally by Galton. Two remarks: (a) Some researchers argue that small sample sizes in particular should satisfy the normality condition by nonsignificant results in the Kolmogorov-Smirnov or Shapiro test. However, in this case, the normality was not rejected but it was *not* proven. (b) Simulation studies have shown that outlier values or bimodality can spoil the statistical test substantially. However, luckily, moderate shape differences of the normal distribution can be harmless.

Many principal hypotheses in the psychotherapy research (and elsewhere) are connected to bivariate methods that investigate some type of association between two variables. There are two basic types of methods: *measures*, which estimate the closeness of association between two variables, and *tests*, which decide if an association exists at all. Basic methods are mentioned in Table 12.5.

Bob, using this table for navigation, looks for methods suitable for his data presented above. To find the association between the session number and the WAI score, he applies the Spearman correlation coefficient. Its value is 0.69—a positive number which was expected, or at least wished for—and the significance of the one-sided hypothesis is $p = 0.014$. This number is smaller than a conventional value, 0.050. Bob is allowed to say that the decreasing level of Alice's complaints over the course of the therapy was confirmed statistically.

The methods in Table 12.5 are generally intended to support the researcher in making decisions regarding the independence versus the dependence of two variables. The dependence question can be asked by a pair of variables of any type.

In special cases, the variables are different instances of the same concept. For instance, Bob is measuring the same WAI score at the beginning of therapy (t1) and the end of therapy (t2). Another example: Bob asks a patient two analogous questions about the patient's relationship to his father and his mother. Bob is asking the analogous question twice or, in statistician terminology, using repeated measurements. On the one hand, Bob can test the association between these two measurements according Table 12.5 again.

Table 12.5 Basic methods for association between two variables

Association	Interval	Ordinal	Nominal	Dichotomous
Interval	Correlation test *Correlation r* Test of rho *Spearman's rho*	[a]	[a]	[a]
Ordinal	Test of rho *Spearman's rho*	Test of rho *Spearman's rho*	[a]	[a]
Nominal	One-way ANOVA Kruskal-Wallis H-test	Kruskal-Wallis H-test	Generalized Fisher's test	[a]
Dichotomous	2-Sample t-test *Effect size d* Mann-Whitney U-test	Man-Whitney U-test	Generalized Fisher's test	Fishers' exact test *association—Yule's Q*

[a]See the symmetric table field
Standard font: tests. *Italics*: *measures*

Table 12.6 Basic methods for repeated measures between two variables

Repeated measurements	Interval	Ordinal	Nominal	Dichotomous
	Pairwise t-test	Wilcoxon text	McNemar test	McNemar test

On the other hand, he can ask a second question, such as: Is there improvement in WAI between the beginning and end of therapy? Are the estimations of the relationship to the father and mother different? He will find appropriate basic tests for these questions in Table 12.6.

Bob has learned the statistical methods from Tables 12.5 and 12.6 by doing-and-trying using the statistical system. Even more importantly, Bob recognized when a question fell outside of the scope of these tables. This will be particularly the case as soon as three or more variables are involved in the analysis concurrently. Multiple repeated measurements on the group of patients, comparison of therapy change between two or more patient groups, investigating psychometrical quality of a questionnaire: these are just few examples of such situations. Bob will ask his consultant L for help in such cases. First after the practical experience and playing with real and fictitious data, he will go to buy a textbook on data analysis (cf. Sect. 12.3.3), and he will likely understand what the people are talking about.

The number of methods mentioned in Tables 12.5 and 12.6 is limited. However, by understanding their nature and using them at the right place and time, and in a sound way, Bob will be able to solve maybe 80 % of his statistical questions.

It is similar to the guitar that Bob started to play. He can play only ten chords, but it sounds good.

12.3.2 Advanced Methods

There exists a wide landscape for quantitative data analysis within psychotherapy process research, including continuous and categorical perspectives as well as a confirmatory or exploratory way of questioning. A metaphoric presentation of this landscape is found in Fig. 12.3. (For a somewhat analogous representation of qualitative data analysis in process research, see Chap. 20; see Chap. 13 for an overview of the application of different procedures of data analysis in quantitative research that involves the psychotherapy process.)

The First Dimension in the Landscape At the beginning of this chapter (Sect. 12.1.2), we described the different variable types that are distinguished by their theoretical range. The simplest variable type was dichotomous; on the opposite pole was the interval-scaled variable

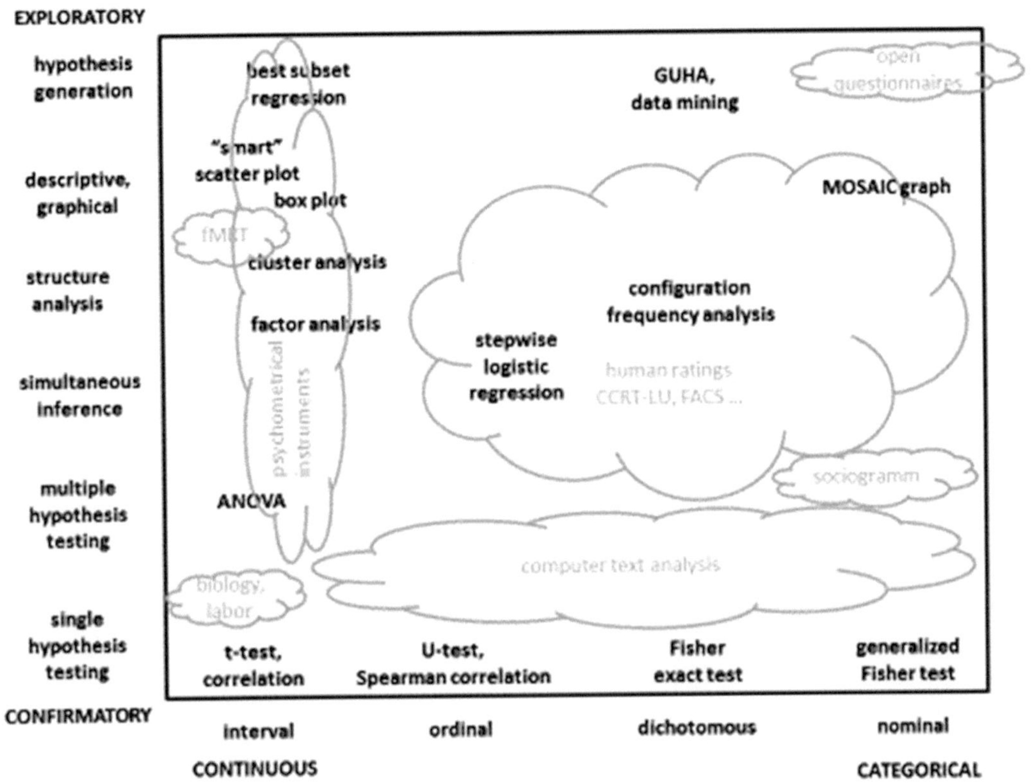

Fig. 12.3 The landscape of psychotherapy research and data analysis methods. The clouds contain different approaches to data collection

type. Some researchers believe that interval-scaled variables represent the most exact and consequently the highest quality standard of measurement. In our opinion, whatever scale is most adequate for observing a particular subject and for the researcher's question is the best choice. The complexity of the variable types constitutes the horizontal dimension, the x-axis in Fig. 12.3.

The Second Dimension in the Landscape The goal of the investigation can be, similar to in this study, the *confirmation* of one a priori stated hypothesis or the *exploration* of the data structure and search for possible new hypotheses. The confirmatory analysis is covered by the classical theory of mathematical statistics, and the need for exploratory data analysis (EDA) was explicitly stated by John Tukey. The realest studies lie somewhere on the continuum between these two poles. In typical empirical studies, more hypotheses are tested, and unexpected other findings are welcome. The orthodox methodology school recognizes only confirmatory studies with a single hypothesis as the research Lege Artis. For this reason, many authors try to keep exploratory parts of their studies secret. One question remains unanswered: Where are the hypotheses being born? (See Pokorny 2010) This confirmatory vs. exploratory continuum represents the second dimension of our landscape, and it is depicted as the y-axis of Fig. 12.3.

Data Analysis Methods As we can see, the basic bivariate methods for *single hypothesis testing*, such as the t-test, correlation, or a Fisher test, are close to the bottom of the figure. These methods are frequently used for testing basic principal hypotheses in empirical studies. As a metaphor, these methods keep themselves safely on the earth.

The next level consists of slightly more complex statistical methods for *multiple hypothesis testing*. These methods are used in research that involves nominal variables with more than two categories, with more than two independent variables, etc. In most cases, we address one general principal hypothesis (such as, "Are the means of these four groups different?") and subsequently pose a simpler a posteriori hypothesis that elucidates the general finding (such as, "Which of possible six group pairs contain two different groups?").

In the last example, we have to consider the *simultaneous inference*, which means comparing three groups, A, B, and C, and testing six a posteriori hypotheses "simultaneously," specifically group pairs AB, AC, BC, BD, and CD. With ten groups, we have to test $10 \times (10 - 1)/2 = 45$ group pairs.

The impact of this problem increases in the subsequent higher levels; finally, we increasingly have an explorative search for possible models and solutions rather than stringent hypothesis testing. This is typically the case with multivariate stepwise methods (linear regression, logistic regression, and discriminant analysis).

Typical multivariate analyses, such as factor analysis ("classical" or "exploratory" factor analysis) or cluster analysis, have a primary goal of finding *structure* in hardly comprehensible data configurations. The findings can be used for building hypotheses in future studies.

Descriptive or graphical procedures try to present the data in a visual "at first glance" way. The prominent example is Tukey's boxplot, originally named "box and whiskers," which enables the checking and presenting of the findings of t-tests and other methods of the variance analysis. The scatterplot does this work for the correlation of two interval-scaled variables; some programs allow this by clicking on dots in the graph to see which case (person, session) is hidden behind each dot. The MOSAIC visualizes the association between two nominal variables.

Finally, there are genuine explorative procedures for the *generation of hypotheses* using a sophisticated, exhaustive search of the vast data material. In the "data analysis heaven" figure, we see methods such as best subset regression or procedures for mining interesting facts from complex databases. The pioneer role within these approaches used the GUHA method ("general unary hypothesis automaton") proposed in the 1960s by Prague mathematician Petr Hájek (cf. Hajek et al. 1966; Hajek and Havranek 1978).

The clouds in Fig. 12.3 note different approaches to collecting data within process research. The positions of clouds in the data analytical landscape indicate the preferable methods in these fields. Because process research is open to original and creative ideas, the correspondence between statistical and psychotherapeutic methods is neither sharply delimited nor constantly fixed as it is by the clouds in the figure.

12.3.3 Where to Read About It

There are many textbooks on methods of statistical data analysis; you can search for a suitable one, looking inside and feeling which one attracts you, or vice versa; let the book find you. Anyway, we would recommend combining the reading with practical experience with a statistical software using real or fantasy data. Reading the theory and waiting for later understanding can be compared to learning languages only by studying grammatical theory. We would like to propose two books oriented to the learning-by-doing or learning-by-trying or learning-by-playing, whatever you want to call it:

- SPSS for Dummies (Griffith 2010) introduces the SPSS application in an easy way, which is characteristic for this book series.
- Discovering Statistics Using IBM SPSS Statistics by Andy Field (2013), a book that is funny, advanced, and readable.

Recent applications of data analysis in the general field of psychotherapy research are reported in a special issue of the journal *Psychotherapy Research* (Lutz and Hill 2009).

12.3.4 Interpretation and the Way Back

A great portion of reports on psychotherapy studies follows the black arrow from the real-life process to the data matrix in Fig. 12.1 (in the sections called *Introduction*, *Method*, and *Sample* or *Material*) and the white arrow from the data matrix to statistical procedures (in the section *Results*); this direction concludes with significant findings. Within the following section *Discussion*, limitations of the study and statistical findings are discussed, and other studies' results are being compared.

The comparison and a look back to the originally studied processes are in many cases not included in the report. We would like at least to briefly advocate the "back-translation" step shown in Fig. 12.1, indicated by the dashed line. We will try to demonstrate it on some fictitious examples:

- Bob has found that Alice has shown a significant improvement on the Working Alliance Inventory scale, and he is eager to start a highly theoretical interpretation of this result. He might be recommended to check the trends of all 12 instrument items: Are nearly all items involved in this change or are just a few? In the latter case, Bob might reinterpret the results.
- After analyzing the affective vocabulary in transcripts of Alice's sessions, Bob has found a significant increase in category 4, joy. Upon inspecting the word occurrences in context, he discovered depressive idioms, such as "Not funny."
- In session 7, there were a dramatically higher number of words marked by the transcribing assistant as "not understandable by transcription." Bob connected this to Alice's resistance, which manifested in unclear communication and also associated it with the minor decrease in the working alliance score. In fact, he was worried about it. A first look into the transcript reveals a remark of the transcribing assistant that says, "The following two minutes are not understandable because of the noise caused by military airplanes."

All three examples are based on situations that really happened. The "way back" is useful for three different roles:

- *The researcher* can check the plausibility of the results and, moreover, gain highly valuable hints for results interpretation and presentation.
- *The therapist* gets clinically comprehensible feedback from the researcher.
- *The patient* can, when the results are communicated, better understand the findings and relate them directly to his personal experiences.

12.4 Statistical Consultation in the Mirror of Psychotherapy

We have outlined that the structures for data acquisition are created by a human, a researcher, and reflect the psychotherapy process. Plurality of perspectives is a natural fact; researchers differ clearly in their opinion of which aspects of the process are substantial for "useful simplification." The design is likely elaborated during discussions with a statistical consultant. We understand the psychotherapy research as more of a manifestation of interpersonal interactions of involved persons than as an "objective" human-independent procedure. Therefore, we try to look at statistical consultation from the perspective of dyadic processes.

Humanistic scientists say that five experts have ten different opinions about one problem. Many of them maintain that in statistics, a part of mathematics, truths are apparent and exactly examinable and that statistical consultants must therefore share the universally true opinions.

Nothing could be less true. Two statistical or methodical consultants will agree that in the standard normal distribution, the mean is 0 and the standard deviation is 1 by definition. When asked what role, if any, it has within process research, they will start to argue, and they will disagree even more about sound strategies for the consultation/support/supervision of their psychotherapy research clients. Not only their opinions but also their attitudes toward and preferences in the working alliance differentiated the consultants. The nature of process research and

Table 12.7 Two prototypes of statistical consultation styles

Consultant prototype 1	Consultant prototype 2
Is critical and destructive	Is critical and constructive
Knows which methods are allowed and which methods are prohibited	Understands the nature of methods and can make his/her judgments independent of authorities
Adapts all problems to [his/her] standard designs	Uses standard designs for standard situations and searches for creative solutions whenever necessary or desirable
Advocates only the confirmatory analysis and prohibits exploratory procedures	Applies confirmatory and exploratory analyses and distinguishes clearly between them
Is not really interested in the problems of the client because he/she is an "objective" expert	Is interested in the client's research and is emotionally involved
And has no time for something such as that	And hence he/she has time problems as well

of the particular researcher leads to different prognoses of the working alliance by different consultants. We have outlined two possible prototypes of statistical/methodical consultation styles in Table 12.7.

This table shows conjectures based on personal experience; we did no such empirical study. Without a success guarantee, its lines can serve a checklist in the search for a suitable research partner.

The last metaphoric comment can help the psychotherapist to understand the human being behind the statistical/methodical consultant. Looking at the process of consultation as a real interaction of two real people, we came to an amazing comparison: The statistical/methodical consultation has certain aspects similar to those acting within psychotherapy or counseling:

- Clients claim to have a small question (what test shall I use here?), but they can have a large problem (the whole data structure is not usable).
- Clients search for help too late.
- Clients do not know exactly and consciously what they are really interested in, but it is possible for the client and therapist to find it together.
- Consultation is addressed not to the problem but to the client.
- The consultant's feelings about the client and the study are essential (countertransference).
- A solution the client does not accept is not a solution.
- No good consultation is without a good helping or working alliance.
- Statistical consultation is an interpersonal relationship.

Conclusion

This chapter aims to outline and discuss the methods of data analysis in the area of psychotherapy process research. We have divided the considerations into two fields. First, thinking about *data structures*, which consist of two subfields of data acquisition and data manipulation, and second, thinking about *procedures* for exploration and confirmation. Our attention was more focused on the data structures than on the data procedures. The reason was that in our opinion, appropriate data structures are essential both for reflecting the research questions and for the sound choice of statistical procedures. We have seen that in both fields, structures and procedures, even the basic options can be sufficient for studies that substantially contribute to process research and that in both fields, a nearly infinite spectrum of advanced method options exists. Finally, we have hopefully shared our opinion that psychotherapy process research can offer a lot for an engaged, curious, and creative researcher.

What about Bob? He already left this chapter. We guess he is studying other chapters of this book now. On his desk he left the following message (Fig. 12.4).

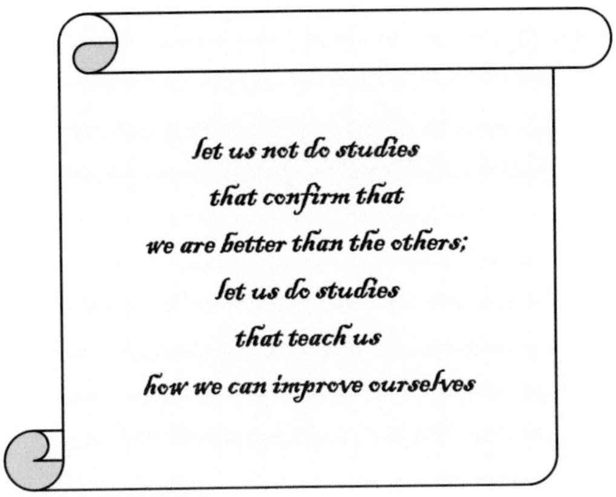

Fig. 12.4 Bob's message

Acknowledgment I am grateful to—in alphabetical order by the given name—*Blerta Bodinaku*, *Kathrin Mörtl*, *Michael Stigler*, and *Omar C.G. Gelo* for their friendly help and discussions.

References

Albani C, Pokorny D, Blaser G, Kächele H (2008) *Beziehungsmuster und Beziehungskonflikte*. Theorie. Klinik und Forschung, Vandenhoeck & Ruprecht, Göttingen

APA (2013) The diagnostic and statistical manual of mental disorders DSM-V. American Psychiatric Association, Washington

Dahl H, Hölzer M, Berry JW (1992) How to classify emotions for psychotherapy research. Ulmer Textbank, Ulm

Field A (2013) Discovering statistics using IBM SPSS statistics. Sage, Thousand Oaks, CA

Griffith A (2010) SPSS for dummies, 2nd edn. Wiley, New York

Hajek P, Havranek T (1978) Mechanizing hypothesis formation. Mathematical foundations for a general theory. Springer, Berlin

Hajek P, Havel I, Chytil M (1966) The GUHA Method of automatic hypotheses determination. Computing 1:293–308

Hill CE, Lambert MJ (2004) Methodological issues in studying psychotherapeutic processes and outcome. In: Lambert MJ (ed) Bergin and Garfield's handbook of psychotherapy and behaviour change, 5th edn. Wiley, New York, pp 55–71

Horvath AO (1981) The working alliance inventory (WAI). Client and therapist forms. http://conferences.jbs.biz/tx_for_homeless_06/presentations/Wednesday,%20Jan%2025/Consumer%20Centered,%20Hohman/Working%20Alliance%20Inventory-Client%20form.pdf

Horvath AO, Greenberg LS (1989) Development and validation of the working alliance inventory. J Couns Psychol 36(2):223–233. doi:10.1037/0022-0167.36.2.223

Kächele H, Mergenthaler E (1983) Computer-aided analysis of psychotherapeutic discourse—a workshop. In: Minsel W-R, Herff W (eds) Methodology in psychotherapy research. Lang, Frankfurt

Luborsky L, Crits-Christoph P (eds) (1998) Understanding transference: the core conflictual relationship theme method, 2nd edn. American Psychological Association, Washington

Lutz W, Hill CE (2009) Quantitative and qualitative methods for psychotherapy research. Special section. Psychother Res 19(4–5):369–615

Orlinsky DE, Howard KI (1967) The good therapy hour. Experiential correlations of patients' and therapists' evaluations of therapy sessions. Arch Gen Psychiat 16:621–632

Orlinsky DE, Rønnestad MH, Willutzki U (2004) Fifty years of psychotherapy process-outcome research: continuity and change. In: Lambert M (ed) Bergin and Garfield's handbook of psychotherapy and behavior change, 5th edn. Wiley, New York, pp 307–392

Pokorny D (2010) Where are hypotheses being born? On exploratory and confirmatory faces of the GUHA method. In: Cintula P, Haníková Z, Švejdar V (eds) Witnesses years. Essays in honour of Petr Hájek. College Publications, London, pp 87–102

R-Project (2014) The R Project for statistical computing. www.r-project.org

SPR (2014) Book of abstracts. Society for psychotherapy research. Proceedings of 45th international annual meeting. SPR, Copenhagen

Stern DN (2004) The present moment in psychotherapy and everyday Life. WW Norton, New York

Stigler M, Pokorny D (2001) Emotions and primary process in guided imagery psychotherapy: computerized text-analytic measures. Psychother Res 11(4):415–431

WHO (2010) International Classification of Diseases (ICD). World Health Organization. http://www.who.int/classifications/icd/en/

Quantitative Approaches to Treatment Process, Change Process, and Process-Outcome Research

13

Omar Carlo Gioacchino Gelo and Stefano Manzo

Contents

Abstract

To understand how and why psychotherapy works, it is necessary to focus on (both) the process of psychotherapy (i.e., what takes place during the treatment) and the relationship between this process and the outcome of psychotherapy (i.e., the treatment's clinical effects). In the present chapter, we provide an overview of three main quantitative research strategies that may be differently used to fulfill this aim. These include treatment *process research* (which investigates what takes place during psychotherapy, regardless of its clinical meaningfulness), *change process research* (which investigates what takes place during psychotherapy, with regard to its clinical meaningfulness), and *process-outcome research* (which investigates the relationship between what takes place during psychotherapy and its clinical effects). We first define the process and outcome of psychotherapy; then, for each research approach proposed, we review the research design, data collection, and data analysis issues; finally, we conclude with suggestions for future research.

13.1 Introduction

The clinical practice of psychotherapy primarily addresses change, which represents both the

O.C.G. Gelo (✉)
Department of History, Society and Human Studies, University of Salento, Via Stampacchia 45, 73100 Lecce, Italy

Department of Psychotherapy Science, Sigmund Freud University, Freudplatz 1, 1020 Vienna, Austria
e-mail: omar.gelo@unisalento.it; omar.gelo@sfu.ac.at

S. Manzo
Animal Research Institute, Via Toledo 148, Napoli, Italy

O.C.G. Gelo et al. (eds.), *Psychotherapy Research*,
DOI 10.1007/978-3-7091-1382-0_13, © Springer-Verlag Wien 2015

therapy's *means* and *end*. In the first case, which is usually described as the *process* of psychotherapy, we address modifications of experiences, behaviors, beliefs, feelings, fantasies, etc. that are faced by the clients and/or therapists during the course of a treatment. In the second case, which is usually referred to as the *outcome* of psychotherapy, we address modifications within those specific domains (affective, cognitive, behavioral, etc.), which represent the target of the intervention and occur as the effect of the therapeutic process.

Since its inception, modern psychotherapy research has focused on the process, the outcome, or their relationship (see Chap. 3). After an initial period when the investigations mainly focused on the outcome, with the aim of demonstrating the *efficacy* of psychotherapy, researchers began to also turn their attention to the process and its relationship with the outcome, with the aim of showing *what* happens during psychotherapy and identifying *why* therapy works, respectively. By doing this, the scientific investigation of psychotherapy has mainly been characterized by a quantitative research approach, although the use of qualitative approaches has been gaining increasing relevance over the last few decades (see Chaps. 9, 12, 14, 20, 26, and 27 for an introduction and overview; see Lambert 2013 for an extensive review).

In this chapter, we focus on three different ways to investigate the psychotherapeutic process, either by itself or in relation to the psychotherapeutic outcome (for a general introduction, see Chap. 9). We distinguish between *treatment process research* (which investigates what takes place during psychotherapy, regardless of its clinical meaningfulness), *change process research* (which investigates what takes place during psychotherapy, with regard to its clinical meaningfulness), and *process-outcome research* (which investigates the relationship between what takes place during psychotherapy and its clinical effects). Our aim is to describe the main *quantitative* approaches which may be used to answer the research questions that are posed by each of these three different types of research. Here, a *quantitative* approach is defined as any approach that exclusively uses statistical data analysis to answer the study's research question (see Chap. 12 for an introduction), regardless of whether qualitative procedures of text analysis may have been used to collect the data (see Chap. 20 for a discussion on this issue).[1] We first define the process and the outcome of psychotherapy; then, for each research type proposed, we describe the research design, data collection, and data analysis issues; finally, we conclude with suggestions for future research. When doing this, we mainly focus on individual therapy (for an overview of quantitative research on group therapy, see Chap. 14).

13.2 The Process and Outcome of Psychotherapy

13.2.1 The Process of Psychotherapy

The *process* of psychotherapy represents anything that can be conceptualized as *a constituent* of the psychotherapeutic treatment; more specifically, it refers to all of the events that, during the course of a treatment, *occur* as part of the therapy sessions and/or may be related to these sessions (Hill and Lambert 2004; Orlinsky et al. 2004). These events may refer to any domain (physiological, affective, cognitive, behavioral, etc.) that is ascribable to the client, to the therapist, and/or to their relationship. This definition is highly inclusive and, thus, analogous to the definition of the *treatment* process that is given by Orlinsky et al (2004); therefore, it should be distinguished from the more specific *change* process, which refers to those specific aspects of the treatment process that represent any clinically meaningful event "through which

[1] Actually, quantitative research may also be described with regard to other aspects that are related to the *research methods* (e.g., data collection, sampling, and research designs) as well as with reference to the *methodological principles* that underlie these methods and the *philosophical worldviews* that are the basis of these methodological principles. However, we believe that, at a very pragmatic and procedural level, considering data analysis is enough to characterize the quantitative approaches to empirical research (see Gelo 2012; Gelo et al. 2008, 2009; Polkinghorne 1983; and Ponterotto 2005 for an articulated discussion; also see Chap. 4).

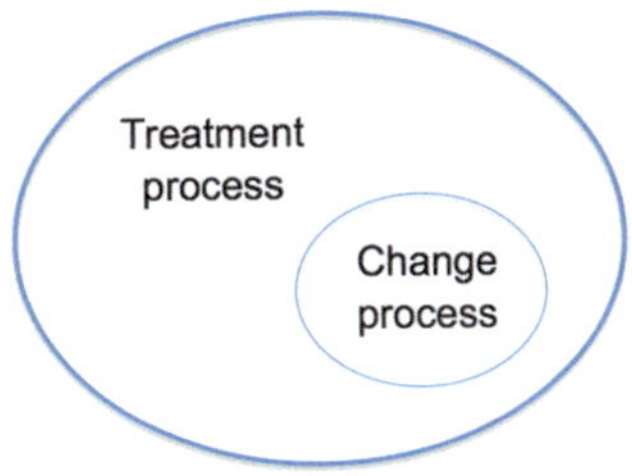

Fig. 13.1 Relationship between the treatment process and the change process

clients or patients are hypothesized to improve" (p. 312; also see Greenberg 1986; Rice and Greenberg 1984) (see Fig. 13.1).

Thus, for example, the client's verbalization of emotions will be considered an aspect of the general treatment process, unless it is theoretically supposed (or empirically shown) to represent a clinically significant aspect of the process; in the latter case, it will be considered an aspect of the change process. In the present chapter, unless otherwise specified, we will refer to the treatment process whenever the more general terms of "process" or "therapeutic process" are used.

An extremely useful heuristic description of the different main facets of the therapeutic process is provided by the Generic Model of Psychotherapy (Orlinsky et al. 2004).[2] These include the following: (1) the *therapeutic contract* (referring to the *organizational* aspects of the process), (2) the *therapeutic operations* (referring to the *technical* aspects of the process, including the client's presentation, the therapist's understanding, the therapist's interventions, and the client's responsiveness), (3) the *therapeutic bond* (referring to the *interpersonal* aspects of the patient-therapist relationship), (4) *self-relatedness* (referring to the *intrapersonal* aspects of this relationship), and (5) *in-session impacts* [referring to the immediate, positive, or negative consequences that any in-session event may have regarding the patient and/or therapist (for this reason, in-session impacts are very similar to what we have described above as the change process)]. It should be noted that, with regard to the distinction that is made above, the first four facets address the treatment process, and the last one addresses the change process.[3]

In the field of quantitative research, several instruments have been developed to assess the different aspects of the therapeutic process (for an example, see Table 13.1; see Elliott 1991; Greenberg and Pinsof 1986; Lepper and Riding 2006; Hill and Lambert 2004 for a review and discussion. See Chap. 20 for an overview of instruments developed to assess the therapeutic process in the field of qualitative research). A few of these measures are considered *micro*-processual because they provide a turn-by-turn output that focuses on *within*-session units that may vary in content from single words to sentences, speaking turns, thought units, and even entire episodes of therapy. Most of them consist of *observational* instruments (mostly in the form of nominal category systems and interval scales) that are applied by a rater (or judge) to session transcripts or audio/video recordings, which allows the construct(s) investigated to be assessed at a moment-by-moment level. In certain cases, these observational instruments may be automatized, with the computer working as a rater alone (e.g., Fertuck et al. 2012; Mergenthaler 1996; Mergenthaler and Bucci 1999) or in combination with a human judge (e.g., Salvatore et al. 2012).

In contrast, *macro*-processual measures use at least one session as a unit of analysis; they

[2] Elaborated with the aim to coherently organize the empirical literature that links the therapeutic process to the outcome (see Sect. 13.3.3 for more details on process-outcome research), it offers a very useful abstract and synthetic representation of what can be considered the main dimensions of the therapeutic process. Beyond this process, the Generic Model of Psychotherapy also encompasses the *input* (i.e., antecedents of the process) and the *output* [i.e., the consequences of the process, which include the therapy outcome (see Sect. 13.2.2)] (see Orlinsky 2009 for a detailed overview).

[3] Actually, a sixth facet exists, *temporal patterns*, which was introduced in the fourth edition of the *Handbook of Psychotherapy and Behaviour Change*. This facet describes a specific way of analyzing one or more process variables and, for this reason, will be introduced later in this chapter (see Sect. 13.3.3.1).

Table 13.1 Example of instruments developed to collect data about the psychotherapy process

Construct assessed	Name of the instrument	Type of instrument	Type of measurement	Perspective of evaluation	Unit studied	References
Relational patterns	Core Conflictual Relationship Themes (CCRT)	Observational	Nominal category system	J	Micro	Luborsky (1998)
	Structural Analysis of Social Behavior (SASB)	Observational	Nominal category system	J	Micro	Benjamin, Rothweiler, and Critchfield (2006)
Therapeutic alliance	Working Alliance Inventory (WAI)	Self-report, Observational	Set of ordinal/ interval scales	C, T, J	Macro, Micro	Horvath and Greenberg (1989)
	Alliance Negotiation Scale (ANS)	Self-report	Set of ordinal/ interval scales	C	Macro	Doran et al. (2012)
	Collaborative Interaction Scale (CIS)	Observational	Set of ordinal/ interval scales	J	Micro	Colli and Lingiardi (2009)
Narrative processes	Narrative Process Coding System (NPCS)	Observational	Nominal category system	J	Micro	Angus et al. (2012)
Innovative self-narratives	Innovative Moments Coding System (IMCS)	Observational	Nominal category system	J	Micro	Gonçalves et al. (2011)
Metacognition	Metacognition Assessment Scale (MAS)	Observational	Set of dichotomous scales	J	Micro	Semerari et al. (2003)
Reflective functioning	Computerized Reflective Functioning Scale (CRF)	Observational	Nominal category system	Com	Micro	Fertuck et al. (2012)
Therapist interventions	Comparative Psychotherapy Process Scale (CPPS)	Observational	Set of ordinal/ interval scales	J	Macro	Hilsenroth et al. (2005)
	Psychodynamic Intervention Rating Scale (PIRS)	Observational	Set of ordinal/ interval scales	J	Micro	Milbrath et al. (1999)
	Comprehensive Psychotherapy Intervention Rating Scale (CPIRS)	Observational	Set of ordinal/ interval scales	J	Micro	Trijsburg et al. (2002)

Symbolization of internal experience	Experiencing Scale	Observational	Set of ordinal/ interval scales	J	Micro	Klein et al. (1986)
	Computerized Referential Activity (CRA)	Observational	Nominal category system	Com	Micro	Bucci and Maskit (2006), Mergenthaler and Bucci (1999)
Defense mechanisms	Defense Mechanism Rating Scale (DMRS)	Observational	Set of dichotomous scales	J	Macro	Perry (1990)
	Defense Mechanism Rating Scales-Q (DMRS-Q)	Observational	Q-sort	J	Macro	Di Giuseppe et al. (2014)
Emotional-cognitive regulation	Therapeutic Cycle Model (TCM)	Observational	Nominal category system	Com	Micro	Mergenthaler (2008, 1996b)
Linguistic content	Automated Co-occurrence Analysis for Semantic Mapping (ACASM)	Observational	Nominal category system	Com + J	Macro	Salvatore et al. (2012)
Dimensions of psychotherapy process	Psychotherapy Process Q-set	Observational	Q-sort	J	Macro	Jones (1985)
	Therapy Session Reports	Self-report	Set of ordinal/ interval scales	C	Macro	Orlinsky and Howard (1986)
	Bern Post-Session Report (BPSR)	Self-report	Set of ordinal/ interval scales	C, T	Macro	Flückiger et al. (2010)
	Session Evaluation Questionnaire (SEQ)	Self-report	Set of ordinal/ interval scales	C, T	Macro	Stiles and Snow (1984)
Intersession experience	Intersession Experience Questionnaire (IEQ)	Self-report	Set of ordinal/ interval scales	C	Macro	Lundy and Orlinsky (1987), Hartmann et al. (2003)
School-independent change processes	Generic Change Indicators (GCI)	Observational	Nominal category system	J	Micro	Krause et al. (2007)

C client, *T* therapist, *J* judge, *Com* computer

mostly consist of *self-report* instruments (mainly in the form of interval scales), which are answered *post*-session by the client and/or therapist, who, thus, retrospectively express their appraisal of the session; in certain cases, they may also consist of *observational* instruments (usually in the form of nominal category systems, interval scales, and Q-sorts), which are applied to session transcripts and/or audio/video recordings but only require one evaluation of the entire session.[4]

13.2.2 The Outcome of Psychotherapy

The *outcome* of psychotherapy represents anything that can be conceptualized as a *clinical effect* of the psychotherapeutic treatment process; more specifically, it refers to those clinically meaningful changes that, during the course of a treatment and/or after its completion, may be observed as *results* of the therapeutic process, as defined above. These changes refer to the client's problematic domains (e.g., physiological, affective, cognitive, or behavioral) that represent the treatment's target, and should be observed outside the treatment situation (Orlinsky et al. 2004).

According to Orlinsky et al. (2004), the therapeutic outcome can be ascribed to the therapeutic *output* (consequences) of a treatment, which consists of "the whole spectrum of changes that may arise as a result of psychotherapy—whether in patients, therapists, their families and associates, or the organizations, institutions, and value patterns of their social milieu" (p. 316); an example of an output for therapists is the professional development that results from their being engaged in a particular treatment (Orlinsky et al. 2004). What distinguishes the more general output of psychotherapy from its outcome is that the latter "is a clinical concept signifying some degree of improvement or deterioration in the patient's condition, as judged from some observer's perspective by some value criterion" (Orlinsky et al. 2004). The several value criteria that may be employed may differ with regard to different clinical theories, personal inclinations, cultural backgrounds, etc. One of the tasks of psychotherapy research is to contribute to the identification of a plausible enough set of criteria that is shared by a specific scientific community.

Regarding the therapeutic process, multiple levels of descriptions are possible for the therapeutic outcome. Similar to Orlinsky et al. (2004), we distinguish between *immediate* outcomes (defined as the client's improvements observed at a *post-session* level), *intermediate* outcomes (defined as the client's improvements observed *over several sessions* of a treatment), and *final* outcomes (defined as the client's improvements observed at a *posttreatment* level). Our position is slightly different than that of other colleagues (e.g., Greenberg 1986; Greenberg and Pinsof 1986; also see Elliott 2010), according to whom the psychotherapy outcome should not be confined to clinical changes in the client's problematic target behaviors observable after at least a single session; according to these authors, in fact, *any in-session clinically meaningful* event may be considered a (micro-)outcome. The careful reader will notice that what Greenberg and colleagues identify as a *micro-outcome* is actually considered an *in-session impact* by Orlinsky and colleagues (see Sect. 13.2.1). It is important to notice here that Greenberg and colleagues ascribe in-session clinically meaningful events to the domain of outcome and that Orlinsky and colleagues ascribe them to the domain of process (which is coherently represented in their Generic Model of Psychotherapy in terms of in-session impacts). This difference is because the outcome, according to the latter authors, "ought to be observed *outside* the patient-therapist relationship" because a treatment is valuable based on how much change it produces in the "patient's ongoing life or personality" (Orlinsky et al. 2004, p. 314; also see Orlinsky and Howard 1978). Thus, although we agree with Greenberg and colleagues that it may be helpful to also focus on micro-outcomes, we consider that this may be done at a post-session level; on the other hand, we consider any clinically

[4] It should be noted that the observational instruments used to collect process data at a within-session level actually make use of qualitative text analysis (see Chap. 20 for more details; see Gelo et al. 2012 for a discussion).

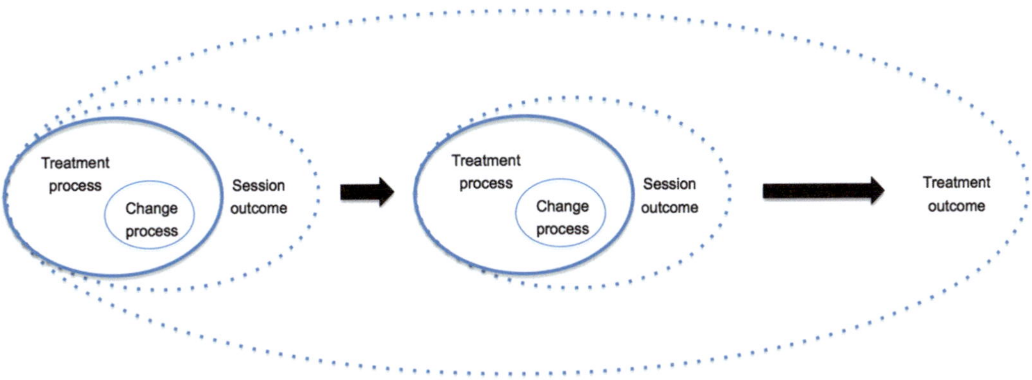

Fig. 13.2 Relationship between the treatment process, the change process, and the outcome over the course of a treatment

meaningful change that occurs within the session "as a distinct aspect of process, which we refer to as in-session impacts" (Orlinsky et al. 2004, p. 314). Figure 13.2 depicts the hypothetical relationship between the treatment process, the change process, and the outcome over the course of a treatment.

Beyond the fact that in-session impacts should be ascribed to either the process or the outcome, which is ultimately a matter of definition and personal evaluation, an important fact is worth noting: when we move from a macrolevel to a micro-level of observation, the distinction between process (what happens in therapy) and outcome (what changes, in clinical terms, as a consequence of the therapy) becomes more arbitrary, vague, and fuzzy; this should not be a surprise because these two concepts are actually heuristic constructs that we separate to describe psychotherapy better. However, ultimately, they are inextricably connected to each other.

Several instruments have been developed to assess outcomes in quantitative research (for an example, see Table 13.2; for a comprehensive overview, see Hill and Lambert 2004. See Chap. 27 for an overview of instruments developed to assess the therapeutic outcome in qualitative research). Traditionally, these instruments may focus on different clinical target domains (e.g., *symptomatology*, *interpersonal relationships*, *personality*, *well-being*, or ad hoc formulated *therapeutic goals*). Most of these instruments used to assess outcomes consist of standardized *self-reports* filled out by clients or *observational* instruments applied by a trained therapist. Usually, it is strongly suggested to assess outcomes that relate to several target domains by using different instruments that are applied from different perspectives.

13.3 Treatment Process, Change Process, and Process-Outcome Research

Depending on whether we are interested in investigating the process (either in the form of a treatment process or a change process) or the relationship between the process and the outcome, we may distinguish between treatment process research, change process research, and process-outcome research. Each of these three main types of research will be described in the following pages with regard to the research design, data collection, and data analysis (see Chap. 3 for an historical overview).

13.3.1 Treatment Process Research

Treatment process research (TPR) may be defined as the scientific investigation of what takes place during psychotherapy, regardless of its clinical meaningfulness.[5] More specifically, TPR focuses

[5] It should be noted that the term of process research may also be used to refer to any kind of research that focuses on the process, either alone (see Chap. 1 and 9) or with

Table 13.2 Example of instruments developed to collect data about the psychotherapy outcome

Name of the instrument	Domain assessed	Type of instrument	Perspective of evaluation	References
Beck Depression Inventory (BDI)	Symptoms	Self-report	C	Beck et al. (1961)
Symptom Checklist-90-R (SCL-90-R)	Symptoms	Self-report	C	Derogatis et al. (1976)
State-Trait Anxiety Inventory (STAI)	Symptoms	Self-report	C	Spielberger et al. (1983)
Dysfunctional Attitudes Scale (DAS)	Vulnerability	Self-report	C	Weissman and Beck (1978)
Clinical Outcome Routine Evaluation-Outcome Measure (CORE-OM)	Symptoms, well-being	Self-report	C	Evans et al. (2002)
Outcome Questionnaire-45 (OQ-45)	Symptoms, interpersonal problems	Self-report	C	Lambert et al. 2004
Inventory of Interpersonal Problems (IIP)	Interpersonal problems	Self-report	C	Horowitz et al. (1988)
Rosenberg Self-Esteem Scale (RSES)	Well-being	Self-report	C	Rosenberg (1965)
Post-Therapy Questionnaire (PTQ)	Treatment goals	Self-report	C	Mintz et al. (1979)
Patient Target Complaint (PTC)	Treatment goals	Self-report	C	Battle et al. (1966)
Hamilton Rating Scale for Depression (HRSD)	Symptoms	Observational	J	Hamilton (1960)
Structured Clinical Interview for DSM personality disorders (SCID-II)	Personality	Observational	J	Spitzer et al. (1990)
Shedler-Westen Assessment Procedure (SWAP-200)	Personality	Observational	J	Shedler and Westen (2007)
Global Assessment Scale (GAS)	Treatment goals	Observational	J	Endicott et al. (1976)
Therapist Target Complaint (TTC)	Treatment goals	Observational	J	Battle et al. (1966)

C client, *J* judge

on the treatment process, as defined above (see Sect. 13.2.1), including "the events—all of the events—that occur as part of therapy sessions, without a priori distinctions between neutral and specifically helpful or hindering events" (Orlinsky et al. 2004, p. 313). Thus, for example, any treatment process described by the Generic Model of Psychotherapy (Orlinsky et al. 2004), with the exception of in-session impacts, may be the object of this type of research. TPR began to be used in the 1930s and was motivated by the interest in "what goes on during a treatment", which was an interest that had been completely neglected by traditional outcome studies of the same period that exclusively focused on the question of "whether the treatment produced clinical effects."

The birth of modern quantitative TPR may be ascribed to electronic recordings of therapy sessions in the early 1930s (e.g., Covner 1942; Lasswell 1935), which was systematized by the work of Carl Rogers (1942) (see Chap. 3). At this

regard to its relationship with the outcome (see Sect. 13.3.3).

time, the general aim of TPR, which would extend to current use, was to develop and apply specific instruments that would be able to measure (in a reliable and objective way) what happens within the therapy sessions (see Dittes 1959; Marsden 1971). The constructs that were often investigated during this period and during the following years relate to the therapeutic relationship, especially from the perspective of person-centered psychotherapy (Rogers 1975, 1957), although instruments were also developed during this time to assess the constructs of different orientations, such as the depth of interpretation in psychoanalysis (Harway et al. 1955) or the quality of an individual's experience in humanistic therapies (Klein et al. 1969). Later, a series of instruments were developed to investigate different constructs from a transtheoretical perspective, including different aspects of the within-session verbal behavior of clients and therapists (Friedlander 1982; Hill 1978; Stiles 1978, 1979; see Elliott et al. 1987 for a review), as well as the structure (Benjamin 1974) and quality (Luborsky et al. 1983; Hartley and Strupp 1983) of the therapeutic relationship (for an overview of the instruments used during this early phase of TPR, see Kiesler 1973). Over these decades, we observe an increasing commitment to the principles of logical positivism and the corresponding logic of justification.

During the 1960s, researchers began to emphasize the importance of investigating the therapeutic process from the perspective of the clients and/or therapists themselves instead of exclusively relying on nonparticipant-observer instruments. To address this aim, a series of instruments began to be developed that asked clients and/or therapists for their appraisals of the sessions. A few of the very first instruments of this type focused on defense mechanisms (Gleser and Ihilevich 1969) and the therapeutic relationship (Barrett-Lennard 1962). These were followed by other instruments that aimed to investigate the disparate facets of the therapeutic process (Orlinsky and Howard 1986) or the therapeutic alliance itself (Horvath and Greenberg 1989),

Finally, over the last three decades, we have witnessed a return of the interests in nonparticipant assessment of the within-session, moment-by-moment aspects of the therapeutic process, with the aim of investigating the micro-dynamics of therapeutic events; this is related to the increasing tendency to integrate the logic of justification and verification with the logic of discovery (see Greenberg 1991; also see Hill 1990, 1994; Mahrer 1988). Both of these events (i.e., the focus on micro-dynamics and the discovery-oriented approach) are responsible for the birth, during the 1980s, of a new type of process research that specifically focuses on in-session change processes (see Sect. 13.3.2).

13.3.1.1 Research Designs

TPR is mainly characterized by a *nonexperimental* approach (also called passive-observational, correlational, or naturalistic[6]), although attempts to use an experimental approach were made in the past) (e.g., Hill and Gormally 1977). In experimental and quasi-experimental approaches, the researcher attempts to establish a *cause-effect relationship* between one specific aspect of the therapeutic process (i.e., the independent variable) and another aspect (i.e., the dependent variable); this is done by manipulating the independent variable to observe its systematic effects within a very *controlled* setting.[7] In contrast, nonexperimental approaches address one or more variables that represent different aspects of the therapeutic process, which are evaluated in significantly *less controlled* settings, either in terms of reciprocal *associations* or by *comparing* them in at least two groups.

An example of experimental TPR is the study conducted by Hill and Gormally (1977), who were interested in determining whether a different combination of the therapist's verbal and nonverbal behavior (independent variable) has a certain effect on the client's affect (dependent

[6] The term naturalistic is often used to describe the approach used by qualitative research (see Chap. 20).

[7] At a very pragmatic level, the difference between an experiment and a quasi-experiment is that in the former case, subjects are randomized to the different conditions, while this is not the case for quasi-experiments. Both include the manipulation of an independent variable.

variable). Clients were randomly assigned to the different possible combinations of the therapist's verbal and nonverbal behavior. This independent variable was manipulated by the researcher who, by means of using different-colored lights located in the consultation room, indicated to the therapists which type of verbal and nonverbal behavior they should display during specific moments of the session. The dependent variable (the client's affect) was assessed by trained judges who rated the session's transcripts with regard to the amount of affect that was verbally expressed by the client.

On the other hand, the work of Williams and Fauth (2005) is an example of a non-experimental study of the relationship between the therapist's in-session self-awareness, its affective and behavioral manifestations, the management strategies employed by the therapist, and the client's perceptions of the therapy process. Subjects were not randomized. Moreover, the researcher was not interested in the causal relationship between an independent and dependent variable, but rather, he was interested in the different associations between a series of process variables. None of these variables were manipulated but rather, they were observed post hoc without external constraints regarding how they naturally occurred within the session.

Deciding which approach to use (experimental vs. non-experimental) is not only a matter of practical possibilities (e.g., controlled experiments may be more complex to arrange) but a matter of personal inclinations regarding what is considered to be more relevant, especially in terms of internal and external validity vs. ecological validity.[8]

TPR makes use of both *cross-sectional* and *longitudinal* designs (see Elliott and Anderson 1994 for a discussion). In the first case, one or more aspects of the therapeutic process are considered with regard to *one specific point in time*, with a focus on the *between* subjects variability. For example, it is possible to compare the total amounts of different forms of the therapist's verbal behavior in treatments of different orientations (e.g., Tomori and Bavelas 2007) or to assess the relationship between the client's defensive functioning and alliance with the therapist's intervention in therapies with a specific orientation (Siefert et al. 2006). It should be noted that although data may be collected at different time points during the treatment (see the longitudinal design below), the design has to be considered as cross-sectional if the analyses are used on data that are aggregated regarding the subjects.

In the case of longitudinal designs, in contrast, one or more aspects of the therapeutic process are considered with regard to their *temporal development*; thus, the focus here is on the *within*-subject variability. For example, it is possible to study how the proportions of therapist interpretations may vary during different phases of the treatment (Hersoug et al. 2003). The single-case design, for which there has been a "widespread resurgence of interest" over the last few years (Hilliard 1993, p. 373; also see Iwakabe and Gazzola 2009), is a specific variant of the longitudinal design that aims to provide an intensive in-depth investigation of one case (Grabhorn et al. 2006); another variant is the multiple case study, where two or more cases are compared (e.g., Dimaggio et al. 2007) see Chap. 20 for a description of single-case design in qualitative research.

One important issue to consider when applying a longitudinal design relates to how many observations should be made over time. Of course, the ideal situation is to have as many observations as possible; however, this very often may be rather energy and time consuming,

[8] Although experimental research presents higher *internal* validity (due to the greater control of confounding variables with regard to the investigated cause-effect relationships) and *external* validity (due to the higher control of sampling procedures that allow the results to be generalized from the sample to the population), non-experimental research presents a higher *ecologic* validity (which addresses the degree to which we may generalize our results to real-life contexts outside the laboratory) due to being characterized by less strict control. Different researchers, who provide different emphasis on either internal and external validity or ecological validity, will, consequently, prefer to use either an experimental or non-experimental approach.

especially when data collection requires the analysis of session transcripts (see Sect. 13.3.1.2). For this reason, several studies use *temporal sampling*, in which the variables of interest are assessed and analyzed only at specific, a priori defined time points (e.g., the first 3, the middle 3, and the last 3 sessions of a treatment; the first 5 min, the middle 5 min, and the last 5 min of each session; see, e.g., Hersoug et al. 2003).

13.3.1.2 Data Collection

Most contemporary psychotherapy TPR addresses *in-session processes*, which include the processes that take place during the treatment sessions. A *within-session* assessment of the variables of interest is a popular way to collect data about these in-session processes. This is done by means of *nonparticipant observational* instruments, which are applied to the session transcripts by trained judges (raters) (see Hill and Lambert 2004 for a discussion; see Mergenthaler and Stinson 1992 for an example of the international transcription standards currently used in psychotherapy research). These instruments may take the form of a set of dichotomous scales [e.g., Defense Mechanism Rating Scale (Perry 1990), Metacognition Assessment Scale (Semerari et al. 2003)] or nominal category systems [e.g., Core Conflictual Relationship Themes (Luborsky 1998); also see Chap. 19; Structural Analysis of Social Behavior (Benjamin et al. 2006); Narrative Process Coding System (see Angus et al. 2012 and Chap. 20)] when the assessment of different aspects of the process is made with regard to whether they are present or not. On the other hand, a set of ordinal or interval scales [e.g., Comparative Psychotherapy Process Scale (Hilsenroth et al. 2005), Psychodynamic Intervention Rating Scale (Milbrath et al. 1999), Comprehensive Psychotherapy Intervention Rating Scale (Trijsburg et al. 2002)] may be used when the rater's assessment of different aspects of the process is made through the use of a Likert scale with regard to their intensity; finally, Q-sorts may also be used [e.g., Psychotherapy Process Q-set (Jones 1985), Defense Mechanism Rating Scales-Q (Di Giuseppe et al. 2014)] when the items that describe different aspects of the process are sorted into a forced distribution.

All of these instruments may focus on the most disparate constructs related to the client, the therapist, and/or both; in most cases, they allow the variables of interest to be assessed at a turn-by-turn level (*micro*-processual assessment), although in other cases the analysis of the transcript is used to produce an overall judgment of the entire session (*macro*-processual assessment) (see Table 13.1 for a few examples). Nonparticipant observational instruments have the advantage of allowing for an assessment of the process that is grounded in the examinations of the audio/video registrations of the session, but this may be very time and energy consuming (thus, with the possible result, e.g., of limiting the sample size).

To overcome a few of these limitations, computer-assisted procedures of text analysis that can be applied to session transcripts have been developed in recent years. In most cases, they follow a top-down approach where words from the therapeutic conversation are deductively ascribed to a priori defined categories; examples include the Therapeutic Cycle Model (e.g., Mergenthaler 1996, 2008), the Computerized Referential Activity (Bucci and Maskit 2006; Mergenthaler and Bucci 1999), and the recently developed Computerized Reflective Functioning Scale (Fertuck et al. 2012). However, Salvatore et al. (2012) recently developed a computerized approach (the Automated Co-occurrence Analysis for Semantic Mapping), which allows the content categories in the patient-therapist conversation to be identified through the use of a bottom-up approach (see Chap. 20 for a discussion of top-down and bottom-up approaches to text-analysis in psychotherapy research).

Another common way to collect data about the in-session psychotherapeutic process is through a *post-session* assessment of the variables of interest. This is done through *participant self-report* instruments (usually in the form of interval scales) that are used to ask the clients and/or the therapist about their subjective appraisals regarding one or more aspects of what happened during the entire session (*macro*-processual assessment). Examples include the Working Alliance Inventory (Horvath and Greenberg 1989), Therapy Session Reports (Orlinsky and Howard 1986), the Bern Post-Session Report (Flückiger et al. 2010), and the Group Climate Questionnaire (MacKenzie 1983; see Hill and Lambert 2004 for a discussion; see Chap. 18 for an overview of research on the process from the perspective of therapists). Similar to the case of nonparticipant observational instruments, participant self-report instruments focus on the most disparate constructs (see Table 13.1 for a few examples). Participant self-report instruments have the advantage of allowing for an assessment of the process from the subjective perspective of the participants, which is not as time and energy consuming as nonparticipant observational instruments (thus, e.g., enabling data to be collected for larger samples).

Although most contemporary TPR over the last few years has addressed in-session processes, TPR has witnessed an increasing interest in *between-session processes;* these are defined as those events that occur during the intervals between at least two treatment sessions and that may be related to what occurred during the latter session. This shift in focus is based on the idea that "patients typically recollect, reflect on, practice, and imaginatively elaborate on experiences they had during sessions with their therapists" (Hartmann et al. 2011, p. 1044) and, thus, extends the therapeutic process beyond the walls of the consultation room. To our knowledge, the only instrument developed for this purpose is the Intersession Experience Questionnaire (Lundy and Orlinsky 1987; Hartmann et al. 2003), which is a client self-report where the participant is asked, before the beginning of a new session, to answer a few questions about his/her experiences that have occurred since the last session.

13.3.1.3 Data Analysis

TPR makes use of a vast array of statistical methods that mainly depend on the research questions posed and the research design that is adopted. To compare one or more process variable across different groups or conditions, chi-squared tests (e.g., Gelo and Mergenthaler 2012), analyses of variance (ANOVA) for independent measures, and t-tests for independent samples (e.g., Jaycox et al. 1998) are usually employed. Correlations are very often used to assess the degree of association between two or more variables (e.g., Michalak et al. 2005), although researchers may prefer to use regression analyses (e.g., Kolden et al. 2005) and path analyses (e.g., Moyers et al. 2005); the latter two have the advantage of allowing inferences of a more causal nature to be made for the investigated variables (see Elliott and Anderson 1994 and Russell and Trull 1986 for a discussion).

In contrast, researchers who are interested in the development of one or more process variables over time typically use an ANOVA for repeated measures and t-tests for paired samples (e.g., Gilles et al. 2007). To overcome a few limitations of these traditional approaches (e.g., very restrictive assumptions, the focus on a group as opposed to an individual, mean change and variance), more complex procedures that use longitudinal data analysis have been developed over the last few years, such as longitudinal hierarchical linear modeling and growth curve analysis (Gallop & Tasca 2009; Tasca & Gallop 2009; Tschacher and Ramseyer 2009; also see Lutz and Knox 2013). These procedures allow to investigate the *shape* of change of one or more process variables over time. For example, by using growth curve analysis, Tasca et al. (2006) found that the engaged group's climate presented a cubic trend in group psychodynamic-interpersonal psychotherapy and that it showed a linear trend in group cognitive-behavioral therapy.

Another very interesting data-analytic approach is the Markovian sequence analysis by Bakeman and Gottman (1997), which allows to assessed the time-lagged relationship between categorical variables. For example, Salvatore et al. (2009) recently analyzed the transcripts of an entire treatment based on the suggestion by Russell and Trull (1986) and were able to identify how the temporal sequence of the content of the therapeutic dialogue changes as a function of the treatment phase.

13.3.2 Change Process Research

Change process research (CPR) can be defined as the scientific investigation of what occurs during psychotherapy, with regard to its clinical meaningfulness; in other words, it investigates the process through which clinically relevant changes occur within psychotherapy. With reference to the Generic Model of Psychotherapy (Orlinsky 2009; Orlinsky et al. 2004), we may assert that CPR is any research that focuses on *in-session impacts*, that is, all of the "clinically relevant consequences" of the treatment process within the therapy sessions (p. 319).

Because we consider the change process (as represented by in-session impacts) to be a subclass of the treatment process (see Fig. 13.1; also see Orlinsky et al. 2004), we view CPR as a subclass of TPR that specifically focuses on those aspects of the treatment process that may be considered to be clinically meaningful. Thus, our definition of CPR is slightly different than that of other authors (e.g., Elliott 2010; Greenberg 1986) who, by ascribing in-session impacts to the domain of (micro-)outcomes, consider CPR to be a form of process-outcome research (see Sect. 13.3.3). For Greenberg (1986), for example, the core of CPR consists in the assessment of in-session impacts within a session (i.e., micro-outcomes) and the identification of the in-session treatment processes that lead to these in-session impacts; moreover, he also asserts that it is necessary to establish a relationship between these in-session change processes and post-session and final outcomes (see Elliott 2010, for an overview of the different qualitative, quantitative, and mixed-methods approaches that may be used for this purpose). We completely agree with Greenberg (1986) that (1) the investigation of the process of change is an essential aspect of understanding how psychotherapy works and that (2) process-outcome relationships should be investigated on different timescales; however, we do believe that these in-session change processes (1) are the objects of process research rather than process-outcome research and that (2) the smallest timescale at which they can be related to an outcome is at the post-session level rather than the within-session level (see Orlinsky et al. 2004, for a similar position).[9]

What constitutes a clinically meaningful process is a clinical-theoretical and/or empirical issue and, thus, may vary from case to case. In quantitative CPR, researchers usually explicitly define "clinically meaningful" a priori based on their clinical theory and clinical experience.[10] As mentioned, we find the reference to the concept of in-session impacts very helpful and instructive for understanding the focus of CPR. In-session impacts represent any clinically relevant consequence of the treatment process that occurs within a session. Usually, researchers tend to focus on clients' in-session impacts, but it is possible to also consider the in-session impacts of the therapist; moreover, both client and therapist impacts may be both positive and negative. As clearly stated by Orlinsky et al. (2004), "patient impacts may be positive ('therapeutic realizations') and/or negative ('harms')—for example, insight vs. confusion, relief vs. distress, encouragement vs. demoralization, self-efficacy vs. dependence. Therapist impacts may be positive ('returns') and/or negative ('costs') accruing from their work investment—for example, self-efficacy vs. frustration, professional growth vs. burnout." (p. 318). Yet, in-session impacts represent "the 'pot of gold' (or 'lead' in the case of negative

[9] We should stress that this difference is of a more heuristic and theoretical/conceptual nature and does not necessarily have practical implications for the practice of psychotherapy research.

[10] In contrast, more complex, mixed-method approaches to CPR, belonging to the so called *significant event approache* (see Elliott 2010 for an overview; also see Rice and Greenberg 1984), make use of a combination of both theoretical and empirical ways to identify significant events. Prototypical examples of this approach include task analysis (e.g., Greenberg 2007; Pascual-Leone et al. 2009), comprehensive process analysis (e.g., Elliott et al. 1994), and assimilation analysis (Stiles et al. 1990).

impacts) at the end of the rainbow where the clinical aspects of therapeutic process collect" (Orlinsky 2009, p. 327).

CPR was born at the same time as TPR at the hands of those researchers who were specifically interested in the clinically meaningful aspects of the process through which clients might be considered to improve. Actually, a pioneering form of CPR may be traced back to Freud's clinical (or narrative) case study, which has spanned from the subsequent decades until recently (see Hilliard 1993; Iwakabe and Gazzola 2009; see Chap. 19 for an example). However, the first "modern" CPR study was conducted by Snyder (1945), a member of Rogers' research group, with the aim of identifying which therapist behaviors led to higher degrees of client insight (Elliott and Farber 2010; see Chap. 3). Since then, several CPR investigations have been conducted that focus on the most disparate constructs, which has led to the development of what have been referred to as the *micro-theories* of therapeutic change (see Lambert, Garfield and Bergin, 2004; see also Rice & Greenberg, 1984).

13.3.2.1 Research Design

CPR is characterized by a *non-experimental* approach; we are not aware of any experimental studies. The research design may be *cross-sectional*, which aims to provide an overall but static picture of the phenomenon that is under investigation. For example, Kolden and colleagues (1996; Kolden et al. 2006) investigated the relationship between different treatment process variables (i.e., therapeutic bond, therapeutic openness-involvement, and self-relatedness) and the client's in-session impacts (i.e., therapeutic realizations) that were assessed early in the treatment. Kolden (1991) followed a similar approach, with data collection occurring at several time points over the treatment but also aggregating all of the collected data. However, most of the designs used in CPR are *longitudinal*, which allows the variables of interest to be investigated over time. The minimal requirement is to repeatedly assess at least one treatment process variable (considered to be an independent variable) and one in-session impact variable (considered to be a dependent variable) over the course of the sessions and/or treatment; three main approaches are, thus, possible.

In one approach, the behavior of the treatment process variable is modeled over time, and the in-session impact variable is used as a criterion measure; the aim is to assess the extent to which the former might show a different time course over the therapy with regard to different values of the latter. For example, Pascual-Leone (2009) was interested in the extent to which the different time courses of clients' emotional processing (the treatment process variable) may impact their level of experiencing (the in-session impact variable); thus, after having divided the sessions of several treatments into high vs. low experiencing, he was able to find that the time course of clients' emotional processing significantly differed between the two groups.

Following a second approach, which is quite widespread and usually known as a *micro-analytic sequential process design* (Elliott 2010), the treatment process and the change process variables are assessed at a turn-to-turn, in-session level (although they might eventually be assessed at a post-session level; see Sexton 1993), with the aim of assessing the extent to which the treatment process variable (i.e., the *antecedent* variable) effectively triggers the in-session impact variable (i.e., the *consequent* variable). For example, it might be possible to test the hypothesis that therapists' supportive strategies will trigger more disclosure from the clients and that interpretive interventions will trigger more emotional disclosures from the clients (Milbrath et al. 1999).

Finally, it is possible to combine both of these approaches to assess, first, the time-lagged sequential dependency between at least two treatment process variables and, then, the extent to which these micro-dynamics are different with regard to the in-session impact variable used as a criterion measure. For example, Safran and Muran (1996) were able to test the hypothesis that client and therapist interactional in-session micro-dynamics differed between the rupture resolution and rupture nonresolution sessions.[11]

It should be noted that change dynamics in CPR may be investigated at an *interindividual* level (i.e., individual change dynamics of either the client or the therapist) and/or an *intraindividual* level (i.e., interactional change dynamics of the therapeutic dyad). In the first case, at least one variable should be related to the client and at least one to the therapist (e.g., Milbrath et al. 1999; Safran and Muran 1996); in the second case, we might focus on variables that are related to either the patient or the therapist. Of course, a combination of these two approaches is possible, with a focus on both the interindividual and intraindividual levels (e.g., Sexton 1993).

13.3.2.2 Data Collection

As mentioned, in CPR, we need to assess at least one treatment variable and one in-session impact variable. With regard to the latter, it should be noted that in order for any process variable to be considered an in-session impact variable, it must be *explicitly* considered to reflect a desirable and clinically meaningful aspect of the therapeutic process. For this to occur, the researcher needs a clinical theory. Thus, generally speaking, any instrument that is able to assess any process variable (see Table 13.1) that is considered by the researcher to be clinically meaningful in the process of change is a good instrument for assessing an in-session impact.

Similar to TPR, data collection in CPR may occur by means of *participant self-report* instruments, which are filled out by the client and/or therapist at a *post-session* level and, thus, provide a *macro*-level assessment. An excellent instrument for this purpose is the Therapy Session Report (TSR; Orlinsky and Howard 1986; see Kolden 1991, 1996; Kolden et al. 2006), which was mentioned previously (see section 13.3.1.2); with reference to the Generic Model of Psychotherapy (Orlinsky et al. 2004), TSR allows for the assessment of different treatment process variables (i.e., therapeutic openness-involvement, the therapeutic bond, and self-relatedness) and in-session impact variables (i.e., therapeutic realizations) from the client's and/or therapist's perspective. The different self-report instruments used to assess the alliance's ruptures and resolution [e.g., the Post-Session Questionnaire (Muran et al. 1992) and the Alliance Negotiation Scale (Doran et al. 2012)] can also be used when these constructs are considered to be in-session impacts (see Safran and Muran 1996). Another interesting example is provided by Owen et al. (2012), who used the Intersession Experience Questionnaire to assess the client's experiences after one session, hypothesized to represent the impact of the alliance in that session (Hartmann et al. 2003).

In addition to self-report measures, a second and more frequently used way to collect data in CPR is by means of *nonparticipant observational* instruments; these allow for a *within-session*, turn-to-turn assessment and may, thus, shed light on the *micro*-processes of change. Examples of instruments that have been used or could be used include the Experiencing Scale (Klein et al. 1986) which assesses the quality of clients' emotional processing; the Depth Scale of the Session Evaluation Questionnaire (Stiles and Snow 1984a, b), which assesses the depth of a therapist's interpretation (see Lingiardi et al. 2011); and the Collaborative Interaction Scale (CIS; Colli and Lingiardi 2009), which assesses the alliance's ruptures and repairs. A series of instruments have recently been ad hoc developed to identify change episodes and assess their different characteristics.[12] Examples of these include the Innovative Moments Coding System (Gonçalves

[11] This work of Safran and Muran (1996) actually represents a more complex design where, prior to the quantitative assessment of the relationship among the variables of interest, a performance model was created following an empirical-rational approach. This is a prototypical example of what Greenberg (2007) calls task analysis.

[12] By doing this, these instruments may be ascribed to the significant event approach (Rice and Greenberg 1984; also see Elliott 2010).

et al. 2011), which identifies different types of exceptions to the client's usual problematic self-narrative, and the Generic Change Indicators (Krause et al. 2007), which assess different types of psychotherapeutic change from a transtheoretical perspective.

Currently, the authors know of no studies that have investigated the change processes at an intersession level.

13.3.2.3 Data Analysis

As for TPR, various statistical procedures may be used within CPR. We will mention a few of them here. Within *cross-sectional* designs, rank and Pearson's correlations may be used to investigate the relationship between the variables of interest (e.g., Lingiardi et al. 2011); however, more complex data-analytic strategies may be employed that allow researchers to make inferences of a more causal nature. An example of these include hierarchical linear modeling (Raudenbush and Bryk 2002), which is able to take into account the *nested* structure of the data (which is often the case in psychotherapy research) (e.g., Owen et al. 2012), multiple regression analysis (Petrocelli 2003; see Kolden 1996), and path analysis (Kline 1998; Quintana and Maxwell 1999; see Kolden et al. 2006). For example, Kolden et al. (2006), by means of path analysis, found a positive reciprocal association between several treatment process variables (collaborative role enactment, empathic resonance, and mutual affirmation) as well as a positive influence of two of these latter (empathic resonance and mutual affirmation) on one change process variable (therapeutic realizations).

On the other hand, when researchers are interested in the temporal development of the variables under investigation, several procedures of *longitudinal* data analysis may be used. In designs that aim to investigate the time course of a treatment process variable with regard to an in-session impact variable used as a criterion variable (see Sect. 13.3.2.1), it is important to first model the time course of the treatment process variable and then see whether it differs with regard to the in-session impact variable; this may also be done by using relatively classic data analysis procedures. An example is the study by Pascual-Leone (2009), who ran a linear regression analysis of the scores of emotional processing (the treatment process variable) onto time for each case in the sample, which allowed him to obtain a series of slopes that indicate the degree of improvement of emotional processing as the session progresses; then, Wilcoxon signed-rank tests were used to assess the degree to which the average slopes of the high vs. low experiencing sessions (the criterion variable) were significantly different. The results showed that emotional processing increases more during sessions that are characterized by a higher level of experiencing.

Other cases, including the micro-analytic sequential process design (Elliott 2010), may use longitudinal data analysis, which aims to model the time-lagged relationship between the variables of interest. When data are categorical, which is very often the case in psychotherapy process research, sequence analysis (Bakeman and Gottman 1997) may be used (see Milbrath et al. 1999; Safran and Muran 1996). For example, Milbrath et al. (1999) ran a series of sequential analyses at different time lags between the frequency of different therapist interventions (the treatment process variable) and the frequency of different clients' verbal reactions (the change process variable) to determine which therapist behavior at a certain point in time triggers which client behavior (for a similar approach, see Sexton et al. 1996).

In the case of continuous variables, time-lagged cross-correlations (e.g., Ramseyer and Tschacher 2011) or a time-series analysis (Hamilton 1994) may be employed (e.g., Sexton 1993; Tschacher and Ramseyer 2009; Ramseyer et al. 2014). For example, the former was used by Ramseyer and Tschacher (2011) to assess the extent to which the amount of nonverbal behavior of the client and the therapist may synchronize over time at different time lags, with either the client or the therapist leading or pacing the nonverbal interaction. Time-series analysis has been applied by Tschacher et al. (2000) to assess the time-lagged relationship between the patient's view of the therapist's contribution, the patient's sense of self-efficacy, the therapist's view of effectiveness, and the therapist's view of the patient's engagement (for a similar approach, also see Brossart et al. 1998; Ramseyer et al. 2014). This approach represents a very valuable way for the *bottom-up* identification of change processes, where the predicted variable at t_{+1} represents the in-session impact variable and the predicting variable at t represents the treatment process variable that triggers the former.

13.3.3 Process-Outcome Research

Process-outcome research (POR) can be defined as the scientific investigation of the relationship between what takes place during psychotherapy and its clinical effects (see Orlinsky et al. 2004; also see Elliott 2010); thus, it focuses on the relationship between the process of therapy (either considered to be the treatment process or the change process; see Sect. 13.2.1) and the therapeutic outcome (see Sect. 13.2.2). The birth of POR, in the 1950s, was motivated by the increasing awareness of researchers that psychotherapy should aim to identify the factors that explain "why psychotherapy works": which aspects of the psychotherapeutic process may be considered to be responsible for the outcome of the treatment? This led to an integration of process research (see Sects. 13.3.1 and 13.3.2) and outcome research (Lambert 2013; also see Chap. 26), with the aim of identifying the aspects of the psychotherapeutic process that are responsible for the outcome of psychotherapy (see Kazdin 2009 for a general discussion on the issue). As stated by Kazdin (2009), "understanding the processes through which treatment operates can help sort through those facets that might be particularly influential in treatment outcome and permit better selection and triage of suitable patients" (p. 418).

Since its inception, a series of reviews regarding the results of POR have been produced [e.g., the work of Meltzoff and Kornreich (1970) and Luborsky et al. (1971)]. In the second edition of the *Handbook of Psychotherapy and Behavior Change*, these results and many other results were systematically organized by Orlinsky and Howard (1978) by means of a theoretically derived scheme that considered psychotherapy to be both a system of actions and a system of experiences. However, the most comprehensive and consistent review of POR findings was conducted by Orlinsky and colleagues between the third and the fifth editions of the same handbook (Orlinsky and Howard 1986; Orlinsky et al. 1994, 2004), where the authors organized the vast and ever-increasing amount of studies over the decades by means of the Generic Model of Psychotherapy (GMP; Orlinsky and Howard 1984; Orlinsky 2009).

The GMP can be considered a "research-based metatheory of psychotherapy" that can "provide a coherent account of research findings in a large number of studies on the relation of varied aspects of therapeutic process to the clinical outcomes attained by patients" (Orlinsky 2009, p. 320). More specifically, it was developed with the aim of (1) identifying the facets of the psychotherapeutic process that have been mostly investigated with regard to the client's outcome and (2) assessing the extent to which each of them may be associated with this outcome. These facets, as mentioned in Sect. 13.2.1, include the therapeutic contract, therapeutic operations, the therapeutic bond, self-relatedness, and in-session impacts; each of these components may be considered to represent a common therapeutic factor across various psychotherapeutic models (see Chap. 11 and 15 for a detailed discussion see also Chap. 3 for a description of the historical development).[13] In summary, self-relatedness, therapeutic realizations (i.e., the client's in-session impacts), and the therapeutic bond have been found to be the aspects of the process that are most consistently associated with treatment outcome.

Finally, in the last edition of *Bergin and Garfield's Handbook of Psychotherapy and Behavior Change*, there has been a shift in emphasis from the common factors represented

[13] It should be noted that, beginning with the fourth edition of the handbook, the GMP was enriched with a sixth dimension, *temporal patterns*. Because these address a specific way of analyzing the process rather than a constitutive conceptual element of it, we will refer to it later when discussing data analysis in POR (see Sect. 13.3.3.3).

by the GMP dimensions to the factors specific to various psychotherapeutic orientations (Crits-Christoph et al. 2013). The authors first summarized and updated the POR findings regarding the relationship between the therapeutic alliance and the outcome; then, they focused on the POR findings related to the major psychotherapeutic orientations. With regard to the first point, they were able to confirm the general finding that the alliance plays a key role in the achievement of a treatment outcome (see Chap. 15). With regard to the latter point, they were able to find relatively consistent support for the fact that emotional arousal in exposure-based behavior therapy for anxiety disorders, the application of "concrete" techniques in cognitive therapy for depression, and the gains in self-understanding in psychodynamic therapies are likely to represent very important ingredients in the achievement of good treatment outcomes (Crits-Christoph et al. 2013)

13.3.3.1 Research Design

Similar to TPR and CPR, POR mostly follows a *non-experimental* approach, although a few *experimental* studies have also been conducted. To be considered experimental, a POR study is required to manipulate the process variable, which is considered to be the outcome predictor (i.e., the independent variable), and randomize the participants to at least two different conditions of this independent variable (see the notion of Randomized Controlled Trial [RCT] in Chap. 26).

A process variable that can be manipulated is represented by the therapist's behavior; for example, in the study by Barrett and Berman (2001), therapists were instructed to either increase or decrease the amount of self-disclosure during their sessions, with the hypothesis being that higher levels of self-disclosure would lead to a better outcome. In addition to procedural complexity and difficulties, this approach has the limitation of actually reducing therapist responsiveness (Elliott 2010; see Stiles et al. 1998 for a discussion). Lambert et al. (2001) provides an interesting example of an experimental POR study, specifically aimed at increasing therapist responsiveness; the authors investigated the extent to which providing therapists with feedback on a client's progress during the course of a treatment would enhance the psychotherapy outcome (also see Harmon et al. 2007). The independent variable (providing the therapist with feedback) was manipulated by creating an experimental (the therapist receiving feedback) and a control (the therapist not receiving feedback) group. Finally, clients were randomized and sorted into the two conditions.

Although some POR studies may be experimental, most of them make use of a non-experimental design, where there is no manipulation of the process variable of interest and no randomization of the subjects to the different levels of the process variable (e.g., Barber et al. 2000; Feeley et al. 1999; Hoffart et al. 2009; Strauss et al. 2006; Weerasekera et al. 2001; Gonçalves et al. 2012; Mendes et al. 2010). It should be noted that any RCT outcome study that either provides an treatment adherence check (e.g., Hogue et al. 2008) or investigates a mediator of treatment effectiveness (e.g., Watson and Bedard 2006; Zuroff et al. 2000) can be regarded as POR (Orlinsky, personal communication; also see Hill et al. 1994). However, in this regard, it is important to stress that this type of POR study, although "embedded" in RCTs, is not experimental because the manipulation does not relate to the process variable that is considered to predict the outcome. For example, the study by Weerasekera et al. (2001) aimed to investigate the extent to which the therapeutic alliance predicted the treatment outcome in client-centered and process-experiential therapy. Although this study is an RCT that contains a treatment manualization, randomization, and adherence check, these procedures affected the treatment administration rather than the therapeutic alliance; for this reason, in regard to the process-outcome link, the study that is described above cannot be considered to be an experimental study.

Different than TPR and CPR, POR exclusively uses *longitudinal* designs because at least the outcome variable is always assessed at two or more time points; moreover, most of these studies use group designs because single-case designs do not allow for an adequate generalization of the results regarding the eventual process-outcome relationship.[14]

Concerning the assessment of *outcome* variables, most POR studies view the process variables as the predictors of the *final* outcome treatment (e.g., Weerasekera et al. 2001; Gonçalves et al. 2012); however, there has been an increasing tendency in recent years to use multiple assessments of *intermediate* outcomes over the course of the treatment. This design offers two advantages. First, it allows us to demonstrate a "*time line* or ordering of the proposed mediator and outcome (i.e., the mediator changes before the outcome)" (Kazdin 2009, p. 420; italics added) and to examine whether the process variable (i.e., the hypothesized mediator) effectively changes before the outcome, which is considered an important prerequisite for demonstrating mediation and mechanisms of change (e.g., Kazdin 2009; Falkenstrom et al. 2013; Hoffart et al. 2009; Kolden 1991, 1996; Kolden et al. 2006; Sexton 1993). Second, it allows for the investigation of process-outcome relationships at different timescales (see Fig. 13.2) (e.g., Klein et al. 2003; Strauss et al. 2006).

Regarding the assessment of *process* variables, the latter are usually assessed at time points that are defined a priori (temporal sampling) (e.g., Klein et al. 2003; Loeb et al. 2005; Sexton 1993; Strauss et al. 2006; Watson and Bedard 2006), although there is an increasing tendency to assess these variables more often, even in every session (e.g., Falkenstrom et al. 2013; Ramseyer et al., 2014), especially when researchers are interested in the extent to which micro-processual aspects of the treatment predict its outcome (Gonçalves et al. 2012; Mendes et al. 2010).

[14] In contrast to quantitative approaches, in qualitative and/or mixed-method approaches, single-case designs within an interpretative, theory-building framework are used more often (see Stiles 2007; Elliott 2010).

13.3.3.2 Data Collection

POR requires the assessment of at least one process variable and one outcome variable (see Sects. 13.2.1 and 13.2.2). Regarding the former, most data collection in POR addresses *in-session* processes, similar to TPR and CPR. In the majority of cases, these are assessed at a *post-session* level by means of *participant self-report* instruments that are completed by either the client and or the therapist (*macro*-processual assessment). The therapeutic alliance is one of the most investigated constructs at this level, although almost all of the aspects of the therapeutic process have been assessed to evaluate their relationship with the outcome [see Orlinsky et al. (2004) and Crits-Christoph et al. (2013) for a review]. These process variables are usually assessed at time points that are defined a priori (temporal sampling); a few studies assess these variables in only one session (e.g., Kolden 1996; Kolden et al. 2006), although there is now the tendency to use a repeated assessment procedure over time (e.g., Feeley et al. 1999; Klein et al. 2003; Loeb et al. 2005; Sexton 1993; Strauss et al. 2006; Watson and Bedard 2006). In certain cases, process variables are even assessed in every session over the entire treatment (e.g., Falkenstrom et al. 2013; Gonçalves et al. 2012; Mendes et al. 2010; Ramseyer et al., 2014). Increasing the amount of assessment time points has the advantage of improving the dependability of the study, which "refers to the adequacy of generalizing over sampling units (e.g., sessions, patients, therapist) to the universe of such units from which the samples were selected" (Crits-Christoph et al. 2013, p. 300).

In-session process variables may also be assessed at a *within-session* level, by means of *nonparticipant observational* instruments (*micro*-processual assessment) (see Table 13.1). Recent examples of these instruments include the Innovative Moments Coding System (Gonçalves et al. 2011), which has been used to assess the extent to which the exceptions to the client's usual problematic self-narrative (i.e., innovative moments) may be predictive of the clinical outcome in different forms of therapy (Matos et al. 2009; Gonçalves et al. 2012; Mendes et al. 2010), and the Generic Change Indicators, which have been used to assess the extent to which different types of change processes that occur at an in-session level may be associated with different treatment outcomes. Computer-assisted text analysis has also been used to assess the extent to which the distribution of different patterns of in-session emotional-cognitive regulation may be predictive of the clinical outcome (Erhard Mergenthaler 1996). Also, in this case, there is an increasing tendency to assess the process variables over the entire course of the treatment, especially when researchers are interested in the extent to which micro-processual aspects of the treatment predict its outcome (Gonçalves et al. 2012; Mendes et al. 2010).

Finally, although most of the data collection in contemporary POR addresses in-session processes, it is possible to assess therapy-related *between-session* processes, based on the hypothesis that they may be predictor of a good outcome in therapy [see Hartmann et al. (2010)].

Regarding the assessment of *outcome* variables, most POR studies view the process variables to be predictors of the *final* outcome treatment (e.g., Weerasekera et al. 2001; Gonçalves et al. 2012); however there has been an increasing tendency over the last few years to use multiple assessments of the *intermediate* outcomes over the course of the treatment. This design offers two advantages. First, it allows process-outcome relationships to be investigated on different timescales (e.g., Ramseyer et al. 2014; Klein et al. 2003; Strauss et al. 2006). Second, it allows the researcher to demonstrate a "*time line* or ordering of the proposed mediator and outcome (i.e., the mediator changes before the outcome)" (Kazdin 2009, p. 420; italics added) and to check whether the process variable (i.e., the hypothesized mediator) changes before the outcome, which is considered an important prerequisite for demonstrating mediation and mechanisms of change (e.g., Kazdin 2009; Falkenstrom et al. 2013; Hoffart et al. 2009; Kolden 1991, 1996; Kolden et al. 2006; Sexton 1993).

Outcome variables can be assessed with a variety of instruments (see Table 13.2 for a few examples). In most cases, *self-reports* completed by the clients are used. The most frequently used self-reports include the Beck Depression Inventory (Beck et al. 1961; e.g., Feeley et al. 1999; Strauss et al. 2006), the Symptom Checklist-90-R (SCL-90-R; Derogatis et al. 1976; e.g., Watson and Bedard 2006), the State-Trait Anxiety Inventory (STAI; Spielberger et al. 1983; e.g., Beutler et al. 2003), the CORE-OM (Evans et al. 2002; e.g., Falkenström et al. 2014), the OQ-45 (Lambert et al. 2004; e.g., Harmon et al. 2007), the Inventory of Interpersonal Problems (IIP; Horowitz et al. 1988; e.g., Watson et al. 2003), and the Rosenberg Self-Esteem Scale (RSE; Rosenberg 1965; e.g., Watson and Bedard 2006).

However, *observational instruments*, which are usually rated by (trained) therapists, may also be used. Examples of these include the Hamilton Rating Scale for Depression (HRSD; Hamilton 1960; e.g., Hawley et al. 2006; Klein et al. 2003), the Structured Clinical Interview for DSM personality disorders (SCID-II; Spitzer et al. 1990; e.g., Strauss et al. 2006), the Global Assessment Scale (Endicott et al. 1976; e.g., Zuroff et al. 2000), and the Therapist Target Complaint (Battle et al. 1966; e.g., Stevens et al. 2007)

13.3.3.3 Data Analysis

Several statistical procedures may be used in POR. The easiest way to determine the association between the process and outcome variables is to employ correlation indices, which often use the values of one or more process variables that are assessed at one point in time (e.g., Feeley et al. 1999; Strauss et al. 2006). In the case where outcome scores are used to build poor vs. good outcome groups, it is possible to use parametric or nonparametric tests to assess the different occurrences of the process variables investigated in the two groups (e.g., Gonçalves et al. 2012).

However, more complex data-analytic procedures may be employed that can overcome the many limitations of purely correlational approaches, such as the ones described. Regression analysis (Montgomery et al. 2012) represents a valuable instrument that allows researchers to make causal inferences regarding one or more independent variable(s) (i.e., the process) and a dependent variable (i.e., the outcome). Thus, for example, it is possible to assess the degree to which different techniques of cognitive therapy predict subsequent symptom change (Feeley et al. 1999) or the degree to which early alliance and rupture-repair episodes predict the final treatment outcome (Strauss et al. 2006). Path analysis (Kline 1998; Quintana and Maxwell 1999) may also be used to test synchronic models of the relationship between different aspects of the psychotherapeutic process and the outcome. For example, Kolden et al. (2006) was able to model the relationships between collaborative role enactment, empathic resonance, mutual affirmation, and therapeutic realizations in regard to both session progress and early outcomes.

The data-analytic approaches described above are characterized by the fact that they disregard the *temporal* dimension of the therapeutic process; this represents a serious limitation because "psychotherapy is inherently dynamic, namely a function of time" (Salvatore and Tschacher 2012, p. 1; also see Chap. 10). Due to this, an increasing number of researchers over the last few decades have begun to systematically "examine outcome as a function of patterns of sequential relations" over time (Orlinsky et al. 2004, p. 320).[15] This has been done by applying *longitudinal* data-analytic procedures and "has produced an important conceptual advance, from a temporally decontextualized synchronic representation of therapeutic process (achieved by averaging across randomly selected process segments) to a truer representation of process as patterns of change or trajectories across sequential time points" (Orlinsky et al. 2004, p. 360).[16]

[15] To account for these results, a sixth dimension, *temporal patterns*, was added to the GMP beginning with the fourth edition of the *Handbook of Psychotherapy and Behavior Change* (Orlinsky et al. 1994, 2004).

[16] Dynamic systems theory (DST) has been recently applied to psychotherapy research in order to explain the dynamic nature of clinical processes. A theoretical and methodological account of this is offered in Chap. 10. See Tschacher, Gelo, Koch, & Salvatore (2014) for some empirical applications.

ANOVAs for repeated measurements can be used to assess the extent to which one or more process variable may present a different time course over the therapy for the good vs. poor outcome groups (e.g., Watson and Bedard 2006; Weerasekera et al. 2001). Another approach includes running a set of regression analyses, which allow the researcher to test whether the independent (process) variable is predictive of the dependent (outcome) variable at each of the different time points considered over the treatment. For example, Loeb et al. (2005) used this strategy to assess whether the therapeutic alliance at sessions 6, 12, and 18 predicted subsequent post-session symptom change (also see Barber et al. 2000; Hartmann et al. 2010).

The approaches described, although valuable in allowing researchers to study the behavior of one or more process variable over time and the relationship of this latter with the outcome, contain certain limitations. For example, problems include their ability to address missing data, their consideration of time as a qualitative variable, and not adequately accounting for intraindividual variability. To address these limitations, several procedures for modeling longitudinal data have been developed in recent years and have been increasingly applied to POR. Two of these procedures include time-series panel analysis (TSPA; Hamilton 1994) and multilevel models (MLMs; Gallop and Tasca 2009; Tasca and Gallop 2009[17]; for further reviews and discussions, see Hayes et al. 2007; Laurenceau et al. 2007).

These two data-analytic approaches share two very important characteristics: they consider time as a quantitative variable and they are able to model interindividual change (level 2 of the analysis) based on the interindividual change (level 1 of the analysis). However, these procedures are also different in certain ways. TSPA focuses on the "multivariate change patterns among longitudinal variables" (Tschacher and Ramseyer 2009, p. 478), whose relationship is analyzed at one or more time lags. These time-lagged associations

[17] MLMs represent a collective group, including, among others, hierarchical linear models, mixed-effects models, random regression models, and growth curve modeling (Tasca and Gallop 2009).

are very useful for POR because they may be considered to approximate causal models (Tschacher and Ramseyer 2009); moreover, as soon as we analyze the data of both the client and the therapist, there is the possibility of modeling their interactional patterns. Once the parameters of the time-lagged relationships between the different process variables have been identified, they may be entered as dependent variables into a regression analysis to assess their predictive power regarding the treatment outcome. For example, Ramseyer et al. (2014) first investigated the multivariate time-lagged relationship between the patient's alliance, the patient's self-efficacy, the therapist's alliance, the therapist's clarification interventions, and the therapist's mastery interventions; then, they were able to assess the extent to which these variables were predictive of the final outcome (see Fisher et al. 2011 for a similar approach).

In contrast, MLMs focus on the univariate change in one or more of the considered process variables, which allows their trajectory over time (i.e., shape of change); to be identified it is then possible to assess the degree to which the modeled trajectories (e.g., linear, quadratic, cubic) may be predictive of the outcome. For example, Tschacher and Ramseyer (2009) determined the time course of the patient's well-being and the patient's therapy motivation over the course of a treatment and then assessed the extent to which this was predictive of the final outcome. In another study, Hoffart et al. (2009) modeled the shape of the change in several common factors over the treatment; they were then able to assess the degree to which the ongoing processes impacted the weekly fluctuations of the outcome.

A very interesting and more elaborate extension of MLMs relates to latent difference score analysis (LDS; McArdle & Hamagami 2001), which may be considered to be a type of dynamic path analysis. LDS combines the features of latent growth curve models and cross-lagged regression models, which allows for the modeling of "dynamic longitudinal growth within a time series while also examining multivariate interrelationships and determinants" (Hawley et al. 2006; p. 932). This data-analytic strategy has been, for example, used by Hawley et al. (2006) to investigate the relationship between perfectionism, depression, and the therapeutic alliance during treatment for depression. The authors first modeled the within-subject change in and growth of perfectionism and depression over the treatment; then, they were able to assess the extent to which the therapeutic alliance may be a determinant of this change (for another application of LDS, see, for example, Gloster et al. 2014).

Finally, we would like to mention an approach that may be very useful when modeling the therapeutic process with categorical data, which is often the case in psychotherapy process research. As mentioned in Sects. 13.3.1 and 13.3.2 regarding TPR and CPR, respectively, sequence analysis (Bakeman and Gottman 1997) may be a very useful tool in assessing the time-lagged relationship between at least two categorical variables. This includes calculating the transition probabilities of the different categorical variables considered. In POR, it is possible to further assess the extent to which these time-lagged relationships may be associated with and/or predictive of outcome. For example, Milbrath et al. (1999), in one of the very few studies that adopted such an approach, found correlations between the combinations of the transition probabilities, the therapist's interventions, and the client's verbal behavior and posttreatment outcome scores.

Conclusion

To fully understand what psychotherapy consists of and how and why it may lead to change, we need to investigate both its process and the relationship between this process and the treatment outcome. In the present chapter, we have provided an overview of three main quantitative approaches that may be useful to reach this aim. Each of them contains its own limitations and strengths. TPR allows us, coherently a discovery-oriented and theory-building approach, to broadly focus on the main ingredients of the psychotherapy process and to examine how they may be related. The relevance of the logic of discovery in exploring what occurs in psychotherapy has been endorsed by various scholars (e.g., Greenberg 1991; Hill 1990, 1994, Mahrer 1988; Meehl 1967, 1978) based on their acknowledgment that the traditional hypothesis-testing approach has so far contributed little to the cumulative body of knowledge in psychotherapy (see Mahrer 1988). However, TPR presents the limitation of not explicitly focusing on clinically meaningful events.

This limitation is actually tackled by CPR, which allows the specific aspects of the treatment process that represent clinically meaningful events to be investigated. A specific focus on the change processes is relevant because this may shed light on the mechanisms through which in-session impacts are formed (Orlinsky et al. 2004). One of the core aspects of the clinical practice of psychotherapy is, in fact, its promotion of clinically meaningful in-therapy performances. However, in addition to the fact that it may be very energy and time consuming, CPR's main limitation lies in the fact that explaining therapeutic gains does not necessarily describe how these gains may be responsible for the positive treatment outcome. This limitation seems to be the main strength of POR, which allows us to investigate the relationship between what occurs in psychotherapy and its clinical outcome. The final aim of psychotherapy is to produce significant clinical changes in the client's problematic target behavior(s); thus, identifying the mechanisms that are responsible for this is fundamental in clinical research (Kazdin 2009). POR also presents limitations. For example, most POR studies focus on only one or a small number of process variables as outcome predictors, which disregards the patterned complexity of the therapeutic process that may be responsible for the outcome. Moreover, most of the time, these process variables are measured at a macro-level (see Sect. 13.2.1), and the outcome is assessed at treatment termination (see Sect. 13.2.2). Thus, both the process and the outcome are observed at a low degree of resolution, which creates a "distance between the process measured and the outcome of therapy" (Elliott 2010, p. 124). Finally, most of the analyses do not allow the way that the relationship between the process and the outcome may vary over time to be taken into account, thus providing results that may be of little clinical relevance (for a discussion, see Stiles 1988; Stiles et al. 1998; Stiles and Shapiro 1989, 1994; Crits-Christoph et al. 2013; Elliott 2010).

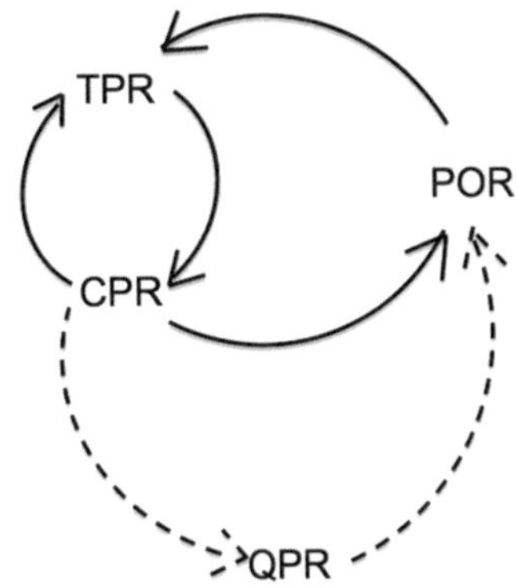

Fig. 13.3 The cycles of treatment process research (TPR), change process research (CPR), process-outcome research (POR), and qualitative psychotherapy research (QPR)

To overcome the limitations of each single approach and emphasize the reciprocal strengths of the approaches, we suggest that it would be profitable to combine them based on what has been labeled "systematic *methodological pluralism*" (Elliott 2010, p. 131, italics added; also see Gelo et al. 2008, 2009; Gelo and Gelo 2012; Slife & Gantt 1999). Clinical reality is too complex to be adequately understood and explained by means of a single approach. What is needed is, instead, "a more balanced approach that brings all available methodological tools to bear on the problem" (Elliott 2010, p. 131). This form of pluralism should be achieved by means of research programs that examine the cycles of the three different approaches presented in this chapter, as shown in the upper part Fig. 13.3.

Starting with TPR may provide meaningful initial insight into the general occurrences in the treatment process of therapy, which may then be examined in greater depth by CPR because it more specifically focuses on possible clinically meaningful events. These results could then be used to inform POR studies, with the aim of establishing meaningful associations between the different aspects of the process that were previously investigated and the outcome. Finally, these results could be used to inform new TPR, as well as CPR, studies, and so on. During each phase of this process, we should oscillate between discovery-oriented and hypothesis-testing approaches; nonetheless, we would suggest gradually but definitively moving toward hypothesis testing as we move from TPR and CPR to POR during the different cycles of the research program. At the very end of this continuum, RCTs should be conducted.

With regard to this process, the following recommendations can be made. (a) Researchers should primarily make use of a *longitudinal* design to assess how the variables of interest change over time. Purely cross-sectional designs are rather useless because psychotherapy is a dynamic phenomenon (see Chap. 10; Salvatore and Tschacher 2012); group comparisons should be made only when they allow researchers to compare the behavior of one or more variable over time (i.e., dynamic patterns in different groups).

(b) Data collection of both process and outcome variables should occur as *frequently* as possible based on the resources that are available; temporal sampling should be avoided when possible. Both the process and the outcome are inherently nonlinear phenomena; thus, when we assess them more often, we are more able to approximate the "real" behavior they show over time (Hayes et al. 2007; Laurenceau et al. 2007).

(c) Data collection of both process and outcome variables should also occur on *different timescales*. Ideally, the process should be assessed both at a within-session level and at a post-session level; similarly, the outcome should be assessed both at a post-session level and at a posttreatment level (Greenberg 1986; Orlinsky et al. 2004). When analyzing the data, the focus should be on the differential relationship between the different variables that are assessed on different timescales.

(d) The data-analytic procedures that are employed should be able to adequately model the behavior of the variables under investigation *over time*; procedures that consider time as a quantitative variable should be preferred (see Fisher et al. 2011; Gallop and Tasca 2009; Tasca and Gallop 2009; Laurenceau et al. 2007; Tschacher and Ramseyer 2009). If we have to address more than one variable, the *reciprocal* relationship between the variables over time should be taken into account. If we intend to observe the behavior of these variables over the treatment phases, the time points should not be defined a priori but should follow a *bottom-up* approach where they are derived from the data.

(e) The data-analytic procedures used should also allow *interindividual* change to be modeled without disregarding *intraindividual* change. This relates to the idea that generalized (i.e., *nomothetic*) knowledge is grounded in individual and context-bounded (i.e., *idiographic*) knowledge (Molenaar and Campbell 2009; Salvatore and Valsiner 2010).

We would like to conclude with a final remark. This chapter has exclusively focused on quantitative approaches; due to this, the considerations made above address a type of *within*-paradigm methodological pluralism. However, we do strongly believe in the importance of between-*paradigm* methodological pluralism as well. Both of these forms of pluralism greatly differ from the dominant methodological *monism*, which characterizes contemporary mainstream psychotherapy research; at the same time, each of them emphasizes slightly different issues. A within-paradigm pluralism advocates to use not only of RCTS but also other, more naturalistic quantitative approaches; A between-paradigm pluralism advocates reliance not only on quantitative approaches but also on qualitative ones (see Chap. 4 for the philosophical underpinnings of such a form of pluralism).

With regard to this form of between-paradigm methodological pluralism, we are convinced that each of the three quantitative approaches reviewed in this chapter should be used in cycles with each other, as well as with qualitative psychotherapy research (QPR; see Chaps. 20, 21, and 27). As shown in Fig. 13.3, we believe that the results that are obtained by the different quantitative approaches should inform QPR, which, in turn, would inform the quantitative approaches as well. A specific qualitative approach that may be very useful in this regard is the *qualitative helpful factors* design (Elliott 2010); this design aims to explore the subjective experiences of clients (and/or therapists) to identify what they have perceived as helpful in the treatment. Once identified, these helpful factors could then more specifically be investigated by means of quantitative approaches.

Moreover, in addition to informing each other, quantitative and qualitative approaches may also be integrated (see Gelo et al. 2008, 2009 for a general discussion). A prototypical example of such a strategy, *recently reviewed by Elliott* (2010), *is the significant events approach*; it is characterized by an integration of quantitative and qualitative methods within a theory-building and interpretive framework, with the aim of investigating clinically relevant moments of the therapy; declinations of this approach include task analysis (Greenberg 2007), comprehensive process analysis (Elliott et al. 1994) and assimilation analysis (Stiles et al. 1990).

We believe that methodological pluralism is an indispensable attitude for any psychotherapy researcher. We hope that the present chapter provides a contribution to how this may be accomplished within quantitative psychotherapy research, with the aim of finding out how and why psychotherapy works.

Acknowledgment We would like to thank David Orlinsky and Marcello Gallucci for their discussions, which helped to inform the contents of this chapter. However, as the authors, we are solely responsible for the content of this chapter.

References

Angus L, Lewin J, Boritz T, Bryntwick E, Carpenter N, Watson-Gaze J et al (2012) Narrative processes coding system: a dialectical constructivist approach to assessing client change processes in emotion-focused therapy of depression. Res Psychother 15(2):54–61. doi:10.7411/RP.2012.006

Bakeman R, Gottman JM (1997) Observing interaction: an introduction to sequential analysis, 2nd edn. Cambridge University Press, Cambridge

Barber JP, Connolly MB, Crits-Christoph P, Gladis L, Siqueland L (2000) Alliance predicts patients' outcome beyond in-treatment change in symptoms. J Consult Clin Psychol 68(6):1027–1032. doi:10.1037/0022-006X.68.6.1027

Barrett MS, Berman JS (2001) Is psychotherapy more effective when therapists disclose information about themselves? J Consult Clin Psychol 69(4):597–603. doi:10.1037/0022-006X.69.4.597

Barrett-Lennard GT (1962) Dimensions of therapist response as causal factors in therapeutic change. Psychol Monogr 76(43):1–36. doi:10.1037/h0093918

Battle CC, Imber SD, Hoehn-Saric R, Stone A, Nash ER, Frank JD (1966) Target complaints as criteria for improvement. Am J Psychother 20:184–192

Beck AT, Ward CH, Mendelson M, Mock J, Erbaugh J (1961) An inventory for measuring depression. Arch Gen Psychiatry 4:561–571. doi:10.1001/archpsyc.1961.01710120031004

Benjamin LS (1974) Structural analysis of social behavior. Psychol Rev 81(5):392–425. doi:10.1037/h0037024

Benjamin LS, Rothweiler JC, Critchfield KL (2006) The use of structural analysis of social behavior (SASB) as an assessment tool. Annu Rev Clin Psychol 2:83–109. doi:10.1146/annurev.clinpsy.2.022305.095337

Beutler LE, Moleiro C, Malik M, Mark Harwood T, Romanelli R, Gallagher-Thompson D et al (2003) A comparison of the Dodo, EST, and ATI factors among comorbid stimulant-dependent, depressed patients. Clin Psychol Psychother 10(2):69–85. doi:10.1002/cpp.354

Brossart DF, Willson VL, Patton MJ, Kivlighan DM Jr, Multon KD (1998) A time series model of the working alliance: a key process in short-term psychoanalytic counseling. Psychother Theory Res Pract Train 35 (2):197–205. doi: 10.1037/h0087645

Bucci W, Maskit B (2006) A weighted dictionary for referential activity. In: Shanahan YJG, Wiebe Q (eds) Computing attitude and affect in text. Springer, Dordrecht, pp 49–60

Colli A, Lingiardi V (2009) The collaborative interactions scale: a new transcript-based method for the assessment of therapeutic alliance ruptures and resolutions in psychotherapy. Psychother Res 19(6):718–734. doi:10.1080/10503300903121098

Covner BJ (1942) Studies in phonographic recordings of verbal material: I. The use of phonographic recordings in counseling practice and research. J Consult Psychol 6(2):105–113. doi:10.1037/h0053878

Crits-Christoph P, Connolly G, Mukherjee D (2013) Psychotherapy process-outcome research. In: Lambert MJ (ed) Bergin and Garfield's handbook of psychotherapy and behavior change, 4th edn. Wiley, New York, pp 298–340

Derogatis LR, Rickels K, Roch AF (1976) The SCL-90 and the MMPI: a step in the validation of a new self-report scale. Br J Psychiatry 128:280–289

Di Giuseppe M, Perry JC, Petraglia J, Janzen J, Lingiardi V (2014) Development of a Q-sort version of the defense mechanism rating scales (DMRS-Q) for clinical use. J Clin Psychol 70(5):452–465. doi:10.1002/jclp.22089

Dimaggio G, Procacci M, Nicolò G, Popolo R, Semerari A, Carcione A, Lysaker PH (2007) Poor metacognition in narcissistic and avoidant personality disorders: four psychotherapy patients analysed using the metacognition assessment scale. Clin Psychol Psychother 14(5):386–401. doi:10.1002/cpp.541

Dittes JE (1959) Previous studies bearing on content analysis of psychotherapy. In: Dollard J, Auld F (eds) Scoring human motives: a manual. Yale University Press, New Haven, pp 325–351

Doran JM, Safran JD, Waizmann V, Bolger K, Muran JC (2012) The alliance negotiation scale: psychometric construction and preliminary reliability and validity analysis. Psychother Res 22(6):710–719. doi:10.1080/10503307.2012.709326

Elliott R (1991) Five dimensions of therapy process. Psychother Res 1:92–103. doi:10.1080/10503309112331335521

Elliott R (2010) Psychotherapy change process research: realizing the promise. Psychother Res 20(2):123–135. doi:10.1080/10503300903470743

Elliott R, Anderson C (1994) Simplicity and complexity in psychotherapy research. In: Russell RL (ed) Reassessing psychotherapy research. Guilford, New York, NY, pp 65–113

Elliott R, Farber BA (2010) Carl Rogers: idealistic pragmatist and psychotherapy research pioneer. In: Castonguay LG, Muran JC, Angus L, Hayes JA, Ladany N, Anderson T (eds) Bringing psychotherapy research to life: understanding change through the work of leading clinical researchers. American Psychological Association, Washington, DC, pp 17–27

Elliott R, Hill CE, Stiles WB, Friedlander ML, Mahrer AR, Margison FR (1987) Primary therapist response modes: comparison of six rating systems. J Consult Clin Psychol 55(2):218–223. doi:10.1037/0022-006X.55.2.218

Elliott R, Shapiro DA, Firth-Cozens J, Stiles WB, Hardy G, Llewelyn SP et al (1994) Comprehensive process analysis of insight events in cognitive-behavioral and psychodynamic-interpersonal therapies. J Couns Psychol 41:449–463. doi: 10.1037/0022-0167.41.4.449

Endicott J, Spitzer RL, Fleiss JL, Cohen J (1976) The global assessment scale: a procedure for measuring overall severity of psychiatric disturbance. Arch Gen Psychiatry 33(6):766–771. doi:10.1001/archpsyc.1976.01770060086012

Evans C, Connell J, Barkham M, Margison F, McGrath G, Mellor-Clark J et al (2002) Towards a standardised brief outcome measure: psychometric properties and utility of the CORE–OM. Br J Psychiatry 180 (1):51–60. doi:10.1192/bjp.180.1.51

Falkenstrom F, Granstrom F, Holmqvist R (2013) Therapeutic alliance predicts symptomatic improvement session by session. J Couns Psychol 60(3):317–328. doi:10.1037/a0032258

Falkenström F, Granström F, Holmqvist R (2014) Working alliance predicts psychotherapy outcome even while controlling for prior symptom improvement. Psychother Res 24(2):146–159. doi:10.1080/10503307.2013.847985

Feeley M, DeRubeis RJ, Gelfand LA (1999) The temporal relation of adherence and alliance to symptom change in cognitive therapy for depression. J Consult Clin Psychol 67(4):578–582. doi: 10.1037/0022-006X.67.4.578

Fertuck EA, Mergenthaler E, Target M, Levy KN, Clarkin JF (2012) Development and criterion validity of a computerized text analysis measure of reflective functioning. Psychother Res 22(3):298–305. doi:10.1080/10503307.2011.650654

Fisher AJ, Newman MG, Molenaar PCM (2011) A quantitative method for the analysis of nomothetic relationships between idiographic structures: dynamic patterns create attractor states for sustained posttreatment change. J Consult Clin Psychol 79:552–563. doi:10.1037/a0024069

Flückiger C, Regli D, Zwahlen D, Hostettler S, Caspar F (2010) Der berner patienten- und therapeutenstundenbogen 2000: Ein instrument zur erfassung von therapieprozessen (The Bern Post Session Report 2000, patient and therapist versions: measuring psychotherapeutic processes). Zeitschrift für Klinische Psychologie und Psychotherapie: Forschung und Praxis 39(2):71–79. doi:10.1026/1616-3443/a000015

Friedlander ML (1982) Counseling discourse as a speech event: revision and extension of the hill counselor verbal response category system. J Couns Psychol 29 (4):425–429. doi:10.1037/0022-0167.29.4.425

Gallop R, Tasca GA (2009) Multilevel modelling of longitudinal data for psychotherapy researchers: II. The complexities. Psychother Res 19(4–5):438–52. doi:10.1080/10503300902849475

Gelo OCG (2012) On research methods and their philosophical assumptions: "raising the consciousness of researchers" again. Psychotherapie and Sozialwissenschaft 14:111–130

Gelo OCG, Mergenthaler E (2012) Unconventional metaphors and emotional-cognitive regulation in a metacognitive interpersonal therapy. Psychother Res 22(2):159–175. doi:10.1080/10503307.2011.629636

Gelo OCG, Braakmann D, Benetka G (2008) Quantitative and qualitative research: beyond the debate. Integr Psychol Behav Sci 42(3):266–290. doi:10.1007/s12124-008-9078-3

Gelo OCG, Braakmann D, Benetka G (2009) Erratum to "Quantitative and qualitative research: beyond the debate". Integr Psychol Behav Sci 43:406–407. doi:10.1007/s12124-009-9107-x

Gelo OCG, Gelo C (2012) Dialogical relationships among scientific paradigms in psychotherapy research. In: Paper presented at the 3rd joint meeting of the society for psychotherapy research, European and UK Chapters, Porto, Portugal

Gelo OCG, Salcuni S, Antonello C (2012) Text analysis within quantitative and qualitative psychotherapy process research: introduction to special issue. Res Psychother 15(2):45–53. doi:10.7411/RP.2012.005

Gilles A, de Roten Y, Drapeau M, Despland JN (2007) Early change in maladaptive defence style and development of the therapeutic alliance. Clin Psychol Psychother 14(2):89–95. doi:10.1002/cpp.521

Gleser GC, Ihilevich D (1969) An objective instrument for measuring defense mechanisms. J Consult Clin Psychol 33(1):51–60. doi:10.1037/h0027381

Gloster AT, Klotsche J, Gerlach AL, Hamm A, Ströhle A, Gauggel S et al (2014) Timing matters: change depends on the stage of treatment in cognitive behavioral therapy for panic disorder with agoraphobia. J Consult Clin Psychol 82(1):141–153. doi:10.1037/a0034555

Gonçalves MM, Ribeiro AP, Mendes I, Matos M, Santos A (2011) Tracking novelties in psychotherapy process research: the innovative moments coding system. Psychother Res 21(5):497–509. doi:10.1080/10503307.2011.560207

Gonçalves MM, Mendes I, Cruz G, Ribeiro AP, Sousa I, Angus L et al (2012) Innovative moments and change in client-centered therapy. Psychother Res 22(4):389–401. doi:10.1080/10503307.2012.662605

Grabhorn R, Stenner H, Stangier U, Kaufhold J (2006) Social anxiety in anorexia and bulimia nervosa: the mediating role of shame. Clin Psychol Psychother 13(1):12–19. doi:10.1002/cpp.463

Greenberg LS (1986) Change process research. J Consult Clin Psychol 54(1):4–9. doi: 10.1037/0022-006X.54.1.4

Greenberg L (1991) Research on the process of change. Psychother Res 1(1):3–16. doi:10.1080/10503309112331334011

Greenberg LS (2007) A guide to conducting a task analysis of psychotherapeutic change. Psychother Res 17(1):15–30. doi:10.1080/10503300600720390

Greenberg LS, Pinsof WM (1986) The psychotherapeutic process: a research handbook. Routledge, New York

Hamilton MA (1960) A rating scale for depression. J Neurol Neurosurg Psychiatry 23(6):56–62

Hamilton J (1994) Time-series analysis. Princeton University Press, Princeton

Harmon SC, Lambert MJ, Smart DM, Hawkins E, Nielsen SL, Slade K et al (2007) Enhancing outcome for potential treatment failures: therapist-client feedback and clinical support tools. Psychother Res 17(4):379–392. doi:10.1080/10503300600702331

Hartley DE, Strupp HH (1983) The therapeutic alliance: Its relationship to outcome in brief psychotherapy. In: Masling J (ed) Empirical studies of psychoanalytical theories. Analytical Press, Hillsdale, NJ, pp 1–38

Hartmann A, Orlinsky DE, Geller JD, Zeeck A (2003) The intersession questionnaire–an inventory for the measurement of patients' processing of psychotherapy between sessions. Psychother Psychosom Med Psychol 53(11):464–468. doi:10.1055/s-2003-43391

Hartmann A, Orlinsky D, Weber S, Sandholz A, Zeeck A (2010) Session and intersession experience related to treatment outcome in bulimia nervosa. Psychother Theory Res Pract Train 47(3):355–370. doi:10.1037/a0021166

Hartmann A, Orlinsky D, Zeeck A (2011) The structure of intersession experience in psychotherapy and its relation to the therapeutic alliance. J Clin Psychol 67(10):1044–1063. doi:10.1002/jclp.20826

Harway NI, Dittmann AT, Raush HL, Bordin ES, Rigler D (1955) The measurement of depth of interpretation. J Consult Psychol 19(4):247–253. doi:10.1037/h0041396

Hawley LL, Ho M-HR, Zuroff DC, Blatt SJ (2006) The relationship of perfectionism, depression, and therapeutic alliance during treatment for depression: latent difference score analysis. J Consult Clin Psychol 74(5):930–942. doi: 10.1037/0022-006x.74.5.930

Hayes AM, Laurenceau J-P, Feldman G, Strauss JL, Cardaciotto L (2007) Change is not always linear: the study of nonlinear and discontinuous patterns of change in psychotherapy. Clin Psychol Rev 27(6):715–723. doi:10.1016/j.cpr.2007.01.008

Hersoug AG, Bøgwald K-P, Høglend P (2003) Are patient and therapist characteristics associated with the use of defence interpretation in brief dynamic psychotherapy? Clin Psychol Psychother 10(4):209–219. doi:10.1002/cpp.372

Hill CE (1978) Development of a counselor verbal response category. J Couns Psychol 25(5):461–468. doi:10.1037/0022-0167.25.5.461

Hill CE (1990) Exploratory in-session process research in individual psychotherapy: a review. J Consult Clin Psychol 58(3):288–294. doi:10.1037/0022-006X.58.3.288

Hill CE (1994) From an experimental to an exploratory naturalistic approach to studying psychotherapy process. In: Russell RL (ed) Reassessing psychotherapy research. Guilford, New York, pp 144–165

Hill CE, Gormally J (1977) Effects of reflection, restatement, probe, and nonverbal behaviors on client affect. J Couns Psychol 24(2):92–97. doi:10.1037/0022-0167.24.2.92

Hill CE, Lambert MJ (2004) Methodological issues in studying psychotherapeutic processes and outcome.

In: Lambert MJ (ed) Bergin and Garfield's handbook of psychotherapy and behaviour change, 5th edn. Wiley, New York, pp 55–71

Hill CE, Nutt EA, Jackson S (1994) Trends in psychotherapy process research: samples, measures, researchers, and classic publications. J Couns Psychol 41 (3):364–377. doi:10.1037/0022-0167.41.3.364

Hilliard RB (1993) Single-case methodology in psychotherapy process and outcome research. J Consult Clin Psychol 61(3):373–380. doi:0022-006X.67.4.578/0022-006X.61.3.373

Hilsenroth MJ, Blagys MD, Ackerman SJ, Bonge DR, Blais MA (2005) Measuring psychodynamic-interpersonal and cognitive-behavioral techniques: Development of the comparative psychotherapy process scale. Psychother Theory Res Pract Train 42 (3):340–356. doi: 10.1037/0033-3204.42.3.340

Hoffart A, Borge FM, Sexton H, Clark DM (2009) The role of common factors in residential cognitive and interpersonal therapy for social phobia: a process-outcome study. Psychother Res 19(1):54–67. doi:10.1080/10503300802369343

Hogue A, Henderson CE, Dauber S, Barajas PC, Fried A, Liddle HA (2008) Treatment adherence, competence, and outcome in individual and family therapy for adolescent behavior problems. J Consult Clin Psychol 76(4):544–555. doi:10.1037/0022-006X.76.4.544

Horowitz LM, Rosenberg SE, Baer BA, Ureño G, Villaseñor VS (1988) Inventory of interpersonal problems: psychometric properties and clinical applications. J Consult Clin Psychol 56(6):885–892. doi:10.1037/0022-006X.56.6.885

Horvath AO, Greenberg LS (1989) Development and validation of the working alliance inventory. J Couns Psychol 36(2):223–233. doi:10.1037/0022-0167.36.2.223

Iwakabe S, Gazzola N (2009) From single-case studies to practice-based knowledge: aggregating and synthesizing case studies. Psychother Res 19 (4–5):601–611. doi:10.1080/10503300802688494

Jaycox LH, Foa EB, Morral AR (1998) Influence of emotional engagement and habituation on exposure therapy for PTSD. J Consult Clin Psychol 66(1):185–92. doi: 10.1037//0022-006x.66.1.185

Jones EE (1985) Manual for the psychotherapy process Q-set. University of California, Berkeley

Kazdin AE (2009) Understanding how and why psychotherapy leads to change. Psychother Res 19 (4–5):418–428. doi:10.1080/10503300802448899

Kiesler DJ (1973) The process of psychotherapy: empirical foundations and systems of analysis. Aldine, Oxford

Klein MH, Mathieu PL, Gendlin ET, Kiesler DJ (1969) The experiencing scale: a research and training manual. Madison, Wisconsin

Klein MH, Mathieu-Coughlan P, Kiesler DJ (1986) The experiencing scales. In: Greenberg LS, Pinsof WM (eds) The psychotherapeutic process: a research handbook. Guilford, New York, pp 21–71

Klein DN, Schwartz JE, Santiago NJ, Vivian D, Vocisano C, Castonguay LG et al (2003) Therapeutic alliance in depression treatment: controlling for prior change and patient characteristics. J Consult Clin Psychol 71 (6):997–1006. doi:10.1037/0022-006x.71.6.997

Kline RB (1998) Principles and practice of structural equation modeling. Guilford, New York

Kolden G (1991) The generic model of psychotherapy: an empirical investigation of patterns of process and outcome relationships. Psychother Res 1(1):62–73. doi:10.1080/10503309112331334071

Kolden GG (1996) Change in early sessions of dynamic therapy: universal processes and the generic model of psychotherapy. J Consult Clin Psychol 64 (3):489–496. doi: 10.1037/0022-006X.64.3.489

Kolden GG, Klein MH, Strauman TJ, Chisholm-Stockard S, Heerey E, Schneider KL et al (2005) Early psychotherapy process and cluster B and C personality pathology: similarities and differences in interactions with symptomatic and interpersonal distress. Psychother Res 15(3):165–177. doi:10.1080/10503300512331387825

Kolden GG, Chisholm-Stockard SM, Strauman TJ, Tierney SC, Mullen EA, Schneider KL (2006) Universal session-level change processes in an early session of psychotherapy: path models. J Consult Clin Psychol 74(2):327–336. doi: 10.1037/0022-006x.74.2.327

Krause MS, Lutz W, Saunders SM (2007) Empirically certified treatments or therapists: the issue of separability. Psychother Theory Res Pract Train 44 (3):347–353. doi: 10.1037/0033-3204.44.3.347

Lambert MJ (2013) The efficacy and effectiveness of psychotherapy. In: Lambert MJ (ed) Bergin and Garfield's handbook of psychotherapy and behavior change, 6th edn. WIley, New York, pp 169–218

Lambert MJ, Whipple JL, Smart DW, Vermeersch DA, Nielsen SL (2001) The effects of providing therapists with feedback on patient progress during psychotherapy: are outcomes enhanced? Psychother Res 11 (1):49–68. doi:10.1080/713663852

Lambert MJ, Garfield SL, Bergin AE (2004) Overview, trends, and future issues. In: Lambert MJ (ed) Bergin and Garfield's handbook of psychotherapy and behaviour change, 5th edn. Wiley, New York, pp 805–821

Lambert MJ, Morton JJ, Hatfield D, Harmon C, Hamilton S, Reid RC et al (2004) Administration and scoring manual for the outcome questionnaire-45. American Professional Credentialing Services, Orem

Lasswell HD (1935) Verbal references and physiological changes during the psychoanalytic interview: a preliminary communication. Psychoanal Rev 22:10–24

Laurenceau J-P, Hayes AM, Feldman GC (2007) Some methodological and statistical issues in the study of change processes in psychotherapy. Clin Psychol Rev 27(6):682–695. doi:10.1016/j.cpr.2007.01.007

Lepper G, Riding N (2006) Researching the psychotherapy process: a practical guide to transcript-based methods. Palgrave Macmillan, Basingstoke

Lingiardi V, Colli A, Gentile D, Tanzilli A (2011) Exploration of session process: relationship to depth and alliance. Psychotherapy (Chic) 48(4):391–400. doi:10.1037/a0025248

Loeb KL, Wilson GT, Labouvie E, Pratt EM, Hayaki J, Walsh BT et al (2005) Therapeutic alliance and treatment adherence in two interventions for Bulimia Nervosa: a study of process and outcome. J Consult Clin Psychol 73(6):1097–1107. doi:10.1037/0022-006x.73.6.1097

Luborsky L (1998) A guide to the CCRT method. In: Luborsky L, Crits-Christoph P (eds) Understanding transference: the core conflictual relationship theme method, 2nd edn. American Psychological Association, Washington, pp 15–42

Luborsky L, Auerbach AH, Chandler M, Cohen J, Bachrach HM (1971) Factors influencing the outcome of psychotherapy: a review of quantitative research. Psychol Bull 75(3):145–185. doi:10.1037/h0030480

Luborsky L, Crits-Christoph P, Alexander L, Margolis M, Cohen M (1983) Two helping alliance methods for predicting outcomes of psychotherapy: a counting signs vs. a global rating method. J Nerv Ment Dis 171 (8):480–491. doi:10.1097/00005053-198308000-00005

Lundy MS, Orlinsky DE (1987) Therapists' experiences of therapy between sessions. In: Paper presented at the 18th annual meeting of the society for psychotherapy research, Ulm

Lutz W, Knox S (2013) Quantitative and qualitative methods in psychotherapy research. Routledge, London

MacKenzie K (1983) The clinical application of a group climate measure. In: Dies RR, MacKenzie KR (eds) Advances in group psychotherapy: Integrating research and practice. International Universities Press, Madison, pp 159–170

Mahrer AR (1988) Discovery-oriented psychotherapy research: rationale, aims, and methods. Am Psychol 43(9):694–702. doi:10.1037/0003-066x.43.9.694

Marsden G (1971) Content analysis studies in psychotherapy: 1954 through 1968. In: Bergin AE, Garfield SL (eds) Handbook of psychotherapy and behavior change, 1st edn. Wiley, London, pp 345–407

Matos M, Santos A, Gonçalves M, Martins C (2009) Innovative moments and change in narrative therapy. Psychother Res 19(1):68–80. doi:10.1080/10503300802430657

McArdle JJ, Hamagami F (2001) Latent difference score structural models for linear dynamic analyses with incomplete longitudinal data. In: Collins LM, Sayer AG (eds) New methods for the analysis of change. American Psychological Association, Washington, pp 137–175

Meehl EE (1967) Theory-testing in psychology and physics: a methodological paradox. Philos Sci 34:103–115

Meehl PE (1978) Theoretical risks and tabular asterisks: Sir Karl, Sir Ronald, and the slow progress of soft psychology. J Consult Clin Psychol 46:806–834. doi:10.1037/0022-006X.46.4.806

Meltzoff J, Kornreich M (1970) Research in psychotherapy. Atherton, New York

Mendes I, Ribeiro AP, Angus L, Greenberg LS, Sousa I, Gonçalves MM (2010) Narrative change in emotion-focused therapy: how is change constructed through the lens of the innovative moments coding system? Psychother Res 20:692–701. doi:10.1080/10503307.2010.514960

Mergenthaler E (1996) Emotion-abstraction patterns in verbatim protocols: a new way of describing psychotherapeutic processes. J Consult Clin Psychol 64:1306–1315. doi:10.1037//0022-006X.64.6.1306

Mergenthaler E (2008) Resonating minds: a school-independent theoretical conception and its empirical application to psychotherapeutic processes. Psychother Res 18(2):109–126. doi:10.1080/10503300701883741

Mergenthaler E, Bucci W (1999) Linking verbal and non-verbal representations: computer analysis of referential activity. Br J Med Psychol 72:339–354. doi:10.1348/000711299160040

Mergenthaler E, Stinson CH (1992) Psychotherapy transcription standards. Psychother Res 2(2):125–142. doi:10.1080/10503309212331332904

Michalak J, Wiethoff M, Schulte D (2005) Therapeutic alliance and behavior inhibition. Psychother Res 15 (3):334–338. doi:10.1080/10503300500091207

Milbrath C, Bond M, Cooper S, Znoj HJ, Horowitz MJ, Perry JC (1999) Sequential consequences of therapists' interventions. J Psychother Pract Res 8(1):40–55

Mintz J, Luborsky L, Christoph P (1979) Measuring the outcomes of psychotherapy: findings of the Penn psychotherapy project. J Consult Clin Psychol 47 (2):319–334. doi:10.1037/0022-006X.47.2.319

Molenaar PCM, Campbell CG (2009) The new person-specific paradigm in psychology. Curr Dir Psychol Sci 18:112–117. doi:10.1111/j.1467-8721.2009.01619.x

Montgomery GH, Peck S, Vining GG (2012) Introduction to linear regression analysis, 5th edn. Wiley, Hoboken

Moyers TB, Miller WR, Hendrickson SML (2005) How does motivational interviewing work? Therapist interpersonal skill predicts client involvement within motivational interviewing sessions. J Consult Clin Psychol 73(4):590–598. doi:10.1037/0022-006X.73.4.590

Muran JC, Safran JD, Samstag LW, Winston A (1992) Patient and therapist postsession questionnaires, Version 1992. Beth Israel Medical Center, New York

Orlinsky DE (2009) The "Generic Model of Psychotherapy" after 25 years: evolution of a research-based metatheory. J Psychother Integr 19:319–339

Orlinsky DE, Howard KI (1978) The relation of process to outcome in psychotherapy. In: Garfield SL, Bergin AE (eds) Handbook of psychotherapy and behavior change, 2nd edn. Wiley, New York

Orlinsky DE, Howard KI (1984) A Generic Model of Psychotherapy. In: Paper presented at the 1st annual meeting of the society for the exploration of psychotherapy integration (SEPI), Annapolis

Orlinsky DE, Howard KI (1986) The psychological interior of psychotherapy: explorations with the Therapy Session Reports. In: Greenberg LS, Pinsof WM (eds) The psychotherapeutic process: a research handbook. Guilford, New York, pp 477–501 (Guilford clinical psychology and psychotherapy series)

Orlinsky DE, Grawe K, Parks B (1994) Process and outcome in psychotherapy—noch Einmal. In: Bergin AE,

Garfield SL (eds) Handbook of psychotherapy and behavior change, 4th edn. Wiley, New York, pp 270–376
Orlinsky DE, Rønnestad MH, Willutzki U (2004) Fifty years of psychotherapy process-outcome research: continuity and change. In: Lambert MJ (ed) Bergin and Garfield's handbook of psychotherapy and behavior change, 5th edn. Wiley, New York, pp 307–392
Owen J, Quirk K, Hilsenroth MJ, Rodolfa E (2012) Working through: in-session processes that promote between-session thoughts and activities. J Couns Psychol 59(1):161–167. doi:10.1037/a0023616
Pascual-Leone A (2009) Dynamic emotional processing in experiential therapy: two steps forward, one step back. J Consult Clin Psychol 77(1):113–126. doi:10.1037/a0014488
Pascual-Leone A, Greenberg LS, Pascual-Leone J (2009) Developments in task analysis: new methods to study change. Psychother Res 19(4):527–542. doi:10.1080/10503300902897797
Perry JC (1990) Defense mechanisms rating scale. Cambridge Hospital, Harvard Medical School, Boston, MA
Petrocelli JV (2003) Hierarchical multiple regression in counseling research: common problems and possible remedies. Meas Eval Couns Dev 36(1):9–22
Polkinghorne DE (1983) Methodology for the human sciences: systems of inquiry. State University of New York Press, Albany
Ponterotto JG (2005) Qualitative research in counseling psychology: a primer on research paradigms and philosophy of science. J Couns Psychol 52(2):126–136. doi:10.1037/0022-0167.52.2.126
Quintana SM, Maxwell SE (1999) Implications of recent developments in structural equation modeling for counseling psychology. Couns Psychol 27 (4):485–527. doi:10.1177/0011000099274002
Ramseyer F, Tschacher W (2011) Nonverbal synchrony in psychotherapy: coordinated body movement reflects relationship quality and outcome. J Consult Clin Psychol 79:284–295. doi:10.1037/a0023419
Ramseyer F, Kupper Z, Caspar F, Znoj H, Tschacher W (2014) Time-series panel analysis (TSPA): multivariate modeling of temporal associations in psychotherapy process. J Consult Clin Psychol, No Pagination Specified. doi:10.1037/a0037168
Ramseyer F, Kupper Z, Caspar F, Znoj H, Tschacher W (2014) Time-series panel analysis (TSPA): multivariate modeling of temporal associations in psychotherapy process. J Consult Clin Psychol. doi:10.1037/a003716
Raudenbush S, Bryk AS (2002) Hierarchical linear models, 2nd edn. Sage, London
Rice LN, Greenberg LS (1984) Patterns of change. Guilford, New York
Rogers CR (1942) Counseling and psychotherapy. Houghton Mifflin, Boston
Rogers CR (1957) The necessary and sufficient conditions of therapeutic personality change. J Consult Psychol 21(2):95–103. doi:10.1037/h0045357
Rogers CR (1975) Empathic: an unappreciated way of being. Couns Psychol 5(2):2–10. doi:10.1177/001100007500500202
Rosenberg M (1965) Society and the adolescent self image. Princeton University Press, Princeton, NJ
Russell RL, Trull TJ (1986) Sequential analyses of language variables in psychotherapy process research. J Consult Clin Psychol 54(1):16–21. doi:10.1037/0022-006X.54.1.16
Safran JD, Muran JC (1996) The resolution of ruptures in the therapeutic alliance. J Consult Clin Psychol 64 (3):447–458. doi:10.1037/0022-006X.64.3.447
Salvatore S, Tschacher W (2012) Time dependency of psychotherapeutic exchanges: the contribution of the theory of dynamic systems in analyzing process. Front Psychol 3:1–14. doi:10.3389/fpsyg.2012.00253
Salvatore S, Valsiner J (2010) Between the general and the unique. Theory Psychol 20:817–833. doi:10.1177/0959354310381156
Salvatore S, Gelo O, Gennaro A, Manzo S, Al Radaideh A (2009) Looking at the psychotherapy process as an intersubjective dynamic of meaning-making: a case study with discourse flow analysis. J Constr Psychol 23(3):195–230. doi:10.1080/10720531003765981
Salvatore S, Gennaro A, Auletta AF, Tonti M, Nitti M (2012) Automated method of content analysis: a device for psychotherapy process research. Psychother Res 22(3):256–273. doi:10.1080/10503307.2011.647930
Semerari A, Carcione A, Dimaggio G, Falcone M, Nicolo G, Procacci M et al (2003) How to evaluate metacognitive functioning in psychotherapy? The metacognition assessment scale and its applications. Clin Psychol Psychother 10(4):238–261. doi:10.1002/cpp.362
Sexton H (1993) Exploring a psychotherapeutic change sequence: relating process to intersessional and post-treatment outcome. J Consult Clin Psychol 61 (1):128–136. doi:10.1037/0022-006X.61.1.128
Sexton HC, Hembre K, Kvarme G (1996) The interaction of the alliance and therapy microprocess: a sequential analysis. J Consult Clin Psychol 64(3):471–480. doi:10.1037/0022-006X.64.3.471
Shedler J, Westen D (2007) The Shedler–Westen assessment procedure (SWAP): making personality diagnosis clinically meaningful. J Pers Assess 89(1):41–55. doi:10.1080/00223890701357092
Siefert CJ, Hilsenroth MJ, Weinberger J, Blagys MD, Ackerman SJ (2006) The relationship of patient defensive functioning and alliance with therapist technique during short-term psychodynamic psychotherapy. Clin Psychol Psychother 13(1):20–33. doi:10.1002/cpp.469
Slife BD, Gantt E (1999) Methodological pluralism: a framework for psychotherapy research. J Clin Psychol 55(12):1–13
Snyder WU (1945) An investigation of the nature of non-directive psychotherapy. J Gen Psychol 33 (2):193–223. doi:10.1080/00221309.1945.10544506
Spielberger CD, Gorsuch RL, Lushene R, Vagg PR, Jacobs GA (1983) Manual for the state-trait anxiety inventory. Consulting Psychologists Press, Palo Alto

Spitzer RL, Williams JBW, Gibbons M, First MB (1990) Structured clinical interview for DSM–III–R—personality disorders (SCID-II). American Psychiatric Press, Washington

Stevens CL, Muran JC, Safran JD, Gorman BS, Winston A (2007) Levels and patterns of the therapeutic alliance in brief psychotherapy. Am J Psychother 61(2):109–129

Stiles WB (1978) Verbal response modes and dimensions of interpersonal roles: a method of discourse analysis. J Pers Soc Psychol 36(7):693–703. doi:10.1037/0022-3514.36.7.693

Stiles WB (1979) Verbal response modes and psychotherapeutic technique. Psychiatry 42(1):49–62

Stiles WB (1988) Psychotherapy process-outcome correlations may be misleading. Psychotherapy 25:27–35. doi:10.1037/h0085320

Stiles WB (2007) Theory-building case studies of counselling and psychotherapy. Couns Psychother Res 7(2):122–127. doi:10.1080/14733140701356742

Stiles WB, Shapiro DA (1989) Abuse of the drug metaphor in psychotherapy process-outcome research. Clin Psychol Rev 9:521–543. doi:10.1016/0272-7358(89)90007-X

Stiles WB, Shapiro DA (1994) Disabuse of the drug metaphor: psychotherapy process-outcome correlations. J Consult Clin Psychol 62:942–948

Stiles WB, Snow JS (1984a) Counseling session impact as viewed by novice counselors and their clients. J Couns Psychol 31(1):3–12. doi:10.1037/0022-0167.31.1.3

Stiles WB, Snow JS (1984b) Dimensions of psychotherapy session impact across sessions and across clients. Br J Clin Psychol 23(1):59–63. doi:10.1111/j.2044-8260.1984.tb00627.x

Stiles WB, Elliott R, Llewelyn SP, Firth-Cozens JA, Margison FR, Shapiro DA et al (1990) Assimilation of problematic experiences by clients in psychotherapy. Psychotherapy 27(3):411–420. doi:10.1037/0033-3204.27.3.411

Stiles WB, Honos-Webb L, Surko M (1998) Responsiveness in psychotherapy. Clin Psychol 5(4):439–458. doi:10.1111/j.1468-2850.1998.tb00166.x

Strauss JL, Hayes AM, Johnson SL, Newman CF, Brown GK, Barber JP et al (2006) Early alliance, alliance ruptures, and symptom change in a nonrandomized trial of cognitive therapy for avoidant and obsessive-compulsive personality disorders. J Consult Clin Psychol 74(2):337–345. doi:10.1037/0022-006X.74.2.337

Tasca GA, Balfour L, Ritchie K, Bissada H (2006) Developmental changes in group climate in two types of group therapy for binge-eating disorder: a growth curve analysis. Psychother Res 16(4):499–514. doi:10.1080/10503300600593359

Tasca GA, Gallop R (2009) Multilevel modeling of longitudinal data for psychotherapy researchers: I. The basics. Psychother Res 19(4–5):429–37. doi:10.1080/10503300802641444

Tomori C, Bavelas JB (2007) Using microanalysis of communication to compare solution-focused and client-centered therapies. J Fam Psychother 18(3):25–43. doi:10.1300/J085v18n03_03

Trijsburg RW, Frederiks G, Gorlee M, Klouwer E, den Hollander AM, Duivenvoorden HJ (2002) Development of the comprehensive psychotherapeutic interventions rating scale (CPIRS). Psychother Res 12(3):287–317. doi:10.1093/ptr/12.3.287

Tschacher W, Gelo OCG, Koch SC, & Salvatore S (2014). Dynamic systems theory and embodiment in psychotherapy research. A new look at process and outcome [Special issue]. Front. Psychol. 5:1089. http://journal.frontiersin.org/ResearchTopic/1744#overview

Tschacher W, Ramseyer F (2009) Modeling psychotherapy process by time-series panel analysis (TSPA). Psychother Res 19(4):469–481. doi:10.1080/10503300802654496

Tschacher W, Baur N, Grawe K (2000) Temporal interaction of process variables in psychotherapy. Psychother Res 10(3):296–309. doi:10.1093/ptr/10.3.296

Watson JC, Bedard DL (2006) Clients' emotional processing in psychotherapy: a comparison between cognitive-behavioral and process-experiential therapies. J Consult Clin Psychol 74(1):152–159. doi:10.1037/0022-006X.74.1.152

Watson JC, Gordon LB, Stermac L, Kalogerakos F, Steckley P (2003) Comparing the effectiveness of process-experiential with cognitive-behavioral psychotherapy in the treatment of depression. J Consult Clin Psychol 71(4):773–781. doi:10.1037/0022-006X.71.4.773

Weerasekera P, Linder B, Greenberg L, Watson J (2001) The working alliance in client-centered and process-experiential therapy of depression. Psychother Res 11(2):221–233. doi:10.1093/ptr/11.2.221

Weissman AN, Beck AT (1978) Development and validation of the dysfunctional attitudes scale: a preliminary investigation. In: Paper presented at the 86th annual convention of the american psychological association, Toronto

Williams EN, Fauth J (2005) A psychotherapy process study of therapist in session self-awareness. Psychother Res 15(4):374–381. doi:10.1080/10503300500091355

Zuroff DC, Blatt SJ, Sotsky SM, Krupnick JL, Martin DJ, Sanislow CA III et al (2000) Relation of therapeutic alliance and perfectionism to outcome in brief outpatient treatment of depression. J Consult Clin Psychol 68(1):114–124. doi:10.1037/0022-006X.68.1.114

14 Current Issues on Group Psychotherapy Research: An Overview

Gianluca Lo Coco, Salvatore Gullo, Claudia Prestano, and Gary M. Burlingame

Contents

G. Lo Coco (✉)
Department of Psychology, University of Palermo, Viale delle Scienze, edificio 15, 90128 Palermo, Italy
e-mail: gianluca.lococo@unipa.it

S. Gullo
N. Cusano University, Via Don Gnocchi 3, 0016, Italy

C. Prestano
University of Palermo, Viale delle Scienze, edificio 15, 90128 Palermo, Italy

G.M. Burlingame
Brigham Young University, 238 TLRB, Provo, UT 84602, USA

Abstract

Recent efforts to improve group psychotherapy have focused on codifying both evidence-based treatments and therapeutic relationships. This chapter reviews the numerous advances in empirical research on group psychotherapy and highlights therapeutic practices ensuing from the evidence. The authors synthesize some of the most crucial development in group psychotherapy research, such as the effectiveness of group treatments, the mechanisms of change of group therapies, the components of group relationship, and issues regarding methodological problems associated with the analysis of group data.

14.1 Introduction: Is Group Psychotherapy Effective?

Group therapies are important resource by the managed care industry and mental health and substance abuse service providers that are pressured by the supply and demand of delivering services which leads to an increasing provision of group treatment. Group treatments have historically been seen as a secondary treatment modality, certainly not on the same level as the gold standard of individual therapy. Fortunately, there is a substantial literature comparing the efficacy of the two approaches that suggests at

O.C.G. Gelo et al. (eds.), *Psychotherapy Research*,
DOI 10.1007/978-3-7091-1382-0_14,

the very least that group psychotherapy is clearly not a second-rate treatment (Bednar and Kaul 1994). Group therapies have been used in a wide range of conditions including anxiety and mood disorders, late-life depression, infertility, adjustment to personal loss, substance abuse, schizophrenia, bipolar disorder, post-traumatic stress disorder, eating disorders, and personality disorders (Burlingame et al. 2003). They have also been used across the lifespan and in differing healthcare settings, including inpatients, day hospitals, and outpatient settings. Group psychotherapy, like individual psychotherapy, is intended to help people who would like to improve their ability to cope with difficulties and problems in their lives. But, while in individual therapy the patient meets with only one person (the therapist), in group psychotherapy the meeting is with a whole group and one or two therapists. There are many kinds of groups in the group psychotherapy field. The techniques used in group psychotherapy can be verbal, expressive, psychodramatic, etc. The approaches can vary from psychoanalytic to behavioral, Gestalt or encounter groups. Moreover, groups vary from classic psychotherapy groups, where process is emphasized, to psychoeducational, which are usually focused on the most common areas of concern (Yalom and Leszcz 2005).

We can affirm that we know far more about what efficacious group treatments for specific patient populations than we did a decade ago (Burlingame et al. 2013). For instance, an important meta-analysis regarding outcome of group and individual therapy found there was virtually no difference between the two (McRoberts et al. 1998). Moreover, one of the latest reviews (Burlingame et al. 2004) examined 107 studies and 14 meta-analysis published between 1990 and 2002. These authors stated that there was "sufficient" evidence to conclude that group psychotherapy is as effective as individual therapy and for clients suffering from severe mental illnesses. Beneficial effects were also found for inpatient group psychotherapy in controlled studies as well as in naturalistic studies (Kosters et al. 2006).

The efficacy indicated by the research results, combined with the relative efficiency of the group modality, makes a powerful argument for more extensive use of groups in service delivery settings.

Most reviews which examined the effect of treatment orientation did not find any significant difference between the outcomes of groups as a result of therapy type. For instance, Piper et al. (2001) found patients with complicated grief improved in both psychodynamic and supportive group treatment; there was no significant difference between therapy types. Blay et al. (2002) found brief psychodynamic group treatment gave clinically and statistically significantly greater benefit than usual clinical care for a mixed diagnosis group at the end of the 8-week treatment, but at follow-up (9–30 weeks post randomization), there was no significant difference. Tasca et al. (2006) found binge-eating patients gained similar benefit from psychodynamic interpersonal therapy and group cognitive–behavioral therapy, both being superior to no-treatment controls at the end of therapy: follow-up data on the no-treatment control group were not available.

Recently, Burlingame and McClendon (2010) tabulated the efficacy and effectiveness of group treatments by patient population and provided categorical recommendations for its application. More specifically, some theoretical orientations "dominate" particular disorders (e.g., group CBT for anxiety disorders), although most show support for a variety of disorders (i.e., mixed). In short, these results provide evidence for the clinical effectiveness of group psychotherapy approaches in a various clinical problems, but not for specific benefits of any particular theoretical approach.

Different studies also examined the relationship between patient characteristics and therapy outcome, and the role of mediating or moderating variables. Overall, the evidence suggests that there may be important effects of age, sex, self-efficacy, treatment duration, and psychological mindedness on clinical outcomes and effects of attachment style and interpersonal distress on group attendance. For example, a significant finding was that the quality of object relations is an important moderator of the impact of treatment type on outcome. Patients with high quality of object relations had better outcomes from interpretive group psychotherapy than from supportive group psychotherapy, and this may be a useful selection criterion for groups (Piper et al. 2001). Lorentzen and Hoglend (2008), in a preliminary report, suggest that patients with more severe pathology (in terms of depression, other psychiatric symptoms, personality disorders, and poor interpersonal functioning) require long-term group psychotherapy to achieve improvements in interpersonal functioning.

Regarding the research on outcome of group psychotherapy, psychodynamic group interventions have been underevaluated, and the number of high controlled studies (i.e., RCTs) is sparse. Several researchers issued a call for the study of psychodynamic group, especially long-term treatments, as a next step in the group treatment literature. Two recent studies that have emerged from Norway seem to be a promising start. Overall, the two prospective naturalistic studies (Wilberg et al. 2003; Lorentzen and Hoglend 2004) suggest that long-term psychodynamic group psychotherapy may be effective for outpatients with personality disorders. Moreover, two recent small studies with eating-disorder outpatients (Valbak 2003; Prestano et al. 2008) suggest that psychodynamic long-term group therapy may be of value for patients with bulimia and anorexia nervosa. However, since neither study employed a control group or a manualized treatment approach that could indicate that psychodynamic principles were being followed, the validity of these results are still open to question.

Finally, although the empirical evidence for the effectiveness of group psychotherapy is strong, it is important to remind that several patients experience no benefit and often drop out from treatment (see Lambert and Ogles 2004). Premature termination rates vary from 20 to 50 % of group members in the extant literature. Most dropouts, which often involve 30–40 % of a therapy group, seem to occur early in the life of a group (Yalom and Leszcz 2005). How to help patients who are at risk for treatment failure? It may be a core question for researchers and clinicians alike involved in group psychotherapy. Recently, a study examined the effects of a feedback intervention directed at both members and leaders of psychotherapy groups held in a university counseling center (Davies et al. 2008). This study adopted the method developed by M. Lambert and colleagues, who found that providing therapists with feedback (using patient self-reported symptom distress) improved outcome for patients predicted to drop out from treatment and reduced deterioration rates (Whipple et al. 2003; Hawkins et al. 2004; Harmon et al. 2007). In the study of Davies and colleagues, the feedback consisted of group climate information using scores from the Group Climate Questionnaire, completed by members after each group session. Unexpected results indicate the feedback intervention had little impact on the therapeutic factors and outcome. However, the authors caution overinterpretation of these results. Specifically, finding may be due to the irrelevance of the feedback provided to patients. Members were given feedback on the group climate which may be of little overall value to them. Moreover, small sample size may have "hidden" the ability to detect reliable effects for feedback on outcome.

Addressing the issues of selection and composition of group may help therapist to reduce dropout rates. Group psychotherapy is indicated for clients who manifest interpersonal difficulties and interpersonal pathology; consequently, the group literature suggested that clients should be excluded from group psychotherapy if they cannot engage in the primary activities of the group (interpersonal engagement, interpersonal learning, and acquiring insight) due to logistical, intellectual, psychological, or interpersonal reasons (Yalom and Leszcz 2005). The *clinical practice guidelines for group treatment* (Bernard et al. 2008) outlined that clients who demonstrate poor psychological mindedness, little self-reflection, poor motivation, high degrees of defensiveness, and denial and who elicit angry and negative reactions from others are at risk of early dropout.

14.2 Mechanisms of Change in Group Treatments

Although previous research has demonstrated the effectiveness of group psychotherapy, the underlying mechanisms by which change is achieved have limited empirical support. In individual treatment, the therapeutic ingredients arise from the interventions of the therapist and the nature of the relationship between therapist and patient. The therapeutic relationship is the ubiquitous mechanism of action that operates across all therapies (Martin et al. 2000). In group psychotherapy, the situation is radically different. The individual patient is interactionally engaged with each member of the group. The individual also experiences the atmosphere of the whole group that results from the mix of all contributions. The qualities specific to group processes create an interactional field that is considerably more complex than that in the individual therapy setting. These features apply mainly to the nature of the interventions and of the therapeutic bond, which now involves the entire group membership and not just the therapist. Greater emphasis is placed on the importance of using the group environment as a focus for experiencing typical reactions involving one's relationships with others. Groups provide a distinctly more real relationship environment in which the complex reactions of the individual may emerge through interaction with a host of protagonists, not just the authority figure of the therapist. To understand the nature of personal problems, the patient must consider the responses of other group members in addition to those of the group leader. Group members express numerous interpretations, ideas, suggestions, and common experiences. This provides each member with a wealth of feedback for consideration.

Regarding dyadic therapies, a number of researchers demonstrated that the nature of therapeutic alliance is the strongest single predictor of outcome in individual psychotherapy. A similar trend is also found in the group literature. However, the concept of therapeutic alliance, and particularly of bond, is more complicated in groups. The closest analogy to the therapeutic bond in dyadic therapy is that of group cohesion, a property of the entire group. There is growing consensus that cohesion is the best definition of the therapeutic relationship in group (Burlingame et al. 2002a, b; Yalom and Leszcz 2005), and it has been described as the "bedrock of the group experience" (Butler and Fuhriman 1983, p. 500). For Yalom and Leszcz (2005), cohesion is not just the primary curative factor in group psychotherapy but a "precondition for other therapeutic factors to function" (p. 55). Cohesion generally refers to the emotional bonds among members for each other and for a shared commitment to the group and its primary task. Moreover, it is the group process variable generally linked to positive therapeutic outcome (Burlingame et al. 2002a, b).

A recent meta-analysis of 40 studies that tested the relationship between cohesion and outcome found overwhelming support for its ability to predict improvement in group members (Burlingame et al. 2011). More specifically, the average weighted correlation between cohesion and outcome was $r = .25$, and five variables (age, theoretical orientation, length, size of group, as well as interventions to enhance cohesion) were shown to moderate the effects of cohesion on improvement in outcome. Groups led by cognitive–behavioral, psychodynamic, and interpersonal orientations produced reliable cohesion-outcome relationships. Group leaders who emphasized member interaction over problem-specific focused groups posted higher cohesion-outcome links suggesting the importance of encouraging member interaction. Cohesion was the strongest predictor of outcome in groups composed of 5–9 members and that lasted more than 12 sessions. Thus, cohesion takes time to build and requires the correct balance of member–member interaction. Finally, groups composed of younger members (college age) produced the largest gains in outcomes when cohesion was present. No differences were found in cohesion ability to predict outcome by setting (inpatient vs. outpatient) or patient

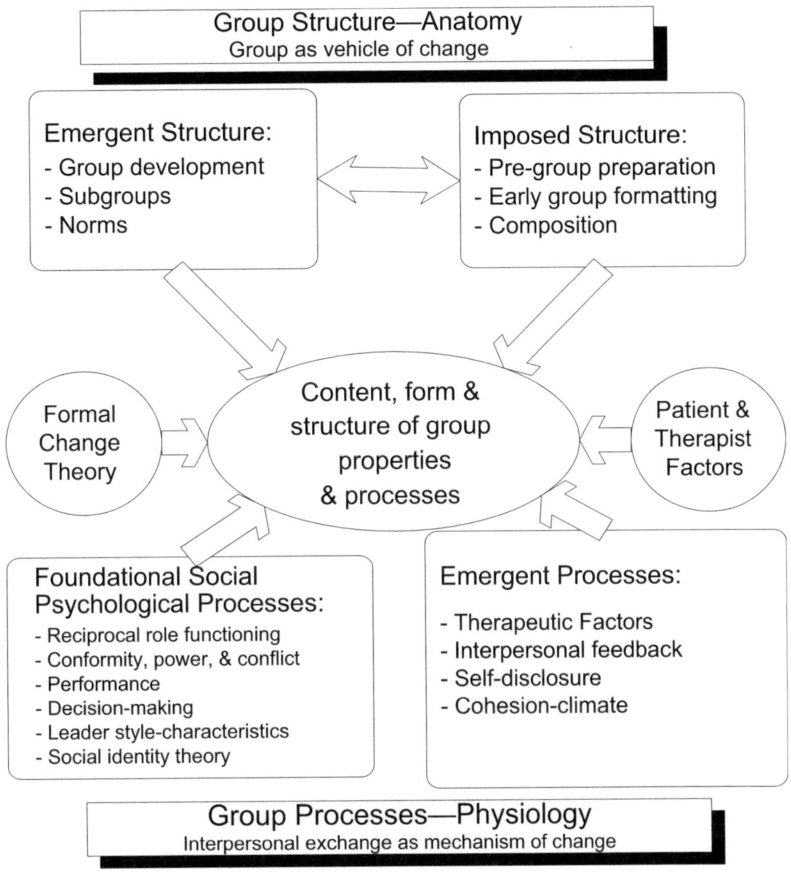

Fig. 14.1 The anatomy and physiology of small-group treatments

diagnosis suggesting that it is a robust group dynamic across diverse settings and populations.

14.2.1 The Process of Group Psychotherapy

Group process generally refers to what happens in the group: a widely used definition of group psychotherapy process describes it as "the study of the group-as-a-whole system and changes in its development, the interactions within the patient and therapist subsystems, the patient and patient (dyadic or subgroup) subsystems, the therapist and therapist subsystem if there are co-leaders, and the way each of the subsystems interacts with and is influenced by the group as a whole" (Beck and Lewis 2000, p. 8).

Recently, Burlingame et al. (2008a) offered an organizing framework to give clinicians and researchers the opportunity to integrate important aspects of the complex system "group" (see Fig. 14.1).

They differentiate between the "anatomy of a small group," which reflects the group structure, and the "physiology of a small group," which reflects dynamic interactions and processes (such as the therapeutic factors, interpersonal feedback, and self-disclosure). The group structure focuses on the group as a vehicle of change and contains an emergent and an imposed facet of the group. The second aspect of group structure, the imposed structure, refers to pre-group preparation and composition and early group formatting. Similar to the *anatomy* of the group, the *physiology* of the group is divided into two parts, the emergent structure and foundational social–psychological processes (e.g., reciprocal role functioning, power, conflict, performance, decision-making, leader style characteristics), and considers the interpersonal exchange as a mechanism of change. Therapeutic factors, interpersonal feedback, self-disclosure, cohesion, and group climate are facets of the emergent process and are often subject matter in research on topic of small-group processes. Great importance is attributed to the leaders of a group, even if their impact is not directly evident most of the time. Helping the group in developing and maintaining a therapeutic milieu that is conducive to beneficial member interaction, with the goal to facilitate changing long-standing behaviors, beliefs, and skills, is a fundamental responsibility of the leader [according to Yalom (1995)]. As a result, the group leader does not only have the responsibility to perceive the emergent processes in the group but also to influence the process of change.

A recent and well-conducted review of relationship constructs on group psychotherapy (Johnson et al. 2008) found that group climate, cohesion, alliance, and empathy had mixed to positive results predicting outcome in group treatment. Moreover, we have well sound measures of these four therapeutic relationship constructs (i.e., the Group Climate Questionnaire, GCQ; the California Psychotherapy Alliance Scale-Group, CALPAS-G; the Working Alliance Inventory, WAI; the Curative Climate Instrument, CCI) which are widely used in group psychotherapy research.

We will show only few key findings about this topic (see Burlingame et al. (2004) and Johnson et al. (2008) for a complete review): the group climate subscales have been associated with levels of other therapeutic factors (Johnson et al. 2006; Kivlighan and Goldfine 1991) and behavioral observations of self-disclosure and therapeutic work. A high level of engagement seems to be associated with other positive aspects of therapeutic relationship and to provide a foundation for other group processes that are considered to be helpful (Castonguay et al. 1998). Several studies have investigated the association between group cohesion and therapeutic improvement and reported beneficial effects in a variety of settings and therapeutic approaches (Budman et al. 1989; Marziali et al. 1997; Ogrodniczuk et al. 2006). Moreover, higher levels of cohesion as well as an increase in cohesion over time were related to symptom improvement (Dinger and Schauenburg 2010). However, some other studies failed to detect a positive association between high cohesion and symptomatic improvement for psychodynamic groups, CBT groups, and different patient populations (e.g., Gillaspy et al. 2002; Lorentzen et al. 2004; Oei and Browne 2006). Cohesion is also widely agreed to be a helpful foundation for other curative factors to operate (Yalom 1995). Group alliance too has been found to predict outcome in psychotherapy groups (Marziali et al. 1997; Strauss and Burgmeier-Lohse 1994; Lorentzen et al. 2004; Lo Coco et al. 2012). Several studies have also found alliance to be related to other therapeutic relationship variables such as cohesion (Budman et al. 1989; Gillaspy et al. 2002; Joyce et al. 2007; Marziali et al. 1997) and empathy (Horvath 1994).

Two of the most neglected areas in group research literature, regarding the study of group therapeutic factors and of group leader interventions, have been improving our knowledge for the last 10 years, by establishing the validity of new group assessment tools.

Regarding the study of therapeutic factors in group treatment, Yalom (1995) suggested that there is a core of therapeutic factors that therapists agree on independent of their therapeutic orientation. His view of the therapeutic factors comprises 11 elements: instillation of hope, universality, imparting information, altruism, the corrective recapitulation of the primary family group, development of socializing techniques, imitative behavior, interpersonal learning, group cohesiveness, catharsis, and existential learning. The broad clinical adoption of this classification of therapeutic factors did not lead to a strong empirical basis for understanding helpful process patterns, because too many divergent and psychometrically questionable measures exist (see Bednar and Kaul 1994). The Therapeutic Factors Inventory (TFI) by Lese and MacNair-Semands (2000) has been designed to assess all of Yalom's factors; it is psychometrically sound and differentially correlates with interpersonal problems of individual members and is sensitive to group development.

Regarding the group research literature on the leader effects on groups, a new measure of group leader interventions, the Group Psychotherapy Intervention Rating Scale [GPIRS; Sternberg S, Trijsburg W (2005) The relationship between therapeutic interventions and therapeutic outcome (Unpublished manuscript)] is promising. The GPIRS evaluates group leaders on the basis of their ability to perform interventions aimed at enhancing mainly group cohesion. The GPIRS is an observer-rated, behavioral measure consisting of 48 items, aimed at assessing three dimensions: (1) *group structuring*, which assesses the leader's ability to establish rules and norms, define therapist and member roles, and address fears regarding self-disclosure; (2) *verbal interaction*, which measures the therapists' ability to perform interventions that have been shown to facilitate the development of therapeutic verbal interactions; (3) *emotional climate*, which includes items assessing the group leader's ability to create and maintain an emotional climate in the group and to perform interventions shown to help create a safe milieu allowing for meaningful self-exploration by group members. Recent findings with the GPIRS (Chapman et al. 2010) support the concept that therapists who implement appropriate structure, facilitate member–member interactions, and interact with a warm and empathic interpersonal style tend to have stronger, more therapeutic groups.

Some recent studies also investigated the role of coleadership in group interventions: the *coleadership team cognition-team diversity model* suggests that group coleaders will be most effective when coleaders share cognitions about the group but are dissimilar in terms of their skill sets and behavior within the group (Miles and Kivlighan 2008). In other words, this model suggests that diversity in leadership style would be associated with more effective group processes because dissimilar coleaders bring complementary skills to the group. A recent study provided empirical data on the relationship between the coleaders and suggested that dissimilarity in how coleaders behave in their group may facilitate positive group member outcomes through the creation of a productive group climate (Miles and Kivlighan 2010). These findings also suggest that the issue of coleader similarity or dissimilarity is more complex than suggested by the coleadership model, because the importance of coleader similarity versus dissimilarity changed as a function of time. The pattern of conflict development found in this study suggests that coleader behavioral dissimilarity may be related to a pattern of decreasing conflict over time.

Finally, the interpretations of empirical studies on the therapeutic relationship are still complicated by two methodological issues (Johnson et al. 2008). The first is that interpretations of therapeutic relationship constructs differ somewhat depending on whether the group or individual is the unit of analysis. The second is that the interpretations of findings for open and closed groups differ (see Kipnes et al. 2002). Moreover, a recent review (Burlingame et al. 2002b) found that two thirds of the literature had focused on a single relationship, member–group. Studies investigating member–member and member–leader relationships were far less frequent. Finally, it is still difficult to compare different studies on group therapeutic relationship because these process variables may be measured by vastly different instruments, and differing findings may be directly due to differing measures and definitions.

14.2.2 A Three-Component Model of Group Relationship

Although there is consensus about the major ingredients of group process mechanisms, there are also a wide variety of conceptualizations of single process components that resulted in a diversity of empirical approaches, leading to difficulties in summarizing the empirical support. Previous research has identified the relationship cultivated by the group setting as cohesion, group climate, alliance, and empathy, which has consistently been linked to patient improvement and low dropout rate (Burlingame et al. 2002b). Although containing important differences, these therapeutic relationships are closely interrelated (Johnson et al. 2005). The process studies that have examined the empirical overlap between cohesion and alliance (see Gillaspy et al. 2002; Marziali et al. 1997; Piper et al. 2007), alliance and empathy (Horvath 1994), and empathy and group climate (Phipps and Zastowny 1988) have suggested that they are highly related to one another.

Johnson et al. (2005) analyzed the associations between different relationship aspects (group climate, cohesion, alliance, and empathy) in group treatment. They found considerable overlap between different relationship measures and came up with three latent variables (positive bonding, positive working, and negative empathy) that best represented the relationship constructs in their data. The first component represents the *positive relational bonds* in the group: the individual member's emotional connection or attachment to the other members of the group, including the therapist and the group as a whole. The second component represents the *positive working relationships* in the group: the individual member's collaborative engagement in therapeutic work with the other members, the therapist, and the group as a whole for the purpose of progressing toward treatment goals. Finally, the third component represents the *negative relationship factors* that may be operating in the group: those aspects of the group process that may adversely affect member attachments or impede the therapeutic work.

Bormann and Strauss (2007) followed Johnson's study by collecting data on the same measures from 15 hospitals in Germany and Switzerland, and the same three factors emerged. Recently, Bakali et al. (2009) in a study from Norway reported a similar 3-factor model. Results from these studies are leading to the development of a composite measure of the group relationship by eliminating items with redundant information or poor fit (Burlingame 2010).

14.3 A Methodological Issue: The Nested Data Structure

Given the complexity of the group treatment, research programs that analyze relationships between characteristics of patients, specific process patterns, mechanisms of change, and outcomes are very composite. Several previous studies have addressed problems associated with the analysis of group data, particularly regarding evaluation of intervention effects (Kenny et al. 2002; Roberts and Roberts 2005). The key issue in the analysis of group data is within-group dependence, because members who are in the same group exercise a mutual influence on each other, which means that individuals who attend the same group are more similar (or dissimilar) to one another than individuals who participate in different groups. This nonindependence can be viewed as a correlation between observations (Kenny et al. 2002) and determines a violation of key assumption of most statistical analyses, increasing the risk of type I errors (Baldwin et al. 2005; Burlingame et al. 1994).

However, there is general agreement among researchers that although the group data structure complicates research design and statistical analyses, it is not simply a methodological nuisance. Of course, mutual influence is often at the heart of group interventions; the group leads numerous opportunities for group members to interact and influence each other. Consequently, in recent years many authors tried to provide a guide to group treatment researchers and developed several methods that are specifically designed to model and analyze group data.

Before illustrating these strategies of analysis, it is important to highlight that correlations within a group can be either positive or negative. Since group members share a common environment, their behaviors and their response to intervention can become more homogenous (positive correlations), especially in long-term group psychotherapy. For example, rates of cohesion, attrition, and attendance can impact outcomes in group treatment (Burlingame et al. 2002a, b). The sharing of environment can also, in opposite way, differentiate members' response to the intervention. As Kenny et al. (2002) suggested, in the group there may be fixed resources (such as time or attention of the leader); thus, for instance, the percentage of time that one member spends talking in a group discussion is inversely proportional to the percentage of time that remains to the other members.

The most common approach to analyzing group data was, for a long time, to consider the individual-as-unit analysis, and ignoring within-group dependence. The 2005 review by Baldwin et al. found that in the 33 studies examined (among those that met criteria for empirically supported treatments, ESTs; Task Force, 1998) none of these studies assessed for dependence in their data.

Behind this article, several others (Baldwin et al. 2008; Imel et al. 2008) have evaluated the extent and variability of dependence in data taken from previously published randomized clinical trials of group psychotherapy. Taken together, these studies found a moderate to large (0.03–0.12) within-group-dependence effect, even if Baldwin et al. reported that the majority of statistically significant results reported in these studies would no longer be significant if one assumed a moderate level of within-group dependence (0.05). On the other hand, statistical effects of within-group dependence are now clear, because it does bias significance tests (Wampold and Serlin 2000), and several authors recommend to assess and report the degree of within-group dependence for all group treatment studies.

Group nonindependence is typically indexed by an intraclass correlation (ICC). There are two methods for estimating the ICC. The first approach uses ANOVA, treating group as the independent variable in a one way, between-subjects ANOVA. The second method uses the correlational method for group data, creating every possible pair of scores in the group and computing Pearson's *r* on these pair of scores.

A relatively new approach in group psychotherapy research is to consider data from small-group research as hierarchically structured. The individual participants are nested within groups; thus, there are two possible levels of analysis in group data: individual (level 1) and group (level 2). Multilevel model (MLM) or hierarchical linear model (HLM) is used to accomplish the nested effect of the groups (Tasca et al. 2009). One of the primary advantages of HLM is that they allow one to simultaneously investigate relationships *within* a particular hierarchical level, as well as relationships *between* or across hierarchical levels. In order to model both within-level and between-level relationships, HLM consists in two stages of estimation (Kenny et al. 1998); the first involves computing an analysis across individuals within each group separately (level 1), and the second involves aggregating the first stage results across groups (level 2). Furthermore, when groups are nested within therapist and clients are nested within groups, the three-level HLM can be used; in this model therapist is level 3, group is level 2, and client is level 1.

Longitudinal data can be also analyzed within the paradigm of multilevel models. In the three-level growth HLM, one can estimate variables at level 1 of the model as a function of time (repeated measurements of group outcome or group process across sessions). At level 2, the level 1 parameters are nested within each person, and at level 3, each person is nested within a group.

It is important to highlight that the magnitude of the nonindependence can fatally reduce the power of the study (Murray and Blitstein 2003). Although the best way to increase power is to plan for within-group dependence when designing a group-based intervention study, a possible solution is to base degrees of freedom on the number of groups because it has little effect on power (if there are sufficient groups or more groups across all conditions).

Beyond the analytic strategies, from the theoretical and clinical perspectives, within-group dependence sets a series of important issues. According to Baldwin et al. (2005), one of these issues is to identify the sources of within-group dependence, as Kenny et al. (2002) tried to do describing three possible sources: the group composition, the common fate, and the mutual influence. Within-group dependence likely reflects psychological and social processes central to group-based interventions and leads one to think it could be important to explore how it changes during the group psychotherapy, how is it associated to the outcome, and how is it related to the process variables (e.g., cohesion).

14.4 The Need to Bridge the Gap Between Science and Practice in Group Psychotherapy

Psychotherapy research has witnessed increased attention for the need to bridge the gap between science and practice. Often the arguments have been that the practitioners were not practicing what researchers had found to be efficacious. It is also worth noting that rarely were practitioners actively informing researchers of the topics to be investigated. Most professional associations underscored the importance of bridging this gap. However, research evidence indicates that in the majority of clinical settings, this has not occurred. In this decade, the "bridging the gap" mantra pertains to evidence-based practice. Results from these evidence-based studies have led to recommendations for best practice based on criteria proposed by a variety of scientific committees (Norcross et al. 2006).

Two documents of the American Group Psychotherapy Association (AGPA) may be representative of the connections between clinical practice and group psychotherapy research, by supporting practitioners in their practice of group psychotherapy. The first is the CORE-revised (CORE-R) battery (Burlingame et al. 2006). The goal of the CORE-R Task Force was to provide clinicians with the best recommendations regarding psychometrically sound and empirically tested selection, outcome, and process instruments that have shown to be of value in the group literature (Burlingame et al. 2008b). The revised CORE (CORE-R) Task Force was charged with reviewing the original recommendations of the CORE battery (which was developed in the 1980s) and advances in the literature in the subsequent two decades so that the CORE-R would be suitable for both clinical practice and research endeavors. The CORE-R is divided into three main sections related to materials and measures that can assist a clinician in: (a) starting a group and/or preparing group members, (b) assessing group member outcomes, and (c) tracking group-level processes. Regarding point a, the CORE-R is primarily focused on the beginning group leader who may be less familiar with how to set up a group and select members. This section identifies empirically and clinically grounded principles for selecting group members and preparing them for treatment in a group format. Regarding the outcome of group member, it is noted that outcome measures allow therapists to supplement their clinical judgment regarding client progress with information about client change derived from formal assessments. The CORE-R Task Force only suggests measures which are brief, comprehensive, easy to administer, optimally free from theoretical biases, sensitive to change (with established reliability and validity), and widely used (i.e., the Outcome Questionnaire [OQ-45], and the Inventory of Interpersonal Problems [IIP]; see Lambert et al. 1996; Horowitz et al. 2000). The process section of the CORE-R relied on the model developed empirically by Johnson et al. (2005), which found three main components of group psychotherapy process (positive bonding relationship, positive working relationship, negative relationship). The analysis of group process may provide clinicians with important distinctions concerning the quality of the group functions and the fostering of a therapeutic environment. This process not only examines the interactions between group members but also the interactions of the therapist and the group itself.

The second document developed by a task force of the AGPA is the *clinical practice guidelines for group psychotherapy* (CPG) which "is intended to be a relevant, flexible, accessible, and practical document that respects practitioners and the clinical context of their work" (Bernard et al. 2008, p. 457). These guidelines are distinct from treatment guidelines, and aim to augment, not to supplant, the clinical judgment of group practitioners. The CPG addressed some core issues of group psychotherapy, such as creating a successful therapy group from the perspectives of clients, therapists, and referral sources; understanding mechanisms of action in group psychotherapy; selection of clients and composition of therapy groups; pre-group preparation and training; group process and development; and therapist's interventions.

Taken together, these two documents support practitioners of group psychotherapy to meet the appropriate demands for evidence-based practice and greater accountability in the practice of contemporary psychotherapy.

Finally, it is noteworthy that despite an increase in qualitative methods and studies, the arrival of qualitative approaches into mainstream research on group psychotherapy remains tentative. We agree with Dattilio et al. (2010) that "information from controlled studies on the efficacy of treatments needs to be complemented by information about the contexts in which the treatments are delivered and the processes set in motion in their delivery. A balanced picture can only be achieved by gathering information by means of a range of methods, both quantitative and qualitative, and synthesizing it reflectively and critically" (p. 436). However, there is still a dearth of research investigating the effectiveness and process of group treatments by means of both quantitative and qualitative methods. The challenge of integrating science and practice in group psychotherapy is still alive.

Conclusion

In summary, this review highlighted some core issues in group psychotherapy research: (a) group psychotherapy has been shown to be effective for a variety of psychological disorders; (b) apart from questions regarding the effectiveness of group treatments, psychotherapy researchers have been interested in mechanisms of change for group therapy, and different components of group process have been investigated; (c) while there are important methodological improvements being made in group psychotherapy research studies, there is still room for improvement—needed improvements may include the use of: (a) some measures tied to past research increasing generalizability between studies, (b) increasingly complex hypotheses that simultaneously test multiple sources to explain outcomes, and (c) increasingly complex analytic models (Burlingame et al. 2004). Although there is much to be done to improve the group psychotherapy literature, much has been accomplished, and important advances are being made.

References

Bakali J, Baldwin S, Lorentzen S (2009) Modeling group process constructs at three stages of group psychotherapy. Psychother Res 19:332–343

Baldwin SA, Murray DM, Shadish WR (2005) Empirically supported treatments or Type-I errors? Problems with the analysis of data from group administered treatments. J Consult Clin Psychol 73:924–935. doi:10.1037/0022-006X.73.5.924

Baldwin SA, Stice E, Rohde P (2008) Statistical analysis of group-administered intervention data: reanalysis of two randomized trials. Psychother Res 18:365–376. doi:10.1080/10503300701796992

Beck A, Lewis CS (2000) The process of group psychotherapy: systems for analyzing change. American Psychological Association, Washington, DC

Bednar RL, Kaul TJ (1994) Experimental group research: can the cannon fire? In: Bergin AE, Garfield SL (eds) Handbook of psychotherapy and behaviour change, 4th edn. Wiley, New York, pp 631–663

Bernard H, Burlingame MG, Flores P, Greene L, Joyce A, Kobos JC et al (2008) Clinical practice guidelines for group psychotherapy. Int J Group Psychother 58:455–542. doi:10.1521/ijgp.2008.58.4.455

Blay SL, Vel Fucks JS, Barruzi M et al (2002) Effectiveness of time-limited psychotherapy for minor psychiatric disorders. Randomised controlled trial evaluating immediate v. long-term effects. Br J Psychiatry 180:416–422

Bormann B, Strauss B (2007) Gruppenklima, Kohasion, Allianz und Empathie als Komponenten der therapeutischen Beziehung in Gruppenpsychotherapien-Uberprufung eines Mehrebenen-Modells. Gruppenpsychother Gr 43:1–20

Budman SH, Soldz S, Demby A, Feldstein M, Springer T, Davis MS (1989) Cohesion, alliance, and outcome in group psychotherapy. Psychiatry 52:339–350

Burlingame GM (2010) Small group treatments: introduction to special section. Psychother Res 20:1–7. doi:10.1080/10503301003596551

Burlingame GM, McClendon D (2010) Sensitivity groups. In: Levine JM, Hogg MA (eds) Encyclopedia of group processes and intergroup relations. Sage, London

Burlingame GM, Fuhriman A, Barlow S (1994) Clinical application of empirical research to the practice of group psychotherapy. Invited presentation to Intermountain Health Care, Salt Lake City, UT

Burlingame GM, Earnshaw D, Hoag M, Barlow SH, Richardson EJ, Donnell AJ, Villani J (2002a) A systematic program to enhance clinician group skills in an inpatient psychiatric hospital. Int J Group Psychother 52(4):555–587. doi:10.1521/ijgp.52.4.555.45523

Burlingame GM, Furhiman A, Johnson J (2002b) Cohesion in group psychotherapy. In: Norcross J (ed) A guide to psychotherapy relationships that work. Oxford University Press, Oxford, pp 71–88

Burlingame GM, Fuhriman A, Mosier J (2003) The differential effectiveness of group psychotherapy: a meta-analytic prospective. Group Dyn Theor Res 7:3–12. doi:10.1037/1089-2699.7.1.3

Burlingame GM, MacKenzie KR, Strauss B (2004) Small group treatment: evidence for effectiveness and mechanisms of change. In: Lambert M (ed) Handbook of psychotherapy and behavior change. Wiley, New York, pp 647–696

Burlingame GM, Strauss B, Joyce A, MacNair-Semands-R, MacKenzie KR, Ogrodniczuk J et al (2006) Core battery–revised. An assessment tool kit for promoting optimal group selection, process and outcome. American Group Psychotherapy Association, New York

Burlingame GM, Strauss B, Borman B, Johnson J (2008a) Are there common change mechanisms for all small group treatments? A conceptual model for change mechanisms inherent in small groups. Gruppenpsychother Gr 44(3):177–241

Burlingame GM, Strauss B, Hwang AD (2008b) La Core-battery-revised dell'American group psychotherapy association. In: Lo Coco G, Prestano C, Lo Verso G (eds) L'efficacia clinica delle psicoterapie di gruppo. Raffaello Cortina, Milan, pp 183–194

Burlingame G, McClendon D, Alonso J (2011) Cohesion in group psychotherapy. In: Norcross JC (ed) A guide to psychotherapy relationships that work, 2nd edn. Oxford University Press, Oxford

Burlingame GM, Strauss B, Joyce AS (2013) Change mechanisms and effectiveness of small group treatments. In: Lambert MJ (ed) Bergin and Garfield's handbook of psychotherapy and behavior change, 6th edn. Wiley, New York, pp 640–689

Butler T, Fuhriman A (1983) Curative factors in group therapy: a review of the recent literature. Small Group Res 14:131–142

Castonguay LG, Pincus AL, Agras WS, Hines CE (1998) The role of emotion in group cognitive-behavioral therapy for binge-eating disorder: when things have to feel worse before they get better. Psychother Res 8:225–238. doi:10.1093/ptr/8.2.225

Chapman CL, Baker EL, Porter G, Thayer SD, Burlingame GM (2010) Rating group therapist interventions: the validation of the group psychotherapy intervention rating scale. Group Dyn Theor Res 14:15–31

Dattilio FM, Edwards DJA, Fishman DB (2010) Case studies within a mixed methods paradigm: toward a resolution of the alienation between researcher and practitioners in psychotherapy research. Psychother Theory Res Pract Train 47:427–441. doi:10.1037/a0021181

Davies DR, Burlingame MJ, Johnson JE, Gleave RL, Barlow SH (2008) The effects of a feedback intervention on group process and outcome. Group Dyn Theor Res 12:141–154. doi:10.1037/1089-2699.12.2.141

Dinger U, Schauenburg H (2010) Effects of individual cohesion and patient interpersonal style on outcome in psychodynamically oriented inpatient group psychotherapy. Psychother Res 20:22–29. doi:10.1080/10503300902855514

Gillaspy JA, Wright AR, Campbell C, Stokes S, Adinoff B (2002) Group alliance and cohesion as predictors of drug and alcohol abuse treatment outcomes. Psychother Res 12:213–229. doi:10.1093/ptr/12.2.213

Harmon SC, Lambert MJ, Smart DM, Hawkins E, Nielsen SL, Slade K, Lutz W (2007) Enhancing outcome for potential treatment failures: therapist-client feedback and clinical support tools. Psychother Res 17:379–392. doi:10.1080/10503300600702331

Hawkins EJ, Lambert MJ, Vermeersch DA, Slade K, Tuttle K (2004) The effects of providing patient progress information to therapists and patients. Psychother Res 14:308–327. doi:10.1093/ptr/kph027

Horowitz LM, Alden LE, Wiggins JS, Pincus AL (2000) Inventory of interpersonal problems (IIP-32/IIP-64). Psychological Corporation, London

Horvath AO (1994) Empirical validation of Bordin's pantheoretical model of the alliance: the working alliance inventory perspective. In: Horvath AO, Greenberg LS (eds) The working alliance: theory, research, and practice. Wiley, New York, pp 109–130

Imel ZE, Baldwin SA, MacCoon DG, Bonus K (2008) Beyond the individual: an investigation of group effects in a mindfulness based stress reduction program. Psychother Res 18:735–742. doi:10.1080/10503300802326038

Johnson JE, Burlingame GM, Olsen J, Davies DR, Gleave R (2005) Group climate, cohesion, alliance, and empathy in group psychotherapy: multilevel structural equation models. J Couns Psychol 52:310–321. doi:10.1037/0022-0167.52.3.310

Johnson JE, Pulsipher D, Ferrin SL, Burlingame GM, Davies DR, Gleave R (2006) Measuring group processes: a comparison of the GCQ and CCI. Group Dyn Theor Res 10:136–145. doi:10.1037/1089-2699.10.2.136

Johnson JE, Burlingame MG, Strauss B, Bormann B (2008) Die therapeutischen Beziehungen in der Gruppenpsychotherapie (Therapeutic relationships in group psychotherapy). Gruppenpsychother Gr 44:52–89

Joyce AS, Piper WE, Ogrodniczuk JS (2007) Therapeutic alliance and cohesion variables as predictors of outcome in short-term group psychotherapy. Int J Group Psychother 57:269–296. doi:10.1521/ijgp.2007.57.3.269

Kenny ME, Lomax R, Brabeck M, Fife J (1998) Longitudinal pathways linking adolescent reports of maternal and paternal attachments to psychological well-being. J Early Adolesc 18(3):104–125. doi:10.1177/0272431698018003001

Kenny ME, Waldo M, Warter E, Barton K (2002) School-linked prevention: theory, science and practice for enhancing the lives of children and youth. Couns Psychol 30:726–748. doi:10.1177/0011000002305004

Kipnes DR, Piper WE, Joyce AS (2002) Cohesion and outcome in short-term psychodynamic groups for complicated grief. Int J Group Psychother 52:483–509. doi:10.1521/ijgp.52.4.483.45525

Kivlighan DM, Goldfine DC (1991) Endorsement of therapeutic factors as a function of stage of group development and participant interpersonal attitudes. J Couns Psychol 38:150–158. doi:10.1037//0022-0167.38.2.150

Kosters M, Burlingame GM, Nachtigall C, Strauss B (2006) A meta-analytic review of the effectiveness of inpatient group psychotherapy. Group Dyn Theor Res 10:146–163. doi:10.1037/1089-2699.10.2.146

Lambert MJ, Ogles BM (2004) The efficacy and effectiveness of psychotherapy. In: Lambert MJ (ed) Handbook of psychotherapy and behaviour change, 5th edn. Wiley, New York, pp 139–193

Lambert MJ, Burlingame GM, Umphress V, Hansen NB, Vermeersch DA, Clouse GC, Yanchar SC (1996) The reliability and validity of the outcome questionnaire. Clin Psychol Psychother 3:249–258. doi:10.1002/(SICI)1099-0879(199612)3:4<249::AID-CPP106>3.0.CO;2-S

Lese KP, Macnair-Semands RR (2000) The therapeutic factors inventory: development of a scale. Group 24:303–317

Lo Coco G, Gullo S, Kivlighan DM Jr (2012) Examining patients' and other group members' agreement about their alliance to the group as a whole and changes in patient symptoms using response surface analysis. J Couns Psychol 59:197–207. doi:10.1037/a0027560

Lorentzen S, Hoglend P (2004) Predictors of change during long-term analytic group psychotherapy. Psychother Psychosom 73:25–35. doi:10.1159/000074437

Lorentzen S, Hoglend P (2008) Moderators of the effects of treatment length in long-term psychodynamic group psychotherapy. Psychother Psychosom 77 (5):321–322. doi:10.1159/000147946

Lorentzen S, Sexton HC, Hogland P (2004) Therapeutic alliance, cohesion and outcome in a long-term analytic group. A preliminary study. Nord J Psychiat 58:33–40. doi:10.1080/08039480310000770

Martin D, Garske J, Davis M (2000) Relation of the therapeutic alliance with outcome and other variables: a meta-analytic review. J Consult Clin Psychol 68:438–450. doi:10.1037//0022-006X.68.3.438

Marziali E, Munroe-Blum H, McCleary L (1997) The contribution of group cohesion and group alliance to the outcome of group psychotherapy. Int J Group Psychother 47:475–497

McRoberts C, Burlingame GM, Hoag MJ (1998) Comparative efficacy of individual and group psychotherapy: a meta-analytic perspective. Group Dyn Theor Res 2 (2):101–117. doi:10.1037//1089-2699.2.2.101

Miles JR, Kivlighan DM (2008) Team cognition in group interventions: the relation between co-leaders' shared mental models and group climate. Group Dyn Theor Res 12:191–209. doi:10.1037/1089-2699.12.3.191

Miles JR, Kivlighan DM (2010) Co-leader similarity and group climate in group interventions: testing the co-leadership, team cognition-team diversity model. Group Dyn Theor Res 14:114–122. doi:10.1037/a0017503

Murray DM, Blitstein JL (2003) Methods to reduce the impact of intraclass correlation in group-randomized trials. Eval Rev 27(1):79–103. doi:10.1177/0193841X02239019

Norcross JC, Beutler LE, Levant RF (eds) (2006) Evidence-based practices in mental health: debate and dialogue on the fundamental questions. American Psychological Association, Washington, DC

Oei TPS, Browne A (2006) Components of group processes: Have they contributed to the outcome of mood and anxiety disorder patients in a group cognitive-behaviour therapy program? Am J Psychother 60:53–70

Ogrodniczuk JS, Piper WE, Joyce AS (2006) Treatment compliance among patients with personality disorders receiving group psychotherapy: What are the roles of interpersonal distress and cohesion? Psychiatry 69:249–261. doi:10.1521/psyc.2006.69.3.249

Phipps LB, Zastowny TR (1988) Leadership behavior, group climate and outcome in group psychotherapy: a study of outpatient psychotherapy groups. Group 12:157–171. doi:10.1007/BF01456565

Piper WE, Ogrodniczuk JS, Azim HF, Weideman R (2001) Prevalence of loss and complicated grief among psychiatric outpatients. Psychiat Serv 52:1069–1074. doi:10.1176/appi.ps.52.8.1069

Piper WE, Ogrodniczuk JS, Joyce AS, Weideman R, Rosie JS (2007) Group composition and group therapy for complicated grief. J Consult Clin Psychol 75:116–125. doi:10.1037/0022-006X.75.1.116

Prestano C, Lo Coco G, Gullo S, Lo Verso G (2008) Group-analytic therapy for eating disorders: preliminary results in a single-group study. Eur Eat Disord Rev 16:302–310. doi:10.1002/erv.871

Roberts C, Roberts SA (2005) Design and analysis of clinical trials with clustering effects due to treatment. Clin Trials 2:152–162. doi:10.1191/1740774505cn076oa

Strauss B, Burgmeier-Lohse M (1994) Prozess-Ergebnis-Zusammenhänge in der analytisch orientierten Gruppenpsychotherapie. Psychotherapeut 39:239–250

Tasca GA, Balfour L, Ritchie K, Bissada H (2006) Developmental changes in group climate in two types of group therapy for binge-eating disorder: a growth curve analysis. Psychother Res 16(4):499–514. doi:10.1080/10503300600593359

Tasca GA, Illing V, Joyce AS, Ogrodniczuk JS (2009) Three-level multilevel growth models for nested change data: a guide for group treatment researchers. Psychother Res 19(4–5):453–461. doi:10.1080/10503300902933188

Valbak K (2003) Specialised psychotherapeutic group analysis: How do we make group analysis suitable for 'non-suitable' patients? Group Anal 36 (1):73–86

Wampold B, Serlin RC (2000) The consequence of ignoring a nested factor on measures of effect size in analysis of variance designs. Psychol Methods 5:425–433. doi:10.1037//1082-989X.5.4.425

Whipple JL, Lambert MJ, Vermeersch DA, Smart DW, Nielsen SL, Hawkins EJ (2003) Improving the effects of psychotherapy: the use of early identification of treatment failure and problem-solving strategies in routine practice. J Couns Psychol 50:59–68. doi:10.1037//0022-0167.50.1.59

Wilberg T, Karterud S, Pedersen G, Urnes O, Irion T, Brabrand J, Haavaldsen G, Leirvag H, Johnsen K, Andreasen H, Hedmark H, Stubbhaug B (2003) Outpatient group psychotherapy following day treatment for patients with personality disorders. J Pers Disord 17:510–521. doi:10.1521/pedi.17.6.510.25357

Yalom ID (1995) The theory and practice of group psychotherapy, 4th edn. Basic Books, New York

Yalom I, Leszcz M (2005) The theory and practice of group psychotherapy, 5th edn. Basic Books, New York

The Process of Change in Psychotherapy: Common and Unique Factors

15

Andrew A. McAleavey and Louis G. Castonguay

Contents

Abstract

As a field, psychotherapy has long been dominated by the different types (or orientations) of psychological therapies in practice. Though there are hundreds if not thousands of different kinds of psychotherapy, in many ways some are quite similar—they share some common factors. In other ways, each orientation may possess some unique elements, or combinations of elements not found in most other kinds of therapy: unique factors. In this chapter, we describe how the theoretical and empirical discussions of common and unique factors have progressed historically, highlighting major contributions in identifying and organizing the influential components and active ingredients of psychotherapy. It can be shown that both common factors and more unique factors can be reliably identified, and that these factors can be linked with outcome, and may both be necessary to the successful application of any psychological therapy. Ultimately, the distinction between "common" and "unique" factors may be a false dichotomy when comparing many face-to-face psychotherapies, because neither common factors nor unique factors can exist without the other. Common factors rely on specific treatments, and unique factors exist in the context of common variables.

A.A. McAleavey (✉)
Department of Psychology, The Pennsylvania State University, 346 Moore Building, University Park, PA 16802, USA
e-mail: aam239@psu.edu

L.G. Castonguay
Department of Psychology, The Pennsylvania State University, 308 Moore Building, University Park, PA 16802, USA

O.C.G. Gelo et al. (eds.), *Psychotherapy Research*,
DOI 10.1007/978-3-7091-1382-0_15, © Springer-Verlag Wien 2015

15.1 The Process of Change in Psychotherapy: Common and Unique Factors

Over the last century we have seen a proliferation of varieties of psychotherapy, many with vastly different scopes and aims. This proliferation seems to have been both a cause and effect of an equally astounding number of researchers, theoreticians, and clinicians specializing and honing their practices in increasingly diverse ways. The increasing demands from governmental, healthcare, and research organizations in recent years have led to pressure on these many camps to demonstrate that their practices are effective, or else suffer the possibility of limited reimbursement, loss of clientele, or both. Despite this increased scrutiny on individual psychotherapies, it has been noted for several decades that many psychotherapies that are theoretically different (at least according to their proponents) in fact share many attributes. Rosenzweig (1936) is often regarded as one of the first to have addressed this issue, and his short article foreshadowed major themes of comparative psychotherapy research to the present: psychotherapies that are different do indeed have many similar features, and these similar features may be responsible in some way for the fact that proponents of many treatments report success. As he wrote: "besides the intentionally utilized methods and their consciously held theoretical foundations there are inevitably certain unrecognized factors in any therapeutic situation–factors that may be even more important than those being purposely employed" (p. 412). Still today, writers concerned with documenting and explaining the effects of psychotherapy have been faced with a central question: Are the effects of diverse psychotherapies due to those elements that make them unique (or specific), or are they better explained by what these diverse approaches share with one another?

While much can be said about the so-called Dodo bird verdict (Luborsky et al. 1975)—the finding that several kinds of psychotherapy produce roughly equivalent outcomes across a range of disorders—which itself is still a focus of hot debate (e.g., Crits-Christoph 1997; Norcross 1995; Wampold 2001), the subject matter of this chapter is only tangentially related to it. Though many authors view outcome equivalence as the main reason to study common factors in psychotherapy, we cheerfully disagree. Regardless of outcome, it is noncontroversial to say that psychotherapies of many origins share several features of process and content, and it follows that better understanding the patterns of these commonalities may be an important part of better understanding the effects of psychotherapy. That is, irrespective of whether some psychotherapies are equivalent to others in symptomatic outcome, understanding what part of clients' improvement is due to factors that are shared by several approaches appears to us to be a conceptually and clinically important question.

In this chapter we will examine the issue of whether common factors can be viewed as empirically and theoretically valuable, or whether they are epiphenomenal to the real work of psychotherapy. That is, are common factors real, and are they important to the therapeutic effect of psychotherapy? It is our distinct impression that the work that is undertaken in psychotherapy is much too complex and nuanced to describe common and unique factors as being mutually exclusive descriptions of psychotherapy process. Instead, we believe that the common and unique factors most likely work symbiotically (and sometimes parasitically) with one another, and it is likely that in any given psychotherapy both common and unique aspects will be present and potentially relevant. Importantly, studying the interaction of common and unique factors in psychotherapy is likely to be a productive path to improve psychotherapy as it is practiced around the world. Thus, in our opinion, the question of whether common or unique effects are more important than the other forecloses on the very reasonable conclusion that both are significant contributors to the therapeutic process, and both require further understanding.

15.2 Common Factors

15.2.1 Common vs. "Nonspecific" Factors

In this chapter we use the term "common factors" to refer to those elements of psychotherapy that are so frequently present in different psychotherapeutic treatments that they cannot be considered to be restricted to one school of psychotherapy (as discussed later, there are also some who have distinguished between common therapeutic factors and the relatively inert common factors). Though the term "common factors" has become increasingly popular, an alternative has also been present in the field: "nonspecific factors." While some authors have used the terms nonspecific and common interchangeably to refer to the construct we intend, "nonspecific" has additional meanings beyond "common," and at times some authors have used it to mean those elements of psychotherapy that are either somehow unspecified at present, inherently unspecifiable and therefore unobservable, or else elements of therapy that are auxiliary to the technical variables that are primarily responsible for producing therapeutic effects (Castonguay 1993). Many authors have suggested that since these statements are not generally true of the common factors anymore, the term "nonspecific" should be dropped from the lexicon entirely (e.g., Castonguay 1993; Castonguay and Grosse Holtforth 2005; Lampropoulos 2000; Omer and London 1989; Weinberger and Rasco 2007). As we will see, increasing evidence supports several common factors as specific contributors to the therapeutic process which have been identified, isolated, and sometimes manipulated, and the use of the term "nonspecific" to describe them constitutes an undeserved continued belittling of these important therapeutic elements.

15.2.2 Identification of Common Factors

Several attempts have been made to describe common factors of psychotherapy, based on the experience and expertise of preeminent researchers and clinicians. These attempts have been made by leaders from all orientations and schools of psychotherapy and differ in terms of scope and detail. Rosenzweig (1936) was certainly one of the first, and in his brief article he identified several possible factors that may operate across diverse therapies, including therapist adherence to a system of treatment, client developing some new understanding based on a coherent model of personality, and several "implicit" factors such as the therapist's personality and catharsis. Since Rosenzweig, several avenues of study regarding common factors have been followed.

In particular, a great debt is owed to several individuals who generated early lists and/or categories of common factors that have influenced later conceptual and empirical efforts. Though we refer later to a few works that have attempted to integrate and synthesize common factors into a single comprehensive and coherent framework, it is important to recognize the contributions of such influential figures as Frank (1961), Marmor (1976), Garfield (1980), Marks and Gelder (1966), Karasu (1986), Prochaska and DiClemente (1984), Sloane (1969), Masserman (1980), and Strupp (1973). These lists stimulated research and theory, with each taking a different approach to the common factors. Frank (1961) and Frank and Frank (1991) contributed a particularly influential list of several common factors and provided a rationale for their effects. Though few contemporary writers have maintained this distinction, Frank usefully divided the common factors into the common features (aspects of the situation, observable components behaviors of the participants, and so on) and common functions (impacts on the client; what the therapy does to the client that is different than ordinary life) of psychotherapy. This distinction itself is an important clarifying element in dialogue regarding common factors, since it highlights what has already been discussed: while many psychotherapeutic treatments share components or observable features (e.g., a helping relationship, a socially sanctioned healing setting), the debates surrounding common factors more frequently surround the question of common functions or impacts (e.g., the significance of corrective experiences and behavior change across treatments). Frank's four common features were a helpful relationship, a healing setting, a rationale or "myth" explaining the client's problems, and a "ritual" implied by the myth that is believed to help solve the problem. The six common functions that he proposed include a decrease in alienation through the therapeutic relationship, expectations of improvement, providing new learning experiences, emotional arousal, enhancing a sense of mastery and self-efficacy, and providing opportunities for practice (Frank and Frank 1991). Although published in a book that is now more than 50 years old, Frank's list has helped to spur one of today's zeitgeists in psychotherapy: identifying, exploring, and explaining factors that cut across different theoretical orientations.

15.2.3 Integration of Common Factors

As the number of lists of common factors has increased, perhaps to the point that these "lists of lists" have become unwieldy (Castonguay 2009), several authors have attempted to organize and understand the common factors by integrating them using empirical and theoretical means. In this chapter we will focus our discussion on a few empirical approaches to documenting common factors and then describe two particularly important systems for understanding common factors that have influenced the field greatly.

One important empirical contribution is the work of Grencavage and Norcross (1990), who systematically reviewed the literature for any mentions of common factors and then divided them into thematically similar categories of common factors. These authors identified 89 distinct factors in 50 published works, which they divided into five categories: client characteristics, therapist qualities, change processes, treatment structure, and therapeutic relationship. These categories were derived from the authors' reading of the theoretical literature and are therefore quite consistent with much of the extant literature itself. Interestingly, only one of these five categories clearly corresponds with Frank's (1961) common functions of psychotherapy, while the rest may be defined as primarily common features.

Tracey et al. (2003) reported a different attempt to understand the varieties of common factors that have been identified, and in this study they used statistical dimension-reduction strategies. These authors took as their starting point the 35 commonalities identified by at least 10 % of the sample reported in Grencavage and Norcross (1990), and they then had experienced professionals and expert researchers rate these common factors for similarities. The resulting data was amenable to scaling and cluster analysis, and rather than the five categories identified by Grencavage and Norcross (1990), Tracey et al. identified three distinct clusters of common factors: bond, information, and structure. This suggests that, in terms of how psychotherapy experts think of common factors, there are essentially three different types of common factors: those related to the therapeutic relationship (e.g., warmth), those related to specific information and conceptual knowledge (e.g., direct feedback), and those related to the roles of psychotherapy (e.g., being a healer). This is a stark departure from the 89 initially found by Grencavage and Norcross (1990) and even compared to the five superordinate categories that they identified. It should be noted that this study suggests that these clusters share features in common, not that they are the same factors.

Common factors have also been identified using methods of factor analysis and self-report measures. In one recent example, McCarthy and Barber (2009) reported the development of the Multitheoretical List of Therapeutic Interventions (MULTI), which is a self-report and observer-rated measure of therapist behaviors. They developed the instrument using input from experts in several orientations of psychotherapy and showed that the subscales of this measure differentiate between seven orientations of psychotherapy and common factors in terms of the reported therapist techniques. On the MULTI, the common factors subscale comprises items on basic helping skills and relationship maintenance behaviors like focused listening and general warmth. Interestingly, in their studies and that of Boswell et al. (2010), the common factors subscale of the MULTI has been rated as more prevalent than any theory-specific subscale across several therapeutic orientations—that is, therapists in these samples typically use common factors as much or more than other techniques, when measured on the MULTI. Similarly, Larsson et al. (2010) reported another effort that identified common factors based on therapist self-report, but rather than reported or rated therapist behaviors, the Valuable Elements in Psychotherapy Questionnaire (VEP-Q) which these authors developed is based on therapists' attitudes about what is most helpful in therapy. The authors showed that the VEP-Q differentiated between cognitive-behavioral and psychodynamic therapists in terms of how much they value orientation-specific mechanisms, but these psychotherapists did not differ on how much they valued the common factors items included in the VEP-Q (which include items on the alliance, empathy, positive regard, and goals of therapy). Interestingly, psychotherapists who were treating more clients valued common factors more, holding all other variables constant. Other studies have also identified commonalities across types of psychotherapy using therapist self-report, for instance, in terms of therapists' intentions across treatment types (e.g., Hill and O'Grady 1985). Such quantitative measures provide evidence that common factors can be empirically identified as specific therapeutic interventions that cut across therapies and that, on the whole, therapists of different orientations seem to value them roughly equally.

Thus, while the number of essential common factors is in question, empirical evidence appears to support that certain aspects of psychotherapy, including both circumstances and processes of therapy, are present in many types of psychotherapy. How we understand these common factors and their operations in psychotherapy, however, is a more difficult question than whether we can simply observe them. Although several authors have offered reviews of common factors and/or models of psychotherapy based on these factors (e.g., Castonguay 2006; Weinberger 1995), two particular systems of understanding have inspired much of the theoretical and empirical work on common factors in recent decades: the Generic Model of Psychotherapy and principles of change.

15.2.3.1 The Generic Model

The work of David Orlinsky, Ken Howard, and their colleagues has been indescribably important to the study of common factors and psychotherapy process more broadly. These authors produced some important early empirical research on sessions of psychotherapy (e.g., Orlinsky and Howard 1967) and have developed a unifying framework by inductively reading the psychotherapy process research literature, known as the Generic Model of Psychotherapy, that has been applied around the world. Since one of the original purposes of this model was to organize the results of psychotherapy research studies, this model has been designed and revised so as to be inclusive of all psychotherapy events as well as extra-therapeutic environments and conditions. Recently summarized by Orlinsky et al. (2004) and Orlinsky (2009), the Generic Model categorizes processes of psychotherapy into six categories: therapeutic contract, therapeutic operations, therapeutic bond, self-relatedness, in-session impacts, and temporal patterns. While these categories are broad, they are designed to describe and organize a complex system of interconnected events, personalities, and interactions. One of the impacts of attempting to inclusively describe all therapeutic context and activities is that the Generic Model inherently provides a framework for both identifying common factors of psychotherapy and identifying ways that theoretical orientations differ from one another. For instance, the therapeutic contract is seen in the Generic Model to be a common factor of psychotherapies. The contract itself may be quite different between a CBT and a psychodynamic treatment for depression, for instance, because in CBT the therapist is typically more didactic and directive than most psychodynamic treatments for depression (as in, for example, Jones and Pulos 1993). From a common factors perspective, however, the fact that the two treatments both create an unwritten contract regarding the role of the participants in therapy may be more significant than the differences between the two: the socialization process required by establishing a therapeutic contract in any particular model of therapy is a useful and necessary component of treatment.

The Generic Model has also inspired empirical research, such as the work of Kolden (1991, 1996) on process (e.g., client openness, therapist interventions, and therapeutic bond) and outcome (e.g., session progress). In addition, several other lines of research inspired by the Generic Model are worth noting, including dose effect and phase models of change in therapy (e.g., Howard et al. 1986, 1993) as well as patient-focused research (e.g., Lambert et al. 2001) and research on therapist effects (e.g., Lutz et al. 2007).

15.2.3.2 Principles of Change

A conceptually different paradigm for understanding common factors was put forward by Goldfried (1980), who suggested the organizing framework of *therapeutic principles* or *strategies of change*. Principles of change are likely, Goldfried suggests, to reveal more commonalities between psychotherapies because they occupy a conceptual middle ground between theories of change (how therapists suppose that meaningful change comes about, which varies widely between therapeutic approaches) and psychotherapy techniques (the interventions derived from or prescribed by the theories of change, which may also vary widely across orientations). Principles, Goldfried suggests, represent somewhat more universal aims of psychotherapies: short-term goals of therapists of nearly all orientations. This is similar to the distinction between tactics and strategies: the former representing the small-scale constituent steps (techniques) which are contextually dependent and different in every situation, whereas the latter represent general intentions or goals in the absence of any specific context (principles) but which may be applied to a situation by using any number of tactics.

Goldfried proposed five common strategies, based on clinical reasoning and a broad reading of the theoretical and empirical literature: providing the possibility of corrective experiences and new behaviors, feedback from the therapist to the client to promote new understanding in the client, promoting an expectation that psychotherapy can be helpful (that is, hope and expectancy that the client will get better), establishing the desired therapeutic alliance and relationship, and promoting ongoing reality testing by the client (Goldfried 1980; Goldfried and Padawer 1982). These principles are not meant to be inclusively descriptive of the events in psychotherapy as the Generic Model is but instead provide two noteworthy contributions with regard to the process of change. First, and as described in more detail later, they challenge the false dichotomy between common factors and unique variables by showing that some elements of therapy can be both transtheoretical (as general strategies of intervention) and unique (as when they manifest in particular ways within specific approaches). Second, they allow therapists to broaden their clinical repertoire by informing them that they can use a wide range of therapeutic procedures to achieve important therapeutic goals such as improving clients' interpersonal functioning. Thus, therapists may be more easily able to assimilate interventions that are not typically emphasized in their preferred theoretical orientation.

Goldfried showed that using principles of change, it is possible to understand why different techniques may have similar (and similarly beneficial) effects. In some ways this is the opposite side of what Messer (1986) described as "choice points" that distinguish the techniques of various therapy orientations. Messer suggested that psychotherapists of different orientations elect interventions in order to pursue theory-specific goals, whereas Goldfried's (1980) concept of principles of change suggests that sometimes the goals that therapists pursue (the clinical strategies) are the same across orientations, but it is the techniques and theory of change that are distinct to a given theory. Goldfried gives the example of psychoanalysts and behavior therapists who have noticed that the simple process of paying close attention to one's thoughts or behaviors often leads to new understandings on the parts of their patients (p. 995). Here, the intention and effect can be identical across two overtly different psychotherapy orientations, whereas the techniques that these psychotherapists use are effectively quite varied (free-associative analysis and daily monitoring of explicit behaviors). Thus, the common factors between psychotherapies may not be obvious on the level of techniques but may emerge when studying a deeper level of strategies and principles.

In fact, one of the lasting legacies of Goldfried's (1980) work has been an increase in empirical investigations of the process of change. The introduction of principles was partially responsible for a de-emphasis on technique as the only relevant process variables, including an increase in the study of the therapist's focus of intervention (Hill 2009). For instance, the Coding System of Therapist Feedback (CSTF, Goldfried MR, Newman CF, Hayes AF (1989) The coding system of therapeutic focus. Unpublished manuscript, State University of New York at Stony Brook) was developed and has been used to rate therapist comments across a range of psychotherapy orientations. Goldfried et al. (1998) used the CSTF to rate pre-defined high- and low-significance segments of psychotherapy sessions by master therapists of either cognitive-behavioral (CBT) or psychodynamic-interpersonal (PI) psychotherapy. They found that orientation was only significantly related to a few foci of intervention (e.g., CBT therapists focused more on between-session experiences, while PI therapists focused more on the therapist themselves) but that clinical significance of the segment was related to many differences. For instance, compared to the nonsignificant segments, during segments they identified as being highly significant therapists focused more on themselves, connections between time periods and people in the clients' life, new information, and the future. There were very few significant interaction effects, which in sum suggests that these therapists did not select different foci of intervention on the basis of their therapeutic orientation alone, but rather, the moments of psychotherapy identified as significant by both groups of therapists tended to have different foci than the less-significant segments. That is, master therapists from different orientations appear to focus on similar topics in general, but in moments of clinical significance, they focus on different topics than their usual while continuing to appear similar to one another. In part because of findings like this, Goldfried's work on principles of change has also been regarded as one of the key catalysts of the psychotherapy integration movement (e.g., Wachtel 2009), which has certainly come to define a major trend in psychotherapy for the last 30 years (Castonguay 2009).

15.2.4 Common Factors and Outcome

While it is clear that common factors of psychotherapy can be identified and studied empirically, the fact that diverse psychotherapies share certain features does not necessarily mean that these features actually promote positive outcomes in psychotherapy. Lampropoulos (2000) discussed this issue in some depth in a thoughtful summary of the difference between "common factors" and "common therapeutic factors," the latter of which is a label he reserved for those commonalities that have been shown to be important to the process of change. Some common factors of psychotherapy may be ubiquitous for reasons other than their efficacy, one example being the typical length of psychotherapy sessions (frequently 45 or 50 min long), which may have started as early as psychotherapy itself but now is often perpetuated more by expectations and demands on participants' time from other activities rather than because it has been clearly demonstrated that 50 min represents an optimal dose of psychotherapy. Though 50 min is a common time, there is no sufficient evidence to say that this common factor produces psychotherapeutic change itself.

Although many common factors now have at least some empirical support as correlates or facilitators of change, many (or possibly most) have not been the focus of enough empirical research to either support or refute the significance of their role. Weinberger and Rasco (2007) provide a similar distinction and concept in what they call "empirically supported common factors." They discuss five such empirically supported common factors: the therapeutic relationship, expectations of treatment effectiveness, confronting the problem (exposure), mastery or control experiences, and attribution of therapeutic outcome. This list is hardly intended to be inclusive but rather to capture those elements of therapy that have been found to be generally beneficial and organize them in a coherent way. Lambert and Ogles (2004) provide a longer list of 32 common factors, divided into three presumed phases of treatment (p. 173). These authors contend that each of these factors has received empirical support in relation to outcome and that the process of therapy progresses in part by the provision of these common factors.

While it is clear that there are numerous reasonable approaches to this topic, in this chapter we will limit our discussion to a less-than-comprehensive discussion of the empirical support for common factors in order to accommodate a discussion of their context. Therefore, we will focus on a subset of the factors that have received recent support and accept the fact that we cannot do justice to certain common factors, despite their importance. The factors that we will touch on are Rogers' facilitative conditions and the therapeutic alliance.

15.2.4.1 Rogers' Facilitative Conditions

One of the most significant conceptualizations of the therapeutic relationship is Rogers' (1957) assertion that genuineness (congruence), accurate empathy, and unconditional positive regard are the necessary and sufficient conditions of therapeutic change (see also Chap. 11). Since this assertion, these facilitative conditions have been the focus of much research. When the American Psychological Association's Division of Psychotherapy Task Force on empirically supported therapeutic relationships organized their findings (Norcross 2002), the significance of Rogers' contribution was clear, as this task force devoted separate reviews to the effects of empathy (Bohart et al. 2002), positive regard (Farber and Lane 2002), and congruence (Klein et al. 2002). Based on these and other literature reviews (e.g., Asay and Lambert 1999; Lambert et al. 1978; Orlinsky et al. 1994), Rogers' (1957) facilitative conditions have been linked to outcome across therapeutic orientations and numerous clinical problems.

These findings have been supported by recent meta-analyses. Specifically, Elliott et al. (2011) reported a meta-analytic effect size (r) of .31 for empathy, Farber and Doolin (2011) reported $r = 0.27$ for positive regard, and Kolden et al. (2011) reported $r = 0.24$ for congruence/genuineness. Conventionally, an r value of 0.10 is considered small, 0.30 is considered medium, and 0.50 is considered large, in the psychological sciences. At first glance, therefore these effect sizes may be unimpressive—they are small to medium sized. However, aside from the fact that numerous factors impact psychotherapy outcomes, creating very "noisy" data, small correlations between process and outcome may be obtained even when the processes under investigation are important to therapy outcome. Stiles (1988) clearly described the confound of therapist responsiveness: a nonsignificant correlation between process and outcome would be expected if the process being investigated was consistently being started and stopped in good outcome cases, modulated by the therapist to fit the client's needs and resources. This is consistent with what Horvath and Luborsky (1993) suggested regarding the alliance (which is discussed below): small overall correlations between the alliance measured at several times in therapy might be small, even smaller than the correlation would be with some specific early sessions, due to the hypothesized rupture-repair cycle that is thought to characterize successful cases of therapy. Thus, though the effect sizes of these correlations are often low, there may be reason to believe that the relatively consistent positive correlations reflect meaningful relationships between therapist facilitative conditions and outcome.

As an example, one prominent study that has influenced much of the subsequent psychotherapy research was that of Sloane et al. (1975), who conducted retrospective assessment with clients of psychodynamic psychotherapy and cognitive-behavioral therapy. Part of this process included asking clients about what aspects of their therapy they perceive to have been most beneficial to their treatment. Perhaps surprisingly, clients in both treatments identified many similar aspects of treatment as useful, nearly all of which were related to the therapy relationship and provision of basic conditions such as an understanding therapist to talk to. This suggests that, at least from the clients' perspective, relationship factors are particularly important to the process of successful therapy across treatments. Since the publication of this investigation, numerous other studies have produced similar findings, suggesting that relationship variables like empathy are related to outcome across many kinds of psychotherapy (e.g., Burns and Nolen-Hoeksema 1992).

More recently, Hoffart et al. (2009) conducted a study of residential group and individual psychotherapy for social phobia. In this study the authors had patients and therapists rate several common factors (including therapist empathy, alliance, and patient expectancies) at multiple times during treatment and also assessed symptomatic outcomes during treatment simultaneously. Using advanced statistical techniques, the authors concluded that there is general support for several common factors influencing subsequent symptomatic improvement, as evidenced for the fact that change in the common factors predicted subsequent decrease in symptoms. The authors also found some support for certain feedback loops from improved symptomatic functioning to stronger ratings of common factors, suggesting that positive therapeutic processes are self-perpetuating with improved outcome.

Drawing conclusions about direct or indirect causation between these relationship variables in psychotherapy is often difficult or impossible due to the frequency of correlational rather than experimental designs in this literature. However, some noteworthy studies have provided the empirical background for such a position. In an early attempt to assess its effect, Morris and Suckerman (1974) conducted an experimental study of therapist warmth. These authors found that systematic desensitization was more effective at reducing snake phobia when conducted by a warm therapist (speaking softly, expressing concern) than by a cold therapist, though the technique itself was delivered in both instances. Interestingly, these results were not consistent across all behavioral techniques tested using similar methods, for instance, Morris and Magrath (1979) reported opposite results for contact desensitization. Unfortunately, very few true experimental studies like these one have been conducted on common factors of therapy, and the reasons for the observed differences are not clear. Despite some limitations in the literature, these and other studies certainly suggest that the continued emphasis on basic therapeutic relationship variables in the clinical and research literature is likely appropriate.

15.2.4.2 The Therapeutic Alliance

Perhaps the most prominent common factor investigated in psychotherapy research is the therapeutic alliance, a multifaceted construct that has been the subject of over 1,000 empirical findings (Orlinsky et al. 2004) and several volumes (e.g., Barber and Muran 2010; Horvath and Greenberg 1994) (see also Chaps. 11 and 16). The therapeutic alliance is clearly related to the provision of the facilitative conditions discussed above, but it has a distinct theoretical history and meaning. The alliance is often defined by Bordin's (1979) tripartite model, encompassing the bond between client and therapist, agreement on the goals of treatment, and agreement on the tasks of treatment. While the alliance is derived from psychoanalytic theory and research (Constantino et al. 2002), in recent decades proponents of most, if not all, psychotherapy orientations have adopted the alliance in some way (Castonguay et al. 2006). The adoption of the therapeutic alliance across psychotherapeutic orientations has come in tandem with two facts: first, that the alliance has been operationalized and studied empirically in many treatments and settings, often correlating with outcome in diverse treatments; and second, the recognition that the therapeutic alliance may differ across therapies both in terms of its role in promoting change and the way that a "good" alliance may appear.

The first fact, that the alliance has been found to be empirically related to outcome in many forms of psychotherapy, has been the subject of the majority of discussion of the alliance. Most studies and meta-analyses in this topic have found that there is a relatively small but significant positive correlation between alliance measured early in therapy and overall symptom outcome: for instance, Martin et al. (2000) found the average correlation to be $r = 0.22$ across the samples they included, and Horvath et al. (2011) found an aggregate effect of $r = 0.275$. This effect size is not overwhelmingly large, but it appears to be a robust and consistent finding in such meta-analyses.

However, there continues to be considerable controversy about what this correlation means. Several authors have pointed out that since the alliance is often measured a few sessions into psychotherapy treatment, whereas outcome is typically assessed by comparing overall change from pre- to post-treatment, it may be the case that the alliance is partially a result of early symptomatic change (e.g., Barber et al. 2010). The intricacies surrounding this issue are complex and deserve attention on their own, but suffice it to say that when researchers have attempted to statistically control for prior symptom change in interpreting alliance-outcome correlations, results have been inconsistent (Barber 2009). This has sparked perhaps the most substantial debate surrounding the alliance: whether it is a cause of therapeutic change, an epiphenomenal result of productive therapy, or a combination of useful precursor and marker of productive psychotherapy. Because of the volume of work on the alliance as it relates to outcome, the equally important investigation of the different roles of the alliance across therapy orientations has been relatively obscured.

Nevertheless, it is worth nothing that proponents of many psychotherapy orientations have reported that the alliance is an important therapy process variable in their preferred orientation, including psychodynamic (Messer and Wolitzky 2010), cognitive-behavioral (Castonguay et al. 2010), and humanistic (Watson and Kalogerakos 2010) psychotherapies. Interestingly, particular orientations also emphasize and use the alliance slightly differently. For instance, Castonguay et al. (2010) and Watson and Kalogerakos (2010) both note that the development of more directive forms of their orientations has required that the relationship and alliance be used by therapists to facilitate adherence to the prescribed processes of the treatment, but these different authors also describe the unique mechanisms through which the alliance may itself be useful in CBT (e.g., as a vehicle for social learning and in vivo behavior-modification techniques) and in humanistic psychotherapy (e.g., facilitating the client's exploration and processing of emotions).

Thus, the relationship variables in diverse psychotherapies share much in common and also differ in meaningful ways. This dynamic interplay between common and unique factors is frequently overlooked, though it has become the focus of research in more recent years (Horvath and Bedi 2002). Because of their constantly and intrinsically enmeshed effects, no discussion of common factors is complete without a discussion of orientation-unique factors as well.

15.3 Unique Factors

Unique factors are those elements of a given type of psychotherapy that are uncommon, absent, or inert in other types of psychotherapy. Like common factors, unique factors can be divided into many different categories, including techniques (e.g., the provision of daily thought records in cognitive therapy), impacts (e.g., insight into the developmental roots and conflictual reproductions of maladaptive patterns in traditional psychoanalysis), mechanisms of change (e.g., increase in reflective functioning in certain psychodynamic approaches), and others. Since unique factors tend to be paid substantial attention in the literature, we will only provide a limited overview of this important topic here. It should be noted first that neither common nor unique factors of psychotherapy operate in the absence of the other (at least in the context of any bona fide psychotherapy), and it will be clear that this distinction between common and unique factors represents a false dichotomy. For example, an important part of the construct of the alliance is a sense of shared goals between client and therapist, but there are no goals without a theoretical forecast (most frequently based on a particular model of change) of what the immediate and long-term objectives ought to be to improve functioning and reduce symptoms.

That being said, it is clear from empirical research that a number of factors emphasized in some psychotherapeutic treatments do have support. One example of an empirically supported unique variable is homework. The incorporation of explicit and cooperatively assigned homework into psychotherapy is largely unique to cognitive-behavioral therapy (though it must be noted that integrative work in other orientations has sometimes incorporated this as well; Nelson et al. 2005). Burns and Nolen-Hoeksema (1991) have shown that client rates of completion of therapist-suggested self-help homework predict outcome of therapy in cognitive therapy for depression. Building on this, Burns and Spangler (2000) used structural equation modeling (SEM) in an attempt to separate the effects of homework on symptoms from the reverse effects and found that homework compliance was generally a more powerful predictor of symptomatic improvement than the other way around in CT for depression. This finding is consistent with theoretical formulations of CBT that suggest that homework assignments can provide opportunities for application of new skills, new opportunities for mastery experiences, generalization of learned behavior outside of the therapy hour, and increased interactions with positively reinforcing stimuli.

However, one of the best experimental designs to test any specific or unique factor in a particular therapy may be a dismantling or component analysis design, rather than the quasi-experimental designs described above. Jacobson et al. (1996) provided an excellent example of such a design, in which they treated major depressive disorder with either complete cognitive therapy or two of its components: cognitive processes aimed at changing automatic thoughts (ATs) or treatment focused solely on behavior activation (BA), which primarily consisted of activity monitoring and planning. In the Jacobson et al. study, as well as a number of subsequent explorations (e.g., Dimidjian et al. 2006), the behavioral activation treatment has been shown to be as effective in treating depression as the full CT treatment. This line of research helps support the notion that increasing enjoyable and therapeutic behaviors in the treatment of depression is an efficacious part of the CBT protocol and therefore that the techniques of providing clients with behavioral homework is a viable unique factor (though, of course, other factors in the BA treatment, including a strong therapeutic relationship, may be active as well).

While much of the published and well-controlled empirical research on psychotherapy has been conducted on cognitive-behavioral therapy, there is also support for certain unique factors from other therapies. For instance, psychodynamic researchers have focused on the technique of interpretation (especially transference interpretations), and a body of work now suggests that interpretations are valuable unique interventions in this orientation. Interestingly, two elements of this intervention have been highlighted in the literature: frequency and accuracy.

There is some evidence suggesting that the overall frequency or concentration of interpretations is either negatively related or unrelated to outcome. Using correlational methods, both Piper et al. (1993) and Schut et al. (2005) found that the overall frequency of interpretation was not positively linked to outcome in psychodynamic psychotherapy. In addition, a recent experimental study of psychodynamic psychotherapy with and without moderate levels of transference interpretations (Hoglend et al. 2006) failed to find differences in outcome between the low transference interpretation and moderate transference interpretation groups. However, they did find that some patient variables moderated the relationship between interpretation and outcome, and subsequent analysis has suggested that, as would be expected by theory, insight mediated the effect of transference interpretations on outcome (Johansson et al. 2010). This finding suggests that interpretations are not always beneficial (so just doing more is not recommended), but when they are used in an appropriate context (and/or with attunement to the client's needs), they can be helpful.

Crits-Christoph et al. (1988) conducted an important study on interpretation accuracy, a variable that would be expected to improve the chances that an interpretation would be effective. These authors found that in cases in which therapists used more accurate interpretations (meaning that the interpretation was relevant to an important conflictual relationship theme, as rated by an independent observer), treatment outcome was better than when interpretations were less accurate. This finding held true when alliance scores were statistically controlled, which is important considering that the interpretations assessed were early in treatment but the outcome was assessed much later. Using similar methods, Crits-Christoph et al. (2010) found that accuracy of interpretation was positively related to outcome in interpersonal therapy for depression but that the opposite was true in cognitive therapy.

Andrusyna et al. (2006) also found support for the use of accurate interventions in a psychodynamic psychotherapy, but in this study the authors examined changes on shorter time spans: large intersession reductions of symptoms, or rather sudden gains. These authors found that in sessions prior to sudden gains (pregain sessions), interpretation accuracy was significantly higher than control sessions. In addition, they found a higher number of accurate interpretations in pregain sessions as compared to control sessions. Taken in total, it seems that accurate interpretation is empirically related to outcome in psychodynamic psychotherapy (but not in cognitive therapy), though the raw frequency of interpretation is less important.

It is clear from these examples that certain psychological treatments contain theoretically identified elements that can be empirically assessed, manipulated, and linked to outcome within their respective treatments and deserve the term "unique factors."

15.4 Common and Unique Factors in Context

While the evidence reviewed here suggests that both unique and common factors operate in psychotherapy, much of the discussion on this topic has either subtly or overtly assumed that only one of these groups of effects is actually essential or that one of them is inherently more important than the other. A closer examination of the issues suggests that even the conception of common and unique variables as separate entities is misguided. As Castonguay (2000) has discussed, this is a false dichotomy. That is, several theoretically unique factors operate in treatments other than the one in which they were developed, and it is more than likely that common factors *always* operate within the context of a unique psychotherapy orientation. Castonguay pointed out the necessity of understanding common factors from an established theoretical orientation, as the case formulation derived from this orientation provides the necessary context for implementing any effective interventions, common or unique. Some empirical basis for this statement has been found. In a recent paper, Tschacher et al. (2012) used results of a survey of psychotherapy research experts to identify potential relationships between common factors and specific psychotherapy techniques. These authors found that each of the 22 common factors they included in their survey was significantly related to orientation-specific techniques in practice, suggesting that the common and unique processes of psychotherapy are systematically linked. Thus, discussing common and unique factors in absence of each other fails to reflect the complex reality of therapeutic change. Castonguay (2011) suggested that the study of two concepts could provide a useful integration of common and unique factors: faux-unique variables and change principles.

Faux-unique variables are those psychotherapeutic processes that are expected to operate within one orientation but may also be present in others, even though the theoretical framework of the other orientations may not account for them. That is, any component of psychotherapy that is claimed to be a "unique" part of a certain psychotherapy orientation may actually be found outside its orientation of origin. These faux-unique variables are not specific or intentional integrations or the result of eclectic practice but rather represent commonalities between treatments that are either not anticipated by theory or are not explicitly included within a therapist's explanation of change. The identification of faux-unique variables has been a hallmark of the integrative movement in psychotherapy for many years. There may be countless examples of identified faux-unique variables in psychotherapy. For instance, Murray and Jacobson (1971) summarized that clear processes of social influence operate in the therapeutic work of Carl Rogers, despite his original theory that his work was explicitly nondirective and exclusively enacted clients' change mechanisms. In addition, the presence (and importance) of transference in behavior therapy has been noted for many years, in spite of many behavior therapists' sense that psychoanalytic constructs are not applicable to their practice (e.g., Rhoads and Feather 1972). Several studies have also shown that emotional deepening and exploration of the past (techniques clearly associated with humanistic and psychodynamic treatments) have been linked with outcome in CBT (see Castonguay 2011).

The near ubiquity of these faux-unique variables provides both promise and disillusionment to psychotherapy researchers: On the one hand, it suggests that if we look close enough, we will find important and nearly universal processes underlying psychotherapeutic change (ultimate common factors). On the other, the observable differences between orientations would be obscured beyond recognition in this exclusively common factors description, and this may not be sufficient to guide the process of psychotherapy, as discussed above. It is difficult to conceive the provision of a stand-alone treatment that comprises all of the common and faux-unique factors of psychotherapies without incorporating any factors that could be identified as truly unique. It is just as hard to believe that any psychological treatment can be accurately described as devoid of any common factors of psychotherapy.

One path forward is provided by the second concept advocated by Castonguay (2000, 2011): Goldfried's (1980) concept of change principles. Focusing on principles can often help delineate *both* the shared and distinct features of an intervention or therapeutic process. For instance, one principle of change identified by Goldfried and Padawer (1982) is the provision of alternative views of self. While therapists from various theoretical orientations have identified this as an important task and/or goal of therapy, the technical procedures that are prescribed to achieve it vary from one orientation to another (e.g., cognitive restructuring, transference interpretation, etc.). Thus, these principles can identify empirically testable and clinically useful commonalities between treatments while simultaneously accounting for real differences between treatments in terms of both the rationale for understanding the principles and the implementation of principles in practice.

Castonguay and Beutler (2006) provide one example of an initiative demonstrating the potential of these principles of change in improving our understanding of the process of change in the context of evidence-based practice. Castonguay and Beutler brought together many influential researchers from diverse orientations to review the research on psychological treatments for four major types of psychopathology (dysphoric disorders, anxiety disorder, personality disorders, and substance use disorders) and develop empirically anchored principles for their treatments. Of the 61 identified principles of change, the task force identified 26 of these principles that may not only cut across treatments for specific disorders but also cut across disorders—that is, principles that are likely to be beneficial when used by therapists of different orientations and when implemented for clients with diverse clinical problems. Some examples include: "Positive change is likely if the therapist provides a structured treatment and remains focused in the application of his/her interventions," and "Therapists should be able to skillfully use "non-directive" interventions" (Castonguay and Beutler 2006, p. 361). These principles are precise enough to provide clinicians with effective guidelines and/or focus of intervention, yet they also reflect strategies that are general enough that they could be implemented by various technical procedures. In doing so, they avoid the "either/or" trap of common versus unique factors and allow for a large repertoire of interventions, fostering a flexible approach to evidence-based practice.

Conclusion

The process of change in psychotherapy is extraordinarily complex. While it is important that we seek to identify the mechanisms of this change, it is equally important that we not lose sight of the variety of factors (and their interactions) involved in therapy, so that we do not oversimplify and unnecessarily limit our ability to both understand why therapy is helpful (when it is) and to further develop and improve our existing treatments as much as possible. There is good evidence to support the assertion that certain common features of several different psychotherapies are beneficial to the process of change across disorders and treatments. Similarly, there is good evidence that some treatments differ meaningfully from others and that certain productive elements of some treatments may be viewed as unique contributions from particular types of psychotherapy.

Based on this, it seems that one important goal of psychotherapy research over the next several years and decades will be to better understand how common and unique processes operate simultaneously, rather than to determine which one is the "true" or best mechanism. Several patterns and conventions may need to change in order to accomplish this goal. For instance, there is a need for more empirical studies that evaluate both common and unique effects in the same cases of psychotherapy, and it is important that we conduct more studies on the same variables in the process of different psychotherapies. Readers may have noted that many of the studies cited in this chapter have been primarily quantitative studies rather than qualitative. This represents another important area for future research: increasing the use of qualitative research methods to investigate common factors, unique factors, and their interactions. Qualitative methods (see Chap. 20) allow for a unique set of research questions and provide researchers with the opportunity to discover new phenomena that may not be easily described in quantitative studies. As an attempt to begin addressing this gap of research, a number of qualitative analyses have recently been published as part of two books focusing on specific common factors: insight or the acquisition of new understanding (Castonguay and Hill 2007) and corrective experiences (Castonguay and Hill 2012).

Future empirical studies, both quantitative and qualitative, are likely to provide the field with helpful information to improve explanatory theories of how and why different factors of psychotherapy are beneficial. In our view, new theories are likely to be most useful if they are based on (and provide expansions to) existing theoretical structures, such as the models of personality and psychopathology that drive our major orientations at present: cognitive-behavioral, humanistic, and psychodynamic theories. That is, in our minds there is no reason to create new models of human functioning from scratch, to prevent reinventing the therapeutic wheel. Using these theories as the lenses through which we view commonalities of psychotherapy, it may be possible that we can better understand how best to help a given client that seeks treatment. In the long run, this is the most important outcome of our collective work as psychotherapy researchers, and the task is monumental. However, by proceeding in ways that will not obscure real differences between treatments while also permitting the recognition of the valuable commonalities, it is our hope that we will be able to achieve this goal sooner rather than later.

References

Andrusyna TP, Luborsky L, Pham T, Tang TZ (2006) The mechanisms of sudden gains in supportive-expressive therapy for depression. Psychother Res 16:526–536

Asay T, Lambert M (1999) The empirical case for the common factors in therapy. In: Hubble M, Duncan B, Miller S (eds) The heart and soul of change. American Psychological Association, Washington, DC, pp 23–55

Barber JP (2009) Toward a working through of some core conflicts in psychotherapy research. Psychother Res 19:1–12

Barber JP, Muran JC (eds) (2010) The therapeutic alliance: an evidence-based approach to practice and training. Guilford, New York

Barber JP, Khalsa S-R, Sharpless BA (2010) The validity of the alliance as a predictor of psychotherapy outcome. In: Muran JC, Barber JP (eds) The therapeutic alliance: an evidence-based guide to practice. Guilford, New York, pp 29–43

Bohart AC, Elliott R, Greenberg LS, Watson JC (2002) Empathy. In: Norcross JC (ed) Psychotherapy relationships that work. Oxford University Press, New York, pp 89–108

Bordin ES (1979) The generalizability of the psychoanalytic concept of the working alliance. Psychotherapy 16:252–260

Boswell JF, Castonguay LG, Wasserman RH (2010) Effects of psychotherapy training and intervention use on session outcome. J Consult Clin Psychol 78: 717–723

Burns DD, Nolen-Hoeksema S (1991) Coping styles, homework compliance, and the effectiveness of cognitive-behavioral therapy. J Consult Clin Psychol 59:305–311

Burns DD, Nolen-Hoeksema S (1992) Therapeutic empathy and recovery from depression in cognitive-behavioral therapy: a structural equation model. J Consult Clin Psychol 60:441–449

Burns DD, Spangler DL (2000) Does psychotherapy homework lead to improvements in depression in cognitive-behavioral therapy or does improvement lead to increased homework compliance? J Consult Clin Psychol 68:46–56

Castonguay LG (1993) "Common factors" and "non-specific variables": clarification of the two concepts and recommendations for research. J Psychother Integr 3:267–286

Castonguay LG (2000) A common factors approach to psychotherapy training. J Psychother Integr 10: 263–282

Castonguay LG (2006) Personal pathways in psychotherapy integration. J Psychother Integr 16:36

Castonguay LG (2009) Marvin goldfried's (1980) american psychologist paper: (re) introducing a classic. Appl Prev Psychol 13:1

Castonguay LG (2011) Psychotherapy, psychopathology, research and practice: pathways of connections and integration. Psychother Res 21:125–140

Castonguay LG, Beutler LE (2006) Common and unique principles of therapeutic change: What do we know and what do we need to know? In: Castonguay LG, Beutler LE (eds) Principles of therapeutic change that work. Oxford University Press, New York, pp 353–369

Castonguay LG, Grosse Holtforth M (2005) Change in psychotherapy: a plea for no more "non-specific" and false dichotomy. Clin Psychol Sci Pract 12:198–201

Castonguay LG, Hill CE (eds) (2007) Insight in psychotherapy. American Psychological Association Press, Washington, DC

Castonguay LG, Hill CE (eds) (2012) Transformation in psychotherapy: corrective experiences across cognitive behavioral, humanistic, and psychodynamic approaches. American Psychological Association Press, Washington, DC

Castonguay LG, Constantino MJ, Grosse Holtforth M (2006) The working alliance: where are we and where should we go? Psychotherapy 43:271–279

Castonguay LG, Constantino MJ, McAleavey AA, Goldfried MR (2010) The therapeutic alliance in cognitive-behavioral therapy. In: Muran JC, Barber JP (eds) The therapeutic alliance: an evidence-based guide to practice. Guilford, New York, pp 150–171

Constantino MJ, Castonguay LG, Schut AJ (2002) The working alliance: a flagship for the "scientist-practitioner" model in psychotherapy. In: Tryon GS (ed) Counseling based on process research: applying what we know. Allyn & Bacon, Boston, pp 81–131

Crits-Christoph P (1997) Limitations of the dodo bird verdict and the role of clinical trials in psychotherapy research: comment on Wampold et al. (1997). Psychol Bull 122:216–220

Crits-Christoph P, Cooper A, Luborsky L (1988) The accuracy of therapists' interpretations and the outcome of dynamic psychotherapy. J Consult Clin Psychol 56:490–495

Crits-Christoph P, Gibbons MB, Temes CM, Elkin I, Gallop R (2010) Interpersonal accuracy of interventions and the outcome of cognitive and interpersonal therapies for depression. J Consult Clin Psychol 78:420–428

Dimidjian S, Hollon SD, Dobson KS, Schmaling KB, Kohlenberg RJ, Addis ME, Gallop R, McGlinchey JB, Markley DK, Gollan JK, Atkins DC, Dunner DL, Jacobson NS (2006) Randomized trial of behavioral activation, cognitive therapy, and antidepressant medication in the acute treatment of adults with major depression. J Consult Clin Psychol 74:658–670

Elliott R, Bohart AC, Watson JC, Greenberg LS (2011) Empathy. Psychotherapy (Chic) 48:43–49

Farber BA, Doolin EM (2011) Positive regard. Psychotherapy (Chic) 48:58–64

Farber B, Lane JS (2002) Positive regard. In: Norcross JC (ed) Psychotherapy relationships that work. Oxford University Press, New York, pp 175–194

Frank JD (1961) Persuasion and healing. Johns Hopkins University Press, Baltimore, MD

Frank JD, Frank JB (1991) Persuasion and healing. Johns Hopkins University Press, Baltimore

Garfield SL (1980) Psychotherapy: an eclectic approach. Wiley, New York

Goldfried MR (1980) Toward the delineation of therapeutic change principles. Am Psychol 35:991–999

Goldfried MR, Padawer W (1982) Current status and future directions in psychotherapy. In: Goldfried MR (ed) Converging themes in psychotherapy. Springer, New York, pp 3–49

Goldfried MR, Raue PJ, Castonguay LG (1998) The therapeutic focus in significant sessions of master therapists: a comparison of cognitive-behavioral and psychodynamic-interpersonal interventions. J Consult Clin Psychol 66:803–810

Grencavage LM, Norcross JC (1990) Where are the commonalities among the therapeutic common factors? Prof Psychol Res Pr 21:372–378

Hill CE (2009) Reaction to goldfried (1980): What about therapist techniques? Appl Prev Psychol 13:16–18

Hill CE, O'Grady KE (1985) List of therapist intentions illustrated in a case study and with therapists of varying theoretical orientations. J Couns Psychol 32:3

Hoffart A, Borge F-M, Sexton H, Clark DM (2009) The role of common factors in residential cognitive and interpersonal therapy for social phobia: a process-outcome study. Psychother Res 19:54–67

Hoglend P, Amlo S, Marble A, Bogwald KP, Sorbye O, Sjaastad MC, Heyerdahl O (2006) Analysis of the patient-therapist relationship in dynamic psychotherapy: an experimental study of transference interpretations. Am J Psychiatry 163:1739–1746

Horvath AO, Bedi RP (2002) The alliance. In: Norcross JC (ed) Psychotherapy relationships that work. Oxford University Press, New York, pp 37–69

Horvath AO, Greenberg LS (eds) (1994) The working alliance: theory, research, and practice. Wiley, New York

Horvath AO, Luborsky L (1993) The role of the therapeutic alliance in psychotherapy. J Consult Clin Psychol 61: 561–573

Horvath AO, Del Re AC, Fluckiger C, Symonds D (2011) Alliance in individual psychotherapy. Psychotherapy (Chic) 48:9–16

Howard KI, Kopta SM, Krause MS, Orlinsky DE (1986) The dose-effect relationship in psychotherapy. Am Psychol 41:159–164

Howard KI, Lueger RJ, Maling MS, Martinovich Z (1993) A phase model of psychotherapy outcome: causal mediation of change. J Consult Clin Psychol 61: 678–685

Jacobson NS, Dobson KS, Truax PA, Addis ME, Koerner K, Gollan JK, Gortner E, Prince SE (1996) A component analysis of cognitive-behavioral treatment for depression. J Consult Clin Psychol 64: 295–304

Johansson P, Hoglend P, Ulberg R, Amlo S, Marble A, Bogwald KP, Sorbye O, Sjaastad MC, Heyerdahl O (2010) The mediating role of insight for long-term improvements in psychodynamic therapy. J Consult Clin Psychol 78:438–448

Jones EE, Pulos SM (1993) Comparing the process in psychodynamic and cognitive-behavioral therapies. J Consult Clin Psychol 61:306–316

Karasu TB (1986) The specificity versus nonspecificity dilemma: toward identifying therapeutic change agents. Am J Psychiatry 143:687–695

Klein MH, Kolden GG, Michels JL, Chisholm-Stockard SM (2002) Congruence. In: Norcross JC (ed) Psychotherapy relationships that work. Oxford University Press, New York, pp 195–215

Kolden GG (1991) The generic model of psychotherapy: an empirical investigation of patterns of process and outcome relationships. Psychother Res 1:62–73

Kolden GG (1996) Change in early sessions of dynamic therapy: universal processes and the generic model of psychotherapy. J Consult Clin Psychol 64:489–496

Kolden GG, Klein MH, Wang CC, Austin SB (2011) Congruence/genuineness. Psychotherapy (Chic) 48: 65–71

Lambert MJ, Ogles BM (2004) The efficacy and effectiveness of psychotherapy. In: Lambert MJ (ed) Bergin & Garfield's handbook of psychotherapy and behavior change. Wiley, New York, pp 139–193

Lambert MJ, DeJulio SS, Stein DM (1978) Therapist interpersonal skills: process, outcome, methodological considerations and recommendations for future research. Psychol Bull 85:467–489

Lambert MJ, Hansen NB, Finch AE (2001) Patient-focused research: using patient outcome data to enhance treatment effects. J Consult Clin Psychol 69: 159–172

Lampropoulos GK (2000) Definitional and research issues in the common factors approach to psychotherapy integration: misconceptions, clarifications, and proposals. J Psychother Integr 10:415–438

Larsson BPM, Kaldo V, Broberg A (2010) Theoretical orientation and therapists' attitudes to important components of therapy: a study based on the valuable elements in psychotherapy questionnaire. Cogn Behav Ther 39:161–172

Luborsky L, Singer B, Luborsky L (1975) Comparative studies of psychotherapies. Is it true that "everyone has won and all must have prizes"? Arch Gen Psychiatry 32:995–1008

Lutz W, Leon SC, Martinovich Z, Lyons JS, Stiles WB (2007) Therapist effects in outpatient psychotherapy: a three-level growth curve approach. J Couns Psychol 54:32–39

Marks IM, Gelder MG (1966) Common ground between behavior therapy and psychodynamic methods. Br J Med Psychol 39:11–23

Marmor J (1976) Common operational factors in diverse approaches to behavior change. In: Burton DA (ed) What makes behavior change possible? Burnner/Mazel, New York, pp 3–12

Martin DJ, Garske JP, Davis MK (2000) Relation of the therapeutic alliance with outcome and other variables: a meta-analytic review. J Consult Clin Psychol 68: 438–450

Masserman JH (1980) Principles and practice of biodynamic psychotherapy: an integration. Thieme-Stratton, New York

McCarthy KS, Barber JP (2009) The multitheoretical list of therapeutic interventions (multi): initial report. Psychother Res 19:96–113

Messer SB (1986) Behavioral and psychoanalytic perspectives at therapeutic choice points. Am Psychol 41:1261–1272

Messer SB, Wolitzky DL (2010) A psychodynamic perspective on the therapeutic alliance: theory, research, and practice. In: Muran JC, Barber JP (eds) The therapeutic alliance: an evidence-based guide to practice. Guilford, New York, pp 97–122

Morris RJ, Magrath KH (1979) Contribution of therapist warmth to the contact desensitization treatment of acrophobia. J Consult Clin Psychol 47:786–788

Morris RJ, Suckerman KR (1974) The importance of the therapeutic relationship in systematic desensitization. J Consult Clin Psychol 42:148

Murray EJ, Jacobson LI (1971) Cognition and learning in traditional and behavioral psychotherapy. In: Bergin AE, Garfield SL (eds) Handbook of psychotherapy and behavior change. Wiley, New York, pp 661–688

Nelson DL, Castonguay LG, Barwick F (2005) Directions for the integration of homework in psychotherapy practice. In: Kazantis N, L'Abate L (eds) Handbook of homework assignments in psychotherapy: research, practice, and prevention. Springer, New York, pp 425–444

Norcross JC (1995) Dispelling the dodo bird verdict and the exclusivity myth in psychotherapy. Psychotherapy 32:500

Norcross JC (ed) (2002) Psychotherapy relationships that work. Oxford University Press, New York

Omer H, London P (1989) Signal and noise in psychotherapy: the role and control of non-specific factors. Br J Psychiatry 155:239–245

Orlinsky DE (2009) The "generic model of psychotherapy" after 25 years: evolution of a research-based metatheory. J Psychother Integr 19:319

Orlinsky DE, Howard KI (1967) The good therapy hour. Experiential correlates of patients' and therapists' evaluations of therapy sessions. Arch Gen Psychiatry 16:621–632

Orlinsky DE, Grawe K, Parks BK (1994) Process and outcome in psychotherapy—noch einmal. In: Garfield SL, Bergin AE (eds) Handbook of psychotherapy and behavior change. Wiley, New York

Orlinsky DE, Ronnestad MH, Willutzki U (2004) Fifty years of process-outcome research: continuity and change. In: Lambert MJ (ed) Bergin and Garfield's handbook of psychotherapy and behavior change. Wiley, New York, pp 307–365

Piper WE, Joyce AS, McCallum M, Azim HF (1993) Concentration and correspondence of transference interpretations in short-term psychotherapy. J Consult Clin Psychol 61:586–595

Prochaska J, DiClemente C (1984) The transtheoretical approach: towards a systematic eclectic framework. Dow Jones Irwin, Homewood, IL

Rhoads JM, Feather BW (1972) Transference and resistance observed in behavior therapy. Br J Med Psychol 45:99–103

Rogers CR (1957) The necessary and sufficient conditions of therapeutic personality change. J Consult Psychol 21:95–103

Rosenzweig S (1936) Some implicit common factors in diverse methods of psychotherapy. Am J Orthopsychiatry 6:412–415

Schut AJ, Castonguay LG, Bedics JD, Smith TL, Barber JP, Flanagan KM, Yamasaki AS (2005) Therapist interpretation, patient-therapist interpersonal process, and outcome in psychodynamic psychotherapy for avoidant personality disorder. Psychotherapy 42: 494–511

Sloane RB (1969) The converging paths of behavior therapy and psychotherapy. Am J Psychiatry 125:877–885

Sloane RB, Staples FR, Cristol AH, Yorkston N, Whipple K (1975) Psychotherapy vs behavior therapy. Harvard University Press, Cambridge, MA

Stiles WB (1988) Psychotherapy process-outcome correlations may be misleading. Psychotherapy 25: 27–35

Strupp HH (1973) On the basic ingredients of psychotherapy. J Consult Clin Psychol 41:1–8

Tracey TJ, Lichtenberg JW, Goodyear RK, Claiborn CD, Wampold BE (2003) Concept mapping of therapeutic common factors. Psychother Res 13:401–413

Tschacher W, Junghan UM, Pfammatter M (2012) Towards a taxonomy of common factors in psychotherapy—results of an expert survey. Clin Psychol Psychother 21(1):82–96

Wachtel PL (2009) The evolving investigation of therapeutic change principles. Appl Prev Psychol 13:30–31

Wampold BE (2001) The great psychotherapy debate: models, methods, and findings. Erlbaum, Lawrence

Watson JC, Kalogerakos F (2010) The therapeutic alliance in humanistic psychotherapy. In: Muran JC, Barber JP (eds) The therapeutic alliance: an evidence-based guide to practice. Guilford, New York, pp 191–209

Weinberger J (1995) Common factors aren't so common: the common factors dilemma. Clin Psychol Sci Pract 2:45–69

Weinberger J, Rasco C (2007) Empirically supported common factors. In: Hofmann SG, Weinberger J (eds) The art and science of psychotherapy. Routledge, New York, pp 103–129

Therapeutic Alliance and Alliance Ruptures and Resolutions: Theoretical Definitions, Assessment Issues, and Research Findings

16

Vittorio Lingiardi and Antonello Colli

Contents

V. Lingiardi (✉)
Sapienza University of Rome, Rome, Italy
e-mail: vittorio.lingiardi@uniroma1.it

A. Colli
Carlo Bo University of Urbino, Urbino, Italy

Abstract

Therapeutic alliance is one of the most important and investigated constructs in psychotherapy research. In this chapter we first discuss the historical development of therapeutic alliance, from psychoanalytic theory to empirical research, and then its measurement and the problematic issues related to it. Then we will focus our discussion on the therapeutic alliance ruptures and resolutions construct, which represents one of the most interesting but, at the same time, controversial issues of contemporary therapeutic alliance research. Finally we propose a brief research agenda about therapeutic alliance ruptures and resolutions.

16.1 Introduction

Therapeutic alliance, also described as the quintessential integrative variable (Wolfe and Goldfried 1988), is probably the most cited "common factor" in psychotherapy and one of the most investigated constructs in psychotherapy research. Just consider that in a recent meta-analysis, Horvath et al. (2011), using as key words alliance, helping alliance, working alliance, and/or therapeutic alliance, found over 7000 published papers on electronic databases. Although the concept has its origins in the psychoanalytic field, its relevance now is recognized across several therapeutic approaches.

O.C.G. Gelo et al. (eds.), *Psychotherapy Research*,
DOI 10.1007/978-3-7091-1382-0_16, © Springer-Verlag Wien 2015

The aims of this chapter are (1) to provide a brief historical review of the construct, (2) to discuss one of the most important aspects of empirical research on therapeutic alliance—its measurement—and the critical aspects related to this topic, and (3) to discuss the therapeutic alliance ruptures and resolutions construct, its measurement, and the critical aspects related to it. In relation to therapeutic alliance ruptures and resolutions, we will discuss the problems related to the construct definition and assessment, and we will present the most relevant research findings. Finally, we will discuss some future directions about therapeutic alliance and therapeutic alliance ruptures and resolutions.

16.2 A Short History of Therapeutic Alliance: From Therapeutic Alliance to Therapeutic Alliance Ruptures and Resolutions

The construct's evolution can be divided into three periods (Lingiardi 2002; De Bei 2006; Hatcher 2010). A first period, of concept definition, starts from first Freud's writings on therapeutic relationship (Freud 1910, 1912) until Greenson's paper (1965) on the three elements of therapeutic relationship: transference, working alliance, and real relationship. A second period, from the mid-1970s to the early 1990s, is characterized by several attempts to measure the construct and to empirically investigate its relationship with therapy outcome. Finally, in the third period, from the 1990s until now, several researchers place a great emphasis on clinical practice (Hilsenroth et al. 2012; Ackerman and Hilsenroth 2001, 2003) and, in particular, on alliance rupture and resolution processes.

16.2.1 First Period: Theoretical Definition

The origins of the concept can be traced in Freud's early writings on transference (Freud 1910, 1912). Although he did not use the term therapeutic alliance, in "Dynamic of Transference" Freud (1912) described a concept that can be assimilated to therapeutic alliance: the unobjectionable positive transference.

Freud divided the transference, in a positive translation, which keeps the patient in treatment, helps overcome doubts, and promotes cooperativeness, and in a negative translation, which interferes with the analytic process and takes the form of resistance. In this way Freud partially resolved the paradox that transference is the vehicle for the expression of the patient's unconscious desires, supplies the underlying emotional force that binds the patient to the doctor, and hence commits him or her to the treatment process but simultaneously powers the patient's resistance to the doctor's influence and, by extension, to the requirements of the treatment (Friedman 1969).

In one of his last publications, Freud specified that the analytic situation is also based on an alliance between the analyst and a more rational and mature part of the patient's ego (Freud 1937). This idea was introduced by Sterba (1934) who first used the term "alliance" and expanded the idea that the patient has a rational, observing capacity with which the analyst can ally against the irrational forces of the patient.

Sterba's conceptualization was the starting point for Zetzel's reflections about alliance. Elizabeth Zetzel (1956), who first introduced the expression "therapeutic alliance," describes a part of the ego of the patient as an "observing ego" that is allied with the analyst. This relationship is based on a real object relation and on a patient's capacity to maintain a significant one-to-one relationship. Differently from Sterba, Zetzel also stressed the contribution of the therapist—not only as a transference object but also as a real person: also, the analyst must ally with the patient. In some way, Zetzel first explicitly recognized the bi-personal and interactive essence of therapeutic alliance (Zetzel 1958).

A cornerstone of the therapeutic alliance definition is represented by Greenson's (1965) paper "The Working Alliance and the Transference Neuroses." In this paper the author introduced the term *working alliance* to stress "the patient ability to work in the analytic situation" (Greenson 1965, p. 157). An innovative part of

Greenson's contribution was to talk directly with his patient about alliance issues and not only as transference or defense manifestations. Greenson describes three levels of the analytic relationship: (1) transference, (2) working alliance, and (3) real relationship. It is important to observe that for Greenson "real" has two different meanings: (a) real as realistic, as opposed to transference deformations, and (b) real as genuine and authentic, as opposed to false (Greenson, 1965, p.235).

16.2.2 Second Period: Empirical Research and the Relationship Between Therapeutic Alliance and Outcome of Treatments

In the mid-1970s, interest in the construct gradually shifted from psychoanalysis to empirical research. In this period the therapeutic alliance crossed the psychoanalytic boundaries and was recognized as a relevant construct across different therapeutic approaches.

Bordin's pan theoretical definition of the alliance as a "mutual understanding and agreement about change goals and the necessary tasks to move toward these goals along with the establishment of bonds to maintain the partners' work" (Bordin 1994, p. 13) stimulated a vast array of research studies on alliance that continue today. The basic idea of Bordin's conceptualization is that (a) every form of therapy has its demands and expectations to patient and therapist ("embedded working alliances") (Bordin 1979, p. 253) and (b) that alliance is strong to the extent that patient and therapist can jointly negotiate the expected work and, especially, are able to negotiate the three elements of therapeutic alliance: tasks, goals, and bond.

From this point of view, Bordin's conceptualization is not only a therapeutic alliance definition but also a pan theoretic theory of psychotherapy process and furnished the basis for more recent contributions on therapeutic alliance, for example, as we will see later in the chapter, Safran and Muran's (2000a) concept of alliance ruptures and resolutions. Bordin's conceptualization, which includes some aspects of Greenson's (1967) and Zetzel's (1956) formulations, represents the major theoretical change about therapeutic alliance since Freud's early contributions: he emphasized the curative aspects of the alliance in itself, without considering it only as a precondition for other "main" curative factors such as interpretation.

In this period, stimulated by the Dodo verdict (Luborsky et al. 1975)—which stated that all psychotherapies, regardless of their specific components, produce equivalent outcomes—several authors focused their work on investigating the influence on therapy outcome of common factors across therapies rather than specific factors [see McAleavey and Castonguay (2015); see also Budge and Wampold (2015)]. Among common factors, therapeutic alliance was one of the most fashionable, probably because its clinical relevance, on one side, and its lack of complexity permitted its operationalization and measurement. Since the mid-1970s, there was a flourishing of alliance measures. It is possible to describe the construct's evolution through the evolution of the measures built to assess it (Elvins and Green 2008). Some of them conceptualized the alliance only as a patient dimension (*Helping Alliance Counting Signs*, Luborsky 1976), others recognized also the therapist contribution to alliance formation (*Working Alliance Inventory*, Horvath and Greenberg 1989), some scales also explicitly evaluated negative therapist contributions (*Vanderbilt Therapeutic Alliance Scale*, Hartley and Strupp 1983) and his/her emotional involvement (*California Psychotherapy Alliance Scales*; Marmar and Gaston 1988).

In this period many researchers investigated the relationship between therapeutic alliance and therapy outcome, taking into consideration several variables such as the perspective of evaluation (patient, therapist, or observer), the time of evaluation (early, middle, late, averaged), and the kind of therapy (psychodynamic, cognitive–behavioral therapy, interpersonal psychotherapy, etc.). The results of this research have been summarized in several meta-analyses (Horvath and Bedi 2002; Horvath and Symonds

1991; Martin et al. 2000; Horvath et al. 2011) that indicated a moderate but consistent relationship between therapeutic alliance and outcome. Summarizing very briefly the results of these meta-analyses, we could say that:

> This result strongly supports the claim the impact of the alliance on therapy outcome is ubiquitous irrespective of how the alliance is measured, from whose perspective it is evaluated, when it is assessed, the way the outcome is evaluated, and the type of therapy involved. (Horvath et al. 2011 p. 13)

16.2.3 Third Period: Bridging the Gap Between Empirical Research and Clinical Practice

Until the 1990s, most research investigated the relationship between therapeutic alliance and outcome. These studies permit us to recognize the importance of aspecific factors for therapy outcome. At the same time, because this research partially neglected the processes and mechanisms implicated in the formation and development of the therapeutic alliance, the results were not very relevant for clinical practice.

Starting from the 1990s, there was a growing interest in the processual aspects of therapeutic alliance and in techniques that could affect its quality and formation (Ackerman and Hilsenroth 2001, 2003) with a greater emphasis on practical aspects of therapeutic alliance construction (Hilsenroth et al. 2012).

At the same time there was a growing interest in the treatment of the kind of patients, such as personality disordered patients, who chronically present problems in the therapeutic alliance. This led to a change in the conceptualization of alliance from a prerequisite to a goal of the treatment (Roth and Fonagy 2004). In this period Safran and Muran begin to elaborate a conceptualization of therapeutic alliance based on rupture and resolution processes (Safran et al. 1990, 1994). The authors, starting from a seminal idea of Bordin who highlighted the importance of "tear and repair" processes (Bordin 1979), redefined therapeutic alliance as an ongoing process of intersubjective negotiation between patient and therapist characterized by the presence of moments of deterioration in the quality of therapeutic alliance (ruptures) and moments in which this tension is resolved (resolutions).

In general, we could say that different research increased the awareness that the alliance represents:

> An emergent quality of partnership and mutual collaboration between therapist and client. As such, it is not the outcome of a particular or typical intervention. Its development can take different forms and may be achieved quickly or nurtured over a longer period of time depending on the kind of therapy and the stage of treatment. (Horvath et al. 2011, p. 11)

Moreover, in this period several authors suggested looking in a different way at the relationship between therapeutic alliance and therapy outcome. As observed by Barber et al. (2010), many researchers who investigated the predictive validity of therapeutic alliance did not examine the possibility that therapeutic alliance was a product of a priori change: some research suggested in fact that therapeutic alliance could actually be a product of a priori symptomatic reduction rather than a prerequisite for change (Barber et al. 1999, 2000; DeRubeis and Feeley 1990; Gaston et al. 1991).

In conclusion, it is important to observe how the emergence from empirical research of some controversial issues about therapeutic alliance and the increasing complexity of clinical questions regarding the construct also suggested the importance of returning to the roots of its conceptualization, trying to give more clarity to its definition boundaries (Horvath 2011; Colli 2011).

16.3 Assessing Therapeutic Alliance: General Issues and Critical Aspects

16.3.1 General Issues

As we already observed, there is a multitude of measures for the assessment of therapeutic alliance. In a review, Elvins and Green (2008) found 34 instruments developed for this purpose. Many

Table 16.1 Core measures of therapeutic alliance

Measure	Background	Dimensions	Form
Working Alliance Inventory (WAI; Horvath and Greenberg 1989)	Pan theoretical. Designed to measure the three dimensions of Bordin (1979) working alliance concept in adults across all types of therapy	1. Bond 2. Goals 3. Tasks	Patient Therapist Observer
California Psychotherapy Alliance Scales Alliance Scales (CALPAS; Marmar and Gaston 1988)	Primarily from a psychodynamic point of view and empirical results of older alliance measures in adult populations	1. Patient Working Capacity (PWC) 2. Patient commitment (PC) 3. Working strategy consensus (WSC) 4. Therapist Understanding and Involvement (TUI)	Patient Therapist Observer
Penn Helping Alliance Scales (PHAS; Luborsky et al. 1983)	Luborsky's (1976) psychodynamic conceptualization of the helping alliance, measuring both Type 1 signs (the patient's experience of the therapist as providing the help that is needed) and Type 2 signs (the patient's experience of treatment as a process of working together toward goals)	1. Type 1 Helping Alliance signs 2. Type 2 helping alliance signs	Patient[a] Therapist[a] Observer[b, c]
Vanderbilt Therapeutic Alliance Scale (VTAS; Hartley and Strupp 1983)	Influenced by the Orlinsky and Howard (1975) self-report instrument and combining psychodynamic and pan theoretical conceptualizations of the alliance	1. Therapist and Patient Contribution 2. Patient/Therapist interaction	Observer

[a]Helping Alliance Questionnaire (HAq-I; Luborsky 1976)
[b]Helping Alliance Global Rating (HAr; Luborsky et al. 1983)
[c]Helping Alliance Counting Signs (HAcs; Luborsky et al. 1983)

scales were designed for use with adult patients. More recently other measures were developed for use with children, adolescents, and in different settings such as family, couple, and group therapy.

In spite of this abundance, the bulk of alliance research is conducted with few core measures (Table 16.1): the Working Alliance Inventory (WAI) (Horvath and Greenberg 1989), California Psychotherapy Alliance Scale (CALPAS) (Gaston and Marmar 1994), Helping Alliance Questionnaire (Haq) (Alexander and Luborsky 1986), and Vanderbilt Psychotherapy Process Scale (VPPS) (O'Malley et al. 1983). If we consider that these four measures accounted for two-thirds of the 201 studies included in the latest published meta-analysis on therapeutic alliance (Horvath et al. 2011), the imbalance between the multitude of therapeutic alliance measures and their effective use becomes evident.

Every measure refers to a different therapeutic alliance conceptualization and as consequence evaluates different dimensions of the construct. In most of the cases, these measures are constructed in three forms—patient, therapist, and observer—based on Likert scales.

The *Working Alliance Inventory* (WAI) (Horvath and Greenberg 1989) is designed to capture Bordin's (1979) pan theoretical conceptualization of the working alliance and consists of three subscales: the goal subscale addresses the extent to which therapy goals are important, mutual, and capable of being accomplished; the task subscale focuses on the participant's agreement about the steps taken to help improve the client's situation; and the bond subscale assesses mutual liking and attachment by focusing on tone of voice, empathy, and comfort in exploring intimate issues. The WAI in the full-length version is composed of 36 items and evaluates therapeutic alliance from the patient, therapist, and observer perspectives.

The *California Psychotherapy Alliance Scale* (CALPAS) (Marmar and Gaston 1988) draws from a psychodynamic perspective, including Freud's concept of the patient's affective bond with the therapist and Bordin's conceptualization. It is composed of four subscales: Patient Working Capacity (PWC), Patient Commitment (PC), Working Strategy Consensus (WSC), and Therapist Understanding and Involvement (TUI). The PC scale items describe the patient's confidence that efforts will lead to change, view of therapy as an important experience, and trust in therapy and therapist. The PWC scale is composed of items measuring the patient's capacity to self-disclose intimate and salient information, to self-observe reactions, and to explore contribution to problems. The WSC scale encompasses the patient–therapist similarity of goals, joint effort, and agreement on how people are helped and how therapy should proceed. The TUI scale reflects the therapist's capacity to understand the patient's point of view and sufferings, to demonstrate a nonjudgmental acceptance of the patient, and to intervene with tact and timing. The CALPAS is composed of 21 items that evaluate the therapeutic alliance from a patient, therapist, and observer perspective.

The *Penn Helping Alliance Scales* (PHAS) (Luborsky et al. 1983; Alexander and Luborsky 1986) are several measures based on Luborsky's conceptualization of alliance and focus on two types of alliance: type 1, which refers to the patient's experience of the therapist as providing the help that is needed, and type 2, which refers to the patient's experience of treatment as a process of working together toward goals. Three main different forms exist: the Helping Alliance Counting Signs (HAcs) (Luborsky et al. 1983) that evaluates the presence of 14 types of patient helping alliance signs (positive and negative) and 18 types of therapist signs (positive and negative) of helping alliance statements; the Helping Alliance Global Rating (HAr) that evaluates the same signs as HAcs but through a rating scale (Luborsky et al. 1983); and the Helping Alliance Questionnaire (Alexander and Luborsky 1986), a 19-item questionnaire that evaluates alliance from patient and therapist perspectives. The HAcs and HAr assess the alliance from the observer perspective, while the HAq-I assesses from the patient and therapist perspectives.

The *Vanderbilt Therapeutic Alliance Scale* (VTAS) (Hartley and Strupp 1983) represents a theoretical blend of dynamic and pan theoretical frameworks. The VTAS consists of 44 items within three subscales: therapist contribution to the alliance, client contribution to the alliance, and client–therapist interactions.

Every measure gives a different emphasis to different aspects of the alliance. The WAI seems to better capture the aspects of generic agreement on tasks and goals; the CALPAS emphasizes the patient's working capacity and also the emotional involvement of the therapist; the PHAS underline the process of change of therapeutic alliance across time, and the VTAS is more focused on the therapist's negative contributions and the quality of client–therapist interactions. Despite their conceptual differences, all of these measures cover two main common core aspects of the construct: the "personal alliance," referring to the interpersonal relationship between client and therapist, and the "task-related alliance," addressing the more contractual aspects of treatment planning and goal orientation (Hougaard 1994) or, in other words, "the personal attachments and collaboration or willingness to invest in the therapy process" (Horvath and Luborsky 1993, p. 564).

Therapeutic alliance research is usually carried out using quantitative methods as the scales mentioned above. Another way to investigate therapeutic alliance makes use of qualitative methods, as post-session interviews or open-ended questionnaires (Bedi and Richards 2011). These methodologies do not produce a quantification of therapeutic alliance and, as consequence, they use qualitative methods of analysis as, for example, consensual qualitative research

(CQR) (Hill 2011; Hill et al. 2005, 1997; see Hill 2015; see also Mörtl and Gelo 2015).

16.3.2 Critical Aspects

Although therapeutic alliance measures, in particular the ones used most often, were developed 25–30 years ago and have been validated and used in much research, they present some problematic aspects.

In order to develop alliance measures, researchers have been using two different approaches, each of which presents some advantages and limitations. One approach is to begin with a theory of the alliance and select or create items considered to reflect the essential concepts of the theory. The second is to begin with a collection of alliance-related items and examine the factor structure of the responses for coherent groupings (e.g., Hartley and Strupp 1983). Concerning the first approach, several therapeutic alliance measures have been developed and structured in different subscales reflecting specific alliance definitions, but this composition is not fully confirmed by factor analysis. The subscale composition of WAI (task, goal, and bond), for example, when confronted with empirical evidence, is not so clear: some research using factor analytic methods reported a two-factor solution with goal and task items loading on one large factor and the bond items loading on another smaller factor (Andrusyna et al. 2001; Hatcher and Gillaspy 2006; Reynolds et al. 1995).

The second approach to constructing therapeutic alliance measures is to develop them by factor analytic methods with a bottom-up logic: in this case, the researcher does not assume an a priori subscale composition but, starting from a wide pool of items and collecting a large number of evaluations, performs a factor analysis in order to observe how the items collapse together in various factors/dimensions that will constitute the subscales of the measure. Although this procedure avoids the pitfalls of an a priori conceptualization, it could be lacking in terms of theoretical coherence in fact, as observed by Hatcher and Barends (2006):

> The alliance concept is further blurred when alliance measures are formed by factoring item pools that include a very wide range of properties of the client, the therapist, and their relationship. Thus, the alliance loses its conceptual moorings and becomes an atheoretical amalgam, the relationship or therapeutic climate. (p. 296)

A second critical point of therapeutic alliance measures is represented by the fact that all of the most important alliance measures contain items that give an overall description of the state of the collaboration between patient and therapist but seem to lack the measurement of specific alliance features characteristic of a therapeutic approach (Hatcher 2010). This bias could lead to a low sensibility of the measures and a low capacity to capture important aspects of the relationship related to a specific therapeutic approach.

Another critical aspect of therapeutic alliance self-report measures is represented by how clients and therapists use the Likert scale to provide their answers. As noticed by Jenkis and Dillman (1997), researchers who create questionnaires do not always know how respondents will answer them. This is also the case of therapeutic alliance. Despite using different instruments to assess the client–therapist alliance, authors of studies frequently comment that both clients and therapists tend to rate the alliance highly (i.e., Hilsenroth et al. 2004; Lingiardi et al. 2005; Tryon and Kane 1995). For example, Hatcher and Gillaspy (2006) found that clients tend not to use the lower 5 points of the 7-point Working Alliance Inventory (WAI) (Horvath and Greenberg 1989). Thus, clients used just the top 30 % of the rating points of the WAI when evaluating the alliance with their therapists. Another study noticed a difference in the use of Likert scale between patients and therapists: clients tended to use only the top 20 % of rating points and therapists only the top 30 % of rating points on alliance measures (Tryon et al. 2008).

The tendency to rate highly by patients and therapists may be explained as a form of a certain loyalty to each other and thus a discomfort with providing lower alliance ratings. This consideration conducts us to the other bias of self-report measures. Researchers in various fields who utilize survey instruments have commented that these measures are prone to response distortions (Lanyon and Goodstein 1997), including those of acquiescence, social desirability, extreme response sets, and dissonance reduction.

16.4 Therapeutic Alliance Ruptures and Resolutions

As we have already observed (see Sect. 16.2.3), we are now in a third phase of therapeutic alliance studies: research is now more focused on the investigation of how patients and therapists build a positive relationship or deal with negative reactions rather than only on the relationship between therapeutic alliance and outcome. From this point of view, the alliance is no longer considered as a static phenomenon and a prerequisite for treatment but as an ongoing co-construction between patient and therapist and an objective of treatments. The study of alliance ruptures and resolutions is a good example of this change in the conceptualization of therapeutic alliance.

Generally speaking, with the term *therapeutic alliance rupture*, we refer to a moment of the therapy characterized by a weakening in the quality of the alliance. Several terms have been used to describe this phenomenon: challenges (Harper 1989a, b), misunderstanding events (Rhodes et al. 1994), impasses (Hill et al. 1996), alliance threats (Bennett et al. 2006), and transference–countertransference enactments (Safran and Muran 2006).

As observed by Safran and Muran (2006), "alliance rupture" is a "very slippery concept" (p. 288); in fact we have different definitions of the construct that reflect different theoretical nuances. The construct has been defined as a tension or breakdown in the collaborative relationship between patient and therapist (Safran et al. 2002), a deterioration in the relationship (Safran and Muran 2000b), and a problem in the quality of "relatedness" or a "deterioration in the communicative process" (Safran and Muran 2006). In our opinion, a particularly clear and useful definition of the construct identifies the alliance rupture as "an impairment or fluctuations in the quality of the alliance between the therapist and client" (Safran et al. 1990, p. 154). To the contrary, alliance resolutions can be defined as the patient's and therapist's willingness to participate in a process of collaborative inquiry about what is going on in the therapeutic relationship (Safran and Muran 2000a, p. 145).

The quality of the therapeutic alliance can be defined as "a function of the degree of agreement between therapist and client about the goals and tasks of psychotherapy that is mediated by the quality of the relational bond between therapist and patient" (Safran et al. 1990, p. 154). To establish the quality of the therapeutic alliance is, in our opinion, the central problem of the definition of the alliance rupture and resolution construct. In fact, in some way this construct requires theorists and researchers to define what they consider a good alliance and what they consider a bad alliance.

Two opposite ways to conceptualize alliance ruptures and resolutions may be identified: the *rational* and the *relational*. If we adopt a rational point of view, we could see a rupture or a breakdown in the collaboration process if a patient does not agree with her/his therapist about a task of therapy (e.g., "I don't think it is important for me to speak about my childhood"). Conversely, if we adopt a relational point of view, the content of the communication (the disagreement) is less important than the way the patient communicates about the disagreement and negotiates it with the therapist. Following a rational approach, we could consider as a sign of collaboration a patient who always agrees with his/her therapist although, from a relational perspective, this agreement could be interpreted as a sign of acquiescence of the patient; conversely, the patient's communication of disagreement with her/his therapist could be interpreted as the patient's need to negotiate his/her need rather than a sign of alliance deterioration.

The *rational* point of view, which is characteristic of standard cognitive therapy and ego psychoanalysis, has its roots in *one-person psychology* and has an implicit assumption that the therapist is the owner of the truth and that therapeutic alliance impasses are derived from patients unwilling to accept what therapists propose to them. On the contrary, from a *relational* point of view, the therapeutic alliance is seen as "an on-going process of intersubjective negotiation" (Safran and Muran 2000a, p. 165), and the objects of this negotiation are the patient's agency and relatedness needs. This model is based on a definition of psychotherapy processes and therapeutic impasses and resistances in light of a *two-person psychology*. From this point of view, any "apparent obstruction in the therapeutic process must be understood as a function of the interaction between the patient and the therapist." For example, "a patient who has difficulty accessing painful emotional material is having difficulty accessing it in a specific relational context" (Safran and Muran 2000a, p. 80). From a relational and interpersonal perspective, resistance is interpreted not only as a patient's character issue but also as the product (at both the conscious and unconscious level) of the interpersonal matrix in which it is produced. Similarly, a therapist's negative contributions to the relationship are interpreted not only as a therapist's problem but also as the product of the interpersonal matrix in which they are produced.

In our opinion, this is the main theoretical feature that differentiates an "old" conceptualization of patient resistance from the more current concept of alliance ruptures and resolutions.

16.4.1 Assessing Alliance Ruptures and Resolutions: General Issues and Critical Aspects

As suggested by Eubanks-Carter et al. (2010a), there are at least three methods for assessing alliance ruptures and resolutions: direct self-report, indirect self-report, and observer-based measures.

16.4.1.1 Direct Self-Report

The main characteristic of direct self-report measures for therapeutic alliance ruptures and resolution assessment is that they directly ask the patient and therapist, through items based on a Likert scale, if alliance ruptures have occurred in the session, of what kind, and how they felt during the session. An example of direct self-report for the assessment of alliance ruptures and resolutions is the Post-Session Questionnaire (PSQ) by Muran et al. (1992). The PSQ consists of several measures assessing session impact and the therapeutic alliance and includes the 12-item version of the Working Alliance Inventory (WAI) (Tracey and Kokotovic 1989), the Session Evaluation Questionnaire (SEQ) (Stiles 1980), and also three direct questions regarding ruptures and their resolution; all items are scaled in a five-point Likert-type format, plus an open-ended description. Another example of direct self-report is the Alliance Negotiation Scale (ANS) (Doran et al. 2012) that evaluates from the patient perspective the degree to which patient and therapist are able to constructively negotiate disagreements about tasks and goals.

The major advantages of this kind of measure are that we can have information from the perspective of patients and therapists and they are quite economical to administer. However, as has been pointed out (Colli and Lingiardi 2009; Westen and Shedler 1999a, b), these kinds of measures can be faulty (a) because of poor self-reflection or any type of bias on either the patient's or the therapist's part and (b) because they use a retrospective (post-session) recollection of the session. For example, using self-reports, patients could not remember the effort made by the therapist to overcome a rupture because they were in an angry state after the session; other patients could acknowledge with difficulty the idea that the therapist did his or her job in creating a negative atmosphere; others might simply dissociate emotionally marked relational episodes after the session. Moreover, these measures could have the same problems of Likert utilization by patient and therapist that we have reported above for therapeutic alliance self-report (see Sect. 16.3.2).

16.4.1.2 Indirect Self-Report

The main characteristic of indirect self-report measures is that they do not specifically assess the presence/absence of alliance ruptures and resolutions. This methodology is similar to direct self-report because the evaluators are patient and therapist, but it differs from direct measures because participants complete measures of the overall alliance such as WAI or CALPAS and the presence of alliance ruptures and resolutions is only inferred through fluctuations in the alliance scores across sessions. This kind of methodology was applied in several studies (Stevens et al. 2007; Strauss et al. 2006; Stiles et al. 2004; Kivlighan and Shaughnessy 2000) that investigated the development pattern of the alliance over time.

The criteria to establish whether a fluctuation can be considered as a rupture or as a resolution are different across studies (Eubanks-Carter et al. 2012). We can divide these criteria into two main groups (for some more strategies see Eubanks-Carter et al. 2012): studies that identified rupture and resolution sequences using criteria based on *shape of change parameters* calculated for each patient's profile of patient report alliance scores (Stiles et al. 2004) and studies that identified rupture and resolution sequences looking for fluctuation in overall alliance scores taking as parameter the *mean standard deviation* (Strauss et al. 2006; Stevens et al. 2007).

The approaches just described may well present some shortcomings. Traditionally, therapeutic alliance measures such as WAI and CALPAS (including their observer versions), which evaluate the therapeutic alliance at a macro-level, seem more suitable for assessing therapeutic alliance as a general factor related to the outcome than for "depicting the idiosyncratic interactional patterns that unfold between patient and therapist" (Charman 2004, p. 18). Because these measures can only study shifts between sessions rather than within the session itself, some rupture events may go undetected (Stevens et al. 2007). In short, these methodologies "described shifts in alliance but did not directly examine in-session transactions. We can only infer that ruptures were captured by our quantitative method" (Strauss et al. 2006, p. 344).

16.4.1.3 Observer-Rated

Considering the limitations we reported above, some researchers have focused their attention on the evaluation of alliance ruptures and resolutions and of alliance and collaboration fluctuation through observer-based/within-session methods. These methods share two important features: (a) they use external raters to evaluate alliance ruptures and/or collaboration fluctuations, and (b) the rater does not give a global evaluation of the session, as happens with other observer measures to evaluate therapeutic alliance, but gives a rating at a within-session level, searching for alliance ruptures and resolutions markers or evaluating shift in collaboration between patient and therapist at a speaking turn level of analysis.

Although there is a proliferation of instruments to assess therapeutic alliance, there is a shortage of measures assessing within-session therapeutic alliance fluctuations and alliance ruptures and resolutions. Some measures are developed to assess alliance ruptures and resolution markers (Eubanks-Carter et al. 2009; Samstag et al. 2000); other measures evaluate exclusively shifts in the patient collaboration (Allen et al. 1984), and some evaluate dimensions, alliance ruptures, and resolution markers and shifts in the collaboration of patient and therapist (Collaborative Interactions Scale [CIS]) (Colli and Lingiardi 2009). Some instruments require session transcripts (Ribeiro et al. 2012; Colli and Lingiardi 2009) and others require videotapes (Rupture Resolution Rating System [3RS]) (Eubanks-Carter et al. 2009).

The utilization of session transcripts for the evaluation of therapeutic alliance ruptures and resolutions is controversial. Evaluating transcripts is very time- and money-consuming. At the same time, the evaluation at a micro process level of every single conversational turn between patient and therapist permits "depicting the idiosyncratic interactional patterns that unfold between patient and therapist" (Charman 2004, p. 18), and this is in line with a relational point of view in which great emphasis is given to micro processes and mutual influences (Siegel 2002). Video recordings have the advantage of giving important information about patient's and therapist's nonverbal communications, helping raters in detecting very subtle tears in the alliance. At the same time, video recordings can be more difficult for clinicians, especially in private clinical practice, and could make patients feel too exposed.

In the last years we have developed a new measure for the assessment of alliance ruptures and resolutions and patient–therapist collaboration fluctuations based on transcript evaluations: the Collaborative Interactions Scale (CIS) (Colli and Lingiardi 2009). The CIS is the result of 10 years of ongoing research on transcript-based investigation of therapeutic alliance and rupture/repair processes. The first version of the scale, formerly known in Italian as IVAT (Indice di Valutazione dell'Alleanza Terapeutica [Therapeutic Alliance Evaluation Index]), was presented at the 2001 conference of the Italian Society for Psychotherapy Research (Colli and Lingiardi 2001). The scale has been revised and tested in several pilot studies (Colli and Lingiardi 2002, 2003, 2005, 2006). The scale is structured into two main scales: one for the evaluation of patient contributions to the process (CIS-P) and one for therapist contributions (CIS-T), each with subscales. The CIS-P is composed of three subscales evaluating patients' positive and negative contributions: the Collaborative Processes scale (CP), the Direct Rupture Markers scale (DRM), and the Indirect Rupture (IRM). The scale, which was largely derived starting from the seminal empirical works of Safran and collaborators on alliance ruptures (Safran et al. 1990, 1994) and at a theoretical level was based on the work of Safran and Muran (2000a), has in our opinion two important characteristics: (1) it evaluates positive and negative contributions of patient and therapist to the quality and construction of the relationship, and (2) it permits study at a micro level of the negotiation process between patient and therapist and depicts the idiosyncratic interactional patterns that unfold between patient and therapist.

16.4.2 Therapeutic Alliance Ruptures and Resolutions: Empirical Findings

The alliance rupture and resolution construct as suggested by Eubanks-Carter et al. (2010, unpublished manuscript) has been investigated principally in four kinds of studies: (a) quantitative process studies, (b) quantitative outcome studies, (c) task analytic studies, and (d) qualitative process studies.

(a) In *quantitative process* research the principal focus is the study of the occurrence of ruptures and resolution in psychotherapy and, in some cases, the link between these processes and therapy outcome. Across several studies the occurrence of alliance ruptures varies from 19 % of the sessions (Eames and Roth 2000) to 100 % (Colli and Lingiardi 2009; Eubanks-Carter et al. 2010a). Withdrawal markers are generally present in every session, while confrontation ruptures are less frequent. A difference has been observed between the perspective of evaluations: therapists tend to report a higher number of ruptures than patients (Eames and Roth 2000; Muran et al. 2009), and external observers tend to report a high number of ruptures compared to patients (Sommerfeld et al. 2008). These results suggest that there is a great variability in the occurrence of alliance ruptures and also that some rupture processes, such as withdrawal ruptures, are physiologically present in every session.

In other research, the authors found a significant association between the occurrence of ruptures and the presence of dysfunctional relational schemas involving the therapist identified by using the CCRT method (Sommerfeld et al. 2008; Luborsky and Crits-Christoph 1998), while in other research the authors found an occurrence of therapist rupture interventions in 31 % of the sessions and a significant correlation between therapist negative intervention and the occurrence of more disruptive patient alliance rupture markers (Colli and Lingiardi 2009). These results seem to confirm two important "relational" ideas: (1) that an alliance rupture is a patient's vehicle for the expression of core relational problems and (2) that alliance is mainly a patient and therapist co-construction.

(b) In *quantitative outcome studies* researchers compared the efficacy of treatments focused on alliance rupture and resolution with other forms of intervention (Muran et al. 2005; Constantino et al. 2008). One study comparing a specific therapeutic alliance rupture-focused intervention, the brief relational therapy (Muran et al. 2005), with short-term psychodynamic therapy and cognitive–behavioral therapy, found significant differences in clinical significance change and dropout rates. It was found that brief relational and cognitive–behavioral models produced more clinically significant change than short-term dynamic psychotherapy, and brief relational therapy had significantly lower dropout rates than the other forms of treatment (Muran et al. 2005). Other researchers evaluated the efficacy of an integrative form of cognitive therapy (ICT) for depression that incorporates specific strategies for addressing alliance ruptures and compared it with a traditional cognitive therapy (CT): Effect size estimates revealed that ICT patients evidenced greater posttreatment improvement and more clinically significant change than CT patients (Constantino et al. 2008). A similar effort to incorporate rupture and resolution strategies into CBT for generalized anxiety disorder was proposed by Newman et al. (2008). The study found that the integrative treatment significantly decreased GAD symptoms, yielding a higher effect size than the average effect size of standard CBT reported in literature. In a recent study, based on a sample of 128 patients randomly assigned to three different time-limited psychotherapies for personality disorders (cognitive–behavioral, brief relational, and short-term dynamic), results indicate that lower rupture intensity and higher rupture resolution are associated with better ratings of the alliance and session quality, and lower rupture intensity predicts good outcome on measures of interpersonal functioning, while higher rupture resolution predicts better retention (Muran et al. 2009).

(c) In *task analytic* studies, researchers analyze the processes involved in producing change (Greenberg 1986). Greenberg (Greenberg 1986; Greenberg and Foerster 1996), using a combination of quantitative and qualitative approaches, pioneered the use of task analysis for the intensive analysis of events in therapy. Greenberg and Foerster (1996) outlined six steps of analysis: (a) select a specific type of problem-solving task and operationalize in-session markers; (b) devise a rational (ideal) analysis of how the problem might be solved using experts (i.e., identify a rationally derived range of strategies for problem solving); (c) carry out an empirical study of actual problem solving; (d) progressively correct the rational model using empirical data (i.e., form a rational–empirical model); (e) refine the model by successively completing rational and empirical analyses; and (f) verify the model by comparing successful and unsuccessful problem-solving tasks to identify the impact on outcome. Thus, task analysis utilizes an observational, inductive, and iterative strategy in which investigators use observations of individuals performing tasks to progressively improve descriptions of how the task can best be performed. In other words, task analysis studies what patient and therapist do, at a micro analytic level, to resolve a task relevant for the process of change in psychotherapy. Safran, Muran, and colleagues, in a series of studies, investigated through task analytic investigation paradigm the process of rupture and resolutions (Safran et al. 1990, 1994; Safran and Muran 1996). These studies permitted the authors to construct a rupture resolution model (Safran and Muran 2000a).

The model consists of four stages. In the first stage the therapist recognizes a rupture and tries to disengage from it by inviting the patient to explore the event. In stage 2, the therapist and patient explore their perceptions of the rupture. In stage 3 the therapist and patient explore avoidance maneuvers in relation to stage 2. Finally, in stage 4 the therapist and patient move toward clarifying the wish or need that underlies the patient's problematic interpersonal behaviors. Safran and Muran (2000a), in accordance with Harper's work, have organized patient ruptures into two main subtypes: withdrawal and confrontation (Harper 1989a, b).

In withdrawal ruptures, "the patient withdraws or partially disengages from the therapist, his or her own emotions, or some aspect of the therapeutic process" (Safran and Muran 2000a, p. 141). Withdrawal markers include patient behaviors such as verbal disengagement (e.g., changing the topic, long silences, or use of vague, abstract language) or a mismatch between affective expression and narrative content. In this kind of marker, the patient indirectly expresses disaffection or disagreement about the tasks or goals of therapy or about the relationship. Withdrawal markers also include patient avoidance maneuvers such as skipping from topic to topic in such a way as to prevent therapist interventions in order to reduce patient anxiety associated with a rupture in the alliance. Another maneuver involves self-esteem-enhancing operations, in which the client may attempt to justify or defend him- or herself during the process of a rupture as a means of boosting a deflated sense of self-worth. As observed by Safran et al. (1990), avoidance maneuvers and self-esteem-enhancing operations can be considered as reflections of what Sullivan (1953) termed "security operations." Conversely, in confrontation ruptures, "the patient directly expresses anger, resentment, or disaffection with the therapist or some aspect of the therapy" (Safran and Muran 2000a, p. 141). Examples of this kind of marker are most evident in the patient's verbal criticisms of the therapist, either as a person or in terms of his or her professional qualifications. These generally appear as hostile or dismissive manners of communication.

Agnew et al. (1994), starting from the work of Safran and Muran and using a task analytic paradigm, tested a psychodynamic interpersonal model of resolution of confrontation ruptures. This model is quite similar to Safran and Muran's but differs from it for a greater focus on linking the alliance rupture to situations outside of therapy and discussing new ways to handle those situations. In the same way, another study that investigated alliance rupture and resolution in cognitive analytic therapy of borderline patients (Bennett et al. 2006) shares many similarities with Safran and Muran's model (2000a) but differs from it for a different way of dealing with the fourth stage: Bennett et al. placed greater emphasis on linking rupture to a preestablished case formulation and to the patient's other relationships.

(d) In *qualitative process* studies researchers have focused their attention on negative experiences, impasse, and misunderstanding events (Hill 2010),[1] with an emphasis on the perceptions of the events by patient and therapist captured by the use of interviews with open-ended questions. Some researchers found that clients had and hid negative feelings about their therapies (Rennie 1994; Regan and Hill 1992) and that experiences of anger toward the therapist occur quite often (Dahlenberg 2004). Rhodes et al. (1994), in a sample of 19 cases characterized by the presence of a misunderstanding event, investigated the differences between the cases in which the misunderstanding event was resolved (11 cases) and the unresolved cases (8 cases).

[1] In this section we gave emphasis to qualitative studies related to alliance ruptures and resolutions, but it is important to underline that there are also several qualitative studies that investigated the construct of "therapeutic alliance" from a qualitative point of view (Bedi and Richards 2011).

The main difference was that in the resolved cases, clients reported a good quality of the relationship before the event (patients felt safe and supported by the therapist); conversely, in unresolved cases clients reported a poor quality of the relationship (therapist was critical, did not remember important facts). In another study, a follow-up to the Rhodes et al. study (1994), therapists interviewed about therapeutic impasses that occurred during therapy reported that the impasse clients had a considerable pathology (such as personality disorder) and interpersonal problems or problematic current intimate or family relationships. Through therapists' interviews it emerged that impasse generally involved a lack of agreement about tasks or goals of therapy and, rather being a single event, thus involved a general disagreement and power struggles related to the way therapy should be conducted (Hill et al. 1996). In another study Hill et al. (2003) investigated the inner experience of therapists working with angry patients. Researchers investigated the different impacts on therapists of patients who directly expressed their anger and patients who did not directly express anger. Not surprisingly, therapists reported more difficulties with the first group (direct expression of anger) than with those who did not express their anger, and quite often therapists tended to respond to client hostility with mutual hostility.

16.4.3 A Brief Research Agenda About Therapeutic Alliance Ruptures and Resolutions

As observed by the interdivisional task force on evidence-based therapy relationships (Norcross and Wampold 2011), alliance ruptures and resolutions represent a promising effective element of the relationship, but we need further research to evaluate their role and importance in contributing to psychotherapy efficacy. In our opinion, future research will have to resolve some problematic points of therapeutic alliance rupture and resolution processes investigation:

(a) *Definition of the construct*: In psychotherapy we have a clear problem of a "Tower of Babel" (Horvath 2011): sometimes we use the same words but with different meanings or conversely we use different terms but with the same meanings. The problem of construct definition is crucial because the definition we adopt influences how we operationalize the construct and what we evaluate. From this point of view, therapeutic alliance but much more alliance ruptures and resolution constructs need additional work to clear similarities and differences among the definitions. For example, looking closer inside and beyond the therapeutic alliance ruptures and resolutions definitions, we can find several constructs such as transference–countertransference enactment, empathic failure, impasses, etc., that are hard to differentiate from it (Safran & Kraus, 2014).

(b) *Evaluation perspective*: Every perspective has its strengths and limits. According to the interdivisional task force on evidence-based therapy, relationship researchers are encouraged to address the observational perspective (i.e., therapist, patient, or external rater) in future studies. Agreement among different perspectives provides a solid sense of established fact; divergence among perspectives holds important implications for construct definition and for practice. For the same reason we think it necessary to also improve studies to evaluate convergent validity between different measures in observer-rated versions.

(c) *Patient characteristics*: Until now research has partially excluded the investigation of the relationship between patient characteristics and different modalities to break the alliance and to repair it. For example, it could be useful to differentiate the stage process model proposed by Safran and Muran in relation to different patients' interpersonal style, such as different attachment styles. It is clinically realistic to think that different attachment styles will lead to different alliance rupture and repair processes. Another variable to take into consideration could be the patient's level of functioning in terms of patient defense level, object relation level, and reflective functioning. For example, with high-functioning patients, it could be useful to focus resolution strategies more on connecting past relational experience to the here and now of the therapeutic relationship (transference interpretations), while with low-functioning patients, it could be useful to limit resolution strategies to the here and now of the relationship or a redefinition of task and goals of therapy or validating strategies.

(d) *Intensive and processual investigation*: Although we have a growing amount of (but still insufficient) research investigating the relationship between alliance ruptures and resolutions and therapy outcome, very few studies investigated the processes through which alliance ruptures are resolved: this kind of research could help us in promoting more effective resolution processes, taking a balance between the need of replication and relationship guidelines and the need to reflect the uniqueness of every patient–therapist dyad.

(e) Statistical analysis: The last point concerns the use of statistical procedures more able to capture the interactive and time-related nature of the alliance, such as time series analysis and growth curve analysis (Tschacher and Ramseyer 2009). We consider it the last point because we strongly believe that the abovementioned points are necessary prerequisites that permit the creation of reliable data to analyze.

Conclusions

In this chapter we gave a short review of what we consider some of the main aspects of therapeutic alliance and research focusing on it, trying to make a journey from the historical therapeutic alliance construct, passing through the evaluation of therapeutic alliance and the problems connected to its measurement, to more recent studies focused on alliance ruptures and resolutions. Considering that the literature about the topic is so wide, we did not examine in detail a lot of several important issues related to therapeutic alliance, such as the relationship between therapist interventions and the formation of therapeutic alliance and the resolutions of therapeutic alliance ruptures (Hilsenroth et al. 2012; Lingiardi et al. 2011), the relationship between therapeutic alliance formation and patient personality (Smith et al. 2013), the problem of the efficacy of psychotherapy training focused on therapeutic alliance building skills in therapists (Safran and Muran 2000a), or the overlaps between therapeutic alliance and other confining constructs such as transference–countertransference (Safran and Muran 2006; Betan et al. 2005; Colli et al. 2014) and real relationships (Gelso 2009a, b; Horvath 2009). As we have seen, therapeutic alliance construct has spread during the years, crossing the boundaries of the psychoanalytic field and becoming a central issue in all therapeutic approaches. Moreover, the construct today cannot be considered a separate variable of the psychotherapy process and must be studied in relation with other variables such as therapists' interventions (Lingiardi et al. 2011) and patient diagnosis (Bender 2005). From our point of view, to study therapeutic alliance in a modern fashion requires maintaining a balanced focus on theoretical, empirical, and clinical issues and a balance between the need to use sophisticated statistical analysis and to perform research that can inform clinicians in their clinical practice.

References

Ackerman S, Hilsenroth M (2001) A review of therapist characteristics and techniques negatively impacting the therapeutic alliance. Psychother Theory Res Pract Train 38:171–185. doi:10.1037/0033-3204.38.2.171

Ackerman S, Hilsenroth M (2003) A review of therapist characteristics and techniques positively impacting the therapeutic alliance. Clin Psychol Rev 23:1–33. doi:10.1016/S0272-7358(02)00146-0

Agnew RM, Harper H, Shapiro DA, Barkham M (1994) Resolving a challenge to the therapeutic relationship: a single-case study. Br J Med Psychol 67:155–170. doi:10.1111/j.2044-8341.1994.tb01783.x

Alexander LB, Luborsky L (1986) The Penn helping alliance scale. In: Greenberg LS, Pinsof WM (eds) The psychotherapeutic process: a research handbook. Guilford, New York, pp 325–356

Allen JG, Newsom GE, Gabbard GO, Coyne L (1984) Scales to assess the therapeutic alliance from a psychoanalytic perspective. Bull Menninger Clin 48 (5):383–400

Andrusyna TP, Tang TZ, DeRubeis RJ, Luborsky L (2001) Factor structure of therapeutic alliance in cognitive behavioral therapy: two independent constructs? J Psychother Pract Res 10:173–178, PMCID: PMC3330646

Barber JP, Luborsky L, Crits-Christoph P, Thase ME, Weiss R, Frank A, Onken L, Gallop R (1999) Therapeutic alliance as a predictor of outcome in treatment of cocaine dependence. Psychother Res 9(1):54–73. doi:10.1080/10503309912331332591

Barber JP, Connolly MB, Crits-Cristoph P, Gladis M, Siqueland L (2000) Alliance predicts patients' outcome beyond in-treatment change in symptoms. J Consult Clin Psychol 68:1027–1032. doi:10.1037/1949-2715.S.1.80

Barber JP, Khalsa SR, Sharpless BA (2010) The validity of the alliance as a predictor of psychotherapy outcome. In: Muran JC, Barber JP (eds) The therapeutic alliance: an evidence-based approach to practice. Guilford, New York, pp 29–43

Bedi RP, Richards M (2011) What a man wants: the male perspective on therapeutic alliance formation. Psychotherapy 48(4):381–390. doi:10.1037/a0022424

Bender DS (2005) The therapeutic alliance in the treatment of personality disorders. J Psychiatr Pract 73–87

Bennett D, Parry G, Ryle A (2006) Resolving threats to the therapeutic alliance in cognitive analytic therapy of borderline personality disorder: a task analysis. Psychol Psychother Theory Res Pract 79:395–418. doi:10.1348/147608305X5835

Betan E, Heim A, Conklin CZ, Westen D (2005) Countertransference phenomena and personality pathology in clinical practice: an empirical investigation. Am J Psychiatry 162(5):890–898. doi:10.1176/appi.ajp.162.5.890

Bordin ES (1979) The generalizability of the psychoanalytic concept of the working alliance. Psychother Theory Res Pract 16:252–260. doi:10.1037/h0085885

Bordin ES (1994) Theory and research on the therapeutic working alliance: new directions. In: Horvath AO, Greenberg LS (eds) The working alliance: theory, research, and practice. Wiley, New York, pp 13–37

Budge SL, Wampold BE (2015) The relationship: how it works. In: Gelo OCG, Pritz A, Rieken B (eds) Psychotherapy research: foundations, process, and outcome. Springer, Heidelberg

Charman D (ed) (2004) Processes in brief psychodynamic psychotherapy: advancing effective practice. Lawrence Erlbaum Associates, Hillsdale, NJ

Colli A (2011) Returning to the roots. A comment on the paper "Alliance in Common Factor Land: A View through the Research Lens". Res Psychother 14 (2):4–11

Colli A, Lingiardi V (2001) Una proposta di valutazione dell'alleanza terapeutica a partire dai trascritti delle sedute: il sistema IVAT. Relazione presentata al Convegno SPR Italia Palermo

Colli A, Lingiardi V (2002) Indice di valutazione dell'alleanza terapeutica. In: Lingiardi V (ed) L'Alleanza terapeutica: Teoria, Ricerca, Clinica. Raffaello Cortina, Milano, pp 212–222

Colli A, Lingiardi V (2003) Valutazione multi-strumentale di una paziente in psicoterapia: La valutazione dell'alleanza terapeutica con l'IVAT. Paper Relazione presentata al Convegno SPR. Italia, Milano

Colli A, Lingiardi V (2005) Valutare i processi di rottura e riparazione dell'alleanza terapeutica: l'IVAT-II. Relazione presentata al V Convegno SPR Italia, San Benedetto del Tronto

Colli A, Lingiardi V (2006) Therapist's interventions adjustment ratio and relational failures: a pilot study on the way therapists break the alliance. Paper presented at the 37th 79 international meeting of the society for psychotherapy research, Edinburgh, Scotland

Colli A, Lingiardi V (2009) The collaborative interactions scale: a new transcript-based method for the assessment of therapeutic alliance ruptures and resolutions in psychotherapy. Psychother Res 19:718–734. doi:10.1080/10503300903121098

Colli A, Tanzilli A, Dimaggio G, Lingiardi V (2014) Patient personality and therapist response: an empirical investigation. Am J Psychiatry 171(1):102–108. doi:10.1176/appi.ajp.2013.13020224

Constantino MJ, Marnell ME, Haile AJ, Kanther-Sista SN, Wolman K, Zappert L et al (2008) Integrative cognitive therapy for depression: a randomized pilot comparison. Psychother Theory Res Pract Train 45:122–134. doi:10.1037/0033-3204.45.2.122

Dahlenberg CJ (2004) Maintaining the safe and effective therapeutic relationship in the context of distrust and anger: countertransference and complex trauma. Psychother Theory Res Pract Train 41:438–447. doi:10.1037/0033-3204.41.4.438

De Bei F (2006) La ricerca sull'alleanza terapeutica. In: Dazzi N, Lingiardi V, Colli A (eds) La ricerca in psicoterapia: Modelli e Strumenti. Raffaello Cortina, Milano, pp 505–534

DeRubeis RJ, Feeley M (1990) Determinants of change in cognitive therapy for depression. Cogn Therapy Res 14:469–482. doi:10.1007/BF01172968

Doran JM, Safran JD, Waizmann V, Bolger K, Muran JD (2012) The alliance negotiation scale: psychometric construction and preliminary reliability and validity analysis. Psychother Res 22:1–10. doi:10.1080/10503307.2012.709326

Eames V, Roth A (2000) Patient attachment orientation and the early working alliance: a study of patient and therapist reports of alliance quality and ruptures. Psychother Res 10:421–434. doi:10.1093/ptr/10.4.421

Elvins R, Green J (2008) The conceptualization and measurement of therapeutic alliance: an empirical review. Clin Psychol Rev 28:1167–1187. doi:10.1016/j.cpr.2008.04.002

Eubanks-Carter C, Muran JC, Safran JD (2009) Rupture resolution rating system (3RS): manual. Beth Israel Medical Center, New York (Unpublished manuscript)

Eubanks-Carter C, Muran JC, Safran JD (2010a) Alliance ruptures and resolution. In: Muran C, Barber JP (eds) The therapeutic alliance: an evidence-based guide to practice. Guilford, New York, pp 74–83

Eubanks-Carter C, Mitchell A, Muran JC, Safran JD (2010) Development of a new observer-based system for rating confrontation and withdrawal rupture markers and rupture resolution strategies. (Unpublished manuscript)

Eubanks-Carter C, Gorman BS, Muran JC (2012) Quantitative naturalistic methods for detecting change points in psychotherapy research: an illustration with alliance ruptures. Psychother Res 22:621–637. doi:10.1080/10503307.2012.693772

Freud S (1958) The dynamics transference. In: Strachey J (Ed. & Trans.) The standard edition of the complete psychological works of Sigmund Freud, vol 12. Hogart Press, London, pp 99–108 (Original work published 1912)

Freud S (1964) Analysis terminable and interminable. In: Strachey J (Ed. & Trans.) The standard edition of the complete psychological works of Sigmund Freud, vol 23. Hogart Press, London, pp 209–254 (Original work published 1937)

Freud S (1975) 'Wild' psycho-analysis. In: Strachey J (Ed. & Trans.) The standard edition of the complete psychological works of Sigmund Freud, vol 11. Hogart Press, London, pp 219–228 (Original work published 1910)

Friedman L (1969) The therapeutic alliance. Int J Psychoanal 50:139–154

Gaston L, Marmar C (1994) The california psychotherapy alliance scales. In: Horvath AO, Greenberg LS (eds) The working alliance: theory, research and practice. Wiley, New York, pp 85–108

Gaston L, Marmar CR, Thompson LW, Gallagher D (1991) Alliance prediction of outcome beyond in-treatment symptomatic change as psychotherapy process. Psychother Res 1:104–13. doi:10.1080/10503309112331335531

Gelso CJ (2009a) The real relationship in a postmodern world: theoretical and empirical explorations. Psychother Res 19:253–264. doi:10.1080/10503300802389242

Gelso CJ (2009b) The time has come: the real relationship in psychotherapy research. Psychother Res 19:278–282. doi:10.1080/10503300902777155

Greenberg LS (1986) Change process research. J Consult Clin Psychol 54:4–11. doi:10.1037/0022-006X.54.1.4

Greenberg LS, Foerster FS (1996) Task analysis exemplified: the process of resolving unfinished business. J Consult Clin Psychol 64(3):439–446. doi:10.1037/0022-006X.64.3.439-

Greenson RR (1965) The working alliance and the transference neurosis. In: Greenson RR (ed) Explorations in psychoanalysis. International Universities Press, New York

Greenson RR (1967) The technique and practice of psychoanalysis. International Universities Press Inc., New York

Harper H (1989a) Coding guide I: IDENTIFICATION of confrontation challenges in exploratory therapy. University of Sheffield, Sheffield, UK

Harper H (1989b) Coding guide II: Identification of withdrawal challenges in exploratory therapy. University of Sheffield, Sheffield, UK

Hartley DE, Strupp HH (1983) The therapeutic alliance: its relationship to outcome in brief psychotherapy. In: Masling J (ed) Empirical studies of psychoanalytical theories, vol 1. Erlbaum, Hillsdale, NJ, pp 1–37

Hatcher RL (2010) Alliance theory and measurement. In: Muran C, Barber JP (eds) The therapeutic alliance: an evidence-based guide to practice. Guilford, New York, pp 7–28

Hatcher RL, Barends AW (2006) How a return to theory could help alliance research. Psychother Theory Res Pract 43:292–299. doi:10.1037/0033-3204.43.3.292

Hatcher RL, Gillaspy JA (2006) Development and validation of a revised short version of the working alliance inventory. Psychother Res 16:12–25. doi:10.1080/10503300500352500

Hill CE (2010) Qualitative studies of negative experiences in psychotherapy. In: Muran C, Barber JP (eds) The therapeutic alliance: an evidence-based guide to practice. Guilford, New York, pp 63–73

Hill CE (2011) Consensual qualitative research: a practical resource for investigating social science phenomena. American Psychological Association, Washington, DC

Hill CE (2015) Consensual qualitative research (cqr) methods for conducting psychotherapy process research. In: Gelo OCG, Pritz A, Rieken B (eds) Psychotherapy research: foundations, process, and outcome. Springer, Heidelberg

Hill CE, Nutt-Williams E, Heaton KJ, Thompson BJ, Rhodes RH (1996) Therapist retrospective recall of impasses in long-term psychotherapy: a qualitative analysis. J Couns Psychol 43:207–217. doi:10.1037/0022-0167.43.2.207

Hill CE, Thompson BJ, Williams EN (1997) A guide to conducting consensual qualitative research. Couns Psychol 25:517–572. doi:10.1177/0011000097254001

Hill CE, Kellems IS, Kolchakian MR, Wonnell TL, Davis TL, Nakayama EY (2003) The therapist experience of being the target of hostile versus suspected-unasserted client anger: factors associated with resolution. Psychother Res 13:475–491. doi:10.1093/ptr/kpg040

Hill CE, Knox S, Thompson BJ, Williams EN, Hess S, Ladany N (2005) Consensual qualitative research: an update. J Couns Psychol 52:196–205. doi:10.1037/0022-0167.52.2.196

Hilsenroth MJ, Peters EJ, Ackerman SJ (2004) The development of therapeutic alliance during psychological assessment: patient and therapist perspectives. J Pers Assess 83:332–344. doi:10.1207/s15327752jpa8303_14

Hilsenroth MJ, Cromer T, Ackerman S (2012) How to make practical use of therapeutic alliance research in your clinical work. In: Levy RA, Ablon JS, Kaechele H (eds) Psychodynamic psychotherapy research: evidence-based practice and practice-based evidence. Springer, New York, NY, pp 361–380

Horvath AO, Luborsky L (1993) The role of the therapeutic alliance in psychotherapy. J Consult Clin Psychol 61:561–573. doi:10.1037/0022-006X.61.4.561

Horvath AO (2009) How real is the "Real Relationship"? Psychother Res 19(3):273–277. doi:10.1080/10503300802592506

Horvath AO (2011) Alliance in common factor land: a view through the research lens. Res Psychother Psychopathol Process Outcome 14(1):121–135

Horvath AO, Bedi RP (2002) The alliance. In: Norcross JC (ed) Psychotherapy relationships that work: evidence-based responsiveness. Oxford University Press, New York, NY, pp 37–69

Horvath AO, Greenberg LS (1989) Development and validation of the working alliance inventory. J Couns Psychol 36:223–233. doi:10.1037/0022-0167.36.2.223

Horvath AO, Symonds BD (1991) Relation between working alliance and outcome in psychotherapy: a meta-analysis. J Couns Psychol 38:139–149. doi:10.1037/0022-0167.38.2.139

Horvath A, Del Re AC, Flückiger C, Symonds D (2011) Alliance in individual psychotherapy. Psychotherapy 48:9–16. doi:10.1037/a0022186

Hougaard E (1994) The therapeutic alliance–a conceptual analysis. Scand J Psychol 35:67–85. doi:10.1111/j.1467-9450.1994.tb00934.x

Jenkis C, Dillman D (1997) Towards a theory of self-administered questionnaire design. In: Lyberg LE et al (eds) Survey measurement and process quality. Wiley, New York

Kivlighan DM, Shaughnessy P (2000) Patterns of working alliance development: a typology of working alliance ratings. J Couns Psychol 47:362–371. doi:10.1037/0022-0167.47.3.362

Lanyon RI, Goodstein LD (1997) Personality assessment, 3rd edn. Wiley, New York

Lingiardi V (2002) L'alleanza terapeutica. Raffaello Cortina, Milano

Lingiardi V, Filippucci L, Baiocco R (2005) Therapeutic alliance evaluation in personality disorders psychotherapy. Psychother Res 15(12):45–53. doi:10.1080/10503300512331327047

Lingiardi V, Colli A, Gentile D, Tanzilli A (2011) Exploration of session process: relationship to depth and alliance. Psychotherapy 48(4):391–400. doi:10.1037/a0025248

Luborsky L (1976) Helping alliances in psychotherapy: the groundwork for a study of their relationship to its outcome. In: Claghorn JL (ed) Successful psychotherapy. Brunner/Mazel, New York, pp 92–116

Luborsky L, Crits-Christoph P (1998) Understanding transference: the core conflictual relationship theme method, 2nd edn. American Psychological Association, Washington, DC

Luborsky L, Singer B, Luborsky L (1975) Comparative studies of psychotherapies. Arch Gen Psychiatry 32:995–1008. doi:10.1001/archpsyc.1975.01760260059004

Luborsky L, Crits-Cristoph P, Alexander L, Margolis M, Cohen M (1983) Two helping alliance methods for predicting outcomes of psychotherapy: a counting signs versus a global rating method. J Nerv Ment Dis 171:480–492

Marmar CR, Gaston L (1988) Manual for the California psychotherapy alliance scale – CALPAS. Department of Psychiatry, University of California, San Francisco (Unpublished manuscript)

Martin DJ, Garske JP, Davis MK (2000) Relation of the therapeutic alliance with outcome and other variables: a meta-analytic review. J Consult Clin Psychol 68:438–450. doi:10.1037/0022-006X.68.3.438

McAleavey AA, Castonguay LG (2015) The process of change in psychotherapy: common and unique factors. In: Gelo OCG, Pritz A, Rieken B (eds) Psychotherapy research: foundations, process, and outcome. Springer, Heidelberg

Mörtl K, Gelo OCG (2015) Qualitative methods in psychotherapy process research. In: Gelo OCG, Pritz A, Rieken B (eds) Psychotherapy research: foundations, process, and outcome. Springer, Heidelberg

Muran JC, Safran JD, Samstag LW, Winston A (1992) Patient and therapist postsession questionnaires, Version 1992. Beth Israel Medical Center, New York

Muran JC, Safran JD, Samstag LW, Winston A (2005) Evaluating an alliance-focused treatment for personality disorders. Psychother Theory Res Pract Train 42 (4):532–545. doi:10.1037/0033-3204.42.4.532

Muran JC, Safran JD, Gorman BS, Samstag LW, Eubanks-Carter C, Winston A (2009) The relationship of early alliance ruptures and their resolution to process and outcome in three time-limited psychotherapies for personality disorders. Psychother Theory Res Pract Train 46:233–248. doi:10.1037/a0016085

Newman MG, Castonguay LG, Borkovec TD, Fisher AJ, Nordberg SS (2008) An open trial of integrative therapy for generalized anxiety disorder. Psychother Theory Res Pract Train 45:135–147. doi:10.1037/0033-3204.45.2.135

Norcross JC, Wampold BE (2011) Evidence-based therapy relationships: research conclusions and clinical practices. Psychotherapy 48:98–102. doi:10.1037/a0022161

O'Malley SS, Suh CS, Strupp HH (1983) The Vanderbilt psychotherapy process scale: a report on the scale development and a process-outcome study. J Consult Clin Psychol 51(4):581–586

Orlinsky DE, Howard KI (1975) Varieties of psychotherapeutic experience: multivariate analysis of patients' and therapists' reports. Teachers College Press, New York

Regan AM, Hill CE (1992) An investigation of what clients and counselors do not say in brief therapy. J Couns Psychol 39:168–174. doi:10.1037/0022-0167.39.2.168

Rennie DL (1994) Clients' deference in psychotherapy. J Couns Psychol 41:427–437. doi:10.1037/0022-0167.41.4.427

Reynolds M, Hatcher R, Hansell J (1995) Exploration of the individual factor structures of three widely used alliance measures (patient versions). Annual meeting of the society of psychotherapy research

Rhodes R, Hill CE, Thompson BJ, Elliott R (1994) Client retrospective recall of resolved and unresolved misunderstanding events. J Couns Psychol 41:473–483. doi:10.1037/0022-0167.41.4.473

Ribeiro E, Ribeiro AP, Gonçalves MM, Horvath AO, Stiles WB (2012) How collaboration in therapy becomes therapeutic: the therapeutic collaboration coding system. Psychol Psychother Theory Res Pract 86:294–314 (2013). doi:10.1111/j.2044-8341.2012.02066.x

Roth A, Fonagy P (2004) What works for whom? A critical review of psychotherapy research, 2nd edn. Guilford, New York

Safran JD & Kraus, J (2014). Alliance Ruptures, Impasses, and Enactments: A Relational Perspective. *Psychotherapy* 51(3):381–387.

Safran JD, Muran JC (1996) The resolution of ruptures in the therapeutic alliance. J Consult Clin Psychol 64:447–458. doi:10.1037/0022-006X.64.3.447

Safran JD, Muran JC (2000a) Negotiating the therapeutic alliance: a relational treatment guide. The Guildford Press, New York

Safran JD, Muran JC (2000b) Resolving therapeutic alliance ruptures: diversity and integration. J Clin Psychol 56(2):233–243. doi:10.1002/(SICI)1097-4679

Safran JD, Muran JC (2006) Has the concept of the therapeutic alliance outlived its usefulness? Psychother Theory Res Pract Train 43:286–291. doi:10.1037/0033-3204.43.3.286

Safran JD, Crocker P, McMain S, Murray P (1990) Therapeutic alliance rupture as a therapy event for empirical investigation. Psychother Theory Res Pract 27:154–165. doi:10.1037/0033-3204.27.2.154

Safran JD, Muran JC, Walner-Samstag L (1994) Resolving therapeutic alliance ruptures: a task analytic investigation. In: Horvath AO, Greenberg LS (eds) The working alliance: theory, research, and practice. Wiley, New York, pp 225–255

Safran JD, Muran JC, Samstag LS, Stevens C (2002) Repairing alliance ruptures. In: Norcross JC (ed) Psychotherapy relations that work: therapist contributions and responsiveness to patients. Oxford University Press, New York, pp 235–255

Samstag LW, Safran JD, Muran JC (2000) Rupture resolution scale and coding manual. Beth Israel Medical Center, New York (Unpublished manuscript)

Siegel DJ (2002) Foreword. In: Cozolino L (ed) The neuroscience of psychotherapy: building and rebuilding the human brain. Norton & Company, New York-London, pp 9–12

Smith S, Hilsenroth M, Fiori K, Bornstein R (2014) Relationship between SWAP-200 patient personality characteristics and patient-rated alliance early in treatment. J Nerv Ment Dis 202(5):372–378

Sommerfeld E, Orbach I, Zim S, Mikulincer M (2008) An in-session exploration of ruptures in working alliance and their associations with clients' core conflictual relationship themes, alliance-related discourse, and clients' postsession evaluation. Psychother Res 18:377–388. doi:10.1080/10503300701675873

Sterba R (1934) Il destino dell'Io nella terapia analitica. Psicoterapia e scienze umane 28(2):109–118 (trad. it.)

Stevens CL, Muran JC, Safran JD, Gorman BS, Winston A (2007) Levels and patterns of the therapeutic alliance in brief psychotherapy. Am J Psychother 61:109–129

Stiles WB (1980) Measurement of the impact of psychotherapy sessions. J Consult Clin Psychol 48:176–185. doi:10.1037/0022-006X.48.2.176

Stiles WB, Glick MJ, Osatuke K, Hardy EG, Shapiro DA, Agnew-Davies R, Annerees A, Barkham M (2004) Patterns of alliance development and the rupture-repair hypothesis: Are productive relationships U-shaped or V- shaped? J Couns Psychol 51:81–92. doi:10.1037/0022-0167.51.1.81

Strauss JL, Hayes AM, Johnson SL, Newman CF, Brown GK, Barber JP et al (2006) Early alliance, alliance ruptures, and symptom change in a nonrandomized trial of cognitive therapy for avoidant and obsessive-compulsive personality disorders. J Consult Clin Psychol 74:337–345. doi:10.1037/0022-006X.74.2.337

Sullivan HS (1953) The interpersonal theory of psychiatry. Norton, New York

Tracey TJ, Kokotovic AM (1989) Factor structure of the working alliance inventory. Psychol Assess 1:207–210. doi:10.1037/1040-3590.1.3.207

Tryon GS, Kane AS (1995) Client involvement, working alliance, and type of therapy termination. Psychother Res 5:189–198. doi:10.1080/10503309512331331306

Tryon G, Blackwell S, Hammel E (2008) The magnitude of client and therapist working alliance ratings. Psychother Theory Res Pract Train 45(4):546–551. doi:10.1037/a0014338

Tschacher W, Ramseyer F (2009) Modeling psychotherapy process by time-series panel analysis (TSPA). Psychother Res 19(4–5):469–481. doi:10.1080/10503300802654496

Westen D, Shedler J (1999a) Revising and assessing Axis II. Part I: Developing a clinically meaningful and empirically valid assessment method. Am J Psychiatry 156:2, 258–272

Westen D, Shedler J (1999b) Revising and assessing Axis II, Part II: Toward an empirically based and clinically useful classification of personality disorders. Am J Psychiatry 156(2):273–285

Wolfe BE, Goldfried MR (1988) Research on psychotherapy integration: recommendations and conclusions from an NIMH workshop. J Consult Clin Psychol 56:448–451. doi:10.1037/0022-006X.56.3.448

Zetzel ER (1956) Current concepts of transference. Int J Psycho-Anal 37:369

Zetzel ER (1958) Psichiatria psicoanalitica. Boringhieri, Torino (Tr. it. 1976)

Positive Emotions in Psychotherapy: Conceptual Propositions and Research Challenges

17

A. Stalikas, M. Fitzpatrick, P. Mistkidou, A. Boutri, and C. Seryianni

Contents

A. Stalikas (✉) • P. Mistkidou • A. Boutri • C. Seryianni
Panteion University of Social and Political Sciences, Psychology Dept., Athens, Greece
e-mail: anstal@panteion.gr

M. Fitzpatrick
McGill University, Faculty of Education, Department of Educational and Counselling Psychology, Montreal, Quebec, Canada

Abstract

In this chapter we discuss the contribution and integration of positive psychology concepts in psychotherapy theory, research, and practice. In the first part we introduce the basic tenets, axioms, and foundational concepts of positive psychology followed by the presentation of the broaden-and-build theory of positive emotions and the research findings that support it. We argue that the broaden-and-build theory contributes to psychotherapy theory and research and practice. We focus on the concepts of broadening, undoing, and building and their potential contribution to psychotherapy. In the last part of the chapter, we focus on the methodological and conceptual research issues that need to be addressed in order to facilitate research initiatives.

17.1 Introduction

After years in which the landscape of psychology was pathology, psychology has begun to cultivate the terrain of the positive (Maddux 2008). A corner of that terrain is the field of positive emotions. The purpose of this chapter is to review what is known about positive emotions in the realm of psychotherapy. We begin with a brief look at positive psychology to establish a context for understanding positive emotions and their role in human functioning. Using a framework called the broaden-and-build theory

O.C.G. Gelo et al. (eds.), *Psychotherapy Research*,
DOI 10.1007/978-3-7091-1382-0_17,

(Fredrickson 1998), we present an understanding of the role of positive emotions in our lives. The research support for that model both outside and within psychotherapy is reviewed. We will also suggest that positive emotions have a generative role of change in psychotherapy and then discuss the psychotherapeutic findings as a framework for considering methodological strategies and challenges for psychotherapy researchers who study positive emotions.

17.1.1 The Growth of Positive Psychology

Prior to World War II, psychology had three missions: curing mental illness, making the lives of all people more fulfilling, and identifying and nurturing talent. In the period following the war, thousands of veterans with psychological problems needed treatment, and psychology responded by shifting its research and treatment emphasis toward curing mental illness (Seligman 1998). The other two important missions—the improvement of normal life and the identification and nurturing of talent—were largely set aside. The question "What is wrong?" guided the thinking of applied psychologists throughout the twentieth century. Diagnostic and measurement methods for disorders such as schizophrenia, depression, anxiety, and alcoholism were developed, and many effective treatments were validated for specific disorders (see Champless and Hollon 1998). Psychotherapists engaged in helping their patients face and overcome struggles. However, the focus of the pathology model on accurate descriptions of specific problems is somewhat incomplete; problems are only part of humankind. This attention to the negative has come at a price. With little research support in the domain of what makes life worth living or how normal people flourish, psychologists must either proceed without an empirical basis or ignore the positive emotions of their clients.

Positive psychology emphasizes the exploration of people's strengths along with their weaknesses. It is the scientific study of optimal human functioning that aims to discover and promote the factors that allow individuals and communities to thrive (Seligman and Csikszentmihalyi 2000). In the twenty-first century, positive psychology has increased in influence; its ideas have grown not only within the psychology community but in the larger society. This growth has probably been fuelled by a confluence of factors, in particular the satiation of pathological models to explain well-being, the increase in pathology in spite of the psychotherapeutic and medical developments for combating it, and the increasing cost of psychological treatments. Theories with alternative depictions of human structure, development, and function, and research developments in areas, such as neuropsychology (e.g., Isen 2002), neurophysiology (e.g., Fredrickson and Levenson 1998; Fredrickson et al. 2000), and psychobiology (e.g., Ashby et al. 1999; Fredrickson and Joiner 2002; Fredrickson et al. 2000; Watson et al. 1988a), have provided alternative conceptual and empirical frameworks.

17.1.2 Positive Emotions: The Broaden-and-Build Model

Fredrickson's (1998) broaden-and-build theory is one prominent and useful theoretical framework situated within the positive psychology domain. Her model has shifted attention to positive emotions and spawned a body of research. Instead of attempting to shoehorn an understanding of positive emotions into existing ideas developed from studying negative emotion, her model is built on the premise that there is a unique evolutionary importance and purpose to positive emotion. Positive and negative emotions are understood to have distinct and complementary adaptive functions, and cognitive and physiological effects (Tugade and Fredrickson 2004, p. 321). The experiences of positive emotions *broaden* a person's thought-action repertoire, meaning that a wider array of thoughts and actions become available (Fredrickson 1998,

2001). This broadening process results in the building of enduring personal and social resources, which can be drawn on when necessary. The resources can be *cognitive*, like the ability to mindfully attend to the present moment; *psychological*, like the ability to maintain a sense of mastery over environmental challenges; *social*, like the ability to give and receive emotional support; or *physical*, like the ability to ward off the common cold. This is the broadening aspect of the theory. People with these resources are more likely to effectively meet life's challenges and take advantage of its opportunities, becoming successful, healthy, and happy in the months and years to come (Fredrickson 2008); this is the *build* element of the broaden-and-build theory.

Fredrickson describes two hypotheses for how positive emotions generate change: the upward spiral and the undoing hypotheses. The upward spiral includes increases in positive emotion that lead to cognitive broadening; increases in cognitive broadening further facilitate the experience of positive emotion. The net result is that of an upward spiral that leads to increases in well-being. The undoing hypothesis refers to the idea that positive emotions reduce the autonomic arousal caused by negative emotions by speeding the recovery from the cardiovascular effects of fear, anxiety, and sadness. Positive emotions loosen the grip that negative emotions hold on thinking; individuals experience a distance that can prompt them to explore alternative thoughts and actions other than those prompted by the initial negative emotion (Fredrickson and Branigan 2005).

17.1.3 Broaden-and-Build Research in General Psychology

These fundamental hypotheses of the broaden-and-build theory have garnered substantial empirical support. Relative to the *broaden* hypothesis, positive emotions have been shown to produce patterns of thought that were notably unusual (Isen et al. 1985), flexible (Isen and Daubman 1984), creative (Isen et al. 1987), integrative (Isen et al. 1991), open to information (Estrada et al. 1997), and efficient (Isen and Means 1983; Isen et al. 1991). Isen and colleagues have also shown that positive emotions increase people's preferences for variety and their openness to new experiences (Kahn and Isen 1993). These cognitive effects of positive emotions have been linked to increases in circulating brain dopamine (Ashby et al. 1999; Isen 2002). Studies examining positive emotions relative to neutral and negative states showed that induced positive emotions widen the scope of people's visual attention (Fredrickson and Branigan 2005; Rowe et al. 2007; Wadlinger and Isaacowitz 2006), broaden their repertoires of desired actions (Fredrickson and Branigan 2005), and increase their openness to critical feedback (Raghunathan and Trope 2002). At the interpersonal level, induced positive emotions increase people's sense of "oneness" with others (Hejmadi et al. 2008), their trust in acquaintances (Dunn and Schweitzer 2005), and their ability to accurately recognize individuals of another race (Johnson and Fredrickson 2005).

Relative to the *build* dimension, the theory suggests that the cognitive broadening accompanying states of positive emotion builds personal resources that expand and improve the ways people cope during crises. Laboratory experiments have shown that positive emotions facilitate attention to, and processing of, important self-relevant information (Reed and Aspinwall 1998; Trope and Pomerantz 1998; for reviews, see Aspinwall 1998, 2001). Consistent with these experimental data are naturalistic studies that also support broaden-and-build processes. Longitudinal studies of bereaved caregivers found that those who experienced positive emotions in the midst of their bereavement were more likely to find positive meaning in their experiences (Moskowitz 2001). Similarly, those who experienced more positive emotions during bereavement were more likely to develop long-term plans and goals. Together with positive emotions, plans and goals predicted greater well-being 12 months after bereavement (Stein et al. 1997; see also Bonanno and Keltner 1997; Keltner and Bonnano 1997). A study of stress and coping among college students linked positive emotions to a style of coping characterized by taking a broad perspective on problems, seeing beyond immediate stressors, and generating multiple courses of action. Positive emotions and broad-minded coping enhance one another; initial levels of positive emotions predicted improvements in broad-minded coping over time and initial levels of broad-minded coping predicted increases in positive emotions over time (Fredrickson and Joiner 2002; see also Fredrickson 2000). This body of work demonstrates that positive emotions do more for people than simply causing them to feel good in the moment. By improving the ways that people cope with adversity, positive emotions also increase the odds that people will feel better and do better in the future. Moreover, as the study by Fredrickson and Joiner (2002) shows, this upward spiral toward improved emotional well-being is linked to the broadened thinking that accompanies positive emotions.

Empirical evidence for the *upward spiral* effect has been largely indirect. Prospective correlational studies have shown that people who, for whatever reasons, experience or express positive emotions more than others show increases over time in optimism and tranquility (Fredrickson et al. 2003), ego resilience (Cohn et al. 2009), mental health (Stein et al. 1997), and the quality of their close relationships (Gable et al. 2006; Waugh and Fredrickson 2006). The first experimental evidence testing the upward spiral hypothesis came from a field experiment with working adults, half of whom were randomly assigned to begin a practice of loving-kindness meditation (Fredrickson 2008). Results showed that this meditation practice produced increases over time in daily experiences of positive emotions, which, in turn, produced increases in a wide range of personal resources: increased mindfulness, purpose in life, and social support and decreased illness symptoms. In turn, these increments in personal resources predicted increased life satisfaction and reduced depressive symptoms.

Relative to the *undoing hypothesis*, research suggests that positive emotions undo the cardiovascular aftereffects of negative emotions. Contentment-eliciting and amusing films produced faster cardiovascular recovery than neutral or sad films (Fredrickson et al. 2000). Laboratory experiments have shown that experiences of positive emotions can quell or undo the lingering cardiovascular effects of these negative emotions. Compared with neutral distractions and sadness, positive emotions produce faster returns to baseline levels of cardiovascular activation following negative emotional arousal (Fredrickson and Levenson 1998; Fredrickson et al. 2000). It is notable that this undoing effect of positive emotions has been demonstrated for high-activation positive emotions such as joy or amusement as well as for low-activation positive emotions such as contentment or serenity. The body of research strongly suggests that positive emotions promote cognitive functioning (Alvarez and Neményy 2001), broaden attention focus (Fredrickson 2001; Fredrickson and Branigan 2005; Isen and Shmidt 2007), and regulate both the psychological and physiological effects of negative emotions (Fredrickson et al. 2000).

Positive emotions also contribute to *valuable life outcomes* (Lyubomirsky et al. 2005) including greater satisfaction and success at work (Losada and Heaphy 2004), greater marital satisfaction (Waldinger et al. 2004), and better coping (Folkman and Moskowitz 2000; Tugade et al. 2004). Research investigating the relationship between positive affects and health has associated positive affectivity with longer life (e.g., Danner et al. 2001; Levy et al. 2002; Ong and Allaire 2005), lower risk of developing a disease (e.g., Cohen et al. 2003; Ostir et al. 2001), survival from life-threatening diseases (e.g., Carver and Scheier 1993; Kubzansky et al. 2001, 2002; Middleton and Byrd 1996; Moskowitz 2003), and reporting of fewer symptoms, less pain, and improved health (e.g., Cohen et al. 2003; Gil et al. 2004; Salovey and Birnbaum 1989) (*for review*, see Pressman and Cohen 2005). Positive emotions are correlated with increased life satisfaction (Schimmack et al. 2004) and a sense of subjective well-being (Hooker et al. 1992; Khoo and Bishop 1997; Sweetman et al. 1993).

While research throughout the twentieth century focused largely on negative emotions, that trend has shifted. Following the lead of Isen and colleagues (for reviews see Isen 2000, 2008), the evidence began to accumulate to indicate that positive emotions function in a different way than negative emotions. An alternative theoretical framework, the broaden-and-build theory of positive emotions (Fredrickson 1998, 2001) has spawned a large body of research. The conclusion that positive emotions are implicated in protecting us during difficulties and enhancing our lives now has a strong empirical base. However, most of this research relates only tangentially to psychotherapy.

17.2 Positive Emotions and Psychotherapy Research

17.2.1 Therapeutic Outcomes of Broadening and Positive Emotion

Fitzpatrick and Stalikas (2008) have suggested that irrespectively of the way they are named in the different treatment modalities, "change events in successful treatment often involve a process of broadening within the client that builds toward successful therapeutic outcomes" (p. 141). Sequences at the level of a change process or change event can be described as common factors in psychotherapy (Grencavage and Norcross 1990). However, a strong evidence base is needed before arriving at the conclusion that broaden-and-build is a therapeutic common factor. Positive emotions may function as generators of change by either directly promoting change or indirectly by facilitating as mediators the psychotherapeutic change process (Fitzpatrick and Stalikas 2008). Research is needed to study how the broadening process undoes or replaces the narrowed or negative perspectives of the individual and if positive emotions build toward change in psychotherapy.

Studies across major therapeutic modalities have already provided strong links between broadening and positive therapeutic outcomes. In the framework of psychodynamic psychotherapies, Gelso et al. (1997) showed that the interaction of transference and emotion insight predicted therapeutic outcome. Kivlighan et al. (2000) have found that increases in insight predicted decreases in target complaints. Alvarez and Neményy (2001) suggested that positive experiences and pleasurable states promote cognitive functioning; introjection, internalization, and sharing of positive experiences were proposed to promote emotional and mental development. In the humanistic tradition, the construct or experiencing came from the work of Carl Rogers and Eugene Gendlin. Experiencing refers to a process of cognitive-affective exploration of feelings related to self or others, in which clients turn their attention inward and attempt to get in touch with the edges of their own personal experience (Gendlin 1996). At higher levels, this cognitive-affective exploration is used to ask questions that challenge current modes of functioning—effectively to broaden the experience of the client. A review of 91 studies examining experiencing in different treatments indicated that higher levels of experiencing related to better therapeutic outcomes (Hendricks 2002). In cognitive and behavioral therapies, cognitive challenging of automatic thoughts and beliefs and modification of core schemata have been linked to positive therapeutic outcome for different types of psychopathology (see Butler et al. 2006). The strong support for the relationship between broadening and outcome in psychotherapy begins to suggest the potential of the broaden-and-build theory within the therapeutic process. However, the role of positive emotions needs further exploration.

Boutri and Stalikas (2009) examined the application of the broaden-and-build model in psychotherapy sessions. For the purpose of the study, they first constructed an instrument for locating the process of broadening in psychotherapy process (Broadening Inventory; Boutri and Stalikas 2005). The instrument consists of 22 statements that describe various manifestations of broadening during the session, at the cognitive, emotional, behavioral, and process levels. At the end of the session, clients were invited to select the statements that accurately describe their in-session experience. Results with 35 psychotherapy sessions indicated several interesting findings: (a) clients experience the process of broadening in therapy sessions; (b) broadening is related to both depth and smoothness of the session, as measured by the Session Evaluation Questionnaire (Stiles and Snow 1984), and thus the quality of the session; (c) broadening is conceptually different, yet related, to in-session therapeutic phenomena such as insight, experiencing, and reflecting and serves a distinct function; (d) the occurrence of the broadening experience during the session is related to the experience of the positive emotion of enthusiasm at the beginning of the session; and (e) broadening leads to the experience of more positive emotions at the end of the session, especially the positive emotions of feeling "strong" and "inspired." Finally, (f) clients' experience of positive emotions at the end of the session leads to the experience of more positive emotions, in general, and more enthusiasm at the beginning of the following session (Boutri and Stalikas 2009). Overall, this early investigation of Fredrickson's model in psychotherapy process provided initial support for several links between broadening and positive emotions and the upward spiral and revealed the importance of broadening to the outcome of the session.

Several studies have suggested that the experience and expression of positive emotions potentially plays an important role in treatment. Pennebaker et al. (1997) investigated the association between the words people use to process their grief in writing interventions and improvement in their physical and mental health. Their findings indicated that those who more frequently used positive rather than negative emotion words in the writings had better mental and physical health; the more frequent use of negative emotion words was associated with poorer outcomes in the subsequent months. Joiner et al. (2001) studied suicidal individuals and found that those who were prone to positive mood showed more positive problem-solving attitudes following treatment of suicidal symptoms and a better response to treatment compared with those less prone to positive moods. Piper et al. (2002) studied complicated grief and found that the experience and expression of positive emotions was associated with positive therapeutic outcome, while the intense expression of negative emotions was related to negative outcomes in short-term group psychotherapy. Mergenthaler (2003) showed that therapeutic change seemed to follow the experience of positive emotions; the experience of only negative emotions was found to be related to negative therapeutic outcome.

The cross-theory support for the importance of broadening to outcome, together with research suggesting that positive emotions also relate to outcome, begins to suggest the potential of the broaden-and-build theory within psychotherapy. For the broaden-and-build theory to have utility in psychotherapy, however, research is needed to link broadening and positive emotion in an upward spiral and to indicate how positive emotions undo or transform negative emotions.

17.2.2 The Upward Spiral and the Undoing Hypothesis in Therapy

17.2.2.1 The Upward Spiral in Therapy

Direct examinations of the broaden-and-build hypothesis have produced preliminary research support of the upward spiral in therapy. Stalikas and colleagues (Seryianni et al. 2004; Stalikas et al. 2004) conducted a series of psychotherapy studies designed to explore the implementation of the key constructs of Fredrickson's theory. With 30 client-therapist dyads, they assessed the emotions of the client before entering the session using the Positive and Negative Affect Scale (PANAS; Watson et al. 1988b). After the sessions, they assessed the therapeutic alliance (Working Alliance Inventory; Horvath and Greenberg 1989) along with the clients' evaluation of the sessions using the Session Impact Scale (Elliott and Wexler 1994) and Session Evaluation Questionnaires (Stiles and Snow 1984). According to their data, clients who reported experiencing positive emotions *before* a session reported higher levels of insight, understanding, and depth in their session (Seryianni et al. 2004). This is the link from PE to broadening. In addition, clients who reported higher broadening levels *during* a session reported higher levels of positive emotions immediately after that session (Stalikas et al. 2004). This is the link in the opposite direction, from broadening to PE. Finally, clients who reported higher depth and alliance in their sessions reported also higher levels of positive emotions before their next session (Seryianni et al. 2004); clients who reported higher positive emotions before the session evaluated alliance and the quality of the session as better (Mertika et al. 2005). Together these data indicate the presence of an upward spiral in psychotherapy.

17.2.2.2 Undoing in Therapy

The other change process of the broaden-and-build model is undoing. Experiencing positive emotions "undoes," counteracts, and minimizes the effects of experiencing negative emotions. Greenberg and Pascual-Leone (2006) have suggested that there are four types of emotional processes that are useful in therapy: emotion awareness and arousal, emotion regulation, active reflection on emotion, and emotional transformation. One of the main outcomes of experiencing negative emotions is their influence on the creation or modification of the emotional schemata, the effects of those new schemata on perceiving and experiencing the self and the world. The modifications lead to changing the perception, experience, and labeling of the emotion. An example of this would be the transformation of the perception of the desire to be close to someone from neediness, weakness, and handicap to desire for intimacy, togetherness, love, and mutual caring.

The work of Leslie Greenberg within the framework of emotion-focused therapy (EFT) provides evidence of emotion transformation. In EFT, a maladaptive emotion state can be transformed by replacing the maladaptive emotion with another, more adaptive emotion. This is not replacing bad feelings with happy feelings or simply looking at the bright side but rather evoking meaningfully embodied alternative experiences that undo perceptions that had been established because of experiencing negative emotions (Greenberg 2008). Research on the in-session resolution of two different kinds of tasks—resolving splits and unfinished business—in emotion-focused therapy (Greenberg 2002) indicated that tasks involving emotional transformation predicted outcome at both termination and 18-month follow-up. The performance of the emotional processing tasks predicted was associated with fewer relapses over the follow-up period (Greenberg and Pedersen 2001), indicating that this undoing of negative affect had impacts on outcome.

Fosha (2004) accelerated experiential dynamic psychotherapy (AEDP) proposes a therapeutic version of emotional transformation. In AEDP, positive emotions function as affective markers that signal that healing transformational processes are at work. Through meta-therapeutic processing—a set of interventions developed for working with emotions, involving alternating waves of experience and reflection—the positive affective experiences that arise as an integral part of healing becomes a sustained focus of experiential exploration. Positive affective states in AEDP do not refer simply to feelings of happiness but rather to experiences that feel *right or true*, even when painful. Positive affective phenomena occurring within the AEDP stages of transformation can include a sense of ease, calm, openness, connection, faith, hope, creativity, enthusiasm, liberation, truth and meaning, competence, agency, initiative, and action (Fosha 2009). These positive emotions instigate a transformational process that can undo the effects of painful experiences.

Research studies offer support for the concept of undoing in psychotherapy across a range of problems. Experiences of positive emotions are momentary. When they accumulate, they undo the impacts of the negative experiences that brought people to therapy and can lead to positive outcomes. In other words, experiencing positive emotions not only initiates the broadening process but changes the maladaptive perspectives, narratives, and meaning making established by experiencing negative emotions.

For people who are grieving, laughter has been found to predict recovery; being able to remember the happy times, to experience joy, serves as an antidote to sadness (Bonanno and Keltner 1997). For people who are depressed, a protest-filled, submissive sense of worthlessness can be transformed therapeutically by guiding them to the desire that drives their protest—a desire to be free of their cages and to access their feelings of joy and excitement for life (Greenberg 2008, p. 96). In women experiencing postpartum depression, instilling an optimistic outlook and attitude had a significant effect in reducing depression (Moraitou and Stalikas 2004). For those who have had a distressing experience, resilience was associated with generating a positive feeling (often through imagery or memory) in order to soothe and combat negative feelings (Whelton and Greenberg 2004). These studies indicate that positive emotions are useful in regulating or transforming emotions in a therapeutic framework.

The growing evidence for the efficacy of positive emotions in the therapeutic context has created momentum. A number of intervention modalities and practices that attempt to harness positive processes in helping people to live better have emerged along this slipstream. While these interventions do not necessarily work directly with positive emotions, they do provide a framework for research initiatives. As positive emotions would be expected to occur with some frequency in these kinds of interventions, they would offer opportunities to study the therapeutic microprocesses in which positive emotions play a role.

17.2.3 Positive Interventions

A range of new clinical approaches within positive psychology offer these opportunities (for a review see Magyar-Moe 2009). In the framework of psychotherapy, these interventions focus not on the reduction of symptoms but on the enhancement of well-being (Fava and Tomba 2009). A number of them focus on the enhancement of positive affect both in clinical and non-clinical populations (Sin and Lyubomirsky 2009). Most of the interventions are oriented to client strengths and are used to overcome problems and enrich lived experiences. Below we highlight several of these approaches and indicate how they actively engage positive emotions to create change.

Hope therapy (Lopez et al. 2000, 2004) is an approach that uses the experience of positive emotions to create and develop hope. In this modality, hope is the active agent of therapeutic change. *Strengths-based counseling* (Smith 2006) also has a hope component. This ten-stage model with elements from a number of different therapeutic modalities draws on emotional strengths, such as insight, optimism, perseverance, perspective, purpose, love of life, and hope. It offers clients feedback that emphasizes their efforts to improve rather than the outcomes of their *efforts. Well-being therapy* (Fava 1999; Fava and Ruini 2003) is based on a multidimensional model of psychological well-being suggested by Ryff (1989). Positive emotions facilitate personal growth, autonomy, positive relations with others, purpose in life, and self-acceptance. *Quality of life therapy* (Frisch 2006) uses positive emotions for finding meaning, attaining goals, and recognizing strengths. This life satisfaction approach encourages clients to find and pursue goals and satisfy their needs and wishes. Positive emotions are linked to meaning making and to the active search for the ingredients that generate life satisfaction. *Strength-centered therapy* (Wong 2006) emphasizes empowerment of clients' character strengths and virtues (Peterson and Seligman 2004). The experience of particular positive emotions helps to identify strengths and virtues. Recognizing and harnessing strengths and virtues also generate positive emotions and increase well-being.

One clinical approach that has begun to accrue research support is *positive psychotherapy* (Rashid 2008). The approach is based on the idea that happiness comes from leading not only a pleasant but an engaged and meaningful life (Seligman 2002). Research studies have indicated that *positive psychotherapy* results in a reduction of depression symptoms and more cases of complete remission of depression in comparison to treatment as usual with or without medication and also leads to increased happiness (Seligman et al. 2006). Group *positive psychotherapy* for college students resulted in reductions of depressive symptoms and increases in life satisfaction over a year (Seligman et al. 2006), and a brief version of group *positive psychotherapy* with children led to increases in well-being (Rashid and Anjum 2007). Many of the homework exercises utilized in *positive psychotherapy* have been validated through a variety of web-based studies conducted by Seligman et al. (2005).

Another therapeutic model that emphasizes the positive is REACH (Recall the hurt, Empathize with the one who hurt you, (offer the) Altruistic gift of forgiveness, (make a) Commitment to forgive, and Hold on to the forgiveness). This model specifically includes a place for negative emotion, helping clients to move toward forgiveness and reconciliation (Worthington 2001). There are at least eight controlled outcome studies assessing its outcome. In the largest and well-designed study, a consortium of Stanford researchers led by Thoresen et al. (2001) randomly assigned 259 adults to either a 9-h forgiveness workshop or to an assessment-only control group. Sizable effects were observed relative to reducing anger and stress and increasing optimism and health as well as forgiveness.

Clearly applications of positive psychological principles are increasing including approaches that actively harness strengths and positive emotions to help clients to effect important changes in their lives. As the aforementioned research findings indicate, there is at least a preliminary support for facilitating beneficial therapeutic processes and contributing to therapeutic outcomes. Some interventions attribute a healing role to experience of positive emotions; others propose that positive emotions facilitate other therapeutic processes such as the creation of meaning, and still others suggest that positive emotions are part of the attainment of well-being and happiness. However, research is preliminary and work still needs to be done to link the processes that engage positive emotions to the promising outcomes. For research to move forward, a number of methodological issues need to be addressed.

17.3 Challenges in Studying Positive Emotions in Psychotherapy

There are several methodological and conceptual issues that make research on positive emotions a substantial challenge. We begin with considering the challenges inherent in defining any emotion and discuss how those definitional issues become increasingly complex when considering positive emotions. Finally, we consider particular issues related to the assessment of positive emotions in psychotherapy.

17.3.1 Definitional Issues

The problems in accurately defining emotions have been extensively reviewed (see Lewis et al. 2008). These problems include issues related to discriminating between different emotions, describing the relationships between emotions, mapping their structure, identifying basic emotions, and grouping emotions with similar qualities. Most emotion theories define emotions as including four components: (a) a specific event that elicits the emotion, (b) an appraisal process of the event, (c) the neurophysiological arousal that accompanies the appraisal, and (d) a specific action tendency or behavioral response (i.e., Frijda 1986; Izard 1977; Panksepp 1982; Plutchik 1980; Rosenberg and Ekman 2000; Tomkins 1984). While the first three components may apply to the definition of a positive emotion, the fourth does not. Experiencing a negative emotion is most often related to an action tendency; experiencing a positive emotion is different. The most common ways of differentiating emotion from mood or affect involve the existence of a perceived triggering event, the duration of the emotional experience, and its intensity. Emotions are closely related to the occurrence of the triggering event. The response to the triggering event is brief and intense and leads to specific actions. Moods, on the other hand, develop in more subtle ways and last for longer periods of time (Fridja 2000).

Despite the vivid scientific dialogue around this definition, emotions and moods are often conflated in research measures along with a variety of other emotion-related constructs such as affect and emotional states, which are sustained and not momentary experiences.

Emotion research is often conducted with reference to emotion models that fit into three categories: (a) models of basic emotions (e.g., Ekman 1992; Otorny and Turner 1990; Panskepp 1992), (b) dimensional approaches, (i.e., Russell 1980; Schimmack and Grob 2000; Watson et al. 1999), and (c) hierarchical approaches (Watson and Clark 1992). Basic emotion research has identified discrete emotional states like anger and fear that can be reliably elicited and identified. Dimensional or circumplex models of emotion suggest that affective states are the end product of a complex interaction of *arousal* (level of activation or alertness) and *valence* (positive and negative) systems (Posner et al. 2005). Research on the valence and arousal systems has consistently suggested two factor solutions for each of these dimensions, dividing valence into positive and negative affect (Anderson and Phelps 2002; Northoff et al. 2000) and arousal into activation and deactivation (Nesse and Ellsworth 2009; Posner et al. 2005). Hierarchical models of emotions constitute the integration of those two traditions, proposing two (Watson and Tellegen 1985) or three (Tellegen et al. 1999) levels of hierarchical structure. For example, in the two-level model, positive and negative valences form the higher order factors, whereas the lower level reveals the content of the mood descriptors in the form of correlated but discrete emotions (Watson and Tellegen 1985).

Fredrickson (1998) proposes that positive emotions and moods are incompatible with these traditional definitions and models. The central idea is that positive emotions are rather diffuse and difficult to differentiate. She draws on a body of literature to assert that positive emotions are not initiated by discernible appraisal processes, are not connected to distinguishable autonomic responses, do not tend to have unique facial configurations, and do not lead directly to specific action tendencies. Positive emotions are even experienced in a less distinctive manner; they tend to be less keenly felt than negative emotions. Effectively, the characteristics that defined the construct of negative emotions are different for positive emotions. This represents a particular challenge with respect to understanding and ultimately measuring positive emotions.

17.3.2 Assessing Positive Emotions in Psychotherapy

The definitional and structural issues highlighted above become methodological issues for psychotherapy researchers. These issues have implications for *what*, *where*, *when*, and *how* to assess positive emotions. However, all of these questions ultimately need to be decided based on the overarching research question of *why* we measure positive emotions. Fitzpatrick and Stalikas (2008) have suggested that in psychotherapy positive emotions have generative qualities that relate to important kinds of broadening processes. The research that we have considered to this point provides evidence to support that suggestion both outside and inside the psychotherapy realms. With the potential generative quality of positive emotions as answer to the why question, we will now consider the what, where, when, and how issues and suggest possible strategies and directions for psychotherapy researchers.

17.3.2.1 What to Measure: Selecting and Developing Instruments

Clearly psychotherapy researchers need validated process measures of both positive emotions and what positive emotions generate—the broadening dimension. Within positive psychology, scales and instruments have been constructed to measure concepts like forgiveness, gratitude, altruism, flow, broadening, compassion, and self-compassion, just to name a few.

Discrete positive emotions can be analyzed separately, can be combined into groups or *families* of emotions that act in similar ways, or can be conjoined to form a general positive emotion variable. Fredrickson (1998), for example, has suggested that there are families of positive emotions including joy, interest, contentment, and love. More specifically, joy is described to share conceptual space with other positive emotional states such as happiness, amusement, mirth, exhilaration, elation and gladness, interest with challenge and intrinsic motivation, and contentment with mild or receptive joy, while love is considered to include a number of discrete positive emotions among which are joy, interest, and contentment.

In measuring positive emotions, researchers also need to take a stand on the issues of whether positive and negative emotions are two independent variables or two opposite poles that function in contrasting ways (Lucas et al. 2009). Depending on the researchers' stance on this issue, positive emotions investigations may look at positive and negative emotions together or measure positive emotions independently. The PANAS (Watson et al. 1988b) is a popular research instrument that can accommodate either strategy (for a review of the issues involved in measuring positive emotion see Larsen and Fredrickson 1999). In PANAS positive emotions can be calculated in two ways: either as the total sum of discrete positive emotion items or as the result of subtracting the total sum of the negative emotion items from the total sum of the positive ones.

Positive emotions alone are particularly difficult to measure because they are diffuse and difficult to differentiate. To study negative emotions, researchers have developed instruments that can tap aspects such as voice quality, paralinguistic characteristics, neurophysiological changes, and facial expressions. If Fredrickson is correct and positive emotions are not connected to distinguishable autonomic responses and do not tend to have unique facial configurations, these strategies will tend to yield little. Foa et al. (2010) have developed a preliminary vocal profile for interest, distinguishing between the vocal acoustical properties of animated and contemplative interest. However, vocal acoustics alone are not sufficient to identify emotions that are relatively subtle. Additional work is needed to complement these parameters in order to make reliable identification possible.

In the context of psychotherapy research, potentially useful process measures include the Client Perceptual Processing Scale (CPPS; Toukmanian (1994, 2004), the Therapeutic Realizations Scale–Revised (TRS-R; Kolden et al. 2000), the cognitive-emotional processing category of the Change and Growth Experiences Scale (CHANGE; Hayes et al. 2006), and the Experiencing Scale (Klein et al. 1986). These are observer-based measures that include aspects of the elaboration that can represent the broadening construct. The Broadening Inventory (Boutri and Stalikas 2005) has been constructed specifically to measure this construct and includes items that tap the cognitive, affective, and behavioral dimensions of broadening separately.

17.3.2.2 How to Measure: Finding Positive Emotions and Selecting Measurement Strategies

As most clients come to therapy with a surfeit of negative emotions, in order to know how positive emotions operate in the therapeutic setting, we need to be able to find them. While positive emotions presumably operate in all therapeutic modalities, therapies that actively prescribe the therapeutic elaboration of positive emotions such as accelerated experiential dynamic psychotherapy (Fosha 2000), process-experiential therapy (Elliott et al. 2004), and emotion-focused therapy (Greenberg 2002) would seem to be good places to readily find examples for study. Given the building component to which positive emotions are theorized to contribute, we also need to examine extra-session processes in order to follow positive emotions in the upward spiral. It will also be important to explore client processes over a longer time frame than the course of the session in order to trace the ongoing role of positive emotion in building necessary resources that support change.

Self-report questionnaires are one way to access client's positive emotions. Most emotion measures include at least a few positive emotions or a general factor of positive emotionality or pleasantness [i.e., Affect Balance Scale (Bradburn and Caplovitz 1965), PANAS (Watson et al. 1988a), modified Differential Emotions Scale (Fredrickson et al. 2003), Mood Adjective Checklist (Nowlis and Green 1957), Affect Grid (Russell et al. 1989), Multiple Affect Adjective Checklist (Zuckerman and Lubin 1985)]. Having clients report on positive emotions raises an important definitional issue. Are positive emotions those that have a pleasant valence or those that lead to approach behavior (Lucas et al. 2009)? The answer to this question will ultimately be embedded in the research question. However, asking clients to report on positive emotions probably will only access experiences that have a positive valence. A further limitation to the self-report strategy is that we can only ask clients to report *after* sessions on what happens in the process. This limits access to positive emotions as they are happening and introduces the possibility that clients are not reporting on the phenomenon itself but on a recreation of it from memory.

Using clinical judges is another common psychotherapy process research strategy. The use of clinical judges allows researchers to review a session at a later time, locate the segments of interest, and investigate them thoroughly, without disrupting the natural course of the session. The method usually entails a set of comprehensive instructions, training of the clinical judges, and a consensus process. The difficulty with this strategy is that positive emotions could be considered as semiprivate phenomena, since they are not necessarily accompanied by observable change in the clients' appearance or specific behavioral responses, thus yielding few valid and observable indices to guide the assessment. A possible way to overcome this obstacle is expert training in identifying specific signs of emotional expression, such as facial muscle movements (i.e., facial action coding system—FACS, Ekman and Friesen 1978), a method that requires extensive training and considerable amount of time. However, the nature of positive emotions represents an ongoing challenge for those interested in investigating this potentially fruitful variable.

17.3.2.3 When to Measure

Deciding the place to focus our investigations is always a challenge to psychotherapy process researchers. It is a particularly salient challenge when the purpose of the research is to relate the emotional experience with other significant therapeutic phenomena. *Events-based* research may hold promise for the investigation of broaden-and-build sequences. This approach draws on the tradition of critical incident research (Flanagan 1954) and of protocol analysis in which specific verbal behaviors or interactions are examined to understand the nature of change (Elliott and James 1989; Greenberg et al. 1996; Greenberg and Pinsof 1986). It requires researchers to isolate "key episodes" in order to gain a better understanding of change processes in clinically meaningful units. Examining therapy events or episodes has three advantages: specificity, richness, and immediacy (Greenberg and Pinsof 1986). Events can be isolated using *markers* of a key process such as in task analysis (Rice and Greenberg 1984; Pascual-Leone et al. 2009). Client input is also extremely valuable in locating key incidents of their own emotional experiences. Combining self-reports with brief structured recall interviews (Elliott 1986) in which clients review recordings of their sessions to identify the place where positive emotions begin or peak would seem to offer a solution to this dilemma. Clients are also capable of providing rich information about the complexity involved in therapy events, increasing our understanding of how particular change processes work in therapy. In addition, immediate post-session reports of events are not contaminated by the subsequent effects of other therapies or life experiences.

17.3.2.4 Integrating the *What, How,* and *When* to Study Positive Emotions

In the previous sections, we separately presented the three basic questions a researcher answers regarding the what, how, and when to study positive emotions in psychotherapy. These answers are not independent from one another since most often decisions regarding the "what" are related to the "how" and the "when." There is a relationship among the choices. Deciding on the "what" to assess creates a conceptual framework regarding the "how" and the "when." For example, if the "what" is the assessment of the frequency of the different types of positive emotions appearing during the session (e.g., joy, interest, pride, etc.), a self-report assessment after the session, and an interpersonal process recall (IPR) procedure represent two very different but acceptable choices. If, however, the IPR interest of the researcher focuses on the agreement between client experiencing and therapist's perception of client experiencing, then the choices regarding how and when to assess are different. Ultimately, the criteria regarding what, how, and when to assess are related to: (a) the aim, goal, or research questions of the study, (b) the nature and assessment of the other variables in the study, and (c) the epistemological foundation and overall design of the research program.

The research questions of the study guide the researcher for the identification of the exact aspect, facet, or content of the variable measured. For example, for research questions aiming in identifying the emotional state of the client before or after a session, assessing overall mood or naming the experience of specific emotions (what) using self-report scales (how) before and after the session (when) is an appropriate choice. On the other hand, research questions aiming in studying carefully selected session segments, or session events for their therapeutic significance and contribution to change (like incidents of client insight, events characterized by high levels of experiencing, etc.), and the possible contribution of positive emotions preceding the onset of the event may use an IPR process (how) where the client recalls-describes right after the session (when), in an either quantitative or qualitative way, the nature, experience, valence, and intensity of the emotions present at that moment (what).

One of the ways to safeguard the statistical validity of a research study is to properly assess the variables under study using valid tools and collecting data for all variables using compatible measurement scales among variables that allow the application of the appropriate statistical analyses. For example, data collected on a nominal measurement scale (e.g., category of emotions) are not compatible for statistical analyses with data collected on an ordinal measurement scale (e.g., number of session).

Finally, the setting where the research will be carried out, the sample size, and the number of variables under study will also influence what, how, and when to assess positive emotions. Large samples allow for complex and multivariable analyses. Small samples and special settings (e.g., prisons) provide unique opportunities for qualitative descriptions.

To date, most research initiatives involving the study of positive emotions fall in the quantitative research strategy. This preference is to be expected, since it is customary to apply quantitative assessment to new concepts aggiungi crossreference con stiles. The quantitative "scrutiny' produces the first wave of research findings and provides for the initial support (or not) of the new concept. In a sense, descriptive quantitative research strategies first establish the presence, variability, and strength of the new concept (in our case positive emotion), followed by the establishment of their relationship with other psychotherapy concepts. Qualitative research strategy initiatives often follow this first wave in an effort to provide better descriptions and conceptual clarity. In addition, positive emotion research was initiated within the domain of social psychology where there is a preference for quantitative research designs.

Given the relatively recent development of concepts such as broadening, positive emotions as generators of change, and the upward spiral, most studies in psychotherapy research focus in providing research support and apply quantitative methodologies. This initial focus on quantitative assessment resulted in the design of several instruments, scales, self-reports, and quantitative rater assessment procedures. Qualitative research initiatives are rare for the moment. As it has been aforementioned, this absence of qualitative studies may reflect the lack of an initial quantitative research framework which can be used as the basis for developing conceptual clarity. Having said that, there are presently several ongoing qualitative projects which study the role of positive emotion in specific therapeutic approaches, with distinct client pathology and from different perspectives (Pagnini 2013; Vandenberghea and Silvestreb 2013; Willutzki 2013).

Conclusion

This chapter has provided a theoretical framework, the broaden-and-build theory, which is a useful model for the operation of positive emotions in psychotherapy. The model represents a way of understanding the operation of positive emotion that is compatible with existing cognitive theory and provides additional insight into change processes that have been largely unexplored in psychotherapy process and outcome research. We have reviewed the preliminary research findings that bear on the role and the value of positive emotions in the therapeutic healing process and found evidence that positive emotions are part of a process that contributes to improved therapeutic outcomes. Some of the clinical approaches associated with positive psychology are presented here in order to orient psychotherapy researchers to the core concepts and variables that need to be understood in research initiatives in this area. Our final goal has been to identify salient research challenges and issues. We believe that the study of positive emotions has the potential to make an important and lasting contribution to our understanding of psychotherapeutic change, a contribution with significant clinical implications. A systematic and sustained focus by psychotherapy researchers is needed to address the conceptual and methodological difficulties and realize this potential.

References

Alvarez A, Neményy E (2001) Frustration and separateness, delight and connectedness: reflections on the conditions under which bad and good surprises are conductive to learning. Kinderanalyse 9:210–228

Anderson AK, Phelps EA (2002) Is the human amygdala critical for the subjective experience of emotion? Evidence of intact dispositional affect in patients with amygdale lesions. J Cogn Neurosci 14:709–720. doi:10.1162/08989290260138618

Ashby FG, Isen AM, Turken AU (1999) A neuropsychological theory of positive affect and its influence on cognition. Psychol Rev 106:529–550. doi:10.1037//0033-295X.106.3.529

Aspinwall LG (1998) Rethinking the role of positive affect in self-regulation. Motiv Emotion 22:1–32

Aspinwall LG (2001) Dealing with adversity: self-regulation, coping, adaptation, and health. In: Tesser A, Schwarz N (eds) The Blackwell handbook of social psychology. Blackwell, Malden, MA, pp 591–614. doi:10.1002/9780470998519.ch27

Bonanno GA, Keltner D (1997) Facial expressions of emotion and the course of conjugal bereavement. J Abnorm Psychol 106:126–137. doi:10.1037/0021-843X.106.1.126

Boutri A, Stalikas A (2005) Development of an instrument for measuring broadening in psychotherapy and application on a Greek sample. Paper presented at the 36th annual meeting of the society for psychotherapy research (SPR), Montreal, Canada

Boutri A, Stalikas A (2009) Positive emotions and broadening: measurement and assessment. Paper presented at the 40th annual meeting of the society for psychotherapy research, Santiago, Chile

Bradburn NM, Caplovitz D (1965) Reports on happiness. Aldine, Chicago, IL

Butler AC, Chapman JE, Forman EM, Beck AT (2006) The empirical status of cognitive behavioral therapy: a review of meta-analyses. Clin Psychol Rev 26:17–31. doi:10.1016/j.cpr.2005.07.003

Carver CS, Scheier MF (1993) Vigilant and avoidant coping in two patient samples. In: Krohne HW (ed) Attention and avoidance: strategies in coping with aversiveness. Hogrefe & Huber, Kirkland, WA, pp 295–319

Champless DL, Hollon S (1998) Defining empirically supported therapies. J Consult Clin Psychol 66:7–18. doi:10.1037/0022-006X.66.1.7

Cohen S, Doyle WJ, Turner RB, Alper CM, Skoner DP (2003) Emotional style and susceptibility to the common cold. Psychosom Med 65:652–657. doi:10.1097/01.PSY.0000077508.57784.DA

Cohn MA, Fredrickson BL, Brown SL, Mikels JA, Conway AM (2009) Happiness unpacked: positive emotions increase life satisfaction by building resilience. Emotion 9:361–368. doi:10.1037/a0015952

Danner D, Snowdon DA, Friesen WV (2001) Positive emotions in early life and longevity: findings from the nun study. J Pers Soc Psychol 80:804–813. doi:10.1037/0022-3514.80.5.804

Dunn JR, Schweitzer ME (2005) Feeling and believing: the influence of emotion on trust. J Pers Soc Psychol 88:736–748. doi:10.1037/0022-3514.88.5.736

Ekman P (1992) Are there basic emotions? Psychol Rev 99:550–553. doi:10.1037/0033-295X.99.3.550

Ekman P, Friesen W (1978) Facial action coding system. Consulting Psychologists Press, Palo Alto, CA

Elliott R (1986) Interpersonal process recall (IPR) as a psychotherapy process research method. In: Greenberg L, Pinsof W (eds) The psychotherapeutic process. Guilford, New York, NY, pp 503–527

Elliott R, James E (1989) Varieties of client experience in psychotherapy: an analysis of the literature. Clin Psychol Rev 9:443–467. doi:10.1016/0272-7358(89)90003-2

Elliott R, Wexler MM (1994) Measuring the impact of sessions in process experiential therapy of depression: the session impacts scale. J Couns Psychol 41:166–174

Elliott R, Watson J, Goldman R, Greenberg LS (2004) Learning emotion-focused therapy: the process-experiential approach. American Psychological Association, Washington, DC

Estrada CA, Isen AM, Young MJ (1997) Positive affect facilitates integration of information and decreases anchoring in reasoning among physicians. Organ Behav Hum Decis Process 72:117–135. doi:10.1006/obhd.1997.2734

Fava G (1999) Well-being therapy: conceptual and technical issues. Psychother Psychosom 68:171–179. doi:10.1159/000012329

Fava GA, Ruini C (2003) Development and characteristics of a well-being enhancing psychotherapeutic strategy: well-being therapy. J Behav Ther Exp Psychiatry 34:45–63. doi:10.1016/S0005-7916(03)00019-3

Fava GA, Tomba E (2009) Increasing psychological well-being and resilience by psycho-therapeutic methods. J Pers 77:1903–1934

Fitzpatrick M, Stalikas A (2008) Positive emotions as generators of therapeutic change. J Psychother Integr 18:137–154. doi:10.1037/1053-0479.18.2.137

Flanagan JC (1954) The critical incident technique. Psychol Bull 51(4):327–358. doi:10.1037/h0061470

Foa C, Fitzpatrick M, Singh Saini A (2010) Toward understanding interest through vocal acoustic analysis. In: Diamond G (chair) Examining emotional arousal or processing in psychotherapy: new methods. Society for psychotherapy research 41st international meeting, Asilomar, CA

Folkman S, Moskowitz JT (2000) Positive affect and the other side of coping. Am Psychol 55:647–654. doi:10.1037/0003-066X.55.6.647

Fosha D (2000) The transforming power of affect: a model for accelerated change. Basic Books, New York, NY

Fosha D (2004) "Nothing that feels bad is ever the last step:" The role of positive emotions in experiential work with difficult emotional experiences. Clin Psychol Psychother 11:30–43. doi:10.1002/cpp.390 (In: Greenberg L (ed) Special issue on emotion)

Fosha D (2009) Positive affects and the transformation of suffering into flourishing. Ann NY Acad Sci 1171:252–262. doi:10.1111/j.1749-6632.2009.04501.x

Fredrickson BL (1998) What good are positive emotions? Rev Gen Psychol 2:300–319. doi:10.1037/1089-2680.2.3.300

Fredrickson BL (2000) Cultivating positive emotions to optimize health and well-being. Prev Treat 3. doi:10.1037/1522-3736.3.1.31a, http://journals.apa.org/prevention. Accessed 20 Jan 2003

Fredrickson BL (2001) The role of positive emotions in positive psychology: the broaden-and-build theory of positive emotions. Am Psychol 56:218–226. doi:10.1037//0003-066X.56.3.218

Fredrickson BL (2008) Promoting positive affect. In: Eid M, Larsen RJ (eds) The science of subjective well-being. Guilford, New York, NY, pp 449–468

Fredrickson BL, Branigan C (2005) Positive emotions broaden the scope of attention and thought-action repertoires. Cogn Emotion 19:313–332. doi:10.1080/02699930441000238

Fredrickson BL, Joiner T (2002) Positive emotions trigger upward spirals toward emotional well-being. Psychol Sci 13:172–175. doi:10.1111/1467-9280.00431

Fredrickson BL, Levenson RW (1998) Positive emotions speed recovery from the cardiovascular sequelae of negative emotions. Cogn Emotion 12:191–220. doi:10.1080/13632752.2012.757097

Fredrickson BL, Mancuso RA, Branigan C, Tugade M (2000) The undoing effect of positive emotions. Motiv Emotion 24:237–258

Fredrickson BL, Tugade MM, Waugh CE, Larkin GR (2003) What good are positive emotions in crises? A prospective study of resilience and emotions following the terrorist attacks on the United States on September 11th, 2001. J Pers Soc Psychol 84:365–376

Fridja NH (2000) The psychologists' point of view. In: Lewis M, Haviland Jones JM (eds) Handbook of emotions, 2nd edn. Guildford, New York, NY, pp 59–74

Frijda NH (1986) The emotions. Cambridge University Press, New York, NY

Frisch MB (2006) Quality of life therapy: applying a life satisfaction approach to positive psychology and cognitive therapy. Wiley, Hoboken, NJ

Gable SL, Gonzaga GC, Strachman A (2006) Will you be there for me when things go right? Supportive responses to positive event disclosures. J Pers Soc Psychol 91:904–917. doi:10.1037/0022-3514.91.5.904

Gelso CJ, Kivlighan DM, Wine B, Jones A, Friedman SC (1997) Transference, insight, and the course of time-limited therapy. J Couns Psychol 44:209–217. doi:10.1037/0022-0167.44.2.209

Gendlin ET (1996) Focusing-oriented psychotherapy: a manual of the experiential method. Guilford, New York, NY

Gil KM, Carson JW, Porter LS, Scipio C, Bediako SM, Orringer E (2004) Daily mood and stress predict pain, health care use, and work activity in African American adults with sickle-cell disease. Health Psychol 23:267–274. doi:10.1037/0278-6133.23.3.267

Greenberg LS (2002) Emotion-focused therapy: coaching clients to work through their feelings. APA Press, Washington, DC

Greenberg LS (2008) Emotion and cognition in psychotherapy: the transforming power of affect. Can Psychol 49:49–59. doi:10.1037/0708-5591.49.1.49

Greenberg LS, Pascual-Leone A (2006) Emotion in psychotherapy: a practice-friendly research review. J Clin Psychol 62:611–630. doi:10.1002/jclp.20252

Greenberg LS, Pedersen R (2001) Relating the degree of resolution of in-session self-criticism and dependence to outcome and follow-up in the treatment of depression. Paper presented at the North American chapter of the society for psychotherapy research, Puerto Vallarta, Mexico

Greenberg LS, Pinsof WM (1986) The psychotherapeutic process: a research handbook. Guilford, New York, NY

Greenberg LS, Heatherington L, Friedlander ML (1996) The events-based approach to couple and family therapy research. In: Sprenkle DH, Moon SM (eds) Research methods in family therapy. Guilford, New York, NY, pp 411–428

Grencavage LM, Norcross JC (1990) What are the commonalities among the therapeutic factors? Prof Psychol Res Pract 21:372–378. doi:10.1037/0735-7028.21.5.372

Hayes AM, Feldman GC, Goldfried MR (2006) The change and growth experiences scale: a measure of insight and emotional processing. In: Castonguay LG, Hill C (eds) Insight in psychotherapy. American Psychological Association, Washington, DC, pp 231–253. doi:10.1037/11532-011

Hejmadi A, Waugh CE, Otake K, Fredrickson BL (2008) Cross-cultural evidence that positive emotions broaden views of self to include close others. Manuscript in preparation

Hendricks MN (2002) Focusing-oriented experiential psychotherapy. In: Cain DJ, Seeman J (eds) Humanistic psychotherapies: handbook of research and practice. American Psychological Association, Washington, DC, pp 221–251. doi:10.1037/10439-007

Hooker K, Monahan D, Shifren K, Hutchinson C (1992) Mental and physical health of spouse caregivers: the role of personality. Psychol Aging 7:367–375. doi:10.1037/0882-7974.7.3.367

Horvath AO, Greenberg LS (1989) Development and validation of the working alliance inventory. J Couns Psychol 36:223–233. doi:10.1037/0022-0167.36.2.223

Isen AM (2000) Positive affect and decision making. In: Lewis M, Haviland-Jones J (eds) Handbook of emotions, 2nd edn. Guilford, New York, NY, pp 417–435

Isen AM (2002) Missing in action in the AIM: positive affect's facilitation of cognitive flexibility, innovation, and problem solving. Psychol Inq 13:57–65

Isen AM (2008) Positive affect and decision processes: some recent theoretical developments with practical implications. In: Haugdvedt CFR, Herr PH, Kardes FR (eds) Hand-book of consumer psychology. Erlbaum, New York, NY

Isen AM, Daubman KA (1984) The influence of affect on categorization. J Pers Soc Psychol 47:1206–1217

Isen AM, Means B (1983) The influence of positive affect on decision-making strategy. Soc Cogn 2:18–31. doi:10.1521/soco.1983.2.1.18

Isen AM, Shmidt E (2007) Positive affect: broadened focus without increased distractibility. Paper presented at the emotions preconference to the annual meeting of the society for personality and social psychology, Memphis, TN

Isen AM, Johnson MMS, Mertz E, Robinson GF (1985) The influence of positive affect on the unusualness of word associations. J Pers Soc Psychol 48:1413–1426. doi:10.1037/0022-3514.48.6.1413

Isen AM, Daubman KA, Nowicki GP (1987) Positive affect facilitates creative problem solving. J Pers Soc Psychol 52:1122–1131. doi:10.1037/0022-3514.52.6.1122

Isen AM, Rosenzweig AS, Young MJ (1991) The influence of positive affect on clinical problem solving. Med Decis Making 11:221–227. doi:10.1177/0272989X9101100313

Izard CE (1977) Human emotions. Plenum, New York, NY

Johnson KJ, Fredrickson BL (2005) "We all look the same to me": positive emotions eliminate the own-race bias in face recognition. Psychol Sci 16:875–881. doi:10.1111/j.1467-9280.2005.01631.x

Joiner J, Thomas E, Pettit J, Perez M, Burns A, Gencoz T, Gencoz F, Rudd D (2001) Can positive emotion influence problem-solving attitudes among suicidal adults? Prof Psychol Res Pract 32:507–512. doi:10.1037/0735-7028.32.5.507

Kahn BE, Isen AM (1993) The influence of positive affect on variety seeking among safe, enjoyable products. J Consum Res 20:257–270. doi:10.1086/209347

Keltner D, Bonnano GA (1997) A study of laughter and dissociation: distinct correlates of laughter and smiling during bereavement. J Pers Soc Psychol 73:687–702. doi:10.1037/0022-3514.73.4.687

Khoo SA, Bishop GD (1997) Stress and optimism: relationships to coping and well-being. Psychologia 40:29–40

Kivlighan DM, Multon KD, Patton MJ (2000) Insight and symptom reduction in time-limited psychoanalytic counseling. J Couns Psychol 47:50–58. doi:10.1037/0022-0167.47.1.50

Klein MH, Mathieu-Coughlan P, Kiesler D (1986) The experiencing scales. In: Greenberg LS, Pinsof WM (eds) The psychotherapeutic process: a research handbook. Guilford, New York, NY, pp 21–71

Kolden GG, Strauman TJ, Gittleman M, Halverson JL, Heerey E, Schneider KL (2000) The therapeutic realizations scale-revised (TRS-R): psychometric characteristics and relationship to treatment process and outcome. J Clin Psychol 56:1207–1220. doi:10.1002/1097-4679(200009)56:9<1207::AID-JCLP7>3.0.CO;2-Z

Kubzansky LD, Sparrow D, Vokonas P, Kawachi I (2001) Is the glass half empty or half full? A prospective study of optimism and coronary heart disease in the normative aging study. Psychosom Med 63:910–916

Kubzansky LD, Wright RJ, Cohen S, Weiss S, Rosner B, Sparrow D (2002) Breathing easy: a prospective study of optimism and pulmonary function in the normative aging study. Ann Behav Med 24:345–353. doi:10.1207/S15324796ABM2404_11

Larsen RJ, Fredrickson BL (1999) Measurement issues in emotion research. In: Kahneman D, Diener E, Schwarz N (eds) Well-being: foundations of hedonic psychology. Russell Sage, New York, NY, pp 40–60

Levy BR, Slade MD, Kunkel SR, Kasl SV (2002) Longevity increased by positive self-perceptions of aging. J Pers Soc Psychol 83:261–270. doi:10.1037/0022-3514.83.2.261

Lewis M, Haviland-Jones J, Feldman Barrett L (2008) Handbook of emotions, 3rd edn. Guildford, New York, NY

Lopez SJ, Floyd RK, Ulven JC, Snyder CR (2000) Hope therapy: helping clients build a house of hope. In: Snyder CD (ed) Handbook of hope: theory, measures, and applications. Academic Press, San Diego, CA, pp 123–150. doi:10.1016/B978-012654050-5/50009-9

Lopez SJ, Snyder CR, Magyar-Moe JL, Edwards LM, Pedrotti JT, Janowski K, Turner JL, Pressgrove C (2004) Strategies for accentuating hope. In: Linley PA, Joseph S (eds) Positive psychology in practice. Wiley, Hoboken, NJ, pp 388–404. doi:10.1002/9780470939338.ch24

Losada M, Heaphy E (2004) The role of positivity and connectivity in the performance of business teams: a nonlinear dynamics model. Am Behav Sci 47:740–765. doi:10.1177/0002764203260208

Lucas RE, Diener E, Larsen RJ (2009) Measuring positive emotions. In: Diener D (ed) Assessing well-being: the collected works of Ed Diener. Social indicators series, vol 39, pp 139–155. doi:10.1007/978-90-481-2354-4_7

Lyubomirsky S, King LA, Diener E (2005) The benefits of frequent positive affect: does happiness lead to success? Psychol Bull 131:803–855. doi:10.1037/0033-2909.131.6.803

Maddux JE (2008) Positive psychology and the illness ideology: toward a positive clinical psychology. Appl Psychol 57:54–70. doi:10.1111/j.1464-0597.2008.00354.x

Magyar-Moe JL (2009) Therapist's guide to positive psychological interventions. Academic Press, San Diego, CA

Mergenthaler E (2003) Shifts from negative to positive emotional tone: facilitators of therapeutic change? Paper presented at the 34th annual meeting of the society for psychotherapy research, Weimar, Germany

Mertika A, Seryianni C, Fitzpatrick M, Stalikas A (2005) Exploring positive affect and broadening in psychotherapy sessions. Paper presented at the 36th annual meeting of the society for psychotherapy research, Montreal, Canada

Middleton RA, Byrd EK (1996) Psychosocial factors and hospital readmission status of older persons with cardiovascular disease. J Appl Rehabil Counsel 27:3–10

Moraitou M, Stalikas A (2004) Positive emotions during the passage to maternity. Vema of Asklipios 2:204–211

Moskowitz JT (2001) Emotion and coping. In: Mayne TJ, Bonanno GA (eds) Emotion: current issues and future directions. Guilford, New York, NY, pp 311–336

Moskowitz JT (2003) Positive affect predicts lower risk of AIDS mortality. Psychosom Med 65:620–626. doi:10.1097/01.PSY.0000073873.74829.23

Nesse RM, Ellsworth PC (2009) Evolution, emotions, and emotional disorders. Am Psychol 64:129–139. doi:10.1037/a0013503

Northoff G, Richter A, Gessner M, Schlagenhauf F, Fell J, Baumgart F, Kaulisch T, Kotter R, Stephan KE, Leschinger A, Hagner T, Bargel B, Witzel T, Hinrichs H, Bogerts B, Scheich H, Heinze H (2000) Functional dissociation between medial and lateral prefrontal cortical spatiotemporal activation in negative and positive emotions: a combined fMRI/MEG study. Cereb Cortex 10:93–107. doi:10.1093/cercor/10.1.93

Nowlis V, Green R (1957) The experimental analysis of mood. Technical report, contract no. Nonr-668 (12). Office of Naval Research, Washington, DC. doi:10.1016/S0001-6918(59)80215-8

Ong AD, Allaire JC (2005) Cardiovascular intraindividual variability in later life: the influence of social connectedness and positive emotions. Psychol Aging 20:476–485. doi:10.1037/0882-7974.20.3.476

Ostir GV, Markides KS, Peek MK, Goodwin JS (2001) The association between emotional well-being and the incidence of stroke in older adults. Psychosom Med 63:210–215

Otorny A, Turner TJ (1990) What is basic about basic emotions? Psychol Rev 97:315–331

Pagnini F (2013) Using mindfulness to increase positive emotion for individuals with amyotrophic lateral sclerosis: preliminary results. Paper presented at the 44th international meeting of the society of psychotherapy research (SPR), Brisbane, Australia

Panksepp J (1982) Toward a general psychobiological theory of emotions. Behav Brain Sci 5:407–467

Panskepp J (1992) A critical role for "affective neuroscience" in resolving what is basic about basic emotions. Psychol Rev 99:554–560

Pascual-Leone A, Greenberg LS, Pascual-Leone J (2009) Developments in task analysis: new methods to study change. Psychother Res 19:527–542. doi:10.1080/10503300902897797

Pennebaker JW, Mayne TJ, Francis ME (1997) Linguistic predictors of adaptive bereavement. J Pers Soc Psychol 72:863–871. doi:10.1037/0022-3514.72.4.863

Peterson C, Seligman MEP (2004) Character strengths and virtues: a handbook and classification. Oxford University Press, New York, NY

Piper WE, Orgodniczuk JS, Joyce AS, McCallum M, Rosie JS (2002) Relationships among affect, work, and outcome in group therapy for patients with complicated grief. Am J Psychother 56:347–362

Plutchik R (1980) A general psychoevolutionary theory of emotion. In: Plutchik R, Kellerman H (eds) Emotion: theory, research, and experience, vol 1, Theories of emotion. Academic Press, New York, NY, pp 3–33

Posner J, Russell JA, Peterson BS (2005) The circumplex model of affect: an integrative approach to affective neuroscience, cognitive development, and psychopathology. Dev Psychopathol 17:715–734. doi:10.1017/S0954579405050340

Pressman SD, Cohen S (2005) Does positive affect influence health? Psychol Bull 131:925–971. doi:10.1037/0033-2909.131.6.925

Raghunathan R, Trope Y (2002) Walking the tightrope between feeling good and being accurate: mood as a resource in processing persuasive messages. J Pers Soc Psychol 83:510–525. doi:10.1037/0022-3514.83.3.510

Rashid T (2008) Positive psychotherapy. In: Lopez SJ (ed) Positive psychology: exploring the best in people, vol 4. Praeger Publishers, Westport, CT, pp 187–217

Rashid T, Anjum A (2007) Positive psychotherapy for children and adolescents. In: Abela JRZ, Hankin BL (eds) Depression in children and adolescents: causes, treatment and prevention. Guilford, New York, NY

Reed MB, Aspinwall LG (1998) Self-affirmation reduces biased processing of health-risk information. Motiv Emotion 22:99–132. doi:10.5005/jp/books/11350_4

Rice LN, Greenberg LS (1984) Patterns of change: intensive analysis of psychotherapy process. Guilford, New York, NY

Rosenberg E, Ekman P (2000) Emotion: methods of study. In: Kazdin AE (ed) Encyclopedia of psychology, vol 3. American Psychological Association/Oxford University Press, Washington, DC, pp 171–175. doi:10.1037/10518-064

Rowe G, Hirsh JB, Anderson AK (2007) Positive affect increases the breadth of attentional selection. Proc Natl Acad Sci U S A 104:383–388. doi:10.1073/pnas.0605198104

Russell JA (1980) A circumplex model of affect. J Pers Soc Psychol 39:1161–1178. doi:10.1037/h0077714

Russell JA, Weiss A, Mendelsohn GA (1989) The affect grid: a single-item scale of pleasure and arousal. J Pers Soc Psychol 57:493–502. doi:10.1037/0022-3514.57.3.493

Ryff CD (1989) Happiness is everything, or is it? Explorations on the meaning of psychological well-being. J Pers Soc Psychol 57:1069–1081. doi:10.1037/0022-3514.57.6.1069

Salovey P, Birnbaum D (1989) Influence of mood on health-relevant cognitions. J Pers Soc Psychol 57:539–551. doi:10.1037/0022-3514.57.3.539

Schimmack U, Grob A (2000) Dimensional models of core affect: a quantitative comparison by means of structural equation modeling. Eur J Pers 14:325–345. doi:10.1002/1099-0984(200007/08)14:4<325::AID-PER380>3.0.CO;2-I, doi:10.1002/1099-0984(200007/08)14:4<325::AID-PER380>3.0.CO;2-9

Schimmack U, Oishi S, Furr RM, Funder DC (2004) Personality and life satisfaction: a facet-level analysis. Pers Soc Psychol Bull 30:1062–1075. doi:10.1177/0146167204264292

Seligman MEP (1998) Building human strength: psychology's forgotten mission. APA Monit 29

Seligman MEP (2002) Authentic happiness: using the new positive psychology to realize your potential for lasting fulfillment. Free Press/Simon and Schuster, New York, NY

Seligman MEP, Csikszentmihalyi M (2000) Positive psychology: an introduction. Am Psychol 55:5–14. doi:10.1037/0003-066X.55.1.5

Seligman MEP, Steen TA, Park N, Peterson C (2005) Positive psychology progress: empirical validation of interventions. Am Psychol 60:410–421. doi:10.1037/0003-066X.60.5.410

Seligman MEP, Rashid T, Parks AC (2006) Positive psychotherapy. Am Psychol 61:774–788. doi:10.1037/0003-066X.61.8.774

Seryianni C, Mertika A, Stalikas A (2004) The relationship between the therapeutic alliance and positive affect in psychotherapy. Paper presented in 2nd European conference on positive psychology, Verbania Pallanza, Italy

Sin LN, Lyubomirsky S (2009) Enhancing well-being and alleviating depressive symptoms with positive psychology interventions: a practice-friendly meta-analysis. J Clin Psychol 65:467–487. doi:10.1002/jclp.20593

Smith E (2006) The strengths-based counseling model. Counsel Psychol 34:13–79. doi:10.1177/0011000005277018

Stalikas A, Mitskidou P, Gazzola N (2004) Positive emotions and psychotherapeutic change: a pilot study. Paper presented at the 35th annual meeting of the society for psychotherapy research, Rome

Stein NL, Folkman S, Trabasso T, Richards TA (1997) Appraisal and goal processes as predictors of psychological well-being in bereaved caregivers. J Pers Soc Psychol 72:872–884. doi:10.1037/0022-3514.72.4.872

Stiles WB, Snow JS (1984) Counseling session impact as viewed by novice counselors and their clients. J Consult Clin Psychol 31:3–12. doi:10.1037/0022-0167.31.1.3

Sweetman ME, Munz DC, Wheeler RJ (1993) Optimism hardiness, and explanatory style as predictors of general well-being among attorneys. Soc Indicators Res 29:153–161. doi:10.1007/BF01077893

Tellegen A, Watson D, Clark LA (1999) On the dimensional and hierarchical structure of affect. Psychol Sci 10:297–303. doi:10.1111/1467-9280.00157

Thoresen CE, Luskin F, Harris AHS, Benisovich SV, Standard S, Bruning B, Evans S (2001) Effects of forgiveness intervention on perceived stress, state and trait anger, and self-reported health. Paper presented at the annual meeting of the society of behavioral medicine, Seattle, WA

Tomkins SS (1984) Affect theory. In: Scherer KR, Ekman P (eds) Approaches to emotion. Erlbaum, Hillsdale, NJ, pp 163–195

Toukmanian SG (1994/2004) Levels of client perceptual processing (lcpp): a measure for psychotherapy process research, revised. Unpublished measure, York University, Toronto, ON

Trope Y, Pomerantz EM (1998) Resolving conflicts among self-evaluative motives: positive experiences as a resource for overcoming defensiveness. Motiv Emotion 22:53–72

Tugade MM, Fredrickson BL (2004) Resilient individuals use positive emotions to bounce back from negative emotional experiences. J Pers Soc Psychol 86:320–333. doi:10.1037/0022-3514.86.2.320

Tugade MM, Fredrickson BL, Barrett LF (2004) Psychological resilience and positive emotional granularity: examining the benefits of positive emotions on coping and health. J Pers 72:1161–1190. doi:10.1111/j.1467-6494.2004.00294.x

Vandenberghea L, Silvestreb RLS (2013) Therapists' positive emotions in-session: why they happen and what they are good for. J Counsel Psychother Res 14:119–127. doi:10.1080/14733145.2013.790455

Wadlinger HA, Isaacowitz DM (2006) Positive mood broadens visual attention to positive stimuli. Motiv Emotion 30:89–101. doi:10.1007/s11031-006-9021-1

Waldinger RJ, Hauser ST, Schul MS, Allen JP, Crowell JA (2004) Reading others emotions: the role of intuitive judgments in predicting marital satisfaction, quality, and stability. J Fam Psychol 18:58–71. doi:10.1037/0893-3200.18.1.58

Watson D, Clark LA (1992) Affect separable and inseparable: on the hierarchical arrangement of the negative affects. J Pers Soc Psychol 62:489–505. doi:10.1037/0022-3514.62.3.489

Watson D, Tellegen A (1985) Toward a consensual structure of mood. Psychol Bull 98:219–235. doi:10.1037/0033-2909.98.2.219

Watson D, Clark LA, Carey G (1988a) Positive and negative affectivity and their relation to anxiety and depressive disorders. J Abnorm Psychol 97:346–353. doi:10.1037/0021-843X.97.3.346

Watson D, Clark LA, Tellegen A (1988b) Development and validation of brief measures of positive and negative affect: the PANAS scales. J Pers Soc Psychol 47:1063–1070. doi:10.1037/0022-3514.54.6.1063

Watson D, Wiese D, Vaidya J, Tellegen A (1999) Two general activation systems of affect. Structural findings, evolutionary considerations, and psychobiological evidence. J Pers Soc Psychol 76:820–838. doi:10.1037/0022-3514.76.5.820

Waugh CE, Fredrickson BL (2006) Nice to know you: positive emotions, self-other overlap, and complex understanding in the formation of new relationships. J Posit Psychol 1:93–106. doi:10.1080/17439760500510569

Whelton W, Greenberg L (2004) From discord to dialogue: Internal voices and the reorganization of the self in process-experiential therapy. In: Hermans H, DiMaggio G (eds) The dialogical self. doi:10.4324/9780203314616_chapter_7

Willutzki U (2013) Strengthening personal resilience: evaluation of an intervention module. Paper presented at the 44th international meeting of the society of psychotherapy research (SPR), Brisbane, Australia

Wong J (2006) Strengths-centered therapy: a social constructionist, virtue-based psychotherapy. Psychother Theory Res Pract Train 43:133–146. doi:10.1037/0033-3204.43.2.133

Worthington EL (2001) Five steps to forgiveness: the art and science of forgiving. Crown Publishers, New York, NY

Zuckerman M, Lubin B (1985) Manual for the MAACL-R: the multiple affect adjective checklist revised. Educational and Industrial Testing Service, San Diego, CA

Psychotherapeutic Process from the Psychotherapist's Perspective

18

Thomas Schröder, David Orlinsky, Michael Helge Rønnestad, and Ulrike Willutzki

Contents

Abstract

Process research began with therapist-reported case studies describing therapeutic practice but conflating data and analysis. Audio recordings of therapy shifted the focus towards a third-party perspective, avoiding previous bias but marginalising therapy participants who alone can supply first-hand reports of the process. Today, both patients' and therapists' experiences remain underrated. We seek to redress the balance, highlighting empirical studies of the therapist's perspective on process that avoid the limitations of early case study research.

Our review starts with the broadest perspective on therapists' experience, using data from a large international study. Analysing self-reports of specific aspects of process experience yielded two dimensions, *Healing* and *Stressful Involvement*, leading to distinct patterns of work experience.

The subsequent section affords a sharper focus, using observations within sessions gathered through structured questionnaires, particularly the *Therapy Session Report*. Completed by both therapists and patients, it allows progressively complex stages of analysing experience, from describing specific facets, via constructing individual profiles from latent patterns, to generating conjoint dimensions, characterising a therapist-patient dyad.

T. Schröder (✉)
University of Nottingham, Nottingham, UK
e-mail: thomas.schroder@nottingham.ac.uk

D. Orlinsky
University of Chicago, Chicago, IL, USA

M.H. Rønnestad
University of Oslo, Oslo, Norway

U. Willutzki
Witten/Herdecke University, Alfred-Herrhausen-Straße 50, 58448 Witten, Germany

O.C.G. Gelo et al. (eds.), *Psychotherapy Research*,
DOI 10.1007/978-3-7091-1382-0_18, © Springer-Verlag Wien 2015

Finally, we exemplify a close-up view by examining therapeutic difficulties, an aspect of therapists' process experience particularly relevant for clinical practice and supervision. Qualitative and quantitative studies have yielded distinct dimensions, individual profiles, and markers for problematic processes.

At all levels we demonstrate the feasibility of moving from therapists' experience-near reports of process to empirically derived dimensions transcending what is accessible to self-awareness, thereby facilitating reflective practice. Investigating process in terms congruent with therapists' own experience helps close the gap between research and practice.

18.1 Introduction

For approximately 50 years, from the earliest days of modern psychotherapies (e.g. Breuer and Freud 1895/2009), essentially the only access that readers had to information about the psychotherapeutic process—that is, psychotherapy as it is really practised—was through case histories written by therapists. Consequently, all knowledge concerning psychotherapeutic process was based on the psychotherapist's perspective. These case histories were impressionistic, in the sense that the observational *data* and the *method* of data analysis were commingled, observations were selectively rather than systematically collected, and methods of data analysis were implicitly applied and reported. In addition, such impressionistic case histories were typically motivated by the writers' desire to validate their treatment procedures, and thus for the most part were theoretically driven and often polemical in tone (Kächele et al. 2008).

A wholly new avenue of access to therapeutic process that bypassed the therapist's perspective altogether opened with the advent of audio recording of therapy sessions in the early 1940s (Porter 1943; Rogers 1942). Psychotherapy process research in the modern sense began at that point, when investigators felt that they finally could hear (and later, see) for themselves 'what really happens' in psychotherapy, without having to depend any longer on the quite probably biased reports written by therapists. This resulted in the accumulation of a large body of systematic and seemingly 'objective' data (i.e. data based on non-participant observation) about therapeutic processes, as observers repeatedly listened to and rated diverse aspects of what could be heard from recordings of conversations between clients and therapists (e.g. Rogers and Dymond 1954; Rubinstein and Parloff 1959) or simply counted the frequency with which certain words or vocalisations occurred (see Marsden (1971) for examples). For more than a decade thereafter, the psychotherapist's own perspective on the psychotherapeutic process was essentially unwanted and unsought.

Not until the early 1960s did dissatisfaction with the limitations of recording-based psychotherapy process research emerge, and a few investigators began to study participants' (mainly clients' but also therapists') experiences of their therapy sessions (cf. Elliott 2008; Elliott and James 1989; Feiffel and Eells 1963; Kamin and Caughlin 1963; Orlinsky and Howard 1967; Snyder 1961; Strupp et al. 1964). The studies conducted by these researchers were based on the premise that clients and therapists, as participant observers, could provide reliable reports of their experiences in therapy which could be systematically collected from them and analysed independently by the investigators, avoiding the limitations inherent in the prior case history literature.

By definition, all empirical studies entail observations, whether formulated quantitatively (in numbers) or qualitatively (in text). Although this chapter focuses primarily on quantitative studies, all of these observations inevitably reflect the perspectives from which they are made. The important distinction is not between 'subjective' and 'objective' but rather between participant and non-participant observation. Participant observers are only in a position to report about first person experiences (of myself) and/or second person experiences (of *you*, my interaction partner). Thus, in observing the therapeutic process, therapists as participant observers are in a position to report their self-perceptions (first person), their perceptions of the client (second person), and their perceptions of interacting in a relationship with their client (first and second person). Similarly, as participant observers, clients are in a position to report their self-perceptions (first person), their perceptions of the therapist (second person), and their perceptions of interacting in a relationship with their therapist (first and second person).

Non-participant observers (as external witnesses to a situation) are only in a position to report on their third person experiences of what others said and did (about *them*), within the further limitations of the observational and recording equipment used. It is, of course, possible to have external raters make judgements about the 'inner' psychological processes of participants in therapy—for example, by using the 'Experiencing Scale' (Klein et al. 1986)—but the data produced are still 'third person' judgements based on non-participant observations of others and are methodologically quite distinct from the 'first person' or 'second person' perspectives of participant observers. This distinction between observational perspectives applies as much to qualitative analyses of text-based data as to quantitative analyses that rely on checklists or rating scales. Indeed, it might be argued that 'what really happens' in psychotherapy may be better viewed in terms of what the participants experience together (first and second person observations) than what external auditors are able to glean from recordings of the speech and movements of the actors (third person observations).

Given the independent if inherently circumscribed validity of each observational perspective, a more comprehensive view is that the three basic observational perspectives complement and supplement one another, each providing access to one aspect of the total situation, and all are together being needed to form a more comprehensive picture of the situation (as classically illustrated in Akira Kurosawa's iconic 1950 film *Rashomon*). Furthermore, researchers must also study the interrelations of these perspectives, which are clearly not identical, so that they can translate between them and make findings based on one perspective accessible to observers from alternate perspectives (see Feiffel and Eells (1963), or Orlinsky and Howard (1975), for some early examples of inter-perspective coordination). It is critically important to include studies of the psychotherapist's perspective on therapeutic process in such inter-perspective 'translations', since therapists cannot apply research findings unless they are framed in terms of phenomena that can potentially be perceived by the therapist (Orlinsky 1994).

In addition, clinicians frequently discuss the process of psychotherapy from their own point of view, be that formally in supervision or case conferences, informally in meetings between colleagues or debriefings between co-therapists, or communally in published case studies or clinical conference papers. Although a few researchers have examined therapists' experiences of psychotherapy, or included therapist measures along with measures based on client and external perspectives, the field of psychotherapy research has continued to focus primarily on clients' or raters' views of process. This chapter aims to shift the focus back to the psychotherapist's perspective and show how that has been and can be done in a systematic, quantitative, and objectively analysed fashion. In principle, such analyses not only reflect therapists' perceptions of psychotherapeutic process but can also reveal patterns of experience that are beyond their immediate awareness (e.g. by correlational and factor analyses).

The studies described in this chapter are organised along a dimension reflecting breadth of focus or *levels of analysis*. As in photography, it ranges from a wide-angle perspective, giving a panoramic, multifaceted picture of therapists' overall experience of therapeutic practice, to a close-up view, focusing in detail on one particular aspect or strand of practice experience. Between these, the intermediate perspective takes phenomena within single sessions or across a series of sessions as the relevant unit of observation. Using the level of analysis concept as its organising principle, this chapter will be presented in three parts: The first takes the broadest view and concentrates on the most comprehensive study of the therapist's perspective undertaken so far, using data from the Development of Psychotherapists Common Core Questionnaire (Orlinsky et al. 1999); the second features the intermediate view, based on the Therapist Session Report (Orlinsky and Howard 1966, 1986) and related instruments; and the third focuses intensively on therapeutic difficulties to exemplify the fine-grained exploration of the therapist's experience of process, using a quantitative approach based on an initial qualitative study.

18.2 Therapeutic Practice: A Panoramic Perspective on Process

Although there have been recent attempts to gather data from large numbers of therapists (see for instance Cook et al. 2010), by far the largest survey of therapists' experience of their work can be found in the data acquired as part of the International Study of the Professional Development of Psychotherapists (ISPDP) conducted by the Collaborative Research Network (CRN)—a group of clinically active researchers who joined together under the auspices of the Society for Psychotherapy Research (Orlinsky et al. 1999). This cooperative venture, which began in 1989 and has continued to the present, set out to investigate therapeutic practice and professional development from the psychotherapist's point of view and to survey the very varied professional and personal characteristics of psychotherapists in many countries. By now, the principal instrument of the ISPDP—the *Development of Psychotherapists Common Core Questionnaire* (DPCCQ)—has been completed by more than 10,000 therapists from a wide range of theoretical orientations, professional backgrounds, and experience levels. Over 30 countries are represented in the current data base, with the largest samples having been collected to date in Australia, Germany, Norway, the United Kingdom, and the United States. The DPCCQ is a comprehensive questionnaire, modelled initially on the concept of an in-depth interview to gather information on therapists' characteristics and experiences including demographics, theoretical influences, training and personal therapy experiences, work settings and modalities, client characteristics and caseload, experience of current therapeutic work, past and current development, and personal life and experience of self. Most of the items have structured response formats (rating scales or checklists), although some open-ended questions requiring qualitative analysis are also included. In the following paragraphs, we summarise the results of initial statistical analyses, as previously reported in book format by Orlinsky and Rønnestad (2005). Based on information from nearly 5,000 therapists, two broad domains of psychotherapists' experience could be discerned, encompassing *therapeutic work* and *professional development*. The first of these is of particular relevance to the topic of this chapter.

Table 18.1 presents a conception of therapists' experience of their practice, based on the structure of the 'generic model' of psychotherapy (Orlinsky 2010; Orlinsky et al. 1994), as this can be interpreted in terms of the DPCCQ. The conceptual model underlying the table is the generic model, while the process concepts in the table (skills, difficulties, etc.) are aspects of therapists' experience empirically surveyed in the DPCCQ. At the top, *input* variables reflect the institutional context and therapeutic objectives characteristic of each respondent's practice, as well as their customary adherence to therapeutic frames. At the bottom, indices of outputs can be found in therapists' satisfaction/dissatisfaction with their work, felt professional growth or depletion, and the nature of client-related experiences between sessions. The realm of therapeutic process is examined in the broad band between inputs and outputs.

Although input and output variables are also surveyed by the DPCCQ, the primary data that constitute the domain of process experience—and will be discussed in this chapter—were supplied by those sections of the DPCCQ that enquire about therapists' self-reported clinical

Table 18.1 Conceptual analysis of therapist's experience of therapeutic practice

Category	Subcategory	Aspects of therapist's experience
Input[a]		Therapist's professional environment: autonomy and support
		Therapist's treatment goals: typical aims with clients
		Therapist's frame management: degree of boundary flexibility
Process	Specific aspects	Therapist's current clinical skills
		Therapist's difficulties in practice a. Professional self-doubt b. Difficult treatment case c. Negative personal reaction
		Therapist's coping strategies a. Constructive coping b. Avoidant coping
		Therapist's manner in relating with clients a. Warm b. Directive c. Guarded d. Organised-effective
		Therapist's feelings in sessions a. 'Flow' b. Boredom c. Anxiety
	Overall experience	Therapeutic work involvement[b] a. Healing involvement (skills, constructive coping, warmth, flow) b. Stressful involvement (difficulties, avoidant coping, boredom, anxiety)
Output[a]		Therapist's work satisfaction a. Satisfaction with one's work as a therapist b. Dissatisfaction with one's work as a therapist
		Therapist's intersession experiences
		Ongoing professional development a. Currently experienced growth b. Currently experienced depletion

[a]For therapists
[b]Derived from specific aspects

skills, therapeutic difficulties and coping strategies, manner of relating to patients, and in-session feelings. These were transformed through item and factor analyses into reliable scales representing specific facets of work experience (Orlinsky et al. 1999; Orlinsky and Rønnestad 2005). Subsequent second-order factor analyses yielded two broad independent dimensions of therapists' overall experience of therapeutic process, integrating and subsuming the DPCCQ item scales and the first-order analytic dimensions constructed from them. One of the overall process experience scales, labelled *Healing Involvement*, was defined by first-order dimensions reflecting a general sense of therapeutic efficacy, skilfulness in current practice, and experiences in sessions of deep personal interest [called 'flow' by Csikszentmihalyi (1990)], in the context of an affirming and committed therapeutic relationship, with infrequent experiences of therapeutic difficulties that, when they occur, are approached by using constructive coping strategies.

By contrast, the second broad dimension described a pattern of experience best characterised for therapists as a *Stressful Involvement*, featuring frequent experiences of therapeutic difficulties that are typically met unconstructively by therapists with defensive or avoidant coping strategies, accompanied by feelings of anxiety and boredom.

Some therapist characteristics surveyed in the DPCCQ emerged as clear predictors of *Healing Involvement*, most notably the breadth of

Table 18.2 Patterns of therapeutic work experience

	Stressful involvement	
Healing involvement	Little	More than a little
Much	Effective practice (n = 1,802, 50 %)	Challenging practice (n = 821, 23 %)
Not much	Disengaged practice (n = 629, 17 %)	Distressing practice (n = 377, 10 %)

Note. Adapted from Orlinsky and Rønnestad (2005). Scales range from 0 to 15; n = 3,629. For Healing Involvement, much >9.55, not much ≤9.55; for Stressful Involvement, little ≤4.75, more than a little >4.75

therapists' repertoires in terms of the variety of theoretical influences they had assimilated and the range and depth of their experience in a number of treatment modalities. Other important variables predicting *Healing Involvement* were therapists' positive work morale and their sense of having adequate support and satisfaction in their work settings. The most important predictors of *Stressful Involvement* were a felt lack of support and satisfaction in the work setting, a sense of having little professional autonomy, having no private practice, and a general sense of demoralisation. The level of *Stressful Involvement* seems to depend more on the therapist's work situation, while the level of *Healing Involvement* was more closely related to therapists' characteristics.

As the two dimensions of work experience are statistically nearly independent of each other, therapists can report high (or low) levels of each simultaneously. This allows for the construction of a simple 2 × 2 contingency table, cross-tabulating two levels of *Healing Involvement* ('much' or 'not much') with two levels of *Stressful Involvement* ('little' and 'more than a little'), yielding four distinct patterns of practice experience, each represented by a significant segment of the highly varied group of therapists in the sample (see Table 18.2).

The largest group, comprising 50 % of therapists, showed a pattern of *Effective Practice*, combining 'much' *Healing Involvement* with 'little' *Stressful Involvement*. The next largest group, comprising 23 % of therapists, also experienced 'much' *Healing Involvement* but 'more than a little' *Stressful Involvement*. They appear to be clearly engaged in their work but have conflicting experiences, so this pattern was named *Challenging Practice*.

Another 17 % of therapists reported only 'little' *Stressful Involvement* but also 'not much' *Healing Involvement*, being apparently untroubled by but also not greatly invested in their work, in a pattern of experience that seemed to reflect an overall sense of *Disengaged Practice*. The smallest group, including only 10 % of the therapists (which unfortunately still numbered in the hundreds), reported experiencing 'more than a little' *Stressful Involvement* and 'not much' *Healing Involvement*—an alarming state of affairs for which the label *Distressing Practice* was chosen. This last group is comparable to one reported by Pope et al. (1987), who found that 10 % of the therapists in their sample described themselves as frequently being too distressed to do their work.

If the *Effective Practice* and *Challenging Practice* groups are combined, it will be seen that almost three out of four therapists experienced 'much' *Healing Involvement*—a position which one might hope and expect to be the norm for flourishing practitioners, but which for nearly a third of them was tempered by a concurrent experience of some *Stressful Involvement*. One might say that therapists in this latter group feel tested but not unduly troubled by their professional practice.

The remaining quarter of the total sample give more cause for concern as they appear to have found no adequate response to the challenges of therapeutic work and are consequently either suffering and running the risk of burnout, or attempting to cope by withdrawing subjectively and potentially heading for professional stagnation.

The question arises whether these findings hold true for different stages over the course of a therapist's career. For the answer, we must turn to a cross-sectional analysis that formed part of the study of professional development (Orlinsky et al. 2001; Orlinsky and Rønnestad 2005). Therapists were differentiated into six career cohorts according to how long they had been practising with real patients since starting their professional training. These were called *novices* (less than 1.5 years in practice), *apprentices* (1.5–3.5 years in practice), *graduates* (3.5–7 years in practice), *established* therapists (7–15 years in practice), *seasoned* therapists (15–25 years in practice), and *senior* therapists (with 25–50 years of practice).

Applying these categories, it emerged that extent of clinical experience was clearly related to practice patterns; for example, while only 40 % of novices were within the *Effective Practice* group, the proportion rose to 60 % among senior therapists. Similarly, only 60 % of novices but 80 % of seniors report 'much' *Healing Involvement*. By contrast, as many as one in five novice therapists experienced a *Distressing Practice*, whereas only 6–7 % of established, seasoned, and senior therapists did so. To some extent, these discrepancies may be accounted for by seriously distressed therapists leaving the profession, but it appears that the accumulation of professional practice offers therapists some degree of protection against distressing work experiences.

There are many other questions that can be asked of the data collected with the DPCCQ, and a number of additional analyses have been and are currently being undertaken (cf. Orlinsky et al. 2010). What they have in common is that they reach beyond a simple reflection of experience as recounted by therapists to a higher level of analysis, thus creating a picture that while grounded in self-report is framed by empirically derived indices of process and practice. For instance, the DPCCQ items that constitute the dimensions of *Healing Involvement* and *Stressful Involvement* have been combined into a self-monitoring scale (Orlinsky and Rønnestad 2005) that allows therapists to assess the quality of their current work involvement in a way that goes beyond what they could readily access through introspection and can be a resource to help them monitor and enhance their development (Duncan 2010).

18.3 Therapy Sessions: A Focused View of Process

Therapists' global experience of their work, as captured by the dimensions of the DPCCQ described in the section above, reflects the entire span of their current practice, aggregated from many treatment cases with many different patients. Each of those cases in turn consists of a number of single sessions. These were studied by Orlinsky and Howard (1967, 1975, 1977) from both the patient's and the therapist's viewpoint using the Therapy Session Report (TSR; Orlinsky and Howard 1966, 1986), and in this section we focus on findings derived from this instrument. The TSR is a 152-item questionnaire, covering 10 facets of experience, endorsed on 3- or 4-point anchored scales. There are parallel versions for both parties in the therapeutic encounter. In the therapist form, six facets of experience encompass therapists' perceptions of their *patients*' topics of dialogue, motives, concerns, feelings, interpersonal behaviours, and self-management, while the remaining four facets comprise therapists' appraisals of their *own* treatment goals, interpersonal behaviours, feelings, and evaluations of session development.

When the TSR is completed by therapists on a session-by-session basis, it can be analysed at successively greater levels of complexity: (1) individual item frequencies to show the relative salience of therapist experiences; (2) factor analysis of the items representing each facet of experience to shed light on the dimensional structure of that particular area; (3) factor analysis of the facet dimensions across the varied facets of experience to reveal the global dimensions of therapist experience in sessions; and if parallel patient TSRs for the same sessions are available, (4) comparisons between the dimensions of therapist and patient experiences to expose dimensions of *conjoint* experience that are not discernible when patients' or therapists' perspectives are separately considered. The following illustrative examples are taken from a study involving 17 therapists treating 32 patients in treatments ranging from 5 to 64 sessions (Orlinsky and Howard 1975, 1977).

Therapists' *aims* in sessions were assessed by 14 TSR items selected on the basis of clinical relevance. Most therapists (more than 85 %) endorsed the following goals for sessions: helping patients to talk about their feelings and concerns, helping patients realistically evaluate their reactions and feelings, and getting a better understanding of the patient. By contrast, only one quarter of therapists endorsed helping patients get better self-control as one of their session aims. The factor structure of this facet shows therapists' objectives of promoting insight and enhancing the therapeutic relationship as the prevalent patterns.

The therapist's *interpersonal manner* with patients was gauged by eight items. Modal experiences were being warm and attentive, which also form one salient first-level factor analytic dimension. Another prevalent pattern first-level dimension for this facet shows therapists to assume expressing relational agency: by talking, expressing feelings, and (to a lesser extent) providing structure for the sessions.

Therapists' perceptions of patient motives were evaluated by 14 items. The motivations in sessions that therapists most frequently reported for patients were (1) wanting to understand the reasons for their problematic feelings and actions and (2) seeking relief from tension or unhappy feelings. The least common session motivation attributed to patients was wanting to evade or withdraw from contact with the therapist, as a form of resistance. Salient dimensions of patients' aims in sessions included (1) a desire for understanding and insight, which is congruent with therapist *aims*; (2) a desire for therapist involvement, which is well matched with therapists' *manner of being*; and (3) the less frequent but factor analytically distinct wish to avoid therapeutic involvement.

Taking all facets of the therapist's in-session experience as the unit of analysis, a second-level factor analysis found these dimensions to generate several broad dimensions. Of the 11 second-level therapist process factors that Orlinsky and Howard (1975) identified, four that have clear clinical relevance are cited here as illustrations of the results obtained:

1. *Depressive Stasis vs. Effective Movement.* Components of the negative pole of this factor include therapists seeing their clients as depressed, not making progress, wanting to gain sympathy, and aiming to obstruct therapy; while viewing themselves as feeling resigned, not being motivated and understanding, and relating in a frank manner. At the positive pole of this dimension, therapists perceive their clients as not depressed, as making progress, as wanting to work on their problems, and as seeking insight; while regarding themselves as being motivated and understanding, relating in a supportive manner, and not feeling resigned.
2. *Uneasy Intimacy.* This factor is characterised by the therapist experiencing an uneasy sense of nurturing warmth with a patient seen as warm and seductive. At the intense end of this dimension, therapists look upon their patients as trusting and warm but also as flirtatious and provocative, while considering themselves tender and close, but also playful and embarrassed.
3. *Engagement with a Patient Perceived as Enthusiastic and Open vs. Reserve with a Patient Seen as Feeling Uncomfortably Involved and Mistrustful.* The engagement pole of this dimension is epitomised by therapists' perceptions of their patients as trusting, relaxed, and relating to them with enthusiastic acceptance; and of themselves as animatedly responsive in return. At the opposite end, therapists experience their patients as mistrustful, embarrassed, and relating with ambivalent involvement; while experiencing a sense of independence in the relationship.
4. *Collaborative Relationship vs. Abiding a Patient Perceived as Assertively Narcissistic.* The constituents of the collaborative pole of this factor are therapists' views of their patients as not feeling good, but wanting to gain insight and relating collaboratively and with mutuality; and of themselves as relating collaboratively and as personally involved

and responsive. Conversely, at the opposing pole, therapists see their patients as feeling good, but as seeking to obstruct therapy by engaging assertively in unresponsive activities; while experiencing themselves as relating with attentive compliance, unresponsive activities, and neither influencing nor being influenced by the patient.

Taken together, scores on the 11 therapist dimensions were used to create a distinctive profile of session experience for each therapist. When a cluster analysis of these profiles was done, two broad patterns of therapists' session experiences were identified, one that brought together various strands of *Helping Experience* and a contrasting one that wove together aspects of *Stressful Experience*—which, quite independently (30 years earlier and with a completely different sample), resemble *Healing Involvement* and *Stressful Involvement* viewed from the 'panoramic' perspective highlighted in the second section of this chapter.

The cluster of therapists whose session dimension profiles defined *Helping Experience* had distinctively high scores on (1) *Progress with a Patient Seen as Responsive and Motivated*, (2) *Active Supportive Involvement with a Patient Seen as Anxious and Communicative*, and (3) *Engagement with an Open, Enthusiastic Patient* and distinctively low scores on (4) *Uneasy Intimacy*, (5) *Erotic Countertransference*, and (6) a *Sense of Failure with a Patient Perceived as Feeling Inferior*. At the heart of this pattern were dimensions in which therapists perceived themselves and their patients in several ways as positively and comfortably engaged in a productive relationship, while avoiding potential pitfalls inherent in a relationship that requires keeping an effective balance between professional and personal aspects of involvement.

By contrast, the cluster of therapists whose session dimensions comprised *Stressful Experience* for therapists included distinctively high scores on (1) *Reserve with an Uncomfortably Involved and Mistrustful Patient*, (2) *Enduring an Assertively Narcissistic Patient*, (3) *Erotic Countertransference*, (4) *Uncaring Detachment*, (5) *Calm Frank Facilitation with a Hostile Withdrawing Patient*, and (6) a *Sense of Failure with a Patient Perceived as Feeling Inferior*. In these, the balance between professional and personal aspects appears to have been lost, such that either therapist or the patient has become overly involved or, perhaps as a defensive reaction, insufficiently involved in their relationship.

So far, we have illustrated three levels of analysis available when focusing on therapists' in-session experiences. Similar to the analysis of panoramic data from the DPCCQ described in the previous section, the most basic level is that of direct self-report, which is experience-near and within the conscious awareness of informants—even though therapists may have been prompted by some questions to focus on aspects of their experience which had hitherto been outside their awareness. Descriptive data, such as those reflecting modal experiences, portray what therapists can readily say about therapeutic process from their perspective. Derived from this, the next level goes beyond simple description by extracting latent patterns of experience. Some factors may be readily recognised by informants, others less so. A third level, generating broadly inclusive dimensions, allows the construction of profiles of therapists' experiences of process within sessions which permit a systematic, empirically grounded examination of variability between therapists.

Finally, an additional level explores intersubjective dimensions of conjoint experience by analysing dimensions of therapist experience together with corresponding dimensions of patient experience derived in a similar fashion. Despite the fact that there is no one-to-one correspondence between patients' and therapists' observational perspectives, these fourth level intersubjective dimensions allow us to determine what the therapist's experience of process nevertheless can actually tell us about the patient's experience, in a way that likely would not be available to observation from the perspective of 'objective' non-participant observers.

Conjoint dimensions of experience were generated by Orlinsky and Howard (1975) by factor analysing a correlation matrix of the 11 dimensions of therapist experience and

11 corresponding dimensions of patient experience. We illustrate the results by describing two of the seven conjoint factors that seem to have special clinical relevance:

Healing Magic Versus Uncomfortable Involvement The patient's contribution to this factor consists of the dimension of *Therapeutic Satisfaction*, which is characterised *inter alia* by patients experiencing themselves as feeling good, getting relief and insight, making progress, and wanting to win their therapist's respect, while viewing their therapists as feeling pleased and effective and being understanding and helpful. This is matched in the therapist's own experience by a high score on *Engagement with a Patient Perceived as Enthusiastic and Open* and a low score on *Uneasy Intimacy*. Orlinsky and Howard (1975) described this somewhat playfully as *Healing Magic*, alluding to the 'placebo' aspect of this highly positive pattern. The negative side of this bipolar dimension was called *Uncomfortable Involvement*, defined by a low score on the patient dimension of *Therapeutic Satisfaction*, and high scores on the therapist's dimensions of *Uneasy Intimacy* and *Reserve with a Patient Seen as Feeling Uncomfortably Involved and Mistrustful*.

The second conjoint dimension showed another bipolar relationship pattern as viewed from an intersubjective perspective. The positive pole of *Therapeutic Alliance vs. Defensive Impasse* combines patient experience dimensions in which the therapist is perceived as *Involved and Helpful* and patient experiences of *Painful Self-Exploration* in a *Collaborative Exploration of Emotionally Significant Relationships* combined with therapist experiences of *Effective Movement* in a highly *Collaborative Relationship*. The negative pole, *Defensive Impasse*, is constituted mainly by patients perceiving their therapist as being *Mean and Attacking*, while the therapist's own experience is that of *Enduring a Patient Perceived as Assertively Narcissistic*. It is notable that each person views the other as the aggressor in this negative therapeutic impasse.

More than three decades have passed since the studies outlined above were undertaken. There have been some further efforts to broadly investigate therapists' and patients' session-by-session experiences with the TSR, notably those by Kolden (1991, 1996), Kolden and Howard (1992) and Saunders et al. (1989). Following this approach, similar instruments were developed to assess aspects of in-session therapeutic process including the Session Evaluation Scales (Stiles and Snow 1984a, b), the Working Alliance Inventory (Horvath and Greenberg 1986), and, in German, the Session Report (Grawe and Braun 1994; Grawe et al. 1990). Recent studies that focus on in-session processes in relation to outcome include Flückiger et al. (2010, 2013) and Lutz et al. (2013).

Complementary to session process measures is another called the Intersession Experience Questionnaire (Orlinsky et al. 1993) which focuses on clients' and therapists' experiences regarding their therapy during the intervals between sessions. An interesting series of studies have been conducted by Hartmann, Zeeck, and their colleagues to explore the relation of intersession process to in-session process and outcome for different types of patients, in different treatment settings (e.g. Hartmann et al. 2003, 2010, 2011; Zeeck et al. 2004, 2006). Schröder et al. (2009) have adapted part of this instrument for use in the DPCCQ.

The potential of this line of enquiry lies in the promise of determining markers of therapist experience that may be indicative of client experiences, as, for instance, if therapists experience *Uneasy Intimacy* combined with *Reserve with a Patient Seen as Mistrustful*, a reasonable working hypothesis they might explore in therapy would be that patients concurrently are experiencing very little *Therapeutic Satisfaction*. We explore the potential of using therapists' experience of difficulties as a marker variable of troublesome process in more detail in the section below.

18.4 Therapist Difficulties: A Close-Up View of One Process Aspect

Again and again, in our analyses of psychotherapists' experiences, one facet emerged as particularly meaningful: the difficulties that psychotherapists encounter in their work with patients. Such episodes are also paramount in psychotherapists' working lives: more often than not, when therapists meet colleagues over coffee, they recount the trials and tribulations from their latest session (within the bounds of confidentiality). That is, they focus on discrete, and often impactful, difficulties they are experiencing with some client during their treatment sessions. It was this common experience which initially led a group of clinician-researchers in the UK to initiate a collaborative study analysing written self-reported accounts of therapists about difficulties in their practice, with the aim of constructing taxonomies of therapist difficulties and coping strategies (Davis et al. 1987a, b). The studies resulted in categories of difficulties (for instance, 'therapist feels... incompetent; ...threatened; ...out of rapport', 'therapist experiences... ethical/moral dilemma; ...painful reality') and of coping strategies (such as 'therapist turns... to patient; ...to others; ...against patient; ...away from difficulty') that could be used reliably to classify narratives of difficulties, such as might be related in supervision or peer consultation (Schröder et al. 1987a, b). Apart from clinical applications, the taxonomies also showed potential for further research. In one development, they were transformed into self-report scales, which provided two facets of therapists' work experience in the DPCCQ that was described in the second section of this chapter. Factor analyses of the 20-item difficulties scale identified three separate dimensions, labelled respectively as (1) *Professional Self-Doubt* [perhaps better named more neutrally as *Professional Uncertainty*, in light of findings recently reported by Nissen-Lie et al. (2012)], (2) *Frustrating Treatment Case*, and (3) *Negative Personal Reaction*—the first of these being the most commonly experienced kind of difficulty.

The work by Davis and collaborators focused on difficulties that psychotherapists experience as persons across all their patients. This is an important perspective, as psychotherapists' personalities and their more or less professional habits contribute to the atmosphere and the process of psychotherapy. Still, it is only one part of the story, in that the difficulties which psychotherapists encounter in their daily practice are partly but not exclusively related to the therapist as a person. Some patients have interpersonal styles or specific problems that interact with their psychotherapists' individual personalities and their ability to deal with these problems. Moreover, the psychotherapist may try to cope with the difficulties in a way that is at least partly specific for the particular patient. Thus, an interaction between patient's and therapist's inputs to the psychotherapeutic process develops which can have a more or less beneficial impact.

To focus specifically on the inputs to difficulties of individual therapist and patient pairs, the 20 DPCCQ items were adapted by Willutzki et al. (1997) for use with each patient that a therapist treats. The items stayed the same, but the entry question was changed to the following stem: 'In your current work with your patient Mr. X, how often do you experience these difficulties...?' Following this perspective, since 1997 about 200 therapists have reflected on the difficulties they encountered in their work with about 1,800 patients.

Factor analyses of all difficulty items extracted three subscales, differentiating between the sources of difficulties as (1) originating from the psychotherapist, experienced as *Professional Self-Doubt*; (2) originating from the patient, experienced as *Difficult Patient*; or (3) deriving from the context, experienced as *Difficult Contextual Factors*. Across all patients and all therapists, *Professional Self-Doubt* was most prevalent, followed by the experience of *Difficult Patients*. Therapists differed substantially from one another, particularly concerning the amount or level of difficulties they reported. Moreover, some reported that they hardly ever experienced their patients as difficult; others rarely regarded the context as a problem in their therapeutic work.

While some therapists generally experienced only few difficulties in their work with patients, most reported mixed patterns, that is, with some patients work seemed fairly easy, whereas others were quite a challenge, leading to much

Professional Self-Doubt and the impression of a very *Difficult Patient*. This work shows that the difficulties a therapist experiences in psychotherapy partly seem to depend on the therapist as a person. Not surprisingly though, difficulties are often influenced by patients' characteristics or are a phenomenon emerging from the particular patient-therapist interaction.

In a separate development, Schröder and Davis (2004) followed up a previous finding which had suggested that therapists may have specific individual difficulty profiles reflecting their professional and personal characteristics (Davis et al. 1987a, b). Two consecutive studies investigated the pervasiveness of difficulty experiences within and between therapists, drawing on written narratives. Using trained, clinically experienced judges, they established reliable distinctions between three different types of difficulty experiences: one that was located in the situation or the specific patient and would be found problematic by most therapists regardless of their level of experience; one that was related to gaps in the therapist's skills, knowledge, or experience and was associated with early career stages; and one that was idiosyncratic and emerged as personally characteristic of the therapist reporting the difficulty. Each of these types of experience might call for a different remedial or supervisory response. For example, situational difficulties require humility and acceptance from the therapist; competence deficits highlight the need for additional training, broadened repertoires, and opportunities for wider experience, while idiosyncratic difficulties are best addressed through reflection and enhanced self-awareness gained either in supervision or the therapist's own personal therapy.

These latter difficulties, which resonated with informants' experiences from their family and social relationships and hence appear characteristic of them as persons as well as professionals, came into sharper focus in a second investigation. In that study, a subsample of 100 English-speaking therapists, mainly drawn from the UK, each provided two accounts of difficulty experiences, one with a 'difficult' and one with a 'not-so-difficult' patient, together with a number of both situation-specific and general self-report measures. Unlike situational difficulties, which were associated with 'difficult' patients, idiosyncratic difficulties were reported equally with both patient types, but were more likely to occur with patients whom therapists saw as similar to themselves. In addition, they had high emotional impact on therapists, evoked in them internal states similar to their worst self-images and appeared related to internalised attachment conflicts. Perhaps most alarmingly, when experiencing such difficulties, therapists reported an inclination to exert hostile control over their clients, even though they did not perceive them as being hostile themselves (Schröder 1998).

The expression 'conscious countertransference reaction' (Torres 1983) goes some way towards capturing both aspects of the experience of such difficulties: On the one hand, therapists know that something has gone awry and thus report the incident as a difficulty; on the other hand, it requires a third-party perspective to capture the full impact of such experiences on the therapist and the therapeutic process, either through use of process measures or the clinical judgement of an external observer (e.g. supervisor reviewing a recorded session). Many supervisors will recognise this constellation from their work with their more open and perceptive supervisees.

One experience that appears to be particularly difficult for therapists to acknowledge is that of shame. As Scheff (1987) observed in a clinical paper, if unrecognised and left unprocessed, shame may lead to critical alliance ruptures with damaging impact on patient engagement and the eventual outcome of therapy. With this in mind, Schröder et al. (2013) developed a typology of difficulty experiences involving self-conscious emotions such as guilt, shame, and humiliation. They demonstrated that raters can reliably detect such feelings in written accounts, using a manual with descriptions and definitions, which in itself can help clinicians to identify and acknowledge shame experiences in supervision or private reflection. To this end, both the above typologies have been incorporated in a self-monitoring form (Schröder 2007), which is currently being evaluated as an aid to reflective practice.

Some valuable lessons can be drawn from this highly focused view of therapy process as seen through the close-up lens of therapists' accounts of difficulties. While therapists may not be particularly reliable in predicting therapy outcomes (Lambert and Shimokawa 2011) or their patients' experiences of process (Orlinsky and Howard 1975; Stiles and Snow 1984a), they are still expert observers of their own experience during therapy sessions and can report on it in considerable detail when prompted. However, they also know more than they can say and their self-report can be enhanced both through standardised measures (like the DPCCQ and TSR) and through the additional understandings generated be a clinically sensitive observer.

A Concluding Thought

What general lessons can we draw from our entire outlook on the therapist's experience of process, ranging from the most general to the most detailed perspective? Answering this, we believe we can say that systematically collected observations from therapists can be used to generate quantitative, empirically derived dimensions and measures of process that can help practitioners reflect upon their own practice, and do so in ways that go beyond what is immediately accessible to their awareness but is nevertheless latent in their experience. Such quantitative investigations of the therapist's experience of process are complemented by qualitative enquiries, mixed method studies, and rigorous case study research (McLeod 2010). In undertaking studies that illuminate psychotherapeutic process from the therapist's perspective, we may also help clinicians to interpret the findings of process research that has been conducted from the separate perspectives of patients and external observers, in ways which make those research findings more accessible to them, and so have a better chance of influencing clinical practice.

References

Breuer J, Freud S (1895/2009) Studies on hysteria. Basic Books, New York, NY

Cook JM, Biyanova T, Elhai J, Schnurr PP, Coyne JC (2010) What do psychotherapists really do in practice? An internet study of over 2,000 practitioners. Psychotherapy 47:260–267. doi:10.1037/a0019788

Csikszentmihalyi M (1990) Flow: the psychology of optimal experience. Harper & Row, New York, NY

Davis JD, Elliott R, Davis ML, Binns M, Francis VM, Kelman JE, Schröder TA (1987a) Development of a taxonomy of therapists' difficulties: initial report. Br J Med Psychol 60:109–119. doi:10.1111/j.2044-8341.1987.tb02720.x

Davis JD, Francis VM, Davis ML, Schröder TA (1987b) Development of a taxonomy of therapists' coping strategies: initial report. Unpublished manuscript, University of Warwick, Coventry, UK

Duncan BL (2010) On becoming a better therapist. American Psychological Association, Washington, DC

Elliott R (2008) Research on clients' experiences of psychotherapy: introduction to the special section. Psychother Res 18:239–242. doi:10.1080/10503300802074513

Elliott R, James E (1989) Varieties of client experience in psychotherapy: an analysis of the literature. Clin Psychol Rev 9:443–467

Feiffel H, Eells J (1963) Patients and therapists assess the same psychotherapy. J Consult Psychol 27:30–318

Flückiger C, Regli D, Zwahlen D, Hostettler S, Caspar F (2010) Der Berner Patienten- und Therapeutenstundenbogen 2000. Ein Instrument zur Erfassung von Therapieprozessen (Bern post-session report for patients and for therapists: measuring psychotherapeutic processes). Zeitschrift für Klinische Psychologie und Psychotherapie 39(2):71–79. doi:10.1026/1616-3443/a000015

Flückiger C, Holtforth MG, Znoj HJ, Caspar F, Wampold BE (2013) Is the relation between early post-session reports and treatment outcome an epiphenomenon of intake distress and early response? A multi-predictor analysis in outpatient psychotherapy. Psychother Res 23(1):1–13. doi:10.1080/10503307.2012.693773

Grawe K, Braun U (1994) Qualitätskontrolle in der Psychotherapiepraxis (Quality control in psychotherapy practice). Z Klin Psychol Psychother 23 (6):657–678

Grawe K, Caspar F, Ambühl H (1990) Die Berner Therapievergleichsstudie: Prozessvergleich. (The Bernese comparative psychotherapy trial: process). Zeitschrift für Klinische Psychologie 19:316–337

Hartmann A, Orlinsky D, Geller J, Zeeck A (2003) Der Inter-Session-Fragebogen (ISF)- Ein Instrument zur Erfassung von psychotherapierelevanten Prozessen zwischen Sitzungen (The Intersession Questionnaire- an inventory for the measurement of patients' processing of psychotherapy between sessions).

Psychother Psychosom Med Psychol 53(11):464–468. doi:10.1055/s-2003-43391

Hartmann A, Orlinsky D, Weber S, Sandholz A, Zeeck A (2010) Session and intersession experience related to treatment outcome in Bulimia Nervosa. Psychother Theory Res Pract Train 47(3):355–370. doi:10.1037/a0021166

Hartmann A, Orlinsky DE, Zeeck A (2011) The structure of intersession experience in psychotherapy and its relation to the therapeutic alliance. J Clin Psychol 67 (10):1–20. doi:10.1002/jclp.20826

Horvath A, Greenberg LS (1986) The development of the working alliance inventory. In: Greenberg LS, Pinsof WM (eds) The psychotherapeutic process: a research handbook. Guilford, New York, NY, pp 529–556

Kächele H, Schachter J, Thomä H (2008) From psychoanalytic narrative to empirical single case research: implications for psychoanalytic practice. Routledge, London

Kamin I, Caughlin J (1963) Subjective experiences of outpatient psychotherapy. Am J Psychother 17:660–668

Klein MH, Mathieu-Coughlan P, Kiesler DJ (1986) The experiencing scales. In: Greenberg L, Pinsof W (eds) The psychotherapeutic process: a research handbook. Guilford, New York, NY, pp 21–72

Kolden GG (1991) The generic model of psychotherapy: an empirical investigation of patterns of process and outcome relationships. Psychother Res 1:62–73

Kolden GG (1996) Effective microprocesses in early sessions of dynamic psychotherapy. J Psychother Pract Res 5:122–131. doi:10.1080/10503309112331334071

Kolden GG, Howard KI (1992) An empirical test of the generic model of psychotherapy. J Psychother Pract Res 1(1992):225–236

Lambert MJ, Shimokawa K (2011) Collecting client feedback. Psychotherapy 48:72–79. doi:10.1037/a0022238

Lutz W, Ehrlich T, Rubel J, Hallwachs N, Röttger M-A, Jorasz C, Mocanu S, Vocks S, Schulte D, Tschitsaz-Stucki A (2013) The ups and downs of psychotherapy: sudden gains and sudden losses identified with session reports. Psychother Res 23(1):14–24. doi:10.1080/10503307.2012.693837

Marsden G (1971) Content analysis studies of therapy: 1954 through 1968. In: Bergin A, Garfield S (eds) Handbook of psychotherapy and behavior change. Wiley, New York, NY

McLeod J (2010) Case study research in counselling and psychotherapy. Sage, London

Nissen-Lie HA, Monsen JT, Ulleberg P, Rønnestad MH (2012) Psychotherapists' self-reports of their interpersonal functioning and difficulties in practice as predictors of patient outcome. Psychother Res 22:1–19. doi:10.1080/10503307.2012.735775

Orlinsky DE (1994) Research-based knowledge as the emergent foundation for clinical practice in psychotherapy. In: Talley F, Butler S, Strupp H (eds) Psychotherapy research and practice: bridging the chasm. Basic Books, New York, NY

Orlinsky DE (2010) The "Generic Model of Psychotherapy" after 25 years: evolution of a research-based metatheory. J Psychother Integr 19:1–23. doi:10.1037/a0017973

Orlinsky DE, Howard KI (1966) Therapy session report, form T. Institute for Juvenile Research, Chicago, IL

Orlinsky DE, Howard KI (1967) The good therapy hour: experiential correlates of patients' and therapists' evaluations of therapy sessions. Arch Gen Psychiatry 16:621–632

Orlinsky DE, Howard KI (1975) Varieties of psychotherapeutic experience. Teachers College Press, New York, NY

Orlinsky DE, Howard KI (1977) The therapist's experience of psychotherapy. In: Gurman AS, Razin AM (eds) Effective psychotherapy: a handbook of research. Pergamon, New York, NY

Orlinsky DE, Howard KI (1986) The psychological interior of psychotherapy: explorations with the therapy session reports. In: Greenberg L, Pinsof W (eds) The psychotherapeutic process: a research handbook. Guilford, New York, NY

Orlinsky DE, Rønnestad MH (2005) How psychotherapists develop. A study of therapeutic work and professional growth. American Psychological Association, Washington, DC

Orlinsky DE, Geller JD, Tarragona M, Farber B (1993) Patients' representations of psychotherapy: a new focus for psychodynamic research. J Consult Clin Psychol 61:596–610

Orlinsky DE, Grawe K, Parks BK (1994) Process and outcome in psychotherapy–noch einmal. In: Bergin A, Garfield S (eds) Handbook of psychotherapy and behavior change, 4th edn. Wiley, New York, NY

Orlinsky DE, Ambühl H, Rønnestad H, Davis J, Gerin P, Davis M et al (1999) The development of psychotherapists: concepts, questions, and methods of a collaborative international study. Psychother Res 9:127–153. doi:10.1080/10503309912331332651

Orlinsky DE, Botermans J-F, Rønnestad MH (2001) Towards an empirically-grounded model of psychotherapy training: five thousand therapists rate influences on their development. Aust Psychol 36 (2):139–148. doi:10.1080/00050060108259646

Orlinsky DE, Rønnestad MH, Willutzki U (2010) The SPR collaborative research program on the development of psychotherapists. In: Norcross J (ed) History of psychology: a century of change, 2nd edn. American Psychological Association, Washington, DC

Pope KS, Tabachnick BG, Keith-Spiegel P (1987) Ethics of practice – the beliefs and behaviors of psychologists as therapists. American Psychologist 42:993–1006

Porter EH Jr (1943) The development and evaluation of a measure of counseling interview procedure. Educ Psychol Meas 3(105–126):215–238. doi:10.1177/001316444300300111

Rogers CR (1942) The use of electrically recorded interviews in improving psychotherapeutic techniques. Am J Orthopsychiatry 12:429–434

Rogers CR, Dymond RF (eds) (1954) Psychotherapy and personality change. University of Chicago Press, Chicago, IL

Rubinstein EA, Parloff MB (eds) (1959) Research in psychotherapy, vol 1. American Psychological Association, Washington, DC

Saunders SM, Howard KI, Orlinsky DE (1989) The therapeutic bond scales: psychometric characteristics and relation to treatment effectiveness. Psychol Assess 1:323–330. doi:10.1037/1040-3590.1.4.323

Scheff TJ (1987) The shame-rage spiral: a case study of an interminable quarrel. In: Lewis HB (ed) The role of shame in symptom formation. Lawrence Earlbaum Associates, London

Schröder TA (1998) Therapists' experience of difficulties in their practice. Doctoral thesis. Accessed from http://wrap.warwick.ac.uk/2922/

Schröder TA (2007) Therapist difficulties self-assessment form. Unpublished manuscript, University of Nottingham, Nottingham, UK

Schröder TA, Davis JD (2004) Therapists' experience of difficulty in practice. Psychother Res 14:328–345. doi:10.1093/ptr/kph028

Schröder TA, Binns M, Davis JD, Davis ML, Elliott R, Francis VM, Kelman JE (1987a) A taxonomy of therapist difficulties. In: Kächele H, Cierpka M, Hölzer M (eds) Society for psychotherapy research, abstracts of the 18th annual meeting. PSZ, Ulm

Schröder TA, Binns M, Davis JD, Davis ML, Elliott R, Francis VM, Kelman JE (1987b) A taxonomy of therapist coping strategies. In: Kächele H, Cierpka M, Hölzer M (eds) Society for psychotherapy research, abstracts of the 18th annual meeting. PSZ, Ulm

Schröder TA, Wiseman H, Orlinsky DE (2009) "You were always on my mind...": therapists' intersession experiences in relation to their therapeutic practice, professional characteristics, and quality of life. Psychother Res 19:42–53. doi:10.1080/10503300802326053

Schröder TA, Gilbert P, McEwan K, Gale C, Irons C (2013) Experiences of shame, humiliation and guilt in psychotherapy: the therapist's tale. Manuscript submitted for publication

Snyder WU (1961) The psychotherapy relationship. Macmillan, New York, NY

Stiles WB, Snow JS (1984a) Counseling session impact as viewed by novice counsellors and their clients. J Couns Psychol 31:3–12. doi:10.1037/0022-0167.31.1.3

Stiles WB, Snow JS (1984b) Dimensions of psychotherapy session impact across sessions and across clients. Br J Clin Psychol 23:59–63

Strupp HH, Wallach M, Wogan M (1964) Psychotherapy experience in retrospect: questionnaire survey of former patients and their therapists. Psychol Monogr 78:11. doi:10.1037/h0093869

Torres MA (1983) Conscious countertransference reactions by beginning therapists in response to patient anger. Unpublished doctoral thesis, Adelphi University, New York, NY

Willutzki U, Hernandez Bark G, Davis J, Orlinsky DE (1997) Client outcome as a function of the therapist's difficulties and coping strategies in the course of psychotherapy: initial results. Paper presented at the 28th international meeting of the society of psychotherapy research, Geilo, Norway

Zeeck A, Hartmann A, Orlinsky DE (2004) Inter-Session-Prozesse – Ein vernachlässigtes Thema der Psychotherapieforschung (Inter-session-processes – a neglected area). Psychotherapie, Psychosomatik & medizinische Psychologie 54(6):236–242. doi:10.1055/s-2003-814790

Zeeck A, Hartmann A, Orlinsky DE (2006) Internalization of the therapeutic process: differences between borderline and neurotic patients. J Pers Disord 20 (1):22–41. doi:10.1521/pedi.2006.20.1.22

From a Psychoanalytic Narrative Case Study to Quantitative Single-Case Research

19

Horst Kächele, Cornelia Albani, and Dan Pokorny

Contents

H. Kächele (✉)
International Psychoanalytic University Berlin, Stromstraße 3, 10555 Berlin, Germany

Sonnenweg 25, 89081 Ulm, Germany
e-mail: horst.kaechele@ipu-berlin.de

C. Albani
SINOVA Hospital Aulendorf, Aulendorf, Germany

D. Pokorny
Department Psychosomatic Medicine and Psychotherapy, Ulm University, Ulm, Germany

Abstract

Narrative case studies concerning the psychoanalytic process date back more than a century; Breuer and Freud were the pioneers of this research path. A great shift in methodology occurred after the development of computers that could work with both text and numbers. On the one hand, it became possible to store detailed, verbatim protocols of therapy sessions. On the other hand, it was possible to analyze derived quantitative data by using sophisticated statistical procedures. This is exemplified in three different methods that analyze different psychoanalytical cases. We conclude by mentioning that research on the psychoanalytic process has to start with clinical experience, which can be used when introducing new observational tools to check for the appropriateness of each tool. This is made possible by the synergetic work of people and processes that were mentioned above.

19.1 The Psychoanalytic Narrative Case Study

Historically, in psychoanalysis' oral tradition and loosely documented cases, vignettes were used as the principal means of reporting the insights that originated from the therapeutic situation. Breuer's (1893–1895) reporting on a young

O.C.G. Gelo et al. (eds.), *Psychotherapy Research*,
DOI 10.1007/978-3-7091-1382-0_19, © Springer-Verlag Wien 2015

lady's (Anna O.) cloudy talking nourished in his colleague Freud the idea that one should tell these clinical observations as stories to accurately depict what had transpired.

Freud was aware of the imperfections of his case histories. In his *Studies on Hysteria*, we detect a note of both amazement and self-justification in his remark that indicated that his case histories "read like short stories" and "lack the serious stamp of science" (Freud 1895, p. 160). Yet, in the very next sentence, he also rejects artistic ambitions: "I must console myself with the reflection that the nature of the subject is evidently responsible for this, rather than any preference of my own" (ibid).

The model that Freud suggested was creatively continued by the growing number of psychoanalysts who reported the discoveries from the consulting room, mainly in the form of case vignettes (e.g., Ferenczi 1927). Until today, in the psychoanalytic literature, the "vignette" is still the primary form of presentation. A vignette is characterized by unity, subtlety, and refinement and serves to illustrate typical psychodynamic connections. In regard to vignettes, the implications for the analyst's therapeutic actions are secondary when compared to this focus of interest. Therefore, they hardly describe how the analyst actually works and what he feels, thinks, and does. Therefore, it seems useful to at least distinguish between *case histories* that focus on the psychodynamic properties of a disorder and *treatment reports* that focus on the technicality of how to perform the therapeutic work.

The genre of treatment reports is clearly characterized by a quantitative increase over the last few decades, which was detailed by Kächele (1981; see also Kächele et al. 2009, Chap. 3). More analysts have been willing to make their clinical work accessible to readers (e.g., Klein 1961; Winnicott 1972; Dewald 1972; Thomä 1961). Providing adequate presentational critical discussion within the profession could be on sound footing.

Thus, psychoanalysis became a narrative science by using narration that led to narrative truth (Forrester 1980; Spence 1982). To highlight the importance of this methodological decision, one has to imagine what the development of chemistry would be like if chemists would have started the habit of providing stories about what they had observed in their test tubes: a science of chemistry based on reported colors, of blue and red and green reactions in the little tubes after having performed a certain experiment. Imagine a science of musicology with musicians sharing their most personal experiences by writing case histories or by letting consumers speak about their emotional involvement after a piano concerto. What is wrong with such an approach? It is possible that a person could build a science of musical experience by collecting a large sample of these reported subjective testimonies. This approach would not work for chemistry, which is why the alchemist tried in vain to find the recipe for how to make gold. One should remember the work of the brothers Grimm, the two professors from Göttingen in Germany, who systematically started out collecting orally transmitted fairy tales. After many decades, a well-developed field of fairy-tale research exists that uses highly sophisticated methods to analyze the available large collections of fairy tales from all over the world (Propp 1928).

Until today, we encountered prominent authors who emphasized that the clinical encounter was best reported via the narrative (Michels 2000). Indeed, there are good reasons for maintaining the tradition of clinical reporting because it conveys the subjective evidence of the reporting person (e.g., a therapist or a patient). Therefore, describing the origin and changing functions of case studies have become a topic that is discussed by qualitatively minded researchers who examine the place of novellas as a scientific form of representation and communication (Frommer and Rennie 2001).

The problem that we face is that in psychoanalysis, each of the diverse psychoanalytic cultures often remains within its own confines and largely ignores case studies from other branches of the discipline (Luyten et al. 2006). Therefore, more research-minded psychoanalysts have explicitly indicated the following:

> Today, the historically fertile narrative procedure of Freud is no longer able to carry the responsibility for the existence of psychoanalysis, even though they still are still a major tool for didactic and identity formation of the members of the analytic community because case stories may be a rich material means of communication (Stuhr 2004, p. 63).

19.2 Empirical Single-Case Studies

In 1971, Wallerstein and Sampson concluded that it was necessary to conduct formalized and systematized examinations of the therapeutic process in psychoanalysis: "Our central conviction is that the informal case study, in spite of its forceful power of conviction, has certain realistic and obvious scientific limitations" (p. 47). In the same year, Luborsky and Spence (1971) asked the psychoanalytic community to provide "specimen cases":

> Ideally, two conditions should be met: the case should be clearly defined as analytic..., and the data should be recorded, transcribed and indexed to maximize accessibility and visibility (1971, p. 426).

A few years later, Hartvig Dahl introduced the term "the specimen hour" (Dahl et al. 1988) to provide for the interested public the transcript of session five of the completely tape-recorded treatment of Mrs. C. This implied that there are not only "specimen dreams" in psychoanalysis, which is a term that Freud coined, but there are also specimen cases that have to be studied in their own rights. In our view, the decisive criterion that should be used to attribute the label "specimen" should be its public accessibility, which allows for critical, nonpartisan discussion. The development of textbanks has become part of this requirement (Mergenthaler and Kächele 1988).

However, the number of papers that call for formalized single-case research far outnumbers the number of papers that report on such detailed single-case studies (Leuzinger-Bohleber 1995).

Single-case studies are not confined to tape recording; any systematic gathering of treatment-relevant material can be used to document a treatment (see Chap. 20 with regard to the possibility of considering the narrative text that is produced by clinicians in regard to their treatment being a form of secondary qualitative data that needs to be further analyzed by using the specific procedures of qualitative data analysis). Detailed clinical case reports are, in our view, necessary and act as a bridge to the more formalized systematic case studies. Given their material qualities, they could have been and still can be the object of more formal empirical studies. A few of the detailed case reports that are mentioned above provide sufficient material that can be used as a starting point in formalized evaluations.

The introduction of tape recording into the psychoanalytic treatment situation opened a new window in the process that was ardently debated for a long time, and for most analysts, it is still controversial. Audio recordings of the psychoanalytic dialogue do pose a number of substantial clinical and ethical problems, although, in regard to scientific reasons, they provide true progress (Kächele et al. 1988). They allow an independent, third-person perspective on the analytic, interpersonal transaction; in regard to the analyst's and the patient's internal modes of experience, they are silent, but ideally, they may be able to provide an estimation of this based on the participant's testimony. The recording of these cases has led to the creation of many theoretical and technical issues.

Overviews of the methodology were presented by Kazdin (1982), Hilliard (1993), Iwakabe and Gazzola (2009), and Fonagy and Moran (1993). The latter summarized the topic succinctly:

> Individual case studies attempt to establish the relationship between intervention and other variables through repeated systematic observation and measurement ....The observation of variability across time within a single case combines a clinical interest to respond appropriately to changes within the patient, and a research interest to find support for a causal relationship between intervention and changes in variables of theoretical interest. The attention to repeated observations, more than any other single factor, permits knowledge to be drawn from the individual case and has the power to eliminate plausible

alternative explanations. (Fonagy and Moran 1993, p. 65)

The most prominent case in the Anglo-American literature is the case of Mrs. C who was treated by Hartvig Dahl (as we know by now). Weiss, Sampson, and their research team (1986) reported on a host of experiments that were performed on the case material. Within this team, G. Silberschatz was an important member who was guided by Dahl in his doctoral dissertation in New York on Mrs. C in 1978. Years later, Dahl presented his FRAMES concept on the material of session five (1988); his colleague Bucci (1988, 1997) approached the case from a different vantage point by identifying emotional structures. Another major work on Mrs. C was the application of the Jones Psychotherapy Process Q-Set (PQS) as a method for systematic inquiry of the whole process (Jones and Windholz 1990).

19.3 Psychoanalytic Process

For many years, the Ulm Psychoanalytic Process Research Study Group has implemented a program that examines the material bases of psychoanalytic therapy. We were and are convinced that only the careful exploration of the patient's interaction with the analyst can illustrate the central aspects of psychoanalytic treatment and enable an empirically driven theory of the process.

However, we encounter a multiplicity of meanings and models regarding the notion of the "psychoanalytic process" (Compton 1990). Opinions differ regarding whether models have to be tested, but language games are useful for those who use these models (Wittgenstein 1921/2014). Our investigations were guided by a working model of the process, which encompasses all of the steps of the process, from the start of a patient/analyst contact to the termination of this relationship. The methodological specificity of the psychoanalytic process is produced by the analytic method, which prescribes a specific discourse—with evenly hovering attention and free association being functional units. The impact of these rules on both of these parts sets a process in motion that transforms the covered processes within the patient (e.g., transference dispositions) into relationship patterns between the patient and the analyst.

In psychoanalysis, similar to other fields of human intervention, theories exist about how the process should be supported empirically; at present, these thoughts are used to a much greater extent as instruments for theory criticism. The process model of psychoanalytic therapy as an "ongoing, temporally unlimited focal therapy with a changing focus," which was described in the Ulm textbook *Psychoanalytic Practice* by Thomä and Kächele (1987, Chap. 9), has been posited as a claim that is based on one's own clinical experience. After all, the aim suggests guidelines regarding how psychoanalytic processes are currently conceived and practiced.

Our starting point for this conception was the awareness of various technical elements, such as working alliance, transference and countertransference phenomena, and resistance, whose combinations then generated the different forms of psychoanalytic therapy. The manifold therapeutic processes that exist in reality between the poles of macroprocess and microprocess reveal fluid boundaries in the macro field, which comprises so-called psychoanalysis proper, analytic psychotherapy, and short therapy in the field of individual therapies (Kächele 2010). These generic descriptions were questioned when the criterion, which is unable to be specified externally, of the "analytical process" was introduced on the basis of variables that concerned the setting. For instance, the extensively published case of Dewald (1972) was described by two out of three training analysts of the American Psychoanalytic Association as being psychoanalysis, but by the third only described it as analytical psychotherapy. Even the use of the couch by no means guarantees that the process will be described as "psychoanalytic" when it exists by virtue of functioning transference/countertransference (Schachter and Kächele 2010). Process models at a micro level, which is formulated, for example, by von Zeppelin (1987) who used the cognitive-affective regulation system for intrapsychic processes, are claimed to be valid for all of the psychoanalytically oriented therapeutic approaches (Kächele 2010).

In its use of the focus concept, the Ulm process model primarily aims to have a medium level of description. The concept of "focus" is semantically quite diffuse because we also speak of "focusing" and may be referring to relatively short-term processes. The focus concept that was introduced by French (1952) formed a part of his cognitively oriented analysis of dreams; this concept was used by Seitz (1966) in the Chicago consensus study, in which French was also involved. Here, the focus came to be seen as the least common multiple, which was understood clinically by the concept of "prevailing transference." An interactive, process-oriented conception of the focus was crystallized from the work that was developed in Malan's focal therapy workshop (1963, p. 272). Our conception of the focus relates to a structure that extends over a longer period of time and involves a longer sequence of sessions. For quite some time, the Ulm Psychoanalytic Process Research Study Group has been working on the empirical identification of such structures. A number of methods at different levels of abstraction from the clinical work have been used for this purpose. It seemed obvious to organize research along poles that stretch from the traditional case history to very formalized methods, which correspond to qualitative approaches and hard-nosed quantitative methods (Kächele 1992; see Chap. 13 for an overview of quantitative approaches to the study of the psychotherapy process).

19.4 Methods

We shall illustrate empirical approaches in regard to our recorded cases:

First, we introduce our method of systematic longitudinal description and Dahl's (1983) evaluation strategy of the therapist's topic index (see Sect. 19.4.1). Second, we refer to the systematic analysis of the method of Core Conflictual Relationship Theme (CCRT; Luborsky and Crits-Christoph 1998) and its Leipzig-Ulm category system (CCRT-LU; Albani et al. 2008) in a longitudinal fashion (see Sect. 19.4.2). Third, we present results that relate to the empirical identification of process phases on the basis of systematic clinical ratings that are given to the first half of another psychoanalytic case (Kächele 2009) (see Sect. 19.4.3). Finally, a future strategy that is based on computer-aided text analysis will be mentioned as an outlook to future sophisticated approaches in psychoanalytic process research.

19.4.1 Systematic Longitudinal Descriptions

Systematic longitudinal descriptions require quite a different way of approaching the clinical material that is in contrast to the episodic, highly selected narrations that are at the heart of vignettes. The decisive feature resides in a preselection of points of interest from the researcher's point of view and of a sampling procedure, which is independent of the clinician's point of view. The raw material may consist of session notes or be available via transcripts. The complex array of interactions of a treatment process is considered with the help of these preset points of view: these clearly represent the researcher's interests. They might vary from case to case. For example, for patient "Christian Y,"[1] anxiety and transference were the key notions; for "Amalia X," hirsutism was the key notion (male type of hairiness), along with the development of her quest for heterosexual relations, that was of prominent interest. The material basis of these systematic descriptions was based on verbatim transcripts of different samples that were created during the history of the purposes of different studies.

First, the contiguous groups of 5 sessions that started the blocks of 50 sessions were transcribed (sample a1 below). Second, the sample (a1) was enhanced by the sample (a2), which led to a joint sample (a) that consisted of the contiguous groups of 5 sessions that started the blocks of 25 sessions. The strategy (b) had the goal of investigating the subsequence of sessions with

[1] Throughout this text, the patients are named in concordance with our procedure that is explained by Thomä and Kächele (1987).

regular distances. In contrast, the strategy (c) targeted the irregular distances; the aim was to exclude the bias that was caused by potentially possible periodically occurring events. Finally, the strategies that were mentioned under strategy (d) were used for particular research questions. The concluding sample of available transcribed sessions is a union of these particular samples.

Sampling Strategies (Examples)

(a) Sessions 1–5, 26–30, 51–55, 76–80, 101–105, 126–130, . . ., 501–505, 513–517.
  (a1) Sessions 1–5, 51–55, 101–105, 151–155, ...
  (a2) Sessions 26–30, 76–80, 126–130, 176–180, ...
(b) Sessions 1, 11, 21, 31, 41, 51, 61, 71, 81, 91, 101, ...
(c) Blocks of limited numbers of sessions that are drawn in random distance from one another out of the total population of sessions.
(d) Selected session segments, such as dreams, were transcribed.

The task of systematically reading the verbatim records of the sessions and then writing up condensed summaries of the content and transactions of the sessions still remains very close to clinical narration. When third party, uninformed people produce these descriptions, we feel that they can procure a fairly reliable perspective of what happened. This clinical-descriptive step permits an evaluation that is under certain formal constraints: the report is no longer dictated by the narrator's epic perspective that characterizes the traditional case study approach. Instead, by using a systematic sample, the assumption is made that repeated descriptions in fixed time intervals capture the decisive processes of change that have occurred.

We have prepared a fairly extensive report on our first case of Christian Y through the joint endeavors of the treating analyst, a second psychoanalyst, and a clinical psychologist who worked together through group discussion (Kächele 2009, Chap. 4). A similar systematic description was prepared for our second research case, patient Amalia X, by two graduate students. They focused on systematic changes of the patient's transference and other aspects of the treatment (Kächele et al. 2009, Chap. 4).

Two medical students succeeded in creating the report regarding the story of Amalia X's analysis by repeatedly reading the 110 sessions that represented one-fifth of the analysis. Therefore, their narrative achieved an acceptable "interreader" reliability according to the treating psychoanalyst and other colleagues who worked with the material (Leuzinger-Bohleber 1989). We think that they have achieved more than narrative truth.

The material that was available after such an effort was generated into a report; the voluminous collected verbatim records (thousands of pages) were elegantly compressed into a readable hundred-page account. Such a booklet can serve many purposes in addition to it being a valuable achievement in itself. It provides easy access regarding the orientation for the whole case, and it is more detailed and more systematic than a traditional case history, which tends to be more novella-like. However, the systematic description record marked the orderly progress of things. One can rearrange the qualitative data by concatenating all of the transference descriptions, and by doing this, one can gain a good view regarding the development of major transference issues, which are investigated through the use of the CCRT. Based on these analyses, the following titles for groups of sessions that were established by the sampling strategy (a, see above) were formulated.

1–5	The analysis as confession
26–30	The analysis as an examination
51–55	The bad, cold mother
76–80	Submission and secret defiance
101–105	Searching for her own rules
116–120	The disappointing father and the helpless daughter
151–155	The cold father and the daughter's desire for identification
176–180	Ambivalence in the father relationship
201–205	The father as seducer or judge of moral standards
226–230	Does he love me—or not?
251–255	Even my father cannot change me into a boy

276–280 The Cinderella feeling
301–305 The poor girl and the rich king
326–330 If you reject me, I'll reject you
351–355 The powerless love to the mighty father and jealousy
376–380 Separation for not being deserted
401–405 Discovery of her capacity to criticize
426–430 I'm only second to my mother, first-born are preferred
451–455 Hate for the giving therapist
476–480 The art of loving consists in tolerating love and hate
501–505 Be first in saying goodbye
513–517 Departure symphony

It is not by chance that these descriptions sound similar to titles of fairy tales. At any given point in treatment, the relationship between the patient and the analyst is couched in a narrative pattern that clinicians are very apt to spot. Systematic clinical descriptions thus rely on the very capacity of narrative accounting, but by using the systematic sampling technique, these accounts change in their nature. Systematic clinical description is a way to recount the treatment in a mixed mode. To introduce some objectivity into the narrative accounts that are based on verbatim records, we recommend using two readers who are to agree about the information in their accounts.

A similar task was performed by other students who went through the video recordings of the 29 sessions of the patient "DER STUDENT" many times and wrote down an account of the treatment in a short form (one page per session) and a long form (three pages per session), which have been distributed within the PEP study group[2] to provide a shared basis for detailed discussion of the results that use different methods (Kächele et al. 1990a, b).

[2] The PEP study group that was directed by Klaus Grawe and Horst Kächele "Psychotherapeutische Einzelfallprozessforschun" investigated two cases, one from Ulm (The Student) and one from Berne (The Forward) with quite a variety of process methods.

19.4.1.1 Topic Index

For the determination of thematic structures, it is necessary to be certain of what is being discussed. An initial convenient approach might be to use the therapist's process notes; however, a more exact observation should be based on the evaluation of video or audiotape recordings by an observer who was not involved in the process. Dahl introduced the method of the Topic Index to psychoanalytic process research in a seminal paper in 1972; this became an important source for our ideas regarding how to organize a working model of focus-oriented process research.

The method of the Topic Index assumes that patterns of thematic work can be represented by configurational analyses of the statistical patterns of single topics that are a part of the conversation. By using the therapist's detailed knowledge of his patient, "the analyst had identified 58 variables of specific interest in the case and had coded the presence of each of these in abbreviated transcripts of 363 sessions" (Dahl 1983, p. 42). Through the use of the statistical technique of factor analysis, Dahl could extract common variability among several of these clinical topics, which were then represented as descriptive mathematical organizations. The six factors then were named, taking into account the leading topics. A graphical representation portrayed the type of information that resulted from this procedure. Thus, the descriptive richness of a clinical case description was replaced by quantitative preciseness, which allowed for the determination of *phases* and *foci*.

It may be of historical interest that the case was treated by an experienced analyst who, for personal reasons, had to stop the treatment, and the patient was handed over to a young female candidate. The findings of Dahl's study clearly demonstrate the downhill course of the treatment.

We first used this approach for a comparative descriptive study of a patient's and her analyst's topics over the course of the psychoanalytic case of Amalia X: again, the two medical students rather than the analyst extracted from the verbatim transcripts the presence or absence of topics in a sample of evenly distributed blocks of five sessions over the whole course of treatment (22 × 5 sessions) and weighted them in a simple fashion. The resulting graph is a map of thematic events and was used for the purpose of descriptively mapping out the expansion of focal themes (Thomä 1975).

We also used this approach for a systematic description of the video-recorded, psychodynamic short-term therapy (DER STUDENT), again by using two external observers who recorded the presence or absence of the tailored topics every 10 min. This procedure led to a fine-grained web of a 5 × 29 session topic index for 10 topics. A first version of the description was supplemented by the therapist's comments (Kächele et al. 1999, Unpublished manuscript).

The summarizing technique regarding the interrelations of the various topics is a special issue that is still open because a correlational approach implies that the correlations between the variables remain stable over time (see Luborsky's comment to the P-technique 1995). Stable correlations only report on the change of factors' scores; however, they miss the aim of treatment, which relates to changing the connections between topics. Therefore, other statistical models have to be used; as Russell and Czogalik (1989) demonstrated, Markov models can be useful for the analysis of the interlinking of thematic sequences.

19.4.2 Core Conflictual Relationship Theme

The second approach for identifying focal areas was first performed by a continuous analysis of the sessions of the case THE STUDENT by using Luborsky's CCRT method, with original category system of Luborsky and Barber. The results showed that ramifications of the wish formulation can be found over the course of the 29 sessions, and these relate to the clinically formulated focus topics (Kächele and Albani 2001). This same strategy was applied after studying a large longitudinal sample of the psychoanalytic case of Amalia X (Albani et al. 2003). The study used the hierarchal system CCRT-LU of relationship categories.

The method of Core Conflictual Relationship Theme (CCRT) was invented in the 1970s by Lester Luborsky, and it was developed by him and his collaborators at Pennsylvania University. The method was intended for analyzing narrative material in therapy session transcripts. Within the relationship episodes, three types of relationship elements were able to be identified and coded, according to the three lists of standard categories. The most frequent elements constituted the core theme.

The development of the system CCRT-LU at the universities of Leipzig and Ulm began with the aim to rectify certain minor discrepancies in the original CCRT category system. This led to the complete redesign of the system structure (Albani et al. 2008; www.ccrt-lu.org)—*logically unified* is the second meaning of the acronym suffix LU. The rich database that was available made it possible to analyze the absolute frequencies of CCRT-LU components, as well as the complex structure of the data.

For the first time, the process of a long-term psychoanalytic therapy was studied with the CCRT method. The relatively large number of reactions on the subject when compared to the reactions for other CCRT studies may be because this was a psychoanalytic therapy and the patient was particularly encouraged to reflect her feelings and thoughts. Though the negative reactions of the objects and of the patient still predominate the final phase of the therapy, a significant increase in the positive reactions of the patient became apparent. The patient also described the reactions of the objects more positively at the end of the analysis, but these changes could not be statistically established. The component "subject-related wishes and reactions of the subject" reveals that over the course of the therapy, the patient was able to expand her freedom of action and acquire new competencies, and her depressive symptoms decreased. Starting in therapy phase VII, Amalia X (out of XXII) was in a position to perceive and express aggressive wishes, and starting in therapy phase XV, these gain relevance in action.

Particularly, when this was contrasted with the dominant feelings of dissatisfaction and fearfulness at the inception of the therapy, the change in Amalia X became apparent.

Alongside the basic theme that was manifested in each of the absolute highest frequency categories ("nuclear conflict"), each of the therapy phases also showed typical categories that characterize thematic foci in the sense of French's *focal conflicts* and that can be operationalized by the CCRT-LU method. Thus, the CCRT-LU method makes it possible to structure this material by content.

In contrast with a clinical description, which uses metaphorical language to highlight a theme according to the subjective assessment of the clinical judges, investigation of the therapy phases by the CCRT-LU method makes a more differentiated (and less subjective) analysis of the themes possible, which is observed in therapy phase III. In the clinical description, the "bad mother" takes center stage, while in the CCRT-LU evaluation, other aspects emerge: "I feel good" (regarding the patient's newly gained/regained freedom of action). While the clinical description is limited to the transference configuration, the CCRT-LU method makes it possible to access interpersonal aspects inside and outside of the therapeutic relationship.

The CCRT method distinguishes different dimensions of relationship elements. This can be a reported reaction (R) that happened or the wish of the patient (W). Reactions are divided into the reaction of other relationship objects (RO) or of the patient—subject (RS). The hierarchical system of CCRT-LU goes a step further: ROS are the reactions of objects towards the subject, while RSO is the opposite; ROO or RSS are self-reactions of objects or subjects.

The strengths, as well as the limits, of the CCRT-LU method stem from its confinement to reports on relationship experiences by the patient herself. In other words, the investigation remains limited to those relationship experiences that the patient perceived and verbalized. The method provides no direct way of focusing on unconscious material or of assessing defense mechanisms at particular transcript points. However, the patients follow—often unconsciously—the repetitive schemas when describing the course of relationships. Hence, the evaluation remains very close to the clinical material, though it does reflect intrapsychic processes in the narratives of the interactions.

In the case of Amalia X, one central relationship pattern was found, which was represented by the most frequent CCRT-LU categories and could be seen as a "basic theme" or Freud's "Klischee" (Freud 1912):

- W: Amalia X wants to be understood by others.
- RO: Others are unreliable, dominant, and refusing.
- RS: She, by herself, responds with anxiety and feelings of guilt and draws herself back.

Moreover, the CCRT-LU category system allows for the determination of specific relationship patterns with different objects, including the instant, repetitive schemes of Amalia X, the teacher, with her school class (Albani et al. 2008):

- WOS: She wants to be accepted and respected by her pupils.
- WSO: She will be a good teacher for them.
- ROS: The pupils are undisciplined and do not respect her.
- RSO: She manages to discipline the class successfully.
- RSS: When reflecting upon this at home, she is depressed and disappointed by herself.

Apart from this, we captured object specific relationship patterns by using alternative methods of analysis (for detailed descriptions, see Pokorny 2008). For instance, similarities in her descriptions between her relationships with her father, her analyst, and her partner were found.

In this way, parallels between the patient's descriptions of her relationship with the therapist and other objects can be examined by using the CCRT method. Thus, the method makes it possible to capture structural aspects of the clinical transference concept. Nevertheless, the interactive aspects of the work on transference and the concomitant countertransference are not captured by the CCRT method.

In regard to the CCRT method itself, it is not possible to clarify how therapeutic changes arise.

On the whole, the relationship between the patient and her therapist seems to have been satisfying and positive for her—no other relationship is described with such a high rate of positive reactions towards the object of interaction.

This study shows that the CCRT method makes it possible to capture clinically relevant interpersonal aspects of the psychoanalytic process from the patient's point of view, which supports the Ulm process model. The analyst's contribution, however, is reflected only in the patient's narratives regarding her relationship with the therapist. Use of the CCRT method provides a way to structure the clinical material, develop clinical hypotheses, and check therapeutic focus during the course of therapy. This method is easily learned for clinical application, and the time that is required in formulating the psychodynamic connections for clinical use is minimal. Therefore, the method can accompany treatment over time.

The CCRT method can also be used to analyze manifest dream contents along the treatment process, which we demonstrated in a study on the psychoanalytic case of a patient with an anxiety neurosis who was called "Franziska" (Albani et al. 2001a, b). Differences between relationship patterns from episodes in dreams and from narratives apart of the dream session could be demonstrated. Relationship patterns in dream episodes revealed wishes more explicitly, and the most frequent responses were characterized by wish fulfillment and satisfying relationship experiences. However, narratives' objects were described as being distant and reluctant, and the patient felt anxious and nervous.

19.4.3 Clinical-Guided Judgments

Our third approach to the identification of thematic foci refers to the application of scaled assessments of clinical concepts in the case of the patient Christian Y (Kächele 2009). The basis of our study consisted of 11 × 5 sessions, which were selected at intervals of 50 sessions. The status of the treatment was evaluated by the systematic description of the process on the basis of the five-session periods. This joint clinical discussion of the research group was preceded by a classification of the 55 sessions, in random order, in accordance with the following clinically relevant concepts, which had to be rated on five-point Likert scales with regard to their intensity and degree of consciousness:

= Positive transference
= Negative transference
= Separation anxiety
= Castration anxiety
= Guilt anxiety
= Shame anxiety
= Diffuse anxiety
= Insight
= Working alliance

Evaluation of this guided clinical rating was carried out by three judges; the therapist was one of these judges. By using the factor analysis, the following five factors were identified:

Factor 1: Working alliance (assessed by rater B and C)
Factor 2: Positive transference as a defense against separation anxiety
Factor 3: Diffuse anxiety with aggressive transference
Factor 4: Working alliance (assessed by the analyst)
Factor 5: Shame and guilt anxiety

On the basis of our detailed clinical knowledge and of the understanding of the course of treatment that was achieved by the research group in the systematic description study, we tentatively formulated four focus-related periods of treatment (we call them "periods" here to distinguish them from "phases" that are described above):

Period 1 (sessions 1–5, 51–55, 101–105): maintenance of defense
Period 2 (sessions 151–155, 201–205): intensification and access to consciousness of the early positive object relation in the transference
Period 3 (sessions 251–255, 301–305, 351–355): alternation of pregenital-positive clinging transference and aggressive distancing in the transference
Period 4 (sessions 401–405, 451–455, 501–505): consolidation of the aggressive transference

Table 19.1 Classification matrix of the discriminant analysis in the case of Christian Y

Observed period	Predicted period 1	2	3	4	Total	Correct
1	**12**	0	2	1	15	80 %
2	2	**6**	1	1	10	60 %
3	3	4	**5**	3	15	33 %
4	5	1	0	**9**	15	60 %
Total	22	11	8	14	55	58 %

Period 1 is characterized predominantly by a friendly attitude on the part of the patient, who approaches the analytical process with a great deal of interest and seemingly good defenses, which is judged based on the verbal exchange within the sessions. The problem of separation emerges only incipiently in the transference; the aggressive transference is predominantly unconscious and not very intense. Feelings of guilt and shame alternate in their intensity.

Period 2 is characterized predominantly by the mobilization of the separation problem in the analytic situation; aggressive aspects of the transference are manifested only in individual sessions.

In period 3, the therapeutic aim of reactivating aggressive impulses in the transference, which underlines the severe anxieties, is achieved for the first time; at the same time, the alternation with a symbiotic-clinging position is marked.

In period 4, one can discern a perceptible decline of the friendly, conciliatory object relation, which is replaced by an openly negative aggressive transference.

It should be noted that this study was performed when the treatment was not yet completed; therefore, future periods are to be expected when the entire course of analysis that lasts for approximately 1,200 sessions is studied.

The clinically derived focus formulations were then checked by a formal algorithm. By using the five factors of the rating investigation, discriminant analysis was used to calculate linear functions by which the membership of the individual session within the four periods can be predicted (see Table 19.1). In this way, each of the 55 h is assigned by the discriminant analysis to one of the four periods. The comparison of the predicted and real period membership confirmed the relative homogeneity of each of the four periods in terms of the sessions that were assigned to them.

The overall rate of the correct prediction, 58 %, is 2.3 times higher than the 25 % that is expected by random rating. With the exception of period 3, we find a dominating type of session in each period; the results of period 3 clearly indicate that all four types of sessions are parsed over this period, which indicates that there was no stable topical preference. Let us note that this prediction was based on the values of the five factors only, which correspond clinically to the focal schemes, which we created based on our joint clinical discussion.

Conclusion

The empirical approaches mentioned in this chapter are just a few examples from the field of single-case methodologies that have been developed over the last few decades. A future step in our endeavor regarding the development of descriptive tools for the identification of focally determined phases in analytic treatments is based on the combination of the clinically derived, through the use of systematic and controlled judgment procedures, ratings of clinically relevant concepts with a more stringently definable computer-assisted content analysis tool (Kächele and Mergenthaler 1983; Mergenthaler 1985; Kächele 1986). We would underscore that the empirical attempt to test psychoanalytic process theories needs descriptive tools that are capable of mastering the large amount of data that is involved in such a task.

We are convinced that psychoanalytic process research has to start from the clinical experience, which can lead to the introduction of new observational tools that can be checked in regard to their appropriateness. Once we are able to go beyond clinical descriptions, we may be in a better position to decide which model of process fits the data best. Then, the clinical issue can be solved regarding what the relationship between the various phases of treatment may be and what its relevance for the ultimate treatment outcome is.

References

Albani C, Kühnast B, Pokorny D, Blaser G, Kächele H (2001a) Beziehungsmuster in Träumen und Geschichten über Beziehungen in einem psychoanalytischen Prozeß (Relationship patterns in dreams and stories about relationships in a psychoanalytic process). ForumPsychoanal 17:287–296

Albani C, Pokorny D, Blaser G, König S, Geyer M, Thomä H, Kächele H (2001b) Zur empirischen Erfassung von Übertragung und Beziehungsmustern - eine Einzelfallanalyse (On the empirical study of transference and relationship patterns – a single case study). Psychother Psychol Med 51:1–10

Albani C, Pokorny D, Blaser G, König S, Thomä H, Kächele H (2003) Study of a psychoanalytic process using the core conflictual relationship theme (CCRT) method according to the Ulm process model. Eur Psychother 4:11–32

Albani C, Pokorny D, Blaser G, Kächele H (2008) Beziehungsmuster und Beziehungskonflikte. Theorie, Klinik und Forschung. Vandenhoeck & Ruprecht, Göttingen

Breuer J (1893–1895) Case I. Fräulein Anna O. In: Breuer J, Freud S (eds) Studies on hysteria. In J. Strachey (eds and trans) The standard edition of the complete psychological works of Sigmund Freud, vol 2. Hogarth Press, London, pp 21–47

Bucci W (1988) Converging evidence for emotional structures: theory and method. In: Dahl H, Kächele H, Thomä H (eds) Psychoanalytic process research strategies. Springer, Berlin, pp 29–49

Bucci W (1997) Pattern of discourse in good and troubled hours. J Am Psychoanal Assoc 45:155–188

Compton A (1990) Psychoanalytic process. Psychoanal Q 59:585–598

Dahl H (1983) On the definition and measurement of wishes. In: Masling J (ed) Empirical studies of psychoanalytical theories. The Analytic Press, Hillsdale

Dahl H (1988) Frames of mind. In: Dahl H, Kächele H, Thomä H (eds) Psychoanalytic process research strategies. Springer, Berlin, pp 51–66

Dahl H, Kächele H, Thomä H (eds) (1988) Psychoanalytic process research strategies. Springer, Berlin

Dewald P (1972) The psychoanalytic process. A case illustration. Basic Books, New York, NY

Ferenczi S (1927 [1964]) Bausteine zur Psychoanalyse (Fundamentals of psychoanalysis), vol 2, Praxis (Practice). Internationaler Psychoanalytischer [Huber], Wien [Stuttgart – Bern]

Fonagy P, Moran G (1993) Selecting single case research designs for clinicians. In: Miller N, Luborsky L, Barber J, Docherty J (eds) Handbook of psychodynamic treatment research. Basic Books, New York, NY, pp 62–95

Forrester J (1980) Language and the origins of psychoanalysis. Macmillan, London

French TM (1952) The integration of behaviour. Basic postulates, vol 1. University of Chicago Press, Chicago, IL

Freud S (1895) Studies on hysteria. In: Strachey J (ed and trans) The standard edition of the complete psychological works of Sigmund Freud, vol 2. Hogarth Press, London

Freud S (1912) The dynamics of transference. SE XII: 97–108

Frommer J, Rennie DL (eds) (2001) Qualitative psychotherapy research. Methods and methodology. Pabst, Lengerich

Hilliard RB (1993) Single case methodology in psychotherapy process and outcome research. J Consult Clin Psychol 61:373–380

Iwakabe S, Gazzola N (2009) From single-case studies to practice-based knowledge: aggregating and synthesizing case studies. Psychother Res 19(4–5):601–611

Jones EE, Windholz M (1990) The psychoanalytic case study: toward a method for systematic inquiry. J Am Psychoanal Assoc 38:985–1016

Kächele H (1981) Zur Bedeutung der Krankengeschichte in der klinisch-psychoanalytischen Forschung (On the relevance of case history in clinical psychoanalytic research). Jahrb Psychoanal 12:118–177

Kächele H (1986) Die Maschinelle Inhaltsanalyse in der Psychoanalytischen Prozessforschung (Computer-based content analysis in psychoanalytic process research). PSZ, Ulm

Kächele H (1992) Narration and observation in psychotherapy research. Reporting on a 20 year long journey from qualitative case reports to quantitative studies on the psychoanalytic process. Psychother Res 2:1–15

Kächele H (2009) Psychanalytische Prozesse. Methodische Illustrationen und methodologische Reflexionen (Psychoanalytic processes. Methodical illustrations and methodological reflections). Munich Electronic Database, München. http://edoc.ub.uni-muenchen.de/10558/

Kächele H (2010) Distinguishing psychoanalysis from psychotherapy. Int J Psychoanal 91:35–43

Kächele H, Albani C (2001) Die Arbeit an einem zentralen Beziehungsmuster als Musterbeispiel klinisch relevanter Empirie (Work on a core conflictual relationship pattern as a sample of clinically relevant research). In: Cierpka M, Buchheim P (eds) Psychodynamische Konzepte. Springer, Berlin, pp 169–190

Kächele H, Mergenthaler E (1983) Computer-aided analysis of psychotherapeutic discourse – a workshop. In: Minsel W-R, Herff W (eds) Methodology in psychotherapy research. Proceedings of the 1st European conference on psychotherapy research. Lang, Frankfurt a. M., pp 116–161

Kächele H, Thomä H, Ruberg W, Grünzig H-J (1988) Audio-recordings of the psychoanalytic dialogue: scientific, clinical and ethical problems. In: Dahl H,

Kächele H, Thomä H (eds) Psychoanalytic process research strategies. Springer, Berlin, pp 179–194
Kächele H, Dengler D, Eckert R, Schnekenburger S (1990a) Veränderung des zentralen Beziehungskonfliktes durch eine Kurztherapie (Change of the core conflictual relationship conflict by a short term therapy). Psychother Psychol Med 40:178–185
Kächele H, Heldmaier H, Scheytt N (1990b) Fokusformulierungen als katamanestische Leitlinien (Focal formulations as guidelines for a follow-up study). Psychother Psychol Med 35:205–216
Kächele H, Scheytt N, Schwendele W (1999) Der STUDENT – eine detaillierte Verlaufsbeschreibung (THE STUDENT – a detailed description of a treatment process). In: Kächele H, Grawe K (eds) PEP-Projekt. http://www.horstkaechele.de/plib/index.php?id=1_23_22 (Unpublished manuscript)
Kächele H, Schachter J, Thomä H (eds) (2009) From psychoanalytic narrative to empirical single case research. Implications for Psychoanalytic Practice. Routledge, New York
Kazdin AE (1982) Single case research designs: methods for clinical and applied settings. Oxford University Press, Oxford
Klein M (1961) Narrative of a child analysis. Hogarth Press, London
Leuzinger-Bohleber M (1989) Veränderung kognitiver Prozesse in Psychoanalysen. Bd 2: Eine gruppenstatistische Untersuchung (Change of cognitive processes in psychoanalyses, vol 2: A group-statistical study). PSZ/Springer, Berlin
Leuzinger-Bohleber M (1995) Die Einzelfallstudie als psychoanalytisches Forschungsinstrument (The single case study as a psychoanalytic research instrument). Psyche – Z Psychoanal 49:434–480
Luborsky L (1995) The first trial of P-technique in psychotherapy research. A still-lively legacy. J Consult Clin Psychol 63:6–14
Luborsky L, Crits-Christoph P (eds) (1998) Understanding transference: the core conflictual relationship theme method, 2nd edn. American Psychological Association, Washington, DC
Luborsky L, Spence DP (1971) Quantitative research on psychoanalytic therapy. In: Bergin AE, Garfield SL (eds) Handbook of psychotherapy and behavior change, 1st edn. Wiley, New York, NY, pp 408–438
Luyten P, Blatt SJ, Corveleyn J (2006) Minding the gap between positivism and hermeneutics in psychoanalytic research. J Am Psychoanal Assoc 54:571–610
Malan DH (1963) A study of brief psychotherapy. Tavistock, London
Mergenthaler E (1985) Textbank systems: computer science in psychoanalysis. Springer, Heidelberg
Mergenthaler E, Kächele H (1988) The Ulm textbank management system: a tool for psychotherapy research. In: Dahl H, Kächele H, Thomä H (eds) Psychoanalytic process research strategies. Springer, Berlin, pp 195–212
Michels R (2000) The case history. With commentaries by S. Pulver, S. B. Bernstein, P. Rubovits-Seitz, I. Szecsödy, D. Tuckett, A. Wilson. J Am Psychoanal Assoc 48:355–375
Pokorny D (2008) Datenanalyse mit ZBKT-LU (Data analysis with the CCRT-LU). In: Albani C, Pokorny D, Blaser G, Kächele H (eds) Beziehungsmuster und Beziehungskonflikte. Theorie, Klinik und Forschung. Vandenhoeck & Ruprecht, Göttingen, pp 174–214
Propp WJ (1928) Morfologia delle fiabe. Einandi, Torino
Russell RL, Czogalik D (1989) Strategies for analyzing conversation: frequencies, sequences or rules. J Soc Behav Pers 3:221–236
Schachter J, Kächele H (2010) The couch in psychoanalysis. Contemp Psychoanal 46:439–459
Seitz P (1966) The consensus problem in psychoanalysis. In: Gottschalk LA, Auerbach AH (eds) Methods of research in psychotherapy. Appleton Century Crofts, New York, NY, pp 209–225
Spence DP (1982) Narrative truth and historical truth: meaning and interpretation in psychoanalysis. Norton, New York, NY
Stuhr U (2004) Klinische Fallstudien (Clinical case studies). In: Hau S, Leuzinger-Bohleber M (eds) Psychoanalytische Therapie. Eine Stellungnahme für die wissenschaftliche Öffentlichkeit und für den Wissenschaftlichen Beirat Psychotherapie. Forum Psychoanal 20:63–66
Thomä H (1961) Anorexia nervosa. Geschichte, Klinik und Theorie der Pubertätsmagersucht. Huber/Klett, Bern/Stuttgart; English (1967) Anorexia nervosa. Yale University Press, New Haven
Thomä H (1975) Prozessbeschreibung mit dem Topic Index (Description of a treatment process using the Topic Index). Vortrag an der Psychosomatischen Klinik, Universität Heidelberg
Thomä H, Kächele H (1987) Psychoanalytic practice, vol 1. Principles. Springer, Berlin; paperback. Aronson, New York, 1994
von Zeppelin I (1987) A process model of psychoanalytic therapy. In: Cheshire N, Thomä H (eds) The self and its symptoms. Wiley, New York, NY, pp 149–165
Weiss J, Sampson H, Group TMZpr (eds) (1986) The psychoanalytic process: theory, clinical observation, and empirical research. Guilford Press, New York
Winnicott DW (1972) Fragment of an analysis. In: Giovaccini PL (ed) Tactics and techniques in psychoanalytic therapy. Hogarth Press, London, pp 455–693
Wittgenstein L (1921/2014) Tractatus logico-philosophicus. Logisch-philosophische Abhandlung. Suhrkamp, Berlin

Qualitative Methods in Psychotherapy Process Research 20

Kathrin Mörtl and Omar Carlo Gioacchino Gelo

Contents

K. Mörtl (✉)
Department of Psychotherapy Science, Sigmund Freud University, Freudplatz 1, 1020 Vienna, Austria
e-mail: kathrin.moertl@sfu.ac.at

O.C.G. Gelo
Department of History, Society and Human Studies, University of Salento, Via Stampacchia 45, 73100 Lecce, Italy

Department of Psychotherapy Science, Sigmund Freud University, Freudplatz 1, 1020 Vienna, Austria

Abstract

This chapter describes a variety of qualitative methods that can be used within psychotherapy process research (PPR). After a general introduction of qualitative PPR, this chapter focuses on research design, sampling, data collection, and data analysis. This chapter offers a dimensional conceptualization, especially for data collection and analysis, which provides organization to the different methods employed to collect and analyze data in qualitative PPR. Finally, quality criteria for this type of research are examined and briefly discussed.

20.1 Introduction

Teaching qualitative research methods in psychology-related fields is often a qualitative endeavor in itself. How do we create a space for the curious mind to understand the nature of this research attitude while providing specific tools so students can leave the classroom and start with a research project?

Teaching is our fascinating work, which motivated us to think deeply about how to introduce methods so that they accompany and

O.C.G. Gelo et al. (eds.), *Psychotherapy Research*,
DOI 10.1007/978-3-7091-1382-0_20, © Springer-Verlag Wien 2015

stimulate students as they develop into academic researchers. This is the starting point of this chapter. First, we present the landscape of the qualitative research field. In a recently published special issue, "Qualitative Researchers at University" (Mörtl 2012), generations of qualitative researchers (graduate students, research assistants, and professors) voice their experiences and perspectives on the practice of qualitative research in the academic setting. They indicate that the following three factors are needed to become a good qualitative researcher:

(1) Knowledge of methodology to master the general principles inspiring and governing qualitative inquiry, which is assured by acquiring an understanding of the theory (philosophy) of science and related historical knowledge
(2) Knowledge of methods to master the ability to select and implement the appropriate research design, sampling, data collection, and data analysis procedures for a specific qualitative project, which is assured by learning many classic and contemporary methods
(3) Nurturing professional relationships to maintain equilibrium between freedom and structure to conduct a project, which is assured by supportive colleagues and supervisors accompanied by critical reflection and discussion within the research project

This chapter contributes to knowledge of the *methods* used in qualitative PPR, though we will also address general methodological issues at the beginning and end of the chapter (for more on these issues, see Frommer and Rennie 2001; Lutz and Hill 2009; McLeod 2011, 2013; Timulak 2008). For an application of qualitative methods to process research, see Chap. 21). We first introduce the reader to qualitative PPR as well as the research design and sampling issues encountered in this type of research. Then, we turn to methods of data collection and data analysis. We conclude by addressing quality criteria within qualitative PPR (for an analogous treatment of qualitative *outcome* psychotherapy research, see Chap. 27). While it may be easier to clearly distinguish between the investigation of the process and outcome using a *quantitative* approach (see, e.g., Chaps. 13 and 26), in qualitative research, processes and outcomes are more often studied with reference to their connections. This is why, unlike in quantitative research, in qualitative research, several overlaps exist between the methods used to investigate the process and those used to investigate the outcome.

20.2 Qualitative Psychotherapy Process Research

20.2.1 Quantitative Versus Qualitative

Quantitative and qualitative[1] approaches are the most widespread empirical research approaches in contemporary social, psychological, and behavioral sciences. At a general and pragmatic level, quantitative research relies on *numbers* to fulfill its research goals, while qualitative research relies on *words* and *language* (Gelo et al. 2012; Hill and Lambert 2004). Nonetheless, these two approaches may be differentiated by the historical, philosophical, and methodological issues about which there is a richly articulated discussion in the scientific community (see, e.g., Gelo 2012; Slife 2004; and Chap. 4).

Our experience as researchers suggests that the blunt categorization of a research approach as *either* qualitative *or* quantitative is void in conducting actual research. For example, complex interpretive text analyses are often supported by frequency calculations, while numerical data must be conceptualized before statistical analyses can be conducted or interpreted. Quantitative and qualitative research approaches should be considered the prototypical extremes of a continuum along which each research project is located. Nonetheless, we consider it useful to summarize the aspects that differentiate these poles.

[1] Quality and quantity were two of Aristotle's ten categories in which quality refers to the nature of an object (What is it? white, black, straight, curved, etc.), while *quantity* refers to the amount of an object or its attributes (How much? two, three, a specific length, etc.). Kant (2002/1788) revised these categories and formulated the following four categories (with three subcategories each): quality, quantity, modality, and relation.

According to Gelo et al. (2008, 2009), for example, the following key terms may be used to describe the quantitative-qualitative dichotomy: nomothetic (generalizing) vs. idiographic (individualizing), explanation (prediction) vs. comprehension (interpretation), deduction (theory driven) vs. induction (data driven), experimental vs. naturalistic, causal validity vs. interpretive validity, and generalizability vs. transferability (see also, Ponterotto 2005). In a standard German textbook on qualitative social research, Lamnek (2010) provides a similar outline with two poles. In addition to the differences described by Gelo et al. (2008), Lamnek distinguishes among the following categories: objective vs. subjective, ahistorical vs. historical, closed vs. opened, predetermined by researchers vs. relevance system of the investigated, distance vs. identification, statistical vs. dynamic procedural, rigid vs. flexible, particular vs. holistic, and high vs. low scales of measurement. McLeod (2011) also distinguishes among paradigmatic vs. narrative approaches. Again, these authors argue that these dichotomies are ideal—or extreme—types along a quantitative-qualitative continuum. They do pinpoint some implicit and explicit differences, but these rigid categories can never do justice to the internal complexity of any method. The properties by which we distinguish quantitative from qualitative research should be considered, although to different extents, complementary, and enmeshed.

Furthermore, quantitative and qualitative approaches can be formally combined through the so-called *mixed-method* research (Gelo et al. 2008, 2009; Hanson et al. 2005). The core idea guiding such an approach is that quantitative and qualitative approaches may be combined either *concurrently* (as in the very popular triangulation approach) or *sequentially* (in which a researcher follows a qualitative and then a quantitative approach, or vice versa) (see Hanson et al. (2005) for a systematic review). Finally, this chapter will clarify that some qualitative methods tend to be more closely associated with quantitative research than others are, especially methods for data analysis.

20.2.2 Qualitative Research

Outlining the field of qualitative research practice is a challenge. In the introduction of the classic *Handbook of Qualitative Research*, Denzin and Lincoln (2005) provide the following definition of qualitative research:

> Qualitative research is a situated activity that locates the observer in the world. It consists of a set of interpretive, material practices that make the world visible. These practices transform the world. They turn the world into a series of representations, including field notes, interviews, conversations, photographs, recordings, and memos to the self. At this level, qualitative research involves an interpretive, naturalistic approach to the word. This means that qualitative researchers study things in their natural settings, attempting to make sense of, or interpret, phenomena in terms of the meanings people bring to them. (p. 3).

The authors continue by stating that qualitative research emphasizes "processes and meanings that are not experimentally examined or measured (if measured at all) in terms of quantity, amount, intensity, or frequency" (p. 10), while quantitative research "emphasizes the measurement and analysis of causal relationships of variables and not processes" (p. 10). Similar outlines can be found in the qualitative method textbooks written by McLeod (2011) and Barker et al. (2002). As McLeod (2011) affirms, "the primary aim of qualitative research is to develop an understanding of how the social world is constructed" through social practices, actions, conversations, and stories, which, in turn, present a *narrative* structure (McLeod 2011, p. 3). Therefore, qualitative research may be placed within a *constructivist-interpretivist* framework (Gelo 2012; Ponterotto 2005), which emphasizes *emphatic participation* and interpretative processes of a *hermeneutic* nature (Rennie 2012) aimed at incorporating the *individual*, *particular*, *in-depth*, and *contextual* nature of meaning (see Rennie (2012) for a meta-methodology of qualitative research).

However, qualitative research is not necessarily characterized by a single paradigm, methodology, theory, method, or discipline (Denzin and

Lincoln 2005; Mcleod 2011; Hill and Lambert 2004; Ponterotto 2005). To the contrary, qualitative projects are often influenced by paradigms besides the constructivist-interpretivist view, are multi-method, and apply more than one interpretive practice on a variety of empirical material depending on the context (see Nelson et al. 1992 cited in Denzin and Lincoln 2005). Polkinghorne (2005) affirms that qualitative research is an "umbrella term" (p. 137), which can include a variety of approaches and methods. Denzin and Lincoln (2005) define the researcher as a "bricoleur" or "quilt maker" who will use, invent, or combine the necessary tools to investigate the phenomenon of interest (see also, McLeod 2011). Taking these considerations to heart, our attempt to map qualitative methods in PPR seems futile and necessarily limited. Nonetheless, it is worth outlining some of the common core aspects of this type of research.

20.2.3 Qualitative Research and the Psychotherapeutic Process

The *psychotherapeutic process* includes all the events occurring either within or between therapy sessions, which include the "actions, perceptions, intentions, thoughts, and feelings of the patient and therapist, as well as the relationship between them" (Orlinsky et al. 2004, p. 313). Thus, *qualitative* PPR investigates these therapy processes, and their eventual contribution to a successful outcome, through qualitative methods.[2]

Notwithstanding the differences that may be observed among the existing approaches, qualitative PPR may be generally characterized by the following: (1) primary use of non-numerical, *languaged* data Polkinghorne 2005; (2) data that are analyzed through *interpretative-hermeneutical* procedures Rennie 2012; (3) provide a deep understanding of participant perspectives on the therapeutic process, their experience during the course of therapy, and the communicative (inter)actions through which this process is shaped (see Lutz and Hill 2009; Lutz and Knox 2013; Frommer and Rennie 2001; McLeod 2011, 2013).

Point (3) highlights the fact that qualitative process research includes several aims at two main degrees of resolution, which we will illustrate using the metaphor of a photographic lens [for an elaborate discussion, see Mörtl and Lamott (2010)]. Qualitative PPR uses a *wide-angle* objective to capture a whole scene and obtain a view of the gestalt of the phenomenon at a *low* degree of resolution. This, which may be called qualitative *macro*-process research, occurs when broad research questions are posed about the *general subjective experiences about the therapy process* of clients, therapists, and, eventually, third parties, such as family members [e.g., "How does the expectation of cognitive behavioral therapy differ in good and poor outcome clients" (Westra et al. 2011) and "Patients' experiences of change in cognitive–behavioral therapy and psychodynamic therapy" (Nilsson et al. 2007)]. A second research strategy *zooms* into the details of an image to visualize as much microscopic detail as possible. This, which may be called qualitative *micro*-process research, occurs when less holistic questions are posed at a *high* degree of resolution about specific phenomena. The focus here is on the way clients and therapists *organize their experiences during the course of the sessions* [e.g., "Narrative processes in the formation of a therapeutic system" (Laitila et al. 2001) and "Clients' subjective experience of significant moments during the exploration of problematic reactions" (Watson and Rennie 1994)] as well as about the properties of the *within-session conversational and dialogical exchange* between the client(s) and therapist (s) [e.g., "How therapists and clients comanage relational disaffiliation" (Muntigl and Horvath 2014)].

Both approaches are qualitative in the more conservative definition provided by Denzin and Lincoln (2005) or Gelo et al. (2008). On the one

[2] Although investigations of the contribution of the therapeutic process to clinical outcomes is known as *process-outcome* research (see Orlinsky et al. 2004), sometimes the term *process* research is used to refer to the investigation of the process as well as of the process-outcome relationship (see Chap. 13).

hand, macroanalytic studies usually make use of data collected through *qualitative interviews* and *open-ended questionnaires* completed after several sessions or the end of the treatment. These data are then analyzed by focusing on the *content* of the collected material as in grounded theory (Chap. 22) or consensual qualitative research (see Chap. 23). On the other hand, microanalytic approaches utilize the data collected mainly by *recording and transcribing therapy sessions*, which are then analyzed with procedures that focus on the *structure* of the transcribed material as in conversational analysis. Some microanalytic approaches involve a second quantitative step. This occurs when transcripts are analyzed through category systems or ratings scales and when the results of an initial qualitative interpretation of transcripts are transformed into frequency counts and then analyzed statistically.

20.3 Research Design

In the method-supervision work, our experience is that students come with a more or less specific research idea. After facilitating a space to think and elaborate more what the specific phenomenon they are interested in, students usually struggle with how to practically design the research study. Gelo et al. (2008) describe the research design as "the plan of actions or structure which links the philosophical foundations and the methodological assumptions of a research approach to its research methods [...], to provide credible, accountable and legitimate answers to the research questions" (p. 272). Research design decisions are sometimes challenging for less experienced students and must be made along the following three dimensions: (1) naturalistic vs. experimental, (2) single case (intensive) vs. group (extensive), and (3) cross-sectional vs. longitudinal.[3] Each dimension is presented as a dichotomy for heuristic reasons but represents a continuum.

20.3.1 Naturalistic Versus Experimental

Naturalistic design refers to the limited degree of control that can be imposed on the research setting and structure. The fundamental assumption of such a design is that the phenomenon is best observed and understood when investigated without *external constraints* or *control*. The natural context of observation is considered essential for a *deeper* and *articulated understanding* rather than a source of *variability to be controlled*. Most qualitative psychotherapy process studies are naturalistic in this sense.[4] *Experimental* designs, on the contrary, are characterized by a high degree of control over confounding variables, which is necessary to make valid causal inferences about the relationship between independent and dependent variables (Barker et al. 2002; Campbell and Stanley 1963; Kazdin 2003). To our knowledge, no qualitative study within PPR has adopted an experimental design, which is not surprising because some qualitative researchers believe that experimental control denatures the object being investigated. However, it is possible that you could use research results on the effectiveness of psychotherapy interventions and manualize their causal link, so therapists can test the hypothesis in an experimental clinical setting. We do not need to mention the ethical implications of such an approach, and hence the reason why there have not been experimental studies in this sense. Nonetheless, studies adopting a mixed-method approach [i.e., studies combining quantitative and qualitative methods; see Gelo et al. (2008, 2009) and Hanson et al. (2005)] may combine a quantitative

[3] Decisions about these three dimensions must also be taken when following a quantitative or mixed-method approach (see Chaps. 12 and 13).

[4] Within the context of quantitative PPR, some authors use the term naturalistic to refer to *non-experimental* research designs. We prefer to reserve the term naturalistic for qualitative research designs and use the term *correlational* or *passive-observational* for non-experimental quantitative research designs.

experimental design with a qualitative naturalistic design (e.g., Palmer and Cochran 1988).

20.3.2 Single Case (Intensive) Versus Group (Extensive)

The next research design decision must be made about adopting a *single-case* (*intensive*) or *group* (*extensive*) design (Barker et al. 2002; Chassan 1979; Swanborn 2010). In qualitative single-case (intensive) designs, the researcher aims for an *in-depth* analysis by reconstructing and understanding an *individual case* ($N = 1$; *within*-case variation). These designs belong to a qualitative subclass of so-called systematic case studies, which distinguishes them from clinical case studies in which no systematic procedure for data collection or analysis is used (Iwakabe and Gazzola 2009, p. 603). An interesting variant is the *multiple-case* design (Yin 2003) in which two or more single-case cases are investigated to highlight differences not only within but also between the cases (e.g., Stiles 2001). In qualitative group (extensive) designs, the researcher is interested in the *in-width* analysis of *several subjects* (*between*-case variation) that may be considered with reference to one or more groups (e.g., Nilsson et al. 2007).[5]

20.3.3 Cross-Sectional Versus Longitudinal

Finally, students have to decide about whether to adopt a *cross-sectional* or *longitudinal* design (Barker et al. 2002; Kazdin 2003). Qualitative cross-sectional designs are used to investigate one phenomenon in one or more groups of subjects at *one specific time*. For this reason, they may also be referred to as *synchronic* designs. Most studies that use qualitative interviews are of this type (e.g., Nilsson et al. 2007). Qualitative longitudinal designs are used to investigate temporal developments and changes over time for a phenomenon of interest in one or more subjects. For this reason, they may also be referred to as *diachronic* designs. Most qualitative studies examining session transcripts or open-ended questionnaires adopt such a design (e.g., Stiles et al. 1991) (Information can be collected from participants that spans time retrospectively, e.g., by asking what happened during the course of a treatment, or prospectively, e.g., by asking what you think will happen during the course of a treatment. As long as this information is collected at a single time, this represents a cross-sectional design.) Qualitative single-case designs are generally, but not always, longitudinal, while group designs are cross-sectional.

20.4 Sampling

Sampling strategies address the selection of the participants to be investigated and the criteria according to which they should be identified. These may be subjects, processes, events, contexts, settings, etc., depending on the nature of the research question. In the following, however, we will talk about participants, as this is usually the reference point in qualitative research sampling techniques. In empirical research, two general classes of sampling strategies can be identified: *probabilistic* and *non-probabilistic* (see Onwuegbuzie and Leech 2007). Probabilistic sampling [e.g., simple random sampling, systematic random sampling, stratified random sampling, and cluster random sampling; see Gliner et al. (2009)] makes use of *randomness* to ensure that each participant in the population of interest faces the same probability of being included in the sample. This type of sampling is considered the gold standard of quantitative research, especially the randomized clinical trial (RCT; Hsu 1989; see Chap. 26), because it maximizes the likelihood of adequate generalizability of the results from the sample to the population. Conversely, non-probabilistic sampling requires that the researcher "purposely" use

[5] The difference between extensive and intensive designs (Sayer 1992) is analogous to the difference between *P-technique* and *R-technique* (Cattell 1952; see Molenaar and Campbell 2009) and is very generally related to the *nomothetic* vs. *idiographic* distinction (see Molenaar 2004; Salvatore and Valsiner 2010).

criteria besides chance to select the units to be included in the sample (Patton 1990). For this reason, it is also referred to as *purposeful* sampling. This type of sampling strategy is the gold standard of qualitative research in psychotherapy and most quantitative process and process-outcome research (see Chap. 12) because it maximizes the collection of rich data and produces a deep understanding of the phenomenon under investigation (Flick et al. 2004; Patton 1990).

Depending on the research purpose of a qualitative study, several types of purposeful sampling strategies may be identified within the qualitative approach as currently applied in PPR (see Flick et al. 2004; Koerber and McMichael 2008; Luborsky and Rubinstein 1995; Onwuegbuzie and Leech 2007; Patton 1990). These may be considered with regard to basically two conditions: (1) you a priori know who you want to sample because they have relevant information regarding your research question, or (2) you are not entirely sure who might give you uncovering insights into a specific phenomenon, and you decide on the way which people have to be selected. In the first case, you may decide to make use, for example, of *convenience* sampling (which selects participants based on their accessibility), *homogeneous* sampling (which selects participants based on commonalities), *maximum variation* sampling (which selects cases based on their being different from each other), and *typical* and *extreme/deviant case* sampling (which selects cases based on their being, respectively, usual or unusual); these strategies of purposeful sampling are typical of most qualitative studies (see Onwuegbuzie and Leech (2007) for a more exhaustive account). In the second case, you will make use of *theoretical* sampling [which selects participants based on the theoretical relevance they show to have during the analysis process which goes parallel to sampling and data collection; Glaser and Strauss (1967); see also Imelda (1997)].[6] Purposeful sampling is also typical of qualitative studies that utilize grounded theory (see also Chap. 22).

20.5 Data Collection

After designing, the next step in a study process is to start collecting the data. At a very general level, *data collection* is the process of systematically gathering information about the phenomena under investigation. (According to its etymology, from the Latin *datum*, something given, data are themselves the result of a process of co-construction among those involved in the research: the one giving information and the one receiving the information. It might even be possible to talk about data *construction* (see Valsiner 2010). In qualitative research, we address *qualitative data*, which are characterized by their non-numerical, *languaged* form. According to Polkinghorne (2005), "languaged data are not simply single words but interrelated words combined into sentences and sentences combined into discourses" (p. 138). Note the two observations. The languaged format can be the *final* format that qualitative researchers examine. In most cases, the data are collected directly in this format through both observation

[6] Theoretical sampling was introduced into the classic grounded theory by Glaser and Strauss (1967). The researcher cannot know whom to interview a priori because the phenomenon is still being explored. Sampling begins with one subject who promises "to maximize the chances that aspects of the phenomenon will emerge clearly in the initial stages" (Dourdouma and Mörtl 2012, p. 99). Then, after having analyzed the data produced by this first subject, the researcher uses this new understanding to decide which subject should be selected as the second case, etc. (see the concept of the *hermeneutic circle*). This process stops when informational and theoretical redundancy (i.e., *saturation*, Morse 1995) is reached. In their first study about awareness of dying (1965), Glaser and Strauss examined the clinical practice with dying patients in medical institutions [interview with Strauss, published in Mey and Mruck (2007)]. Led by their personal experience with dying relatives, they began with an implicit hypothesis that influenced their sampling. They began with a premature infant station and progressed to a cancer station, which provided them with a broader understanding of the phenomenon of interest. During their fieldwork, they documented new theoretical insights that influenced the subsequent collection, which is the principle of theoretical sampling (Legewie and Schervier-Legewie 2004, p. 72).

and self-reporting (see below in this section). Qualitative researchers may also be interested in *pictorial* or *video* information. Once collected, this information must be translated into a languaged format to be analyzed (see Przyborski and Slunecko 2012). Sometimes this means transcribing the data, but also if you apply computer techniques which do not make transcription necessary, the categories that you will develop during the analysis will, so to say, create languaged data on a secondary level.

Turning now to the specific methods of how to collect the data, within the domain of PPR, qualitative researchers are usually interested in two main types of phenomena: patient or therapist *subjective experiences* related to in-therapy processes and the *communicative (inter)actions* shaping these processes (see Rennie 2012). Different strategies and procedures of data collection may be used depending on the interests of the researcher (see Fig. 20.1, x-axis) [see Elliott et al. (2001), Lutz and Hill (2009), McLeod (2011, 2013), Timulak (2008). For an account in clinical psychology, see Barker et al. (2002)]. Researchers interested in in-therapy communicative (inter)actions primarily utilize qualitative *observational* methods through which they produce a narrative account of *naturally occurring talk and (inter)action*, such as recording psychotherapy sessions. However, researchers interested in patient or therapist subjective experiences primarily utilize *self-reporting* methods to elicit *personal (spoken or written) accounts* of their inner state of affairs from the subjects, such as qualitative interviews and questionnaires. In some cases, a *combination* of these methods may be used.

However, these different strategies and procedures for data collection may also vary by their degree of *structuredness* (i.e., less structured vs. more structured; see Fig. 20.1, y-axis). We define the structuredness of a data collection method with regard to two main aspects: the degree of *standardization* of the information sought (i.e., the extent to which the composition of a method is always the same and thus imposes constraints) and the *degree of freedom* in how the information is gathered (i.e., the extent to which a method is flexible and the data obtained can be more freely produced by the participants).[7] Thus, some of the methods of data collection described above are less structured, while others are more structured (see Fig. 20.1, y-axis).

These different strategies and procedures of qualitative data collection both allow the researcher to gather data in the form of *languaged text* (compared to quantitative data collection methods, which allow data collection in the form of *numbers*; see Chap. 12), which will be then analyzed through specific data analysis procedures. The less structured the data collection, the more possibilities for data analysis. On the contrary, the more structured the data collection, the more confined the choice of data analysis method (e.g., if a highly structured open questionnaire produces one-sentence answers, an in-depth qualitative analysis will not be feasible).

20.5.1 Qualitative Observation

There are two main ways of producing textual data through observation in qualitative PPR (on the use of observation in qualitative outcome research, see Chap. 27). One prominent method consists of *audio* or *video recording therapy sessions*. These represent a specific case of social interaction in its natural occurrence, which may be of great interest to researchers. Audio and video recordings have become more popular during the last decade due also to technical developments. Video recordings often yield the richest data because they capture the spoken words as well as body language, tone, speed, etc. Some of the data-analytic methods focus on clinically meaningful processes, may utilize these tools. Nonetheless, many researchers prefer to obtain *verbatim transcripts* from the audio and video recordings according to transcription standards (e.g., Mergenthaler and Stinson 1992; Jefferson 2004) that allow transcription not only

[7] The distinction is usually made between *open-ended* (i.e., with low constraints) and *closed-ended* (i.e., with high constraints) modalities of data collection (see Barker et al. 2002).

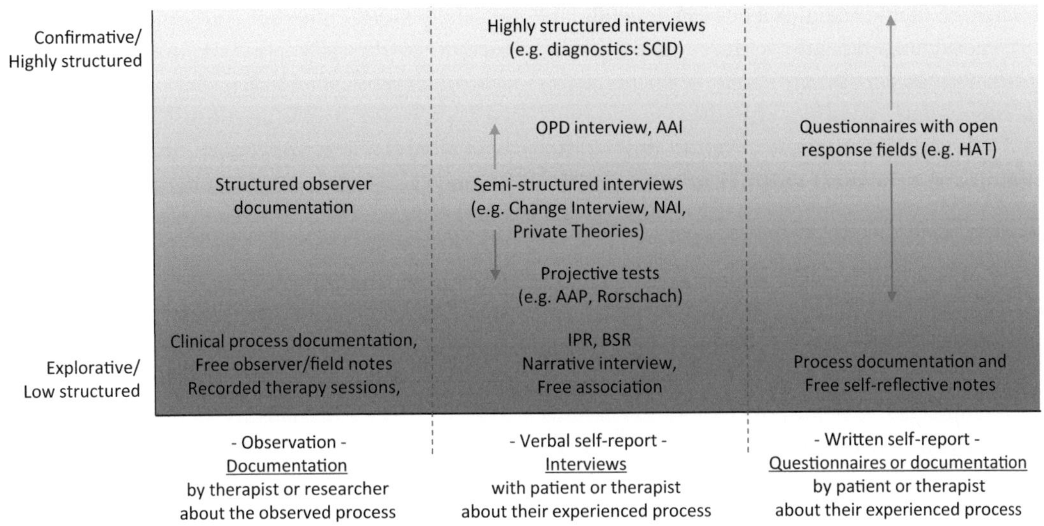

Fig. 20.1 Qualitative data collection methods map. *Arrows* indicate that the application of the relating methods can vary in a specific range. Methods mentioned in the map (from *top left* to *bottom right*): *SCID* Structured Clinical Interview for DSM-IV, *OPD* Operationalized Psychodynamic Diagnostics, *AAI* Adult Attachment Interview, *NAI* Narrative Assessment Interview, *AAP* Adult Attachment Pro- jective, *IPR* Interpersonal Process Recall, *BSR* Brief Structural Recall, *HAT* Helpful Aspects of Therapy

of linguistic but also of para- and extralinguistic speech features to different degrees. This method, although extremely time and energy consuming, may represent an advantage for researchers specifically interested in the in-depth analysis of the conversational structure of a patient-therapist talk but is also used to analyze clinically meaningful processes. Depending on the research interests, recordings may be produced of one, several, or all sessions of one or more treatments.

Audio and video recording psychotherapy sessions and their eventual verbatim transcriptions represent the least structured way of collecting languaged data. Other low structured strategies of qualitative observation exist, which are very similar to *field observation* in traditional ethnographic studies. This is the case, for example, when the researcher following an *open-ended* strategy takes *notes* or keeps *diaries* regarding different aspects of the therapeutic process (see Fig. 20.1, y-axis). This method represents a second, less widespread method of collecting data in PPR through qualitative observation (of naturally occurring contexts). When, as in most of these cases, the researcher is the therapist, this type of observation is a special case of *participant observation* (Barker et al. 2002; Flick et al. 2004), which is frequently used in narrative/clinical case studies (see Barker et al. 2002; Iwakabe and Gazzola 2009). Finally, many languaged documents reflecting the activity of the clinician as observer, such as medical termination reports in a psychiatric institution, are examples of data collected through more structured qualitative observation.[8] Data collected in this way are usually analyzed through content analysis and sometimes depict the subjective experiences of the therapist as a participant observer.

20.5.2 Qualitative Self-Reports

While in the natural sciences observation is the only way of collecting data about a phenomenon,

[8] When the researcher employs data previously collected by someone else for purposes other than those of the study in which the researcher is currently engaged (such as reports collected with diagnostic or documentary aims), these data are *secondary* (or *archival*) data. *Primary* data represents information collected for the first time by the researcher for that study.

in the human and social sciences in general, and in the psychotherapeutic sciences in particular, asking the subject directly about the phenomenon of interest is possible. In these *self-report* methods, the participant is asked to provide the information of interest to the researcher (Barker et al. 2002). The advantage of asking the participant about his/her inner experiences directly is that you will get accounts that might not have been explicit in the observation, for example, experiences in moments of silence and in general feelings and thoughts that are not expressed to the therapist and stay unspoken of on the recording. It should be thus noted that the difference between textual data collected by means of, respectively, qualitative observational and qualitative self-report methods is a difference of perspective: the perspective of the observer/researcher in the first case vs. the perspective of clients and/or therapists in the second case. *Qualitative* self-report methods are characterized by *open-ended* questions, which prompt the subject to provide a *languaged* answer about the investigated issue.[9] Depending on whether these questions are posed within a conversational context, we may distinguish between methods that produce *spoken* accounts (i.e., qualitative interviews) and methods that produce *written* accounts (i.e., qualitative questionnaires and other written accounts) (see Fig. 20.1, x-axis).

20.5.2.1 Qualitative Interviews

Qualitative interviews may vary by their degree of structuredness (Barker et al. 2002; Knox and Burkard 2009; Patton 1990; see Fig. 20.1, y-axis): the less structured the interview protocol used by the interviewer, the more *explorative* and *idiosyncratic* the process of data collection (as in the case, for example, where a researcher is *flexibly* interested in the *elaborate* exploration of a *few* issues), and, consequently, the more *articulated* and *in-depth* the collected subjective experiences.

The most unstructured and explorative method is free association. A more concrete but still explorative method is the *narrative interview* [Schütze (1983); see also McLeod (1997)] in which the interviewee is simply invited to narrate (i.e., to tell a story) the phenomenon of interest (see Fig. 20.1). The interview protocol consists of one opening question (e.g., "Tell me about moments of silence in your psychotherapy") and then allows the interviewee to structure the narration (see Kvale 1996). These methods not only allow content analysis but also a structural analysis of the given data, because of the way a participant decides to narrate his story in his very unique way. The researcher will not direct the participant and will not introduce a priori formulated themes.

At an intermediate level of structuredness are *semi-structured interviews*, which are among the most commonly used methods of data collection in qualitative PPR. The protocol is organized around a relatively small number of topics, which represent the main issues of interest to the researcher. For each topic, an open-ended question is prepared. Nonetheless, depending on the course taken during the interview, both the formulation and sequence of the questions may be changed in a flexible and creative way by the interviewer (Knox and Burkard 2009). The more topics you include in a protocol, the less articulated and in-depth the information collected. Consistent with the notion of qualitative research as bricolage (Denzin and Lincoln 2005; McLeod 2011), the researcher can tailor ad hoc interview protocols consistent with the specific project and research questions (e.g., Williams and Levitt 2007). Nonetheless, some researchers have proposed standardized semi-structured interviews to increase the comparability of results. A prototypical example is the *Change Interview* (Elliott et al. 2001), which includes eight questions exploring the client's subjective experience: (1) "how was being in therapy"; (2) "what has changed"; (3) "which were the causes of the changes (both inside and outside the therapy)"; (4) "what was helpful about the therapy"; (5) "what was hindering about the therapy"; (6) "what was difficult but OK"; (7) "what was missing from the treatment"; (8) "what has it

[9] On the contrary, *quantitative* self-report methods are characterized by *closed-ended* questions, whose answers are recorded on a scale, generating thus *numerical* data (see Chap. 12).

been like to be involved in this research"; and, as a final question, (9) "what are the suggestions for the therapy of the study." Although the Change Interview is usually considered a data collection instrument used in qualitative *outcome* research (see Chap. 27), because it explores not only client experiences about *what* changed but also *why* it might have changed, it is also a method of qualitative data collection for *process* research [for an example of a semi-structured interview that may be used for qualitative psychotherapy outcome research, see the *Narrative Assessment Interview* (Hardtke and Angus 2004; see Chap. 27)].

At the highest level of structuredness is the *structured qualitative interview*, which is characterized by a fixed set of questions that is usually much larger than a semi-structured interview. The questions are always posed in the same order by the interviewer. Moreover, although the formulation of the question may be open-ended, the answer is recorded by the interviewer in a closed-ended format. As stated by Knox and Burkard (2009), structured qualitative interviews "have the potential advantage of greater uniformity across respondents but inhibit the uncovering of participants' rich and unique experiences, especially those that lie outside the bounds of the interview questions themselves." This is likely one reason why this type of interview is not popular in psychotherapy process (and outcome) research, while they find a broader application in clinical psychology, especially for diagnostic purposes (e.g., the interview of the *Operationalized Psychodynamic Diagnosis* (OPD-2; OPD Task Force 2007) and the *Structured Clinical Interview* of the DSM-IV).

Let us recapitulate the three main aspects in learning how to do qualitative research. We said it needs knowledge about the methodology (especially in designing the research), knowledge in methods (especially in data collection and analysis), and the third aspect: the professional relationships which influence all levels in the study process. There is one more ingredient that we need to underline at this point—the choice of data collection method—that will have a huge influence on which method students will use: the student himself/herself. Using an explorative data collection method, such as the narrative interview, is accompanied with uncertainty and the necessity of a high level of flexibility during the interview. More anxious or inexperienced students will ask for more structure and more guidelines by their supervisor. Our experience as supervisors is that students need a good portion of support and training if they want to use open and explorative methods. Too many guidelines intended to be supportive will lead to a bad application of an explorative method. However, for some students it might be more fitting and appropriate to use structured methods that give them a sense of security. In the end, the quality of a good research project will be judged by how valid and reliable a student succeeded to collect and analyze the data. Without confidence and a good amount of fun for the respective student, the results will be impaired. This means the choice of method also needs to be considered as a personal choice, thus supervisors need to take into consideration which methods fit to the student, to avoid under- or overestimating their specific talents; and this, again, refers to the importance of the interpersonal level that makes a good qualitative researcher: the relationship between supervisor and student.

20.5.2.2 Qualitative Questionnaires and Other Invited Written Accounts

While qualitative interviews are used to generate spoken accounts from participants by asking questions within a conversational context, a second subset of self-report methods may be used to ask the participants to produce *written* accounts within a *non-conversational* context.

The first way to do this is through *qualitative questionnaires*. A questionnaire consists of "a structured series of written questions, which usually generate written responses" (Barker et al. 2002, p. 97). In qualitative questionnaires, questions are *open-ended*, so that the respondent may provide *languaged* answers about the issue of interest to the researcher.[10] The number of questions may vary depending on the researcher's interests and focus and range from a couple (*semi-structured* qualitative questionnaires) to several questions (*structured* qualitative questionnaires) (see Fig. 20.1, y-axis). Two observations should be made. First, the less structured and the more fill-in space on the sheet of paper participants have to answer, the more *explorative* and *idiosyncratic* the process of data collection gathering client or therapist subjective experiences in a more *articulated* and *in-depth* way. Second, qualitative questionnaires collect data that are less articulated and in-depth because the context of a questionnaire is non-conversational and no follow-up or clarification questions can be posed.

Process researchers usually develop ad hoc qualitative questionnaires depending on their research interests, although some standardized versions have been proposed (for the use of qualitative questionnaires in qualitative outcome research, see Chap. 27). This is the case, for example, with the *Helpful Aspects of Therapy (HAT) Form* (Elliott et al. 2001; Llewelyn et al. 1988), developed within the *event paradigm* of psychotherapy change process research (Elliott and Shapiro 1988a; Greenberg 1986; Rice and Greenberg 1984) to identify and explore change-enhancing (i.e., helpful) events within one or more therapy sessions. The most used version (see Elliott et al. 2001) includes seven questions administered to the client after one or more therapy session: (1) what was the most helpful for him/her during the considered session, (2) why it was considered helpful, (3) how helpful it was, (4) about the session in which the helpful event occurred, (5) about how long the session was, (6) the nature of any other eventually helpful events in the session (with a rating of its helpfulness), and (7) the nature of any hindering event that might have occurred within the session (with a rating of its hindrance).[11]

Beyond qualitative questionnaires, other forms of invited written accounts may be used to ask clients or therapists about their subjective experiences in therapy. For example, clients or therapists may be asked to take *extensive notes*, maintain *diaries*, or engage in *creative writing tasks* about the relevant treatment.

Qualitative questionnaires and other invited written accounts are not frequently used in qualitative PPR (with the former preferred to the latter). They represent valid alternatives to qualitative interviews, especially when collecting data from larger samples. Finally, the data collected through such methods are mostly analyzed by data analysis that focuses on the content in a structured way.

20.5.3 Tape-Assisted Recall

Another approach to collecting data about participant's subjective experiences in the process of psychotherapy is to use *tape-assisted recall methods*, also known as *Interpersonal Process Recall* [IPR; Elliott (1986), Elliott et al. (2001); also see the *Unstructured Recall* introduced to counseling and psychotherapy research by Rennie (1990)], which uses self-report methods combined with session tape recordings. This method overcomes the limitations of a retrospective *free* recall in which the subjects must rely upon their memories of what happened during one or more sessions of the treatment as in the traditional application of self-report methods. Instead, the researcher provides participants with *retrieval cues*, which facilitate a more valid and

[10] On the contrary, *quantitative* questionnaires are characterized by *closed-ended* questions in which the subject must mark an answer on a scale to generate *numerical* data (see Chap. 12).

[11] Questions (3), (6), and (7) are also answered on a Likert scale (1 = extremely hindering to 9 = extremely helpful). Thus, technically, the HAT form is a *mixed-method* questionnaire, that is, a specific method for data collection (self-report) where the information of interest is gathered both in a languaged and numerical format. Because most of the focus is on the information collected in a qualitative format, we included it in this chapter.

articulated recall of their subjective experiences about the session under investigation.

In IPR, "tapes of therapy sessions, or parts of sessions, are played back for the participant while the researcher assists in eliciting descriptions of the experiences and perceptions of particular conversational events" (Elliott et al. 2001, p. XXX). The researcher plays the segments of the tape that are of interest, stops, replays the segment of interest, and prompts the participant to talk about their experience (thoughts, intentions, emotions, etc.) in that moment of therapy as well as reflect upon them retrospectively. The participant is thereby encouraged to place himself/herself back in the conversational moment to avoid a solely abstract reevaluation of the episode and to distinguish between the "here and now" and the "there and then." This stimulates a more complex, articulated retrieval of his/her subjective experience of the episode (Elliott et al. 2001). IPR is thus a valuable method of linking reported subjective experiences to observed (inter)actions (Elliott et al. 2001).

A particular form of tape-assisted recall is the *Brief Structural Recall* (BSR; Elliott and Shapiro 1988b; Elliott et al. 2001), which was developed to collect data to be further analyzed by comprehensive process analysis (CPA; Elliott 1989; Elliott et al. 2001). The peculiarity of BSR is that the tape of the session is used in combination with the HAT to locate the event of interest more clearly. Instead of reviewing the entire session, the significant event is first identified through HAT and the researcher is then able to find this event on the tape. Then, a semi-structured qualitative interview is usually conducted with the participant. In its simplest version, this interview is conducted with the client and focuses on the *context of the event*, the *major processes involved*, and the *effects of these processes on the client*. In more elaborate and structured versions, the same domains are explored with the therapist, especially the within-session behavior, to obtain a detailed picture of the sequential interaction of the two during the sessions and the associated subjective experiences. For IPR, quantitative measures focusing on such domains may also be used to provide for the possibility of triangulation.

20.6 Data Analysis

20.6.1 Interpretation and Methodical Hermeneutics

Before we will go into the specific analysis methods in PPR, we will again approach this section with a methodological and historical framework. In empirical research, *data analysis* is generally defined as the process of elaborating previously collected data to answer the research question(s) posed by the investigator. In *qualitative* research, this elaboration uses *interpretative* processes governed by the principles of *methodical hermeneutics* (Rennie 2012) applied to *languaged* data (Polkinghorne 2005) (on the contrary, *quantitative* data analysis makes use of *mathematical* calculations based on *probabilistic* principles applied to *numerical* data; see Chaps. 12 and 13). Interpretation is defined as the process through which a subject (in our case, the qualitative researcher) *ascribes a meaning* to a string of text according to its *semantic*, *syntactic*, or *pragmatic* components. According to this definition, meaning is much broader than is conveyed exclusively by the *content* of a text; it involves *structural* and *contextual* aspects. Thus, ascribing meaning is a process of semantic, syntactic, and pragmatic *categorization* [i.e., to establish a relationship among the elements of the text and classes that share attributes at a semantic, syntactic, or pragmatic level (see Gambier et al. 1997)].

The *logical* and *procedural rules* governing how valid meanings can be ascribed to texts are provided by methodical hermeneutics, which is a theory and methodology of interpretation (Sandage et al. 2008; Seebohm 2004) that originated during the Greek Enlightenment and later spread through philology, textual criticism, and exegesis. In modern times, Schleiermacher (1768–1834) extended it beyond theological texts into other texts, and Dilthey (1833–1911) extended it beyond texts into human behavior and cultural products—thus paving the way to a conception of hermeneutics as the methodological foundation of the *human* sciences rather than the *natural* sciences (Sandage et al. 2008). Methodical hermeneutics should be distinguished from *philosophical* hermeneutics, which was initiated in modern times by Heidegger (1884–1976) and continued by others such as Gadamer (1900–2002), in that it is more concerned with the *existential implications* of considering humans interpretative beings (Sandage et al. 2008).

Rennie (2012) demonstrated that qualitative data analysis may be considered to be ruled by the principles of methodical hermeneutics through the following propositions: (a) Qualitative data analysis entails the application of the *hermeneutic circle* to texts about subjective experiences or (inter)actions according to which interpretation emerges from the reciprocal, cyclical, and spiral interaction among the *parts* and the *whole* of the text, the *investigator (pre)assumptions* (what he already knows), and the *characteristics of the text* (what can be found in the text). (b) The use of the hermeneutic circle implies a cycling among *education* [i.e., the initial clarification of the meaning of a text prior to logical analysis based on the analyst's embodied experience; Rennie and Fergus (2006; Suppe, 1999, p. 253)], *deduction* (i.e., the inferences of particular instances with reference to a general law or principle), *induction* (i.e., the inference of a general law from particular instances), and *abduction* (the inference to the best explanation from a single, often unexpected, instance) (see Chap. 6; see also Haig 2008; Salvatore and Valsiner 2010). (c) The *validity* (also called *credibility*;) of the interpretation of the text under examination is supported through *demonstrative rhetoric*, which consists of the investigator (s) persuasion through arguments grounded in the text, that is, by providing examples supporting the results of the performed analysis. (d) To enhance the demonstrative rhetoric used to support the validity of the analysis, *disclosed reflexivity* is used, which consists of the investigator making explicit the perspective(s) and assumptions that frame the analysis. Disclosed reflexivity is strictly interconnected with *bracketing*, that is, the temporary setting aside of these assumptions to avoid an (over)imposition of the researcher's meanings onto the research process (Fischer 2009). (The last two propositions are not always applicable to qualitative data analysis exhibiting a high degree of structuredness. In those cases, the validity of the analysis is supported by the calculation of quantitative indexes (e.g., inter-rater reliability; Gelo et al. 2012).

These four propositions are sustained by a *relativistic* ontology and *transactional* epistemology ascribed to the *constructivist-interpretivist* paradigm, which in turn provides a philosophical foundation for the *human* sciences (Gelo 2012; Polkinghorne 2005; Ponterotto 2005; see also Chap. 4). One major implication is that the human sciences involve a *double hermeneutic*, a subject-subject relationship (i.e., the investigator interpreting the interpretations of the subject being investigated).[12]

20.6.1.1 A Map of Methods

In the current landscape of qualitative PPR, many, sometimes very different, approaches exist to analyze data with these aims. In this chapter, we place some of the most relevant approaches on a *map* (see Fig. 20.2), which was inspired by our teaching. In our qualitative research methods courses, students often miss a pragmatic (and hence reductive) overview of methods to provide a basic orientation of the field. Inspired by an open discussion during the *42nd Annual Meeting of the Society for*

[12] The *natural* sciences are sustained by a *realist* ontology and *objectivistic* epistemology that can be attributed to the (post-)positivist paradigm. These are involved in a *single hermeneutic*, that is, a subject-object relationship (i.e., the investigator interpreting the objects being investigated).

Psychotherapy Research held in Bern in 2011,[13] we recognize that a pragmatic map cannot fully acknowledge all the existing approaches; however, it does simplify the complex range of qualitative data analysis just as a roadmap simplifies terrain by neglecting the full complexity of the land. We hope that our map is elaborate enough to account for the historically "big methods" as well as newer "patchwork methods." Our attempt to create this map is a qualitative project in itself.[14]

All existing different approaches to qualitative data analysis in PPR are concerned with the following: (1) a process of *segmentation* through which the text to be analyzed is divided into parts (segments) of various length (lines, meaning units, conversational turns, etc.) representing the units of analysis; (2) a process of *coding* consisting of sorting and categorizing the text through codes, where a code represents "a word or short phrase that symbolically assigns a summative, salient, essence-capturing, and/or evocative attribute for a portion of language-based [...] data" [Saldaña (2013, p. 3); for the concept of coding as essentially a process of categorization, see Patton (1990), Saldaña (2013)]. We will add a couple of remarks about the definition of "code" and "category" later.

Notwithstanding these very basic similarities, the existing approaches are quite different (and the differences may be analyzed) along two main dimensions: (1) *bottom-up vs. top-down* and (2) *content vs. structure*. Our map (see Fig. 20.2) describes the differences among the approaches to qualitative data analysis in PPR with reference to these two dimensions.

Bottom-up vs. top-down The *bottom-up* vs. *top-down* dimension (see y-axis of Fig. 20.2) refers to the general approach to text/data analysis.[15] *Bottom-up* approaches are *data* driven, that is, the coding process is driven by the investigated data, and the resulting categories *emerge* post hoc as products of the analysis. They are of an *inductive* and *abductive* nature (Lipscomb 2012; Reichertz 2004b; see also Chap. 6), reflexive, flexible, and communicative. Thus, they fully exploit the *discovery-oriented* potential of text analysis and are traditionally qualitative. The methods following such an approach may focus on the *content,*

[13] We thank Clara Hill, Denise Deffey, Bill Stiles, John McLeod, and all the participants for their important contributions.

[14] Based on our research experience and review of the literature (methodology and methods textbooks and empirical articles in select journals in psychotherapy research), we present a conceptualization of qualitative methods. In this sense, this chapter is a qualitative study, and we contextualize this study by disclosing our motivations for writing this chapter. The primary author, Kathrin Mörtl, has been engaged with qualitative methods for 11 years. She has been a lead investigator in ten related projects and accompanied many others as a second coder or auditor in her supervisory work with students. She has lectured about qualitative methods in Germany, Austria, Canada, and France and has conducted workshops on computer-assisted qualitative research as an official ATLAS.ti trainer for North America. Kathrin Mörtl and Omar C.G. Gelo met in Ulm, where they conducted different research projects in the Department of Psychosomatic Medicine and Psychotherapy. He has worked with quantitative text analyses on metaphors, developing a special interest for methodology and epistemology in the years following his PhD. He has supervised students in the application of various psychotherapy process and outcome research methods and has cooperated and published with various colleagues in the field that are interested in how methods are applied in psychotherapy research. The two have worked together for years and bridged the qualitative and quantitative shores in their specific and collaborative work. For both, their international cooperations have opened an understanding of "different qualitative cultures," which are reflected in the maps. Nevertheless, the conceptualization must be understood as product of a circumscribed research community (psychology, psychotherapy process, hermeneutics, academia, medical, and psychosomatic institutions, Europe and North America) and research era (between post-positivism and constructivism). Gaps between coordinates of the maps will occur naturally, are inevitable, and hopefully motivate the reader to think about these issues and become part of a reflective, informed research community.

[15] Lepper and Riding (2006) differentiate PPR into general theory testing (the coding approaches) and microtheory building (the discourse approaches) (p. 4). Our method map locates specific methods differently. For example, we neither equate discourse with theory building nor consider grounded theory to be a discourse strategy. The presented conceptualization is clearly distinct not least because Lepper and Riding (2006) include both quantitative and qualitative approaches in PPR.

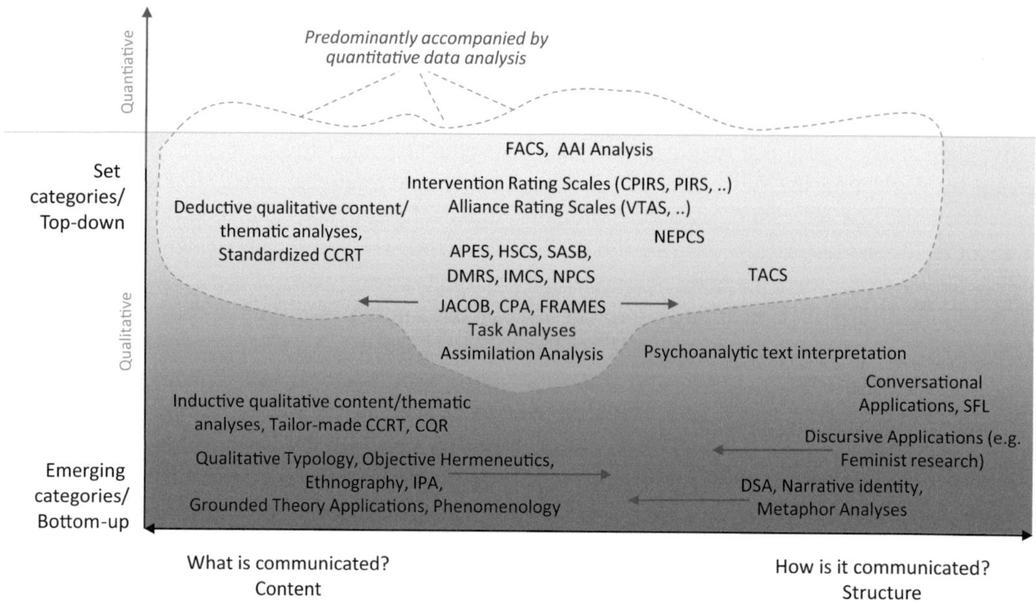

Fig. 20.2 Qualitative data analysis methods map. *Arrows* indicate that the application of the relating methods can vary in a specific range. Methods mentioned in the map are as follows (from *top left* to *bottom right*): *FACS* Facial Action Coding System, *AAI* Adult Attachment Interview Analysis, *CCRT* Core Conflictual Relationship Themes, *CPIRS* Comprehensive Psychotherapeutic Intervention Rating Scale, *PIRS* Psychodynamic Intervention Rating Scale, *VTAS* Vanderbilt Therapeutic Alliance Scale, *NEPCS* Narrative-Emotion Process Coding System, *TACS* Therapeutic Activity Coding System, *APES* Assimilation of Problematic Experiences Scale, *HSCS* Heidelberg Structural Change Scale, *SASB* Structural Analysis of Social Behavior, *DMRS* Defense Mechanism Rating Scale, *IMCS* Innovative Moments Coding System, *NPCS* Narrative Process Coding System, *JAKOB* JAKOB narrative analysis, *CPA* comprehensive process analysis, *FRAMES* fundamental, repetitive, and maladaptive emotion structures, *CQR* consensual qualitative research, *IPA* interpretative phenomenological analysis, *SFL* systemic functional linguistics, *DSA* dialogical sequence analysis

structure or both (see below) and are located at the bottom of our map.

The *top-down* approaches are *theory* driven, that is, the coding process is driven by the researcher's theoretical considerations prior to the analysis, and the categories employed during the analysis are defined a priori by the researcher and organized in a so-called category system. They are of a *deductive* nature, standardized, and rigid. They are thus often used within quantitative studies. The methods following such an approach may focus on the *content* or a combination of *content and structure* but rarely exclusively on the structure of a text (see below). They are located at the top of the map.

In the middle of the top-bottom axis of our map, we located methods that are mainly bottom-up but theory driven to some extent as well as methods that use either bottom-up or top-down techniques.

Content vs. structure The *content* vs. *structure* dimension (see x-axis of Fig. 20.2) relates to the aspect that the methods of text/data analysis address. Methods addressing the *content* depict *what* is communicated by focusing on the *semantic* aspects of the text under investigation. Applied to data collected through self-reports or session transcripts, they allow inferences about the *subjective experiences* of the participants (in the first case) or the *clinical processes* taking place during the treatment (in the second case). Methods focusing on content may be related to categories such as struggles with autonomy, fights with husbands, support of the therapist, fear, maladaptive emotion, and client struggles with guilt. Methods focusing on the content are located in the left part of our map.

On the contrary, methods addressing *structure* depict *how* things are communicated by focusing on the *syntactic* and *pragmatic* aspects of the investigated text. Mostly applied to session transcripts, they allow inferences about how the *conversational and communicative (inter)actions* of participants shape the therapeutic process. For this reason, such methods may be related to categories such as argumentative talk, avoidant response, fragmented story, rejecting therapist intervention, repair sequence, etc. Methods focusing on the structure are located to the right of the map.

Our map (see Fig. 20.2) displays some of the major approaches to qualitative data analysis used in PPR. In the following, we present a selection of these methods based on our knowledge and competences. To facilitate reader understanding, we connect our description of the method to a practical text example, which was analyzed using the presented methods. We sent a short text to representative researchers for each method to invite them to provide an example analysis for this chapter. The text is an episode taken from an original therapy session. However, it has been summarized and modified to provide a dense but comprehensible and manageable text segment. This is the 9th therapy session (of 19 sessions) with Sarah, a client treated throughout the York Depression Study I by a female therapist (Greenberg and Watson 1998). In the middle of this session, Sarah is talking about a man she is interested in whom she met a few months ago.

(. . .)
Therapist: So you get some mixed messages from this man, or you perceive them as mixed.
Sarah: Yeah. Oh it's (10 second pause). I guess one of the things was like when we were talking once about relationships, friendships, uh, he just, he goes, well, I am glad that we are just good friends. And I couldn't really, I didn't really want to comment on it because it was just like, what's going on here?
Therapist: You're just stunned, sort of like a slap in the face.
Sarah: Yeah, literally. It's almost like the same way as with my father.
Therapist: Somehow, I'm not completely; I'd like to understand better what feels like your father when these things happen?
Sarah: Um, like . . . I really . . . I really, well you know it's the same like here I'm trying to let him know like what I'm up to, like how I feel about things, and, like, he turns around like either ignores it or talks against it (sigh). I mean, I like this man; I would like to spend time, more time together . . ., and like, he literally undermines it because, I mean, now like after he has said this, there is no way on earth that I'm going to admit that I care.
(. . .)

Not all invited analysts could conduct the required analysis. In some other cases, this short text did not provide enough information.[16] Especially for some bottom-up methods, an analysis of a micro-segment is unfeasible due to the lack of contextual information. Hill's method of *consensual qualitative research* (CQR; see Chap. 23), for example, would require more than one therapy session to create specific domains that are compared as does Stiles' *assimilation analysis* (Stiles 2001; Stiles and Angus 2001; Stiles et al. 1990). Although this limits the selection of data-analytic methods presented in this chapter, we hope the examples underline our differentiation of the two dimensions described above. For a deeper understanding of the specific

[16] We thank the following researchers for responding to our invitations: Michael Buchholz (metaphor analysis), Philipp Mayring (qualitative content analysis); Brigitte Boothe (JAKOB); Xiaorong Zhou (CCRT); Emily Bryntwick and Tali Boritz (NPCS); Alessandra Vicari (AAP); David Rennie (grounded theory); Clara Hill and Sarah Knox (CQR); Michael Constantino (SASB); Georgia Lepper (conversation analysis); Fabiano Molinaro (CPIRS); Joerg Frommer and Gerald Poscheschnik (psychoanalytic text interpretation); Gabriele Lucius-Hoene (positioning analysis); Bill Stiles, Isabel Caro, Hugo Schielke, and Carol Humphreys (APES); and Paula Miceli (phenomenology).

approaches, we refer the reader to the appropriate handbooks and coding manuals.

20.6.2 Bottom-Up Approaches

Among bottom-up approaches, we distinguish between those that are strongly data driven and those that are theory driven.

20.6.2.1 Bottom-Up and Data-Driven: The BIG 4

Typical methods employing a bottom-up and strongly data-driven approach include *grounded theory*, *phenomenology*, *qualitative types*, and *objective hermeneutics*. The first three focus mainly on the content of the text under investigation, while the fourth may also consider some structural aspects. For this reason, they may be differently located at the bottom of our map (see Fig. 20.2).

20.6.2.1.1 Grounded Theory

Grounded theory (GT) has become a methodology (Mey and Mruck 2007; Dourdouma and Mörtl 2012) that includes different GT methods of analysis (see also Chap. 22). Still, these different methods share common ground: they start with a research question that aims to uncover the structure of a specific phenomenon, categories are created (emerge) throughout the text analysis, and the conceptual work yields results that go beyond pure description of contents. However, the idea of GT (as a methodology) has yielded different contemporary GT applications (methods). Due to a historical schism between Glaser and Strauss, there are rather different approaches. To describe the specific coding strategies common in all GT approaches, we cite Mey and Mruck (2007), who give a thourough summary of the common and separate voices of Glaser and Strauss:

> The basic idea of a grounded theory methodology—as outlined in the concept-indicator-model by Glaser (1978, p. 62) picked up by Strauss (1991, pp. 54)—is the following: based on the data about the phenomenon of interest (e.g., interview segments, protocols, documents of any type, but also, following Glaser's dictum 'all is data', statistics about a specific social events), a term/denomination (code) is assigned to specific incidents. Through this assignment, the data itself becomes a set of indicators that describe an implicit concept that is denominated by the code. Throughout the subsequent coding work and constant comparisons, codes are condensed to theoretically relevant concepts. These are condensed to categories that then lead to the formulation of a core category. This core category is connected to all the categories in ways that need to be defined. Thus, a relational network is established that in turn constitutes the (new substantive) theory. (p. 25[17])

Below we list some typical procedures in GT applications:

- *Identification of meaning units:* The researcher chooses text segments (quotations) that are relevant to the phenomenon. These meaning units vary in length (by project) but are usually a couple of sentences long (depending on the individual coding style of the researcher; this can take the form of line-by-line coding or coding entire pages of the material).
- *Open coding:* Labeling quotations by forming first codes[18] in the form of paraphrases that remain close to the text (low abstraction).
- *Memo-ing:* Writing memos (notes) is essential to GT. Memos can refer to quotes, categories, and conceptualizations and can be directed towards theoretical considerations.
- *Constant comparison:* New understanding emerges by constantly comparing existing codes and categories. Codes, categories and later concepts are created in comparison to one another. This is an essential method or attitude in interpreting the data.
- *Axial coding:* Connecting codes and possibly categories. This step might include a more theoretical procedure, including concepts and ideas that extend beyond the data. It is

[17] This segment was translated from German to English by Kathrin Mörtl.

[18] Codes were traditionally compared to categories in grounded theory: codes often resembled paraphrases of quotation that were low in abstraction, while categories implied interpretation and were usually more abstract. Nowadays, some authors avoid the term code and talk of first- and second-order categories (thus admitting that the creation of a label (coding) includes interpretation).

important not to force a foreign theory or network onto the material.

- *Selective coding:* In later steps of the analysis, specific categories that have been connected to each other become central. This leads to a more selective process that zooms into specific aspects of the material. It is important not to exclude important information that may emerge during the later phases of the analysis.
- *Conceptualization:* The term used to describe the final steps in analysis in which the formation of a concept can result in one grounded theory or a set of core categories.[19]

Analysis Using Grounded Theory (Conducted by Kathrin Mörtl, Sigmund Freud Private University Vienna)

The text segment taken from the Sarah case is defined as one meaning unit. If the therapy transcript was available as a whole, the meaning unit would likely be larger and there would be a set of meaning units. Because this is a transcript from a psychotherapy session, including an interaction between therapist and client, we include both perspectives in our analysis.

Memo 1: Including the therapist and client talk in our analysis means that we will interpret the segment as the client's experience even if the therapist introduced a thought and the client responded positively. For example, in Quotation 2 (see below), the therapist interprets what the client has said and offers a metaphor ("this must have felt like a slap in the face"). Sarah answers with "yes, literally." Therefore, the "slap in the face" can be categorized as her experience even when explicitly offered by the therapist. This understanding is based on the idea of therapy (and experience and experienced change process) as co-construction. This idea can be found in narrative theory. In psychoanalysis, one would argue that the therapist is noticing the client's experience and voicing it (making some possibly unconscious experience conscious through interpretation). This co-construction will serve as a basic principle of my analysis of the text. However, if the client does not notice an offer or answers affirmatively but does not elaborate, we will not include that as the client's experience. This specific method of analysis will require further discussion and complex text segments will need further memo-ing and reflection.

Quotation 1:

Therapist: So you get some mixed messages from this man, or you perceive them as mixed.

Sarah: Yeah. Oh it's (10 second pause). I guess one of the things was like when we were talking once about relationships, friendships, uh, he just, he goes, well, I am glad that we are just good friends. And I couldn't really; I didn't really want to comment on it because it was just like, what's going on here?

Therapist: You're just stunned, sort of like a slap in the face.

Sarah: Yeah, literally.

Assigned Open Codes:

- Mixed messages are confusing.
- Mixed messages disappoint/hurt and make her withdraw.

Quotation 2:

Sarah: It's almost like the same way as with my father.

Therapist: Somehow, I'm not completely; I'd like to understand better what feels like your father when these things happen?

Sarah: Uhm like . . . I really . . . I really, well you know it's the same like, here I'm

(continued)

[19] To offer an adequate differentiation between the later GT applications by Glaser on the one hand and Strauss and Corbin on the other hand, we refer to a comparison of coding procedures presented by Mey and Mruck (2007, p. 26ff). While Glaser (1978) differentiates between *grounded* coding (open coding and selective coding) and *theoretical* coding, Strauss and Corbin (1990) understand the techniques as interconnected, including open coding, axial coding, and selective coding. A more elaborate account on GT techniques and its developments was published by Dourdouma and Mörtl (2012).

trying to let him know like what I'm up to, like how I feel about things, and, like, he turns around like either ignores it or talks against it (sigh). I mean, I like this man; I would like to spend time, more time together ..., and like, he literally undermines it because, I mean, now like after he has said this, there is no way on earth that I'm going to admit that I care.

Assigned Open Codes:

- Experiences with men and father are similar/the same (disappointing).
- When she tries to open up to men she is being ignored or talked against.
- Men are undermining her wish to be close and trusting.
- His mixed messages (saying he wants to be friends) are rejections.
- Being rejected makes her withdraw completely—also from her own feelings/wishes(!).

Axial Coding: The open codes are sequential and one open code or experience that leads or causes the next experience.

Memo 2: This text is a nice example of a narrative sequence that exemplifies how Sarah makes sense of her reaction based on retrospectively conceptualizing the situation—a situation that led to her complete withdrawal from a man she was interested in. I have to note that I am thinking about narrative theory a lot while reading this text—I was reading and preparing classes about narrative theory and therapy, so this clearly influences me right now. I will need to reflect on this once categories are created or more text material is available for comparison. Additionally, the idea of sequences reminds me of the sequential models formulated in task analysis (and my preoccupation with this also needs to be bracketed - excluded - from further conceptualization).

Formulated Categories (Higher Abstraction) and Subcategories

- <u>Receiving a mixed message is painful.</u>
  - (Property or subcategory): Mixed messages are confusing.
  - Mixed messages disappoint/hurt and make her withdraw.
- <u>No attempt to clarify when confused.</u>
  - Mixed messages disappoint/hurt and make her withdraw.
  - Being rejected makes her withdraw completely—also from her own feelings/wishes(!).
- <u>Opening up to men (father and men) is risky.</u>
  - When she tries to open up to men, she is being ignored or talked against.
  - Men are undermining her wish to be close and trusting.
  - His mixed messages (saying he wants to be friends) are rejections.
  - Experiences with men and father are similar/the same (disappointing).
- <u>Withdrawing from men and own feelings when ignored.</u>
  - Mixed messages disappoint/hurt and make her withdraw.
  - Being rejected makes her withdraw completely—also from her own feelings/wishes(!).

Memo 3: I need to note that Sarah is talking about a *fear* of rejection. Even when the man described their relationship as "just good friends," Sarah never clarified what he meant by being friends; neither did she disclose her own interest to him—out of fear to be rejected. Who knows what could have happened if she would have. It

(continued)

is important here to understand this meaning unit as anticipated rejection (triggered by the early experience with the father—see Quotation 2). (I will try to not include a psychoanalytic perspective of projection, although it is in my mind, being psychoanalytically informed myself). The word "trigger" might be capturing this phenomenon of current experience and past experience well, also expressing the sequential order of events here. Also this fear is completely hindering her from the (risky but possible) experience of being loved and being close to someone or also loving someone and actively stepping close to someone herself. This must be compared to other meaning units though (constant comparative method) right now we only talk about this very short text segment.

Selective Coding: There is no selective coding step because there is not enough data to yield a selective focus during the analysis process. Condensing the categories, axial coding, and memos, the following grounded theory is formulated.

Formulation of Core Category/ Grounded Theory:

"When Sarah's fear of rejection is triggered by men, she withdraws from relationships and her own wish to be close."

The procedures described above are inherent in all applications of GT but are not exclusive to GT. To the contrary, these techniques can be found in all bottom-up approaches described in the previous section and are located at the very bottom of our map. Moreover, GT is clearly concerned with the content (see Fig. 20.2). The data analysis work (reading through the texts, understanding, forming first categories, creating categories of higher order, understanding and acknowledging the hermeneutic circle, and establishing a conceptualization of the phenomenon) in GT, phenomenology, objective hermeneutics, and qualitative typology is very similar. Hence, the following approaches are based on the principles described in GT and will not be repeated. While the principles are similar, the language is different at times. For example, while some methods talk about phenomena, others talk about interactions.[20] We will complete this thought at the end of the section.

20.6.2.1.2 Phenomenological Analysis

Giorgi (1997, Giorgi and Giorgi 2003) describes the empirical *descriptive phenomenological psychological method*, which is based on the philosophical considerations of Husserl (1970/1910) and Merleau-Ponty (1962/1945). The following description of phenomenology is based on a book chapter by Giorgi and Giorgi (2003), which provides an exemplary guide to phenomenological analysis. In phenomenology, the researcher tries to grasp the essence of a phenomenon "from the point of view of the behaving organism" (Giorgi and Giorgi 2003, p. 243 quoting Snygg 1941). To do so, the researcher follows certain steps in the methodical application of phenomenology:

- *Read for a sense of the whole:* The researcher must provide an overview of all the material. Using the attitude of phenomenological reduction, the researcher will grasp the basic sense of the phenomenon in this first step.
- *Establishing meaning units:* Here, the researcher creates units every time he/she experiences a novel meaning while reading the text.
- *Transformation of meaning units into psychologically sensitive expressions:* Every day expressions in the text are transformed into psychologically informed expressions. The balance between staying with the described experience and using abstract psychological

[20] One might think that a translation of terms in different methods might be sensible. However, this is not as easy as it may sound. Simple translation would be simplistic because it could not incorporate some basic methodological differences that are reflected by the use of specific language. This cannot be discussed in depth in this chapter. For more reading, we refer the reader to Roth (2005).

terms is crucial during this phase. This is achieved by maintaining an attitude of free imaginative variation.

- *Determination of the structure:* At this stage, the researcher establishes the structure of the phenomenon by describing it with its essential aspects, excluding nonessential aspects found in the analysis.
- *Poststructural analysis:* Based on the empirical information of the structure of the phenomenon, the researcher must consider the complexity of the phenomenon under investigation, take a step back, review the material as a whole, and then form careful generalizations about the phenomenon.[21]

As with GT, phenomenology is clearly concerned with the content of the text.

20.6.2.1.3 Qualitative Types

Based on Max Weber's ideal types, Kluge (1999, 2000) presents the *Empirically Grounded Construction of Types and Typologies*. In her 2000 article, Kluge provides a short overview of the different applications that use qualitative types (e.g., ideal types, empirical types, structure types, and prototypes) by referring to experts in this field (Gerhardt 1991; Haupert 1991). Based on the content, typologies group specific aspects that are as similar as possible into one type (low internal heterogeneity) and that differ from another type as strongly as possible (high external heterogeneity) (in this way, types are similar to categories). Although not highly diffused in qualitative process research, qualitative types can often, but not exclusively, be observed when researchers describe different types of biographies (Buchholz et al. 2008; Kuehnlein 1999). Hug and Poscheschnik (2010) introduce it as follows (p. 154): "Researchers interested in biographies might see that some people tell their life stories as if they themselves had no impact on their life at all. Life happens to them. Others believe that they have total control over their lives in the decisions they make. This produces two types: victim of one's fate and architect of one's fortune." Kluge (2000) described four steps of the analysis:

- *Development of relevant analysis dimensions:* Systematic analysis of attributes/properties as described in the GT approach by Strauss and Corbin (1990).
- *Grouping cases and analysis of empirical regularities:* By carefully examining all possible combinations of attributes within cases, the researcher forms groups of cases. Similar cases that are grouped must sufficiently differ from other groups of cases.
- *Analysis of meaningful relationships and type construction:* Based on the groups of cases, the researcher will now form groups of typical attributes that present meaningful relationships among similar cases. Types are constructed and are defined by the presence and absence of specific attributes.
- *Characterization of constructed types:* Each type must be defined by their constituting attributes.

In successive analysis, more cases are assigned to types, which will be modified by integration or disassociation of emerging attributes. In the end, cases are assigned to a

[21] Another type of analysis that is explicitly based on the phenomenological method developed by Giorgi is *interpretative phenomenological analysis* (IPA). This method is rather popular in the UK, and described by Smith (1997, Smith and Osborn 2008). Just as Giorgi's phenomenology, IPA tries to grasp the essence of a phenomenon from the perspective of the participants (Smith and Osborn 2008, p. 54) but acknowledges the interpretive act immanent in the analysis and thus introduces the perspective of the researcher to the phenomenon. This method seems similar to GT in its application. Procedures for IPA include [according to Smith and Osborn (2008, p. 66ff)] reading of the text, free textual analysis by forming meaning units, and commenting on units. Comments can be summaries or paraphrases. In later stages, the comments become more abstract as they are compared and modified with each new analyzed case. Comments will be linked in terms of sequences, differences, contradictions, etc. The comments are transformed into concise phrases to capture the essence of the text (also called themes). Examining this practice (and the introduction of interpretation to Giorgi's phenomenology), IPA might share a broader methodological base with GT than with phenomenology, but we leave this judgment to the informed reader and leaders in each method.

specific type although the individual case never shares all aspects of just one type [hence Weber's *ideal types* (Weber 1972)].

20.6.2.1.4 Objective Hermeneutics

With reference to the left-right axis of our map (see Fig. 20.2), *objective hermeneutics* (Oevermann et al. 1979) is located at the bottom middle between content and structure, which suggests an approach that focuses on both what is communicated and how something is communicated. The aim is to reconstruct the objective meaning of an interaction dismissing the subjective intention the actor might have had (Reichertz 2004a, p. 290). Like GT, objective hermeneutics has evolved as a method. In the beginning, the primary objectives of analysis were textual protocols of everyday interaction, but the method is currently applied to paintings, architecture, and criminal activity (Reichertz 2004a, p. 290). While classically material is recorded in its original occurrence, contemporary projects also involve interviews. Unlike the many variations of GT, objective hermeneutics has preserved some of its classic procedures, such as the single-case design (one influencing factor here might be that objective hermeneutics is applied by a rather exclusive and consistent group of researchers, especially in German-speaking countries). The typical procedures include three phases that are summarized by Lamnek (2010):

- *Fine analysis:* The context and type of a specific interaction are coded, focusing on the content: what happens before the interaction, paraphrasing the interaction, and explicating the intent, motives, and function of an interaction. Explication of general correlations among these aspects and comparison with further cases is another important aspect.
- *Sequential analysis:* The interactions are analyzed systematically following the specific sequential occurrence. The structure of narration (how and when is it said during the interaction) is central.
- *Structural analysis:* The focus here is how the specific sequential contents are presented in the interactions, e.g., biographical events over time, what happened in the beginning, and what happened at the end (how and when it occurred in the subjective narration, not the interaction).

The specific techniques for the three phases are described similarly or even based on GT techniques: open coding, creation of meaning units, higher aggregated concepts that bind together partial meaning units, and interpretation being falsified, modified, and extended (Reichertz 2004a, p. 291f). However, the next steps in analysis soon switch to the structure of narration (the "how" was something said), thus being allocated in the middle of our content-structure axis. According to Oevermann et al. (1979), the analysis cannot be conducted by one researcher but requires a research team. The researchers control and inspire each other, and through intense discussions and arguments, they will uncover the objective meaning structures of a social event.

The actual analytical work in each method of the bottom-up BIG 4 is similar: reading the text and providing an interpretive framework for the emergence of categories that are later conceptualized. What clearly differentiates the methods is an epistemological criterion. Without diving into issues of methodology and philosophy of science (see Chap. 4; Gelo 2012; Ponterotto 2005; Slife 2004), we must address the issue of epistemology briefly. How do researchers using a specific method think about knowledge? What do they know about the phenomenon at the end of their analysis? Did they present *one possible* conceptualization or the *only true* conceptualization? A grounded theoretician will say that the same analysis on the same phenomenon undertaken by a different person might yield a different grounded theory. This would not mean that these two different theories are contradictory or invalid but that two theories have illuminated the phenomenon better than one. Objective hermeneutics as performed by a group of researcher may capture the objective reality [or more accurately, the objective meaning possibilities; Lamnek (2010)] of an interaction. All irrelevant aspects have been excluded through group discussions, which also excluded any subjective blind-spot interpretations provided by a single researcher. The results of a phenomenological analysis resemble the essence of the phenomenon. According to this view, the results will be similar if two researchers conduct an analysis of the same phenomenon. In a qualitative typology, the results do not claim to describe or explain the specific case but to elicit abstract but typical structural aspects among many cases. The types are empirically constructed; however, the individual, naturally occurring case never equals an ideal type but represents an assortment of aspects from different types. The reader might identify positivist (we uncovered the true meaning), post-positivist (we approximated the true meaning), and constructivist (we uncovered one structural meaning but there is no empirical and individual true meaning) inclinations that are more or less inherent to the BIG 4 methods (see Ponterotto 2005).

20.6.2.2 Bottom-Up, Partially Theory-Driven Approaches

Some approaches are bottom-up and are more (but not exclusively) theory driven than the BIG 4. These approaches are characterized by the fact that in the process of creating categories from the analysis, the researcher is influenced by a specific theoretical framework. There are several approaches of this type, which are used in PPR. In this chapter, we focus on *metaphor analysis*, *JAKOB narrative analysis*, *discourse analysis*, and *conversation analysis*. For other relevant methods of analysis that can be described by this type, such as psychoanalytic text interpretation (Leithäuser and Volmerg 1988), *comprehensive process analysis* (Elliot 1984), *assimilation analysis* (Stiles and Angus 2001), and *task analysis* (Greenberg 1992), we refer the reader to the existing literature (please note that in these three examples, especially in the last two, the qualitative conceptualization may be intertwined with quantitative aspects).

20.6.2.2.1 Metaphor Analysis and JAKOB Narrative Analysis

These methods focus on both the content (what is communicated) and structure (how something is communicated) of the text under investigation. They are located in the middle of the x-axis of our map (see Fig. 20.2). In *metaphor analysis* (Buchholz 1993, 2003), researchers examine the specific use of metaphors that resemble creative cognitive accomplishments. In *JAKOB narrative analysis* (Boothe et al. 2010; Boothe 2000), the investigator is interested in how the description of the narrated self changes over time. Both approaches are clearly influenced by a constituting theory based on which they will analyze the material. While metaphor analysis uses a set of theoretical assumptions borrowed from linguistic and cognitive theory (Lakoff and Johnson 1980), JAKOB narrative analysis is grounded in a psychoanalytic framework.[22] However, the circumscribed theoretical frame of reference can still be the starting point for a hermeneutic analysis where the categories emerge as result of the analysis itself. The two following example analyses begin with a brief theoretical depiction made by the analyst. Let us begin with metaphor analysis.

Metaphor Analysis (Conducted and written by Michael B. Buchholz, University of Hildesheim and International Psychoanalytic University Berlin)

It is an interesting adventure to analyze such a short piece of a therapeutic dialogue when qualitative researchers normally use more.

My method is the analysis of metaphor. A few words about the method. A metaphor is not only a linguistic thing. George Lakoff and Mark Johnson have convinced me that metaphor is an object of interest for

(continued)

[22] JAKOB (acronym that stands for "actions and objects") analysis has evolved since 1989 and produced different applications. While the present example is rather intuitive and inductive, another form of JAKOB is highly structured and standardized: the autoJAKOB is conducted via a computer program that operates with set dictionaries. The automatically yielded results are statistically analyzed; therefore, autoJAKOB is a method consistent with the top-down coding paradigm.

the cognitive sciences. A metaphor belongs to the cognitive domain because by the use of metaphor, we structure how we experience the world. This shift from linguistics to cognition is highly important because we can learn that people have embodied experiences, which are termed by other concepts. Metaphors have a source domain and a target domain. In the classical example, "Achilles is a lion," Achilles is the target domain. The target is conceptualized in terms of another concept that is embodied in the sense of having a sensory or imaginative experience. In the more complex conceptual metaphor, argument is war, the argument is the target domain that is conceptualized by the experience of war. Thus, we can understand why people speak of defeating or fighting an enemy while engaged in a scientific argument. Arguments often are understood as war. The small word "as" achieves a very important meaning because it often designates this conceptualization of a target in terms of a source domain, which stems from embodied experience.

With this very brief information, we turn to the dialogue. The first metaphor is used by the therapist: "mixed messages." The source domain is the experience and/or imagination of some "mixed" substance, which is transferred to the target domain: messages. Sarah begins to analyze this condensed version of her experience with "this man." She adds that she could not "comment on it," which is a next metaphor showing the beginning of a process of self-exploration why she herself could not have her own standing. The therapist offers the next metaphor: this man's messages might have been experienced by Sarah "like a slap in the face." This is a strong embodied metaphor responded to by Sarah with "literally," which we commonly use when, strictly speaking, the correct formulation is "metaphorically." She had not been beaten. She experienced the man's messages "like" a slap in the face.

The whole construction of this embodied experience is then expanded to a more complex metaphor, which is not explicitly formulated. One could describe it like "the experience with this man (target domain) is the same 'as' the experience I had with my father (embodied source domain)." The therapist pushes her a little bit by uttering that she is not "completely" informed. She does not have the full picture of this metaphorical equation that brings "man" and "father" together in a way that makes this experience analyzable as transference—the ancient Greek meaning of *metaphorein* is the same as "transference" which means literally "bringing something from one place to another place." This is what a metaphor does. The therapist's push brings Sarah to explore this metaphorical relationship between "man" and "father" a little bit more, and so she can begin to tell scenarios with these two important figures. So, she can bring before her mind one scenario (with the "man") and the other scenario (with her father) to compare both experiences. This active comparison—which must be considered a basic cognitive activity—brings her to create a new metaphor of being "undermined." The source domain allows one to conclude that she imagines something breaks down like a hill or a building being "undermined." Having concluded this imagining, she is on the way to developing her own standing.

This analysis shows a process of differentiation—to differentiate between father and man—and a process of integration in developing a new standing for both experiences. The integrative process is accompanied by a new metaphor. This analysis further shows how much of a

(continued)

short therapeutic dialogue is structured by the use of metaphors. However, what cannot be decided due to the paucity of material is the degree of adaption to the therapist's experiences or other variables that influence the process. Additional material would enable differentiation of a genuine therapeutic process from a more superficial self-adaptation to another person's expectations.

Let us turn to JAKOB narrative analysis [for more details about narrative approaches, see Labov and Waletzky (1997), McLeod (1997) Joshua].

JAKOB Narrative Analysis (Conducted and written by Brigitte Boothe, University of Zuerich)

When patients tell a story during psychotherapy sessions, it is both mutual interaction between patient and therapist and a presentation of personal experience. The patient calls up and recreates a biographic occurrence and places it before a listener, enacting it verbally in the perspective of wish fulfillment and anxiety coping. JAKOB narrative analysis, situated in the field of psychoanalytical and narrative analytical research, is an encoding-supported qualitative instrument for systematic reconstruction of verbal everyday narratives in the context of psychotherapeutic processes.

The goals are as follows:

(1) Reconstruction of the narrative dynamics of a patient's narrative (according to the following dimensions: reenactment, stage direction, subdivision of segments, dramaturgical coding, social integration, and rules of the narrative)
(2) Formulation of psychodynamic hypotheses (according to the following dimensions: wish/anxiety/defense and conflict dynamics). The unit of analysis is a patient's narrative, which is defined as a self-contained verbal account with a beginning, middle, and end, in transcript material from therapy sessions. The method combines two levels: a first level of lexical analysis of the story organization and its communicative function *(narrative dynamics)* and a second level in which the narrative is understood as psychodynamic compromise formation between wish and anxiety themes and defense mechanisms and is stated as a conflict *(conflict dynamics).*

Narratives in the JAKOB analysis are understood as episodic courses of action that are fixed in space and time and construct a progression with start, story development, and outcome. The persons providing the accounts are a type of stage director setting up the scene with figures (characters), props, and backdrops and stage their own actions and the actions of the other figures. In the role of storyteller, the patients perform a scene and present themselves as actors in this scene—that is, as a narrating ego or ego figures. For the analysis, the narrative text is subdivided into individual segments (simple sentences or subject/predicate combinations) as seen in the example narrative. We label the segments of the narrative phases *start* (SD), *development* (ED), or *outcome* (EG). The *starting conditions* are the segments that initiate the dramaturgical development in the narrative and introduce the figures, actions, and backdrops. These terms are used for determining the rules of the narrative.

The narrative episode's **starting conditions** (SD segments 2–3) are:

"one of the things was like
we were talking once about relationships, friendships, uh."

The segments of **story development** (ED segments 4–6) take the dramatic events further:

"he just, he goes well,

(continued)

I am glad
that we are just good friends."

Then, the action sequence comes to an **episodic ending** (outcome, EG segments 7–9):

"And I couldn't really; I didn't really want to comment on it
because it was just like,
what's goin on here?"

The episode starts (segments 2 and 3) with the ego figure and the man in conversation. The theme of the talk is friendship and relationship. Before the story begins, the reader is oriented towards Sarah's emotional interest in the male protagonist.

Special attention to the *starting conditions* of a story reveals expectations for the best and worst end of the story in the narrator's horizon. Expectancies are of high importance for the narrator's interpretation and evaluation of the situation. The best end of "just good friends" would be the transformation of the communicative theme (relationship) into interactive reality (ego and alter in love). The worst end of "just good friends" is total communicative failure and refusal of the ego figure by the male protagonist.

In the *center* of story developments (segments 4–6), a direct citation of the male protagonist is placed: *I am glad/that we are just good friends.* Just good friends is in the given context a formulation of restriction and demarcation.

The episodic *ending* (outcome, segments 7–9) presents the ego figure remaining without open response, not willing to answer with an open response; she reacts astonished: *what's going on here?*

In the beginning of the story, a dyad is presented; a "we" is in dialogue. The development of the story presents the male protagonist as sole actor, decisive and determining. The story ends with an agency-reduced ego figure leaving the dialogical space. Being confronted with the male protagonist's *just friends* declaration, the ego figure withdraws in silence.

The male protagonist's demarcation and refusal of intimacy is evaluated in the following passages. First the therapist, in identification and sympathy with the narrator, offers a dramatic evaluative outcome formulation: *you're just stunned, sort of like a slap in the face.* He construes the male protagonist using the metaphor of physical attack as humiliating offender; so, the male protagonist's declaration of friendly distance turns into violating, morally disqualified behavior. For Sarah, the path is prepared to articulate herself as violated, ignored, and refused, and indeed, encouraged by the therapist, she expands the refusal experience of the actual episode to her childhood experience with a father who did not want to "know like what I'm up to, like how I feel about things."

All the same, Sarah is not "just stunned, sort like a slap in the face." She is not unable to comment but "didn't really *want* to comment." She *decides* not "to admit that I care." In the refusal narrative, she enacts dependence and demandingness, but she is not completely victimized.

The male protagonist is narratively construed as the ambivalent, loved, and hated object, which plays a central role in the depressive conflict.

Let us take a second look at these two examples. While the researchers do analyze the content of the material, they prominantly consider the structure of narration too: consider the structure of narration. Buchholz notes that the therapist is pushing, and Sarah reacts in an active production of a new metaphor. Boothe notes that Sarah is encouraged by the therapist. These structural aspects extend beyond the analysis of the content and help the researchers understand and conceptualize the analyzed text. At the same time the presented analysis is data driven (understanding emerges from the text) as well as analyzed in a specific theoretical framework that has an influence on how this understanding is conceptualized later.

Another group of partly theory-driven, bottom-up approaches zooms into the structure of narration (how something is communicated). The two primary methods focusing on the structure of a text are *conversational analysis* and *discourse analysis*, which are placed on the right side of our map (see Fig. 20.2). Poscheschnik (2010) differentiates them from content methods as follows: "In comparison to other [content] analysis methods that focus on the thoughts and experiences of the individuals, conversational and discourse analyses focus on the exchange between individuals. Thus, they are directed towards social processes" (p. 158[23]). Rennie (2012) further describes these methods as *discursive* (contrary to methods focusing on the content, which are described as *experiential*), which are "applied to the study of pragmatics or function of language-use" to investigate the "assumptions people use implicitly when interacting" (p. 385).

20.6.2.2.2 Discourse Analysis

There are different forms of *discourse analysis*, but most practices are associated with the critical discourse of Foucault [see overview article by Diaz-Bone et al. (2007)]. In discourse analysis, researchers are interested in understanding controversial exchanges of groups of people who are embedded in a specific societal context. Social perspectives, opinions, prejudices, and media representation are typical research interests. Prominent discourse research includes studies of feminism, gender, identity, and minorities. In psychotherapy research, discourse analyses are often found when "the institution" takes a key position in the research question. Especially in forensic psychotherapy and psychiatry, the institution plays a major role [see the forensic work on group psychotherapy of sex offenders in jail by Buchholz et al. (2008)]. However, discourse analyses are not prominent in contemporary PPR. Additionally, discourse analytic applications are manifold, and published projects often lack an exact description of specific coding techniques because coding strategies are emerging (Poscheschnik 2010, p. 160). Because of this, discourse analysis is located at the very bottom of our map (see Fig. 20.2). This method is not feasible with a short summary, and we refer the interested reader to the extensive theoretical literature in this field (e.g., Parker 1998; Potter and Wetherell 1987).

20.6.2.2.3 Conversation Analysis

Conversational analyses (CA) have been increasingly applied by psychotherapy researchers in the last decade (see Madill et al. 2001; Peräkylä et al. 2008; Lepper 1967). In its original form (Sacks 1972), CA focused on specific actions in everyday situations [close to the practices of ethnomethodology elaborated by Garfinkel (1967)] and analyzed text segments in detail by considering each sentence and each turn in a speech act. The transcription of a CA must be very specific with regard to paraverbal aspects of language [e.g., guidelines by Jefferson (2004)]: pauses, intonation, and overlapping speech are just some indicators that are necessary for CA. In the field of psychotherapy and counseling, several authors have begun to investigate the clinical process through CA [e.g., see Chaps. 24 and 25; Muntigl et al. 2012; Muntigl and Horvath 2014; for a comprehensive overview of exemplary CA psychotherapy process and outcome studies, see Peräkylä et al. (2008)]. Typical CA categories describe question-answer behaviors (turn by turn) between two or more participants. Applied to psychotherapy, this means that the researcher examines therapist interventions and client respones (and vice versa). As Peräkylä et al. (2008, p. 13) summarize, "with the help of qualitative analysis of numerous instances of

[23] Translated from German into English by the first author, Kathrin Mörtl.

such actions, conversation analysts seek to explicate in detail how these actions are performed and responded to: what type of words and syntactic structures are involved in them, what type of presuppositions about the participants are created through them, and how the participants align or misalign while producing them." Categories are usually created throughout the coding procedure (emerging) but follow a specific theoretical guideline for language and social interactions. CA methods, hence, can be found in the middle of our y-axis, a bit higher than the discourse analytic methods described above. Typical conversational features considered during CA include turn taking, sequence organization, repair, word selection, action formation (see Chap. 24), attitudinal stance, and affiliation (Muntigl et al. 2012; Muntigl and Horvath 2014). These CA categories are relevant for the investigation of interpersonal processes occurring within the sessions. More specifically, typical CA categories could be labeled: accepting or rejecting a therapist's intervention, client's resistance, therapist's reformulation, transference-interpretation, and relational ruptures and resolutions. CA is still on the right side of our map but a bit higher than discourse analysis (see Fig. 20.2).

20.6.2.3 Bottom-Up and/or Top-Down Approaches

While the above methods clearly are bottom-up approaches, some methods can be applied according to either a bottom-up *or* top-down approach (this means that each of these methods exists as a bottom-up and a top-down approach). In this section, we present *Qualitative Content Analysis* and *Core Conflictual Relationship Themes.*

20.6.2.3.1 Qualitative Content Analysis

Qualitative Content Analysis (QCA; Elo and Kyngäs 2008; Mayring 2000) is a foundational method in qualitative data analysis focusing on the content of a text. Because of this focus, we direct the reader to the left side of our map (see Fig. 20.2). In English literature, QCA is sometimes referred to as thematic analysis (Braun and Clarke 2006), while the term "quantitative content analysis" or, simply, "content analysis" refers to QCA procedures that provide frequency counts and allow for statistical calculations. In this chapter, we consider QCA and thematic analysis as synonyms, but some differences may be observed, especially concerning the units of analysis (see Braun and Clarke 2006).

Inductive QCA Inductive QCA represent a *bottom-up* (i.e., *data*-driven) approach to the analysis of content. In this approach, the coding process usually takes place at *different levels of increasing abstraction.* The analysis of a rather *descriptive* nature begins at a *low level of abstraction* by focusing on *small segments* where codes (also called first-level codes) are developed to denote the meaning of the single segment. This is done through wording as close as possible to the text (analogous to open coding in GT). Then, the analysis of a more *interpretative* nature takes place at successively *higher levels of abstraction* where codes that are higher in abstraction (second level, third level, etc.) are progressively developed to denote commonalities among lower-level codes. (Although the analysis at lower levels of abstraction is considered rather descriptive, it already involves interpretation according to the hermeneutical nature of any text interpretation, as described before). This process (which is analogous to what GT analysts call *constant comparison*) stops when *saturation* is reached: when the emerged categories present informational redundancy (i.e., no new categories are generated by further cycles of analysis) (Lincoln and Guba 1985; Morse 1995; see also Strauss and Corbin 1990). Finally, the categories must be *conceptually linked* by articulating the relationship among them and demonstrating how this answers the research question(s) (analogous to what GT researchers call *axial coding*). The validity and credibility of the analysis is supported by *demonstrative rhetoric*, which may be achieved through peer review, group discussion, or supervised discussion.

The process of bottom-up QCA is not *linear* but *circular*. This means that to reach increasingly high levels of abstraction in coding, it is necessary to review the categories being identified and the text cyclically and reformulate them as necessary. Although this method is called inductive to stress the process of generating categories in a bottom-up, data-driven way, *abductive* processes also play a relevant role, especially in the revision of category (see Lipscomb 2012). Finally, the general principles governing this method may be considered to ground all the bottom-up approaches described above as well as the data-analytic procedures used in qualitative *meta-analysis* (see Timulak 2009). Because of the characteristics described above, inductive QCA is located at the very bottom of our map in the left corner (see Fig. 20.2).

In his book, *Qualitative Content Analysis*, Mayring (1990) described a model of this analysis (from selecting the material to differentiating the formulation of the research question and to defining the unit of analysis). Let us examine how Mayring analyzed the Sarah segment.

Analysis of an Inductive QCA (Conducted and written by Philipp Mayring, University of Klagenfurt)

Definition of Categories: Reactions of person S (emotional, cognitive, or behavioral) to the mentioned man

Level of Abstraction: Direct formulations (not only affirmations of interviewer questions) on a concrete level

C1: Unwillingness to discuss (comment) his reactions—line 4 and line 14

C2: Uncertainty about motives of his reaction—line 5

C3: Appraisal of ignorance of my feelings—line 12

C4: Thinking that he talks against me—line 12

C4: Appraisal of undermining my offer—line 13

A frequency analysis is possible (C1 is most frequent), but this makes sense only in large text corpora. In a second step, a theory-driven formulation of the main categories and frequency analysis is possible, e.g., emotion-centered categories and communication-centered categories.

A couple of observations may be made with regard to the example above. First, the author, before beginning with the analysis, explicitly defines what he is interested in and the level of abstraction at which the content addresses it. This helps the analyst maintain focus. Then, the author proceeds with the open coding of the text, which results in labels that allow him to refer to the content Sarah spoke by lines. Here, the author calls a category (C1, C2, etc.) what another author might call a first-level code. The inductive analysis stops here because of the brief text. With more textual material, it would have been possible to obtain more first-level codes, to group and label them according to similarities and differences, to revise them when necessary, and to identify conceptual relationships among the different identified categories. Moreover, it should be noted that Mayring explicitly suggests that a different, theory-driven approach might have been possible. This leads us to the second type of QCA.

Deductive QCA Deductive QCA represents the *top-down* (i.e., *theory*-driven) approach to the analysis of content (Elo and Kyngäs 2008; Mayring 2000). In this approach, the coding process consists of applying to the text under investigation a *previously* developed category system, which may be eventually organized at different levels of abstraction (i.e., containing main categories and subcategories). The theory allows the researcher to define the content of the categories that the text must be searched for and their abstraction level. Once developed, the category system is applied to *bigger* or *smaller segments* (depending on the research aims and the degree of resolution) to collect portions of texts, which may be ascribed to each category. The validity and credibility of the analysis is supported, as in bottom-up QCA, by *demonstrative rhetoric*. Another approach is *quantitative* and provides the frequency of occurrence of the different categories, which will be then analyzed statistically (the methods described below are a typical example of this approach). In this case, *quantitative indexes of agreement* among the different analysts must be calculated (e.g., interrater agreement). At the end of his analysis, Mayring suggests how the example might be first analyzed deductively and then subjected to frequency analysis.

Deductive QCA also entails a *circular* process, though more constrained than in inductive QCA. In fact, in this case, the text may require more than one reading, with the possibility of eventually modifying previous coding across different rounds of analysis. *Abductive* inference may help in this process. Moreover, the general principles governing deductive QCA may be considered to ground all top-down methods, which we will describe in the next section. Because of these characteristics, deductive QCA is located at the very top of our map in the left-upper corner (see Fig. 20.2).

These two approaches to QCA may be combined. For example, it is possible to *embed* an inductive QCA within a main, dominant deductive QCA as in the inductive articulation of a deductively obtained set of categories. In this case, after having deductively coded the text with regard to some a priori defined categories, we might decide to inductively articulate the content of each of these categories based on the text that has been previously coded to them. Another possibility is to apply each of the two variants in *sequence*. For example, we might first use inductive QCA to develop a category system, which might be then used for deductive QCA in other studies or on related material of the same study.

20.6.2.3.2 Core Conflictual Relationship Themes

The *Core Conflictual Relationship Themes* (CCRT) approach is an example of how the general principles governing both deductive and inductive QCA may be implemented to analyze a clinically relevant concept. In fact, the CCRT method is deeply grounded in the psychodynamic concept of *transference*, but it can be applied to any *relationship episode* (RE) and observed in therapy sessions of all therapy schools, as well as interviews, novels, poems, movie dialogues, etc. Within the context of PPR, a RE is defined as "a part of a session that is a relatively discrete episode of explicit narration about relationships with others or with the self" (Luborsky 1998, p. 16). To be applied, CCRT requires the following: (1) the *segmentation* of the text into REs, (2) the identification of the *components* of the RE, and (3) the *coding* of the identified REs with regard to the relational properties of the patient-therapist interaction. Some classical and recent developments exist, which differ with regard to 2 and 3. In the classical CCRT formulation (Luborsky 1998), within a RE, it is possible to identify the following components: a subject who expresses a *wish* (W, e.g., "I want to..."), a *response of the other* (RO, "The other does..."), and a *response of the self* (RS, "I do..."). Once these components have been identified within the different REs, each must be coded through a *standardized* category system (Crits-Christoph and Demorest 1988; Barber et al. 1998), which includes 96 categories. Of these, 35 are specific to W and further organized into 8 clusters (which include wishes "to be independent and have individuality," "to hurt and control others," "to be controlled and hurt," "to withdraw," "to be close," "to be loved and understood," "to feel good," and "to achieve"); 30 are specific to RO and further organized into 8 clusters (according to which the others are viewed as "strong and independent," "controlling," "upset," "bad," "rejecting," "helpful," "liking others," and "understanding"); and 31 are specific to RS and further organized into 8 clusters (according to which the subject feels "open and helpful," "unreceptive to others," "respected," "in opposition to others," "self-controlled and confident," "helpless," "disappointed," and "anxious or ashamed"). The coding may occur at the level of the single categories or general clusters. A second way to apply a CCRT analysis is the *tailor-made* method based on the inductive creation of W, RO, and RS categories (hence tailor-made). In this case, after having identified the REs and considered them with regard to their components, the researcher must formulate a code that adequately describes the content of the components of that RE. This is a clear example of applying the CCRT according to a bottom-up approach, contrary to the top-down approach followed when applying the standardized category system. For this reason, the standardized CCRT is placed on the upper-left corner of our map, while the tailor-made application on the left side but a bit below (see Fig. 20.2). Finally, some researchers combine the approaches and first apply the tailor-made method and then translate tailor-made categories into standard categories.

A more recent development is the CCRT-LU (Albani et al. 2008; Pokorny 2014; see www.ccrt-lu.org), which differs from the classical approach in the composition of the RE; the Ws are further divided into *wishes of the other* (WO) and *wishes of the self* (WS). Moreover, each wish (WS and WO) and response (RO and RS) is further differentiated into the following categories:

WOO	Wish of the other directed towards himself/herself
WOS	Wish of the other directed towards the Self
WSO	Wish of the self directed towards the other
WSS	Wish of the self directed towards himself/herself
ROO	Response of the other to himself/herself
ROS	Response of the other to the self
RSO	Response of the self to the other
RSS	Response of the self to himself/herself

Second, a different category system is offered, which produces 120 categories that are valid for every component of the RE; these 120 categories are then organized into 30 clusters (see Albani et al. (2008) and www.ccrt-lu.org for more details).

The exemplary analysis of our Sarah text below includes both tailor-made and standardized applications of the CCRT-LU.

Analysis Using the CCRT-LU Method (Conducted by Xiaorong Zhou, Ulm University)

Relationship	Component	Text	Tailor-made category	Standardized category	Keyword
RE1 *Object:* that man	WSO	I guess one of the things was like when we were talking once about relationships, friendships	Talk about relationships, friendships	Being curious, interested, active, motivated, open; being motivated	Being open
	ROS	He goes well	He talked as what I have wished	Explaining, communicating, having a talk, expressing, convincing	Communicating
	ROS	"I am glad that we are just good friends"	I am glad	Letting oneself go, being spontaneous, developing freely, being happy, feeling well, enjoying, having fun	Feeling happy
	ROS	"I am glad that we are just good friends"	We are just good friends	Dominating, asserting, repressing, degrading, subjugating, disadvantaging, controlling, testing someone, being strict	Rejecting
	RSO	And I couldn't really; I didn't really want to comment on it	I couldn't and didn't want to comment on it	Being angry, being enraged, being frustrated by something	Being frustrated by something
	RSS	It was just like, what's going on here?	Doubting about her own perception	Being passive, doubting, persisting, stagnating, worsening	Doubting
	RSS	It was just like, what's going on here?	Feeling stunned	Being shocked, being horrified, feeling caught in the act	Being shocked
RE2 *Object:* father	ROS	It's almost like the same way as with my father	My father also make me stunned	Being shocked, being horrified, feeling caught in the act	Being shocked
	WSO	I'm trying to let him know like what I'm up to, like how I feel about things and, like	I wish my father could know me	Being close, intimate, accepting; providing for	Being close
	ROS	He turns around like either ignores it	He ignores it	Unnerving, disheartening, devaluating, being disinterested, ignoring	Ignoring
	ROS	Or talks against it (sigh)	He talks against it	Opposing, competing, being stubborn, disputing	Opposing
	RSO	I mean, I like this man	I like this man	Liking; being liked, likeable; having a friendship; understanding one another	Liking
	WSO	I would like to spend time, more time together	I want to spend more time together	Letting oneself go; being spontaneous, happy; developing freely; feeling well; enjoying; having fun	Enjoying
	ROS	He literally undermines it	He undermines it	Being insensitive, destructive, unreasonable, uncontrolled; having no understanding	Being destructive
	RSO	I mean, now like after he has said this, there is no way on earth that I'm going to admit that I care	There's no way on earth that I'm going to admit that I care	Being distrustful	Being distrustful

This type of CCRT-LU application would usually be further analyzed quantitatively using statistical strategies to test specific hypotheses (e.g., changing specific categories over the course of therapy, pre-post treatment, in relation to a specific relationship, comparison among diagnostic groups or good vs. poor outcomes, etc.). However, a qualitative conceptualization (e.g., types of wish-response in anorexic clients) is conceivable. Considering this idea, the testing of hypothesis, we transition to the methods that are exclusively top-down approaches.

20.6.3 Top-Down Approaches

The methods we describe in this final section represent the instantiation of a specific type of deductive QCA in which the researcher, after having coded the text into different a priori categories, uses statistical tools to answer the research question. For this reason, these methods combine aspects of traditionally qualitative (the coding process itself) and quantitative (the transformation in frequencies and use of statistics) research [see Gelo et al. (2012) and Lamnek (2010) as presented in the introduction]. The core component that justifies their inclusion in a qualitative method map is that hermeneutic interpretive practices must be conducted for the deductive coding required by these methods; however, the fact that the results of the coding process are transformed into frequency counts also places these methods in the domain of quantitative research.

More than in any other described section in this chapter, we are faced with a number of specific methods each providing its own coding manual characterized by rather strict rules for the coding process, assessment of validity, and assessment of reliability in terms of inter-rater reliability. Examples of these methods include the *Core Conflictual Relationship Themes* (standard categories) (Luborsky 1998), the *Structural Analysis of Social Behavior* (SASB, Benjamin 1974), the *Vanderbilt Therapeutic Alliance Scale* (VTAS; Hartley and Strupp 1983), the *Defense Mechanism Rating Scale* (DMRS; Perry 1990), the *Psychodynamic Intervention Rating Scale* (PIRS; Milbrath et al. 1999), the *Metacognition Assessment Scale* (MAS; Semerari et al. 2003), the *Narrative Process Coding System* (NPCS; Angus et al. 1999), the *Assimilation of Problematic Experiences Scale* (APES; Stiles 2001), the *Innovative Moments Coding System* (IMCS; Gonçalves et al. 2011), the *Therapeutic Activity Coding System* (TACS; Krause et al. 2009), and many others [actually, almost any of the *observational methods* typically applied to transcripts within *quantitative* PPR may belong to this group of methods; see Gelo et al. (2012) for a discussion].

Because of these characteristics, these methods are located at the top of our map (see Fig. 20.2). Some of them clearly focus on the text *content* (e.g., standardized CCRT), being thus located on the upper-left part of the figure. Other methods may eventually take more into account also structural aspects of the text (e.g., SASB, MAS, VTAS, PIRS, IMCS, NPCS, APES, NEPCS, TACS), and can thus be found more in the upper-middle and upper-right part of the figure. Coding is usually done on a *nominal* scale, and the text is assessed for either the presence or absence of the category under scrutiny, which usually results in mutually exclusive coding (e.g., CCRT, IMCS, TACS, NPCS, DMRS) or an *ordinal* scale that ranks categories by intensity on a Likert scale (e.g., APES, VTAS, PIRS).

In some cases, such as the CCRT or the APES, the interpretive practices connected to the top-down coding do not necessarily serve the production of a dataset that is further analyzed statistically [when APES is used within a more general qualitative approach, it is called *assimilation analysis* (see Stiles and Angus 2001)]. This is an interesting example of the fact top-down methods can yield results that are either "quantified" or further "qualified.

In the remaining pages of this section, we focus on three methods: *Therapeutic Activity Coding System*, *Narrative Process Coding*

System, and a variant, the *Narrative-Emotion Process Coding System*.

20.6.3.1 TACS

The Therapeutic Activity Coding System (TACS; Krause et al. 2009) was developed to analyze the verbal activity of therapists and clients during clinically relevant episodes within the therapeutic process. The TACS represents a particular case in which a conversational analysis can be applied with a top-down category system approach. Therefore, it is located at the top right corner of our map (top-down approach focusing on the text structure with some inclusion of content). Their category system differentiates among following aspects that are coded (explicitly) qualitatively for each single turn and segment while a coding-score sheet is created. The results are usually analyzed statistically:

- *Basic forms*: Agreement, assertion, denial, question, and direction
- *Intention*: Exploring, attuning, and resignifying
- *Technique*: Justification, self-disclosure, confrontation, advice, imagery, information, interpretation, narration, labeling, paradox, reflection, reinforcement, summary, and role-playing
- *Content/domain*: Actions, ideas, and affect
- *Content/reference*: Self, present other, third party, therapeutic relationship, relationship with third party, and neutral

The first two aspects (basic forms and intention) focus on the structure, the last two (content/domain and content/reference) focus on the content, while the third aspect (technique) focuses on both.

Let us see what a TACS coding procedure looks like based on our Sarah segment. By providing this top-down approach, we hope to provide a sufficient snapshot of conversational aspects that may be applied according to a top-down approach or in combination with more traditional content-related aspects. The coding sheet is presented only for the first part of Sarah's text segment to limit the length of the chapter.

Analysis Using the TACS (Conducted and written by Marianne Krause, Pontificia Universidad de Chile)

The following considerations must be kept in mind when coding with TACS (for more details see the manual at www.psychotherapyandchange.org): (A) Texts are coded by two independent coders. (B) Each turn or segment should be coded considering the context of the conversation. Therefore, before analyzing a therapeutic interaction, the text to be coded must be read entirely. Likewise, to code the first turns of the episode, the context of what has been said in previous turns should be kept in mind. (C) The usual unit for coding with TACS is the speaking turn, except when we find two or more different basic forms and/or communicative intentions in one speaking turn. In this case, it will be divided in as many segments as needed. In the example, this is the case of most of the speaking turns. Techniques, domain, and reference are not used to fragment speaking turns. (D) If a segment is linguistically incomplete, only the basic form is coded (see, e.g., speaking turn 2, segments 1 and 2). If it is not understandable, it is not coded. (E) Some segments have no specific communicational technique to be coded (e.g., segments 1 and 2 of speaking turn 2).

As we can see in Table 20.1, the most used basic form in this therapeutic exchange is *assertion*. Only in one segment (turn 5, segment 2) does the therapist ask a *question* and only in two segments (turn 2, segment 1 and turn 4, segment 1) does the client *agree* with the therapist's

(continued)

Table 20.1 The episode coded with TACS (first part of the segment)

Turn	Segment	Participant	Verbalization	Basic form	Intention	Technique	Domain	Reference
1	1	Therapist	So you get some mixed messages from this man	Assertion	Attuning	Reflection	Affect	Present other (client)
1	2	Therapist	Or you perceive them as mixed	Assertion	Exploring	Labeling	Ideas	Present other
2	1	Sarah	Yeah	Agreement	–	–	–	–
2	2	Sarah	Oh it's (10-second pause)	Assertion	–	–	–	–
2	3	Sarah	I guess one of the things was like when we were talking once about relationships, friendships, uh, he just, he goes, well, I am glad that we are just good friends	Assertion	Exploring	Narration	Actions	Relation with a third party
2	4	Sarah	And I couldn't really; I didn't really want to comment on it because it was just like, what's going on here?	Assertion	Exploring	Justification	Affect	Self
3	1	Therapist	You're just stunned, sort of like a slap in the face	Assertion	Attuning	Reflection	Affect	Present other
4	1	Sarah	Yeah, literally	Agreement	–	–	–	–
4	2	Sarah	It's almost like the same way as with my father	Assertion	Resignifying	Interpretation	Ideas	Relation with a third party
5	1	Therapist	Somehow, I'm not completely; I'd like to understand better	Assertion	Attuning	Self-disclosure	Ideas	First person (therap.)
5	2	Therapist	What feels like your father when these things happen?	Question	Exploring	–	Affect	Neutral

statement. The basic form *question* is only used by the therapist, while *agreement* is only used by the client.

On the level of communicative intentions, there is more diversity in this episode. *Exploring*, which is slightly more present than the other forms of communicative intention, is present when the therapist asks for more information and when the client provides more information about her relationship with the man she is interested in. In between this sequence of *explorative* verbalizations, the therapist *attunes* (speaking turns 1, 3, 5, and 6), reacting to the emotional content Sarah is communicating and using the technique *reflection* (turns 1 and 3), for feeding back to the understanding of her emotions, or *self-disclosing*, when the therapist shows her surprise and lack of understanding after the client's *self-interpretation* (turn 5). The client also talks with the communicative intention *attuning* when she explains her feelings towards the man to the

(continued)

therapist (segment 6), trying to *justify* how these relate to her actions. The communicative intention *resignifying* is introduced by the client, together with a *self-interpretation* as technique, when she establishes the association she perceives of her experience with the man and her previous relational experiences with her father (turn 4, segment 2). She seems to be constructing a new meaning (at least for the therapist it seems to be new) by associating meanings that correspond to two different contexts in her life. Later, in segment 6, she explores these meanings by explaining them to the therapist.

When coded with the fourth dimension of the TACS, the domain of communicative contents, this episode appears balanced among *ideas*, *affect*, and *actions*. The client and therapist talk about the actions involved in the client's relationship with a man, her feelings towards him, her understanding (*ideas*) of the event, and how this relates to previous experiences.

We can observe that the dimension reference is also characterized by diversity. The client talks about herself (*first person*) as well as about her *relation with a third party* (the man she is emotionally involved with and her father). In segment 6, she focuses completely on the other person's behavior. The therapist's verbalizations—as it is usual in therapy—focus mostly on the *present other*, the client. Only once, when the client's communication surprises the therapist, she shifts to herself, using the *first person* to inform the client about her astonishment. Finally, the *neutral* reference is used twice, when therapist and client step back (by using the terms *what* and *it* in the last segment of turn 5 and the first segment of turn 6) to examine the new association that the client has established.

Usually a more elaborate single-case conceptualization would follow these first steps, but given the short text example and the lack of comparison to other text segments, this is as much as the TACS analysis can demonstrate.

After the coding procedure presented above, TACS researchers usually conceptualize how the protagonists communicate and what that means in terms of the psychotherapeutic progress over time (e.g., changes in conversational practice in good outcome cases, etc.). This might be supported by frequency tables and comparisons of occurrences. The qualitative conceptualization of results yielded by standardized, a priori category systems is not often discussed but is very much possible and must be acknowledged in our method map.

20.6.3.2 The NPCS and NEPCS

The *Narrative Process Coding System* (Angus et al. 1999, 2012) and the newly developed *Narrative and Emotion Process Coding System* [manual in process; see relating publication by Boritz et al. (2011)] are two other examples of methods not usually considered qualitative because the results are usually conceptualized statistically. They focus both on the content and structure of the text, but contrary to the TACS, this focus is more on the former than on the latter. Moreover, a first stage of the analysis involves bottom-up procedures (despite the presence of this inductive part, these methods are located in the purely top-down approaches because the inductive procedure has a role for the segment identification and denomination, while the categories addressed during the main analysis are defined a priori). Therefore, both are found at the top of our method map but below and to the left of the TACS (see Fig. 20.2).

The *Narrative Process Coding System* (NPCS; Angus et al. 1999; Angus et al. 2012) includes the analysis of the following perspectives: the narrated *topics* (content), the relationship focus (content) and narrative *process modes* (content and structure). Topic segments are similar to the meaning units in grounded theory or domains in consensual qualitative research (for the latter, see Chap. 23). A topic is (1) a description or overview of a specific content area or (2) a detailed elaboration of different facets of a specific content area (Angus et al. 2012). The text analyst organizes the therapy transcript into topic segments that are at least four lines long. Usually, as shown in previous research, the segments consist of 30 complete sentences (ranging from 10 to 133; Angus et al. 2012). Each topic segment is then inductively captured in a topic category and deductively coded for a relationship focus (e.g., self with father, self with mother, boyfriend, men in general, or self).

According to the narrative theory implied in the NPCS, stories can be narrated in three different narrative process modes: *external*, *internal*, or *reflexive*. These three mode categories are set and clearly defined. Mode categories can be applied to text segments that are at least four lines long, and they can comprise a topic segment or change inside of a topic segment. Attention is directed towards mode shifts. The following definitions are taken out of the NPCS manual [see also the related publication by Angus et al. (1999)]:

(1) External: When the individual provides a description of an event that (1) is a general overview of an event or autobiographical memory narrative, (2) highlights a specific incident or event (past or present), or (3) provides information about external events.
(2) Internal: When the individual provides a descriptive elaboration of experienced emotions or bodily felt sensations or feelings, the narrative sequence is coded as internal. It is a description of how one feels in relation to one's self and others.
(3) Reflexive: The individual focuses on the reflexive or interpretive analysis of event descriptions or descriptions of subjective experiences. The individual attempts to understand his/her own feelings regarding self, others, or events.

The *Narrative-Emotion Process Coding System* (NEPCS) was developed by Boritz et al. (2011) and builds upon the NPCS while introducing a completely new set of categories that focus on the type of narration. The system is currently under development but so far consists of the following categories:

(1) The same old story (characterized by stuckness in old patterns)
(2) The empty story (narration with low/missing expressed emotion)
(3) The unstoried emotion (expression of emotion without verbal narrative presentation)
(4) The competing plotlines (two competing stories/interpretations of an event that facilitate confusion)
(5) The fragmented story (fragmented, unclear, hard to understand story)
(6) Abstract story (vague and over-generalized story)
(7) Discovery story (a new understanding or experience is introduced)

Let us now turn to the NPCS and NEPCS analysis of the Sarah segment.

Analysis Using NPCS and NEPCS (Conducted and written by Tali Boritz, York University, Toronto)

(1) NPCS

Topic: Receives mixed messaged from a man and feels rejected

Relationship Focus: Self and man (father)

Narrative Mode

Reflexive: The whole text segment is coded as reflexive as Sarah and her therapist try to make meaning of the experienced situation. The peak of the reflexive is the metaphor (which often points to a reflexive mode) when the therapist and Sarah understand the experienced event as a "slap in the face" (co-constructed reflexive meaning making). Sarah interprets her behavior and links it to past experiences with her

(continued)

father, which is also an indicator of the reflexive mode. In line 3, she starts a short external narrative describing what she and the man talked about ("when we were talking once about relationships, friendships, uh, he just, he goes, well, I am glad that we are just good friends. And I couldn't really; I didn't really want to comment on it because it was just like, what's going on here?"). This external narrative is too short to be coded, however (three lines).

(2) NEPCS

The NEPCS is usually conducted as a minute-by-minute video-coding tool. Without the video, it is very hard to code this. Nonverbal aspects such as tone, gesture, and nature of pausing cannot be determined through a transcript but can be important when differentiating fragmented from abstract and abstract from discovery stories. For the purpose of illustration, however, the following three NEPCS codes were assigned to the segment:

Types of Narration

Fragmented Story (Lines 1–6): Sarah describes a fragmented, unclear, or hard to understand narrative during which she appears to be struggling to understand and articulate an experience, as indicated by the following defined coding rules:

(1) The narrative lacks clear beginning, middle, and end.
(2) The situational/relational context is only partially elaborated.
(3) The fragmented description of subjective experience (internal state) of protagonists and antagonists.
(4) Pausing and/or disrupted speech as client attempts to articulate an internal experience.

Discovery Story (Lines 7–9): (A short flicker of this is found in the middle.) There is an important linkage between the current relationship with the man and the past relationship with her father; however, she does not stay with the story, which makes it too short to code and thus part of the fragmented story. In the minute-by-minute coding with the video file, this part could be coded more precisely.

Abstract Story (Lines 10–14): Sarah's emotional state and narrative expression is presented in a generalized or vague manner. The client may talk about his or her own feelings or self-relevant ideas but with little or no evidence of exploration or discovery. The content of the story holds together loosely as indicated by the following defined coding rules:

(1) Narrative incoherence. Lack of depth in reflection or examination of one's thoughts, feelings, and behaviors.
(2) The content is self-description that is superficial, abstract, generalized, or intellectualized. Little reference is made to the speaker's feelings or internal perspective. The segment may include the ideas, attitudes, opinions or moral judgments, wishes, preferences, aspirations, or capacities of the speaker from an external or peripheral perspective.
(3) Emotion is depersonalized. If the client is emotionally aroused, it is evident from his/her manner not from her words. If the client mentions her feelings, she treats them abstractly, impersonally, as objects.

The first part of the NPCS (the categorization of topics) is an inductive content analysis. The NEPCS reminds us of conversation analysis techniques that capture the method of narration (how is something communicated? abstract? fragmented?). Then, aspects of the content are considered with aspects of the structure (is the narration internal, external, or reflexive?). Hence, there are specific steps in both methods that are clearly qualitative. However, when we examine actual NPCS and NEPCS projects, we can see that the results (as shown in the example above) are further conceptualized through sophisticated statistical analysis. The researchers are usually not interested in formulating a qualitative conceptualization of one or more single cases. Quite contrary, the coding systems are used to encode considerable amounts of data (e.g., six complete short-term therapy cases, which consist of approximately 60 sessions or approximately 1,400 pages of text material, preferably more). In the presentation of the results, the text becomes less important than the numbers and statistical indices (as in all methods included in this section). In fact, the discussion focuses on the interpretation of statistical values (e.g., significantly more internal-reflexive shifts in good outcome clients or flexibility in expressed story types predicts good outcomes, etc.). This is why the NPCS and NEPCS (with the other methods of this section) are often labeled as quantitative. However, it is possible that a researcher would further analyze the coded results of the NPCS and/or NEPCS in terms of qualitative typology of narrative modes across sessions, thus offering a qualitative conceptualization that would pursue the initial qualitative coding.

20.7 Quality Criteria

After we have mapped these various qualitative analysis methods in PPR, we will now turn to one last important aspect in conducting qualitaitve research that researchers need to consider science, *quality criteria* are the principles or standards with regard to which we may evaluate the quality and trustworthiness of the research process. Over the last decades, qualitative researchers have acknowledged the need for emancipation from quality criteria borrowed from quantitative research and pushed forward more appropriate criteria (e.g., Altheide and Johnson 1994; Elliott et al. 1999; Kvale 1996; Lincoln and Guba 1985; Morrow 2005; Packer and Addison 1989; Rennie 2012; Seale 1999; Stiles 1993; Williams and Morrow 2009). These criteria, though elaborated at a general level in psychology and related social sciences, may apply to the field of qualitative psychotherapy process research as well. For example, Rennie (2012) stated that *demonstrative rhetoric* (i.e., the ability to persuade through arguments grounded in text examples) and *disclosed reflexivity* (i.e., the ability to make explicit the assumptions grounding the study) are two essential aspects of good qualitative research.

Stiles (1993) distinguished between quality criteria addressing the (1) *trustworthiness of observations and data* and (2) *trustworthiness of the interpretations or conclusions drawn from the data* (which resemble the concepts of reliability and validity, respectively). The first includes the researcher's disclosure of his/her orientation and assumptions, internal processes, sociocultural context in which the research takes place, intensive engagement with the data, iterative cycling between interpretation and data, use of examples to ground interpretations, and description. The second includes triangulation, inner coherence of interpretation, uncovering, participant feedback, fostering change in participants as well as the researchers, and consensus among researchers. More recently, Elliott et al. (1999) developed a set of seven guidelines specific to qualitative research: (1) owning one's perspective, (2) situating the sample, (3) grounding in examples, (4) providing credibility checks, (5) coherence, (6) accomplishing general vs. specific research tasks, and (7) resonating with readers. Morrow (2005) provides the following criteria: (1) social validity, (2) subjectivity and reflexivity, (3) adequacy of data, and (4) adequacy of interpretation. Finally, Williams and Morrow (2009) recently suggested the following criteria: (1) integrity of data, (2) balance between participant meaning and researcher interpretation, and (3) clear communication and application of the findings.

Lincoln and Guba presented their position on quality criteria in their excellent outline of quality criteria in qualitative research (Lincoln and Guba 1985; see also Seale 1999) and suggested a translation of terms from conventional quantitative inquiry into naturalistic qualitative inquiry (see Morrow 2005) for a discussion on how different paradigmatic underpinnings of qualitative research (post-positivism, constructivist-interpretivist, and postmodern/critical/ideological) may sustain different sets of quality criteria. We present these quality criteria with regard to the main questions to which they refer.

How can qualitative researchers accomplish the following:

(1) Convince that their analyses *really* capture the phenomenon (traditionally referred to as *internal validity* in quantitative research, translated to *credibility* in qualitative research)
(2) Be certain their results are transferable to other subjects and contexts outside their sample and research situation (traditionally referred to as *generalizability* or *external validity*, translated to *transferability*)
(3) Assure that the *same* study design investigating the same subjects yields the same results (traditionally referred to as *replicability* or *reliability*, translated to *dependability*)
(4) Demonstrate that their results are not a *singular isolated* product of their own perspectives and motivations (traditionally referred to as *objectivity*, translated to *confirmability*)

In terms of (1) *credibility*, Lincoln and Guba (1985) advise researchers to check their results with the participants and, if necessary, adjust some interpretations [e.g., clients may be asked to rate their resonance with specific clusters on a 7-point Likert scale; see Williams and Levitt (2007)]. Bracketing, that is, the researcher's self-reflexive disclosure of his/her assumptions and ability to set them aside temporarily during the research process, is another way to increase the credibility of a qualitative study (Fischer 2009). In terms of (2) *transferability*, researchers must provide a rich description of results to convince the reader that results may be applied to other subjects and contexts. This is a rather careful statement by Mayring (1990), who understands Lincoln and Guba (1985) in the context of their famous claim: the only generalization is that there is no generalization. Mayring claims that generalizability (as part of transferability) is allowed and makes sense if the researchers (a) generalize results within the same context (e.g., institutions, countries, therapy approach, etc.), (b) extend their sample to other cases and compare the results, and (c) use time series within single cases and generalize as typical patterns (e.g., intervention-reaction series). (3) *Dependability* is achieved when researchers document the strategy of the analysis and the decisions made during the data analysis process and make the conceptualization of their categories transparent. For example, in grounded theory, this crucial step in the research process is called memo-ing.

The fourth issue, (4) *confirmability*, is the most controversially discussed topic in qualitative research. As anticipated, confirmability addresses the classical issue of reliability and the question of whether qualitative researchers need proof that their results are not arbitrary but can withstand statistical reliability measurements. Elliott et al. (1999) presented publishing guidelines for qualitative research and this issue has been considered in their section on providing credibility checks. In both works, Lincoln and Guba (1985) and Elliott et al. (1999) state that assuring this aspect require the inclusion of *auditors*. Auditors are usually researchers who are somewhat familiar with the research question but are not involved in the actual analysis. Thus, they can serve as an outside perspective to help the main researchers to correct their interpretations and present more trustworthy results. Usually, the results are discussed with this auditor (e.g., a supervisor or colleague) for clarity, but the achieved expertise in the phenomenon of the major researcher or group of researchers is not questioned [examples include an analysis on emotional pain by Bolger (1999) and therapist somatic phenomena in therapy by Shaw (2004)]. In addition to auditing, there are other ways to assure the dependability of a project (compare Elliott et al. 1999). Qualitative projects with one main researcher will document and make transparent their insights throughout the *hermeneutic circular process*. Another method is the *systematic consensual agreement* in which two or more researchers are required to arrive to agree on the results obtained individually, thus presenting credible/dependable results (e.g., see the analysis of therapists' dreams about their clients conducted by Spangler et al. (2009); see also Schielke et al. (2009) and Chap. 23). Lamnek (2010) introduces the practices of *peer reviewing* (reviewing categories and results within the research group) and the *peer debriefing* (reviewing categories and results with experts outside the research group). The use of statistical *inter-rater reliability* calculations must be discussed carefully. Statistical inter-rater agreement checks should only be applied when appropriate to the research aim (e.g., calculation of Krippendorff"s alpha or Cohen's kappa; Mörtl and Wietersheim 2008). It can make sense, for example, to test if another person can be trained in the reliable coding of a specific top-down category system to see if categories and coding rules for categories are comprehensive and clear enough. Inter-rater agreements should not be applied as naive proof of objectivity and are mostly inappropriate for bottom-up approaches.

The implementation of the above quality criteria is highly dependent on how the researcher understands science, his/her personal attitudes, and the research environment within which he/she works. For a deeper and more articulated discussion of the different conceptions of quality criteria in qualitative research, we refer the reader to the extensive existing literature to which we provided citations throughout this section.

Conclusion

In this chapter, we describe the main characteristics of qualitative methods that can be applied in PPR. This description was provided with an awareness of the following: (a) quantitative and qualitative methods and research should be considered ideal types located at the extremes of a continuum, and we should be careful when making sharp delineations between them; (b) contrary to quantitative research, in qualitative research, the methods used to investigate the therapeutic process largely overlap with those used to investigate therapeutic outcomes (see Chap. 27).

We have provided a description of qualitative methods in our field at the level of research design, sampling, data collection, and data analysis. We presented a map of methods and then systematically deconstructed it by stating that methods could be located at different places on the map. At this point, we hope to have confused the reader well enough. As in every qualitative study, there is a point of chaos in which the researcher must lean back, reflect upon all of the gathered information, however coherent or contradictory, and answer the research question. We will do so now. Our desideratum was to present qualitative methods in our field; to do so we had to answer the following question.

When Is a Psychotherapy Process Research Method Qualitative?

A method can be labeled qualitative when the researchers (1) are applying traditional qualitative coding strategies (open coding, inductive categories, documenting reflection in the coding process, etc.) **and/or** (2) conceptualize their found categories clearly qualitatively (without reducing the relationship between categories solely to a numeric-statistical level).[24]

Looking closer, the definition including two aspects beholds a third argument: the researcher. It is not the coding system that makes a method qualitative. It is how the researcher makes use of it. We have demonstrated that set category systems can involve a huge amount of interpretation and reflection (as in the CCRT or the TACS) or

[24] This will hopefully remind the reader of Denzin and Lincoln's definition we presented in the introduction of this chapter. The new twist in the definition is the "or" criterion of the two aspects which now includes specific qualitative methods in psychotherapy process research that would have not been captured by Denzin and Lincoln's definition, namely most of the afore described top-down apporaches.

can be applied rather descriptively by sticking to a few precise definition rules (as in the NPCS or NEPCS). It is the researcher as a person, in a specific context, with a specific aim, and with a manner of interpreting how specific methods might and should be used who shapes a qualitative project. Researchers, including ourselves, tend to avow themselves as either qualitative or quantitative scholars as do academic institutions, supervisors, and journals. Thus, whenever we categorize a method as qualitative, we must consider who shaped or invented this method, who applies it, and when and where it is published. It is not surprising that sometimes projects that, for example, are not "purely" qualitative might lean towards the qualitative pole in one publication or conference talk and then lean towards the quantiative pole in another. At the end of the research day, the choice is the researcher's. Confronted with considerable amounts of complex information, how content is he/she to trust his/her ability to obtain results in a qualitative or a quantitative way? Will the conceptualization consist of listening to themselves to carve out the relationship among specific categories intuitively and empirically? Will the researchers trust their eyes when examining their categories out on the table, making connections, and assuring their accuracy in the empirical coding? Will the researcher choose to reduce complexity into numeric values, put them into tables, and trust the abstract statistical calculations?[25]

Finally, a study is not only influenced by these ideal scientific choices but also by other real-life choices, namely, available resources (Mörtl and Lamott 2010): In addition to (wo) manpower, money, and time, the availability of interviewees is crucial. Finally, the research design and sampling depend on contextual and interpersonal support from the research project team, supervisor, and people and structures in the field under investigation who establish the contact between you and your sample.

Acknowledgments We wish to thank the participating qualitative researchers who contributed their exemplary analyses: Michael Buchholz, Brigitte Boothe, Mariane Krause, Philipp Mayring, Xiaorong Zhou, and Tali Boritz. Additionally, this chapter would not have been possible without the people who shaped our understanding of qualitative research. Thanks to David Rennie for the supportive and enlightening discussions of methodology, Franziska Lamott for the insightful collaboration in our projects, and Horst Kaechele and Joern von Wietersheim for their challenging comments and support to go abroad. We also want to acknowledge two institutions that facilitated this work: the German Research Council (DFG) provided a postdoctoral scholarship and the Society of Psychotherapy Research (SPR) provided a platform for international exchange.

References

Albani C, Pokorny D, Blaser G, Kaechele H (2008) Beziehungsmuster und Beziehungskonflikte. Theorie, Klinik und Forschung. Vandenhoeck & Ruprecht, Goettingen

Altheide DL, Johnson JM (1994) Criteria for assessing interpretive validity in qualitative research. In: Denzin NK, Lincoln YS (eds) Handbook of qualitative research. Sage, Thousand Oaks, CA, pp 485–499

Angus L, Levitt H, Hardtke K (1999) The narrative processes coding system: research applications and implications for psychotherapy practice. J Clin Psychol 55(10):1255–1270

Angus L, Lewin J, Boritz T, Bryntwick E, Carpenter N, Watson-Gaze J, Greenberg LS (2012) Narrative processes coding system: a dialectical constructivist approach to assessing client change processes in emotion-focused therapy of depression. Res

[25] Although we introduced this chapter by stating that we would not venture into the depths of methodology, the philosophically informed reader will spot a parallel that inspired our closing remarks: the basic differences between quality and quantity that were outlined by Aristotle and then Kant and Hegel. In Hegel's Doctrine of Being (part of his Encyclopedia Logic, 1969/1917), quality refers to the immediacy of the determinate being (through contrasting and limiting one category to mark the beginning of another), while quantity by definition is insensitive to quality and refers to the reduction of the experience of being (by neglecting everything but the count and testing units against each other).This differentiation can be directly associated with the outlined techniques in qualitative and quantitative research and, furthermore, characterize two different research attitudes.

Psychother Psychopathol Process Outcome 15 (2):54–61. doi:10.7411/RP.2012.006

Barber JP, Crits-Christoph P, Luborsky L (1998) A guide to the CCRT standard categories and their classification. In: Luborsky L, Crits-Christoph P (eds) Understanding transference: the core conflictual relationship theme method, 2nd edn. American Psychological Association, Washington, DC, pp 43–54

Barker C, Pistrang N, Elliott R (2002) Research methods in clinical and counseling psychology. Wiley, London

Benjamin LS (1974) Structural analysis of social behavior. Psychol Rev 81:392–425

Bolger E (1999) Grounded theory analysis of emotional pain. Psychother Res 9(3):342–362. doi:10.1080/10503309912331332801

Boothe B (2000) Manual der Erzaehlanalyse JAKOB. Zuerich

Boothe B, Grimm G, Hermann M-L, Luder M (2010) JAKOB narrative analysis: the psychodynamic conflict as a narrative model. Psychother Res 20(5):511–525

Boritz T, Angus L, Monette G, Hollis-Walker L (2011) Narrative and emotion integration in psychotherapy: investigating the relationship between autobiographical memory specificity and expressed emotional arousal in brief emotion-focused and client-centred treatments of depression. Psychother Res 21 (1):16–26

Braun V, Clarke V (2006) Using thematic analysis in psychology. Qual Res Psychol 3(2):77–101

Buchholz MB (1993) Metaphernanalyse. Vandenhoeck & Ruprecht, Göttingen

Buchholz MB (2003) Metaphern der Kur. Psychosozial Verlag, Giessen

Buchholz MB, Lamott F, Mörtl K (2008) Tat-Sachen. Narrative von Sexualstraftaetern. Psychosozial Verlag, Giessen

Campbell DT, Stanley JC (1963) Experimental and quasi-experimental designs for research. Houghton Mifflin, Boston, MA

Cattell RB (1952) The three basic factor-analytic designs: their interrelations and derivatives. Psychol Bull 49:499–520

Chassan JB (1979) Research design in clinical psychology and psychiatry, 2nd edn. Wiley, New York, NY

Crits-Christoph P, Demorest A (1988) A list of standard categories, 2nd edn. University of Pennsylvania School of Medicine, Philadelphia, PA, Unpublished Manuscript

Denzin NK, Lincoln YS (2005) The SAGE handbook of qualitative research, 3rd edn. Sage, Thousand Oaks, CA

Diaz-Bone R, Bührmann AD, Encarnación GR, Schneider W, Kendall G, Tirado F (2007) The field of Foucaultian discourse analysis: structures, developments and perspectives [52 paragraphs]. Forum Qual Soc Res 8(2):Article 30. http://nbn-resolving.de/urn:nbn:de:0114-fqs0702305

Dourdouma A, Mörtl K (2012) The creative journey of grounded theory analysis: a guide to its principles and applications. Res Psychother Psychopathol Process Outcome 15(2):96–116

Elliot R (1984) A discovery-oriented approach to significant change events in psychotherapy: interpersonal process recall and comprehensive process analysis. In: Rice LA, Greenberg LS (eds) Patterns of change. Guilford, New York, NY, pp 249–286

Elliott R (1986) Interpersonal process recall (IPR) as a PPR method. In: Greenberg LS, Pinsof WM (eds) The psychotherapeutic process: a research handbook. Guilford, New York, NY, pp 249–286

Elliott R (1989) Comprehensive process analysis: understanding change process in significant therapy events. In: Packer MJ, Addison RB (eds) Entering the circle: hermeneutic investigation in psychology. SUNY Press, Albany, NY, pp 165–184

Elliott R, Shapiro DA (1988a) Clients and therapists as analysts of significant events. In: Toukmanian SG, Rennie DL (eds) Psychotherapy process research: paradigmatic and narrative approaches. Sage, Newberry Park, CA, pp 163–186

Elliott R, Shapiro DA (1988b) Brief structured recall: a more efficient method for studying significant therapy events. Br J Med Psychol 61:141–153. doi:10.1111/j.2044-8341.1988.tb02773.x

Elliott R, Fischer CT, Rennie DL (1999) Evolving guidelines for publication of qualitative research studies in psychology and related fields. Br J Clin Psychol 38:215–229. doi:10.1348/014466599162782

Elliott R, Slatick E, Urman M (2001) Qualitative change process research on psychotherapy: alternative strategies. In: Frommer J, Rennie DL (eds) Qualitative psychotherapy research: methods and methodology. Pabst Science, Lengerich, Germany, pp 69–111

Elo S, Kyngäs H (2008) The qualitative content analysis process. J Adv Nurs 62:107–115. doi:10.1111/j.1365-2648.2007.04569.x

Fischer CT (2009) Bracketing in qualitative research: conceptual and practical matters. Psychother Res 19 (4–5):583–590. doi:10.1080/10503300902798375

Flick U, Kardoff E, Steinke I (2004) A companion to qualitative research. Sage, Thousand Oaks, CA

Frommer J, Rennie DL (eds) (2001) Qualitative psychotherapy research: methods and methodology. Pabst Science, Lengerich

Gambier Y, Gile D, Taylor C (eds) (1997) Conference interpreting: current trends in research. Proceedings of the international conference on interpreting. John Benjamins, Amsterdam

Garfinkel H (1967) Studies in ethnomethodology. Prentice-Hall, Englewood Cliffs, NJ

Gelo OCG (2012) On research methods and their philosophical assumptions: "raising the consciousness of researchers" again. Psychotherapie & Sozialwissenschaft 14(2):111–130

Gelo OCG, Braakmann D, Benetka G (2008) Quantitative and qualitative research: beyond the debate. Integr Psychol Behav Sci 42(3):266–290. doi:10.1007/s12124-008-9078-3

Gelo OCG, Braakmann D, Benetka G (2009) Erratum to "Quantitative and qualitative research: beyond the debate". Integr Psychol Behav Sci 43(4):406–407. doi:10.1007/s12124-009-9107-x

Gelo OCG, Salcuni S, Colli A (2012) Quantitative and qualitative text analysis in psychotherapy process research: introduction to special issue. Res Psychother Psychopathol Process Outcome 15:46–54. doi:10.7411/RP.2012.005

Gerhardt U (1991) Typenbildung. In: Flick U et al (eds) Handbuch Qualitative Sozialforschung. Grundlagen, Konzepte, Methoden und Anwendungen. Psychologie Verlags Union, München, pp 435–439

Giorgi A (1997) The theory, practice and evaluation of the phenomenological method as a qualitative research procedure. J Phenomenol Psychol 28:235–260

Giorgi AP, Giorgi BM (2003) Chapter 13: The descriptive phenomenological psychological method. In: Camic PM, Rhodes JE, Yardley L (eds) Qualitative research in psychology: expanding perspectives in methodology and design. American Psychological Association, Washington, DC, pp 243–273

Glaser B (1978) Theoretical sensitivity. Sociology Press, Mill Valley, CA

Glaser B, Strauss A (1967) The discovery of grounded theory. Aldine, Chicago, IL

Gliner JA, Morgan GA, Leech NL (2009) Research methods in applied settings: an integrated approach to design and analysis, 2nd edn. Routledge, New York, NY

Gonçalves MM, Ribeiro A, Mendes I, Matos M, Santos A (2011) Tracking novelties in PPR: the innovative moments coding system. Psychother Res 21:497–509. doi:10.1080/10503307.2011.560207

Greenberg LS (1986) Change process research. J Consult Clin Psychol 54(1):4–9

Greenberg LS (1992) Task analysis: identifying components of intrapersonal conflict resolution. In: Toukmanian SG, Rennie DL (eds) Psychotherapy process research. Sage, Thousand Oaks, CA, pp 22–50

Greenberg LS, Watson J (1998) Experiential therapy of depression: differential effects of client-centered relationship conditions and process experiential interventions. Psychother Res 8:210–224

Haig B (2008) Scientific method, abduction, and clinical reasoning. J Clin Psychol 64:1013–1018. doi:10.1002/jclp.20505

Hanson WE, Creswell JW, Plano Clark VL, Petska KP, Creswell JD (2005) Mixed methods research designs in counseling psychology. J Couns Psychol 52:224–235

Hardtke K, Angus L (2004) The narrative assessment interview: assessing self-change in psychotherapy. In: Amgus L, McLeod J (eds) The handbook of narrative and psychotherapy: practice, theory, research. Sage, Thousand Oaks, CA

Hartley D, Strupp H (1983) The therapeutic alliance: its relationship to outcome in brief psychotherapy. In: Masling J (ed) Empirical studies of psychoanalytic theories, vol 1. Erlbaum, Hillsdale, NJ, pp 1–27

Haupert B (1991) Vom narrativen Interview zur biographischen Typenbildung. In: Garz D, Kraimer K (eds) Qualitativ-empirische Sozialforschung. Konzepte, Methoden, Analysen. Westdeutscher, Opladen, pp 213–254

Hegel GWF (1917/1969) Book 1: Doctrine of being. In: Hegel GWF (ed) Science of logic. Humanity Books, Amherst, NY

Hill CE, Lambert M (2004) Methodological issues in studying psychotherapy processes and outcomes. In: Lambert MJ (ed) Bergin and Garfield's handbook of psychotherapy and behavior. Wiley, New York, NY, pp 84–135

Hsu LM (1989) Random sampling, randomization, and equivalence of contrasted groups in psychotherapy outcome research. J Consult Clin Psychol 57 (1):131–137

Hug T, Poscheschnik G (eds) (2010) Empirisch Forschen. UTB, Konstanz

Husserl E (1970/1900) Logical investigations I & II. Humanities Press, New York, NY

Imelda TV (1997) Sampling in qualitative research. Purposeful and theoretical sampling; merging or clear boundaries? J Adv Nurs 26(3):623–630. doi:10.1046/j.1365-2648.1997.t01-25-00999.x

Iwakabe S, Gazzola N (2009) From single case studies to practice-based knowledge: aggregating and synthesizing case studies. Psychother Res 19:601–611

Jefferson G (2004) Glossary of transcript symbols with an introduction. In: Lerner G (ed) Conversation analysis: studies from the first generation. John Benjamins, Amsterdam, pp 13–31

Kant I (2002/1788) Critique of pure reason. Hackett, Indianapolis, IN

Kazdin A (2003) Research design in clinical psychology, 4th edn. Allyn & Bacon, Needham Heights, MA

Kluge S (1999) Empirisch begründete Typenbildung. Zur Konstruktion von Typen und Typologien in der qualitativen Sozialforschung. Leske und Budrich, Opladen

Kluge S (2000) Empirically grounded construction of types and typologies in qualitative social research [14 paragraphs]. Forum Qual Soc Res 1(1):Article 14. http://nbn-resolving.de/urn:nbn:de:0114-fqs0001145

Knox S, Burkard AW (2009) Qualitative research interviews. Psychother Res 19(4–5):566–575. doi:10.1080/10503300802702105

Koerber A, McMichael L (2008) Qualitative sampling methods. A primer for technical communicators. J Bus Tech Commun 22:454–473

Krause M, Valdes N, Tomicic A (2009) Therapeutic activity coding system – procedure manual. Fondecyt Project No 1080136, Chilean Research Program Psychotherapy and Change. Unpublished Manuscript. www.psychotherapyandchange.org

Kuehnlein I (1999) Psychotherapy as a process of transformation: analysis of posttherapeutic autobiographic narrations. Psychother Res 9(3):274–288

Kvale S (1996) InterViews: an introduction to qualitative research interviewing. Sage, Thousand Oaks, CA

Labov W, Waletzky J (1997) Narrative analysis: oral versions of personal experience. Journal of Narrative and Life History 7(1–4):3–38

Laitila A, Aaltonen J, Wahlström J, Angus L (2001) Narrative process coding system in marital and family therapy: an intensive case analysis of the formation of a therapeutic system. Contem Fam Ther 23 (3):309–322

Lakoff G, Johnson M (1980) Metaphors we live by. Chicago University Press, Chicago, IL

Lamnek S (2010) Qualitative social research, 5th edn. Beltz, Weinheim

Legewie H, Schervier-Legewie B (2004) Interview with Anselm Strauss. „Forschung ist harte Arbeit, es ist immer ein Stück Leiden damit verbunden. Deshalb muss es auf der anderen Seite Spaß machen". In: Mey G, Mruck K (eds) Grounded theory reader (HSR Suppl 19). ZHSF, Cologne, Germany, pp 69–79

Leithäuser T, Volmerg B (1988) Psychoanalyse in der Sozialforschung. Eine Einführung am Beispiel einer Sozialpsychologie der Arbeit. Westdeutscher, Opladen

Lepper G (1967) Categories in text and talk. A practical introduction to categorization analysis. Sage, London

Lincoln YS, Guba EG (1985) Naturalistic inquiry. Sage, Beverly Hills, CA

Lepper G, Riding N (2006) Researching the psychotherapy process. A practical guide to transcipt-based methods. Palgrave Macmillan, Hampshire/New York

Lipscomb M (2012) Abductive reasoning and qualitative research. Nurs Philos 13(4):244–256. doi:10.1111/j.1466-769X.2011.00532.x

Llewelyn SP, Elliot R, Shapiro DA, Hardy G, Firth-Cozens J (1988) Client perceptions of significant events in prescriptive and exploratory periods of individual therapy. Br J Clin Psychol 27:105–114

Luborsky L (1998) A guide to the CCRT method. In: Luborsky L, Crits-Christoph P (eds) Understanding transference: the core conflictual relationship theme method, 2nd edn. American Psychological Association, Washington, DC, pp 15–42

Luborsky MR, Rubinstein RL (1995) Sampling in qualitative research. Rationale, issues, and methods. Res Aging 17(1):89–113. doi:10.1177/0164027595171005

Lutz W, Hill CE (2009) Quantitative and qualitative methods for psychotherapy research: introduction to special section. Psychother Res 19(4–5):369–373. doi:10.1080/10503300902948053

Lutz W, Knox S (eds) (2013) Quantitative and qualitative methods in psychotherapy research. Routledge, London

Madill A, Widdicombe S, Barkham M (2001) The potential of conversation analysis for psychotherapy research. The Counseling Psychologist 29:413–434. doi:10.1177/0011000001293006

Mayring P (1990) Qualitative Inhaltsanalyse. Grundlagen und Techniken, 2nd edn. Deutscher Studien, Weinheim

Mayring P (2000) Qualitative content analysis [28 paragraphs]. Forum Qual Soc Res 1(2):Article 20. http://nbn-resolving.de/urn:nbn:de:0114-fqs0002204

McLeod J (1997) Narrative and psychotherapy. Sage, London

McLeod J (2011) Qualitative research in counselling and psychotherapy, 2nd edn. Sage, London

McLeod J (2013) Qualitative research: methods and contributions. In: Lambert MJ (ed) Bergin and Garfield's handbook of psychotherapy and behavior change, 5th edn. Wiley, New York, NY, pp 49–84

Mergenthaler E, Stinson C (1992) Psychotherapy transcription standards. Psychother Res 2:125–142

Merleau-Ponty M (1962/1945) The phenomenology of perception (Trans. C. Smith). Humanities Press, New York, NY

Mey G, Mruck K (2007) Grounded theory methodology – Bemerkungen zu einem prominenten Forschungsstil. In: Mey G, Mruck K (eds) Grounded theory reader (HSR Suppl 19). ZHSF, Cologne, Germany, pp 11–39

Milbrath C, Bond M, Cooper S, Znoj HJ, Horowitz MJ, Perry JC (1999) Sequential consequences of therapists' interventions. J Psychother Pract Res 8(1):40–54

Mörtl K (2012) Qualitative Forscher/innen an der Universitaet. Psychotherapie und Sozialwissenschaft 14(2):5–13, Special Issue

Mörtl K, Lamott F (2010) Wie wird Veränderung in der Psychotherapieforschung gemessen? Ein Plädoyer für triangulierende Forschung. Psychotherapie und Sozialwissenschaft 12(2):95–102

Mörtl K, Wietersheim JV (2008) Client experiences of helpful factors in a day treatment program. Psychother Res 18(3):281–293

Molenaar PCM (2004) A manifesto on psychology as idiographic science: bringing the person back into scientific psychology, this time forever. Measurement 2(4):201–218

Molenaar PCM, Campbell CG (2009) The new person-specific paradigm in psychology. Curr Dir Psychol 18 (2):112–117

Morrow SL (2005) Quality and trustworthiness in qualitative research in counseling psychology. J Couns Psychol 52(2):250–260. doi:10.1037/0022-0167.52.2.250

Morse JM (1995) The significance of saturation. Qual Health Res 5:147–149

Muntigl P, Horvath AO (2014) The therapeutic relationship in action: how therapists and clients comanage relational disaffiliation. Psychother Res 24:327–345. doi:10.1080/10503307.201310.1080/10503307.2013.807525

Muntigl P, Knight N, Horvath AO, Watkins A (2012) Client attitudinal stance and therapist-client affiliation: a view from grammar and social interaction. Res Psychother Psychopathol Process Outcome 15 (2):117–130. doi:10.7411/RP.2012.012

Nilsson T, Svensson M, Sandell R, Clinton D (2007) Patients' experiences of change in cognitive-behavioral therapy and psychodynamic therapy: a qualitative comparative study. Psychother Res 17 (5):553–566. doi:10.1080/10503300601139988

Oevermann U, Allert T, Konau E, Krambeck J (1979) Die Methodologie einer „Objektiven Hermeneutik" und ihre Allgemeine Forschungslogische Bedeutung in den Sozialwissenschaften. In: Soeffner HG (ed) Interpretative Verfahren in den Sozial- und Textwissenschaften. Enke, Stuttgart, pp 352–434

Onwuegbuzie AJ, Leech NL (2007) A call for qualitative power analyses. Qual Quan 41:105–121. doi:10.1007/s11135-005-1098-1

Orlinsky DE, Rønnestad MH, Willutzki U (2004) Fifty years of psychotherapy process-outcomes research: continuity and change. In: Lambert MJ (ed) Bergin and Garfield's handbook of psychotherapy and behavior change. Wiley, New York, NY, pp 307–393

Packer MJ, Addison RB (1989) Evaluating an interpretive account. In: Packer MJ, Addison RB (eds) Entering the circle: hermeneutic investigation in psychology. SUNY Press, Albany, NY, pp 275–292

Palmer S, Cochran L (1988) Parents as agents of career development. J Couns Psychol 35:71–76

Parker I (ed) (1998) Social constructionism, discourse and realism. Sage, London

Patton MQ (1990) Qualitative evaluation and research methods, 2nd edn. Sage, Newbury Park, CA

Peräkylä A, Antaki C, Vehviläinen S, Leudar I (eds) (2008) Conversation analysis and psychotherapy. Cambridge University Press, Cambridge

Perry JC (1990) Perry's defense mechanism rating scale. In: Vaillant GE (ed) Ego mechanisms of defense: a guide for clinicians and researchers. American Psychiatric Press, Washington, DC, pp 253–259

Pokorny D (2014) Website des CCRT-LU, online resource, www.ccrt-lu.org

Polkinghorne DE (2005) Language and meaning: data collection in qualitative research. J Couns Psychol 52:137–145

Ponterotto JG (2005) Qualitative research in counseling psychology: a primer on research paradigms and philosophy of science. J Counsel Psychol 52(2):126–136. doi:10.1037/0022-0167.52.2.126

Poscheschnik G (2010) Qualitative Auswertungsmethoden. In: Hug T, Poscheschnik G (eds) Empirisch Forschen. UTB, Konstanz, pp 150–162

Potter J, Wetherell M (1987) Discourse and social psychology: beyond attitudes and behaviour. Sage, London

Przyborski A, Slunecko T (2012) Learning to think iconically in the human and social sciences: iconic standards of understanding as a pivotal challenge for method development. Integr Psychol Behav Sci 46 (1):39–56. doi:10.1007/s12124-011-9159-6

Reichertz J (2004a) Objective hermeneutics and hermeneutic sociology of knowledge. In: Flick U, von Kardorff E, Steinke I (eds) A companion to qualitative research. Sage, Thousand Oaks, CA, pp 290–295

Reichertz J (2004b) Abduction, deduction and induction in qualitative research. In: Flick U, von Kardorff E, Steinke I (eds) A companion to qualitative research. Sage, Thousand Oaks, CA, pp 159–164

Rennie D (1990) Towards a representation of the client's experiences of the psychotherapy hour. In: Lietaer G, Rombauts J, von Balen R (eds) Client centred and experiential psychotherapies in the nineties. Leuven University Press, Leuven, pp 155–172

Rennie DL (2012) Qualitative research as methodical hermeneutics. Psychol Methods 17(3):385–398

Rennie DL, Fergus KD (2006) Embodied categorizing in the grounded theory method: methodical hermeneutics in action. Theory Psychol 16:483–503. doi:10.1177/0959354306066202

Rice LN, Greenberg LS (eds) (1984) Patterns of change: intensive analysis of psychotherapy practice. Guilford, New York, NY

Roth W-M (2005) Textbooks on qualitative research and method/methodology: toward a praxis of method [63 paragraphs]. Forum Qual Soc Res 7(1):Article 11. http://nbn-resolving.de/urn:nbn:de:0114-fqs0601111

Sacks H (1972) An initial investigation of the usability of conversational data for sociology. In: Sudnow DN (ed) Studies in social interaction. Free Press, New York, NY, pp 31–74

Saldaña J (2013) The coding manual for qualitative researchers, 3rd edn. Sage, London

Salvatore S, Valsiner J (2010) Between the general and the unique. Theory Psychol 20:817–833. doi:10.1177/0959354310381156

Sandage SJ, Cook KV, Hill PC, Strawn BD, Reimer KS (2008) Hermeneutics and psychology: a review and dialectical model. Rev Gen Psychol 12:344–364

Sayer A (1992) Method in social science: a realist approach, 2nd edn. Routledge, London

Schielke HJ, Fishman JL, Osatuke K, Stiles WB (2009) Creative consensus on interpretations of qualitative data: the Ward method. Psychother Res 19 (4–5):558–565. doi:10.1080/10503300802621180

Schütze F (1983) Biographieforschung und narratives interview. Neue Praxis 13:283–293

Seale C (1999) Quality in qualitative research. Qual Inq 5:465–478

Seebohm TM (2004) Hermeneutics method and methodology. Kluwer, Dordrecht

Semerari A, Carcione A, Dimaggio G, Falcone M, Nicolo G, Procaci M et al (2003) How to evaluate metacognitive function in psychotherapy? The Metacognition Assessment Scale and its applications. Clin Psychol Psychother 10:238–261

Shaw R (2004) The embodied psychotherapist: an exploration of the therapists' somatic phenomena within the therapeutic encounter. Psychother Res 14(3):271–288

Slife BD (2004) Theoretical challenges to therapy practice and research: the constraint of naturalism. In: Lambert MJ (ed) Bergin and Garfield's handbook of psychotherapy and behavior change, 5th edn. Wiley, New York, NY, pp 44–83

Smith JA, Osborn M (2008) Interpretative phenomenological analysis. In: Smith JA (ed) Qualitative psychology: a practical guide to methods, 2nd edn. Sage, London

Smith JA, Flowers P, Osborn M (1997) Interpretative phenomenological analysis and health psychology. In: Yardley L (ed) Material discourses and health. Routledge, London, pp 68–91

Spangler P, Hill CE, Mettus C, Guo AH, Heymsfield L (2009) Therapist perspectives on the dreams about clients: a qualitative investigation. Psychother Res 19:81–95

Stiles WB (1993) Quality control in qualitative research. Clin Psychol Rev 13:593–618. doi:10.1016/0272-7358(93)90048-q

Stiles WB (2001) Assimilation of problematic experiences. Psychother Theor Res Pract Train 38(4):462–465

Stiles WB, Angus L (2001) Qualitative research on clients' assimilation of problematic experiences in psycho- therapy. In: Frommer J, Rennie D (eds) Qualitative psychotherapy research: methods and methodology. Pabst Science, Lengerich, pp 111–126

Stiles WB, Elliott R, Llewelyn SP, Firth-Cozens JA, Margison FR, Shapiro DA, Hardy G (1990) Assimilation of problematic experiences by clients in psychotherapy. Psychother Theor Res Pract Train 27 (3):411–420. doi:10.1037/0033-3204.27.3.411

Stiles WB, Morrison LA, Haw SK, Harper H, Shapiro DA, Firth-Cozens J (1991) Longitudinal study of assimilation in exploratory psychotherapy. Psychotherapy 28:195–206

Strauss A, Corbin J (1990) Basics of qualitative research: grounded theory procedures and techniques. Sage, Newbury Park, CA

Strauss A (1991) Grundlagen qualitativer Sozialforschung. Datenanalyse und Theoriebildung in der empirischen soziologischen Forschung. Muenchen, Fink

Swanborn G (2010) Case study research: what, why and how. Sage, London

Task Force OPD (2007) Operationalized psychodynamic diagnosis OPD-2: manual of diagnosis and treatment planning. Hogrefe & Huber, Bern

Timulak L (2008) Research in psychotherapy and counselling, 2nd edn. Sage, London

Timulak L (2009) Meta-analysis of qualitative studies: a tool for reviewing qualitative research findings in psychotherapy. Psychother Res 19:591–600. doi:10.1080/10503300802477989

Valsiner J (2010) Why simple lessons from history are recurrently forgotten: the bubble of "epistemic markets". Revista de Historia de la Psicologia 31 (1):81–94

Watson JC, Rennie DL (1994) Qualitative analysis of clients' subjective experience of significant moments during the exploration of problematic reactions. J Couns Psychol 41(4):500–509. doi:10.1037//0022-0167.41.4.500

Weber M (1972) Wirtschaft und Gesellschaft. Grundriß der verstehenden Soziologie, 5th edn. Mohr, Tuebingen

Westra H, Aviram A, Barnes M, Angus L (2011) Therapy was not what I expected: a preliminary qualitative analysis of concordance between client expectations and experience of cognitive behavioural therapy. Psychother Res 20(4):436–446

Williams DC, Levitt HM (2007) A qualitative investigation of eminent therapists' values within psychotherapy: developing integrative principles for moment-to-moment psychotherapy practice. J Psychother Integrat 17(2):159–184

Williams EN, Morrow SL (2009) Achieving trustworthiness in qualitative research: a pan-paradigmatic perspective. Psychother Res 19(4–5):576–582. doi:10.1080/10503300802702113

Yin RK (2003) Case study research, design and methods, 3rd edn. Sage, Newbury Park, CA

Applications of Qualitative and Mixed-Methods Counseling and Psychotherapy Research

21

David L. Rennie and Jörg Frommer

Contents

Abstract

Method: A review is made of qualitative and mixed-methods research applications to counseling and psychotherapy based on 208 articles published between 2003 and mid-2010 in both English-language and German-language journals, 21 in all.

Results: The applications of these studies are sorted into five topics: (1) clients' experience of counseling and therapy; (2) practitioners' experience of counseling and psychotherapy; (3) counseling and psychotherapy process and outcome; (4) supervision, training, and professional development; and (5) professional practice issues, the public view of counseling and psychotherapy, and practitioners' self-care. The studies under each of these topics are tabulated, giving the outlet of each study, its focus, the country of origin, sample size, and method used. From each table studies originating from either Germany or Scandinavia, on the one hand, and other countries, on the other hand, are selected to illustrate the range of applications made within each topic.

Discussion: It is noted that during the period surveyed there has been an increasing emphasis of objectivity, in a variety of ways, reflecting a shift toward positivism. Implications of this development are discussed.

David L. Rennie was deceased at the time of publication.

J. Frommer (✉)
Otto-von-Guericke University, Magdeburg, Germany
e-mail: joerg.frommer@med.ovgu.de

O.C.G. Gelo et al. (eds.), *Psychotherapy Research*,
DOI 10.1007/978-3-7091-1382-0_21, © Springer-Verlag Wien 2015

21.1 Introduction

The field of counseling and psychotherapy has contributed substantially to the rise of qualitative research (Rennie et al. 2002). Several years ago, together with colleagues, the present authors published companion reviews of the production of such research in the Anglo-North American (Rennie 2004) and German-speaking countries, including Scandinavia (Frommer et al. 2004). The focus of the reviews was mainly on epistemology (theory of knowledge), methodology (theory of method), and method. We found that the work in the USA and Canada had been inclined toward modernist objectivism, while to some extent the work in the UK had been influenced by the British postmodern, critical psychological movement (e.g., Billig 1987). It was also apparent that in the German-speaking countries, in addition to psychotherapy research done in departments of psychology, psychosomatic medicine departments also had contributed to qualitative studies, while departments of counseling had not played a significant role in this field of research. In addition we observed that Qualitative Content Analysis (Frommer 1996; Kracauer 1952), Ideal Type Analysis (Gerhardt 2001), Objective Hermeneutics (Oevermann et al. 1979), and the Autobiographical Narrative Interview method of inquiry and analysis (Schütze 1981, 1983, 1984), all of which were developed in the German-speaking region, had been used almost exclusively there.

In those reviews, we mentioned applications mainly to illustrate methodology and methods. In this limited way, among the applications addressed were, for example, the study of metaphor in therapy (Angus and Rennie 1988); the therapeutic alliance (Bachelor 1995); how transition objects work (Arthern and Madill 1999); the assimilation model (Stiles and Angus 2001); categorization of client's pauses during conversation with a therapist (Levitt 2001); diagnostic first interviews with patients (Frommer 1996; Frommer and Faller 1994); research on psychosomatic syndromes (Faller 1998); the characteristics, functions, and evaluation of narrative (Boothe et al. 1999); nonverbal interaction (Streeck 1999); and follow-up research (Kühnlein 1999).

In the present review, we reverse figure and ground by paying more attention to applications than to methodology and methods and by organizing applications in a different way than we did before. We now sort them into five topics: (1) the client's experience of counseling and psychotherapy; (2) the practitioner's experience of counseling and psychotherapy; (3) counseling and psychotherapy process and outcome; (4) supervision, training, and professional development; and (5) professional practice issues, the public view of counseling and psychotherapy, and practitioner's self-care. Correspondingly, methods are now addressed within the various applications rather than the other way round.

21.2 Method

As in the previous reviews, we have selected journals which we consider to be most centrally related to counseling and psychotherapy research. Because the year 2002 marked the end of our earlier surveys, we have now looked at articles published between 2003 and mid-2010 and have extracted all pertinent articles in every issue of the journals. The result is a total of 208 articles taken from 16 journals published in English and 5 published in German. Among these journals, the top five sources were *Counselling and Psychotherapy Research*, which yielded 28 % of the articles, followed by *Psychotherapy Research* (19 %), *Psychology and Psychotherapy* (9 %), the *British Journal of Guidance and Counselling* (9 %), and the *Journal of Counseling Psychology* (7 %). Except for German medical journals, we have not included journals in disciplines unrelated to counseling and psychotherapy, nor have we paid much attention to qualitative research journals, although we have taken one article from *Qualitative Research in Psychology*. The journals addressed are listed in Appendix A. When going through the issues of each journal, we used every article that reported an application of either a qualitative or mixed methods. We take a qualitative method to be the discovery-oriented analysis of verbal text, with the results being presented in such text. If numbers are used at all, it is to indicate the frequencies of constituents of the returns. The methods are intensive and typically necessitate the study of fewer individuals than is customary in quantitative research (Rennie 2012). Alternatively, mixed-methods research involves a combination of qualitative and quantitative methods (see, e.g., Gelo et al. 2008, 2009). This is done in a variety of ways. It may take the form of a type of content analysis wherein the meanings of a sample of textual material are conceptualized as categories or themes; whence, following this step, new textual material is assigned to a single given category or theme (in contrast with qualitative methods, which allow the assignment of a given passage of text to more than one category/theme), thereby producing frequencies that are analyzable statistically. Alternatively, and more typically, the mixed-methods approach entails the application of either interviews or participant observation yielding returns that are analyzed qualitatively, combined with the use of questionnaires judged to bear on the phenomenon of interest—questionnaires that yield numerical scores. Well-known examples of this approach in psychotherapeutic change research are assimilation analysis (Stiles et al. 1990), task analysis (Greenberg 2007), and hermeneutic single-case efficacy design (Elliott 2002).

Among the materials we examined were some English-language articles written by researchers in countries where English is not the first language, including, of course, Germany and Scandinavia (the German-speaking countries addressed in the present review). In the interest of continuing to distinguish between relevant researches coming from the latter region vis-à-vis elsewhere, we have demarcated what we call the "English-language region" (ELR) which includes articles published in English regardless of the country of origin *except* for those coming from Germany and Scandinavia (which we now call the Germany and Scandinavian region, or GSR for short). As for the *non*-English articles originated in the latter region, we used only those written in German. Overall, although the present review is comparatively more thorough than the previous ones, it is not exhaustive and we apologize to authors neglected.

The question arose as to what to do with the resulting 208 articles. We suppose that ideally we might have attempted to synthesize them. But we worried that to do so in the space available would ablate meaning. Thus, we have decided to strike a balance between comprehensiveness and detail. For comprehensiveness, we tabulate sufficient information to enable readers to identify articles of interest and to locate them in the volume and issue of the journal in which they were published. We do this in lieu of listing them in the References section of the chapter; only articles cited in the body of the chapter are listed there. For detail, we select from each table an article produced in each of the ELR and the GSR. It is important to note that, in some cases, a given article crossed boundaries between the five topics, especially in terms of the first and third topics. In such an instance, we have had to make a choice about where to place it.

21.3 Results

As indicated, the overall results are listed in tabular form. The acronyms for the journals in the first column of each table can be found in Appendix A, while the acronyms and abbreviations of terms found in the other columns are provided in a legend beneath each table.

As can be seen in the Focus column of every table, many interesting and important aspects of counseling and psychotherapy have been reported in the literature. It is also evident in the *Method* column that many qualitative research methods have been used. Some are established methods, while others are fashioned by the individual researcher as when, for example, the procedure of Constant comparative analysis is extracted from the Grounded Theory method. In order to distinguish established and fashioned methods, in the tables we use uppercase first letters to signify the former (e.g., Grounded Theory) and uppercase first letter to the first word only to indicate the latter (e.g., Constant comparative analysis).

In general the regional differences in methodology and methods observed in our previous reviews still apply. In the GSR there has been a comparatively somewhat greater emphasis of hermeneutic methods. There has also been comparatively more partiality to mixed methods, such as a mix of conversation analysis and a quantified method of textual analysis, where the latter was originated in Germany by Mergenthaler (1996). As for the ELR, we observe a slight shift among Americans toward an increasing emphasis of indicators of reliability, particularly the use of research teams where consensus among team members is conditional for the development of categories. This procedure is the hallmark of the Consensual Qualitative Research method developed in the USA by Hill et al. (1997), which has been gaining in popularity there. Meanwhile, British researchers have been comparatively partial to Interpretative Phenomenological Analysis, which Smith (1996) developed in England, while in other respects continuing to be more influenced by postmodern thought in the conduct of research, compared to researchers in other countries.

21.3.1 Clients' Experiences of Counseling and Psychotherapy

The results coming under this heading are given in Table 21.1. Many aspects of clients' experience of counseling and psychotherapy can be seen in the 63 studies assigned to this topic. Most frequent have been studies of the experience of a given approach to therapy, followed by the client's experience of the relationship with the therapist. Next have been studies of therapeutic experiences of psychotics and of lesbian, gay, bisexual, and transgender (LGBT) clients. In terms of locale, although 11 countries appear in the table, most of the studies came out of the UK, the USA, and Canada, in that order, while the number of German vs. Scandinavian studies listed in the table is about equal. Most commonly used were the Grounded Theory method (e.g., Strauss and Corbin 1998), mixed methods, Thematic Analysis (e.g., Braun and Clarke 2006), and fashioned methods (see above). Behind them there is another cluster made up of Interpretative Phenomenological Analysis (Smith 1996), Consensual Qualitative Research (Hill et al. 1997), and phenomenological methods.

The study we have selected from the ELR studies listed in this table was conducted in Canada by Bachelor et al. (2007). This was a mixed-methods study of clients' experiences of client-therapist collaboration in psychotherapy. As such it is a useful addition to the literature on the working alliance (Bordin 1979) from the client's perspective. The data consisted of written reports given by 30 non-screened clients drawn from three treatment settings. Categories of experience were developed consensually from a subsample of these reports. The frequencies of these categories across the entire set of reports were then tallied, in expression of content analysis which, in keeping with the North American tradition, had a quantitative component (cf. Qualitative Content Analysis developed by Kracauer (1952) and used in the GSR, as is evident in some of our tables). Employed as well were rating scales assessing symptoms, interpersonal relationships, the psychotherapy alliance, and motivation for psychotherapy.

The most important understanding developed was that there were three modes of collaborative involvement, from the client's perspective: *active*, where the client took the lead; *mutual* where the client valued give-and-take; and *dependent* where the practitioner was given the lead. These modes are amply illustrated with quotations. For example, a participant who was judged by researchers to exemplify the mutual mode observed:

> I found myself incapable of expressing verbally what I felt about my situation and the changes I wanted. My therapist then proposed this activity [drawing]...I quickly associated [the] colors, forms, and textures with which I felt and could then express this to my therapist who was better able to understand me. My fears and anxiety, when faced with difficult situations, are extremely

Table 21.1 Clients' experiences of counseling and psychotherapy

Authors	Focus	Country	*N*	Method
English-language region				
Abba et al. (2008) PR (1)	Responding mindfully to distressing psychosis	UK	16	Grounded theory
Audet and Everall (2003) CPR (3)	Experience of Ts self-disclosure	CAN	9	Phenomenological psychological method
Bachelor et al. (2007) P (2)	Cs' collaboration in therapy	CAN	30	Mixed
Bedi et al. (2005) P (3)	Perception of critical incidents	CAN	40	Mixed
Bedi et al. (2006) JCP (1)	Cs' perspective on counseling alliance formation	CAN	31	Mixed
Berg et al. (2008) PR (3)	Cs' perspectives on medical adherence in CBT for depression in HIV	USA	14	Consensual thematic analysis
Bohart and Byock (2005) THP (3)	Experiencing Carl Rogers	USA	2	Vicarious, empathic, ethnographic, interpretive
Bury et al. (2007) PP (1)	Young people's experience of psychoanalytic therapy	UK	6	Interpretative phenomenological analysis
Carey et al. (2007) CPR (3)	Experience of psychological change in therapy	AUSTRL	27	Framework approach
Chang and Berk (2009) JCP (4)	Experience of cross-racial therapy	USA	16	Consensual qualitative research
Clarke et al. (2004) PP (1)	Experience of change processes in cognitive therapy	UK	5	Grounded theory
Daw and Joseph (2007) CPR (4)	Ts' experience of personal therapy	UK	48	Interpretative phenomenological analysis
Dilks et al. (2010) BJCP (1)	Managing the impact of psychosis	UK	75	Grounded theory
Farber et al. (2004) JCP (3)	Experience of self-disclosure	USA	21	Mixed
Gardner et al. (2009) CPR (1)	Cs' experience of traumatic dreams before, during, and after therapy	UK	5	Tacit thematic analysis
Goodlife et al. (2010) PR (4)	Experience of person-based CT for distressing voice	UK	5 FGs	Grounded theory
Grove (2003) CPR (2)	Gay men's and lesbians' experience of therapeutic help	UK	2 FGs	Constant comparative analysis
Grove and Blasby (2009) CPR (4)	Therapeutic encounter in same-sex couple counseling	UK	9	Thematic Analysis
Hamill et al. (2008) PR (5)	Contribution of therapeutic letters to CAT	UK	8	Thematic analysis
Hanson (2005) CPR (2)	Experience of T disclosure and nondisclosure	CAN	18	Mixed
Harris et al. (2006) PP (1)	Depressed couples' experience of Ts support	UK	9 cpls	Interpretative phenomenological analysis
Henretti et al. (2008) PR (3)	Cs' experience of moments of sadness in therapy	USA	10	Grounded theory
Hodgetts et al. (2007) CPR (3)	Exp of borderline Cs in dialectical behavior therapy	UK	5	Interpretative phenomenological analysis
Huband and Tantam (2004) PP (4)	Pathways to experience of therapy for self-wounding	UK	10	Grounded theory and thematic analysis

(*continued*)

Table 21.1 (continued)

Authors	Focus	Country	*N*	Method
Israel et al. (2008) PR (3)	(+) and (−) therapy experiences of LGBT clients	USA	42	Mixed
King et al. (2006) CPR (3)	Motives for and experience of online counseling	AUSTRL	5 FGs	Consensual qualitative research
Klein and Elliott (2006) PR (1)	Experience of change in process-experiential therapy	USA	10	Mixed
Knox (2008) CPR (3)	Cs' experience of relational depth	UK	14	Grounded theory
Knox et al. (2005) PR (3)	Perspectives on addressing spirituality and religion in therapy	USA	12	Consensual qualitative research
Knox et al. (2009) P (3)	Experience of giving gifts to T	USA	9	Consensual qualitative research
Levitt et al. (2004) JcP (1)	Transformational experience of insight	USA	9	Grounded theory
Mair (2003) CPR (1)	Gay men's experiences of therapy	UK	14	Thematic analysis
Manthei (2007) CPQ (1)	(+) and (−) experiences of counseling	NZ	20	Structured thematic analysis
Martindale et al. (2009) PP (4)	Experiences of confidentiality and informed consent	UK	FG + 12	Interpretative phenomenological analysis
Mayers et al. (2007) CPP (4)	How Cs with religious/spiritual beliefs exp therapy	UK	10	Consensual Thematic Analysis
McGowan et al. PP (4)	Factors in the outcome of CBT for psychosis: C and T views	UK	4 Ts + 8 Cs	Mixed
McMillan et al. (2006) PCEP (4)	Counselor-clients' experience of relational depth	UK	10	Grounded theory
Messari and Hallam BJCP (2)	Experience of CBT for psychosis	UK	5	Discourse analysis
Midgley et al. (2006) PP (2)	Adults' views of the outcome of child psychoanalysis	UK	27	Interpretative phenomenological analysis
Mosher and Stiles (2009) P (4)	Assimilation of experience of the therapist	USA	5	Mixed
Murphy (2009) CPR (1)	Experience of CCT for severe sexual abuse	UK	1	Thematic analysis
Pain et al. (2008) BJCP (2)	C & T exp of case formulation in CBT for psychosis	UK	13 Cs + 5 Ts	Mixed
Pixton (2003) CPR (3)	Experience of gay affirmative therapy	UK	17	Grounded theory
Quereshi (2007) PP (3)	Black male's experience of interracial therapy	SPAIN	1	Hermeneutic phenomenology
Roe et al. (2006) PP (4)	Reasons for terminating therapy	Israel	84	Consensual coding
Timulak (2007) PR (3)	Meta-analysis of C-identified (+) events	SR	7 studies	Tacit thematic analysis
Ward (2005) JCP (4)	African-Americans' experience of therapy	USA	13	Grounded theory
Ward et al. (2008) CPR (2)	Experience of counseling for myalgic encephalitis	UK	25	Thematic analysis
Westra et al. (2010) PR (4)	Clients' expectations and CBT	CAN	18	Consensual grounded theory
Williams and Levitt (2008) PR (3)	Experience of difference with Ts	USA	12	Grounded theory
Wright (2005) CPR (2)	Experience of writing therapy	UK	1	Tacitly reflexive narrative analysis

(*continued*)

Table 21.1 (continued)

Authors	Focus	Country	*N*	Method
Germany and Scandinavian region				
Binder et al. (2009) CPR (4)	Cs' experiences and reflections, successful therapy	NRWY	10	Desc and Hermeneutic phenomenology
Binder et al. (2010) PR (3)	Cs' description of "good outcome" in psychotherapy	NRWY	10	Hermeneutic phenomenology
Conrad and Auckenthaler (2010) PS (1)	Cs' explanation of failure of outpatient psychotherapy	GER	20	Grounded theory
Dundas et al. (2009) CPR (2)	Cs' contributions in cognitive therapy	NRWY	32	Thematic analysis
Lammott et al. (2009) FPA (2)	Sexual offenders reflect on their crimes and biographies	GER	10	Qualitative content analysis
Lilliengren and Werbart (2005) P (3)	Cs' views of (+) and (−) factors in psychoanalysis	SWEDN	22	Grounded theory and qual content analysis
Lindner (2010) PPMP (8)	Psychodynamic hypothesis for suicidality in elderly men	GER	5	Ideal type analysis
Mackrill (2007) CPR (4)	Connection between therapy and Cs exp in other contexts	DNMK	4	Tacit thematic analysis
Mackrill (2008) CPR (3)	Cs' pretreatment change in psychotherapy	DNMK	4	Tacit thematic analysis
Mörtl and Wietersheim (2008) PR (3)	Cs' views of (+) aspects of a day treatment program	GER	26	GT and qualitative content Analysis
Philips et al. (2006) PP (1)	Young adult patients' characteristics at the termination of psychoanalysis	SWEDN	134	Mixed
Plecity et al. (2009) PPMP (9/10)	Cs' experience of art therapy	GER	15	Qualitative content analysis

C client, CBT, cognitive-behavior therapy, CCT, client-centered therapy, Cntry, country, cpls, couples, counselor-client, counselors who were clients, CT, cognitive therapy, CAT, cognitive analytic therapy, desc, descriptive, FG, focus group, GT, Grounded Theory, (+) and (−), helpful and hindering, qual, qualitative, SR, Slovak Republic, T, therapist. For the acronyms of the journals in the first column, see Appendix A

> difficult to share while at the same time feeling understood. My therapist understood and these images are presently addressed and compared with other situations (p. 183).

The main significance of this study is that it now appeared that, in general, clients contribute more actively to the therapeutic relationship than had been thought in the light of earlier studies (e.g., Bachelor et al. 2007; Bedi 2006). In this latest study, it was only clients with the most serious psychological difficulties who depended passively on their therapists to do the therapeutic work.

From the GSR, the study we have chosen reflects a prominent program of qualitative psychotherapy research, namely, the Young Adult Psychotherapy Project (YAPP) conducted by Andrzej Werbart and colleagues (e.g., Philips et al. 2006) of the Institute of Psychotherapy in Stockholm, Sweden. The research program as a whole has involved a naturalistic, prospective mixed-methods approach program entailing, on the one hand, the use of psychometric measures like the Symptom Checklist-90 (SCL-90) (Derogatis 1994), expert rating scales like the Global Assessment of Functioning (GAF; American Psychiatric Association 1994), and interviews, on the other. A sample of 134 patients was used, all of whom were treated with a psychodynamic approach whether in an individual or group setting. The data used for the qualitative part of the study were collected through the use of a method of inquiry called *private theories interview*, developed by Werbart and Levander (2005, 2006). Coming out of this inquiry is a report on 22 interviews conducted at the end of therapy (Lilliengreen and Werbart 2005), which we focus on here.

The report reflects focus on narratives, on examples and episodes bearing on the patients' theories of pathogenesis and therapy, and on their problem formulations and descriptions of changes during and after therapy, including helpful and hindering aspects. Assisted by the software ATLAS.ti (Muhr 2004), the audiotaped and verbatim transcribed interviews were analyzed in the following steps: (1) *focusing on the patient's reports on curative and hindering aspects;* (2) *creating condensates* by reducing the utterances to their essential meaning without losing relevant aspects (a procedure seen as a supplementation of the Grounded Theory method (e.g., Strauss and Corbin 1998) with the application of more precise rules taken from Qualitative Content Analysis (Kracauer 1952)); (3) *coding and conceptualization* entailing open coding, comparisons of codes pursuant to the development of categories which were also compared leading to higher-order categories; and, last but not least (4) *building a theoretical model,* which in this study consisted of 9 categories and 16 subcategories (as another modification of the Grounded Theory method, a core category was not conceptualized).

In this model, *talking about oneself, having a special place and relationship*, and *exploring together with the therapist* are experienced by patients as curative factors, leading to *new relational experiences* and *expanding self-awareness*. Hindering aspects are represented by the categories *Talking is difficult*, and *Something was missing in therapy*, properties of *Self-knowledge is not enough*. For example,

> Of course by meeting and talking about it, going over it, or looking at what happens everyday, one has become a little more aware and sees that it is the same thing that recurs. But I can't really see that I have received any actual help in how I should deal with it. I don't really feel better, unfortunately. (Lilliengreen and Werbart 2005, p. 332)

Both kinds of aspects, of course, are contextualized in the interaction with the therapist.

21.3.2 Practitioners' Experiences of Counseling and Psychotherapy

The 36 articles we have assigned to this topic are given in Table 21.2. Among the many topics addressed under this heading have been the practitioners' experiences of the therapeutic relationship, their views of the roles of spirituality and prayer in counseling and psychotherapy, and their experience of taking risks. In the main, Consensual Qualitative Research, fashioned methods, the Grounded Theory method, Thematic Analysis, and Interpretative Phenomenological Analysis were used. Eleven countries are represented, led by the UK and the USA.

The selected ELR study bearing on this topic was conducted in the USA, directed to European-American therapists' experiences of therapist self-disclosure (TSD) in cross-cultural counseling (Burkard et al. 2006). Therapist self-disclosure was defined as "therapist statements that reveal something personal about therapists" (Hill and Knox 2002, p. 256). Eleven credentialed therapists representing various forms of therapy were recruited. In preparation for a forthcoming interview, they were asked to reflect on the following topics: (1) their overall training in TSD; (2) TSD training in cross-cultural counseling; (3) the quality of the relationship prior to a recalled TSD event; (4) when in the session, the TSD had been offered; (5) the antecedents of the event; (6) the event itself; and (7) its effect. Most of the participants chose TSD events occurring with clients with whom they had good relationships, and these were events that in the participants' judgment had had good outcomes. Except for when a participant was in therapy with one of the four members making up the main research team, the

Table 21.2 Practitioners' experiences of counseling and psychotherapy

Authors	Focus	Cntry	N	Method
English-language region				
Alleyne (2004) CPR (1)	Black identity and workplace oppression	UK	30	Heuristic thematic analysis
Atkins et al. (2004) BJGC (4)	Experience of working with older Cs	UK	7	Heuristic research
Burkhard et al. (2006) JCP (1)	Euro-Amrcn T self-disclosure in cross-cultural cnslng	USA	11	Consensual qualitative research
Carew (2009) CPR (4)	Theoretical background and Ts' attitudes to T self-disclsr	UK	4 FGs	Thematic analysis
Christianson et al. (2009) BJGC (2)	School counselors' experience of client suicide	CAN	12	Consensual qualitative research
Constantine et al. (2004) CPQ (4)	Ts' experience of multicultural counselors	USA	8	Consensual qualitative research
Cooper (2005) CPR (2)	Ts' experiences of relational depth	UK	8	Thematic analysis
Crossley et al. (2005) PP (3)	Counselors' exp of addressing their Cs' spirituality	UK	8	Grounded theory
de Oliveira et al. (2009) JPI (3)	Dealing with upsetting in-session experiences	Brazil	4	Grounded theory
Dunphy et al. (2009) THP (4)	Experience of counseling the bereaved	AUSTRL	2	Thematic analysis
Gubi (2009) CPR (2)	Ethical problems in the use of prayer in cnslng and therapy	UK	8	Interpretative phenomenological analysis
Hewitt et al. (2004) BJGC (4)	Exp of counselors working alone in higher education	UK	8	Thematic analysis
Hill et al. (2008) P (3)	T immediacy in brief therapy: case study II	USA	20	Mixed
Johnson et al. (2007) PR (4)	Exp of working with clients with spiritual problems	USA	12	Consensual qualitative research
Kasper et al. (2008) P (3)	T immediacy in brief therapy: case study I	USA	1	Mixed
R. Knox (2007) BJGC (3)	Experiencing risk in person-centered counseling	UK	8	Heuristic thematic analysis
S. Knox et al. (2003) JCP (2)	Ts' responses to receiving gifts	USA	12	Consensual qualitative research
McPherson et al. (2006) CPR (4)	Working with treatment-resistant depression	UK	4	Interpretative phenomenological analysis
Milner et al. (2003) CPR (2)	How counselors make assessments	UK	18	Tacit thematic analysis
Pugh et al. (2009) PP (3)	Experience of working with an interpreter	UK	10	Interpretative phenomenological analysis
Shaw (2004) PR (3)	Embodied experiencing when conducting therapy	UK	14	Grounded theory
Smith (2003) BJGC (2)	Counselors' fears	UK	10	Constant comparative method
Spangler et al. (2009) PR (1)	Ts' perspectives on their dreams about Cs	USA	8	Consensual qualitative research
Symons et al. (2005) CPR (1)	Managing ethics in psychodynamic counseling	UK	10	Grounded theory
Vivino et al. (2009) PR (2)	(+) and (−) factors in compassion	USA	14	Consensual qualitative research
Westland et al. (2009) PP (4)	Experiences of working with self-deceptive Cs	UK	4	Interpretative phenomenological analysis

(*continued*)

Table 21.2 (continued)

Authors	Focus	Cntry	N	Method
Wright (2009) BJGC (1)	Unfinished business in feminist thnkng in cnslng practice	NZ	1	Tacit autoethnography
Yarrow et al. (2009) CPQ (2)	Exp of working with male sexual trauma survivors	UK	32	Interpretative phenomenological analysis
Germany and Scandinavian region				
Binder et al. (2008a) EJPC (1)	Ts' exp of chllngs in establishing a therapeutic bond	NRWY	9	Modified hermeneutic phenomenology
Binder et al. (2008b) CPR (4)	Ts' exp of alliance ruptures in psychotherapy	NRWY	9	Desc and hermeneutic phenomenology
Davidsen (2009) PP (2)	GPs' processes of understanding patients	DNMK	14	IPA and hermeneutic phenomenology
Lilliengren and Werbart (2010) P (4)	Ts' view of (+) and (−) factors in PA with young adults	SWEDN	16	Grounded theory
Moltu et al. (2010) PR (3)	Ts' recall of successfully resolved impasses with Cs	NRWY	12	Hermeneutic phenomenology
Rober et al. (2008) PR (1)	Ts' reflections during individual therapy sessions	BLGM	12	Grounded theory
Smith et al. (2007) C	Ts' reactions in self-experienced difficult situations	NTHLDS	26	Mixed

C, client, chllngs, challenges, cnslng, counseling, Cntry, country, desc , descriptive, disclsr , disclosure, Euro-Amrcn, European-American, exp, experience, FG, focus group, indvdl, individual, GP, general practitioner, GT , Grounded Theory, (+) and (−) , helpful and hindering, Hrmntc , Hermeneutic, IPA , Interpretative Phenomenological Analysis, PA, psychoanalysis, Pnmlgy , Phenomenology, SD, self-disclosure, T, therapist, thnkng, thinking. For the acronyms of the journals in the first column, see Appendix A

participants were assigned randomly to the members. Each participant was interviewed about the seven topics and given a follow-up interview 2 weeks later.

The resulting transcripts were analyzed with the Consensual Qualitative Research method (Hill et al. 1997). A procedure of this method is conceptualization of domains of experience, whereupon open-ended inquiries are made in terms of these domains. In this study, the domains were set by the seven questions. Also in keeping with the method, analysis of participants' reports pertinent to each domain led to categories conceptualized consensually by a research team. These categories were appraised by an auditor; and the appraisal was taken into account in a further consensus. This team then cross-checked the resulting categories against transcripts left in reserve. The cross-checking was appraised by the auditor and this appraisal was fed into the conceptualization iteratively until consensus of everyone was achieved.

Resulting from this procedure were 18 categories distributed among the seven domains. In keeping with another feature of the method, the applicability of each category to the 11 participants was judged to be either "typical" (applied to at least half of them) or "variant" (applied to at least two but fewer than half); in this study, no category was "general" (applicable to all participants).

An example of a TSD event is the following report of what one participant recalled saying to a client:

> I, too, have witnessed racial discrimination here [on campus], and I have sat with clients who have described such experiences in the classroom, in the residence hall, and in other situations. So I do believe these barriers do exist. I also sense that it was important for you to know my perspective [as a European American person] and whether I believed you that discrimination has occurred for you on this campus.

The participants reported that they had been given little if any training in TSD either generally or in cross-cultural counseling, although TSD had been supported and modeled by their supervisors. The participants recalled that the TSD event had been stimulated either by clients' coping with racism/oppression, therapists' concern about the therapeutic relationship, or their concern that one or more members of their clientele perceived them as complicit in racism. As examples of other returns, among the reasons for using a TSD had been the desire to enhance the counseling relationship; the TSD itself had included the therapists' sharing of their struggles with racist feelings; and an effect of the TSD had been to normalize the client's experience, in the therapist's judgment.

The authors of the study observe that its scope was limited by the preponderance of participants' selection of a client with whom they had a good relationship and for whom their focus on a TSD event that seemed to have had a good effect. The researchers also observe that the reasons the participants gave for their self-disclosures did not necessarily match the disclosures themselves. The investigators call for further inquiry to get a fuller picture. That said, they reasonably conclude that it does seem that TSD is useful, and they encourage faculty members and supervisors to discuss the use of self-disclosure in cross-cultural counseling.

From the GSR, the study we have selected also addressed the psychotherapy relationship. Binder et al. (2008a) interviewed nine psychotherapists from outpatient child and adolescent psychiatric services in Bergen, Norway, focusing on the relationship's specific aspects. The clients of these therapists were between 13 and 18 years in age. The therapists' treatment approaches are described as psychodynamic, systemic, humanistic existential, and/or eclectic. The interviews were semi-structured. A modified hermeneutic phenomenological method was used for data analysis. This method is derived in part from the form of hermeneutics known as philosophical hermeneutics (e.g., Gadamer 1992/1960), a prominent feature of which is the concept of the fusion of a text's and its reader's horizons of understanding, and in part from the Descriptive Phenomenological Psychological method (e.g., Giorgi 1985; Giorgi 2009; Giorgi and Giorgi 2003). Taking these in turn, the philosophical hermeneutic component accordingly prescribes researchers to be concerned with the horizon of the interviewee and to attempt a fusion of that horizon with that of the researcher's taken-as-given assumptions which, now, are reflected upon (Binder et al. 2008b, p. 240). Regarding the Descriptive Phenomenological Psychological method, the transcribed interviews were read carefully; passages of text, called "meaning units" (Giorgi 1979, p. 83), were parsed out of the text as a whole; the passages were transformed into statements relating to the research questions; and the psychological structure of the participants' experience was described.

In the first part of their study, the authors explored how therapists establish a bond with their clients, the bond being one of the three constituents of the working alliance suggested by Bordin (1979). They ascertained that the bond was achieved by (1) transforming the problem into something that can be worked on together, (2) finding a feasible therapist role, (3) motivating the client, (4) establishing a frame for joint meaning making, and (5) handling ambivalence (Binder et al. 2008a). The second part of the study was concerned with problems regarding the working alliance, focusing on the question of how therapists react when they perceive ruptures in the bond and how they handle disagreements about the second and third elements of Bordin's model—goals and tasks. Five strategies used by therapists to restore the alliance when ruptured are described: In the first strategy, the goal is to explore the rupture from the client's point of view. For example,

> I am treating a 17-year old girl who has been physically abused by her boyfriend. It was a really tough kind of violence, so she was rather traumatized when she started up here at the age of 16. For most of the time, she has been ambivalent to treatment. Her ambivalence seems to be strongly related to her doubting if she has the necessary strength to confront and to go further into the things that she has been through ... She seems to think that if she does not go into it, she will just forget it. I think that at one point we were in fairly good contact, but she was afraid of going into things in a way ... and then she wanted to

> come only every third week, and then once a month . . .now she says that she wants to think over whether she is interested at all, and wants to wait for a couple of months . . . (p. 241).

The other strategies for repairing ruptures were as follows: (2) confirming ambivalence and handling it as a choice, (3) establishing a language for fluctuations in clients' experience of motivation and distress, (4) interpreting "not wanting therapy" as a sign of autonomy needs and self-protection, and (5) exploring the reason for the rupture from the therapist's point of view. In their discussion of these results, the main point the authors make is that some of the therapists who were interviewed interpreted such phenomena in the context of specific aspects of individual adolescent development, whereas others understood them as a result of interpersonal dynamics in the client-therapist relationship (Binder et al. 2008b).

21.3.3 Counseling and Psychotherapy Process and Outcome

This is our third topic, with 55 articles sorted into it and listed in Table 21.3. There it can be seen that qualitative researchers have studied the process and outcome of many approaches to therapy, especially cognitive-behavior therapy, person-centered and experiential therapies, and psychoanalytically oriented therapies. The experience and impact of therapies on those suffering from several disturbances and psychological disorders have come under examination as well. In addition, the studies have given attention to clients' and therapists' personal accounts of experience and have provided detailed analyses of their conversations with each other—studies that often have interesting implications for the working alliance.

In this line of research, the mixed-methods approach has played an important role, as in, for example, the application of assimilation analysis (Stiles et al. 1990; see above). The Grounded Theory method has been employed to a fair extent as well, followed by conversation analysis and a motley group of other methods. Fourteen countries are represented in the table, led by the UK, the USA, and Germany.

The article selected from the ELR reports a study done in the UK by Fitzpatrick et al. (2010) on participants' experiences of the effects of an 8-week course in mindfulness-based cognitive therapy (MBCT; Segal et al. 2002). We feel that clients' experience of cognitive therapies has been given insufficient attention and so are attracted to this study. The participants in it suffered from Parkinson's disease. To aid his understanding of the MBCT course, the first author of the study took one of its offerings. Twelve people (average age 66) were interviewed before and after another offering of the course. In the post-treatment interview, they were asked about their experience of both the course in general and specific mindfulness techniques.

Interpretative Phenomenological Analysis (IPA; Smith 1996; Smith and Osborne 2003) was applied to the transcribed interviews. Fitzpatrick read the transcripts several times, making note of interesting comments out of which themes were conceptualized. Those themes developed in the analysis of the initial transcripts were used iteratively to guide the interpretation of later transcripts. Also, eight of the transcripts were analyzed by the second author.

The authors make the point that, in keeping with IPA, the latter analysis was done to appraise the coherence and transparency of the first author's interpretation; it did not involve independent coding by the second author pursuant to consensual agreement on themes. The themes coming out of the analysis were compared with the themes described in other studies of people's experience of Parkinson's disease (e.g., McDonald et al. 2003; Nijohf 1995).

Four major themes were gleaned from the participants' accounts: (1) changing patterns of coping (this is constituted of three sub-themes, which we do not include here); (2) the role of mindfulness in consolidating existing coping skills in the context of loss, "You have to be mindful with Parkinson's anyway"; (3) group support in the context of loss and a society that stigmatizes difference, "It was like one big

Table 21.3 Counseling and psychotherapy process and outcome

Authors	Focus	Cntry	N	Method
English-language region				
Boyd (2007) *CPR* (2)	Impact of Ts dream on a deaf C	UK	1	Tacit narrative analysis
Brinegar et al. (2006) *JCP* (2)	Building a meaning bridge	USA/ CAN	2	Mixed
Brinegar et al. (2008) *PR* (6)	"Lisa" and the assimilation model	USA	1	Mixed
Caro (2004) *CPQ* (4)	Linguistic change in linguistic therapy of evaluation	SPAIN	6	Mixed
Caro Gabalda (2005) *CPP*	Convergence of voices in linguistic thrpy of evaluation	SPAIN	1	Mixed
Carvalho et al. (2008) *CPR* (3)	Recovery from paranoid personality disorder	PRTGL	1	Mixed
Daniel and McLeod (2006) *CPR* (4)	PCT counselors' evaluations of their effectiveness	UK	6	Grounded theory
Detert et al. (2006) *PR* (4)	Assimilation in good and poor outcome in brief therapy for mild depression	UK/USA	8	Mixed
Dilks et al. (2008) *PP* (2)	Therapy processes in psychosis	UK	6	Grounded theory
Elliott et al. (2009) *PR* (4)	Study of experiential therapy for panic/phobia	USA	1	Mixed
Fitzpatrick et al. (2010) *PP* (2)	Parkinson Cs' experience of mindfulness-based CT	UK	12	Interpretative phenomenological analysis
Gazzola et al. (2004) *JPI* (4)	T interpretations and C processes in 3 therapies	CAN/ GRC	4 session x 3 therapies	Consensual qualitative research
Glaesner (2008) *CPQ* (4)	(+) and (−) factors in forgiveness	Kenya	15 Ts	Thematic analysis
Goodrich and Hardy (2009) *PR* (1)	Patterns of sudden gains in CBT	UK	5	Mixed
Hayward and Fuller (2010) *CPP*	Perspectives of various stakeholders on Cs who hear voices	UK	9	Interpretative phenomenological analysis
Henry et al. (2005) *CPQ* (2)	Loss and mourning in immigration	USA	3	Mixed
Humphreys et al. (2005) *CPQ* (2)	Assimilation of anger by C with dissociative identity disorder	USA	1	Mixed
S. Knox et al. (2008) *PR* (2)	Attainment of insight in dream sessions	USA	2	Mixed
Levitt et al.(2006) *JCP* (3)	Principles of what Cs find helpful in therapy	USA	26 Cs	Grounded theory
Levitt and Williams (2010) *PR* (3)	Therapy principles derived from Ts' values	USA	14 Ts	Grounded theory
Lysaker et al.(2007) *CPR* (2)	Relationship and technique in a 22-month integrative therapy of schizophrenia	USA	1	Mixed
Macdonald et al. (2007) *PP* (2)	C & T interaction in an alcohol service	UK	3 Ts, 6 Cs	Mixed

(*continued*)

Table 21.3 (continued)

Authors	Focus	Cntry	N	Method
Madill et al. (2005) *PR* (4)	Interactional positioning and narrative self-construction in psychodynamic-interpersonal therapy	UK	4	Narrative analysis
McGowan et al. (2005) *PP* (4)	Cs' and Ts' views of the outcome of CBT for psychosis	UK	4 Ts, 8 Cs	Grounded theory
Neimeyer etal. (2006) *JcP* (2)	Integration of traumatic loss	USA/ SPAIN	1	GT analysis of 12 T sessions
Orchowski et al. (2009) *PR* (3)	Emotional disclosure by survivors of intimate partner assault	USA	2	Mixed
Siegel et al.(2010) *PR* (4)	Change in affective scripts	USA	1	Mixed
Spong (2007) *BJGC* (3)	Counselors talk about influencing Cs	UK	6 FGs	Discourse analysis
Strong (2005) *BJGC* (4)	Understanding in counseling	CAN	6 Ts, 11 Cs	Ethnomethodology and conversation analysis
Strong and Nielson (2008) *CPR* (4)	Constructive conversations	CAN	18 Ts, 32 Cs	Constant comparative method
Timulak and Elliott (2003) *PR* (4)	Empowerment events in PET	SR	9 Cs; 12 events	Tacit thematic analysis
Van Vliet (2008) *JCP* (2)	Shame and resilience in adulthood	CAN	139	Grounded theory
Vlasto (2010) *CPR* (1)	Ts' views of + and – effects of group vs. indvdl cnslng	UK	9	Grounded theory
D. Williams and Levitt (2007) *PR* (1)	Principles for facilitating agency in therapy	USA	14 Ts	Grounded theory
D. Williams and Levitt (2007) *JPI* (2)	Ts' negotiating value conflicts with Cs	USA	14 Ts	Grounded theory
R. Williams et al. (2009) *CPR* (2)	Processes in in-line counseling	AUSTRL	85 Cs	Mixed
Yurdakul et al. (2009) *PP* (4)	Perceived changes associated with autogenic training	UK	12	Grounded theory
German and Scandinavian region				
Brandestini et al. (2010) *PS* (1)	Ts' expltn of psychoanalysis in intake interviews	SWTZLD	5 Ts; 8 Cs	Qualitative content analysis
Depperman et al. (2008) *PS* (1)	Process of therapy termination if the "Amalie" case	GER	1	Conversation analysis
Grande (2007) *PPMP* (2)	Dysfunctional relationship patterns in T-C interaction	GER	1	Mixed
Grothe (2005) *ZPPM* (1)	Indication for regular psychotherapy vs. short-term intervention for acutely traumatized Cs	GER	30	Mixed case study
Jakobsen et al. (2007) *PS* (1)	Understanding therapeutic process	SWTZLD	2	Comparative case analysis
Lepper and Mergenthaler (2005) *PR* (4)	Therapy group cohesion	UK/GER	7 (group)	Mixed
Lepper and Mergenthaler (2007) *PR* (5)	Interactional level of therapeutic collaboration	UK/GER	1	Mixed

(*continued*)

Table 21.3 (continued)

Authors	Focus	Cntry	N	Method
Lepper and Mergenthaler (2008) *PR* (6)	Idntfcn and analysis of clin sgnfcnt interactions	UK/GER	1	Mixed
Mackrill (2008) *BJGC* (4)	Interplay between Cs' strategies and Ts' responses	DNMK	1	Tacit thematic analysis
Nilsson et al. (2007) *PR* (5)	Quality of change in CBT vs. psychodynamic thrpy	SWEDN	3	GT and qualitative content analysis
Overbeck et al. (2004) *PPMP* (2)	Effect of a combined treatment of OCD	GER	32	Case study and fMRI
Peräkylä (2004) *PR* (3)	Ts' interpretations linking domains of Cs' exp	SWTZLD	1	Conversation analysis
Ruff and Leikert (2003) *PS* (2)	Transfer of changes thru therapy to everyday life	GER	6 Cs (3 Ts)	Ideal Type Analysis
Saladin and Grimmer (2009) *PS* (1)	WA and cooperation in psychoanalytic intake intrvws	SWTZLD	15	Conversation analysis
Schouler-Ocak et al. (2008) *PPMP* (3/4)	Influence of culture-specific factors on trauma-focused therapy	GER	7	Case study
Storm (2010) *FPA* (3)	Trtmnt of an eating disorder in parent-infant thrpy	GER	2	Case study
Streeck (2009) *PS* (1)	Control, projective identification, and course of action in therapeutic conversation	GER	1	Conversation analysis
Viklund et al. (2010) *PR* (2)	Handling disagreement in T-C interaction	SWEDN	7 dyads	Conversation analysis

C, client; CBT, cognitive-behavior therapy; clin, clinically; exp, experience; Cntry, country; expltn, explanation; idntfcn, identification; GRC, Greece; GT, Grounded Theory; (+) and (−), helpful and hindering; indvdl, individual; intrvws, interviews; PCT, person-centered therapy; PET, process-experiential therapy; PRTGL, Portugal; sgnfcnt, significant; SPN, Spain; T, therapist; thrpy, therapy; trtmnt, treatment. For the acronyms of the journals in the first column, see Appendix A

family kind of thing, because we all have something in common"; and (4) the dualism of experience of Parkinson's compared to mindful meditation, "Very calm and peaceful, yeah you're sort of on a different level."

As indicated by the attention given to it by the researchers, the first theme was the most salient and so we shall focus on it to give a sense of what the researchers came to understand. The participants reported that upon the onset of their illness, they had tended to withdraw from social activities. It had been embarrassing for them to be in company when their hands were shaking, and to go to dinner when they could not use cutlery adequately. Having taken the MBCT course, 5 of the 12 participants reported being able to confront embarrassing situations they had previously avoided, one remarking:

> I was coping with things before but I'm coping better. I don't like going among people to dine, because my hands are not good. My husband has to cut the meat up if I have meat but it was my 70th birthday...and that's [i.e., the MBCT intervention] given me the courage to go, where one time I wouldn't have...I would have backed out of these things but I felt good just being one of the party. I felt so relaxed with and I had fish so no one had to cut it up.

Among other returns, the participants reported that the course reduced worry about their symptoms, which had had the happy effect of reducing the symptoms themselves. Throughout their report of the outcome of the course, the authors support their themes with similar ones reported in the literature (e.g., Mackenzie et al. 2007; Mason and Hargreaves 2001), to compensate for having addressed just one MBCT group and in the absence of a control group.

In contrast with the ELR, in the GSR, systematic studies on process factors contributing to good outcome are still limited in psychotherapy research. One of the reasons for this might be that, compared to those in the ELR, researchers in the GSR are more inclined to endorse the argument that, although qualitative research provides access to the dimensions of meaning and experience, it does not enable the exact prediction and statistical generalization characteristic of quantitative research methods. In this regard, it is not surprising that cooperation among qualitative and quantitative researchers in joint projects has taken place, exemplifying this form of mixed methods.

One of these projects listed in Table 21.3 was a joint British-German one involving a combined qualitative conversation analysis and software-based quantitative content analysis of text provided by clients engaged in psychotherapy. The aim of this study by Lepper and Mergenthaler (2005) was to identify and describe crucial moments bearing on cohesion in psychodynamic group therapy. The subject matter was the transcript of session 9 of such a therapy, involving a group of seven women suffering from eating disorders. In Mergenthaler's part of the study, employed was a computer-assisted text analysis program based on standardized dictionaries, the words of which denote *emotional tone* on the one hand and *abstraction* on the other. The program counts the frequencies of words in blocks of 150 words and relates them to each of these two categories. It also represents the relationships graphically. The *Therapeutic Cycles Model* developed by Mergenthaler (1996) differentiates four patterns of discursive activity: *relaxing* (low emotion and low abstraction), *experiencing* (high emotion and low abstraction), *reflecting* (low emotion and high abstraction), and *connecting* (high emotion and high abstraction). Lepper's contribution to the study was inspired by the method of conversation analysis as developed by Harvey Sacks (see Silverman 1998), and introduced to psychotherapy research by Madill and Barkham (1997) and Streeck (Frommer et al. 2004; Streeck 2004). This method involves analysis of conversations from one speaking turn to the next, by both drawing on and developing categories and procedural rules of turn-taking. It thus is directed to how the interacting persons construct coherent talk. Questions such as *What is being talked about?* are addressed in the context of questions like *Who is talking? How are the speakers linking their contributions to previous turns? How do they handle and repair breaks in conversation? How are joint topics developed in dialogues and multiparty talks?* And so on.

In his model, Mergenthaler hypothesizes that the ideal therapeutic cycle is defined by a sequence of relaxing, experiencing, connecting, reflecting, and again relaxing. As a minimum condition for a successful therapeutic cycle, he identifies the presence of connecting within the frame of relaxing. Accordingly, he expected the conversation analytic part of the present study to confirm that:

> The three components of topic coherence – content, participation, and sequential structure – would be at their richest in the cycles, that is, that cycles would be topic rich, participation would be high, and tying between word blocks would be high (Lepper and Mergenthaler 2005, p. 440).

Lepper's qualitative research part of the study supported this hypothesis in that she provides evidence that the cycles indeed are indicators of high levels of therapeutic engagement, identified through conversation analysis as interaction sequences with high topic coherence, which are interpreted as markers of high group cohesion. Another contribution of the conversation analytic component of this study was its use to focus on deviant cases characterized by sequences of abstraction and emotion which did not support the therapeutic cycle. Lepper shows that in Word Blocks 28 and 29 of the transcript, a therapeutic cycle was interrupted when a client who had the floor in the group suddenly exited from the topic of feelings to the abstract and the distant topic of economic climate. In this situation, the therapist interrupted this departure to restore the client's preferred topic "your feelings" (p. 440), whence a multiparty including the group members addressed the client's defensiveness, thereby bringing the cycle successfully to an end, as recorded in Blocks 36–38 of the transcript.

21.3.4 Supervision, Training, and Professional Development

This is our fourth topic, summarized in Table 21.4. Among the 26 studies listed there, half were focused on supervision, a third on training, and the remainder on professional development. The three most frequently used methods were Consensual Qualitative Research, authoethnography, and Grounded Theory. Noteworthy are the contribution of UK researchers to this topic (a little over half of the studies) and the dearth of studies of it in the GSR. The British interest comes especially from the large British Association for Counselling and Psychotherapy, most members of which have backgrounds in the fields other than psychology and have been moving toward making their discipline a regulated profession: This group has been responding to encouragement to do research by taking up qualitative research methods and applying them to their own work (Rennie 2004). The result sometimes has been a personal account of experience, enabled especially through the use of autoethnography and heuristic research methods. We have selected from the table a study from the UK illustrating such engagement of subjectivity.

In this account of becoming a counselor and counselor trainer, Meekums (2008) tells her story of being afflicted with polio when she was three, of her close relationship with her father who massaged her legs tirelessly making them well and who supported her thereafter, of being bullied by peers when an early teen, and of having a passion for dancing. In her account, these experiences are used to illustrate her embodied experience of herself both emotionally and as an agent. Drawing on her poems, on reflections written on scraps of paper, and on archived photographs and other memorabilia, she observes that she has the multiple identities of a wounded dancer, an embodied wordsmith, and a passionate scientist. She provides tables listing the key events and activities making up the timelines of each of these identities.

Meekums engaged both postmodern theory (Beckett and Hager 2002) and theory about the role of embodied experiencing as a source of wisdom (e.g., Corrigal et al. 2006; Lakoff and Johnson 1980). In terms of method, she incorporated ethnography (Sparkes 2002), autoethnography (Berger 2001), the use of reflexivity in inquiry (Richardson 2000), the researchers' use of experiential indwelling (Moustakas 1990), and narrative inquiry (Etherington 2003; McLeod 1997). These influences collectively were integrated into an application of her version of autoethnography, seen as an analysis of one's embodied life situated in culture.

In the article, she illustrates with a poem what it was like at the age of three to be a patient in an isolation ward when she had the polio. The opening lines of the poem are the following:

> My body hurts
> It can't be mine
> It doesn't move
> When I tell it to
> I call the nurse
> *Nurse*
> *Nurse*
> No sound comes out
> I turn my head
> Outside, a tree
> My sister waits
> My lovely sister
> Waves at me
> I long to touch her plaited hair (p. 293)

She includes other poems about being bullied, feeling oppressed sexually when 13 because of the way she dressed, and what it meant to be a girl. She also provides a series of memories of her relationship with her father from when he was 45 to 85. The overall point of the article is summed up in the following passage:

> The stories I narrate here show that, despite the gender discourses, class discourses and peer abuse that worked to disempower me and hold me down and back, I learned that I was indeed strong and

Table 21.4 Supervision, training, and professional development

Authors	Focus	Cntry	N	Method
English-language region				
Bang and Park (2009) TCP 8	Korean SVRs' experiences in clinical supervision	Korea	11	Grounded theory
Benson et al. (2005) QRIP (2)	How clinical supervisors evaluate trainees	USA	15	Dimensional analysis
Burkard et al.(2006) JCP (3)	SVR responsiveness in cross-cultural supervision	USA	13	Consensual qualitative research
Chen (2004) CPQ (2)	Exp of cultural transition in non-Western TRNRs	UK	1	Narrative analysis
Crocket et al. (2009) CPR 2	Informing supervision through research	NZ	6	Mixed
de Stefano et al. (2007) CPR (1)	Trainees' impasses and impact of group supervision	CAN	8	Consensual qualitative research
Gazzola et al. (2007) BJGC (2)	SVSEEs' broadening and narrowing experiences	CAN	10	Consensual qualitative research
Goddard et al. (2008) PP (2)	Ts' views of informed consent and therapy	UK	9	Interpretative phenomenological analysis
Gubi (2007) CPR (2)	CLRs using prayer in cnslng exp of supervision	UK	19	Interpretative phenomenological analysis
Hess et al. (2008) PR (4)	Interns' nondisclosure in supervision	USA	14	Consensual qualitative research
Hill et al. (2007) PR (4)	Exp of novice TRNRs in a beginng graduate class	USA	5	Consensual qualitative research
Hoffman et al. (2005) JCP (1)	SVRs' views of the impacts of varieties of feedback	UK	15	Consensual qualitative research
Knox et al. (2008) PR (5)	SVRs' reports of the effects of SVR S-D on SVSEEs	USA	16	Consensual qualitative research
Lees (2003) CPR (2)	Developing T self-understanding through research	UK	1	Tacit autoethnography
McKenzie-Mavinga (2005) CPR (4)	Understanding black issues in counselor training	UK	3	Tacit autoethnography
Meekums (2008) BJGC (3)	Embodied narratives in becoming a cnslng trainer	UK	1	Autoethnography
Moore and Ray (2009) CPQ (4)	Cnslng psychologists' constructions of themselves	UK	8	Discourse analysis
Murphy (2005) CPR (1)	Exp of mandatory personal therapy in training	UK	5 FGs	Constant comparative analysis
Nelson et al. (2008) JCP (2)	Working with conflict in clinical supervision	USA	12	Grounded theory and CQR
Paris et al. (2006) JMFT (1)	Mrrg and fmly therapy interns' exp of growth	USA	19	Grounded theory
Pattison (2003) CPR (2)	Exp of TRNRs in an international training program	UK	12	Grounded theory
Robson et al.(2006) CPR (3)	Reflections on a telephone supervision relationship	UK	2	Thematic analysis
Turner et al. (2008) CPR (3)	Impact of C work on trainee therapists	UK	2	Heuristic research
Valance (2004) BJGC (4)	TRNRs' perceptions and supervision impact on Cs	UK	19	Phenomenology[a]
Van Rijn et al. (2008) CPR (4)	Training in transactional analysis	UK	11	Mixed

(*continued*)

Table 21.4 (continued)

Authors	Focus	Cntry	N	Method
West et al. (2004) CPR (2)	SVR and SVSEE experience of supervision	UK	3 dyads	Heuristic research
German and Scandinavian region				
Jacobsen (2007) CPR (1)	Parallel processes in therapy and supervision	DNMK	1	Exploratory single case
Will (2006) FPA (2)	Psychoanalytic competences in training and practice	GER	30	Qualitative content analysis

beginng, beginning; C, client; cnslng, counseling; CLR, counselor; exp, experience; Cntry, country; CQR, Consensual qualitative research; fmly, family; FG, focus group; GT, Grounded theory; mrrg, marriage; S-D, self-disclosure; SVSEE, supervisee; SVR, supervisor; T, therapist; TRNR, trainer. For the acronyms of the journals in the first column, see Appendix A

[a]Following McLeod (1994)

> capable both physically and socially. This can be summarized in terms of first their relevance to me as a counsellor/psychotherapist and then their relevance to me as a counsellor trainer. The wounded healer stories link me powerfully with the world of counselling, but perhaps the powerful body stories link me with the world of the trainer, who must embody a leadership role (p. 298).

In her conclusion, Meekums observes that it is her hope that she has achieved Richardson's (2000) criteria of contribution to understanding, aesthetic merit, reflexivity, emotional or intellectual impact, and lived experience. She also hopes that her narrative speaks powerfully to others in the way that novels and poems can.

Turning to the GSR, on the whole, little attention has been given to the topic of training and professional development, especially in psychoanalytic contexts. Nevertheless, in an ongoing study organized by psychoanalytic training candidates of the German Psychoanalytic Society (DPG), investigators have tried to address, through a systematic inquiry, the issue of supervision. The research questions that were asked have to do with (1) how supervisor and supervised candidate match, (2) influences of the social and institutional frame, (3) types of supervision styles co-constructed by the supervision dyad, (4) satisfaction/dissatisfaction of supervision work, (5) crises and collapse, and (6) helpful/blocking relationship experiences in supervision. The research participants are supervisors as well as supervised training candidates. Both standardized and open-ended questionnaires are used (Nagell et al. 2009). Data analytic methods and results are forthcoming.

21.3.5 Professional Practice Issues, the Public View of Counseling and Psychotherapy, and Practitioners' Self-Care

The 26 articles bearing on this our final topic are shown in Table 21.5. They address an interesting assortment of studies on matters such as ethics, referrals, perceptions of counseling and psychotherapy in the public domain, lifestyles of practitioners, and cultural and migration factors in immigrants' therapy. Among the three constituents of the topic, professional practice issues make up half of the studies, public views of counseling and psychotherapy account for over a third, while a few have been directed to practitioners' self-care. A variety of methods were used, the most common being Thematic Analysis and versions of the Grounded Theory method. Seven countries are represented, dominated by the UK.

An ELR study selected under this topic is one from the UK bearing on its National Health Service (NHS). We have chosen it as a good example of how qualitative research can be carried into action in the field. At the time of this study (Snape et al. 2003), its lead author was a physician interested in mental health who worked in

Table 21.5 Professional practice issues, the public view of counseling and psychotherapy, and practitioners' self-care

Authors	Focus	Cntry	N	Method
English-language region				
Athanasiades (2008) BJGC (3)	Factors affecting self-referral in the workplace	UK	11	Grounded theory
Ballinger et al. (2007) CPR (3)	Social class and counseling	UK	9 (group)	Cooperative inquiry
Ben-Ari and Somer (2004) CPP (p. 126f)	Aftermath for the C of T–C sex	UK	14	Consensual constant comparative analysis
Boulton et al. (2007) CPR (3)	Ss' views of their school peer cnslng for bullying	ISRAEL	99	Mixed
Cocksedge et al. (2006) CPR (2)	GPs' views of referring patients to counselors practicing in primary care	UK	28	Grounded theory
Cormack (2009) CPR (2)	Homeless young people's views of counseling	UK	2 FGs[a]	Grounded theory
Cromarty et al. CPR (3)	How 2ndary school cnslrs work with other prfssnls	UK	4 FGs	Thematic analysis
Dhillon et al. (2003) CPR (1)	Implications for therapy of South Asian men's reports on their acculturation and ethnic identity	UK	32	IPA
DiGiorgio et al. (2004) JPI (3)	How Ts integrate EMDR into their orientations	USA	3	Consensual qualitative research
Evans et al. (2008) BJGC (3)	High school cnslrs' reflections on support and self-care	NZ	6	Tacit thematic analysis
Grafanaki et al. (2005) CPQ (1)	Role of leisure in the life of cnslrs and psychlgsts	CAN	10	Consensual constant comparative analytic procedure of GT
Jennings et al. (2008) PR (5)	Psychotherapy expertise in Singapore	USA and SNPR	9	Grounded theory
Manthei (2006) BJGC (4)	Cs' experience of seeking counseling	NZ	20	Structured thematic analysis
Millar (2003) CPR (1)	Men's exp of considering counseling	UK	10	Grounded theory
Newman and Nolas (2008) CPR (3)	Exp with NVR as an approach with violent youth	UK	FG	Discourse analysis
Quinn et al. (2009) BJGC (4)	Students' exp of mental health support in higher education	UK	12 + FG + web space	Thematic analysis
Reynolds et al. (2008) CPQ (3)	Narratives of therapeutic art-making in the context of marital breakdown	UK	3	Narrative analysis
Rizq et al. (2008) BJGC (2)	Meaning and sgnfcnc for Ts of their personal thrpy	UK	9	IPA
Snape et al. (2003) CPR (3)	Ps' accounts of why they didn't take up a referral	UK	49	Tacit thematic analysis
Thériault et al. (2006) CPQ (4)	Sources of feelings of incompetence in experienced Ts	CAN	8	Grounded theory

(*continued*)

Table 21.5 (continued)

Authors	Focus	Cntry	N	Method
Timlin-Scalera et al. (2003) JCP (3)	Help-seeking among white male high school			
students, parents, and staff	USA	26 + 4 + 5	Grounded theory	
German and Scandinavian region				
Behrens and Calliess (2008) PPMP (3/04)	Culture- vs. migration-related factors in therapy	GER	55	Qualitative content analysis
Erhardt et al. (2010) PS (1)	Match between conflict and structure diagnosis and OPD ratings	GER	19	Mixed
Klöß-Rotmann et al. (2009) FPA (1)	Gender prototypes in psychoanalytic case reports	GER	5	Mixed
Küchenhoff et al. (2004) ZPMP (3)	Discrepancies between C and expert ratings regarding environmentally related disorders	GER	61	Mixed
Trosbach and Geister (2010) PPMP (3/4)	Relatives' views of life with an OCD patient	GER	22	Grounded theory

[a]C, client; cnslng, counseling; cnslrs, counselors; Cntry, country; EMDR, Eye Movement Desensitization Reprocessing; FG, focus group; IPA, Interpretative Phenomenological Analysis; GP, general practitioner; GT, Grounded Theory; NVR, nonviolent resistance; OCD, obsessive-compulsive disorder; OPD, Operationalized Psychodynamic Diagnostics; prfssnls, professionals; psychlgsts, psychologists; 2ndary, secondary; SNPR, Singapore; sgnfcnc, significance; S, subject; T, therapist; thrpy, therapy. For the acronyms of the journals in the first column, see Appendix A

primary care in the National Health Service (NHS); the other authors were a counselor, an experienced qualitative researcher, and an academic with research interest in counseling in primary care. The study addressed why people do not take up physicians' referrals to counseling. Participants were recruited through 18 NHS counseling organizations providing services either in general practitioner surgeries or psychology clinics. The researchers conducted five pilot interviews, in the light of which they arranged for the organizations to send out 224 invitation letters to people for whom between a month and a year had elapsed since they had failed to engage their appointment. This procedure resulted in interviews with 17 people and receipt of written comments by 27 others. More women than men responded. The questions asked covered 10 topics such as: knowledge, previous experience and information about counseling, stigma, medication, urgency, and both waiting times and timing of appointments. The interviews lasted up to 50 min. A Thematic Analysis was applied to the transcripts of the 5 pilot interviews, the 17 additional ones, and the written comments sent in by the 24 other participants. No details are given on how this analysis was conducted.

In the researchers' understanding, the main reason participants gave for not following through on the appointment had to do with *time*. Waiting time had been a big concern: This could be as long as a year, but for people urgently wishing an appointment, even 10 days had been too long. Having the appointment scheduled in working hours had also been problematic because for some participants it had been embarrassing to have to explain to their employer why they would have to leave work for a couple of hours. In addition, among the themes other than time were: positive impact of the referral consultation, lack of information, self-image, views of counseling, and organizational aspects. The investigators illustrate constituents of these themes. For example, in terms of the theme of time, during the waiting period, some people either had sought counseling elsewhere or had done something constructive such as exercise or work, while others had felt unsupported, let down, and uncertain. Thus, when reflecting on having been given no information about how long he or she would have to wait, a participant remarked,

> That's a big thing and for them to say, "Right, well we're going to refer you" and even if you've just received a letter saying you're on the waiting list and then that's it, it's like, "Hello, do you know I'm here?" Have they remembered me? (p. 241).

The researchers observe that several revelations were rather surprising given what the literature had led them to expect. These surprises included people's sense of responsibility for their own recovery, how active many people were while waiting for the appointment, people's need for information, and the extent to which getting a referral in and of itself was therapeutic. A notable feature of this study is that it was carried forward into action research wherein the first author both informed her fellow physicians of the results and took steps to institute changes in the practices of the clinic where she worked.

Finally, from Germany comes a report on a mixed-methods study using written treatment records of 55 psychiatric day-clinic patients of Hannover University, addressing the impact of migration backgrounds on diagnostic processes and therapy (Behrens and Calliess 2008). These researchers differentiated between what they call "culture-related" and "migration-related" aspects. The former were influences of specific values, behavior norms, and religious attitudes of the ethnic community to which a person belonged, while the latter were effects of moving from one country to another (e.g., absence of family members, problems with legal status). The data analysis was conducted within the framework of categories developed deductively from the above theoretical preconceptions. In the interest of inter-rater reliability, the researchers tried to ensure that attribution of verbal data to categories was free from idiosyncratic influences of the raters' individuality. Results presented quantitatively showed that aspects due to migration such as feelings of loss of home country and conflicts regarding wishes of going back to it caused nearly twice as many problems as did aspects due to culture, such as either conflicts about the traditional gender roles or religious convictions.

21.4 Discussion

As reflected by the entries in the tables organizing the returns from our survey, among our five topics, according to our categorization of the 208 articles, qualitative research and mixed-methods research have been applied most to the study of the processes and outcomes of counseling and psychotherapy and to clients' experiences of engagement in treatment. Following these applications, roughly equal attention has been given to practitioners' experiences of engaging in treatment; matters bearing on supervision, training, and professional development; and professional practice issues, the public view of counseling and psychotherapy, and practitioners' self-care. To some extent, there have been differences between what we have called the English-language region and the German-Scandinavian region. This disparity is most apparent in the studies coming out of Britain, where there has been comparatively more application of qualitative research to training and supervision, reflecting the emergence of counseling and psychotherapy there as a professional discipline separate from psychology and related disciplines. In contrast, in the GSR, the study of supervision and training falls behind the study of counseling and psychotherapy process and outcome, by a large margin.

The emphasis given to clients' experiences of treatment and to the process and outcome of counseling and psychotherapy maintains the role qualitative research has played in illuminating clients' agency in the production of treatment effects. Such findings in our view help to explain the common finding that although all forms of counseling and psychotherapy have been demonstrated to be more effective than no treatment, to a surprising extent they are not differentially effective among themselves (e.g., Wampold 2001). Correspondingly, we would hope that someday in the future research findings such as these will be taken into account when practice-based evidence of treatment is assessed (cf. Cahill et al. 2010).

In terms of methodology, we observe a continuation of a swing toward objectivism reflected in the concern for inter-judge agreements in terms of qualitative research methods in and of themselves, as in the Consensual Qualitative Research method, for example, as well as in the increasing mixing of qualitative and quantitative methods. In this respect, the willingness of British researchers to disclose their own experiences of various topics is a welcome stand against this tide. After all, it is the revelation of the subjective involvement in experience and action that is the forte of qualitative research, and it would be unfortunate if, over the long run, it should get diluted in response to perceived cultural calls for objectivity. As an example of this drift, in the study by Behrens and Calliess (2008) described above, these researchers took pains to ensure that the development of categories from verbal data was free from idiosyncratic influences of the raters' individuality. In the process, the study that was announced and begun as a qualitative enterprise shifted to a quantitative or "semiquantitative" (Frommer and Faller 1994) study, seeking a foothold in numbers even though understanding of subjectivity is in demand. An alternative approach would have been to apply a content analysis more adherent to phenomenology and hermeneutics, resulting in educed categories organized by, perhaps, Weber's "ideal type" concept, an alternative that may have led to deeper results—deeper, but with the appearance of being more subjective, which is the rub.

The matter of appearances brings into play, of course, rhetoric and, going with it, the given audience to which it is addressed. Entrance into subjectivity, be it the author's own and/or that of someone whom the author is addressing, may resonate with readers, including practitioners, more than does a report of the same phenomenon taken from a more external stance. Alternatively, the same subjectivity may be frowned upon by power brokers in society, whether journal reviewers and editors under the sway of objectivism or government policy makers worried about fiscal accountability.

Another feature of qualitative research that goes against the grain of rhetoric suitable for its power-broker audience is its particularity. Its sensitivity to context makes for precision of meaning, but at the expense of constrained generality. Still, that same particularity enhances the possibility that the reader may relate to the understanding which this kind of qualitative research provides, making it persuasive on this ground.

In conclusion, our review indicates that the application of qualitative and mixed-methods research to a variety of topics in counseling and psychotherapy continues to burgeon, and many interesting and informative understandings have been the result. In many quarters, but not all, there has been a drift toward an increased positive valuing of objectivity. It is our hope that this drift does not go so far as to compromise the richness of the understandings of the meaning of experience and action that qualitative research can provide.

Acknowledgements We are grateful for the help by Mathias Wahl and Swantje Ferchow, members of Jörg Frommer's current students' research group, who supported the German and Scandinavian literature search and manuscript formatting.

Appendix A: List of Journals and Their Acronyms

British Journal of Clinical Psychology (BJCP)
British Journal of Guidance and Counselling (BJGC)
Clinical Psychology and Psychotherapy (CPP)
Counselling Psychology Quarterly (CPQ)
Counselling and Psychotherapy Research (CPR)
European Journal of Psychotherapy and Counselling (EJPC)
Forum der Psychoanalyse (FPA)

Journal of Constructivist Psychology (JcP)
Journal of Counseling Psychology (JCP)
Journal of Marital and Family Therapy (JMFT)
Journal of Psychotherapy Integration (JPI)
Psychotherapy (P)
Psychology and Psychotherapy: Theory, Research and Practice (PP)
Psychotherapie, Psychosomatik,Medizinische Psychologie (PPMP)
Psychotherapy Research (PR)
Psychotherapie und Sozialwissenschaft (PS)
Qualitative Research in Psychology (QRIP)
The Counselling Psychologist (TCP)
The Humanistic Psychologist (THP)
Zeitschrift für Psychosomatische Medizin und Psychotherapie (ZPMP)
Zeitschrift für Psychotraumatologie und Psychologische Medizin (ZPPM)

References

American Psychiatric Association (1994) Diagnostic and statistical manual of mental disorders, 4th edn. American Psychiatric Association, Washington, DC

Angus LE, Rennie DL (1988) Therapist participation in metaphor generation: Collaborative and non-collaborative styles. Psychotherapy 25 (4):552–560. doi:10.1037/h0085381

Arthern J, Madill A (1999) How do transitional objects work? The therapist's view. Br J Med Psychol 72:1–21

Bachelor A (1995) Clients' perception of the therapeutic alliance: a qualitative analysis. J Couns Psychol 42 (3):323–337. doi:10.1037/0033-3204.44.2.175

Bachelor A, Laverdière O, Gamache D, Bordeleau V (2007) Clients' collaboration in therapy: self-perceptions and relationships with client psychological functioning, interpersonal relations and motivation. Psychother Theory Res Pract Train 44:175–192. doi:10.1037/0033-3204.44.2.175

Beckett D, Hager P (2002) Life, work and learning: practice in postmodernity. Routledge, London

Bedi R (2006) Concept mapping the client's perspective on counseling alliance formation. J Couns Psychol 53:26–35. doi:10.1037/0022-0167.53.1.26

Behrens K, Calliess IT (2008) Migration biography and culture as determinants of diagnostic and therapeutic processes in mentally ill immigrants: A systematic differentiation based on a qualitative content analysis of treatment courses. Psychother Psychosom Med Psychol 58:162–168

Berger L (2001) Inside out: Narrative autoethnography as a path towards rapport. Qual Inq 7:504–518

Billig M (1987) Arguing and thinking: a rhetorical approach to social psychology. Cambridge University Press, Cambridge

Binder P-E, Holgersen H, Nielsen GH (2008a) Establishing a bond that works: a qualitative study of how psychotherapists make contact with adolescent patients. Eur J Psychother Couns 10:55–69

Binder P-E, Holgersen H, Nielsen GH (2008b) Re-establishing contact: a qualitative exploration of how therapists work with alliance ruptures in adolescent psychotherapy. Couns Psychother Res 8:239–245

Boothe B, von Wyl A, Wepfer R (1999) Narrative dynamics and psychodynamics. Psychother Res 9:258–273. doi:10.1080/10503309912331332751

Bordin E (1979) The generalizability of the psychoanalytic concept of the working alliance. Psychother Theory Res Pract 16:252–260

Braun V, Clarke V (2006) Using thematic analysis in psychology. Qual Res Psychol 3:77–101. doi:10.1191/1478088706qp063oa

Burkard AW, Knox S, Groen M, Hess SA, Perez M (2006) European- American therapist self-disclosure in cross-cultural counseling. J Couns Psychol 53:15–25. doi:10.1037/0022-0167.53.1.15

Cahill J, Barkham MB, Stiles WB (2010) Systematic review of practice-based research on psychotherapies in routine clinical settings. Br J Clin Psychol 49:421–453. doi:10.1348/014466509X470789

Corrigal J, Payne H, Wilkinson W (eds) (2006) About a body: working with the embodied mind in psychotherapy. Routledge, London

Derogatis LR (1994) Symptom-Checklist-90-R: administration, scoring and procedures manual, 3rd edn. National Computer Systems, Minneapolis

Elliott R (2002) Hermeneutic single-case efficacy design. Psychother Res 12(1):1–21. doi:10.1080/713869614

Etherington K (ed) (2003) Trauma, the body and transformation: a narrative inquiry. Jessica Kingsley, London

Faller H (1998) Krankheitsverarbeitung bei Krebskranken [Coping by patients with cancer]. Verlag für Angewandte Psychologie, Göttingen

Fitzpatrick L, Simpson J, Smith A (2010) A qualitative analysis of mindfulness-based cognitive therapy (MBCT) in Parkinson's disease. Psychol Psychother Theory Res Pract 83:179–192. doi:10.1348/147608309X471514

Frommer J (1996) Qualitative Diagnostikforschung: Inhaltsanalytische Untersuchungen zum psychotherapeutischen Erstgespräch. [Qualitative research into diagnostics: Content analysis investigations of psychotherapeutic intake interviews]. Springer, Berlin

Frommer J, Faller H (1994) Introduction. In Faller H, Frommer J (eds) Qualitative Psychotherapieforschung. Grundlagen und Methoden [Qualitative psychotherapy research: Basics and methods]. Asanger, Heidelberg, pp 9–12

Frommer J, Langenbach M, Streek U (2004) Qualitative psychotherapy research in German-speaking countries. Psychother Res 14:37–55. doi:10.1093/ptr/kph004

Gadamer H-G (1992) Truth and method (2nd rev. ed.: Weisheimer J, Marshall DG, Trans.). Crossroad, New York, NY (Original work published 1960).

Gelo OCG, Braakmann D, Benetka G (2008) Commentary: Quantitative and qualitative research: beyond the debate. Integr Psychol Behav Sci 42(3):266–290. doi:10.1007/s12124-008-9078-3

Gelo OCG, Braakmann D, Benetka G (2009) Erratum to "Quantitative and qualitative research: Beyond the debate". Integr Psychol Behav Sci 43(4):406–407. doi:10.1007/s12124-009-9107-x

Gerhardt U (2001) Idealtypus. Zur methodologischen Begründung der modernen Soziologie [Ideal type: Towards a methodological foundation of modern sociology]. Suhrkamp, Frankfurt

Giorgi A (1979) The relationship among level, type, and structure and their importance for social science theorizing: a dialogue with Schütz. In: Giorgi A, Knowles R, Smith D (eds) Duquesne studies in phenomenological psychology, vol 3. Duquesne University Press, Pittsburgh, pp 81–96

Giorgi A (ed) (1985) Phenomenology and psychological research. Duquesne University Press, Pittsburgh

Giorgi A (2009) The descriptive phenomenological method in psychology: a modified Husserlian approach. Duquesne University Press, Pittsburgh

Giorgi AP, Giorgi BM (2003) The descriptive phenomenological psychological method. In: Camic PM, Rhodes JE, Yardley L (eds) Qualitative research in psychology: expanding perspectives in methodology and design. American Psychological Association, Washington, DC, pp 243–273

Greenberg LS (2007) A guide to conducting task analysis of psychotherapy change. Psychother Res 17:15–30. doi:10.1080/10533006007203 90

Hill CE, Knox S (2002) Self-disclosure. In: Norcross JC (ed) Psychotherapy relationships that work: therapist contributions and responsiveness to patients. Oxford University Press, London, pp 255–265

Hill CE, Thompson BJ, Williams EN (1997) A guide to conducting consensual qualitative research. Couns Psychol 25:517–572. doi:10.1177/0011000097254005

Kühnlein I (1999) Psychotherapy as a process of transformation: analysis of posttherapeutic autobiographic narrations. Psychother Res 9:274–288. doi:10.1080/10503309912331332761

Kracauer S (1952) The challenge of qualitative content analysis. Publ Opin Quart 16:631–642

Lakoff G, Johnson M (1980) Metaphors we live by. University of Chicago Press, London

Lepper G, Mergenthaler E (2005) Exploring group process. Psychother Res 15:433–444. doi:10.1080/10503300500091587

Levitt H (2001) The sounds of silence in psychotherapy: categorization of clients' pauses. Psychother Res 11:295–309. doi:10.1080/713663985

Lilliengreen P, Werbart A (2005) A model of therapeutic action grounded in the patients' view of curative and hindering factors in psychoanalytic psychotherapy. Psychother Theory Res Pract Train 42:324–339. doi:10.1037/0033.42.3.324

MacKenzie MJ, Carlson LE, Munoz M, Speca M (2007) A qualitative study of self-perceived effects of mindfulness in a psychosocial oncology setting. Stress Health 23:59–69. doi:10.1002/smi.1120

Madill A, Barkham M (1997) Discourse analysis of a theme in one successful case of brief psychodynamic-interpersonal psychotherapy. J Couns Psychol 44:232–244. doi:10.1037/0022-0167.44.2.232

Mason O, Hargreaves I (2001) A qualitative study of mindfulness-based cognitive therapy for depression. Br J Med Psychol 74:197–212

McDonald WM, Richard IH, DeLong MR (2003) Prevalence, etiology, and treatment of depression in Parkinson's Disease. Biol Psychiatry 54:363–376

McLeod J (1994) Doing counselling research. Sage, London

McLeod J (1997) Narrative and psychotherapy. Sage, London

Meekums B (2008) Embodied narratives in becoming a counselling trainer: an autoethnographic study. Br J Guid Couns 36(3):287–301. doi:10.1080/03069880802088952

Mergenthaler E (1996) Emotion-abstraction patterns in verbatim protocols: a new way of describing psychotherapeutic processes. J Consult Clin Psychol 64:1306–1315. doi:10.1037/0033-3204.42.3.324

Moustakas C (1990) Heuristic research: design, methodology and applications. Sage, London

Muhr T (2004) ATLAS.ti users guide. Software for qualitative data analysis, management, and model building. http://www.atlasti.com/uploads/media/atlman_02.pdf

Nagell W, Steinmetzer L, Fissabre U, Handrich M (2009) Das Beziehungserleben – Beziehungserfahrung in der Supervision und deren Einfluss auf die psychoanalytische Identitätsfindung des Ausbildungskandidaten. [Relationship experience – How relationships are experienced in supervision and how this affects the formation of psychoanalytical identity in training candidates]. Forum der Psychoanalyse 25:53–65

Nijohf G (1995) Parkinson's Disease as a problem of shame in public appearance. Sociol Health Illness 17:193–205. doi:10.1111/1467-9566.ep10933391

Oevermann U, Allert T, Konau E, Krambeck J (1979) Die Methodologie der objektiven Hermeneutik und ihre allgemeine forschungslogische Bedeutung in den Sozialwissenschaften [The methodology of objective hermeneutics and its general importance for the logic of research in the social sciences]. In: Soeffner HG (ed) Interpretative Verfahren in den Sozial- und

Textwissenschaften [Interpretive techniques in the social- and text analysis sciences]. Metzler, Suttgart, pp 352–434
Philips B, Wennberg P, Werbart A, Schubert J (2006) Young adults in psychoanalytic psychotherapy: patient characteristics and therapy outcome. Psychol Psychother Theory Res Pract 79:89–106. doi:10.1348/147608305X52649
Rennie DL (2004) Anglo-North American qualitative counseling and psychotherapy research. Psychother Res 14:37–55. doi:10.1093/ptr/kph003
Rennie DL (2012) Qualitative research as methodical hermeneutics. Psychol Methods 17(3):385–398. doi:10.1037/a0029250
Rennie DL, Watson KD, Monteiro A (2002) The rise of qualitative research in psychology. Can Psychol 43:179–189. doi:10.1037/h0086914
Richardson L (2000) Writing: a method of inquiry. In: Denzin NK, Lincoln YS (eds) Handbook of qualitative research. Sage, London
Schütze F (1981) Prozessstrukturen des Lebensablaufs [Process structures of course of life]. In: Matthes J (ed) Biographie in handlungswissenschaftlicher Perspektive [Biography under a action theory perspective]. Sozialwissenschaftliches Forschungszentrum der Universität Erlangen-Nürnberg, Nürnberg, pp 67–156
Schütze F (1983) Biographieforschung und narratives interview [Research in biography and narrative interviews]. Neue Praxis 13:283–293
Schütze F (1984) Kognitive Figuren des autobiographischen Stegreiferzählens [Cognitive figures of autobiographical off the cuff narrations]. In Kohli M, Robert G (eds) Biographie und soziale Wirklichkeit. Neue Beiträge und Forschungsperspektiven [Biography and social reality: New contributions and research perspectives]. Stuttgart, Metzler, pp. 78–117.
Segal Z, Williams JMG, Teasdale JD (2002) Mindfulness-based cognitive therapy for depression. Guilford, New York
Silverman D (1998) Harvey Sacks: social science and conversation analysis. Oxford University Press, New York
Smith JA (1996) Beyond the divide between cognition and discourse: using interpretative phenomenological analysis in health psychology. Psychol Health 11:261–271. doi:10.1080/08870449608400256
Smith JA, Osborne M (2003) Interpretative phenomenological analysis. In: Smith JA (ed) Qualitative psychology: a practical guide to research methods. Sage, London, pp 51–80
Snape C, Perren S, Jones L, Rowland N (2003) Counselling – why not? A qualitative study of people's accounts of not taking up counselling appointments. Couns Psychother Res 3(3):239–245. doi:10.1080/14733140312331384412
Sparkes A (2002) Telling tales in sport and physical activity: a qualitative journey. Human Kinetics, Leeds
Stiles WB, Angus LE (2001) Qualitative research on clients' assimilation of problematic experiences in psychotherapy. In: Frommer J, Rennie D (eds) Qualitative psychotherapy research: methods and methodology. Pabst Science, Lengerich, pp 112–127
Stiles WB, Elliott R, Llewelyn SP, Firth-Cozens JA, Margison FR, Shapiro DA, Hardy G (1990) Assimilation of problematic experiences by clients in psychotherapy. Psychotherapy 27(3):411–420. doi:10.1037/0033.27.3.411
Strauss A, Corbin J (1998) Basics of qualitative research: grounded theory procedures and techniques, 2nd edn. Sage, Thousand Oaks
Streeck U (1999) Acting out, interpretation and unconscious communication. Int Forum Psychoanal 8:135–143. doi:10.1080/0803370699436456
Streeck U (2004) Auf den ersten Blick: Psychotherapeutische Beziehungen unter dem Mikroskop [At the first glance: Psychotherapeutic relationships under the microscope]. Klett-Cotta, Stuttgart
Wampold BE (2001) The great psychotherapy debate: models, methods and findings. Lawrence Erlbaum and Associates, Mahwah
Werbart A, Levander S (2005) Understanding the incomprehensible: private theories of first episode psychotic patients and their therapists. Bull Menn Clin 69:103–136
Werbart A, Levander S (2006) Two sets of private theories in analysands and their analysts: Utopian versus attainable cures. Psychoanal Psychol 23:108–127. doi:10.1037/0736-9735.23.1.108

Interpretation-Driven Guidelines for Designing and Evaluating Grounded Theory Research: A Constructivist-Social Justice Approach

22

Heidi M. Levitt

Contents

Abstract

This chapter is meant as guidance for not only investigators designing qualitative research projects but for reviewers assessing manuscripts using qualitative methods. An *interpretation-driven* approach to design and review of qualitative research is proposed as an alternative to the approach of setting in stone rules that consist of *procedure-driven* prescriptions. It walks the reader through the process of considering the design of an individual study and its coherence with the epistemology of the researcher(s). This approach emphasizes the centrality of the role of interpretation that is best evaluated in relation to an epistemology, within the context of the specific study characteristics, and in service of the scientific, practice, and/or social justice goals at hand. It presents context-sensitive guidelines for researchers and reviewers to use in designing and evaluating qualitative research studies. Within the chapter, there is a specific focus on grounded theory (e.g., Glaser and Strauss, The discovery of grounded theory. Aldine, Chicago, 1967); however, many of the principles put forward to guide study design and research review may be relevant across qualitative methods.

H.M. Levitt (✉)
University of Massachusetts Boston, Boston, MA, USA
e-mail: heidi.levitt@umb.edu

O.C.G. Gelo et al. (eds.), *Psychotherapy Research*,
DOI 10.1007/978-3-7091-1382-0_22, © Springer-Verlag Wien 2015

22.1 Developing Interpretation-Driven Guidelines for Constructivist-Social Justice Qualitative Research

The purpose of this chapter is to outline an approach to method design and assessment that upholds the scientific integrity of the interpretive process within qualitative approaches to research—with a specific focus on grounded theory method (e.g., Glaser and Strauss 1967). I use the term *interpretation-driven* to describe the approach because I am advocating that privileging the interpretive process requires consideration of the coherence between methods and epistemology with reference to the specific characteristics and goals within an individual project—as will become clear. This initiative is a response to the development of qualitative approaches that are *procedure-driven*—that is, guided by rules that privilege the integrity of a method when assessing research.

Interpretive judgments are important across both qualitative and quantitative approaches in ensuring that methods selected are appropriate for the questions being asked and in deciding upon the meanings of findings. In quantitative research, however, the process of identifying patterns across numeric data is relinquished to mathematical procedures. This mathematical aspect of analysis renders procedure-driven rules necessary to preserve the integrity of the calculations so that the resultant findings are valid. For instance, a statistical method requires a certain number of participants to have the power required to be informative—regardless of the researchers, participants, or the study context at hand.

In contrast, qualitative methods have their process of pattern identification located in the subjective interpretation of data—and so these procedure-driven assessments may be inappropriate when applied to qualitative methods because they mistake the nature of the process of pattern identification. Instead, study rigor should more accurately be assessed with a central focus upon the interpretive process that can best be understood as it is located within a given method, question, research goals, study characteristics, and epistemologies at play. The integrity of qualitative research then depends upon *adapting the procedures* within a method so as to best enable the interpretive process.

The task of developing interpretation-driven guidelines is complicated for a number of reasons. In a field where qualitative research (i.e., "human science" as distinguished by their epistemology from "natural science"; see Rennie 1997) is still new to many editors and reviewers, it can be helpful to have some direction on assessing these methods. Procedural-driven guidelines can be easier to apply because researchers and reviewers do not need to consider theoretical and contextual factors and do not need to develop sophistication in their thinking about methods. They can seem friendly and accessible. At first blush it may seem reasonable that good rules developed for one qualitative method should generalize to all.

For the process of initially learning qualitative research approaches, procedural guidelines can be helpful as a deeper understanding of epistemology might only emerge after they are engaged in analysis. For instance, I have written papers myself that include recommendations for teaching grounded theory to graduate students (Levitt et al. 2013). Some sets of guidelines are written with a stronger understanding of the epistemological underpinnings of qualitative research practice and address either qualitative research on whole (e.g., Elliott et al. 1999) or grounded theory methods more specifically (e.g., Fassinger 2005; Dourdouma and Mörtl 2012). In general, these guidelines allow for the development of professional standards, create a common language, communicate practices, and expedite assessments of research.

Although useful for those purposes, if taken as procedural prescriptions, these approaches can dictate practices rather than generate sets of considerations that need to be weighed together to best meet the multiple goals of research within an epistemological context. Their danger is not only in discouraging complex thinking in reviewers but in discouraging the submission and acceptance of qualitative research that uses nontraditional epistemologies and/or constructivist-feminist methods (see Frieze 2008 for an example of such a journal policy). In this paper, I argue that procedural recommendations or requirements encourage incoherent research that is judged superficially, constrain the evolution of methods in the field, and, thus, work against the goals of empirical research itself.

In this chapter, I put forward an alternative way of assessing research design—as an expression of an epistemological stance in relation to study characteristics and aims. The epistemology is *constructivist* as it views people as forming the meanings that make their world intelligible via methods like language, narrative, and personal constructs (e.g., Neimeyer 2009; Raskin and Bridges 2008). Also in this perspective, method is thought to serve scientific goals (as opposed to science being defined by sets of procedure-related decisions) as well as other goals, such as clinical, didactic, or social justice goals. My approach to research tends to have a social justice orientation that needs to be understood as having implications for research methods. For instance, social justice (i.e., feminist or multicultural) research tends to investigate and shift into focus marginalized experiences and so research may be used to serve both the goals of generating knowledge and of liberation—which at times might be at odds. Stiles (see Chap. 8) in this book offers a complimentary discussion in which he divides research goals differently (i.e., as developing theories, enriching understandings, or collecting evidence) but describes how each purpose can influence the strategies of research and frameworks of understanding that work. Although these considerations are focused upon the use of grounded theory within a constructivist-social justice framework, many can be adapted for use with other methods or epistemologies. I will begin by describing my journey as a qualitative researcher and my own epistemology to provide some context for what follows.

22.2 Situating the Interpretation-Driven Approach

22.2.1 Methodophily Versus Methodolatry

In qualitative research methods, it is incumbent upon researchers to provide information on their relevant personal perspectives, histories, and philosophies as a framework within which readers can assess their inquiry. In that tradition, I am providing some historical context to frame the development of my own expertise in qualitative methods. I first began using qualitative methods in graduate school (e.g., Levitt 1999). It was in the not-too-distant time before qualitative method courses existed in many North American psychology programs, but I learned about these methods from my mentors in the York University Psychology Department. They were pioneers in these approaches—Lynne Angus (e.g., Angus et al. 1999), Leslie Greenberg (e.g., Greenberg 2007), and David Rennie (e.g., Rennie 2000)—who introduced me to a variety of qualitative methods as well as developing my appreciation for psychotherapy process research (see Rennie 2010 for a history of this particularly innovative department).

The lingering impact of David Bakan's (1967) early work at York was clear. His insightful perspective on statistics and research methods contributed to a climate in which alternative methods could be explored and developed. In particular, his cautions about "methodolatry" in our field have become classic—that is, our becoming so attached to a method (e.g., the clinical trial) that it begins to dictate research agenda instead of being one of many tools that can be used to answer theory-driven questions dictated by researchers (see Gelo 2012; Slife and Gantt 1999 for critiques of the former process). When set down in procedural terms, methods can be reified and take on a life of their own that can become disconnected from goals of science—to know and learn. Instead, aspects of the methods can be tailored to the questions, resources, the epistemology of the investigators, and purposes at hand.

While I continue to be interested in exploring many qualitative methods [see Rennie and Frommer (2015) and Mörtl and Gelo (2012)], I have become particularly attached to grounded theory—perhaps because I have found it flexible enough to be used across many topics of interest to me. It is a method that has allowed me to explore other people's intimate experiences of struggle and making meaning of their world. I have had peak intellectual moments using this method—asking monks about their experiences of developing wisdom in India (Levitt 1999), learning about psychotherapy clients' unspoken experiences in sessions and eminent therapists' experiences of guiding therapy (e.g., Levitt 2001; Levitt and Williams 2010), and working to understand the ways gender is constructed within gay, lesbian, and transgender cultures (e.g., Levitt and Hiestand 2004). Each time I conduct a study, I feel privileged to talk with participants about topics that fascinate me and to learn from their experiences. Whenever I lecture on qualitative methods, I like to impress upon students how joyful and stimulating this research can be. Really—what could be better than being engaged in understanding the inner workings of a compelling subject and then having the opportunity to generate new understandings from those discussions?

I have used grounded theory in the context of three programs of study. My work on domestic violence and faith has included studies that examined the perspectives of perpetrators, survivors, and religious leaders (e.g., Levitt and Ware 2006). My research on gender has focused on sexual orientation identities and minority stressors (e.g., Levitt and Hiestand 2004). And my psychotherapy work has explored a variety of common factors from both clients' and therapists' perspectives (e.g., Levitt and Williams 2010). Over the last 15 years, I have authored or coauthored approximately 50 publications rooted in qualitative analyses, including over 30 projects using grounded theory methods, and have supervised many others. The methods have included content analysis, narrative analysis, metaphor analysis, task analysis, hermeneutic analysis, and grounded theory.

As well, I have taught a variety of methods in qualitative research courses for graduate students (e.g., phenomenology, Wertz 2005; discourse analysis, Gergen and McNamee 2000; consensual qualitative research, Hill et al. 2005). In my course, I survey different qualitative methods, but I guide the students through an intensive grounded theory class project that begins in the first class and runs through the semester. Together, we publish our joint project at the end of the semester (see Levitt et al. 2013 for a detailed description of this course).

This chapter has provided the opportunity to reflect upon my use of grounded theory and the ways I have conceptualized study design. When reviewing my work, I find that I have made quite different interpretation-driven decisions, depending on qualities of the participants, research context, or study topic. In the chapter, I consider the points where in using the method I have made decisions about my method design, and unpack those choices. I proceed to explicate this decisional process—both to stimulate consideration around the elements of the method and to interrogate my constructivist-social justice epistemological approach and its expression in relation to my study goals. Although my research has a scientific purpose broadly, often my psychotherapy research also is directed by the goal of developing clinical recommendations, whereas my domestic violence and gender research also is driven by the goal of advocacy.

22.2.2 Ontological and Epistemological Considerations

It is my ambition that this essay can aid other researchers in tailoring grounded theory designs that are best suited for their own studies and can guide reviewers and consumers of research to consider the role of their own ontological and epistemological beliefs, aims, and study characteristics when assessing research. There are a variety of approaches from which researchers have used grounded theory methods from post-positivist to critical constructivist approaches (e.g., Fassinger 2005). While Morrow (2005) provides a concise and insightful overview of the way criteria shift when moving between postpositive, interpretive constructivist, and critical ideological paradigms, the present paper describes specific ways that method can be adjusted within an epistemological framework given different study characteristics and research aims. It is toward that end that I present a description of my own constructivist-social justice, ontological, and epistemological approach.

Most often in psychology, researchers categorize these positions in terms of competing perspectives envisioned on continua (e.g., Fletcher 1996; Gelo 2012; Guba and Lincoln 1994; Ponterotto 2005). On a spectrum from naïve realism, in which one true fixed reality is directly apprehendable, and relativism, in which reality is grasped through our own understandings and meanings, I adopt a constructivist-social justice approach in which I study understandings of experience as shaped by social and cultural processes and values, often in the form of structural and systemic forces. To some extent, I have developed this ontological approach through my research on gender and sexual orientation and learning from participants how they experienced parts of their own identities as given and inalterable but as having expressions shaped by their context (e.g., Levitt and Hiestand 2004).

On a spectrum in which on one end inquiry is seen as objective and dualist, in which scientists intellectually can observe the truth, and on the other it is understood as subjective and transactional, in which embodied researchers engage with participants to cocreate findings, I see the epistemic task as inherently subjective, interactive, and embodied. By this I mean that our subjectivity, along with our values, blind spots, and biases, is the unavoidable lens through which data are interpreted. The investigator helps participants to articulate their experience, but this cocreation is limited as the exploration is rooted in the participants' sense of the phenomenon of interest, which might be experienced as entirely created or as having roots in historical, social, or biological realms.

In this approach to methodology, the interpretive task is central and the assessment of the reflexive process of analysis is valued. For instance, the guidelines I put forth convey more faith in analyses that are conducted by researchers who become deeply immersed in a data set (e.g., lived experiences, intensive study) than in analyses conducted by less-engaged observers who can arrive at agreement. At the same time, the data communicate the participants' engagement and experience of their reality. As a result, the principles I put forth in the guidelines emphasize obtaining data that are as clear and useful as possible and keeping analyses grounded to maximize the returns from the information therein. Maintaining the balance between these two tensions then becomes the central concern during method design and evaluation for investigators and reviewers. The approach I have adopted is congruent with the methodical hermeneutic approach that Rennie (2000) argued situates grounded theory as a synthesis of relative and realist epistemologies—as an interpretive analysis (relativist aspect) of empirical participants' reports of their experiences in the world (realist aspect).

In addition, the principles reflect social justice and pragmatist approaches to method. A social justice epistemology is present in that I am using my inquiry with an objective to bring into focus marginalized experiences with the aim of raising consciousness and repairing practices that maintain social biases (e.g., Fine 2012; Harding 1986) and an awareness that my process of inquiry itself can be fundamentally influenced by these biases. In my own approach to research, I incorporate insights from several different feminist and multicultural epistemologies: (1) I have been influenced by feminist standpoint epistemologies (e.g., Harding 1998, 2011) in that I tend to start my inquiry process in research focused upon the standpoint of those who have lesser power with the understanding that marginalized groups may have perspectives that usefully can lead to understanding (e.g., clients in therapy, marginalized sexual orientation groups, victims of violence). (2) At the same time, I do not assign epistemic privilege to minority groups (e.g., Bar On 1993; Longino 1993) by confining my research to their perspectives or assigning them sole authority on a subject, but seek to study how those experiences interact with those who have more power and with systems (e.g., therapists, dominant sexual orientation groups, religious authorities). (3) While I am interested in examining and situating my own position as a researcher as it interacts with my reflexive process (e.g., Code 1996), I tend to be interested in understanding communities as generators of understanding in relationship to their own experiences and needs. I see individual participants as members of communities that are shaped by privileging and oppressive forces and that are not monolithic themselves and are in flux over time (see Diamond 2006; Levitt 2006).

A pragmatic framework toward study design is at play because the constraints of the study characteristics (i.e., qualities of the phenomenon, participants, and researchers) are considered in terms of their implications for method, and the effects of methods, in turn, are evaluated in terms of their implications for praxis in light of the research goals (e.g., Peirce 1958). That is, throughout the principles described in this paper, I consider how different method-related decisions influence the processes of gathering clearly articulated useful data, training analysts who are positioned to conduct a thorough analysis, and conducting assessments of research that do not compromise a grounded process of theory creation. These decisions are made to maximize both the epistemic coherence and the practical returns of each study. For instance, I recognize that method-related ideals may need to be altered to give voice to participants who are marginalized and face barriers to research participation. By generating research that is not well represented in the literature, these studies can serve both research and advocacy goals. This is one example of one way in which epistemological beliefs can guide method. The following principles are articulations of rationales for making such decisions.

22.3 Developing Principles for Grounded Theory Research

To make the principles that follow easier to locate, they are organized within the context of the components of a method section in a research paper (see Table 22.1). Within each component, common questions from graduate students or investigators new to grounded theory are addressed, and responses are presented to highlight the ways epistemological and study-specific factors influence design. In the course of answering these questions, I will provide a description of how and when I conduct grounded theory (as opposed to other qualitative or quantitative methods) and formulate the principles that have driven some of my own study design decisions.

Before describing principles, however, it can be helpful to provide a brief overview of grounded theory methods and purposes. There are a number of variants of grounded theory method (e.g., Charmaz 2006; Dourdouma and Mörtl 2012; Glaser and Strauss 1967; Rennie and Fergus 2006; Rennie et al. 1988; Corbin and Strauss 2008). They can be based within multiple epistemologies and use different procedures and terms.

Across grounded theory approaches, however, are the following typical procedures: (1) At first, the interview text is divided into units that capture meanings being conveyed (Rennie et al. 1988, recommend using meaning units, a construct borrowed from phenomenology for this process; Giorgi 2009). (2) As the units are created, labels are assigned to each unit to reflect the meaning therein. (3) Using a process of constant comparison, the researchers then compare the meaning units to one another and create categories to reflect the commonalities identified (i.e., *open* coding). As the data can be sorted into as many categories as are relevant to its content during this analysis, the categories are *not* independent of one another. (4) As initial level categories are formed, they are compared to one another and higher-order categories reflect the commonalities therein (i.e., *axial* coding). By repeating this process with each layer of categories and incorporating new data (i.e.,

Table 22.1 Principles of interpretation-driven research design and evaluation

Domain	Relevant questions	Interpretation-driven guidelines
Deciding upon a method of analysis	Question 1: Is my question consistent with a grounded theory method?	1. To decide if a method (e.g., grounded theory) is appropriate, the researchers consider whether the question *aims* to develop a model of common experiences of one experience (might use grounded theory alone) versus to conduct a comparison of experiences between groups of participants or for purposes beyond understanding participants' experiences (might use other methods or adapt grounded theory methods to meet this aim)
	Question 2: Is a grounded theory analysis too intensive considering the data I will collect?	2. The scientific *goal* of the analysis (i.e., an in-depth understanding of the components of an experience) and the characteristics of both the phenomenon (i.e., complexity) and the participants (i.e., ability to clearly articulate their experience) should be considered when justifying a grounded theory analysis
Participants	Question 3: Which types of difference are most important in participant recruitment?	3. Diversity within participants is sought out to clarify likely differences in experiencing that appear *most relevant* to the subject at hand. Typically, this includes considering how cultural factors may be influential throughout the analytic process, as their impact might be difficult for investigators to assess, and seeking out participants with relevant cultural diversity characteristics
Investigators/ interviewers	Question 4: How does one decide who should be conducting the interviews?	4. Decide who should conduct interviews *after weighing together* the need for interviewing skills, the knowledge needed on a subject matter, and the influence of cultural oppression and disparity upon the participants' ability to disclose and articulate information clearly
Recruitment	Question 5: Should a screening be conducted before the interview?	5. Conduct screening interviews if it is difficult to know if the participants are able to *describe usefully* the topic of interest, because the topic is unclear or uncertain, the participants are suspect, or if their *safety needs* to be secured
Data collection procedure	Question 6: Should I analyze interview or written data?	6. Grounded theory methods can be adapted for the analysis of written data, but analysts should keep in mind the *benefits and costs* of this choice when designing studies
	Question 7: How do I structure my interview? Do I have a main question?	7. When writing your interview protocol, consider the *scientific goal* of your analysis. If your goal is to develop a theoretical model of one phenomenon, design your question protocol to elaborate a central question and use a method of analysis designed for this purpose (such as grounded theory or phenomenology), but if your goal is to shed light on a number of discrete subtopics, create separate groups of questions and conduct an analysis designed for that purpose (such as content analysis or theme analysis)
Measures	Question 8: When should I give measures to participants?	8. Within the confines of the qualitative research, measures likely will rarely have the power to provide useful statistical knowledge due to the small datasets used. They can be useful, however, to provide information that can better *describe* your participants to aid in generalization (i.e., transferability), theoretical sampling, and data interpretation

(*continued*)

Table 22.1 (continued)

Domain	Relevant questions	Interpretation-driven guidelines
Data analysis: adaptations of grounded theory	Question 9: Do I really need so many categories or hierarchy levels?	9. Detailed hierarchies typically are useful *when* researchers are new to grounded theory, when the data is complex and findings are hard to organize or defend, and when results are intended to be used as the basis for future analyses
	Question 10: Should I have a core category?	10. A core category can be developed when it furthers the understanding of the phenomenon being studied, but is not useful when it creates a level of commonality that *distracts* from a more meaningful plurality in the findings
	Question 11: Should I use multiple analysts?	11. Multiple analysts are *not necessary* but are especially helpful when they provide method, topic, or culturally based experiences that will allow for a *more complex interpretation* of the data at hand. These different factors all are considered and weighed together. Ideally, one ends up with an analysis in which one is confident in the meaning units created, the ability of the investigators to conduct the method and interpret the data, and the depth of analysis and its applicability
Assessments of research checks	Question 12: Should I use inter-rater checks or external auditor checks on coding?	12. Within a grounded theory analysis of a complex topic, the use of inter-rater reliability and external auditor checks is not desirable when it *hinders the scientific integrity* of the research—that is, to create fine-tuned categories that represent complex and contextualized data. The researchers can demonstrate to their readers the rigor of their methods by describing that qualitative methods tend to contain intrinsic checks and by supplementing these with additional checks that are consistent with the epistemology at hand
	Question 13: How many participants do I need to interview to reach saturation?	13. Saturation can be demonstrated by showing that new meaningful categories are not generated when adding a new interview; however when the data is *complex*, it is recommended that saturation be tested further
Assessments of research checks	Question 14: What credibility checks should I use? How should I conduct participant checks?	14. *Interview checks* help investigators to assess both the comprehensiveness of the interview and the influences of cultural or interpersonal differences on it
		15. *Consensus* should be conducted in a way that recognizes the differing forms of methodological and interpretative expertise of the investigators, is sensitive to differences in power between investigators, and is open to incorporating multiple perspectives on a dataset
		16. *Memoing* can be used to record thoughts, theories, and method decisions and to recognize and limit the influence of investigators' biases and processes upon the data
		17. *Participants' feedback* with regard to:
		(a) *Efficiency in obtaining written feedback*: It can maximize the response of participants because a second interview is not required, but can limit the ability to receive detailed responses—especially if the participants find written expression challenging

(*continued*)

Table 22.1 (continued)

Domain	Relevant questions	Interpretation-driven guidelines
		(b) *Depth of feedback*: Feedback from participants or others who you think might help you shed light on the questions that remain about your findings, given the purpose of the research at hand (see Sect. 22.5.1 for more on how I might use nonparticipant reviewers' feedback)
		(c) *Social justice goals*: Obtaining feedback from participants is ideal; however, researchers committed to a constructivist-social justice framework should recognize that all participants typically are not able and should not be expected to provide feedback and that this feedback is supplementary
		(d) *Conflicts between participants' feedback and your interpretation*: Feedback from participants can enrich investigators' understanding of data; however, feedback needs to be reconciled with the investigators' interpretations of patterns from across the participants and the hierarchy. If we cannot reconcile the feedback with our interpretation, we typically present the feedback alongside of our interpretation so that readers can assess this discrepancy themselves

selective coding), a hierarchical structure of categories is developed. Finally, a core category is conceptualized, representing a central connection between categories at the apex of this hierarchy. (5) Throughout this process of data analysis, participant recruitment is being conducted strategically to enrich the developing theory (this process being called "theoretical sampling"). (6) When new categories no longer appear to be forthcoming from the addition of new interviews into the hierarchy, the analysis is thought to have reached the point of saturation signifying that the data collection is comprehensive. Grounded theory analyses usually require a smaller number of participants than quantitative studies—often saturating with approximately 6–20 interviews. These studies can analyze a wealth of data, however, as interviews typically range from 1 to 2 h and can easily result in 30–80 transcript pages of data per interview, replete with rich description about a phenomenon containing meanings and distinctions generated by the participant. (7) Throughout this process of analysis, memoing or note-taking is used to record shifts in hypotheses and conceptualizations in an attempt to record and restrict the influence of a priori ideas upon the analytic process as well the influence of theories that develop during the analysis.

Increasingly, these grounded theory procedures are imported into other methods—perhaps to add clarity to qualitative methods that have been described within vague or conflicting approaches—even when the purpose of the method is not to generate a theory. Because there are so very many different qualitative methods and versions thereof, it may be that it is easier for researchers to appeal to grounded theory methods that are familiar to many readers and reviewers and are often clearly defined. In particular, processes of constant comparison, of developing lower- and upper-level categories (although usually not a complete hierarchy), and of saturation are combined with other qualitative methods to strengthen the process of data analysis. For instance, a content analysis might be conducted in a way that uses a process of constant comparison to create a structure of initial and higher-order categories to answer multiple questions even though a central theory is not being formed (e.g., Kannan and Levitt 2009).

22.4 Method

22.4.1 Deciding Upon a Method of Analysis

22.4.1.1 Is My Question Consistent with a Grounded Theory Method? (Question 1)

Answer: Advisors often spend a good deal of time helping their students decide upon a method to use in a given project. Although grounded theory might demand too much effort in some instances, it can also be too limiting, depending on one's objectives. Grounded theory focuses on identifying the commonalities among participants. That is, although differences can be noted between subsets of participants, the method functions by creating categories that are based upon commonalities within these subsets. Grounded theory also tends to be focused more upon the content of participants' speech and what they can report experiencing than focused upon the structure or context of their reports, although this is not a hard line [see Mörtl and Gelo (2015)]. There are four main considerations that I have found helpful in identifying the primary research goals and selecting appropriate method for given projects.

1. It might be preferable to conduct a quantitative statistical analysis at times when the primary research question is to *compare mean or modal responses* across groups or to *verify specific* a priori *hypotheses* within groups. Generally, I prefer to begin a program of study with a qualitative analysis to discover meanings intrinsic to a group and then assess the theory developed using quantitative methods (see Gelo et al. 2008, 2009 for other arguments for mixed-methods research). There are times, however, when a theory is already well developed and it makes sense to begin by evaluating or validating an existing theory with a quantitative method. As a corollary of this approach, there are times when a quantitative data analysis leads to questions that can best be resolved through a qualitative inquiry.
2. In contrast, when the primary purpose of an analysis is to *collect or compare responses to separate main questions*, it might be preferable to conduct a content or thematic analysis (e.g., Braun and Clarke 2006). In the process of conducting such an analysis, methods might be imported from grounded theory (i.e., open coding, constant comparison)—for instance one might decide to create a few levels of categories for each response set without creating a complete hierarchy. The development of an extensive hierarchy and a core category would not make sense in this case because the research goal is not the development of a theory of one phenomenon. (To see an example, I have incorporated grounded theory methods within a content analysis when wanting to compare developing feminist therapists' training needs with their program experiences; Kannan and Levitt 2009.)
3. If the primary goal is to *develop in-depth theories about one question from different perspectives*, it might be necessary to conduct complete qualitative analyses with multiple sets of participants. These analyses could result in separate hierarchies with core categories and then the hierarchies being subjected to a secondary analysis to compare and contrast the similarities and differences between them. For instance, I have used this approach when comparing clients' and therapists' experiences of challenges to clients' beliefs in therapy sessions (Williams and Levitt 2008b) or when conducting research on how victims, perpetrators, and faith leaders experience faith as influencing domestic violence (e.g., Knickmeyer et al. 2003; Levitt and Ware 2006; Levitt et al. 2008).
4. Finally, when a *purpose of the research is to identify patterns that extend beyond the participants' experiences* (*but are about one question and within one perspective*), it can be helpful to conduct a secondary analysis within a hierarchy to glean trends and differences—an analysis of the analysis. This goal usually occurs when researchers are interested in the data for a secondary purpose, such as developing guidelines for practice.

To give an example, in conducting research on eminent therapists' experiences of directing the process of therapy, we developed a hierarchy grounded in our participants' experiences but then wanted to develop principles for practice that focused clinicians on key decision-making points in their sessions (e.g., Levitt and Williams 2010). Some of these decision points were not described in any of the therapists' experiences directly because they were derived by our noticing the different types of description between groups of therapists. For instance, CBT therapists were more likely to position the change moment *outside* of the therapy exchange (e.g., in homework exercises, experiments) and psychodynamic and humanistic therapists tended to locate the change moment *within* the therapy exchange. This structural difference allowed us to make sense of the comparably stronger focus on the relationship by the humanistic and psychodynamic and the comparably stronger focus on designating homework and motivating clients to complete it by CBT therapists. While it allowed us to develop multiple principles for treatment, they were not grounded in the experiences in either group of therapists but the comparison of groups within the hierarchy for the purpose of identifying practice-relevant decisions.

Our importing of a hermeneutic analysis of the differences across these approaches allowed us to conduct this secondary work due to its attunement to both contextual and covert factors (see Rennie 2000 on the view that grounded theory is a form of methodical hermeneutics itself). Hermeneutic analyses can allow for exploration across both content and structure of an identified pattern in data, with a particular attention to the pre-understandings and philosophies underlying that pattern (e.g., Packer and Addison 1989). We have used this method when looking at conflicting client experiences in therapy as well (e.g., Levitt et al. 2006). When clients' responses conflicted, the context and assumptions within the interview text were examined closely to provide differential guidance on *when* or *under what conditions* an intervention might be helpful. The driving consideration across these points is: *To decide if a method* (e.g., *grounded theory*) *is appropriate, the researchers consider whether the question aims to develop a model of common experiences of one experience* (*might use grounded theory alone*) versus *to conduct a comparison of experiences between groups of participants or for purposes beyond understanding participants' experiences* (*might use other methods or adapt grounded theory methods to meet this aim*).

22.4.1.2 Is a Grounded Theory Analysis Too Intensive Considering the Data I Will Collect? (Question 2)

Answer: There are times when the intensive analyses in grounded theory are not necessary. The time that goes into building a hierarchy is worthwhile when the results that are produced are complex, rich, and shed light on processes that would otherwise be difficult to conceptualize or to do so in a manner that has fidelity to the experience of the event. Sometimes, however, this level of focus is simply not necessary to obtain useful results and would create undue labor. In my advising on method, I especially caution students when: (1) the study question is relatively simple to answer (for instance, studying participants' reactions to different course structures); (2) the participants have not had a long or in-depth experience that would have complex enduring associations or meanings (for instance, in a study on participants' reactions to a one-session intervention); (3) the participants do not have a great deal of insight or cannot communicate that insight in detail (e.g., if conducting a study on young children's experiences of rewards or punishments); or (4) results in the form of a detailed hierarchy are not necessary for the purpose of the analysis (e.g., detailed hierarchies may not be necessary for intervention development or for generating dialogues between groups of people).

Typically, I have an estimated length of time for the interviews, which I revise as they are conducted. That said, it is hard for me to imagine that interviews shorter than an hour in length can produce new data that might result in a useful analysis. Similarly, when considering conducting this form of analysis with written text, it is important to have not only a sufficient quantity to find overlapping meanings but a quality of depth that would make an intensive analysis worthwhile. If the participants can communicate the entirety of their experience in 15 min or in a paragraph, you likely will not have the depth of information to make this analysis worthwhile. The principle in this case is: *The scientific goal of the analysis* (i.e., *an in-depth understanding of the components of an experience*) *and the characteristics of both the phenomenon* (i.e., *complexity*) *and the participants* (i.e., *ability to clearly articulate their experience*) *should be considered when justifying a grounded theory analysis*. This being said, grounded theory methods can be used when these conditions are not met, but other methods (e.g., phenomenology, narrative analysis, or discourse analysis) [see Mörtl and Gelo (2015)] might produce similar results with greater ease and in a more applicable format.

22.4.2 Participants

22.4.2.1 Which Types of Difference Are Most Important in Participant Recruitment? (Question 3)

Answer: Differences among participants are seen as a *strength* in grounded theory approaches as researchers seek to diversify sources of information to develop results that are as rich and encompassing as possible. The method of *theoretical sampling* in grounded theory asks researchers to review their emerging theory within the developing hierarchy to identify gaps and then seek to recruit participants whose differences in perspective can best enrich the theory (Glaser and Strauss 1967; see Chap. 8). The logic underlying this participant sampling method is different than in quantitative studies, which have as a goal the estimation of probability and so tend to use larger numbers of participants and procedures like random or representational. I find it helps for me to consider the pool of participants that I wish to understand and the different perspectives therein that would result in a useful theory.

I typically find that I am in a difficult position when I explain to reviewers of my work not only why this diversity is important in this method, but how choices are made in the recruitment process. A challenge is that, given that grounded theory requires a relatively small set of participants, it is often *impossible* to have a reasonable number of participants from every type of diversity in one's sample (e.g., race, gender, sexual orientation, ability, age, ethnicity, sex, therapeutic orientation, therapeutic issues, time since therapy ended, length of time in therapy). As a result, choices have to be made in each study. By consulting the research and theoretical literature on the question at hand, I often can identify some factors that might be most likely to influence the question being investigated. For instance, if I am conducting a study on clients' experience of differences from their therapists, then forms of differences between the clients and therapists likely would be a form of diversity that I would work hard to obtain in my participants (e.g., Williams and Levitt 2008a). In contrast, if my goal is to understand how therapists guide clients through sadness, then differences in psychotherapy orientation might be a primary form of diversity that is sought, as therapists most often understand their methods of delivering treatment via their psychotherapy orientations. That being said, it still may be hard for me, as a white, middle class, able-bodied, Jewish, femme lesbian to conceptualize how other cultural backgrounds might affect the experience I am researching, and because the literatures often do not include discussions of cultural factors, there typically are secondary forms of diversity that I would seek. In the course of interviewing participants, I continue to consider which types of cultural factors (or other factors) might be important and then can seek to recruit those participants (in keeping with the concept of theoretical sampling; Glaser and Strauss 1967). The principle at hand here is: *Diversity within participants is sought out to clarify likely differences in experiencing that appear most relevant to the subject at hand. Typically, this includes considering how cultural factors may be influential throughout the analytic process, as their impact might be difficult for investigators to assess, and seeking out participants with relevant cultural diversity characteristics.* This check stems from a social justice approach to research in which there is an effort to represent and include perspectives that might be marginalized if not deliberately considered and integrated into the theories put forward by psychologists.

22.4.3 Investigators/Interviewers

At times, research may benefit from having one primary or sole interviewer. In other studies, interviewing may be shared between a few researchers or across a large research group. The interview is the most important moment of a qualitative research study. If it does not go well and rich data are not obtained that shed light on the subject, the analysis will not be fruitful no matter how wonderful the methods of analysis. Researchers are required to think on the spot within an interview context to clarify data and direct the interview focus. For each study then, decisions need to be made on who will be interacting with the participants and gathering data.

22.4.3.1 How Does One Decide Who Should Be Conducting the Interviews? (Question 4)

Answer: The following three factors may be useful to weigh together when deciding who should conduct interviews within a given study:

1. *Interviewing skills.* All interviewers who I work with undergo qualitative interview training in which they observe and perform role-plays, and receive feedback, before they conduct their own interviews. Usually, their interviewing skills improve dramatically after obtaining feedback on their first few interviews, so I ask students to transcribe and critique their first interviews within 3 days of conducting them and then we review them together. When the participants are highly verbal and self-reflective and are likely to have already talked with others about the experience under investigation, it is not as important to have interviewers who are as highly skilled. In contrast, interviewing skills become particularly important either when conducting interviews on topics that are difficult to discuss or when participants have difficulty articulating their experience. For instance, using interviewers with a higher level of interviewing skills might be more important when asking depressed clients about their experiences of sadness in psychotherapy (e.g., Henretty et al. 2008) than when asking people about their experiences of curiosity (Levitt et al. 2009).
2. *Knowledge about the subject.* There are different advantages and costs when interviewers are either naïve or expert about a subject at hand. I prefer to have investigators who tend to be naïve about the phenomenon under focus when I think it will prompt interviewees to unpack their experience of it more. For instance, an expert psychotherapist might be more likely to explicate change processes when talking to a graduate student than to another experienced psychotherapist (e.g., Levitt and Williams 2010). In contrast, expertise is particularly important when the question at hand requires subtle differentiations to be made and when the participants need more guidance to focus on a less familiar topic. For instance, I was the primary interviewer in a study of psychotherapeutic wisdom, as I had more therapy experience than my coinvestigator and felt better able to guide participants to clarify the nature of this ambiguous concept (e.g., Levitt and Piazza-Bonin 2011).
3. *Power (Im)balance.* Another factor I consider is how power differentials might influence the interview. The impact of cultural oppression and disparity on participants' comfort with disclosure can be important to consider. For instance, when interviewing men who had committed domestic violence, I chose to have the graduate student investigator act as the primary interviewer (although she

observed me conducting the initial interviews and I attended most of the interviews; Levitt et al. 2008). I reasoned that it could be difficult for these men (some of whom were men of color and all of whom had lower socioeconomic means) to talk about perpetrating abuse to a white person of professional and economic privilege, but, alternatively, talking to a younger female student might allow them to speak more openly. In another study, I conducted the interviews of butch and femme lesbians on their gender experience because I was part of that community and was trusted. Participants repeatedly told me that they would not have confided in an interviewer who was outside of their community.

The study-level principle that can be distilled is: *Decide who should conduct interviews after weighing together the need for interviewing skills, the knowledge needed on a subject matter, and the influence of cultural oppression and disparity upon the participants' ability to disclose and articulate information clearly*. After considering all three factors, we decide upon the types of training that are necessary, and who is best equipped to perform the interviews. These decisions can change as investigators receive more training and as the circumstances shift. For instance, in the wisdom project mentioned, two of the interviews I had conducted were accidentally deleted and had to be repeated. Having conducted the first interview, I worried that it would be difficult for participants to elaborate on their thoughts again with me and so the graduate student coinvestigator conducted the second interview as a more naïve interviewer could better gather these data.

22.4.4 Data Collection

22.4.4.1 Recruitment

The main question I have encountered relating to participant recruitment is if screening should be conducted before an interview.

22.4.4.1.1 Should a Screening Be Conducted Before the Interview? (Question 5)

Answer: A screening process to decide whether or not to include participants in a project before an interview can be important to implement when (1) the criteria for participation might be unclear (e.g., what does it mean for domestic violence to be "resolved"); (2) participants might be opting in who are unqualified to participate (e.g., wanting to get course credit in a subject pool); or (3) when there are issues around safety that needed to be addressed (e.g., interviewing women who had experienced domestic violence and needing to ensure that they would be safe; Knickmeyer et al. 2003). For instance, when studying psychotherapy phenomena that I am confident routinely occur (e.g., silences), I will not conduct screening if I am prepared to compensate participants for their time on the chance that the phenomena do not occur in the given session that we are examining (in which case I might ask instead about the lack of silence). In this case, the principle is: *Conduct screening interviews if it is difficult to know if the participants are able to describe usefully the topic of interest, because the topic is unclear or uncertain, the participants are suspect, or if their safety needs to be secured.*

22.4.4.2 Data Collection Procedure

There are two questions I most often encounter that relate to data collection.

22.4.4.2.1 Should I Analyze Interview or Written Data? (Question 6)

Answer: Sometimes an analyst only has access to written data—as is the case with analyses of historical documents or archived data. Although grounded theory usually entails a semi-structured interview protocol that is organized around one central question (the question whose answer is the theory being developed), written analyses can lead to productive research as well. Although the analysis written data can be wonderful for certain purposes (e.g., item development, analysis of historical documents), there are disadvantages to be kept in mind. Since the purpose of the interview typically is to help the investigators to develop an understanding and accurate interpretation of a complex individual's experience, there are often idiosyncratic clarifying questions asked in each interview that are difficult to ask within a written format. Also, interview questions can be changed across and within interviews as the researchers' understandings become more complex, and they notice gaps in their understanding. As a result, I prefer to conduct interview research when possible. Here the principle is: *Grounded theory methods can be adapted for the analysis of written data, but analysts should keep in mind the benefits and costs of this choice when designing studies.*

22.4.4.2.2 How Do I Structure My Interview? Do I Have a Main Question? (Question 7)

Answer: I consider the results I am seeking. If I am looking to develop a theory of how episodic disengagement in psychotherapy is experienced (Frankel and Levitt 2008), my main question will be "What is the experience of disengagement in psychotherapy for clients?" and the sub-questions will be variations of this main question (e.g., their experiences, before, during, and after these moments). In contrast, if the goal of my project is not to produce a singular theory but to answer a set of questions, I would use another method that is meant to explore multiple themes—like content or theme analysis. In this process, I might use some grounded theory procedures within those analytic approaches. For instance, I might divide the data and conduct separate analyses to answer the different questions and develop only a couple of levels of a hierarchy (e.g., how do feminists understand psychotherapy, what training do they receive, how satisfied are they with their training; Kannan and Levitt 2009). I would structure my interview protocol in this case to provide thorough answers to each main question and my results would be written in a corresponding format. Here, the principle being used is: *When writing your interview protocol, consider the scientific goal of your analysis. If your goal is to develop a theoretical model of one phenomenon, design your question protocol to elaborate a central question and use a method of analysis designed for this purpose (such as grounded theory or phenomenology), but if your goal is to shed light on a number of discrete subtopics, create separate groups of questions and conduct an analysis designed for that purpose (such as content analysis or theme analysis).*

22.4.5 Measures

At times, participants are asked to complete measures within a qualitative research paradigm. Because the number of participants is necessarily small, valid statistical analyses or comparisons cannot be conducted because the analyses would have little power. Reviewers become confused at times about this practice and often researchers have to defend this procedure.

22.4.5.1 When Should I Give Measures to Participants? (Question 8)

Answer: Measures for descriptive purposes most often are given in order to situate a given sample of participants. Giving measures, whether they are given within a mixed-methods data set or collected as part of a solely qualitative analysis, can provide a better sense of a sample's characteristics and can contribute toward the interpretation of the data and theoretical sampling—the process by which additional participants are recruited to flesh out a theory under development (Glaser and Strauss 1967). For instance, if I am conducting a study on psychotherapy clients' experiences, I might be interested to know if I have variation in my sample in the clients' experiences of alliances or therapy outcome (e.g., Levitt et al. 2006). I have found that I often face criticism when including measures, however. Some reviewers have criticized my use of these measures as catering to quantitative psychology and others have wanted statistical analyses conducted which do not make sense because of the small number of participants in most qualitative analyses. The principle at hand is: *Within the confines of the qualitative research, measures likely will rarely have the power to provide useful statistical knowledge due to the small data sets used. They can be useful, however, to provide information that can better describe your participants to aid in generalization* (i.e., *transferability*), *theoretical sampling, and data interpretation.*

22.4.6 Data Analysis: Adaptations of Grounded Theory

The method of analysis that I use is sourced, with variation, in that developed by David Rennie and his colleagues (e.g., Rennie et al. 1988). I base my work in this approach mainly because of the unmatched depth of its philosophical framework (Rennie 2006; Rennie and Frommer 2015). Although this is the prototypical design that I use, there are variations that come into play depending on different design features. [For a description of common problems that I see when supervising the work of new investigators to grounded theory and tips on how to troubleshoot them, see Levitt et al. (2013)]. Questions I often encounter when consulting about method design are whether grounded theory would be the best method to use and how to go about the process of analysis.

22.4.6.1 Do I Really Need So Many Categories or Hierarchy Levels? (Question 9)

Answer: There are many approaches to qualitative analyses, such as phenomenology (Giorgi 2009), content analyses (e.g., Schilling 2006), theme analysis (Braun and Clarke 2006), and versions of grounded theory (see Rennie and Frommer 2015), that do not entail the development of extensive hierarchies. In contrast, I favor the development of comprehensive hierarchies in most cases but in particular for graduate students and new investigators (i.e., emerging out of typically between 30 and 80 lowest-level categories, depending on the complexity of the phenomenon under study and culminating in 2–8 categories at the level below the core category). The reasons I recommend this process are that: (1) The process of moving between category levels seems to encourage creativity and prevents novel ideas from becoming lost in a large analysis. I ask students not to create categories that simply restate the participants' words, but initial categories that stick close to the language of the participants but emphasize the novel, interesting, or the metaphoric concepts in that language—and then moving gradually into more abstract categorization. (2) I find that the process of creating initial categories and moving up slowly helps graduate students learn to think in a complex way about their topic and to have confidence in their thinking. It can be challenging to learn what a strong theory might sound like in the absence of this process. Often I find that if students begin creating higher-order categories too quickly, the categories end up reflecting their questions rather than the answer provided. The category titles (e.g., "Types of Client Disengagement") are not as creative and do not provide answers to the questions being explored (cf. "Disengagement as Moderating Distress Toward Continued Exploration of Sensitive Experiences: Constructive Affect Regulation"; Frankel and Levitt 2008). (3) I find that I can better defend my analyses if I can explain clearly their foundation when I send my work out for review. For instance, when a reviewer asks about a concept, I can easily describe the concepts that led to its development. (4) The results can translate more easily into future analyses when a multilevel hierarchy is formed. For instance, the detail can help in the process of item development for a quantitative measure and can be helpful in the development of a manual to guide raters for coding qualitative variables (e.g., Levitt and Frankel 2004). Because it can be hard to tell how a program of research may develop over time, the process of creating a hierarchy can allow for many options after the initial project is completed. (5) Because I tend to approach my research with feminist and social justice aims, the development of more gradual and complex hierarchies makes it more likely that my findings will remain true to the experiences of my participants. If I jump to an abstract level too quickly, it is more likely that my own cultural biases will hold sway. That said, the more familiar investigators are with both grounded theory and with the subject at hand, the more likely they will be able to move more quickly between levels of analysis and still produce creative meaningful findings. (6) Although having many lower-level categories can be helpful for all these reasons, I find that having more than seven or eight categories at the level below the core category makes the resultant theory unwieldy, difficult to communicate, and obscures the central or dominant features at play. As a result, I work toward having this number become as small as possible while remaining true to the structure of the data. When considering the creation of a hierarchy, the study-level principle I offer is that: *Detailed hierarchies typically are useful when researchers are new to grounded theory, when the data is complex and findings are hard to organize or defend, and when results are intended to be used as the basis for future analyses.*

22.4.6.2 Should I Have a Core Category? (Question 10)

Answer: The core category is formed at the very top of the hierarchy and is the key category in the analysis. In general, a core category is recommended as it articulates the theory that is being put forth and distilling this understanding really is the point of the analytic process. At the same time, there are analyses where a core category might be counterproductive. It may be that within the process of analysis, it becomes clear that commonalities do not exist beyond a certain point. For instance, in my analysis of silences in psychotherapy (Levitt 2001), the central finding was that, although our field had tended to lump silences together in research studies, my analysis suggested there were seven quite distinct processes that led to silences. To develop a core category did not make sense as it would only obfuscate this finding of difference. There may be times as well when, even if a core category is developed, the more important level is the next level of the hierarchy which might outline different processes or types in a phenomenon (e.g., distinct clinical interpretations of disengagement; Frankel and Levitt 2008) that could have theoretical or clinical utility (Dourdouma and Mörtl 2012). The principle at play is: *A core category can be developed when it furthers the understanding of the phenomenon being studied, but is not useful when it creates a level of commonality that distracts from a more meaningful plurality in the findings.*

22.4.6.3 Should I Use Multiple Analysts? If So, How Should I Assign Epistemic Privilege? (Question 11)

Answer: Traditionally, grounded theory is conducted by one investigator (Glaser and Strauss 1967), although increasingly multiple investigators or research teams collaborate in projects. In most of my research, I prefer to have a single investigator or primary and secondary analyst, but I also have conducted research within large teams (e.g., Levitt et al. 2009). The advantage of having a smaller number of investigators is twofold. First, a primary or sole investigator conducts all the interviews and so has not only the experience of hearing the participants' words, but their attitudes, self-presentation, and a host of other meanings that can be lost when only transcripts are used. Also, the process of interviewing can lead an interviewer to *care* about participants and to become invested in safeguarding their stories—which I find increases his/her commitment to a highly attuned analysis and, interestingly, to separating out his/her biases from the analysis. In this way, an interviewer can develop an intimate connection with the data, be well positioned to conduct an analysis with high fidelity to the participants' experiences, and be more likely to advance the understanding of the experience.

On the other hand, there are times when having multiple perspectives on a data set is inherently worthwhile, but only if they are committed to meeting regularly together and focusing intensively on the research over a stretch of time. There are strategies that can be used to improve communication across large teams and to build a sense of caring and investment together. Also, training is an important part of academic research so often I am working with groups of student-investigators who do not have a great deal of experience in either psychotherapy, gender studies, or in qualitative analysis, and working closely together is crucial. Although I use a consensus model, I am careful to consider and discuss the role of epistemic privilege in relation to these factors:

1. *Data analysis experience*. The process of learning to conduct interviews and divide them into units and develop a hierarchy is one that requires close supervision. Typically, I indicate to students when to seek feedback, and, at each point I work closely with them, review initial efforts until I believe that they can continue independently. I give detailed feedback on my students' first interviews, first unitized transcripts, initial categories, and the level of categories below the core category. I usually meet with the student each week to review his/her progress. This level of supervision is the minimal level that students receive. If the only area of expertise that I bring is method of training, my reviews of their work are focused more on the method decisions and less upon the interpretations. I am not so much seeking consensus in interpretation as helping them to make distinctions in the data and to represent or code their data in a way that will result in a useful analysis. To the degree that my experience is greater than theirs, I am more likely to engage in more co-analysis of the data (see point 3 below).
2. *Interview experience*. As can be seen in the preceding section on interview considerations, it may be that the person conducting the analysis is not the best choice as interviewer but there may be insights that the interviewer still has to contribute to the analysis. In this case, I will work with the students to impart to them the meanings and reactions that were communicated in the interview process. These reactions do not necessarily override other interpretations of the data but we look at the data together and work to find interpretations that make sense to us both given our different experiences of the data. In other words, we use a process of consensus to aid our analysis in this case and I work to add my experience of the interviewing to the interpretation (or ask the student to do this when the student was the interviewer). When conducting class analyses, this guideline is explicit—that the student who conducted an interview gains priority in interpretation because of that lived experience.
3. *Experience with the subject*. More typically I am confident that the students can divide the text into the meaning units with supervision, but have some concerns about their ability to interpret the data and draw out all the important distinctions therein. In these cases, I review the data being coded each week and then conduct intensive reviews of the analysis periodically, acting as a co-analyst. I save the prior version of the analysis and then make note of changes I make during my review. When I meet with the students again, we discuss the changes together and if they disagree with a change, we discuss our interpretations with an eye toward reaching consensus. Typically, this process takes the form of representing both of our understandings as there can be aspects of the data that we are attending to differentially but are both important. If we have a strong disagreement and can see the rationale for each other's perspectives, we can inevitably find a way to give voice to the pieces that are important to us both—often with a statement that includes a caveat or a "when-if" clause.
4. *Different cultural experiences*. It can enrich a data set when the interviewers bring to the analysis lived experiences that can refine their interpretation of the data. For instance, when I was conducting research on lesbian gender, having a co-analyst who identified as a butch lesbian allowed us to have discussions that were helpful in developing a more highly attuned analysis (e.g., Levitt and Hiestand 2004), and when conducting analyses on gay male communities, it was similarly useful to have gay male coinvestigators (Manley et al. 2007). Here the idea is to invite coinvestigators who have specific experiences relevant to a phenomenon. I do not think that having investigators of the same cultural

background as a participant group is necessary (or often possible as people may have many different cultural identities), but it can be helpful especially when the group is one that is systemically oppressed in ways that are difficult for the participants to express and/or the investigator to understand. A process of co-analysis can be particularly useful as well in thinking through how to make the results of an analysis applicable in the real life context of different groups of people.

In integrating these points, the study-level principle that emerges is: *Multiple analysts are not necessary but are especially helpful when they provide method, topic, or culturally based experiences that will allow for a more complex interpretation of the data at hand.* These different factors all are considered and weighed together. Ideally, one ends up with an analysis in which one is confident in the meaning units created, the ability of the investigators to conduct the method and interpret the data, and the depth of analysis and its applicability.

22.5 Assessments of Research Checks

Grounded theory entails an empirical process of gathering data from sources that are knowledgeable on the topic and who are able to shed light on the subjective experience of a given phenomenon. Rennie (2000) argued that this method along with all forms of qualitative research (Rennie 2012) is best understood in terms of a methodical hermeneutic methodology (theory of method). He drew upon and modifies Peirce's (1965) theory of inference when proposing a logic of interpretation involving the cycling of education and conceptualization of meaning, abduction, deduction, and induction (cf. Rennie 2000, 2012), wherein in the latter moment evidence is recruited from the text in support of a given conceptualization, whether a category, theme, or structure, etc. In Rennie's view, the cycling of these logical moments makes qualitative research sufficient unto itself. Thus, it can be derived from this formulation that when other checks on rigor are used, these should be understood as supplemental rather than necessary.

Over time, criteria have been recommended for assessing rigor in qualitative research that are congruent with the epistemological paradigm at hand (see Morrow's 2005 review). For instance, assessing the "trustworthiness" or "credibility" (e.g., Elliott et al. 1999) of the research emphasizes the role of the researchers' and readers' faith in an interpretive analysis, rather than the capacity of a method to apprehend an existing truth. Often cited are Lincoln and Guba's (1985) criteria to assess trustworthiness that parallel natural science criteria: *transferability* (like external validity) to indicate the applicability of findings across contexts, *credibility* (like internal validity) to refer to readers' confidence in the truth of the findings by demonstrating depth of engagement and convincing interpretations, *dependability* (like reliability) to suggest whether similar themes could be found by other analysts, and *confirmability* (like objectivity) to indicate the degree to which the analysis is grounded in the data and unaffected by bias.

In addition, other criteria have been developed for assessing trustworthiness within nonrealist research paradigms (see Guba and Lincoln 2005; Morrow 2005). Among others, these included assessing *historical situatedness* and *erosion of ignorance* in critical (e.g., feminist) research, assessing *trustworthiness* and *authenticity* within constructivist research, and assessing *congruence* and *practical knowing* in participatory research. Across all three of these paradigms, they also recommend the criteria of assessing the potential of the research to stimulate *action* in response to the new understandings developed. Although I will not review all the criteria of assessing research quality across paradigms, I will discuss how I adapt methods for studies in relation to criteria that are relevant for my research (i.e., within a constructivist-social justice framework).

22.5.1 Should I Use Inter-rater Checks or External Auditor Checks on Coding? (Question 12)

Answer: In the quest to strengthen qualitative research processes, researchers often seek to augment their methods to establish the credibility of their analyses. Two methods that are sometimes utilized to assess intersubjective agreement are the quantitative documentation of inter-rater reliability on the process of coding or unitizing text and the incorporation of qualitative checks from auditors who are external to an analysis and do not engage in the inductive process. There are a number of reasons why typically I am reluctant to utilize either of these methods:

1. *Quantitative inter-rater agreement is rarely possible or desirable*. Quantitative indices of inter-rater reliability may be especially useful in a quantitative (or natural science) epistemology because the logic of a deductive comparison requires that the data be coded in a similar fashion for statistical analyses. Typically this coding is comprised of a limited set of responses—such as a scale from 1 to 7 or a set of qualitative labels [see Pokorny (2015) and Gelo and Manzo (2015)]. This reduction of complexity is necessary and useful because it allows for the identification of trends across average experiences. The purpose of this coding is to capture a process within a limited set of possibilities for statistical trend identification and hypothesis verification. [And I use these methods myself in my psychotherapy process measure research, e.g., Stringer et al. (2010).]

   In contrast, inter-rater reliability of induction-based coding is virtually impossible, however, when using traditional forms of grounded theory (and many other qualitative methods) as they use large numbers of categories with units that can be assigned to multiple categories (e.g., Glaser and Strauss 1967). (To make this more concrete—some of my analyses have had over 1,600 meaning units with separate labels, over 75 lowest-level categories, and included over 13 hierarchy levels.) Quantitative indices of inter-rater agreement are applicable to a vastly smaller number of categories than these and have no place in such complex categorizing where the ontological commitment is to the production of an interpretation based upon the understanding of complex and contextualized subjective processes.
2. *Inter-rater reliability or external auditor checks within this context could compromise the integrity of the analyses*. A danger of these methods is that they could result in the watering down of analyses to make fine distinctions more accessible to someone less intimate with the data at hand. Qualitative analyses result from an intensive engagement with data, and investigators often take a year to design a study and complete interviewing and then a second in analysis and writing to develop the necessary level of understanding. It could compromise the strengths of the research method—that is, attunement, especially to ambiguity, context, and complexity (sacrificing authenticity) for the sake of a form of rigor that is intrinsic to the logic of a quantitative context.

   Since the logic of this approach is sufficient to itself, I am reluctant to include supplemental checks that may compromise the trustworthiness of an interpretation by asking an investigator with a high level of commitment and understanding of their data to adjust interpretations for the sake of obtaining agreement with an investigator who may not share the same investment in or knowledge. It would be inconsistent with a constructivist epistemology that prioritizes the development of attuned interpretation (e.g., authenticity), as well as a feminist epistemology that is concerned with reducing biases stemming from superficial understandings (e.g., an erosion of ignorance).
3. *The need for these checks is not coherent with a constructivist-social justice ontology*. External audits and inter-rater checks may hinder the scientific goal of these analyses, which is not to produce one theory that is replicable by every analyst, but one that is trustworthy. Qualitative analyses have a different scientific

goal than quantitative ones. They are used to shed light upon data that contain multiple meanings, contradictions, ambiguities, and subjective complexities and to create understandings that accurately represent these qualities. These understandings or theories then can be evaluated and subjected to quantitative evaluation but that typically entails separate studies—as developing a model of a phenomenon itself is a substantial scientific contribution that requires considerable work, and it is rarely possible to present both analyses credibly in one journal article (e.g., Levitt 2001; Frankel et al. 2006).

To elaborate a bit on that point, a core premise of grounded theory is that many different valid understandings can emerge from different perspectives on the same data (e.g., Charmaz 2006; Fassinger 2005; Glaser and Strauss 1967). For instance, the same set of data could lead to a theory explaining clients' rationale for withholding information from therapists or explaining the ways clients develop trust. Both might be grounded in the data and be valid and productive contributions. Feminist approaches also hold that multiple perspectives may be valid—for instance, people may have very different experiences of an event depending on their position in terms of power and privilege (e.g., Code 2006; Harding 1998). Being able to position oneself within the standpoint of participants is key for interpretation. This understanding also means that qualitative analysis is not a completely relative process in which *any* interpretation could be valid. There are definite limits to the theories that can be produced from any one piece of text as it needs to be interpreted in relation to the concepts, perspectives, and meanings that are contained therein. And for an idea to become a dominant theme in an analysis, it would need to be repeated across sections of texts and participants, further limiting possibilities. The purpose of the coding is to interpret and articulate patterns so that a useful understanding can be developed.

This said, I have used external reviewers to shed light on the limits of an analysis or provide perspectives on how analyses can best be useful within a context—especially one with which I am less familiar. For instance, in research on legal wisdom (e.g., Levitt and Dunnavant 2014), two legal consultants advised us on how our findings could be used by or presented to lawyers and judges. They shared an external source of expertise that we lacked and educated us but did not directly evaluate or alter our analysis. If reviewers or auditors are used to strategically provide advice or context for the researchers to consider alongside of their analyses (and to accept or reject as it fits with their interpretation of the data), this process would be more in keeping with my approach. The use of an internal auditor when researchers are seeking another check is another innovative possibility (see Hill et al. 2005 on this evolution in consensual qualitative research; see also Chap. 23).

In making decisions about the type of co-analysis and supervision to provide, the principle distilled from this discussion is: Within a grounded theory analysis of a complex topic, the use of inter-rater reliability and external auditor checks is not desirable when it *hinders the scientific integrity* of the research—that is, to create fine-tuned categories that represent complex and contextualized data. The researchers can demonstrate to their readers the rigor of their methods by describing that qualitative methods tend to contain intrinsic checks and by supplementing these with additional checks that are consistent with the epistemology at hand.

22.5.2 How Many Participants Do I Need to Interview to Reach Saturation? (Question 13)

Answer: In grounded theory method, data collection continues until the categories are "saturated," that is, until further categories that add to or change the meaning of the analysis do not appear to be forthcoming (Glaser and Strauss 1967). Achieving saturation enhances rigor and trustworthiness by suggesting that the theory is comprehensive and thereby develops a basis for generalization of the theory. Typically, I like to collect at least two interviews that have not produced new categories in the hierarchy. As a general rule, I expect that the number of interviews should be related in some way to the level of complexity that might be expected in the data. For instance, I might be satisfied that saturation was reached within a data set of five interviews that examined the ways that clients interpreted therapists' minimal encouragers (e.g., "Mhm" and "Hm") within sessions. I would be unlikely to be satisfied with a claim that saturation was reached within a data set of eight interviews if the question being analyzed was all the processes by which psychotherapeutic change occurred. I would be suspicious that the last participant might just have been someone who was not very verbal or adept at explaining his/her experience and might want more sessions to be added to see if saturation holds. Usually grounded theory analyses seem to contain a minimum of about five interviews for this reason. The study-level principle is: *Saturation can be demonstrated by showing that new meaningful categories are not generated when adding a new interview; however, when the data is complex, it is recommended that saturation be tested further.*

22.5.3 What Credibility Checks Should I Use? How Should I Conduct Participant Checks? (Question 14)

Answer: Increasingly, grounded theory researchers are incorporating a variety of checks to assess the trustworthiness of their analysis and establish its rigor. These checks should be selected with consideration to the purpose and features of the study at hand. Typically, I use four kinds of checks on my credibility:

1. *Interview check*. I conduct a check on my interview process. Usually participants are asked a series of questions to determine whether or not their experience was fully represented at the end of each interview (e.g., Was there anything that wasn't asked about that feels significant about your therapy experience?) and to assess the effects of any cultural or interviewer-participant differences on the interview (e.g., Is there any way that my being a white woman might have influenced the interview?). This process provided the opportunity to collect information that might have been omitted. The principle here is: *Providing an interview check helps investigators to assess both the comprehensiveness of the interview and the influences of cultural or interpersonal differences on it.*
2. *Consensus*. Usually but not always, I work with coinvestigators to conduct analyses and we use a method of researcher consensus. I seek consensus only with investigators who have some level of intimacy with the data and hierarchy (see the previous section on the use of external auditors). We typically meet weekly throughout the entire study to talk about and review together the interviewing and the analysis. Throughout these discussions, I keep in mind the level of and type of expertise being brought by each researcher through that process (see section 22.4.6.3 for more discussion).

   Also, because of power differences between graduate student collaborators and myself, I encourage differences of opinion overtly and seek to include different perspectives within the hierarchy as opposed to representing only one interpretation of a unit. For instance, a segment of text might be coded as representing both the importance of connection and emotion. Irreconcilable conflicts have not occurred yet and I believe that this is not simply a result of my holding more power but a process of ensuring that all perspectives on the analysis are considered in light of the data and incorporated in a way that respects the investigators' sources of interpretative and methodological expertise. In this process, the principle is: *Consensus should be conducted in a way assigns epistemic privilege to the differing forms of methodological and interpretative expertise of the investigators, is sensitive to differences in power between investigators, and is open to incorporating multiple perspectives on a dataset.*

3. *Memoing*. Memoing, a form of note-taking in grounded theory (Glaser and Strauss 1967) sometimes used in other qualitative methods, is sometimes seen as a fourth type of check but sometimes seen as part of the process of data analysis. In this process, researchers act to take notes to record the hypotheses they are creating, the coding they are engaged in, and the methods they are using. It allows them to self-reflect upon the process of making meaning of the data and upon any consensus process. It acts as a form of "fallible bracketing" (Rennie 2000) as, although researchers realize that their perspectives unavoidably influence their analysis, they become aware of biases they hold and decide upon ways of restricting their influence on the data analysis increasing the credibility of the analysis. Memoing can be used to assist with the guideline for qualitative research offered by Elliott et al. (1999) called "owning your perspective." The principle at play is: *Use memoing to record thoughts, theories, and method decisions and to recognize and limit the influence of investigators' biases and processes upon the data.*
4. *Participant feedback*. The fourth check I tend to use is a check on the analysis and its fidelity to participants' experiences. This process can take different forms, such as follow-up interviews or mailing summaries of the results to participants and requesting written feedback. At other times, both methods might be used or something in-between. Often this decision is made based upon the researchers' evaluation of competing goals and restraints of a given project. The following are issues I consider when deciding how to seek and use feedback:
   (a) Efficiency in obtaining written feedback. When I am conducting an analysis as part of a classroom didactic experience, however, I often ask students to email written summaries of the main categories and request quantitative and qualitative feedback from the participants whom they interviewed. This process allows us to obtain quick responses from participants before the semester ends and is influenced by the didactic aim to provide the students with the experience of seeking feedback and writing results. It maximizes the chance that participants will respond but at the expense of the resulting feedback usually being more concise. On the other hand, when seeking feedback from eminent therapists who are very busy but also very adept at providing written descriptions of their work, emailing summaries of findings for feedback might maximize the return without much cost. It may be necessary to contact individuals whose feedback is unclear for additional discussion. The principle at hand is: *Written feedback can maximize the response of participants because a second interview is not required, but can limit the ability to receive detailed responses—especially if the participants find written expression challenging.*
   (b) Depth of feedback. When analyses are complex and researchers have many remaining questions about a hierarchy, asking a subset of the participants to engage in longer second interviews or feedback discussions is more useful—providing a greater depth to feedback. For instance, when I conducted two companion grounded theory projects on butch and femme lesbians—I had a butch, a femme, and an androgynous-identified lesbian provide feedback on all three categories in intensive interviews (1–2 h each). Although the butch and femme women were participants in the study, the androgynous woman provided an external perspective (that provided more contexts on the community but was not a

check on the analysis). Having an in-depth conversation with women who see these identities from different perspectives was useful in answering some of my questions and helping me to make sense of some of the differences and commonalities across the separate hierarchies. I would frame the principle here as: *Seek feedback from participants or others who you think might help you shed light on the questions that remain about your findings, given the purpose of the research at hand* (see Sect. 22.5.1 for more on how I might use nonparticipant reviewers' feedback).

(c) Social justice goals. In my research, I always seek participant feedback (i.e., member checking) as it provides me with helpful feedback on my interpretation of data and, in keeping with my feminist concerns, helps me move beyond the limits of my own cultural understandings. Although desirable, often participants' feedback from all participants is neither possible nor necessary and may not serve feminist ideals (cf. Frieze 2008, 2013). A complicating problem is that a grounded theory study can take a length of time to complete and it may be impossible to track down all the participants without invading participants' privacy—so then ironically the strength of the analysis may lead to *fewer* participants who can give feedback in the end. In other words, it is more coherent within a constructivist epistemology to prioritize the depth of interpretation over agreement in feedback from participants who have engaged in the analysis of the entire set of data under analysis—as the assessment of the analysis is in a strong inductive process rather than in supplemental feedback checks.

In particular, it is harder to obtain feedback when studying populations that have fewer resources, protect their identities more (e.g., may not give out contact information as easily), are reticent to participate in research, are transient, or are members of minority groups with stressors in their own lives that limit their time for research participation. It is coherent with a social justice perspective to have the voices from these groups presented in the literature rather than to insist upon feedback from all participants (see Fine 2011).

Also, experienced researchers realize that it is rare that grounded theory findings result in stark disagreements with participants because the analysis is grounded so entirely in participants' interviews. In my experience the vast majority of feedback responses take the form of affirmations, clarifications of minor points being made, or suggestions on how ideas can be framed. While these responses are helpful, the main results of a study are rarely questioned. The principle here is: *Obtaining feedback from participants is ideal; however, researchers committed to a constructivist-social justice framework should recognize that all participants typically are not able and should not be expected to provide feedback and that this feedback is supplementary*. Because the central form of rigor and trustworthiness in grounded theory is the strength of the induction-based analysis, supplemented as judged helpful by credibility checks, member checking is only one of the many ways in which the research can be assessed.

(d) Conflicts between participants' feedback and your interpretation. Typically, we use the feedback from participants to fine-tune the hierarchy or expand our understanding of the phenomenon. We often make adjustments in our analysis after receiving participant feedback but ultimately we are using the feedback to enrich my understanding rather than to veto my interpretation. Although the participant may have authority over his or her own experiences, we have access to the experiences of all the data across the participants and have conducted a study looking for patterns within it that privileges our interpretation of those patterns. Still, as is the process of a hermeneutic circle, the new piece of information can influence our understanding of the whole analysis, and our understanding of the analysis can influence our understanding of the feedback. The principle here is that *Feedback from participants can enrich investigators' understanding of data; however, feedback needs to be reconciled with the investigators' interpretations of patterns from across the participants and the hierarchy*. If we cannot reconcile the feedback with our interpretation, we typically present the feedback alongside of our interpretation so that readers can assess this discrepancy themselves.

22.6 Meta-principles of Interpretation-Driven Research Design and Evaluation

Reviewing these guidelines, there are many ways in which the specific qualities within a project can radically influence the design of that study. Still, I am certain that there are principles that are missing from the guidelines because they have not been relevant to my program of research as of yet. From a review of the principles created, the following four meta-principles were created to guide research design and evaluation for grounded theory research, but can be extended to other forms of research as well (see Table 22.2):

1. The qualities of *phenomena* under study need to be considered particularly in terms of: seeking diversity within participants, deciding upon the degree of detailed coding needed within a hierarchical structure, deciding if a core category is helpful, selecting the number of transcripts used to establish saturation, and choosing procedures.
2. The qualities of *investigators* involved need to be evaluated, especially in terms of selecting interviewers and analysts, deciding how to respond to the limits of their cultural perspectives, deciding how to involve external reviewers, and structuring of a process of consensus and assigning epistemic privilege.
3. The qualities of the *research participants* need to be appraised when deciding upon the need for screening, the necessity and structure of feedback checks, and the methods with which they might engage (e.g., grounded theory).
4. *Scientific, clinical, and social justice goals* of a given analysis (e.g., are the goals to produce a theory, develop an intervention, and/or to give voice to an underrepresented or marginalized group) need to be considered when selecting a process of analysis, making decisions about measures, designing credibility checks, and deciding upon the necessity and structure of feedback.

From this perspective, creating a set of rules for all qualitative research can be seen as problematic (see Levitt et al. 2005, on the function of principles versus rules). While rules can be inflexible and focused on behaviors across settings, principles allow for flexibility and focus more on intentionality and rationales for adapting decisions across contexts. It does not recognize that qualitative research designs tend to be situated within epistemologies that require understandings of rigor and trustworthiness that are relevant to the qualities of the participants, researchers, phenomena, and research goals. In contrast, interpretation-driven considerations of research design, research consumption, and review, such as those developed in this chapter, allow for a flexibility that can best serve clinical, advocacy, and scientific aims.

Conclusion

In summary, conceptualizing the design and evaluation from interpretation-driven approach has a number of benefits for qualitative research. First, it allows for an appropriate assessment of qualitative studies in which

Table 22.2 Meta-principles of interpretation-driven research design and evaluation

Relevant topic	Interpretation-driven guidelines
Phenomena	The qualities of phenomena under study need to be considered particularly in terms of: seeking diversity within participants, deciding upon the degree of detailed coding needed within a hierarchical structure, deciding if a core category is helpful, selecting the number of transcripts used to establish saturation, and choosing procedures
Investigators	The qualities of investigators involved need to be evaluated, especially in terms of selecting interviewers and analysts, deciding how to respond to the limits of their cultural perspectives, deciding how to involve external reviewers, and structuring of a process of consensus and assigning epistemic privilege
Participants	The qualities of the research participants need to be appraised when deciding upon the need for screening, the necessity and structure of feedback checks, and the methods with which they might engage (e.g., grounded theory)
Project goals	Scientific, clinical, and social justice goals of a given analysis (e.g., are the goals to produce a theory, develop an intervention, and/or to give voice to an underrepresented or marginalized group) need to be considered when selecting a process of analysis, making decisions about measures, designing credibility checks, and deciding upon the necessity and structure of feedback

procedures within methods are adapted to serve a contextualized interpretive process, rather than using a procedure-driven approach that privileges rules associated with decontextualized methods. Second, an interpretation-driven framework can allow one to adopt a pragmatic approach to the characteristics and constraints of a study while considering the effects of method decisions upon scientific, clinical, and social justice goals. As well, it can allow researchers to consider how best to generate results that lead to a depth of understanding that also have fidelity to the experiences of participants. Although this chapter is focused upon grounded theory, researchers can extend the principles to other methods of qualitative research. Instead of solidifying sets of procedural rules that are insensitive to the processes and components at play, interpretation-driven principles guide researchers and reviewers to an understanding of method as an expression of epistemology that is shaped as it serves scientific, practice, and social justice goals. Researchers then are not reduced to technicians who blindly serve a method but become advocates of understanding, developers of treatments, and scientists.

Acknowledgement The author would like to thank David Rennie and Omar C.G. Gelo for sharing their thoughts in response to this chapter.

References

Angus L, Levitt H, Hardtke K (1999) The narrative processes coding system: research applications and implications for psychotherapeutic practice. J Clin Psychol 55(10):1255–1270. doi:10.1002/(SICI)1097-4679(199910)55:10<1255::AID-JCLP7>3.0.CO;2-F

Bakan D (1967) On method: toward a reconstruction of psychological investigation. Jossey-Bass, San Francisco, CA

Bar On BA (1993) Marginality and epistemic privilege. In: Alcoff L, Potter E (eds) Feminist epistemologies. Routledge, New York, pp 83–100

Braun V, Clarke V (2006) Using thematic analysis in psychology. Qual Res Psychol 3:77–101. doi:10.1191/1478088706qp063oa

Charmaz K (2006) Constructing grounded theory: a practical guide through data analysis. Sage, Thousand Oaks, CA

Code, L (1996) What is natural about naturalized epistemology? Am Philos Q 33:1–22

Code L (2006) Ecological thinking: the politics of epistemic location. Oxford University Press, Oxford

Corbin J, Strauss AL (2008) Basics of qualitative research: grounded theory procedures and techniques, 3rd edn. Sage, Thousand Oaks, CA

Diamond LM (2006) Careful what you ask for: reconsidering feminist epistemology and autobiographical narrative in research on sexual identity development. Signs J Women Cult Soc 31:471–491. doi:10.1086/491684

Dourdouma A, Mörtl K (2012) The creative journey of GTA: a guideline to its principle and application. Res Psychother Psychopathol Process Outcome 15:96–106. doi:10.7411/RP.2012.010

Elliott R, Fischer CT, Rennie DL (1999) Evolving guidelines for publication of qualitative research studies in psychology and related fields. Br J Clin Psychol 38:215–229. doi:10.1348/014466599162782

Fassinger RE (2005) Paradigm, praxis, problems, and promise: grounded theory in counseling psychology. J Couns Psychol 52:156–166. doi:10.1037/0022-0167.52.2.156

Fine ML (2011) Troubling calls for evidence. Fem Psychol 22:3–19. doi:10.1177/0959353511435475

Fine ML (2012) Resuscitating critical psychology for 'revolting' times. J Soc Issues 68:416–438. doi:10.1111/j.1540-4560.2012.01756.x

Fletcher GJO (1996) Realism versus relativism in psychology. Am J Psychol 109:409–429. doi:10.2307/1423014

Frankel ZF, Levitt HM (2008) Clients' experiences of disengaged moments in psychotherapy: a grounded theory analysis. J Contemp Psychother 39:171–186. doi:10.1007/s10879-008-9087-z

Frankel ZF, Levitt HM, Murray DM, Greenberg LS, Angus LE (2006) Assessing psychotherapy silences: an empirically derived categorization system and sampling strategy. Psychother Res 16(5):627–638. doi:10.1080/10503300600591635

Frieze IH (2008) Publishing qualitative research in sex roles. Sex Roles 58:1–2. doi:10.1007/s11199-007-9376-0

Frieze IH (2013) Guidelines for qualitative research being published in sex roles. Sex Roles 69:1–2. doi:10.1007/s11199-013-0286-z

Gelo OCG (2012) On research methods and their philosophical assumptions: raising the consciousness of researchers again. Psychother Sozialwiss 2:111–130

Gelo OCG, Manzo S (2015) Quantitative approaches to treatment process, change process, and process-outcome research. In: Gelo OCG, Pritz A, Rieken B (eds) Psychotherapy research: foundations, process, and outcome. Springer, Heidelberg

Gelo OCG, Braakmann D, Benetka G (2008) Quantitative and qualitative research: beyond the debate. Integr Psychol Behav Sci 42:266–290. doi:10.1007/s12124-008-9078-3

Gelo OCG, Braakmann D, Benetka G (2009) Erratum to "Quantitative and qualitative research: beyond the debate". Integr Psychol Behav Sci 43(4):406–407. doi:10.1007/s12124-009-9107-x

Gergen KJ, McNAmee S (2000) From disordering discourse to transformative dialogue. In: Neimeyer RA, Raskin JD (eds) Constructions of disorder: meaning-making frameworks for psychotherapy. APA, Washington, DC, pp 333–349

Giorgi A (2009) The descriptive phenomenological method in psychology: a modified Husserlian approach. Duquesne University, Pittsburgh, PA

Glaser B, Strauss A (1967) The discovery of grounded theory. Aldine, Chicago

Greenberg LS (2007) A guide to conducting a task analysis of psychotherapeutic change. Psychother Res 17:15–30. doi:10.1080/10503300600720390

Guba EG, Lincoln YS (1994) Competing paradigms in qualitative research. In: Denzin NK, Lincoln YS (eds) Handbook of qualitative research. Sage, London, pp 105–117

Guba EG, Lincoln YS (2005) Paradigmatic controversies, contradictions and emerging confluences. In: Denzin N, Lincoln YS (eds) The sage handbook of qualitative research. Sage, London, pp 191–215

Harding S (1986) The science question in feminism. Cornell University Press, Ithaca, NY

Harding S (1998) Is science multi-cultural? Postcolonialisms, feminisms, and epistemologies. Indiana University Press, Bloomington, IN

Harding S (2011) The postcolonial science and technology studies reader. Duke, Durham, NC

Henretty JR, Levitt HM, Mathews SS (2008) Clients' experiences of moments of sadness in psychotherapy: a grounded theory analysis. Psychother Res 18:243–255. doi:10.1080/10503300701765831

Hill CE, Knox S, Thompson BJ, Williams EN, Hess SA, Ladany N (2005) Consensual qualitative research: an update. J Couns Psychol 52:196–205. doi:10.1037/0022-0167.52.2.196

Kannan D, Levitt HM (2009) Challenges facing the developing feminist psychotherapist. Women Ther 32:406–422. doi:10.1080/02703140903153377

Knickmeyer N, Levitt HM, Horne SG, Bayer G (2003) Responding to mixed messages and double binds: religious oriented coping strategies of Christian battered women. J Relig Abuse 5:55–82. doi:10.1300/J154v05n02_03

Levitt H (1999) The development of wisdom: an analysis of Tibetan Buddhist experience. J Humanist Psychol 39(2):85–104. doi:10.1177/0022167899392006

Levitt HM (2001) The sounds of silence in psychotherapy: the categorization of clients' pauses. Psychother Res 11(3):295–309. doi:10.1080/713663985

Levitt H (2006) Butch, Femme, Bear and Leatherman: a programmatic exploration of gender identities within gay and lesbian subcultures. In: Kam-shing YIP (ed) Psychology of gender identity: an international perspective. Nova Science, Hauppauge, NY, pp 105–121

Levitt HM, Frankel Z (2004) Pausing inventory classification system (PICS) manual, 2nd Revision. Unpublished manuscript, University of Memphis

Levitt H, Hiestand K (2004) A quest for authenticity: contemporary butch gender. Sex Roles 50:605–621. doi:10.1023/B:SERS.0000027565.59109.80

Levitt HM, Piazza-Bonin EB (2011) Wisdom-based approaches to therapy: challenging the dominant psychotherapy culture. Unpublished master's thesis, University of Memphis, Memphis, TN

Levitt H, Ware K (2006) "Anything with two heads is a monster": religious leaders perspectives on marital equality and domestic violence. Violence Against Women 12(12):1–22. doi:10.1177/1077801206293546

Levitt HM, Williams DC (2010) Facilitating client change: principles based upon the experience of eminent psychotherapists. Psychother Res 10:337–352. doi:10.1080/10503300903476708

Levitt HM, Neimeyer RA, Williams D (2005) Rules vs. principles in psychotherapy: implications of the quest for universal guidelines in the movement for empirically supported treatments. J Contemp Psychother 35:117–129. doi:10.1007/s10879-005-0807-3

Levitt HM, Butler M, Hill T (2006) What clients find helpful in psychotherapy: principles for facilitating change. J Couns Psychol 53:314–324. doi:10.1037/0022-0167.53.3.314

Levitt HM, Todd-Swanger R, Butler JB (2008) Male perpetrators' perspectives on intimate partner violence, religion, and masculinity. Sex Roles 58:435–448. doi:10.1007/s11199-007-9349-3

Levitt HM, Williams DC, Cifci-Uruk A, Kannan D, Obana M, Smith B, Wang MC, Plexico LW, Camp J, Hardison H, Watts A, Wonch W (2009) The experience of depth curiosity: the pursuit of congruence despite the danger of engulfment. J Constr Psychol 22:187–212. doi:10.1080/10720530902915093

Levitt HM, Dunnavant B (2014) Judicial wisdom: the process of forming wise decisions. J Construct Psychol (in press)

Levitt HM, Ippolito MR, Kannan D (2013) Teaching qualitative methods using a research team approach: publishing grounded theory projects with your class. Qual Res Psychol 10:119–139. doi:10.1080/14780887.2011.586101

Lincoln YS, Guba EG (1985) Naturalistic inquiry. Sage, Newbury Park, CA

Longino H (1993) Subjects, power and knowledge: description and prescription in feminist philosophies of science. In: Alcoff L, Potter E (eds) Feminist epistemologies. Routledge, New York, pp 101–120

Manley E, Levitt HM, Mosher C (2007) Understanding the bear movement in gay male culture: redefining masculinity. J Homosex 53:89–112. doi:10.1080/00918360802103365

Mörtl K, Gelo OCG (2012) Qualitative research methods. In: Gelo OCG, Pritz A, Rieken B (eds) Psychotherapy research: general issues, process and outcome. Springer, Vienna/New York

Morrow SL (2005) Quality and trustworthiness in qualitative research in counseling psychology. J Couns Psychol 52:250–260. doi:10.1037/0022-0167.52.2.250

Mörtl K, Gelo OCG (2015) Qualitative methods in psychotherapy process research. In: Gelo OCG, Pritz A, Rieken B (eds) Psychotherapy research: foundations, process, and outcome. Springer, Heidelberg

Neimeyer RA (2009) Constructivist psychotherapy: distinctive features. Routledge, New York

Packer MJ, Addison RB (1989) Entering the circle: hermeneutic investigation in psychology. State University of New York Press, Albany

Peirce CS (1958) A neglected argument for the existence of god. In: Wiener PP (ed) Values in a Universe of chance: Selected writings of Charles S. Peirce. Stanford University Press, Stanford, CA

Peirce CS (1965) Collected papers of Charles Sanders Peirce. The Belknap Press of Harvard University Press, Cambridge, MA

Pokorny D (2015) Quantitative data analysis in psychotherapy process research. Structures and procedures. In: Gelo OCG, Pritz A, Rieken B (eds) Psychotherapy research: foundations, process, and outcome. Springer, Heidelberg

Ponterotto JG (2005) Qualitative research in counseling psychology: a primer on research paradigms and philosophy of science. J Couns Psychol 52:126–136. doi:10.1037/0022-0167.52.2.126

Raskin JD, Bridges SK (eds) (2008) Studies in meaning 3: constructivist psychotherapy in the real world. Pace University, New York

Rennie DL (1997) Methodical hermeneutics and humanistic psychology. Humanist Psychol 35:1–14. doi:10.1080/08873260709336693

Rennie DL (2000) Grounded theory methodology as methodical hermeneutics: reconciling realism and relativism. Theory Psychol 10:481–502. doi:10.1177/0959354300104003

Rennie DL (2006) The grounded theory method: application of a variant of its procedure of constant comparative analysis to psychotherapy research. In: Fischer CT (ed) Qualitative research methods for psychologists: introduction through empirical studies. Elsevier, Boston, MA, pp 59–78

Rennie DL (2010) Humanistic psychology at York University: retrospective: focus on clients' experiencing in psychotherapy: emphasis of radical reflexivity. Humanist Psychol 38:40–56. doi:10.1080/08873261003635856

Rennie DL (2012) Qualitative research as methodical hermeneutics. Psychol Methods 17(3):385–398. doi:10.1037/a0029250

Rennie DL, Fergus KD (2006) Embodied categorizing in the grounded theory method: methodical hermeneutics in action. Theory Psychol 16:483–503. doi:10.1177/0959354306066202

Rennie DL, Frommer J (2015) Applications of qualitative and mixed-methods counseling and psychotherapy research. In: Gelo OCG, Pritz A, Rieken B (eds) Psychotherapy research: foundations, process, and outcome. Springer, Heidelberg

Rennie DL, Phillips JR, Quartaro GK (1988) Grounded theory: a promising approach to conceptualization in psychology? Can Psychol 29:139–150. doi:10.1037/h0079765

Schilling J (2006) On the pragmatics of qualitative assessment: designing the process for content analysis. Eur J Psychol Assess 22:28–37. doi:10.1027/1015-5759.22.1.28

Slife BD, Gantt E (1999) Methodological pluralism: a framework for psychotherapy research. J Clin Psychol

55:1453–1465. doi:10.1002/(SICI)1097-4679(199912)55:12<1453::AID-JCLP4>3.0.CO;2-C

Stringer JV, Levitt HM, Berman JS, Mathews SS (2010) A study of silent disengagement and distressing emotion in psychotherapy. Psychother Res 20:495–510. doi:10.1080/10503301003754515

Wertz FJ (2005) Phenomenological research methods in counseling psychology. J Couns Psychol 52:167–177. doi:10.1037/0022-0167.52.2.167

Williams DC, Levitt HM (2008a) Clients' experiences of difference with therapists: sustaining faith in psychotherapy. Psychother Res 18:256–270. doi:10.1080/10503300701561545

Williams DC, Levitt HM (2008b) When constructs collide: constructivist research on when and how to challenge clients. In: Raskin JD, Bridges SK (eds) Studies in meaning III. Pace University Press, New York

Consensual Qualitative Research (CQR): Methods for Conducting Psychotherapy Research

23

Clara E. Hill

Contents

Abstract

In this chapter, I describe the background and methods used in consensual qualitative research (CQR). Specifically, I describe the original CQR method used in interviews (CQR-I). Then I describe CQR-M (CQR modified to use with short, simple data) and CQR-C (CQR applied to case studies). I close the chapter with a comparison or the similarities and differences between the three CQR methods.

23.1 Consensual Qualitative Research Methods for Conducting Psychotherapy Process Research

Qualitative methods are ideal for providing a rich, in-depth description of the process and outcome of psychotherapy. Researchers obtain a deep understanding of psychotherapy by listening to stories that participants tell about their experiences or by having judges observe and integrate many sources of data. Qualitative

C.E. Hill (✉)
Department of Psychology, University of Maryland, College Park, MD 20742, USA
e-mail: cehill@umd.edu

O.C.G. Gelo et al. (eds.), *Psychotherapy Research*,
DOI 10.1007/978-3-7091-1382-0_23,

research is also particularly suited for investigating infrequently occurring phenomena within psychotherapy (e.g., misunderstandings; Rhodes et al. 1994) because large samples are not needed and for studying complex phenomena that are not easily defined or quantified and thus are not appropriate for quantitative methods (e.g., compassion; Vivino et al. 2009). In addition, qualitative methods are well suited for studying new areas for which there is little known, and hence there is little basis for knowing what to predict or assess (e.g., clients' feelings about talking about money in therapy). On the other hand, qualitative methods are not good for determining significant differences between groups (e.g., differences between types of treatment) or causality (e.g., linking process to outcome).

In this chapter, I describe consensual qualitative research (CQR). My colleagues and I developed this approach (Hill et al. 1997) based on our integration of grounded theory (Strauss and Corbin 1998), phenomenology (Giorgi 1985), and comprehensive process analysis (Elliott 1989) approaches. We later modified CQR (Hill 2012; Hill et al. 2005) based on our experiences using CQR and a review of the corpus of CQR studies. We developed this approach to provide a clear, rigorous, easily understandable, and teachable research method that could be learned and conducted by ourselves and others. In this chapter, I describe how we have used CQR with interview data (CQR-I), how we can modify it for use with simpler interview or written data (CQR-M), and how we can extend the model for examining data from psychotherapy cases (CQR-C).

23.2 Consensual Qualitative Research: Interview

CQR is a descriptive, inductive research method based on data collected through interviews involving open-ended questions and a semi-structured format. This method is particularly good for investigating inner experiences that are not easily observable to outsiders (e.g., clients' perceptions of therapist anger, therapists' perceptions of relational interventions). Researchers remain open to what the data reveal and ask questions rather than pose directional hypotheses (which imply that they know what to expect from the data). The data involve words (rather than numbers) from participants telling narratives and providing descriptions about their experiences. A small number of cases (typically 8–15) are studied in depth, usually involving one or two interviews for each case. The researchers articulate and bracket (i.e., set aside) their biases and expectations before interviewing participants and stay as close as possible to the participants' words and meanings when they analyze the data (see also Williams and Morrow 2009).

In the analyses, researchers make sense of the parts of the transcribed interviews by being immersed in all the information known about the case (e.g., in understanding a client's need to give a gift to her therapist, it is important to be aware of what has gone on before in the course of the therapy; see Knox et al. 2009). At least three judges (the primary team) examine the data at each step of the analysis so that multiple perspectives are obtained. Judges use their clinical intuition to make sense of the data and discuss their judgments with each other at each step to consensually arrive at the best understanding of the data, always aware that they are constructing an understanding of the data rather than uncovering "truth." Thus, consensus among researchers is a key method for integrating multiple perspectives. In addition, one or two auditors examine the primary team's data analysis to offer additional perspectives and serve as a protection against groupthink. A final feature is that researchers return to the raw interview data repeatedly to resolve disputes and make sure that their interpretations are as accurate as possible. This analysis process is labor intensive and requires a great deal of trust within the team, as well as a willingness to work together collaboratively; judges have to be willing and able to assert their opinions and work with the team to resolve disputes amicably.

Table 23.1 shows the major steps involved in CQR. For detailed descriptions of all the steps for

Table 23.1 Steps of data collection and data analysis in CQR

1. Develop research questions
2. Conduct and transcribe interviews
3. Develop domains
4. Construct core ideas for each case within each domain
5. Audit of domains and core ideas for each case
6. Cross-analyses: develop categories within domains across all cases
7. Audit of cross-analyses

using CQR, I urge readers to first read Hill et al. (1997, 2005), and Hill (2012). I then recommend reading a number of published studies that have used CQR (e.g., Gelso et al. 1999; Hill et al. 2000, 2003; Knox et al. 2003; Ladany et al. 1997; Vivino et al. 2009) to get a model for the application of the method, the range of questions asked, and methods followed. In the next sections of this chapter, I focus only on a broad description of the major steps: creating and implementing the interview, developing domains, constructing core ideas/audit, and conducting a cross-analysis/audit. Throughout the description of the steps, I illustrate the approach by describing a study in which we interviewed therapists-in-training about their experiences of a corrective relational experience in their own personal therapy (Knox et al. 2012).

23.2.1 The Interview

We usually have only a few (6–10 per hour) scripted, open-ended questions in each interview to enable researchers to gain consistent information across individuals so that we can look for emerging themes across cases. In addition, we use unscripted probing (e.g., "Tell me more about...") to gain in-depth information about each individual's unique experiences, as well as to allow unexpected information to emerge. It also helps greatly for interviewers to do at least two pilot interviews prior to collecting the data for the study, both to allow the researchers to refine the interview and to train interviewers to be consistent.

A key to the interviewing process is for the interviewer to develop a research alliance with the interviewee so that the interviewee trusts that it is safe to reveal personal information. The interviewer builds this alliance through remaining nonjudgmental about what the interviewee says, probing to make sure that the interviewee has said as much as possible about the topic, restating the verbal content to allow the interviewee to hear what he or she has been saying, and showing genuine interest and curiosity about the interviewee as a person. In addition, interviewers need to attend to the emotional tone of what interviewees say to be able to pick up on the key elements and help interviewees express themselves deeply, especially about topics that are difficult to explore and to disclose about to others. Trained therapists who are skilled in interviewing and have a deep understanding of psychotherapy constructs are ideal to use as interviewers.

For example, in the Knox et al. (2012) study on corrective relational experiences, we asked the following scripted interview questions: (a) Tell me about your therapy. (b) Tell me about your relationship with your therapist. (c) Now let's talk about a specific corrective relational experience (CRE)—or a particular time in therapy when you felt a distinct shift and you came to understand your relationship with your therapist in a new and unexpected way. What led up to this event? (d) Describe the event itself. (e) What were the consequences of the event? (f) How did our interview affect you? Many unscripted probes were also used, depending on what the interviewee said, to help the participant further explore the CRE. For more thoughts about interviews, consult Burkard et al. (2012).

I should note that although typically we have used telephone interviews, we have sometimes used other data collection methods. For example, in our first study (Rhodes et al. 1994), we asked participants to write their responses to our questions. Unfortunately, we found the responses to this method to be rather "thin," in that participants did not open up as much as they might have with a supportive, probing interviewer. On the other hand, when we used a journal format where novice therapists wrote in a journal each week for a semester and then sent their journals via email to two readers who read and provided feedback (Hill et al. 2007b), we got a wealth of rich data. In another variation, Kim et al. (2004) conducted an "interview" via email with Asian students and thought that this method might be preferable to face-to-face or telephone interviews for populations who are easily shamed by discussion of sensitive topics.

23.2.2 Domains

Domains are topic areas or ways that the interview content can be organized into meaningful sections or topics (see also Thompson et al. 2012). Domains can be determined either by clustering the interview questions or by examining the data to see what domains emerge. Regardless of the method used, researchers modify the domains extensively to fit the emerging data as they proceed through the steps of the CQR process. In the Knox et al. (2012) study, we eventually arrived at five domains: (a) the general background of the therapy, (b) the antecedent to the event, (c) the event itself, (d) the consequences of the event, and (e) the effects of interview. I should note that determining the domains in this study was particularly straightforward as the data fell nicely into a sequential pattern, but it has not proven as easy to determine domains in other studies. We have particularly struggled with identifying domains when there was not a clearly defined research question, the interview protocol was poorly constructed (e.g., confusing questions, lots of closed questions that did not elicit exploration), or the interview was poorly done (e.g., the interviewer did not probe enough for details to clarify participants' experiences, the interviewers did not connect with the interviewees on an emotional level), or participants were not knowledgeable about the topic.

23.2.3 Core Ideas/Audit

With the core ideas, researchers summarize the content within a domain for an individual case (again see also Thompson et al. 2012). Core ideas are akin to abstracts or summaries in that they are shorter and more concise than what the participant has said. For example, if the participant spoke for several minutes and provided several examples to illustrate a point, the primary team might summarize this information into two or three sentences that convey the essence of what the person was communicating. The purpose of the core ideas, then, is to distill what the participant has said to its essence, remove redundancies, and clarify meanings (this latter purpose is particularly important for developing good data for next step of analyzing data across cases). Importantly, primary team members have to understand the whole case to create the individual core ideas, for they must understand the participant's words within the context of everything the person has said. Core ideas are written in a relatively neutral language (not using a lot of jargon or slang that can be misinterpreted out of context) that can be understood across cases, but they use the participants' language as much as possible so as not to go beyond or lose the richness of the data.

In the Knox et al. (2012) study, an example can be found of interview data that was placed in the domain of the event itself. The dialogue between the interviewer and participant went as follows (P stands for participant, I for interviewer):

P: It [the therapy] was something that I really, really looked forward to. There was no time that I ever thought, "Oh, I have to go talk." Even though sometimes at the end of the sessions there were awful feelings of some of the things that we talked about, I always felt that it was a safe environment where I was definitely being heard and he encouraged me to write as well, which I found very beneficial.

I: Kind of a journal type of thing?

P: Yeah, and now I have all those journal notes so I can look back and see where I was and where I am now, and that helps as days get foggy.

I: So it sounds like he was really supportive, gentle, but very action-oriented.

P: Yes. And he was very emotive, like he wasn't afraid to say, "When you said that, I got chills; I'm sitting here feeling tears welling up in my eyes." You know he wasn't afraid to share those or say those things. And I think that was very beneficial for me too, because, although I have an excellent relationship with my husband—he's really, really caring and compassionate—to have someone other than him say those things, it's kind of like "Okay, so this abusive thing that happened in my past, I can't really generalize it until I'm in [the situation]."

The primary team constructed the following core idea for this interview data: *Therapist validated that the participant's abuse experiences were real and awful (therapist said he "got chills" and "felt teary" hearing it), which was especially important coming from a man other than the participant's husband.* Note that the core ideas were written specifically to reflect the "event" domain, with other information in the raw data not emphasized.

Once the domains and core ideas for all of the individual cases have been constructed by the primary team, these are audited (see also Ladany et al. 2012). In this audit, the auditors carefully read the constructed core ideas and the raw data and provide feedback about the adequacy of the domain coding; the accuracy, completeness, and wording of the core ideas; and whether there is anything missing from the rest of the case. The auditors' comments are considered carefully by the primary team, with this auditing process repeating until all are satisfied that the data have been captured as faithfully as possible (often many iterations are necessary for researchers first learning the method),

23.2.4 Cross-Analysis/Audit

We now look for patterns or themes across cases. To do this, the primary team members individually examine all of the core ideas within a given domain *across* cases to see what commonalities emerge, and then we meet as a primary team to discuss these patterns and come to consensus about the categories that capture these patterns or themes. The auditor(s) reviews these initial categories and provides feedback. Once we have a stable category structure (i.e., one that fits the data from successive cases without new categories emerging when new cases are added; note that the term "saturation" has also been used to describe this stability), we assign each core idea within each domain to one or more categories; during this process, the category structure usually evolves even more. The auditor checks the classification of each core idea, and the revision process continues until all are satisfied that the final structure adequately and efficiently reflects the interview data.

This final stage of the analysis (the cross-analysis) is very creative and requires a thorough immersion in the data. Metaphorically, it is like moving from the trees to the forest (i.e., moving from describing the individual twigs on the branches of the trees to describing the different sections of the forest). Of course, finding coherence in the data depends on having selected a good sample, having asked good questions in the interview, having probed deeply to learn in-depth information from each participant, and having developed clear core ideas. This stage typically involves considerable tinkering (i.e., modification, reexamination, reworking) until a clear picture emerges. There is no preset category structure that researchers seek; rather, they attempt to describe what emerges as clearly and elegantly as possible.

The auditors now examine the cross-analysis (both the category structure and the core ideas that fit into each category) and provide feedback about its adequacy, coverage, and elegance. As auditors immerse themselves in the data, they hopefully provide another perspective on how the data can be structured. As before, several iterations of this audit/reconsideration by the primary team may occur until all are satisfied that they have characterized the data as faithfully as possible.

We then characterize categories by the frequency with which they reflect what the participants in the sample have said, doing so to depict the representativeness of categories for the sample (which is especially important when communicating the results given that sample sizes often vary across studies). Those categories that apply to all or all but one of the participants are considered *general*, those that apply to more than half and up to the cutoff for general are *typical*, and those that apply to at least two and up to the typical cutoff are *variant*.

In the study described above about corrective relational experiences (Knox et al. 2012), several categories and subcategories emerged from the cross-analysis for the domain of the event itself (one of the five domains identified in the data). For the first category (type of CRE), three variant subcategories were identified: resolution of rupture, rescue of client, reassurance/normalization. For the second category of participants' actions during events, there were two typical subcategories (explored thoughts and feelings, asserted self or feelings) and one variant category (dissociated/avoided/felt vulnerable). For the third category of therapists' action during events, there was one typical (empathized/reflected/accepted) and five variant subcategories (became active/directive, used immediacy, invited exploration, responded to rupture, reassured/normalized). Thus, these categories and subcategories provided a rich way of describing the experiences of participants' CREs in our sample.

23.2.5 Advantages and Disadvantages of CQR-I

One advantage of CQR-I is that it allows researchers to investigate both inner experiences and infrequently occurring events in great depth. In addition, because words are closer than numbers to clinical phenomena, it enables us to more closely parallel how participants think. This approach also allows results to emerge from the data inductively, which is particularly important when little is known about an area. Furthermore, judges can use their clinical wisdom and include context rather than being forced to use preestablished categories that do not necessarily fit the data. It also allows for multiple perspectives on the data, which should lead to a better understanding of the phenomenon. In this way, it is a psychotherapist-friendly research methodology because therapists can readily identify with the methods (being like case conferences) and apply the results to practice. Finally, this approach is more rigorous than many other qualitative methods in that it uses a semi-structured interview protocol, a number of judges and auditors, and consensus among team members.

A disadvantage is the inevitable bias on the part of the judges given that they are using their clinical judgment to examine data. Although we try to minimize bias in CQR through the use of multiple judges and auditors, it is important to remember that each research project takes place within the context of a certain culture and that the research team has theoretical preferences and evolves a certain way of thinking about the data. The resulting findings are thus constructed rather than representing "truth." Another concern is that this method takes a long time and can become tedious. Furthermore, implementing the method can be difficult (especially for researchers new to this method) because it is not possible to spell out all of the "rules" for the varying circumstances that arise in different studies. Relatedly, it can be difficult to conceptualize data, especially if interviews did not yield rich data (either because of the interview or the way in which it was implemented). In addition, and of relevance to the next section of this chapter, this approach can be applied only to interview data.

Another disadvantage that has been raised frequently in the literature is that it has been difficult to aggregate findings across studies (see Hill et al. 2005). Given that small samples are almost always used, questions are often raised about the broader meaning or generalizability of such findings. Recently, however, some of these concerns have been addressed by advances in qualitative meta-analysis (also called meta-synthesis). These methods (see Hill et al. 2012; Timulak 2009) allow researchers to compare results across studies. In effect, these methods are similar to the cross-analyses in CQR in that researchers look across the findings to determine which elements are consistent across studies. Such methods should help us make advances by providing ways to aggregate results across studies.

A couple of things about CQR could be considered to be advantages or disadvantages depending on one's perspective and philosophy of science (see also Stahl et al. 2012). The first involves causality: Because CQR is a descriptive approach, it cannot produce evidence about causality. For those whose philosophical approach leans toward the phenomenological, thick description is an advantage; for those of a more mechanistic inclination, such inability to determine causality is a negative. The second thing involves the amount of structure in the CQR approach. Those from quantitative backgrounds may perceive that clearly delineated steps as advantageous because this method is rigorous and replicable; those from other qualitative approaches may view the rigor as "rigor mortis" (i.e., too rigid). Because our research teams have fallen in the middle ground of these quantitative and qualitative traditions, we have found CQR to be a reasonable compromise between rigor and relevance.

23.3 Consensual Qualitative Research: Modified

Sometimes we have smaller, less complicated data sets and want to modify the extensive procedures used in CQR. For example, in a current study (Spangler et al. 2014), we asked 134 students in helping skills classes to write a brief one- to two-page reflection paper about their experiences in learning the skill of immediacy; they responded to questions about the most and least helpful components of training, difficulties involved in learning immediacy, and cultural influences on learning immediacy. Answers were brief, and so the full CQR method seemed unnecessary.

For the Spangler et al. study, two authors went through about 30 of the papers and consensually created domains from the data (based on the four questions and a domain that emerged from the data about recommendations for future training) and categories within these domains, thus preserving the discovery-oriented, exploratory nature of qualitative research. Then six of the authors met together and consensually coded another approximately 30 papers, modifying the system substantially to reflect the additional papers. Finally, two to three authors consensually coded the remaining papers using these categories.

Thus, the essential feature of consensus remained the same, as did the idea of categories within domains emerging from the data, but we eliminated the core idea coding and the auditing because the data were relatively simple and straightforward. This CQR-M method (see also Spangler et al. 2012), then, is ideal for simple data that does not require extensive interpretation or understanding of context. Furthermore, it is ideal for large data sets with relatively small amounts of information for each case.

23.4 Consensual Qualitative Research: Cases

In CQR-C, we apply the principles of consensual qualitative methods to sessions or cases of psychotherapy (see also Jackson et al. 2012). In CQR-C, as in CQR, we rely on consensus among a team of judges and auditors. Because in this approach to CQR, we are not doing interviews in which we ask the participant specific questions about the topic of interest; however, we cannot directly impose from CQR the structure of coding the data into domains, core ideas, and cross-analyses. Instead, in CQR-C, researchers pose questions that they want to answer and then go searching for evidence in transcripts or videotapes of psychotherapy sessions to answer these questions.

The development of CQR-C has by no means been as linear or systematic as it is by necessity presented here. In fact, it has been more of a process of pushing the boundaries in each study to allow us to devise methods for analyzing the data. It is only at this point looking back over a few studies that we can begin to draw parallels between the two methods and articulate the commonalities and underlying principles. In this section, then, my goal is to describe our experiences conducting several studies in which CQR-C began to emerge; I use these studies to illustrate the emerging CQR-C method.

23.4.1 How Do Clients Gain Insight Through Dreamwork?

We (Hill et al. 2007a; Knox et al. 2008) were interested in examining how insight develops in dreamwork (the question we posed of the data) using the Hill (2004b) dream model, given that one of the goals of this dream model is the development of insight. Our goal was to examine the contributions of a number of factors (e.g., dream salience; the therapeutic relationship; client characteristics such as readiness or eagerness for insight, involvement, and psychological mindedness; therapist characteristics such as adherence and competence using the model, lack of countertransference, and therapist skills) that had been found in previous studies on dreamwork and psychotherapy to contribute to insight gains. In Hill et al. (2007a), we selected a single, 90-min session in which there were large insight gains from a larger sample of 157 cases (Hill et al. 2007c). In Knox et al., we selected another case with large insight gains and similar demographics so that we could see if the results would replicate; in addition, we selected a case with minimal insight gains so that we could look for differences between cases with insight gains and cases without insight gains. We also had access to post-session ratings from Hill et al. (2007c) by the clients, therapists, and trained observers. For the studies described here (Hill et al. 2007a; Knox et al. 2008), two judges (the primary team) first listened to the tape of each session several times and familiarized themselves with its content. They then reviewed the session and all the accompanying session ratings and looked for evidence of the facilitating and inhibiting factors noted above and also looked for evidence for other contributing factors that had not been mentioned in the previous literature (the written evidence was somewhat equivalent to the development of core ideas). Furthermore, because the judges identified therapist skills as contributing to insight in this initial review, they also consensually coded skills using an established measure of therapist skills (Hill 2004a). Four auditors then reviewed the tape and evaluated the primary team's written claims of evidence, indicating whether they agreed or disagreed with each claim and its accompanying evidence (e.g., the auditors challenged the claim that one of the clients was resistant given that this seemed like a leap from the data). The primary team then reexamined all of their decisions based on the auditors' feedback. The audit/

reconsideration process was repeated until all researchers were confident in the conclusions.

In Knox et al. (2008), we then compared the findings from the two cases that had insight gains to determine if there were similarities between them, and we then contrasted these two cases with the no-insight case to look for differences. We thus draw conclusions about facilitating and hindering factors (somewhat equivalent to a qualitative meta-analysis). Results suggested that the dream needed to be at least moderately salient to the dreamer; there needed to be a good bond between the therapist and client; clients needed to have positive attitudes toward dreams and a lack of overwhelming affect; and therapists needed to be competent using the model, have small amounts of positive countertransference that they could manage (i.e., feel similar to the client in a positive way), and use probes for insight in the session.

We were pleased with our first effort at applying consensual qualitative methods to case material because it allowed us to ask interesting questions of existing data that could not be answered by just looking at the quantitative evidence. The method felt rigorous in that we continually returned to the data and challenged ourselves to make sure we had sufficient evidence for our findings, and it also felt creative because we allowed ourselves to look for unanticipated contributors to insight. In this way, we remained uninvested in what we found (e.g., we were not trying to prove a theory) but were open to what the data revealed. Having a team of six judges also brought many different perspectives and allowed us to describe and understand the data better. Finally, it was beneficial for judges to be thoroughly immersed in the data by both listening to the tapes and reading the transcripts closely many times.

23.4.2 Problems and Action Ideas Revealed During Dreamwork

In Sim et al. (2010), we sought to learn if there were differences between first- and second-generation Asian clients in their discussion of their dreams. Specifically coming from the Hill (2004b) three-stage model of dreamwork, we wondered whether clients from these two groups would differ in the problems they discussed and the action ideas they suggested. From a larger study of 90 90-min dream sessions with East Asian college student clients and East Asian therapists, Sim et al. identified the seven available sessions with first-generation (born in Asia and having lived in the USA for 9 years or less) female Asian students and randomly selected seven sessions (from 19 available) with female Asian students who were at least second generation (born and living currently in the USA). A team of judges listened to the entire session and wrote down every instance in which a problem (e.g., interpersonal concern, career concern) or action idea (e.g., study harder, communicate more clearly) was revealed as the client explored the dream during the session. For each problem or action idea (equivalent to domains in CQR-I), judges constructed core ideas via consensus. Then an auditor provided feedback to the judges about the adequacy of the selection of events and the wording of the core ideas for problems and action ideas. The judges then searched for more evidence either to bolster their claims or to support the auditor's suggested changes. Finally, we did a cross-analysis to determine themes within and across groups.

Interpersonal issues and academic/post-graduation/career issues were typical for both groups, but first-generation Asians more often disclosed concerns related to immigration/culture/adjustment and distress related to physical health issues than did second-generation Asian-Americans. In terms of action ideas, both groups typically proposed interpersonal behavioral changes, but first-generation Asians proposed changes in their thoughts and feelings more often than did second-generation students.

This study posed a different challenge than that presented by the previous studies (Hill et al. 2007a; Knox et al. 2008): We were essentially trying more explicitly to apply the steps of CQR to case data. For example, we specified ahead of time the domains of interest (i.e., problems or action ideas) in which we were interested, sought to find such episodes in the session, then constructed core ideas from the transcribed data that captured those episodes, and finally completed a cross-analysis of each domain's core ideas. Given that this approach was not as direct as asking an interviewee specific questions, identifying the episodes in sessions took more effort, but constructing the core ideas and performing the cross-analysis were relatively straightforward.

23.4.3 Case Studies of Immediacy

Kasper et al. (2008) investigated a case of brief psychotherapy (12 sessions) with a therapist reputed to use immediacy (discussion in the here and now about the here-and-now relationship between the therapist and client) paired with a client who had interpersonal concerns. We first tried more traditional quantitative process methods of having trained judges reliably code each therapist and client statement into different types of immediacy. We quickly were disillusioned with the ability of these codings to capture the richness of the data. Two of us then reviewed all 12 sessions and identified the immediacy events; for each event (broader than the statements used earlier), we consensually coded different types of immediacy (e.g., drew parallels between external and therapy relationships) and identified the effects of immediacy (e.g., allowed the client to talk more openly about immediate feelings). At the end of the whole data analysis, we asked the therapist to provide feedback about the results and write-up. This method yielded rich data and helped us understand the process within events, the effects of immediacy, and the evolution of the relationship across the course of the 12 sessions of therapy.

Taking this method a step further in a second 17-session case study (Hill et al. 2008) with a different interpersonally oriented psychotherapist and a client with interpersonal concerns, a team of five judges listened to tapes of the entire case and identified all immediacy events. We then transcribed all these events, but investigated in more depth only the seven events that seemed to us to be the most salient or impactful. For each of the seven events, we consensually identified the context preceding the event, the therapist and client actions during the event, and the effects of the immediacy interventions. We also constructed a conceptualization of the immediacy event based on all the information in the case. We then summarized findings across events. At the end, the therapist provided extensive feedback on the findings from his perspective of having been involved in the case; this feedback enabled the primary team to reevaluate their thinking and nascent conclusions. The dialectic between the different perspectives (team versus therapist) provided a better understanding of the data.

A comparison of the two cases revealed that the Kasper et al. therapist more often used challenging forms of immediacy that helped break down the client's defenses, whereas the Hill et al. therapist more often used supportive forms of immediacy that helped build the client's fragile ego. Negative effects of immediacy were found only in the first case. We also found that immediacy facilitated negotiation of the therapeutic relationship and provided a corrective relational experience in both cases, with other effects specific to the individual cases.

These studies were different from the studies described above (Hill et al. 2007a; Knox et al. 2008; Sim et al. 2010) in that we had a lot more data about each of the cases (12 or 17 sessions of an entire brief therapy versus a single dream session), which helped provide richness to the data. We started with a question about how immediacy operated in psychotherapy and tried a number of approaches to answer this question. Eventually, we felt that we learned more from the data in the Hill et al. study than the Kasper et al. study, given that we first immersed ourselves in the entire case to get an understanding of the context and then we then went back and examined each immediacy event and consensually constructed an understanding of the antecedents, the process, and the outcome. We liked examining the second case in this way because it allowed us to conceptualize the effects of immediacy within the context of the case, much like clinicians do during case conferences.

23.4.4 Corrective Relational Experiences in the Treatment of Anorexia Nervosa

In this study (Berman et al. 2012), we examined three cases of brief therapy (17–19 sessions) with one female therapist using acceptance and commitment therapy (ACT) to treat three individual female clients with anorexia nervosa. A team of judges first identified all relational events (any time that both therapist and client were discussing their relationship) in each case and then consensually identified the therapist and client actions within these events. The therapist then provided extensive feedback on these codings, which the team considered again by consensus; several iterations of this process between researchers and therapist occurred until there was mutual agreement. We then formulated more global conceptualizations of the three cases in terms of the context of the therapy, patterns during relational events, effects of the relational work, client contributions to the relational work, and therapist contributions to the relational work, using a modification of the Ward method (Schielke et al. 2009). With this method, each team member independently developed a conceptualization of each case. When we met, each person presented her/his ideas and others questioned her/him so that we could get a full accounting of what each person thought. Next, we each independently rewrote our conceptualizations, now borrowing from and integrating what they liked from all the ideas. This process continued until our ideas began to merge, and we then wrote a shared conceptualization. The therapist provided extensive feedback to the team about the conceptualization, which the team used to make modifications. The therapist also wrote a separate rebuttal to provide her own ideas about the case because her ideas differed from the rest of the team given differing theoretical orientations (the therapist had used a behavioral approach; the team members were more interpersonally oriented).

Results suggested that one of the clients responded positively to relational work, one was neutral, and the third had a negative response. We speculated that the one client responded positively to relational work because she was mature, psychologically minded, had a solid sense of self, and had previous experiences with interpersonal therapy. In contrast, the other two clients were more resistant and afraid of confrontation. In terms of therapist interventions that predicted a positive response to relational work, therapist empathy and invitations to explore emerged as helpful. In contrast, therapist psychoeducation and direct guidance seemed to hinder relational work (i.e., the clients did not explore when the therapist used these interventions). Interestingly, although the same therapist treated all three cases, she was clearly different in the relationships with the three clients (e.g., in the negative case, the therapist adhered strictly to the manual and seemed baffled and frustrated with the client; in the positive and neutral cases, the therapist was more open and flexible).

This study demonstrated a nice progression from the two earlier case studies on immediacy in that we were able to use many of the same methods (immersing ourselves in the data by watching all sessions, identifying the relational events, coding the therapist and client actions). We were pleased to learn about the Ward method (Schielke et al. 2009) while we were in the midst of the study, because it helped us think of a new way of approaching the data (having researchers independently conceptualize the data and then come together to nondefensively present ideas with others listening and probing) rather than initially working through to consensus. It also helped us move from an event-level analysis to examining each case from a case-level perspective (e.g., looking at the general effects of relational work across the entire case). In this study, compared to the Kasper et al. (2008) and Hill et al. (2008) case studies, we involved the therapist at a much earlier time in the process. Having the therapist's input was beneficial (albeit occasionally difficult when there were disagreements) because the dialectic provided more perspectives about the data and often forced us to go back and make sure of our interpretations of the data.

23.4.5 Summary of CQR-C

Although CQR-C is still emerging, we can note some consistencies across studies and begin to develop some preliminary guidelines for how to use this method. Researchers first need to sit with the data and think carefully about what it is that they want to know. We found that it helped to watch the entire case before we formulated completely how to approach the data. By immersing ourselves in the data, we were clearer about what we wanted to address more systematically. Clear questions are crucial or else researchers can get bogged down with the wealth of information. After identifying the questions, we go into the data and search for evidence and always look for counterevidence (although crucial to the data analysis, this step is still a little hard to describe and likely varies from study to study). Having multiple perspectives (often 4–5 judges and also therapist input) enables us to look at the data from many directions. We then go on to look for similarities across events or cases. Of course, I should also note that different methods are needed for each study because the questions are somewhat different, hence the need to creatively adapt the method as you go along.

Our experiences in the Berman et al. (2012) study suggest that consensus can be achieved through two different methods. Either all the judges can sit together and construct a consensus opinion or individual team members can independently construct their ideas and then come together to expand on their ideas in a nonjudgmental setting that fosters full explication and integration of various ideas. Both approaches can work and may depend on the research question and the team dynamics. For example, a team with strong hierarchical organization among members (e.g., students who do not feel that they can argue with professors) might be better off using the latter method than using the group consensus method.

23.4.6 Advantages and Disadvantages of CQR-C

An advantage of CQR-C is that it allows researchers to study sessions and whole cases of psychotherapy, which is particularly important in situations when we have access only to archival data, when participants cannot provide answers (e.g., how did something come about?), or when we cannot ethically question participants (e.g., they might be too fragile). Another advantage is that it allows researchers to integrate various types of data (e.g., analysis of transcripts and videos of sessions, self-report process and outcome measures from participants, and codings by judges trained to reliability). A disadvantage of CQR-C is that it is not as well developed as CQR and is thus more difficult to conduct and teach.

23.5 Similarities Across CQR, CQR-M, and CQR-C

Although the steps for CQR-C are not yet as straightforward as those for CQR (and CQR-M), there are several consistencies across methods.

23.5.1 Triangulation

In all three methods, we often have supporting assessment data (e.g., pre-post measurement of change, ratings of satisfaction) that can be used as additional sources of information. Having multiple sources of information often helps clarify results.

23.5.2 Domains/Questions

The equivalent of domains in CQR and CQR-M is questions in CQR-C. Thus, in CQR and CQR-M, researchers first develop research questions that they want to answer and then construct questions to help them get answers. They then examine the data yielded from the interviews/questionnaires and construct domains. In contrast, in CQR-C, researchers develop research questions that they want to answer and then go searching for evidence in transcripts or videotapes of psychotherapy sessions. Regardless of the approach, researchers begin with clear questions about what they want to know from the data. Moreover, in all three types of CQR, the answers are also not limited to the initial questions. Rather, as researchers immerse themselves in the data, other questions/answers may emerge.

23.5.3 Core Ideas/Evidence

In CQR, researchers consider all data coded within a domain and write core ideas that summarize the essence of what the participant has said. In CQR-M, the step of writing core ideas is not necessary since the data are brief and straightforward (although it is useful to have a large sample). In CQR-C, researchers search all the available data for evidence to answer their questions; they write a summary of their conclusions along with a record of which raw data were used to reach that conclusion. In both CQR and CQR-C, researchers extract meaning from the data based on their understanding of all the available data.

23.5.4 Auditors

Although CQR relies heavily on using auditors, the auditing process is less often used in CQR-M and CQR-C although larger primary teams are often used to compensate for not using auditors. The auditor(s) examines all the raw data that pertain to the domain/question and determine if the constructed core ideas/evidence adequately reflect the raw data. The auditor(s) provide detailed feedback to the primary team; several iterations are often necessary to resolve discrepancies between the perspectives of the team and auditor(s). We have experimented with the structure of the primary team—auditor format; we have occasionally had larger teams in which members rotated these roles. In addition, in CQR-C, sometimes the therapist has been involved in the analyses and served as a counterpoint with a different perspective. In contrast, in CQR-M, auditors are often not needed because the data is relatively straightforward, but it is helpful to use multiple judges to make sure that all the data is being addressed in a consistent manner (and certainly auditors could be used to add another layer of trustworthiness).

23.5.5 Cross-Analyses

In CQR, we look for consistent themes in core ideas across episodes/events within cases and across cases. In CQR-C, whether we do this step depends on the study. In some studies (e.g., Hill et al. 2007a, b, c; Kasper et al. 2008), we did only one session/case, and these were interesting studies all by themselves. We later compared the session/case with other sessions/case, respectively (Knox et al. 2008; Hill et al. 2008), although this would not necessarily need to be done. In CQR-M, we simply summarize frequency across categories.

23.5.6 Consensus

Consensus is central to all three CQR methods. Having multiple perspectives clearly leads to richer understandings of the data, and using a consensus method allows us to come to some agreement without being forced into arbitrary agreement such as would be required if we had to determine inter-rater reliability. Of course, it is always important to watch for discrepancies among judges and to use such discrepancies to further refine the data analyses.

Conclusions

Consensual qualitative methods are ideal research strategies for investigating some questions, particularly those related to inner experiences or the complexities of the therapy process not easily captured by self-report measures. Although such methods require considerable time and patient attention to detail, they can be quite rewarding avenues to understand the therapy process and outcome.

Over time, having used many different quantitative and qualitative research methods, I increasingly value this consensual qualitative method. In the past, I used traditional quantitative process approaches, which required trained judges to force their ideas into prescribed categories, limiting clinical judgment and forcing judges to think alike. The qualitative approach of sitting with several people and trying to understand the data in great depth is not only liberating and fun but also provides a more clinically meaningful perspective on the data.

I should note that CQR methods are neither the only nor necessarily the best approach to studying all questions about psychotherapy. For some research questions (e.g., What is the comparative efficacy of different types of psychotherapy? How many head nods are there in sessions?), quantitative methods are clearly superior to qualitative methods. In addition, other qualitative methods (e.g., conversational analysis) are also useful and perhaps more appropriate for specific questions. Finally, qualitative methods are still evolving and thus may undergo important and continued development. But qualitative methods clearly have a place in psychotherapy research in that they allow us to describe interesting and complex phenomena in a rich and clinically meaningful way.

Acknowledgement I express my appreciation to the many people who have helped in the development of these qualitative methods and more specifically to those who reviewed a draft of this paper: Rachel Crook-Lyon, Melissa Goates-Jones, Shirley A. Hess, Sarah Knox, Nicholas Ladany, Wonjin Sim, Barbara J. Thompson, and Elizabeth Nutt Williams.

References

Berman M, Hill CE, Liu J, Jackson J, Sim W, Spangler P (2012) Relational events in acceptance and commitment therapy for three cases with anorexia nervosa. In: Castonguay LG, Hill CE (eds) Transformation in psychotherapy: corrective experiences across cognitive-behavioral, humanistic, and psychodynamic approaches. American Psychological Association, Washington, DC, pp 215–244

Burkard AW, Knox S, Hill CE (2012) Data collection. In: Hill CE (ed) Consensual qualitative research: a practical resource for investigating social science phenomena. American Psychological Association, Washington, DC, pp 83–102

Elliott R (1989) Comprehensive process analysis: understanding change process in significant therapy events. In: Packer MJ, Addison RB (eds) Entering the circle: hermeneutic investigations in psychology. SUNY Press, Albany, NY, pp 165–184

Gelso CJ, Hill CE, Rochlen A, Mohr J, Zack J (1999) Describing the face of transference: psychodynamic therapists' recollections of transference in successful long-term therapy. J Couns Psychol 46:257–267. doi:10.1037/0022-0167.46.2.257

Giorgi A (1985) Sketch of a psychological phenomenological method. In: Giorgi A (ed) Phenomenology and psychological research. Duquesne University Press, Pittsburgh, PA, pp 8–22

Hill CE (2004a) Helping skills: facilitating exploration, insight, and action, 2nd edn. American Psychological Association, Washington, DC

Hill CE (ed) (2004b) Dream work in therapy: facilitating exploration, insight, and action. American Psychological Association, Washington, DC

Hill CE (ed) (2012) Consensual qualitative research: a practical resource for investigating social science phenomena. American Psychological Association, Washington, DC

Hill CE, Sim W, Spangler P, Stahl J, Sullivan C, Teyber E (2008) Therapist immediacy in brief psychotherapy: case study II. Psychother Theor Res Pract Train 45 (3):298–315. doi:10.1037/a0013306

Hill CE, Thompson BJ, Williams EN (1997) A guide to conducting consensual qualitative research. Couns Psychol 25:517–572

Hill CE, Zack J, Wonnell T, Hoffman MA, Rochlen A, Goldberg J, Nakayama E, Heaton KJ, Kelley F, Eiche K, Tomlinson M, Hess S (2000) Structured brief therapy with a focus on dreams or loss for clients with troubling dreams and recent losses. J Couns Psychol 47:90–101. doi:10.1037/0022-0167.47.1.90

Hill CE, Kellems IS, Kolchakian MR, Wonnell TL, Davis TL, Nakayama EY (2003) The therapist experience of being the target of hostile versus suspected-unasserted client anger: factors associated with resolution. Psychother Res 13:475–491. doi:10.1093/ptr/kpg040

Hill CE, Knox S, Thompson BJ, Williams EN, Hess S, Ladany N (2005) Consensual qualitative research: an update. J Couns Psychol 52:196–205. doi:10.1037/0022-0167.52.2.196

Hill CE, Crook-Lyon RE, Hess S, Goates-Jones MK, Roffman M, Stahl J, Sim W, Johnson M (2006) Prediction of session process and outcome in the Hill dream model: contributions of client dream-related characteristics and the process of the three stages. Dreaming 16:159–185. doi:10.1037/1053-0797.16.3.159

Hill CE, Knox S, Hess S, Crook-Lyon R, Goates-Jones M, Sim W (2007a) The attainment of insight in the Hill dream model: a single case study. In: Castonguay LG, Hill CE (eds) Insight in psychotherapy. American Psychological Association, Washington, DC, pp 207–230

Hill CE, Sullivan C, Knox S, Schlosser L (2007b) Becoming psychotherapists: the experiences of novice therapists in a beginning graduate class. Psychother Theory Res Pract Train 44:434–449. doi:10.1037/0033-3204.44.4.434

Hill CE, Tien HL, Sheu H-B, Sim W, Ma Y, Choi K-H, Tashiro T (2007c) Predictors of outcome of dream work for East Asian volunteer clients: dream factors, anxious attachment, Asian values, and therapist input. Dreaming 17:208–226. doi:10.1037/1053-0797.17.4.208

Hill CE, Sim W, Spangler P, Stahl J, Sullivan C, Teyber E (2008) Therapist immediacy in brief psychotherapy: case study II. Psychother Theor Res Pract Train 45 (3):298–315. doi:10.1037/a0013306

Hill CE, Knox S, Hess SA (2012) Qualitative meta-analyses of consensual qualitative research studies. In: Hill CE (ed) Consensual qualitative research: a practical resource for investigating social science phenomena. American Psychological Association, Washington, DC, pp 159–171

Jackson JL, Chui HT, Hill CE (2012) The modification of consensual qualitative research for case study research: an introduction to CQR-C. In: Hill CE (ed) Consensual qualitative research: a practical resource for investigating social science phenomena. American Psychological Association, Washington, DC, pp 285–303

Kasper L, Hill CE, Kivlighan D (2008) Therapist immediacy in brief psychotherapy: case study I. Psychother Theor Res Pract Train 45:281–287. doi:10.1037/a0013305

Kim BSK, Benner BR, Liang CTH, Asay PA (2004) A qualitative study of adaptation experiences of 1.5-generation Asian Americans. Cult Divers Ethnic Minor Psychol 9(2):156–170. doi:10.1037/1099-9809.9.156

Knox S, Hess S, Williams EN, Hill CE (2003) Here's a little something for you: how therapists respond to clients gifts. J Couns Psychol 50:199–210. doi:10.1037/0022-0167.50.2.199

Knox S, Hill CE, Hess S, Crook-Lyon R (2008) Case studies of the attainment of insight in dream sessions: replication and extension. Psychother Res 18:200–215. doi:10.1080/10503300701432242

Knox S, DuBois R, Smith J, Hess SA, Hill CE (2009) Clients' experiences giving gifts to therapists. Psychother Theory Res Pract Train 46:350–361. doi:10.1037/a0017001

Knox S, Hess S, Hill CE, Crook-Lyon RE, Burkard AW (2012) Corrective relational experiences of therapists or therapists-in-training. In: Castonguay LG, Hill CE (eds) Transformation in psychotherapy: corrective experiences across cognitive-behavioral, humanistic, and psychodynamic approaches. American Psychological Association, Washington, DC, pp 191–214

Ladany N, O'Brien K, Hill CE, Melinkoff D, Knox S, Peterson D (1997) Sexual attraction toward clients: a qualitative study of psychotherapy predoctoral interns. J Couns Psychol 44:413–424. doi:10.1037/0022-0167.44.4.413

Ladany N, Thompson BJ, Hill CE (2012) Cross-analysis. In: Hill CE (ed) Consensual qualitative research: a practical resource for investigating social science phenomena. American Psychological Association, Washington, DC, pp 117–134

Rhodes R, Hill CE, Thompson BJ, Elliott R (1994) Client retrospective recall of resolved and unresolved misunderstanding events. J Couns Psychol 41:473–483. doi:10.1037/0022-0167.41.4.473

Schielke HJ, Fishman JL, Osatuke K, Stiles WB (2009) Creative consensus on interpretations of qualitative data: the Ward method. Psychother Res 19:558–565. doi:10.1080/10503300802621180

Sim W, Hill CE, Chowdhury S, Huang T, Zaman N, Talavera P (2010) Problems and action ideas discussed by first- and second-generation female East Asian students during dream sessions. Dreaming 20:42–59. doi:10.1037/a0018993

Spangler PT, Liu J, Hill CE (2012) Consensual qualitative research for simple qualitative data: an introduction to CQR-M. In: Hill CE (ed) Consensual qualitative research: a practical resource for investigating social science phenomena. American Psychological Association, Washington, DC, pp 269–284

Spangler PT, Hill CE, Dunn MG, Hummel A, Walden T, Liu J, Jackson J, Ganginis HV, Salahuddin N (2014) Training Undergraduate students to use immediacy. The Counseling Psychologist 42:729–757

Stahl JV, Taylor NE, Hill CE (2012) Philosophical and historical background of consensual qualitative research. In: Hill CE (ed) Consensual qualitative research: a practical resource for investigating social science phenomena. American Psychological Association, Washington, DC, pp 21–32

Strauss A, Corbin J (1998) Basics of qualitative research: grounded theory procedures and techniques, 2nd edn. Sage, Thousand Oaks, CA

Thompson BJ, Vivino BL, Hill CE (2012) Domains and core ideas. In: Hill CE (ed) Consensual qualitative research: a practical resource for investigating social science phenomena. American Psychological Association, Washington, DC, pp 103–116

Timulak L (2009) Meta-analysis of qualitative studies: a tool for reviewing qualitative research findings in psychotherapy. Psychother Res 19:591–600. doi:10.1080/10503300802477989

Vivino B, Thompson B, Hill CE, Ladany N (2009) Compassion in psychotherapy: the perspective of psychotherapists nominated as compassionate. Psychother Res 19:157–171. doi:10.1080/10503300802430681

Williams EN, Morrow SL (2009) Achieving trustworthiness in qualitative research: a pan-paradigmatic perspective. Psychother Res 19:576–582. doi:10.1080/10503300802702113

Conversation Analysis and Psychotherapy Process Research

24

Anna Madill

Contents

A. Madill (✉)
School of Psychology, University of Leeds, Leeds LS2 9JT, UK
e-mail: a.l.madill@leeds.ac.uk

Abstract

Applied conversation analytic research seeks to understand the ways in which conversational practices are modified in order to fulfill institutional aims. Psychotherapy is one such institution, and in recent years, a research literature has developed in which conversation analysis has been applied to psychotherapy interaction. This chapter provides an overview of the five main features of talk-in-interaction of interest in conversation analysis: turn-taking, sequence organization, repair, word selection, and action formation. An extract from psychotherapy interaction is explored in relation to each of these five features of talk. The analytic lens of conversation analysis and its conceptualization of key phenomena are different in many respects to that of traditional psychotherapy research. Moreover, when directed towards psychotherapy, selection of material has been, in the main, in accordance with conversation analytically informed, as opposed to therapy-informed, observations. The result is that conversation analytic research may seem psychologically shallow to the psychotherapy community: too removed from basic assumptions about human subjectivity and mute on questions of experiential change which are likely of interest to therapists. However, this therapy-neutral orientation may be a significant strength in allowing conversation analysis to complement and enhance process

O.C.G. Gelo et al. (eds.), *Psychotherapy Research*,
DOI 10.1007/978-3-7091-1382-0_24,

research through revealing what psychotherapy may not notice about itself.

24.1 Introduction

A fundamental aspect of psychotherapy, the "talking cure," is that it is a conversation. This is not to overlook nonverbal aspects of the psychotherapeutic process or forms of therapy that focus on the extra-discursive, such as dance therapy. But it is probably fair to say that in most psychotherapies the client-therapist dialogue is an important tool for facilitating change. Developments in psychoanalysis, such as the Lacanian theory and psychotherapy (e.g., Lacan 1968), have built on the growing significance awarded language in the creation of human subjectivity. And, with the "turn to language" in the social sciences during the 1970s, psychotherapy saw analogous developments in variant approaches such as narrative, re-authoring, and conversational methods (Hobson 1985; White and Epston 1990). Hence, in understanding the processes of psychotherapy, a focus on the language used and the transformational potential of the therapy dialogue has a long history.

Conversation analysis developed in the 1960s in North American sociology, the first publications appearing in the early 1970s (e.g., Sacks 1972), and can be defined as a rigorous approach to discovering the ways in which talk-in-interaction is choreographed. The aim of basic research is to understand how ordinary everyday conversation is organized as a self-regulating system. This is a particularly exciting field since discoveries relating to the fundamentals of conversational exchange are still to be made. Conversation analysis continues to grow in popularity and has crossed into disciplines such as psychology and linguistics. There is also a developing field of applied research in which conversation analytic discoveries and methodology are used to understand how talk functions in institutional contexts (e.g., Heritage 2005). In such contexts, interlocutors speak as incumbents of institutional identities with the obligations, responsibilities, and expectations these entail: patient–doctor, witness-policewoman, and pupil–teacher. Moreover, in institutional talk, conversations are a medium in and through which the work of an organization can be conducted, such as making a diagnosis, interrogating a suspect, or teaching a class. Hence, applied conversation analytic research seeks to understand the ways in which conversational practices are modified in order to fulfill institutional aims. Psychotherapy is, of course, one such institution (Morris and Chenail 1995).

Conversation analysis has a unique place in the cluster of methods generally considered qualitative (Madill and Gough 2008). It is avowedly empirical and has a claim to being relatively atheoretical in the sense of (a) eschewing a theory of subjectivity (e.g., not accounting for talk at the level of individual predisposition) and (b) being primarily inductive and data driven. However, arguably, like all methods, conversation analysis has theoretic elements in positing a way of approaching talk-in-interaction. But unlike some other data-driven approaches, such as grounded theory, conversation analysis is foundational (assumes that objective principles can be established) and progressive (seeks to build a corpus of knowledge from established facts). Conversation analysis is therefore not interpretivist. Conversation analysis also differs from grounded theory and other popular methods such as interpretative phenomenological analysis in that no attempt is made to categorize the content of the data with a view to theorizing how participants understand particular social processes or their own experiences. Nor is conversation analysis social constructionist, as are variants of (micro-) discourse analysis which often draw on conversation analytic methods (e.g., Edwards and Potter 1992). Unlike discourse analysis, conversation analysis, in general, is not concerned with how sociocultural meanings are mobilized to create the phenomena which furnish our world and hold individuals in place as particular kinds of subjects. In fact, in many ways, conversation analysis is closer to a natural science than human science approach through taking the stance that rigorous empirical observation and application of the correct method will reveal the (normative) rules of conversational exchange [see Lepper (2015)]. Given this, conversation analysis defies easy placement in paradigmatic schematics as outlined and examined in, for example, Madill and Gough (2008).

Ideal data for conversation analysis are naturally occurring interactions: that is, conversations which have occurred in the conduct of everyday life unaffected by the interests of researchers. Much of the earliest conversation analytic research was based was audio-recorded, overheard telephone conversations on shared party lines. Today informed consent is required from participants but it is not impossible to collect, what is for all intents and purposes, unselfconscious conversation. For example, archives of psychotherapy interaction exist which have been collected with consent for research purposes (e.g., the Second Sheffield Psychotherapy Project: Shapiro et al. 1990; Madill et al. 2001). Moreover, clients and therapists are often willing to release audio and sometimes video recording of their interactions for conversation analytic research (see, e.g., the collection in Peräkylä et al. 2008). Conversation analysis of recorded material requires detailed transcription, particularly of aspects of interaction already demonstrated of importance such as intonation, audible intake of breath, and length of silence. Jeffersonian transcription conventions have been designed for this (see http://www.sscnet.ucla.edu/soc/faculty/schegloff/) and are under constant development (e.g., Hepburn and Potter 2007). Depending on the aims of the study, a relatively small amount of data can be enough to demonstrate the occurrence of an exchange pattern. On the other hand, a large corpus of material can be scoured for multiple examples of a phenomenon (e.g., apologies).

Conversation analysis requires knowledge of an increasingly large corpus of established findings and a high degree of skill operationalizing its analytic procedures. Moreover, like other specialist fields, conversation analysis utilizes a technical vocabulary which can be, at first, rather opaque: adjacency pairs, conditional relevance, repair, etc. However, once familiar with the basic concepts, a good conversation analytic paper can be, in it thoroughness and precision, a beautifully eloquent articulation of the complex, usually tacit, skills of conversational exchange—"largely seen but unnoticed" (Kozart 1996, p. 366). Its painstaking empiricism assures that analytical insights are evidenced in the data and it is often incredible how much can be gleaned from a series of relatively short extracts of dialogue. Typically, the sequence of analysis would entail identification of a conversation phenomenon of interest, the collection of a series of instances of that phenomenon from available conversational data, cross-comparison of these instances in order to determine the common practices through which the phenomenon is regulated (informed by current knowledge regarding interactional exchange), and finally the presentation of a carefully evidenced and argued case for the pattern discovered using detailed analysis of examples of real conversational data.

With its intensive microanalytic focus, conversation analysis is compatible with the change process paradigm as it has been developed in psychotherapy research. Psychotherapy process research is interested in how therapy gets done. Early process research usually made the attempt to be representative in the selection of therapy segments for analysis and hence had generally used random or systematic sampling strategies. Building on works such as those of Gurman (1973) and Rice and Greenberg (1984), more recent process research perceived that all parts of therapy are not the same and that client change is likely to occur at particular important junctures. It is therefore argued that an economical and productive research strategy is to focus research on these key points or, what became known as, significant events (Greenberg 1991). Methodologically, this has entailed intensive analysis of key therapy events using task analysis (e.g., Greenberg 1984), sequential analysis (e.g., Mahrer et al. 1984), and comprehensive process analysis (e.g., Elliott 1984), among others. Intensive process analyses tend to use qualitative language-oriented methods, view the therapeutic dialogue as a communication event, and focus on the development of meaning as it occurs between client and therapist. In recent years a research literature has developed in which conversation analysis has been applied to psychotherapy interaction. However, in the main, this research has been more clearly furthering the aims of conversation analytic research (i.e., understanding conversation employed as an institutional practice) as opposed to understanding and developing psychotherapeutic techniques.

Five main features of talk-in-interaction are identified in conversation analysis as of crucial importance in understanding how conversations work: turn-taking, sequence organization, repair, word selection, and action formation. Depending on the phenomenon of interest, one or two of these features may predominate in any particular analysis. In the following sections I provide an overview of these five features of conversational exchange. Each is illustrated with commentary on an extract of psychotherapy interaction from published conversation analytic research.

24.2 Turn-Taking

It is easy to overlook the importance of the seemingly trivial observation that interlocutors take turns to speak during conversation. It is usual for there to be one beat of silence between speaker turns, which translates to about the length of a spoken syllable. Speaker change is choreographed between interlocutors as a conversation progresses, and conversation analysis has identified normative rules that speakers use as a resource for managing this process.

Central to turn-taking is the phenomenon of a turn-constructional unit (TCU). Normally a speaker has the right to one TCU only before a transition relevance place opens up and another speaker can take the floor. Recipients are able to anticipate the ending of a TCU since it is hearable, in context, as adequately complete. Adequate completion can be judged using three main criteria. The first, and most important, relates to pragmatics. TCUs complete an action: that is they do something in the talk, such as make a request. The second relates to prosody. TCUs sound complete in the way in which they are intonated. The third is syntactic. TCUs are grammatically complete within the conversational context in which they are spoken. Nonverbal cues, such as gaze directed towards the next speaker, also help signal the end of a TCU. Recipients monitor ongoing talk for the projectable ending of the current speaker's TCU and the opening of a transition relevance place in order to take turns at talk in smooth progression of the conversation.

The normative rules of turn-taking are a resource for managing and understanding conversation. For example, they allow recognition of different kinds of silence, each with a range of different interactional significance. Mid-TCU pauses belong to the current speaker and, since the TCU is not complete, do not signal the end of the speaker's turn. Hence, if a recipient attempts to speak during a mid-TCU pause, it is likely to be treated as problematically interruptive. Such pauses may function, for instance, to secure a person's gaze as indication that he or she is willing to converse (see Repair, Sect. 24.4). When a sequence of turns is complete in that a series of conditionally relevant actions is fulfilled (e.g., a question-answer sequence), a lapse in the conversation may occur (see Sect. 24.3). Lapses are not necessarily problematic for the interlocutors. More problematic are inter-turn silences occurring after the end of a speaker's turn during sequences which are not yet complete (e.g., after a question and before some answer has been provided). Conversation is conducted so as to minimize such gaps since they are hearable as belonging to the next speaker who, for some reason, is not supplying their turn.

Speakers can, of course, continue speaking beyond the end of their TCU. The right to do so is achieved interactionally. At the end of a TCU, a speaker may produce a rush through which provides no time for the next speaker to start their turn at the projected turn-transition point. On the other hand, a speaker may indicate during their TCU that a multi-TCU turn is required. This can be done, for example, through structuring the turn around a list of items, all of which need to be expanded upon before the work of the turn is complete. Hearers collaborate with multi-TCU turns through indicating that they are giving up the right to take the floor through using continuers such as "mm" or "uh huh" at turn relevant points. These are not turns in and of themselves but indicators to the current speaker that the recipient is still listening.

A common strategy, which has been the subject of particular analytic interest, is where a speaker indicates the need for multi-TCU in order to tell a story. Storytelling is likely important to psychotherapy interaction as extended sequences of troubles telling are often elicited from clients by therapists (Pain 2009). When a story has reached a point of recognizable completion, one way in which a recipient may indicate cognizance of this is through offering some kind of assessment. In therapy, this may be provided by the therapist by way of a therapeutic formulation or interpretation.

Analysis of the following extract from brief eclectic psychotherapy makes use of the observation that silence following the end of one speaker's turn, when allocatable to the next speaker—that is, an inter-turn gap—is accountable and highly problematic. Wynn and Wynn (2006) provide this extract within a more extended analysis of failures of empathy in psychotherapy. They argue that such turn-withholds are an important way in which failure to bring off empathy is achieved interactionally through interruption of the smooth progressivity of the conversation.

Example 1 [Excerpt 8 from Wynn and Wynn (2006)][1]

1. T it must be quite. . .hurtful not to. . .not to feel the will to live. . .
2. T that wi[ll]
3. P [hmm] ((patient looks away from the therapist))
4. T that lies in. . .lacking that will? I think that must do something with you?
5. (7 s)
6. T do you know what it does with you?
7. (2 s)
8. P no I don't know
9. (5 s)
10. P then I become insecure with this work with assistance and insecure
11. P if I will manage working from eight to four

At line 4, the therapist has, in context, adequately completed her turn. Moreover, she has asked a question so the sequence is still underway as she has yet to receive some kind of answer. Hence a transition relevance space has opened up and the silence at line 5 belongs to the client who can therefore be heard as withholding her turn. Given that the norm is one beat of silence between turns, a 7-s gap is extremely long. This inter-turn gap can therefore be analyzed as signaling a problem in the interaction. This problematic interactional pattern is repeated over lines 6–7. The therapist issues a reformulated version of her prior question in a further hearably complete TCU which is, once again, followed by an interactionally long silence belonging to the client. The client eventually does provide a relevant, although blocking, response in a hearably complete TCU. The client's response provides some kind of answer to the therapist's question and so completes the series of conditionally relevant actions underway. The following 5-s silence is therefore a lapse in the conversation, in which the therapist could but is not obliged to speak, after which the client continues with a change of topic and new sequence.

There are many more observations that could be made of extract 1. The above commentary, however, allows us to see how some of the silences in this extract, i.e., on lines 5 and 7, are in places in which the next speaker, the client, is expected to talk. These are therefore analyzable as turn-withholds and, hence, indicators of interactional problems. In a more extended analysis, Wynn and Wynn argue that the specific

[1]As translated in the original from Norwegian. The authors describe their transcription conventions as a simplified version of that developed by Jefferson and provide a key in Appendix A of their paper.

interaction problem here is a failure to bring off empathy.

24.3 Sequence Organization

As touched on in the previous section, turns at talk come in series which build up coherent sequences. Interestingly, conversation analysis draws attention to action, as opposed to topic per se, as the most analytically useful resource for identifying how conversations are organized into sequences (see, e.g., Bercelli et al. 2008). That is, a sequence is recognizable as such through having completed a series of conditionally relevant actions, such as making and receiving a response to an invitation.

The most basic and minimal kind of sequence consists of two turns at talk in the form of an adjacency pair. An adjacency pair consists of a first pair part (FPP) issued by one speaker initiating an action followed immediately by an appropriate second pair part (SPP) issued by a second speaker completing that action. Hence, a particular kind of FPP makes a particular kind of SPP conditionally relevant and the second speaker is accountable if she or he fails to offer an appropriate type of response. The technology of the adjacency pair is therefore linked to the turn-taking systems because an FPP makes the issues of an SPP by a second speaker a relevant next action.

The actions performed in conversation are not all the same social valence. This is oriented to by speakers and captured in conversation analysis by the concept of preference organization. Preference is a continuum linked to the degree of social delicacy associated with performing particular actions: that is, the relative potential of the action to create interactional difficulties. Dispreferreds tend to block, rather than to progress, the action of the sequence and can make vulnerable the interlocutors' relationship: for example, an SPP declining rather than accepting an invitation. Dispreferreds are avoided, if possible, or delayed in their production. Hence, they tend to appear towards the end of a turn, can be presaged with a silence, hesitation, or lexical marker such as "well" and may include a warrant or explanation. In contrast, preferred actions tend to be performed immediately and directly.

It would be odd to conceptualize conversation as consisting only of short sequences of adjacency pairs. And observation of talk-in-interaction shows that, although sequences are organized around a base adjacency pair, longer sequences relevant to performing this core action are produced. Expansions around a base adjacency pair can consist of pre-sequences, insert sequences, and/or post-expansion sequences.

Some kinds of action initiated in FPPs are potentially problematic for social relations and are, themselves, dispreferred. These include, for example, requests since they can put an imposition on the recipient. Hence, dispreferred FPPs often involve a pre-sequence which checks out the likely response of the recipient to the projected action. Pre-sequences can be responded to by the recipient with a go-ahead (intimating that a preferred response to the projected action may be forthcoming), block (which stops the action progressing), or hedge (e.g., seeking further information before an SPP is supplied). The recipient's response to the pre-sequence influences the trajectory of the subsequent talk. For example, a pre-request projecting the possibility that a request is about to be made will be heard as such by an interlocutor. The preferred response is one that heads off any potential interactional difficulty. Hence, the most preferred response to a pre-request is that the recipient makes the relevant offer so that the request itself does not have to be made. A blocking or, possibly, hedging response to the pre-request allows a speaker to avoid progressing with the request as there are indications that it may be refused. Interestingly, then, conversation analysis allows analysis of where a base adjacency pair integral to the action of a sequence is, in actual fact, never performed.

Preference organization calls for the production of a relevant SPP as soon as possible following the FPP. However, sequences can be inserted between the FPP and SPP interrupting, but recognizably related to, the action underway. Insert sequences come in two main types: those that orient to the FPP and those that orient to the SPP. Post-first insert expansions most commonly consist of repair initiations in which a second speaker requires some clarification of the FPP before being able to produce an appropriate SPP (see Sect. 24.4). Pre-second insert expansions project forward in the conversation and consist commonly of the second speaker requesting additional information necessary to producing the SPP.

The final place at which a base adjacency pair can be expanded is after the issue of the SPP. Minimal post-expansions consist of what is known as sequence closing thirds. The speaker of the FPP receives an SPP and then finishes the sequence in the third turn with a minimal response such as an acknowledgement token like "okay," change of state token like "oh," or brief assessment of the sequence. Longer post-expansions occur, in particular, when a dispreferred SPP is given and often account for and soften their impact. These can consist of extended post-sequence self-talk-like musings (which appear to be an opportunity for a speaker to "have the last word"), a new FPP which continues the sequence (indicating that the action has not yet been completed, e.g., a question topicalizing the SPP as worthy of further discussion), a repair initiation (indicating a problem in the talk), or a rejection of the SPP.

To bring post-expansions to a close, speakers collaborate typically in the following series of turns. The first speaker provides an assessment, summary, or aphoristic formulation of the upshot of the sequence (which projects its closure). A second speaker agrees (which provides the go-ahead for closure). A third turn (sequence closing third) is produced consisting of a closing token or brief assessment following which there is, possibly, the initiation of a new sequence. This kind of sequence closing sequence and initiation of a new one is illustrated in the following extract (which is from either cognitive or relational-systemic therapy).

Bercelli et al. (2008) observe that therapists make both formulations and reinterpretations in response to client-narrated events and examine the organization of sequences in which these two different kinds of action occur. In formulations, therapists offer a candidate understanding of what the client has meant in her or his previous talk. Hence, in terms of sequence, formulations are contingent on the prior talk, which usually consists of sequences of questions and answers providing the information on which the therapist's formulation is based. Formulations are also the FPP of a sequence closing sequence and, as such, make conditionally relevant an SPP. Bercelli et al. note that a preferred SPP response to a formulation is a confirmation. Alternative, but less preferred, SPPs are disconfirmations or reformulations. Example 2 illustrates an FPP formulation, followed by an SPP confirmation, and followed by a sequence closing third and initiation of a new sequence.

Example 2 [Extract 2 in Bercelli et al. (2008)][2]

```
1. Cl:  [no, there] and then I saw my father
        who::: who
2.      hm:: (.) was protecting my mother.
3.      (0.3)
4. Cl:  and n[ot
5. Th:       [you read this thing as (0.3)
6.      protecting your mum=
7. Cl:  =yes
8. Th:  okay explain to me how.
```

The therapist issues an FPP formulation in lines 5–6 in which he offers a candidate understanding of the client's prior talk. She responds immediately and directly in line 7 with a preferred SPP confirmation. Bercelli et al. note that this kind of minimal confirmation token "yes" is the most common such response to therapist formulations in their corpus. The minimal post-expansion, and sequence closing third (line 8 "okay"), is also one of the most common ways in which therapists close such formulation sequences. Then, with the issue of an FPP question, the therapist goes on to initiate the next

[2] As translated in the original from Italian. The transcription conventions for Examples 2, 3, and 4 in the present chapter are described as based on the Jefferson system, and a key is provided on pages 198–199 of Peräkylä et al. (2008).

action and, hence, new sequence. Bercelli et al. contrast formulation sequences, such as this, to reinterpretation sequences in which therapists are observed to offer more of their own perspective on client-narrated events. They argue that reinterpretation FPPs make relevant a much wider range of client SPPs than do formulation FPPs and provide an analysis of the implications of this for therapy interaction.

24.4 Repair

One common type of insert or post-expansion sequence performs the action of repair. In repair attention is drawn to some trouble source in the talk and so occurs when a speaker indicates an (ostensible) problem in speaking, hearing, or understanding. Repair is designed to be heard as correcting, covers a very broad range of phenomena, and is integral to conversation as a self-regulating system. The mechanisms involved are highly organized and sensitive to both linguistic and social considerations.

There are four types of repair. In self-initiated self-repair, the speaker of the trouble source both indicates a problem in her or his own talk and resolves that problem. In self-initiated other-repair, the speaker of the trouble source indicates a problem in her or his own talk but an interlocutor resolves that problem. The pattern is reiterated for the final two types of repair: other-initiated self-repair and other-initiated other-repair.

The preference is for self-repair. In order to clear up misunderstandings quickly, the norm is to issue repair as close as possible to the trouble source. Hence, repairs are often done during the turn in which the trouble source occurs or quickly following in the turn-transition space before another speaker takes the floor. Self-repairs can correct errors but can also be used to reformulate a turn in order to express something more clearly or fine-tune, or redesign, it to perform a particular action (e.g., to mitigate further a dispreferred). Hence, self-repair includes operations such as redoing part of the turn with the insertion of an additional word or phrase. Repair in the form of a recycled turn beginning may have an interactional function such as securing a person's gaze as a sign of their willingness to act as recipient to the talk. Another common place for self-repair is in the turn immediately following that of the next speaker, even if this next speaker has indicated no ostensible trouble in hearing or understanding.

Following the norm of doing repair as close as possible to the trouble source, other-repair is by far most commonly issued in the turn following the trouble source. The recipient may just make a straightforward correction. However, this may not be possible and repairing someone else's talk can be risky socially. So, even if the repair is other-initiated, it is usually designed to allow self-completion. This can be achieved, for example, by the recipient drawing attention to the problem in a mitigated way (such as asking a question) so that resolution is passed back to the original speaker. Hence, where two speakers are involved in a repair, they can make use of the adjacency pair system consisting of an FPP repair initiation followed by an SPP repair solution. Conversation analysis provides detailed analysis of further positions in which repair can be performed in relation to the trouble source and the features commonly associated with such repairs.

Rae (2008) provides an analysis of repair sequences in psychotherapy in which he argues that therapist-initiated repairs containing lexical substitutions are a resource that can be used to prompt clients to describe their feelings in a more explicit or freer way. The following extract illustrating this process is from a person-centered counseling session.

Example 3 [Extract 5 in Rae (2008)]
07. Cl: I am surviving and I am
08. Th: But it feels (.) doesn't feel right
09. Cl: It feels a little uncomfortable
10. Th: Or a lot uncomfortable.
11. Cl: It feels a l(hoh)ot unc(huh)omfortable actually

In line 10, the therapist initiates a repair through proposing a correction to how the client feels. The lexical substitution he uses is to change the client's word a "little" to the word a "lot." He therefore suggests a refinement, specifically an upgrade, to the way in which the client has described her feelings. As a proposed correction, this therapist-initiated repair orients to the preference for self-repair and the repair completion itself is bounced back to the client. Hence, in the turn immediately following (line 11), the client responds with the repair completion in which she accepts the therapist's corrective upgrade. Interestingly, Rae notes that individuals are usually considered to have privileged access to their own feelings. In Example 3 we can see how this often taken-for-granted theory of mind can be problematized in therapy interaction. Antaki et al. (2007) suggest that such claim of expertise about the experience of others may be part of what "doing therapy" is about. However, we still might be surprised to see such therapist recasting of the client's feelings within a client-centered session. Conversation analysis shows how this process can be performed through the everyday practices of repair.

24.5 Word Selection

Word selection is an important aspect of conversational exchange. For example, word selection as an aspect of repair was illustrated in Example 3 above in which the therapist substituted the word a "lot" for the client's word a "little" and in doing so suggested an alternative, more expansive, characterization of her feelings. Such observations reveal the importance of word choice for interlocutors and how attention to the words used, when alternatives are available, is a useful analytic resource for understanding what is being achieved through talk.

A particularly interesting aspect of word selection and focus of conversation analytic work is the way in which persons (and objects and places) are referred to in talk. English-type languages provide dedicated terms, pronouns such as "you" and "I," to allow reference to persons. Different languages provide alternative possibilities, such as the lexically indexed singular-plural and formality differences in French between "tu" and "vous" (although there are colloquial ways of referring to groups of recipients in English such as "yous-all"). Pronouns, in the main, can be considered to be the reference simpliciter: that is, the simple solution allowing speakers to refer to each other and to third parties (she, he, they) during conversation.

When interlocutors use anything other than the reference simpliciter, it suggests that something over-and-above simple reference is being done. Alternatives to the reference simpliciter to refer to the current speaker or recipient include use of third person (e.g., "she" rather than "I" or "you"), use of one's own or the recipient's proper name, but also using the reference simpliciter "I" or "you" with attention-drawing prosody. Such person referencers invite analysis of what is being achieved by this word selection at this point in the conversation.

There are numerous options for referring to non-present third parties, each with different kinds of interactional implication. Conversation analysis identifies two useful sets of overlapping differentiations. First, is the use of locally initial or locally subsequent reference. Locally initial forms tend to be used on first mention of a particular third party. These include proper names, descriptors (e.g., my son), or categories (e.g., one of my colleagues). Once this has been established, reference to this person can be made using a locally subsequent reference such as "she," "he," or "they." Second is the use of recognitional or non-recognitional reference. Recognitionals indicate to the recipient that he or she knows that third party and can, through the description offered, figure out who that person is (e.g., use of the person's name). Non-recognitional person reference indicates to the recipient that he or she does not know that particular third party. These include descriptions such as "someone," "this person I met," and "a guy."

Person reference, particularly non-recognitionals, can be done using a membership categorization device (MCDs). MCDs go beyond person reference and display culture through additional actions such as description since they make use of categories of person found in particular social settings. Categories of person cluster together into types (e.g., youth subcultures), teams (such as family members mother, father, son, etc.), and sequences (e.g., young, middle aged, old). Categories bring with them a stock of cultural associations and assumptions and so can be a shorthand for typifying an individual more broadly. Moreover, given that a person can be categorized in many different ways, it becomes relevant to analyze what a particular MCD is achieving at the point it is used in a conversation.

The following example illustrates use of a zero-person reference by a therapist during group therapy for addicts. Central to the Minnesota model used in this therapy is the idea that for successful outcome the client must both admit to being an addict and identify with the other group members. Halonen (2008) provides an analysis of how zero-person reference can help facilitate both aims.

Example 4 [Extract 3 in Halonen (2008)][3]

01. Th2: well how about in the morning when let's say 0 has
02. drunk more in the evening and in the morning when
03. you wake up so, like when there is a hangover and,
04. like you go

Prior to this extract, the client addressed had not yet produced a description of himself as an alcoholic. The therapist then produces a story in which aspects of this client's own account of his drinking are typified as addict-like. In producing her description, the therapist uses first a zero-person construction (line 1). This is not a reference simpliciter and so invites analysis of what it achieves over-and-above simple person reference. A zero-person construction leaves the person reference open. Hence, the recounted behavior is framed as something familiar to addicts in general. In her next two person references, the therapist seemingly addresses the client directly: "you wake up" (line 3) and "you go" (line 4). Use of the recipient reference simpliciter "you" closely following the open zero-person construction implies that the client's behavior, too, is typical of the established addict-like pattern. In English, the pronoun "you" can also be used as an open category of people in general (where the word "one" would be more formally correct). The person reference "you" in lines 3 and 4 therefore may open the possibility of both linking the specific client's behavior with problematic drinking and describing problematic drinking in a way in which the group members in general can identify. This extract, however, is a translation and Halonen does not comment on whether this ambiguity is also present in the original Finnish. However, using further examples of zero-person construction, she argues that this kind of zero-person reference in the context of group therapy does allow individuals to talk about their own addictions in a way recognized as not unique to the speaker but general to members of the group.

24.6 Action Formation

It has been made clear throughout that talk-in-interaction is a form of social action in that conversationalists do things with their utterances. This section highlights and pulls together action formation as glossed in previous sections and then considers conversational closings as an important "doing" of relevance to psychotherapy interaction.

The fundamental building block for performing social actions in conversation is the adjacency pair. That is, after a first pair part (FPP) initiating an action, the turn-taking system makes conditionally relevant from a recipient a certain kind of second pair part (SPP) which is responsive to that action. Action is important for the turn-taking system also in that, along with syntactic and intonational features, a turn-constructional unit (TCU) is hearably complete when, in context, it completes an action (e.g., makes a question). Speaker change then becomes the relevant next action.

[3] As translated in the original from Finnish.

In conversation there is a preference for progressivity: that is, for moving forward with, or accomplishing, the action projected by the FPP (e.g., invitation-acceptance). However, turns at talk may do, or respond to, more than one action at a time. For example, membership categorization devices (MCDs) may do description as well as person reference. Sequences of adjacency pairs, along with their pre-, insert-, and post-expansions build and close around the performance of an action. And conversation analysis demonstrates that the completion of an action is a more useful way of conceptualizing sequence than is topic: that is, considering what the talk is doing rather than what it is purportedly about.

Where in a sequence a turn is positioned and how it is designed are resources for analyzing what the turn is doing. For example, insert sequences between an FPP and SPP may be doing repair and/or possibly presage a non-preferred SPP through breaking the contiguity between the adjacency pairs—as do design features such as mitigations, hesitations, and weak agreements. In self-repair, the action performed in a turn can be refined or modified through, for example, substituting or adding a word. Moreover, in other-initiated repair, a recipient may indicate a problem in understanding the action being performed in prior talk.

One important action relevant to talk-in-interaction which has been studied in conversation analysis is the act of closing a conversation. Closing requires interlocutors to disengage from the turn-taking system. In practice they need to do two things. First, interlocutors need to check that nothing more needs to be talked about in this conversation. Second, they need to design turns that occasion no further talk but to do so without making their relationship vulnerable. So, interestingly, the act of closing a conversation is achieved by passing up opportunities to do something. This is performed through a particular set of sequences.

The first observation is that closings cannot occur at any point in a conversation. They must occur within closing implicative environments. These environments can be created when a topic is closed down in such a way that it appears that nothing more is to be said on it. This includes making of arrangements for future interactions, providing an overarching summary or assessment which implies that the talk on that topic is complete, offering an appreciation for the opportunity to have interacted, back references to prior topics which suggest that conversational topics have been exhausted, and announcements of closure in which external circumstances are invoked to account for the need to move into terminating the conversation.

Closing the conversation then becomes a possible next action and the interlocutors may move into a pre-closing sequence. Pre-closing sequences consist of an adjacency pair which performs the action of checking if anything more needs to be talked about. In successful closings, the pre-closing FPP and SPP consist of each participant passing up the opportunity to raise further matters for discussion. A second action then follows in which the participants agree to end the conversation. In English, this terminal sequence usually consists of an adjacency pair exchange of goodbyes.

As in ordinary conversations, therapists face the problem of ending sessions in a way that does not damage their relationship with clients. This can be particularly difficult in group therapy, as in the following extract, when clients are engaged in multiparty talk. This example is taken from the ninth of 53 sessions of group psychodynamic psychotherapy for seven women diagnosed with an eating disorder and illustrates interactional achievement of a closing implicative environment.

Example 5 [Final Extract in Lepper and Mergenthaler (2005)][4]

1. P3: Sure but my mum knows about it—hers doesn't.
2. P5: To have a problem + if you have a problem

[4]As translated in the original from Spanish. The authors describe their transcription conventions as the Spanish version of the psychotherapy transcription standards as outlined in Mergenthaler and Gril (1996).

or—if you fail like she said—
3. and you stay there—that's not right but if you have a problem and you try to
4. find a solution like you did by coming here searching for help—why would
5. your mum feel that everything goes wrong? On the contrary okay, she looks
6. for help.
7. T: Well—very + well.
8. P9: I must go to see the doctor at ten.

Clients P3 and P5 are exchanging turns at talk towards the end of the session. Then, in line 7, the therapist produces a brief assessment "well very well." We know that turns projecting the end of a sequence often take the form of a brief assessment, summary, or aphoristic formulations of the gist so far since their production implies that the previous talk has been adequately concluded. In line 7 the therapist also passes up the opportunity to continue the sequence or to introduce a new topic. She therefore prepares the way for another interlocutor, client P9, to move the conversation more formally into a closing implicative environment. P9 does so through an announcement of closure in which she makes reference to external circumstances, an appointment with "the doctor at ten," as imposing an end to the conversation. Hence, in sequence terms, P9 provides the go-ahead for closure. In their more extensive analysis of extracts, Lepper and Mergenthaler argue that therapists fail to tie their turns strongly to the pervious talk as a way to end sequences and, in the above example sessions, in a deliberate manner.

24.7 Discussion

In outlining the main features of talk-in-interaction of interest in conversation analysis—turn-taking, sequence organization, repair, word selection, and action formation—it appears that the analytic lens and conceptualization of key phenomena is different in many respects to that of traditional psychotherapy research. Moreover, as mentioned earlier, even though a literature has developed on conversation analysis of therapy interaction, selection of material has been, in the main, in accordance with conversation analytically-informed, as opposed to therapy-informed, observations. It is therefore pertinent to ask if the projects of conversation analysis and of psychotherapy research can cohere? And one of the most experienced and methodologically informed psychotherapy researchers, Bill Stiles,[5] does caution that "CA concepts cannot be inserted unchanged into gaps in therapy theory. Therapists and conversation analysts must learn each other's theories and make adjustments if the product is to be mutually useful" (Stiles 2008, p. 2).

One important issue is that conversation analysis is agnostic to the psychological theories that inform psychotherapy and its interventions and which frame most traditional psychotherapy research. Conversation analysis approaches dialogue as intersubjectivity in action: that is, how interlocutors produce a shared understanding of the matter at hand in their talk, and true it its ethnomethodological roots, just as it is the talk and associated observations that is available to speakers, conversation analysis limits its observations strictly to this material. What are in other fields considered "internal" (emotions, motivations, the unconscious, etc.) are analyzed as they are constituted in and through the interaction and conversation analysis refuses to comment on the experience of interlocutors (Forrester and Reason 2006). This may seem psychologically shallow to the psychotherapy community: too removed from basic assumptions about human subjectivity and mute on questions of experiential change which are likely of interest to therapists. Moreover, conversation analysis could be considered naïve methodologically if it ignores the vast corpus of psychotherapy theory and research which could help target episodes of therapy for microanalysis.

This therapy-neutral orientation may, however, be a significant strength in allowing conversation analysis to complement and enhance

[5] See also, for example, Chap. 8 in this volume.

process research through revealing what psychotherapy may not notice about itself (Antaki et al. 2007). In particular, Georgaca and Avdi (2009) argue that conversation analysis is useful for illustrating "the intricate micro-processes through which psychotherapeutic technique is pursued (...), throw light on unacknowledged therapist competencies and illuminate the elements that differentiate successful from unsuccessful implementation of therapeutic techniques" (p. 241). In fact, conversation analysis may be the method *par excellence*[6] for raising to awareness tacit skills of both therapist and client in progressing the therapeutic project: fine-grained, moment-by-moment, making the ordinary appear extraordinary (Kozart 1996). At the very least, the orientation and observations of conversation analysis may have potential to hone therapists' skills of attention during their training (Forrester and Reason 2006).

For example, as outlined above, Rae (2008) noticed that lexical substitutions (e.g., exchanging the word a "lot" for a "little") can be used by therapists to prompt clients to describe their feelings in a more expansive manner. Traditional therapy researchers may too make this, seemingly mundane, observation. However, as a conversation analyst, Rae recognizes it as an important conversational phenomenon—a repair—and to bring into play an extensive literature on how repair works in conversation which sheds light on how this therapy technique is used and responded to by clients. Moreover, person-neutral reference was identified by Halonen (2008) as a potentially nonthreatening way of helping clients to acknowledge problematic behavior and to facilitate identification with other clients during group therapy. Such attention to word selection and its importance in bringing off social actions is central to conversation analysis and, again, connects an easy-to-overlook therapy intervention to a relevant, and extensive, research literature.

Kozart (1996) reminds us that conversation analysis of institutional talk is not new and that the growing conversation analytic literature on psychotherapy is positioned within a wider literature on medical discourse more generally. The specific focus on therapy interaction, however, has developed to the extent that it has warranted review. Georgaca and Avdi (2009) provide a useful overview highlighting how conversation analysis has contributed to understanding the processes through which therapy is accomplished in practice and in assessing the role of the therapist. In particular, studies are noted to have focused on therapist formulations of client's talk, use of specific interactional formats, and of idiomatic expressions as important aspects of the therapeutic process. Although published too recently to be included in Georgaca and Avdi's review, Bercelli et al.'s (2008) analysis of the contrast between therapist formulation sequences and reinterpretation sequences, described above, contributes further to this theme, and Vehviläinen et al. (2008) draw attention to sequence organization as a particularly important "site at which many therapy-relevant phenomena happen" (p. 188).

Conclusion

Conversation analysis of therapy talk has, as yet, hardly scratched the surface and the possibilities for future research are exciting. Vehviläinen et al. (2008) suggest that, in particular, there is potential for more analysis of client, as opposed to therapist, actions, and examination of the extent to which the phenomena identified in conversation analytic research are general or specific to different types of therapy. My own suggestion is that there is potential also for conversation analysis to be informed to a greater extent by traditional psychotherapy research without losing its relatively atheoretical stance. This may be accomplished, for example, through accepting for analysis episodes of therapy interaction

[6]In this respect, conversation analysis represents the far end of the scale in terms of microanalysis of talk-in-interaction. Some forms of discourse analysis which draw heavily on conversation analysis may fulfil a similar function, but "discourse analysis" as a term encompasses a range of methods, some of which are highly theoretical (e.g., Foucauldian) and which seek to explicate the presence and use of macro-cultural resources on the scale of "grand narratives."

deemed significant from the viewpoint of psychotherapeutic theory. The link to what therapists find important is therefore strengthened while the usefully distinct orientation to the material provided by conversation analysis can be maintained. For example, as described above, Wynn and Wynn (2006) acknowledge the theoretical and psychological importance of empathy in therapy while exploring what different types of empathy and, indeed, empathy failures look like interactionally through, for instance, the technology of turn-taking.

This chapter has offered an introduction to conversation analysis and the ways in which it has contributed and is likely to continue to contribute to psychotherapy research. It has been suggested that, although their projects may differ, the "noticings" facilitated by a conversation analytic approach are being demonstrated to offer something unique and interesting to psychotherapy researchers and practicing therapists.

Acknowledgment I am most grateful to Professor Celia Kitzinger (University of York, UK) for her inspirational instruction on conversation analysis. I extend huge thanks also to Dr. Sonja Ellis (Sheffield Hallam University, UK) for her support and for her extremely helpful comments on an earlier draft of this chapter. Anna Madill is Chair of Qualitative Inquiry and Deputy Head of the School of Psychology, University of Leeds, UK (https://leeds.academia.edu/AnnaMadill). She cofounded and is former chair of the British Psychological Society Qualitative Methods in Psychology Section and is associate editor of the British Journal of Clinical Psychology.

References

Antaki C, Barnes R, Leudar I (2007) Members' and analysts' interests: 'formulations' in psychotherapy. In: Hepburn A, Wiggins S (eds) Discursive research in practice: new approaches to psychology and interaction. Cambridge University Press, Cambridge, pp 166–181

Bercelli F, Rossano F, Viaro M (2008) Client's responses to therapists' reinterpretations. In: Peräkylä A, Antaki C, Vehviläinen S, Leudar I (eds) Conversation analysis and psychotherapy. Cambridge University Press, Cambridge, pp 43–61

Edwards D, Potter J (1992) Discursive psychology. Sage, London

Elliott R (1984) A discovery-oriented approach to significant change events in psychotherapy: interpersonal process recall and comprehensive process analysis. In: Rice LN, Greenberg LS (eds) Patterns of change: intensive analysis of therapeutic process. Wiley, New York

Forrester M, Reason D (2006) Conversation analysis and psychoanalytic psychotherapy research: questions, issues, problems and challenges. Psychoanal Psychother 20:40–64. doi:10.1080/02668730500524229

Georgaca E, Avdi E (2009) Evaluating the talking cure: the contribution of narrative, discourse, and conversation analysis to psychotherapy assessment. Qual Res Psychol 6:233–247. doi:10.1080/14780880802146896

Greenberg LS (1984) Task analysis: the general approach. In: Rice LN, Greenberg LS (eds) Patterns of change: intensive analysis of psychotherapy process. Guilford, New York, pp 124–148, Chapter 4

Greenberg LS (1991) Research on the process of change. Psychother Res 1:3–16

Gurman AS (1973) Instability of therapeutic conditions in psychotherapy. J Couns Psychol 20:16–24. doi:10.1080/10503309112331334011

Halonen M (2008) Person reference as a device for constructing experiences as typical in group therapy. In: Peräkylä A, Antaki C, Vehviläinen S, Leudar I (eds) Conversation analysis and psychotherapy. Cambridge University Press, Cambridge, pp 139–151

Hepburn A, Potter J (2007) Crying receipts: time, empathy and institutional practice. Res Lang Soc Interact 40:89–116. doi:10.1080/08351810701331299

Heritage J (2005) Conversation analysis and institutional talk. In: Fitch K, Sanders RE (eds) Handbook of language and social interaction. Lawrence Erlbaum, Mahwah, NJ, pp 103–147

Hobson RF (1985) Forms of feeling: the heart of psychotherapy. Tavistock Publications, London

Kozart MF (1996) A sociological perspective on the therapeutic alliance: ethnomethodology and conversation analysis. Psychotherapy 33:361–371. doi:10.1037/0033-3204.33.3.361

Lacan J (1968) The language of the self: the function of language in psychoanalysis. Translated by A. Wilden. Johns Hopkins University Press, Baltimore, MD

Lepper G (2015) A pragmatic approach to the study of therapeutic interaction: towards an observational science of psychotherapy process. In: Gelo OCG, Pritz A, Rieken B (eds) Psychotherapy research: foundations, process, and outcome. Springer, Heidelberg

Lepper G, Mergenthaler E (2005) Exploring group process. Psychother Res 15:433–444. doi:10.1080/10503300500091587

Madill A, Gough B (2008) Qualitative research and its place in psychological science. Psychol Methods 13:254–271. doi:10.1037/a0013220

Madill A, Widdicombe S, Barkham M (2001) The potential of conversation analysis for psychotherapy research. Couns Psychol 29:413–434. doi:10.1177/0011000001293006

Mahrer AR, Nifakis DJ, Abhukara L, Sterner I (1984) Microstrategies in psychotherapy: the patterning of sequential therapist statements. Psychotherapy 21:465–472. doi:10.1037/h0085990

Mergenthaler E, Gril S (1996) Descriptión de las reglas para la transcriptión de sesiones de psicoterapai. Revista Argentina de Clinica Psicológica 5:163–176

Morris GH, Chenail RJ (eds) (1995) The talk of the clinic: explorations in the analysis of medical and therapeutic discourse. Lawrence Erlbaum, New Jersey

Pain J (2009) Not just talking: conversation analysis. Harvey Sacks' gift to therapy. UKCP, Karnac Books, London

Peräkylä A, Antaki C, Vehviläinen S, Leudar I (eds) (2008) Conversation analysis and psychotherapy. Cambridge University Press, Cambridge

Rae J (2008) Lexical substitution as a therapeutic resource. In: Peräkylä A, Antaki C, Vehviläinen S, Leudar I (eds) Conversation analysis and psychotherapy. Cambridge University Press, Cambridge, pp 62–79

Rice LN, Greenberg LS (eds) (1984) Patterns of change: intensive analysis of psychotherapy process. Guilford, New York

Sacks H (1972) An initial investigation of the usability of conversational data for doing sociology. In: Sudnow D (ed) Studies in social interaction. Free Press, New York, pp 31–74

Shapiro DA, Barkham M, Hardy GE, Morrison LA (1990) The second Sheffield psychotherapy project: rationale, design and preliminary outcome data. Br J Med Psychol 63:97–108. doi:10.1111/j.2044-8341.1990.tb01603.x

Stiles WB (2008) Foreword: filling the gaps. In: Peräkylä A, Antaki C, Vehviläinen S, Leudar I (eds) Conversation analysis and psychotherapy. Cambridge University Press, Cambridge, pp 1–4

Vehviläinen S, Peräkylä A, Antaki C, Leudar I (2008) A review of conversational practices in psychotherapy. In: Peräkylä A, Antaki C, Vehviläinen S, Leudar I (eds) Conversation analysis and psychotherapy. Cambridge University Press, Cambridge, pp 188–197

White M, Epston D (1990) Narrative means to therapeutic ends. W. W Norton & Company, New York

Wynn R, Wynn M (2006) Empathy as an interactionally achieved phenomenon in psychotherapy: characteristics of some conversational resources. J Pragmat 38:1385–1397. doi:10.1016/j.pragma.2005.09.008

25 A Pragmatic Approach to the Study of Therapeutic Interaction: Toward an Observational Science of Psychotherapy Process

Georgia Lepper

Contents

G. Lepper (✉)
University of Exeter, Exeter, UK
e-mail: georgia@lepper.co.uk

Abstract

Psychotherapy research has revealed the centrality of relational factors, such as the alliance, in psychotherapy process. This chapter places these findings in the context of contemporary research in developmental psychology, and in the discipline of pragmatics, the study of human communication in its immediate context. It proposes the adoption of the natural observational methods used in these disciplines for the multidisciplinary study of therapeutic interaction. A review of the relevant background is followed by a demonstration of this analytic approach. The chapter concludes with suggestions for a multimodal programme of research into relational processes in psychotherapy.

25.1 Introduction

> "The alliance is not a class of behaviours which can be specified and counted; rather, the alliance is a consequence of responsive behaviours." (Stiles et al. 1998)

The relational aspects of psychotherapy process have been recognized both in clinical practice and in formal research as a significant element in the therapeutic process, starting with the recognition of the importance of the "alliance" by the earliest psychotherapy researchers. 40 years of psychotherapy research has

O.C.G. Gelo et al. (eds.), *Psychotherapy Research*,
DOI 10.1007/978-3-7091-1382-0_25, © Springer-Verlag Wien 2015

demonstrated that the alliance is the most important common factor in successful outcomes [for thorough reviews see Horvath (2006), Lambert (2004), and Wampold (2001)]. Much of the formal research has sought to identify variables and enable measurement, so that significant elements of the alliance can be captured, measured and linked to outcomes (see Chap. 16). A number of measuring devices have been developed, focussing variously on the therapist's, the client's and sometimes an observer's rating of the alliance. Stiles and his colleagues, in the study from which the above quote is taken, demonstrated that it is, however, impossible to reliably identify countable "classes of behaviours".

It is becoming clear that while the focus of research on measurable variables has enhanced the general profile of alliance effect, it has been at the expense of a clear definition of what exactly contributes to it (Horvath 2005). What specific interactions of therapist and client can be identified as contributing to the overall alliance? How can we translate these findings into practical guidance relevant to training and supervision? Horvath wonders whether it might be possible to "identify a limited range of relationship processes that are most facilitative in achieving [an effective alliance]" (Horvath 2005, p. 262). The shift of focus of attention from "variables" to "responsive behaviours" (Stiles et al. 1998) opens up a new range of potential methods for the observation of the therapeutic relationship, and the therapeutic process which is facilitated through the alliance between therapist and client. Such an approach also contains the potential to bridge the gap between the kinds of research which favour distributional findings (generalizations about populations of clients and events) and methods which might reveal what those processes actually look like in the consulting room. "Responsive behaviours" are micro events, observable at the level of turn-by-turn interaction, which structure the overall sense-making activity of the participants. They include non-verbal as well as verbal actions and communications.

The following chapter explores a methodological approach by which the interaction of the therapist and client can be studied in close detail. Its perspective is grounded in a domain of enquiry known broadly as "pragmatics": the study of human communication in its immediate context. Historically, pragmatics originated in the philosophy of Charles Pierce but later developed into an empirical discipline which crosses the domains of sociology, psychology, and linguistics. Its foundational proposition is that knowledge and meaning are grounded in human action and relating and that individual development and the social order are created through the actions of persons in relation. It follows that the detailed study of human interaction, at the level of the talk, can reveal the processes by which a meaningful, intersubjectively shared world is co-produced. [For a general introduction to the philosophical and empirical dimensions of the field of pragmatics, see Mey (1999).]

The perspective taken by this chapter is that the "responsive behaviours" referred to by Stiles are those which generally underpin human sociality. They include physiological, cognitive and interactional components which are linked in a complex system of communicative actions which is universally observable in human interaction (Enfield and Levinson 2006). The methodological approach outlined in this chapter starts from the premise that "responsive behaviours" are observable at the level of turn-by-turn interaction between therapist and client. It seeks to propose an observational science of psychotherapy process, whose findings can be linked to the wider mappings provided by other methods of enquiry in order to establish what kinds of therapeutic interactions are linked to good outcomes, while providing evidence with direct relevance to clinical practice.

The chapter begins with a brief review of findings from the developmental literature, which has demonstrated the foundational aspects of interaction in the affective and cognitive development. It is followed by a review of the findings from the field of pragmatics which bear upon how psychotherapeutic interaction can be studied at the level of the speaking turn. Some significant phenomena of interaction, with significance for psychotherapeutic process, will be illustrated with the detailed analysis of an episode from a session, while issues of sampling and study design are addressed. Finally, the chapter will conclude with some suggestions for further research, integrating this approach with existing process research models we already have to hand.

25.2 An Interactional Model of Human Mind and Language

In recent years, collaboration between social scientists, the study of everyday language (pragmatics) and developmental psychology has resulted in a new, multidisciplinary approach to the study of human sociality (Hendriks- Jansen 1996; Enfield and Levinson 2006). This chapter makes the case for the application of the findings emerging from these studies to the study of psychotherapy interaction. Common to this interdisciplinary approach is the use of naturalistic observational strategies derived from the methods of ethology in order to study human development:

> [Developmental investigators] tried to observe infants' behaviour in the context in which it naturally occurred, deferred analysis and theoretical speculation until they had built up a solid descriptive base, and examined in great detail a particular type of behaviour rather than searching for evidence of a central law that might unify diverse behavioural phenomena. (Hendriks- Jansen 1996, p. 251)

The chapter proposes to demonstrate the application of this methodological strategy to the study of therapeutic interaction. The following sections present some of the background to an emerging interpersonal model of the development of cognition and language, and then some of the findings from the field of pragmatics, upon which an observational study of psychotherapeutic interaction could be undertaken.

25.2.1 Interaction in Human Development

Human affect and cognition develop in a social and cultural context. The infant, genetically endowed with the capacity for imitation (Meltzoff 2005), enters the world helpless and dependent, yet powerfully able to engage caregivers in interactions which will form the basis of cognitive and affective development and language. Observational studies have demonstrated that far from being the passive recipient of maternal care and attention, the newborn infant is already an active agent in engaging his or her caregiver's responsive actions. Early observations of behaviours underpinning the development of social communication include the burst-pause-burst pattern of feeding interactions (Kaye 1982), in which mothers respond to their infants feeding pattern with a "turn", jiggling the infant in order to "encourage" feeding, believing that their jiggling encourages the infant to suck, though "in fact jiggling *reduces* the likelihood of the beginning of a new burst and it is only the *cessation* of jiggling that encourages the infant to resume sucking" (Hendriks- Jansen 1996, p. 264). Early lip and tongue movements and mirroring engaged in between infants and their caregivers (Trevarthen 1977) and species typical activity patterns, such as the rhythmical stereotypical activities such as kicking and hand waving, are "read" by caregivers to interpret the infants mood and "intentions" (Tronick 2007). Interpersonal coordinated patterns of activity, scaffolded by caregiver responsiveness, are observable at a very early age. Mothers read intentions into their infants' spontaneous patterns of activity (kicking, crying, smiling, cooing), name them and respond to them, creating a foundational interpretive environment in which the developing infant learns to communicate her wishes, desires and needs. Primary turn-taking activity, initiated by the infant and responded to by the primary caregiver, provides the foundation for the development of a sense of self and agency in the social world of human communication (Knox 2010).

Starting from these foundational observations, Levinson (2006) proposes a model in which a multidisciplinary study of human interaction can be situated; he calls it "the interaction engine". It starts with, but is by no means sufficiently accounted for by, the capacity for *attribution of intention*, or mind reading. Added to this is the ingredient of *mutual salience for us right now*—the immediate context—or *common ground* of the interaction which is a basic requirement for cooperative actions. Human interaction is driven by *Gricean intentions*: "intentions that drive behaviours whose sole function is to have an effect by virtue of having their intentions recognized" (p. 54). It is basic to human communication that intentions are expected and recognized and responded to. Rules which guide cooperation are also required. All of these are empirically observable as a universal set of practices—turn taking, sequential patterns and repair strategies which form the basic platform for complex, multimodal human communication. They are emergent properties of our genetic inheritance (Knox 2010). It is these observable actions which provide the raw data of model building for a science of human interaction.

The "interaction engine" locates a field of enquiry at a juncture at which developmental, cognitive and social sciences meet. The psychotherapy research we have is a model which primarily focuses on the properties of individual subjects. The shift to a multi-person perspective presents new challenges and offers new opportunities. In the following section, the methods of the discipline of pragmatics are introduced as a practical method, with an existing large body of findings, by means of which the turn-taking properties of persons in interaction are studied using observational methods.

25.2.2 Doing Things with Words

"How to do things with words" is the title of a series of seminal lectures on everyday language by Austin (1975), which launched a new discipline: ordinary language philosophy. Austin proposed a radical change in the way that we think of the phenomenon of language. We think of words as representing "things" (nouns), actions (verbs) or qualities (adverbs or adjectives). We may look them up in dictionaries to find out what they mean. Austin proposed a different perspective on words. It starts from the view that words are resources used in the act of talking. Language is action, and we do things with words. Austin's work was followed by the major contributions of Searle (1969) and Wittgenstein (1968), who developed a philosophical model of meaning grounded in use. Habermas (1987) incorporated this philosophical revolution into his theory of communicative action. Subsequently, empirical research, grounded in this foundational idea, has built a substantial descriptive model of *how* everyday language works. It describes *how* speakers create "meaning" in relation to the context in which the interaction takes place and *how* speakers relate to each other at the level of the turn. Starting from this point of view, we can observe how the dynamics of human communication work, and how the social world in which we live is created through our communicative acts. On this view, the "common ground", or context, shared by speakers is the resource for mean-making, at the same time as it is in a continuous state of creation and renewal by speakers' actions on a turn-by-turn basis. The "common ground" of communicative action accounts for both stability and plasticity (and therefore the possibility of change) at the level of both the social and the psychological.

The early development of the discipline of linguistics was shaped by the distinction made by Saussure (1974) between "*langue*" and "*parole*". For Saussure, language was characterized by two dimensions: formal rules, or "*langue*", and "*parole*", the (to him) debased form of "*langue*" which was the feature of everyday talk—often ungrammatical, evidently inconsistent and imperfect. Linguistic research first focussed its attention on "*langue*", generating disciplines which studied grammar, syntax and phonetics. The phenomena of "*parole*" remained unstudied until the 1960s when researchers began to turn their attention to naturally occurring talk. Labov and Waletzky (1967), challenging the conventional view that everyday talk such as dialect was a "debased" form of language, studied the narratives of inner-city teenagers and developed a model of the formal properties of oral storytelling. Sacks et al. (1974) began to observe how everyday conversational interaction works, turning analytic attention toward the "pragmatic" aspects of language: the turn-by-turn actions of everyday talk and how speakers co-construct meaningful exchanges, building what he termed a "natural observational science of social life". Other investigators—Schiffrin (1987), Levinson (1983, 2006) and more recently, cognitive linguists (e.g. Slobin 1996; Verhagen 2005)—have explored how lexical resources contribute to meaning making at the level of situated interaction.

25.2.3 Turn Taking

One of the most important contributions to the discipline of pragmatics was developed in the 1960s. Through a decade-long series of observations of naturally occurring interactions (recorded on the newly invented portable tape recorder), Sacks (1992) built the foundations of the study of turn-by-turn interaction, which came to be known as Conversation Analysis (CA). He showed that turns are constructed in such a way that they link to the previous turn and create the possibility for the next turn, through observable "rules of use". He called this phenomenon "recipient design". A detailed introduction to CA and its foundational study of the underpinning mechanisms of everyday talk can be found in Chap. 24 of this volume.

The evidence of early, prelinguistic turn-taking behaviours, subsequently observed by developmental psychologists, provides further evidence for the insight of Sacks into the foundations on which human conversation is built. Infants begin with biological disposition to imitation and turn taking, and through interactions with caregivers, these innate behavioural dispositions are shaped into routine activity patterns, mutually engaged in by infants and their caregivers (Trevarthen 1977). The activity patterns which generate talk precede the emergence of language in both species and individual development (Hendriks- Jansen 1996) and underpin "intersubjectivity".

A substantial literature of observational studies of turn taking now exists as a resource for the researcher seeking to study the interactions of people in specific contexts—those seeking to understand psychotherapeutic interaction, for example (see Enfield and Levinson (2006) for some examples from different disciplines). At the same time, other researchers contributing to the general field of pragmatics were investigating other phenomena of interest.

25.2.4 Lexical Devices

> "Linguistic expressions are primarily cues for making inferences, and understanding does not primarily consist in deciding the precise content of the expressions, but in making inferences that lead to adequate next (cognitive, conversational, behavioural) moves." (Verhagen 2005, p. 22)

In addition to turn taking, analytic attention can focus on the linguistic resources used by speakers to manage their talk. Here the focus is on the way lexical resources are used to generate the immediate context in the turn-by-turn dynamic of the talk. These may include substantive words (e.g. nouns—named things, or verbs—actions) which, as pragmatic resources, create easily recognized collections of categories. For example, "mother", "father", "baby", "sister" and "brother" belong to the category "family" and will be heard in that context, unless there is a specific qualification built into the utterance (Lepper 2000). Deictic words ("now", "before", "over there") point the hearer to the relevant location, in time or space, of an utterance (Schegloff 1972a); so-called verbal markers, such as "well", "you know" and "I mean" signal to the hearer how to interpret what is to follow (Schiffrin 1987); and syntactical forms shape the inferential potential of an utterance, providing for the next move in the ongoing talk. Negation is an important case of syntactical organization, by means of which inferences are made about the intended direction of the utterance. Depending on the syntactic structure, negation can be overt or concealed (Verhagen 2005).

Another important category of syntax significant for the purposes of researching everyday interaction is mental state language. Developmental linguistics has shown that 3-year-olds begin to incorporate mental state words into their vocabulary, prior to the acquisition of mastery of false belief understanding, and children who have achieved false belief understanding show higher levels of mental state language (Bartsch and Wellman 1995). Bartsch and Wellman propose that mental state language indexes the richness of children's social interaction. Their findings had further support in the observations of Ruffman et al. (2002) which showed that the mothers' use of mental state terms predicts false belief ability in their children. Mothers mediate their children's entry into the recognition of their own and others' mental states. Further studies of mental state language (Diessel and Tomasello 2001; Verhagen 2005; Peyers 2006) have also implicated the use of complementary clauses ("know, wish or believe *that* ...") as key elements in the acquisition of false belief capacity. The capacity to communicate intersubjectively about a thought or belief requires a rich language foundation of both vocabulary and syntax, built through interactions.

25.2.5 Narrative

Of much interest to developmental research in recent years has been the phenomenon of narrative. Bruner (1990) argued the case for the centrality of narrative in the development of cognition and the self, against the computational model of cognition then in its ascendency, and this tradition of research has informed a rich vein of psychotherapy research. These developments are comprehensively reviewed by Angus and McLeod (2004).

Pragmatics brings another perspective to this study: the production of narratives in talk and their properties in the organization of meaning making in the turn-by-turn process of interaction. The research of Labov and Waletzky (1967) revealed structural properties of oral narrative which make them "hearable". Sacks, in his own study of naturally occurring conversations, noted that storytelling is a ubiquitous phenomenon in everyday talk and that speakers typically announce the upcoming telling in order to signal that a story, and a longer than normal turn, is to follow. They alert hearers with prefacing remark, which precedes and sets the scene for the story to follow. Core elements of an oral narrative prototypically include at least one temporal sequence (first/then) and finish with an evaluative sequence, which signals the end of the story, and also summarizes the point of the story (Labov 1997). Sacks also observed that stories are often followed by "second stories" which function to link to the point of the first story and perhaps to extend it in a subsequent turn (Sacks 1992). Decades of subsequent research have identified the complex operations involved in oral storytelling in naturally occurring conversation (a thorough review of this strand of research can be found in a special edition of *Narrative and Life Stories*, *Vol 7*, 1997).

Pragmatics, like CA, shares with grounded theory, and other qualitative methods, a concern for meaning as a product of human communicative actions. It differs, however, in its methodological approach. As noted by Madill (p. 500 in this volume), "CA is closer to a natural science than a human science approach through taking the stance that rigorous empirical observation and application of correct method will reveal the (normative) rules of conversational exchange". All of the disciplines outlined in this multimodal approach to human communication share this methodological perspective. With this in mind, the strategies for sampling and data analysis used by pragmatics researchers are outlined in the following section. This is followed by a demonstration of an analysis in the pragmatic tradition.

25.3 Getting Started

25.3.1 Approaching the Analytic Task

A major challenge for observational research is: *How* does the researcher establish that the observations made reliably represent significant population of phenomena? On this claim, the confidence in the emerging description will be based. How does the researcher identify relevant elements of interest in order to subject them to intensive scrutiny? There are two aspects of talk in interaction to take into account: local (turn taking) and distributional (where does the sample fit into the overall structure of the talk).

The first task in describing naturally occurring talk is to identify *local* patterns of activity—for example, turn-taking sequences, or lexical sequences of interest—across a dataset. All examples are retrieved and compared across the dataset. The *distribution* of the examples is then examined in the overall context of the talk, as a model of the dialogic process is gradually assembled and tested through the investigator's iterative analytic attention. In the case of deductive, theory testing research, statistical analysis assures the validity of generalization through the application of standardized tests, in which the balance of probability is assured to be confirmed or disconfirmed by the relative frequency of cases: the identified phenomenon was present in 99 % or 95 % of cases, so a safe inference can be made from the sample to the whole population. In the case of observational methodology, with its description-building strategy, "saturation of the data" is essential: all cases must be accounted for (Silverman 2006). What happens when something is observed which doesn't fit the pattern? Central to observational method is the treatment of a "deviant case". A deviant case, once found, must be re-analysed and incorporated into the emerging description in order for that description to be credible. Building an adequate description is a circular process; the guiding theoretical backdrop (in this case, the primacy of turn-by-turn interaction in the construction of meaning) sensitizes the investigator to singular instances for analysis, generating further observations which in turn may develop, alter or enrich the theoretical model (see Salvatore et al. (2010) for a full discussion of abduction).

25.3.2 Analysing the Data

The first principle of observational research is the collection of relevant observations by means of which to build adequate descriptive power. Researchers in pragmatics have evolved a number of strategies for the collection of data.

25.3.2.1 Collect a Wide Sample of Data from Different Contexts

Pragmatics researchers have collected samples of talk in every kind of social setting. Schiffrin (1987) collected hundreds of recordings of everyday conversations between friends, family members and colleagues. Sacks recorded and analysed in great detail hundreds of examples of talk from many different settings, including some group psychotherapy sessions with adolescent boys (it was easier in those days). The availability of adequate observational technology is crucial to observational science. The invention and refinement of the microscope enabled the development of cell biology. The explosion of research into naturally occurring language, starting in the 1950s and 1960s, was enabled through the availability of good-quality portable tape recorders. Different forms of data are made available through different observational technologies. Some new observational instruments available to psychotherapy researchers will be discussed in the final section of this chapter.

25.3.2.2 Find All Examples of an Object of Interest Across a Dataset

This is the usual method of sampling employed by pragmatics researchers across all the subdisciplines. The analysis proceeds through comparative analysis of all instances with a view to building a working explanatory model of the observed phenomena. An early example was Sacks' study of the opening sequences of telephone conversations. Schegloff (1972b) later elaborated on this research, assembling 500 examples of opening sequences of conversations. He found one deviant case which contradicted his emerging rules of use, and returned to his dataset to reconstruct his model of the underlying rules by which speakers negotiate the opening of a conversation. Often, however, it is found that close examination of the deviant case is a variant which confirms the emerging description.

In a study of everyday social encounters, Schiffrin (1987) observed the use of "discourse markers"—words which function as markers of speakers' intentions in the course of a conversation. Working from her large dataset of recorded examples of everyday talk, she was able to demonstrate *how* speakers project their intentions and manage the inferences to be made from their utterance, using stock phrases such as "well", "you know" and "I mean"—phrases whose meaning lies entirely in their strategic use as markers of speaker intentions. Verhagen (2005), focussing on syntactic resources in order to explore the process of intersubjectivity, draws on examples from a wide variety of published data, from live conversations, and occasionally illustrates a point with a constructed example for the purpose of comparing possible versions.

25.3.2.3 Compare the Samples Which Are Identified with Existing Findings

Much studied sequences, for example, discourse markers or syntactic structures, whose underpinning rules of use are already well understood, can then be further explored to examine how they are used as strategies in interaction. An example is question and answer sequences, subject of many of Sacks' (1992) early observations. Heritage (2002) built on these observations with a detailed study of negative interrogatives, showing how speakers use these devices to communicate hostile intentions. Questions and answers are powerful pragmatic devices by means of which speakers pursue interactional aims. The question constrains what can happen in the next turn: an answer is preferred, and failure to answer is "accountable". Hearers will usually adopt some kind of strategy to avoid answering a question if they don't want to, while still taking a turn (otherwise there will be a rupture). A common device is "I don't know", which may be about the state of knowledge of the recipient, but more typically is a means of taking a turn without complying with the request for an answer. Questions are deployed in highly structured settings such as police interviews, legal proceedings and in clinical discourse. Professionals typically have rights to ask questions not acceptable in everyday settings and to expect answers. Their clients, in contrast, have limited rights to ask questions.

25.3.3 Comparative Study or Single Case Study?

All of these methods of sampling rely on the comparative study of phenomena across a dataset to describe the basic mechanisms by which language is used as a resource to do interactional work. A study can be designed seeking to explore one phenomenon in many different sites—across cases, for example. In a study of the client's attitudinal stance, Muntigl et al. (2012a, b) identified several linguistic markers of attitudinal stance and, using a CA approach, compared examples across a dataset of diverse therapeutic models. Another strategy might be to study a single case, examining the way in which a pragmatic phenomenon of interest, already well understood, evolves in the interaction between a single dyad over time (for a discussion and example of single case design, see Chap. 19). The following example of a pragmatic analysis comes from a single case study design.

25.4 A Pragmatic Analysis of an Episode of Interaction

The analysis which follows emerged from a single case study which I undertook with Sumi Kato (2008). The objective of that study was to explore the phenomenon of "mitigation" and "face" (Levinson 1983) in psychotherapy discourse. In the course of the analysis, we noticed an unusual use of the phrase "I mean". This discovery provided the platform for a second, more fine-grained analysis of the text. Through this iterative process of deepening analysis, we sought to develop a richer understanding of the interactional processes in the therapy.

25.4.1 Phase 1: Identification of a Phenomenon of Interest

In the first phase of the case study, Sumi Kato (2008) analysed the full text of eight sessions of a brief psychodynamic psychotherapy, one of a comparative study of CBT and psychodynamic psychotherapy for depression (the Sheffield II depression study) using the subcategories of Systemic Functional Linguistics (Eggins 2004). All subcategories for psychological language were counted as a first step in mapping the linguistic features of the talk across all eight sessions. Sumi Kato noticed that the use of the phrase "I mean" was used in an exceptional way by the client. Unable to decide what significance this might have, we excluded this phrase from the Systemic Functional Linguistics description of the discourse and set it aside for further analysis. It was in this way that "one type of behaviour in one situation" was identified for the present analysis.

25.4.2 Phase 2: Comparison of Samples

Having identified the phrase "I mean" as an object of interest, I used this discovery as the basis for a second study, set within the framework of the single case, about which we already knew a lot from our first analysis of the text. First, I turned to the pragmatics literature to identify existing findings. "I mean" is a marker, in English, not so much of meaning, but of the speaker's intentions. It is a marker of intersubjective "work" (Schegloff 1992)—a signal to the hearer about how to hear what is to follow. In everyday use, it has been shown to have the following functions (Schiffrin 1987):

1. Marks a "self repair": it tells the hearer that a reformulation of a previous statement follows
2. Marks the speakers' intentions about how the previous talk should be interpreted
3. Marks a distance between what was said and what is upcoming

Turning to the text of the psychotherapy, I first recovered all examples of the phrase "I mean" and compared them to the everyday usages Schiffrin discovered.

Here are two examples of the typical uses of "I mean" identified by Schiffrin in the dialogue between this therapist and client:

Session 2

C is it all psychosomatic or, (laughs) I thought, your first thought would be, / (inaudible) (laughs) that would be your first reaction. you know, psychosomatic,

T yeah

C I mean I'm not saying it isn't, I don't know,

In this exchange, the client offers an opening for an "interpretation" of her symptoms (she is offering to participate in the task at hand in the setting of a therapy session). She is also ascribing thoughts and intentions to the therapist (she wonders what his first thought would be). The therapist (not sure what her intentions are?) responds non-committally, leaving the conversation hanging. The client offers a "self-repair", using the phrase, "I mean", mitigating (softening) the impact of her assertion, and also adds the phrase "I don't know". In order to sustain the turn-by-turn sequence, she mitigates the force of her utterance (Caffi 1999).

Here is a different kind of repair:

Session 3

T (pause 11 s) you know, it feels, maybe that, maybe it's not safe, to get upset with me. (pause 6 s) .

C no I wouldn't, s- I mean I don't distrust you mistrust you or anything like that. I don't feel that. (pause 7 s) I suppose what it is again is, admitting, to myself and to other; to somebody else.

The therapist has responded to previous talk by the client with an inference about the client's mental state: "maybe it feels that". She is the privileged "knower"/"feeler", as a subject. In clinical practice, just as in everyday conversation, the dialogical partner can make inferences about what the other "knows", "feels" or "intends". Notice the long pause before he delivers his turn. He also "mitigates" the impact of what he says by using the phrase "maybe", giving the client the opportunity to "know" something he doesn't know. Again, she uses the phrase "I mean"—she is recasting her previous talk, offering a "repair" to what he may have inferred from what she said—that she doesn't trust him. Schegloff (1992) proposes that this kind of "third position repair" as a foundational sequence in intersubjective coordination.

Both of these examples demonstrate how the phrase "I mean" is being used to regulate intersubjective inferences and interpretations from one turn to the next.

A third example demonstrates an atypical variant of the client's use of "I mean":

Session 2

T you don't want people to know, but you also, but you do want, you do want to be looked after.

C oh yes. yes. yes, *I mean* the friend who rang today, *I mean* she was, erm, really smashing, *I mean* she she she knew, *I mean*, well you know friends, if they're friends they understand don't they, it's not that that concerns me, it's er, you know the reaction of, of (work) you know, er "something wrong with her mind"" sort of thing, you know, T mm hm

C sort of, er, I didn't, I didn't sort of think...

In this example, the client inserts "I mean" as a preface to a string of sentence-phrases of her narrative about "the friend" who "knew", who "understood". With each "I mean", she alters the meaning slightly, moving away from the therapist's interpretation (inference) that she both doesn't want people to know (about her illness) but at the same time wants to be "looked after". As in example 2, she rejects his interpretation (inference about her subjective state). However, whereas in example 2, she offers an interpretation of her own, in example 3, while on the surface accepting his suggestion ("Oh yes, yes, yes"), she then changes the emphasis, stepwise, through the use of the interjected "I mean" away from the proposed inference about her wanting to be "looked after". Here "I mean" marks a distance between what came before and what is to come. Her turn ends with an evaluation: "not wanting people to know". The therapist declines to take a turn, leaving the client to find a way keep the talk alive.

In the first phase of this study, Sumi Kato provided a "mapping" of the psychological language in use in a single case, using the method of Systemic Functional Linguistics. In the course of that mapping, a "deviant case" emerged: an apparently idiosyncratic use of the phrase "I mean"—a verbal marker about which some things are already known from the work of Schiffrin (1987). The next step in deepening the observation of this phenomenon was to examine it in some detail to see what interactional work it is doing in the turn-by-turn interaction.

25.4.3 Phase 3: Analysis of an Episode

Having identified through a comparative analysis some of the features of the use of "I mean" as it occurs in the overall text, the next phase of the analysis turned to the first substantive therapeutic "moves" in this therapy, an episode which occurred at the beginning of the second session. Methodologically, the challenge was to identify a "discourse unit" which has relevance to the object of inquiry, the pragmatic use of "I mean". Issues of clinical significance also needed to be considered. The episode was chosen as a discourse unit because it is a co-produced narrative evaluation sequence (Labov and Waletzky 1967) which follows a story told by the client about an event which occurred in the week since the first session. Clinically, it was significant, as the theme of her illness is introduced, and this theme had, in a previous analysis of this case, been identified as a major topic in the therapy (Lepper and Mergenthaler 2007). The client recounts that during the week since the first session, she fainted at work, then went to her doctor and was referred for medical investigations. The excerpt begins with her candidate evaluation—what did she mean to convey by the narrative. The two speakers then go on to co-produce an extended interpretation of the meaning of the events, with many overlaps and repairs, ending in a failure to agree on the interpretation of the narrative. The episode ends with a breakdown in the talk—a rupture (Muran et al. 2009).

Table 25.1 Text sample

1	C	so, really (4) since I've seen you last time, it's been rather a/
2	T	/rather a grim/
3	C	/a traumatic I mean I haven't been back to / (work place) yet you see. I mean I was all set to go, everything was ready on / (day of week) night. there was no thought that I, you know, I wonder whether it is psychosomatic, you know, because I'd been worrying about,
4	T	/yes
5	C	/what I told you.
6	T	that's right, you were, building up, worry about + doing that
7	C	whether that .. it was reaction, it wasn't sort of, I didn't, I'd been into (work place) I saw you on the (day) I went into (work place) on (day) and again on (day) and, put some more displays up and sort of got everything ready. so my room was all ready to walk into, because I knew I wouldn't be able to go in on the (place)
8	T	mm, mm
9	C	with having relations, you know, for the (celebration) . so I knew I was going, that I had to do it on the (day) and (day) . and I chatted with the (boss) and, I felt perfectly at ease when I was in there.
10	T	mm
11	C	but you know, I think well,
12	T	Well
13	C	is it all psychosomatic or, (laughs) I thought, your first thought would be, (inaudible) (laughs) that would be your first reaction, you know, psychosomatic,
14	T	Yeah
15	C	I mean I'm not saying it isn't, I don't know,
16	T	Right
17	C	but, you see I mean, I, I.
18	T	but it happily built up, over the, over the party,
19	C	yes, I mean well,
20	T	and so can you tell me how it really, how the, how your fainting related in time to when you were due to come here, were you due to come here the next day, or
21	C	No
22	T	No

Note Full CA transcription conventions are not used here. The use of the "/" indicates an overlapping turn. Standard transcription conventions can be found in Ten Have (1999, Appendix A)

The episode set out in Table 25.1 begins with an evaluation of the point of the story, which is signalled by the markers "so" and "really" (C1) "So...instructs the hearer to recover a conclusion (an inference, a claim) which has already been presented" (Schiffrin 1987, p. 223). It is also a signal to the hearer that a turn can be taken. "Really" emphasizes the significance of the telling. In response to these markers, the therapist takes a turn, overlapping and providing an evaluative response (T2): "a grim time", to which in yet another overlap, the client upgrades the evaluation from "grim "to "traumatic" (C3). Together, the speakers agree that she has had a bad experience. However, the evaluation is not quite complete because the client returns to her telling, to provide yet another evaluative element. It comes in the form of an indirect question.

> P a traumatic. *I mean* I haven't been back to / (work place) yet you see. *I mean* I was all set to go, everything was ready on / (day) night. there was no thought that I, you know, I wonder whether it is psychosomatic, you know, because I'd been worrying about

The "I mean" which prefaces the next sentence proposes a reformulation of the previous utterance. Another "I mean" follows immediately, followed by a "you know". The phrase "you know" serves to mark "meta-knowledge about shared (either speaker/hearer or general) knowledge... and ...marks information whose importance is its relation to other information in the discourse and to the overall point of the entire story" (Schiffrin 1987, p. 284).

The client seems to be introducing two possible topics—and "troubles": her "worrying" generated by the previous session and the nature of the event (was it psychosomatic?). She invites her hearer to focus on the point of the story, but then offers two candidate versions: "worry" and "psychosomatic". Two uses of "I mean" and two of "you know" lend a turbulent quality to the production of this utterance; and two potential themes, or topics, are put forward. "Worrying" is clearly a communication about her (internal) mental state; "psychosomatic", on the other hand, suggests her inference that this would be the presupposition of the therapist. The "you know" creates "common ground" between them. The common ground of "psychosomatic" carries a heavy load: to categorize an illness as "psychosomatic" carries implications of "not real" and has moral implications as an interpretation of the reported events which has implications for the subsequent course of the talk:

> "Pragmatic presuppositions not only concern knowledge, whether true or false: they concern expectations, desires, interests, claims, attitudes towards the world, fears, etc." (Caffi 1994, p. 324)

The therapist's overlapping "yes" suggests his attentive response to the client's "you know" as she completes her evaluation (C5). He then (T6) responds to the evaluation now completed, taking up the theme of "worry": "that's right, you were, building up, worry about doing that". "That's right" confirms his attention, and by adding an elaboration—"you were building up worry" links the hearing response closely to end of previous utterance and to the previous narrative. In his turn the therapist opts to go with the "internal state" element of the evaluation, while the other category offered as common ground—"psychosomatic"- is not responded to. The work of co-evaluation now breaks down as the client continues her narrative with additional details which add little of substance to the evaluation already begun (C7). The therapist responds with a neutral continuer (T8), leaving the client with the task of keeping the conversation going, which seems to aim in the direction of a disagreement (C9): she "felt perfectly at ease"—implying not "worried" (an indirect negation of the previous turn). The therapist responds with a non-committal token—"mm"—declining to take the next turn (T10).

So while the interaction proceeds in the conventional way (first speaker produces an utterance containing the marker "you know" which leads the hearer to focus on something), there is an element of ambiguity: is it to be "worry" which is the point of the story, or is it to be the categorization of her symptoms as "psychosomatic"? What is to be the common ground of their talk? The client prefaces her next communicative move with three pragmatic markers and creates a communicative imperative (no escape!).

P but you know, I think well,/

"But" marks the upcoming utterance as proposing a contrast and a return to the point the speaker wanted to make. It is used "when the content of what is said contrasts with speakers perception about how their talk will be taken as a portrayal of self—and when those perceptions clash with their sense of what would constitute a suitable self for presentation to hearers" (Schiffrin 1987, p. 158).

The next phrase in the utterance—"you know"—marks the presumption of shared knowledge, or common ground, which is embedded in the telling of the narrative and its evaluation—that it is a "psychological" narrative ("worried"; "psychosomatic").

With the production of "I think", an upcoming mental state predicate should be expected but before that clause is produced, there is a further pragmatic marker—"well". "Well" signals moves that are in some way "dispreferred" (Pomerantz 1984) signalling more interactional trouble to come. Note that the "well" is echoed in the overlapping utterance of the therapist, who perhaps has heard the threat of an upcoming disagreement, and with "well" the two briefly postpone the next move. What is marked here is clearly an argument—a disagreement about how the evaluation sequence will proceed.

The client continues her utterance (C13), which comes in the form of a direct question—"Is it all psychosomatic", followed by the completion of the "I think" predicate of the previous utterance—"I thought, your first thought would be, / (inaudible) (laughs) that would be your first reaction, you know, psychosomatic."

The production of a direct question, referring back to the indirect "wondering" of the first turn of her evaluation, is followed by a laugh. Perhaps it is a response to a short pause, but more probably it mitigates the direct and confrontational nature of the question, which pursues her communicative objectives in the face of the T's retreat from the topic. The question is followed by the explicit inference about what is in the other's mind—the anticipated "that" of the mental predicate "I thought your first thought would be". Given the long delay in delivering this inference-rich utterance, it becomes clearer what is at stake: a contest of inferences and meanings which constitute an acceptable self in the eyes of the other (the therapist's "first thought").

The therapist's response, a non-committal "yeah" (T14), satisfies the turn-taking imperative, but fails to meet the requirement posed by a question: an answer. In doing so he creates an interactional impasse—a rupture in need of repair. The repair is provided by the client in the next turn (C15):

P I mean I'm not saying it isn't, I don't know, I, I...

In its form of a double negative, this utterance is entirely a pragmatic move, aimed repairing the breakdown in the talk. In its double negative form, the communicative intention of the previous utterance is not negated, but "hedged" (Caffi and Janney 1994). It doesn't mean that she is retracting the inference. Nor does the use of "I don't know" here refers to the speaker's knowledge state; rather it serves the pragmatic function of "indicating speaker uncertainty and mitigating polite disagreement in conversation" (Bybee and Scheibman 1999, p. 585), in the service of repairing the rupture.

In his next turn (T16) the therapist postpones a substantive response to either the question or the repair, suggesting doubt about which way to go. "Right" can be heard as (1) intersubjective agreement, (2) an intention to take up an offer of a turn, (3) a partial repair or (4) an attempt to postpone uptake of next turn. That this is a purely pragmatic turn, and doesn't propose agreement, can be seen in the P's response: (C18) "but, you see I mean, I....". She hears it as a postponement and continues the repair sequence, offering another contrastive "but" as a candidate for re-establishing the sequential order. Her repair offer is finally taken up on the next turn, with the therapist echoing the contrastive "but" as he returns to the narrative, rephrasing an evaluation of the event:

T but it happily built up, over the, over the party,

He collaborates in the repair, offering a candidate evaluation to link to previous narrative and provide an explication with the oddly chosen adverb "happily"—referring to an element of "surprise" in the account: everything seemed to be going so well and then all of sudden this happened. What did it mean? However, notice that he prefaces his turn with "but": a hearable expectation of ongoing disagreement.

P yes, I mean well,

With a growing string of "I means", P continues the still incomplete repair sequence. Also, we see another "well". In the context of this repair, "well" shows the speaker's "aliveness to the need to accomplish coherence despite a temporary inability to contribute to [it]" (Schiffrin 1987, p. 126). It becomes clearer that the pragmatic devices in use are serving the function of conducting an "argument" about how to go forward, at the same time as maintaining a commitment to the ongoing interaction. The potential disagreement can be seen operating at multiple levels: (1) at the level of "common ground"—the social context of the interpretation of an "illness" as "psychological"; (2) at the level of inference—of the other's intentions, expectations and judgments and their implications for the stability of the talk.; and (3) at the level of the self, my experiences, intentions and wishes. This exchange demonstrates the local means through which the speakers strive to sustain communicative collaboration while pursuing their own communicative objectives.

> "Any utterance is multiply determined by what I have seen or experienced, my communicative purpose in telling you about it, and the distinctions that are embodied in my grammar". (Slobin, p. 75)

The therapist returns to his agenda (the events leading up to the session) which he raises in the next turn, in the form of a question (T20). The response is a bald "no", and there is nowhere to go. The therapist echoes the "no" in turn T22. This episode—an evaluation of the presented narrative—ends in open disagreement.

From a pragmatic perspective, the telling of the story is a different matter than the contents of the story. How it was told, and how the participants evaluated that telling, provides another dynamic perspective on the therapeutic interaction. All therapists, of whatever theoretical persuasion, face the same dilemma: to attend to the content of the client's story, being led by it and then trying to transform it through the therapeutic process. Much therapeutic attention is directed at the content of the client's talk. Could it be that it is not only the content but also the process of the telling which needs attention?

25.4.4 Discussion

> "Engaging in cognitive coordination comes down to, for the speaker ... an attempt to *influence* someone else's thoughts, attitudes or even immediate behaviour. For the addressee it involves finding out what kind of influence it is that the speaker ... is trying to exert, and deciding to go along with it or not". (Verhagen 2005, p. 10)

Every speaker, in every communication with another person, must construct and sustain a series of inferences about the other's communicative intentions in order to keep the talk going. Sometimes this is straightforward, and at other times, in every kind of setting, there are ambiguities. Speakers use pragmatic devices to manage how inferences are going to be made and interpretations of their meaning taken.

On the evidence of this episode, a contest of inferences seems to be underway. What "I mean" and what "you think" provide the framework for this contest. Resources brought into play actively by the client are both pragmatic and lexical—she uses talk to do some kind of interactional work. "I mean", though apparently mitigating the force of her questions, also operates to conceal her intentions. She wonders what "you think". She is on the one hand a cooperative player in the task of interpretation; on the other, on the evidence of the therapist's avoidance of the topic, she is making interactional "trouble" for him by putting the question "is it all psychosomatic?" on the table. There is an argument concealed under the apparent compliance which the frequent use of "I mean", as a mitigator, might suggest.

The pragmatic means used by these speakers to conduct this "argument" are the learned rules of conversational interaction. This translates into an interactional problem: how do therapist and client negotiate agreement and disagreement about the way forward in the ongoing context of the session? Muran et al. (2009) have demonstrated that early ruptures to the alliance, and their repair, are significantly linked to outcomes. Rupture and repair events constitute a relationship process which has been demonstrated to be significant in the therapeutic process (for a full discussion, see Colli and Lingiardi (2009); Chap. 16). This analysis of an episode which results in a rupture demonstrates a practical means by which ruptures, and their repair, can be studied in detail using the findings and techniques of pragmatics.

25.5 Widening the Observational Field

This chapter set out to demonstrate that we have some powerful methods available to us in the search for a deeper understanding of the psychotherapy process at the level of the interaction between therapist and client. It has focussed on one component of human communicative interaction—the pragmatic study of the talk. A truly multidisciplinary model of psychotherapy process research should ultimately include both linguistic and extralinguistic phenomena. This final section of this chapter looks at how pragmatics might be integrated with observational methods in the psychotherapy process research which we are already familiar with in order to bring the dimension of the local sequential order of the therapeutic interaction into relationship with a wider picture of the process.

25.5.1 A Question of Method

> "[Early turn-taking is] an emergent phenomenon that itself serves as the scaffolding or dynamic context for more advanced patterns of behavior. It may be thought of as the cradle of meaning. Turn-taking is initiated by burst-pause-burst in sucking, but it depends for its emergence on the mother's folk-psychological stance". (Hendriks-Jansen 1996, p. 277)

The theoretical position supporting the project of an observational approach to human communicative interaction is posed in this claim by Hendriks-Jansen, placing turn taking, with its origins in activity patterns at the prelinguistic level, at the heart of human communicative interaction. It was noted that it was the development of the hand-held, portable tape recorder that made possible the development of Conversation Analysis, with its focus on everyday talk. The following sections propose ways in which some recent observational instruments developed for use in psychotherapy research could be used to widen the scope of research into the turn-taking processes in therapeutic interaction. These particular approaches have been chosen because they represent a variety of observational strategies. They offer the investigator into therapeutic interaction a means of locating significant interactional events in the therapeutic process at different levels, both linguistic and paralinguistic.

25.5.2 Facial Expression of Emotion

An important domain of psychotherapy research in recent years has looked at the function of facial expression of emotion in the regulation of affect in interpersonal communication. Developmental psychology has demonstrated the foundational importance of facial expression in the developing infant's discovery of the world through the actions of his or her caregiver (e.g. the "still face" experiments, Tronick 2007). Much work was undertaken by Krause, using the Facial Actions Coding System (FACS) method of analysis to explore interpersonal regulation of affect in the therapeutic dyad (a good example is a study of an unsuccessful behavioural therapy by Dreher et al. 2001). FACS has also extensively used by Banninger-Huber and colleagues to observe the coordination of facial expression in the psychotherapy process (see Benecke et al. 2005). Facial expression is an important component of turn-by-turn interaction. The FACS method is an observational tool ideally suited to the intensive study of emotion behaviours in the therapeutic interaction. Communication of emotion at the level of verbal interaction has been intensively studied by Caffi and Janney (1994). A research question could be asked is: How does the behavioural level of emotion regulation relate to the sequential order of the spoken interaction? For an example of this approach, see Muntigl et al. (2012a, b).

25.5.3 Motion Energy Analysis

A specifically developed technology for the observation of dyadic interaction, the Motion Energy Analysis (MES) (Ramseyer and Tschacher 2011) produces a quantification of the gestural activity patterns of speakers, generating a mapping of the co-ordination of their gestures in the interaction. Clinical significance is predicated on findings from neuroscience and other disciplines, pointing to the foundational properties of synchronous behaviours. The authors point out that these observations do not constitute an exclusive role in empathy and the formation of the "therapeutic bond" and that "it is still a hypothesis that the mechanism of "imitation breeds liking" that has been found in social psychology may be at work in psychotherapy" (p. 344). This methodological caution locates this work firmly in the observational model. A next question might be to ask: What is happening at moments of synchrony at the level of the turn-by-turn interaction? Are synchronous behaviours observable examples of interactional activity patterns? The findings of developmental psychology would suggest a close connection between the two.

25.5.4 Therapeutic Cycles Model

Another potential observational tool already available is the Therapeutic Cycles Model. Using a statistical content analysis technique, the TCM produces a graph of the verbal patterns in therapeutic interaction, which have also been demonstrated to occur more generally. It maps clinical patterns in the therapeutic discourse, over time (single sessions, groups of sessions, whole cases). In a series of single case studies (Lepper and Mergenthaler 2005, 2007, 2008), we have explored features of the therapeutic interaction identified by the TCM (e.g. "connecting moments") at the level of the turn-by-turn interaction, seeking to ask the question: What patterns of activity are happening at the level of the interaction when clinical significant events, identified by the TCM, occur?

25.5.5 Discourse Flow Analysis

A more recent, observational method is Discourse Flow Analysis (DFA), another computer-assisted analytic strategy which produces a model of the content of the discourse (Salvatore et al. 2010) and seeks to map sense-making strategies. It is a quantitative method, which generates a map of a session or sessions, producing, like the TCM, a time series representation of discursive properties of the interaction. In a study using DFA, Nitti et al. (2010) note the highly abstract nature of these methods and its limited sensitivity to contextual features of language. Researchers could use DFA to map large amounts of data, with its potential for identifying significant features of the discourse, which could then be studied in detail in the immediate context of the clinical interaction, using pragmatic methods of analysis.

Conclusion

We do already have substantial evidence that psychotherapy is beneficial, and some clear indications of what elements in the process are significant (Lambert 2004). Less clear is what happens at the level of the therapeutic interaction. This chapter has proposed that the possibility of a rigorous observational study of psychotherapeutic interaction, with the potential to produce the kinds of advances made in developmental psychology and linguistics, using similar methods, is available to us at the current stage of development of psychotherapy research. It has the potential benefit of bringing the disciplines of research to inform the clinical practice of psychotherapy at a relevant level of detail. What happens in the here and now of the session, as we talk with our clients? What can be learned by close observation of patterns of communicative action? What implications do these observations have for clinical theory? Detailed analysis of the interactional processes at the heart of the therapeutic relationship has direct relevance for day-to-day clinical practice and training and for robust theory building.

Acknowledgements I would like to acknowledge my indebtedness to my colleagues Dr. Jean Knox and Dr. Sumi Kato both of whom have made important contributions both to the analysis and to my thinking in this chapter.

References

Angus LE, McLeod J (2004) A handbook of narrative and psychotherapy: practice, theory and research. Sage, London

Austin J (1975) How to do things with words. Oxford University Press, Oxford

Bartsch K, Wellman HJ (1995) Children talk about the mind. Oxford University Press, Oxford

Benecke C, Peham D, Banninger- Huber E (2005) Nonverbal relationship regulation in psychotherapy. Psychother Res 15(1):81–90. doi:10.1080/10503300512331327065

Bruner J (1990) Acts of meaning. Harvard University Press, Cambridge, MA

Bybee J, Scheibman J (1999) The effect of usage on degrees of constituency. Linguistics 37(4):575–596

Caffi C (1994) Pragmatic presupposition. In: Asher RE, Simpson JMY (eds) Encyclopaedia of language and linguistics, vol 6. Pergamon, Oxford, pp 3320–3327

Caffi C (1999) On mitigation. J Pragmat 31(7):881–909

Caffi C, Janney RW (1994) Toward a pragmatics of emotive communication. J Pragmat 22:325–373

Colli A, Lingiardi V (2009) The collaborative interactions scale: a new transcript-based method for the assessment of therapeutic alliance ruptures and resolutions in psychotherapy. Psychother Res 19(6):718–734. doi:10.1080/10503300903121098

Diessel H, Tomasello M (2001) The acquisition of finite complement clauses in English: a corpus based analysis. Linguistics 12:97–141

Dreher M, Mengele U, Krause R, Kammerer A (2001) Affective indicators of the therapeutic process. Psychother Res 11(1):99–117. doi:10.1080/713663855

Eggins S (2004) An introduction to systemic functional linguistics. Continuum International Publishing Group, London

Enfield NJ, Levinson SC (2006) Roots of human sociality: culture, cognition and interaction. Berg, Oxford

Habermas J (1987) The theory of communicative action, vol 2. Polity Press, Cambridge

Hendriks-Jansen H (1996) Catching ourselves in the act. MIT Press, Cambridge, MA

Heritage J (2002) The limits of questioning: negative interrogatives and hostile question content. J Pragmat 34:1427–1446. doi:10.1016/S0378-2166(02)00072-3

Horvath A (2005) The therapeutic relationship: research and theory. Psychother Res 15(1–2):3–7. doi:10.1080/10503300512331339143

Horvath A (2006) The alliance in context: accomplishments, challenges, future directions. Psychother Res 43(3):258–263. doi:10.1037/0033-3204.43.3.258

Kato S (2008) Anxiety arousal and it mitigation in psychotherapy interaction from the perspective of territory of information. Presentation to the International Conference of the Society of Psychotherapy Research, Barcelona

Kaye K (1982) Organism, apprentice and person. In: Tronick E (ed) Social interchange in infancy. University Park Press, Baltimore, pp 183–196

Knox J (2010) Self-agency in psychotherapy: attachment, autonomy and intimacy. W.W. Norton, London

Labov W (1997) Some further steps in narrative analysis. J Narrat Life Hist 7:395–415

Labov W, Waletzky J (1967) Narrative structures. In: Helm J (ed) Essays in the verbal and visual arts. University of Washington Press, Seattle, pp 12–44

Lambert M (ed) (2004) Bergin and Garfield's handbook of psychotherapy and behavior change. Wiley, New York

Lepper G (2000) Categories in text and talk. Sage, London

Lepper G, Mergenthaler E (2005) Exploring group process. Psychother Res 15(4):433–444. doi:10.1080/10503300500091587

Lepper G, Mergenthaler E (2007) Therapeutic collaboration: How does it work? Psychother Res 17 (5):576–588. doi:10.1080/10503300601140002

Lepper G, Mergenthaler E (2008) Observing therapeutic interaction in the "Lisa" case". Psychother Res 18 (6):634–645. doi:10.1080/10503300701442001

Levinson S (1983) Pragmatics. Cambridge University Press, Cambridge

Levinson S (2006) The human "interaction engine". In: Enfield NJ, Levinson S (eds) Roots of human sociality. Berg, Oxford, pp 39–69

Meltzoff A (2005) Imitation and "other minds": the "like me" hypothesis. In: Hurley S, Chater N (eds) Perspectives on imitation: from neuroscience to social science, vol 2. MIT Press, Cambridge, MA, pp 55–77

Mey J (1999) Pragmatics: an introduction. Blackwell Publishers, Oxford

Muntigl P, Knight N, Horvath A, Watkins A (2012a) Client attitudinal stance and therapist-client affiliation: a view from grammar and social interaction. Res Psychother Psychopathol Process Outcome 15 (2):117–130. doi:10.7411/RP.2012.012

Muntigl P, Knight N, Watkins A (2012b) Working to keep aligned in psychotherapy: using nods as a dialogic resource to display affiliation. Language and Dialogue, Dialogue and Representation, pp 9–27 (19). doi:10.1075/ld.2.1.01mun

Muran JC, Safran JD, Gorman BS, Samstag LW, Eubanks-Carter C, Winston A (2009) The relationship of early alliance ruptures and their resolution to process and outcome in 3 time limited psychotherapies for personality disorder. Psychother Res Theory Pract Train 46(2):233–248. doi:10.1037/a0016085

Nitti M, Ciavolino E, Salvatore S, Gennard A (2010) Analyzing psychotherapy process as intersubjective sensemaking: an approach based on discourse analysis and neural networks. Psychother Res 20(5):546–564. doi:10.1080/10503301003641886

Peyers J (2006) Constructing the social mind: language and false-belief understanding. In: Enfield N, Levinson S (eds) Roots of human sociality: culture, cognition and interaction. Berg, Oxford

Pomerantz A (1984) Agreeing and disagreeing with assessments: some features of preferred/dispreferred turn shapes. In: Atkinson J, Heritage J (eds) Structures of social action: studies in conversation analysis. Cambridge University Press, Cambridge, pp 57–101

Ramseyer F, Tschacher W (2011) Nonverbal synchrony in psychotherapy: coordinated body movement reflects relationship quality and outcome. J Consult Clin Psychol 79(3):284–295. doi:10.1037/a0023419

Ruffman T, Slade L, Crowe E (2002) The relation between children's and mother's mental state language and theory-of-mind understanding. Child Dev 73(3):734–751. doi:10.1111/1467-8624.00435

Sacks H (1992) Lectures in conversation, vol 1, 2. Blackwell, Oxford

Sacks H, Schegloff E, Jefferson G (1974) A simplest systematic for the organization of turn-taking for conversation. Language 50:696–735

Salvatore S, Gelo OCG, Gennaro A, Manzo S, Al Radaideh A (2010) Looking at the psychotherapy process as an intersubjective dynamic of meaning making: a study with discourse flow analysis. J Constr Psychol 23(3):195–230. doi:10.1080/10720531003765981

Saussure F (1974) Course in general linguistics. Fontana, London

Schegloff EA (1972a) Notes on a conversational practice: formulating place. In: Sudnow D (ed) Studies in social interaction. Free Press, New York, pp 75–119

Schegloff EA (1972b) Sequencing in conversational openings. In: Gumperz J, Hymes D (eds) Directions in sociolinguistics. Holt Rineheart and Winston, New York, pp 346–380

Schegloff E (1992) Repair after next turn: the last structurally provided defense of intersubjectivity in conversation. Am J Sociol 98:1295–1345

Schiffrin D (1987) Discourse markers. Cambridge University Press, Cambridge

Searle J (1969) Speech acts: an essay in the philosophy of language. Cambridge University Press, Cambridge

Silverman D (2006) Interpreting qualitative data: methods for analyzing talk, text and interaction, 3rd edn. Sage, London

Slobin DI (1996) From "thought and language" to "thinking for speaking". In: Gumperz J, Levinson S (eds) Rethinking linguistic relativity. Cambridge University Press, Cambridge, pp 70–96

Stiles WB, Agnew-Davis R, Hardy GE, Barkham M, Shapiro D (1998) Relations of the alliance with psychotherapy outcomes: findings in the second Sheffield psychotherapy project. J Consult Clin Psychol 66 (5):791–802

Ten Have P (1999) Doing conversation analysis: a practical guide. Sage, London

Trevarthen C (1977) Descriptive analyses of infant communicative behaviour. In: Schaffer H (ed) Studies in mother-infant interaction: proceedings of Loch lLomond symposium. Academic, New York, pp 227–270

Tronick E (2007) The neurobiological and social-emotional development of children. Norton, New York

Verhagen A (2005) Constructions of intersubjectivity: discourse, syntax and cognition. Oxford University Press, Oxford

Wampold BE (2001) The great psychotherapy debate: models, methods, findings. Lawrence Erlbaum, Hillsdale, NJ

Wittgenstein L (1968) Philosophical investigations. Basil Blackwell, Oxford

Part III

Psychotherapy Outcome Research

Quantitative Psychotherapy Outcome Research: Methodological Issues

26

Christian Gold

Contents

Abstract

This chapter reviews methodological issues in quantitative psychotherapy outcome research. In the era of evidence-based medicine, it is vital for researchers to understand the methodological details that ensure the validity of outcome studies. By re-examining some "classical" examples of psychotherapy outcome studies, this chapter explains the relative strengths and merits of different research designs. It discusses why control groups are needed; why large sample sizes are crucial but cannot replace other design aspects; why designs can be ranked according to their internal validity; and how internal validity can be ensured without neglecting external validity. Both efficacy and effectiveness studies can use randomised controlled trial designs; however, the relevance of all design aspects to usual practice is emphasised more in effectiveness trials. This concerns participants, interventions, control conditions and outcomes. Interventions are often applied

C. Gold (✉)
GAMUT, Uni Research Health, Uni Research, Lars Hilles gate 3, 5015 Bergen, Norway
e-mail: christian.gold@uni.no

O.C.G. Gelo et al. (eds.), *Psychotherapy Research*,
DOI 10.1007/978-3-7091-1382-0_26, © Springer-Verlag Wien 2015

more flexibly in effectiveness trials. This chapter places most emphasis on design aspects because, in contrast to statistical analyses, they are more basic; they cannot be corrected after completion; and they are a precondition for a correct analysis. However, some basic principles for statistical analysis, as well as common pitfalls, are also explained briefly. In summary, this chapter should enable the reader to make informed decisions to design outcome studies that are clinically relevant and methodologically sound.

This chapter reviews some basic and some neglected methodological issues in quantitative outcome research. Psychotherapy outcome research now finds itself situated in the context of evidence-based medicine (EBM). In this context, the demand for high-quality evidence appears to be stronger than ever before, and although EBM has not really created any new methodologies, it has highlighted strongly some of the methodological details that need to be observed for studies to be internally valid. Following a brief historical overview, the chapter starts by explaining and discussing the justification of the so-called hierarchy of evidence, which has been much discussed and which places randomised controlled trials (RCTs) at the top of the hierarchy. The need for and adequacy of RCTs has been questioned by many psychotherapy researchers, and this discussion is briefly summarised.

Having reviewed the basic reasoning behind a hierarchy of research designs, the mathematical reason behind the need for large sample sizes is then explained. While this may be less controversial in psychotherapy research, it is important to understand because large samples are so difficult to achieve and particularly in order to avoid misinterpretations of underpowered studies. A common misunderstanding and source of controversy, the alleged need for restrictive therapy manuals in RCTs, is reviewed, as is the much used but not always fully understood difference between efficacy and effectiveness. The difficulty and importance of choosing outcome measures that are relevant for all parties involved is explained on the background of current discussions in both psychotherapy research and EBM. Issues that are somewhat neglected in psychotherapy research while receiving much attention in EBM are reviewed, such as allocation concealment and intention-to-treat analysis. Finally, I discuss the statistical analysis of outcome studies. While there are often several ways how a given study may be analysed, there are some common errors and ways how they should not be analysed. In summary, this chapter should enable the reader to make informed decisions to design studies in ways that are clinically relevant and methodologically sound.

26.1 Psychotherapy Outcome Research in the Era of Evidence-Based Medicine

26.1.1 The Origins of Psychotherapy Outcome Research

Systematic quantitative research into the outcome of psychotherapy (from now on in this chapter simply referred to as outcome research) began in the 1950s and was to a large extent provoked by a negative report that questioned whether psychotherapy had any positive effects (Eysenck 1952; see Chap. 3). Eysenck's review would in today's terminology be called a meta-analysis (even though today's meta-analysis methods are much more sophisticated; see Sect. 26.2.4): Statistical reports from hospitals and psychotherapy institutes, together including more than 7,000 patients, were drawn together quantitatively to form a summary statistic on the percentage of patients improved. This statistic was compared to the percentage of improved patients in state mental hospitals where no psychotherapy was given—a kind of "standard care" condition (see Sect. 26.8). The percentage of improved patients was lower with psychotherapy than without and lower with intensive psychoanalytic therapy than with typically less intensive eclectic psychotherapy. The author concluded that there was no evidence that psychotherapy contributed to improving patients beyond the standard treatments provided at that time. The review had a number of shortcomings, some of which were noted by the author and most of which will be interesting to discuss in this chapter that concerns the methodology of outcome research.

The field of psychotherapy outcome research has exploded in 60 years since that report, and many studies and reviews have shown much more favourable results. Numerous comprehensive overviews have been published summarising the findings of psychotherapy outcome research to date (e.g. Cooper 2008; Lambert 2004; Roth and Fonagy 2005; Wampold 2001). These overviews have led to the conclusion that psychotherapy is effective and that no school of psychotherapy is generally more effective than another. However, the search for the best methodologies and the debate on the right interpretation of this massive body of literature continue until today. It is also interesting in itself that a negative report stands at the beginning of the development of a highly productive research field.

Let us now turn to some of the methodological weaknesses of Eysenck's review:

- Unclear and subjective measurement of outcome: This is a limitation that the author acknowledged. At that time there was little consensus on diagnostic criteria or measurement of clinical outcomes, so it was difficult to judge across studies what was meant by "improved". Very much has changed since then. Thousands of scales have been developed and validated for all kinds of populations, domains and purposes. Problems of objectivity, reliability and validity can be seen as solved when choosing one of these validated instruments. However, one still has to choose the most appropriate tool and schedule for measurement. Today, there almost seems to be the opposite problem: Which one should I choose among the many scales available? This will be addressed later in this chapter (see Sect. 26.7).
- Limited comparability of "experimental" and "control" groups: None of the studies Eysenck had included was experimental in the sense that participants were allocated to different treatment conditions in a *fair* and *unbiased* way. Each study had only one treatment condition that was applied to all participants. They were uncontrolled studies, either prospective or retrospective. Medical researchers often call this type of studies "case series" (Sect. 26.2.2). The problem with the comparison across studies, as Eysenck had attempted, is that it is unknown how similar or dissimilar the patients were and if or how they may have differed in their prognosis. The author did acknowledge this limitation (but less explicitly or less emphasised than the previous one). He argued that a possible bias was more likely to occur in favour of psychotherapy because patients at state mental hospitals were likely more severely disturbed and therefore (he argued) less likely to improve. It is impossible to verify this claim. Only a mechanism that ensures unbiased allocation of clients to groups can solve this problem. This chapter will review in detail why such fair assignment to conditions is important and also how difficult it is to achieve in practice (see Sect. 26.2).
- Possible confounding in the length of follow-up: Improvement rates were reported in the original studies over 1 or 2 years and sometimes over unclear time periods. If improvement can occur at different time points and this varies across patients (a very likely assumption), this will be important to take into account as a possible confounding variable. Modern statistical methods are now available that enable controlling for confounding variables. But practitioners starting to think about research may still think in terms of numbers of sessions and not consider the time scale in the first place.
- Researcher allegiance/bias: The author makes his negative bias towards psychotherapy clear from the outset. Personal bias may have

influenced the way he selected studies and variables, the way he made choices when data were missing, the analyses methods he chose and the interpretation of the results. Researcher allegiance has been shown to influence the results of outcome studies quite drastically (Luborsky et al. 1999), but it is ubiquitous—some have said that the only ones who have no bias are those who know nothing about the subject. Striving for objectivity and transparency in methods and making bias explicit may be the only solutions that exist.

– Sample size and statistical test power: No statistical tests were applied in the Eysenck review, so the question of test power does not arise. However, the sample size was rather large in this early review: $n = 8{,}053$ in the "experimental" groups only (760 in psychoanalytic and 7,293 in eclectic psychotherapy). A later section in this chapter (Sect. 26.4) will highlight why sample size is important (and why large samples make it possible to detect what smaller samples can't). The present example is a reminder that large sample size alone is by no means a guarantee for an unbiased sample. It is true that the *random* error becomes smaller when sample size increases; but the *systematic* error (bias in the study design, in the selection, allocation, attrition of participants and detection of outcomes) does not.

26.1.2 Evidence-Based Medicine

The term evidence-based medicine (EBM) has become popular since the 1990s. In an influential paper it was defined as "conscientious, explicit, and judicious use of current best evidence in making decisions about the care of individual patients" (Sackett et al. 1996, p. 71). Although this definition of EBM does not explicitly refer to any study design, the EBM movement has become largely about randomised controlled trials (RCTs) and systematic reviews/meta-analyses of RCTs. It is implied in the definition of EBM that some types of studies may be more likely than others to represent the "best" evidence. Another interesting observation that can be made is that the definition refers to "individual" patients. They need not necessarily be defined primarily or exclusively by means of a medical diagnosis. Although Sackett most likely had mainstream medicine in mind when formulating it, his definition is open to medical as well as non-medical interventions. For the discussion in psychotherapy, it is important to note that it does not necessarily imply "medicalising" interventions or reducing clients to their diagnosis or to passive recipients of treatment: The definition speaks of care, not of treatment, and of individuals, not of medical diagnoses. (Sometimes the term "evidence-based practice" is used to refer to the same principles applied to non-medical interventions. In this chapter the more common term EBM will be used, but with non-medical interventions in mind.) Another point that is often made is that the definition refers to the "judicious" use of the evidence. This is opposed to a restrictive, "cookbook" approach where prescriptions and referrals are only based on research evidence, not considering individual circumstances and subjective elements in the decision process. The definition may therefore imply that the use of EBM to restrict the freedom of clinicians and patients is a misuse of EBM, not an appropriate application of it. Relatedly, it may also be noted that there is nothing in this definition to imply anything about the interventions themselves, for example, that they should be standardised or manualised. This is a point that we will return to later.

During the last two decades, the EBM movement has certainly served to increase researchers' and clinicians' focus on and attention to RCTs. It has extended to most countries and areas of health care. EBM has become so strongly associated with RCTs that it almost seems necessary to remind readers that RCTs were not invented by it. Early examples of controlled trials can be found throughout history (one of the earliest "trial reports" can be found in the Bible, at the beginning of the Book of Daniel, comparing the health outcomes of a vegetable diet and a meat diet). However, it was not until well into the twentieth century that their methodology started to be refined and elaborated tremendously. Most steps taken have had the purpose of reducing bias and improving the reliability and credibility of the results. Regardless of whether or not one may see psychotherapy as a "medical" intervention, it is probably quite important for all who are interested in evaluating the outcome of psychotherapy to keep up-to-date with the methodological developments in clinical trials.

26.1.3 Evidence-Based Medicine and Psychotherapy Outcome Research

To what extent, one may ask, are the two worlds of EBM and psychotherapy outcome research related to each other? *The Handbook of Psychotherapy and Behavior Change* (Lambert 2004), regarded by many as one of the most authoritative sources on psychotherapy research, does not have "evidence-based medicine" or "evidence-based practice" as an index entry. But it has an entry: "evidence-based treatment—see empirically supported treatment". "Empirically supported treatment" (EST) is a term coined and used in the USA that describes a controversial recent trend in health-care policy that restricts the services of psychotherapists to such therapies that have demonstrated efficacy for a given disorder. Criticism of EST includes that it standardises and "medicalises" psychotherapy more than necessary and more than what would be beneficial for psychotherapy clients. Treatment manuals, for example, play a central role in the definition. Like EBM, EST is also about using the evidence from RCTs, but it also includes other elements that are not necessarily a part of EBM. Current criticism from psychotherapists addresses mostly these other elements, such as therapy manuals and disorder-specific treatments and not so much randomisation per se; but it may have indirectly led some to be sceptical of RCTs in general as well.

Conversely, it is of course also legitimate to ask how much space there is for psychotherapy research within EBM organisations. The Cochrane Collaboration, a worldwide organisation aimed at producing systematic reviews and meta-analyses of RCTs across all fields of health care, is seen by many as one of the spearhead organisations of EBM. It is organised into about 50 "Review Groups" (Higgins and Green 2008), of which five are concerned with mental health. The primary organisation is therefore by clinical problem, which is often (but not always) a medical diagnosis. The type of intervention has a secondary role; given the much larger number of pharmaceutical trials, it is not surprising that these are more prevalent there than psychotherapy. (Some years ago, however, the Cochrane Collaboration decided that they would not accept any support from the pharmaceutical industry for their work, in order to secure its independence.) There is also limited recognition and understanding of the specific issues in psychotherapy research, simply because psychotherapy is too marginal within mainstream medicine. The Cochrane Collaboration has also established "Fields" to address broader issues that exist across a range of clinical problems, such as issues linked to a certain type of intervention. However, a behavioural medicine field has been the closest to psychotherapy so far, and so it can probably be said that a lack of understanding is mutual and dialogue is difficult. On the other hand, some issues may be less problematic within the EBM culture than one might expect. To mention two examples that are controversial in psychotherapy research: there is nothing in the *Cochrane Handbook* (Higgins and Green 2008) that requires therapy manuals (see Sect. 26.5) and standard care control groups are seen as equally acceptable as placebo control groups (see Sect. 26.8). The one element that is considered very important is proper random allocation to groups (see Sects. 26.2, 26.3, 26.9 and also 26.10). This is important to understand for researchers planning to conduct psychotherapy outcome research that will be acceptable within the framework of EBM.

26.2 What Is the Hierarchy of Evidence and How Is It Justified?

26.2.1 The Hierarchy of Evidence

Hierarchies of evidence (the plural is more correct as there is not only one version) attempt to rank different research designs according to their likely reliability in answering questions about treatment effects. With the proliferation of EBM, they have become rather widespread. The hierarchy is often shown as a pyramid, which also illustrates that the most reliable designs (at the narrow top of the pyramid) are more rare than the less reliable (and less expensive) designs. RCTs and/or systematic reviews of RCTs are always ranked at the top, then different observational and quasi-experimental designs follow, and at the bottom is anything from unverified expert opinion to biological mechanisms as tested in cells or rats, for example. Some versions also include qualitative research on one of the lower levels (Else and Wheeler 2010; see also Chap. 27). In the psychotherapy research literature, such hierarchies have been reviewed by Cooper (2008, p. 181) and by Roth and Fonagy (2005, p. 18). But why is the rank ordering as it is? How is this hierarchy of evidence justified?

26.2.2 Evolution of Research Designs

Instead of a seemingly fixed hierarchy it may be more useful to think of an "evolution of comparative methodology" (Berger 2005, p. 3). This evolution is likely to have started with the *single-case study*: "applying [the intervention] to a single subject, and noting if this subject appeared to improve or deteriorate" (p. 3; Table 26.1). Such a study would be sufficient as an evaluation of intervention effects if "the natural history of a disease is known with absolute certainty, and there is literally no variation across patients" (Berger 2005, pp. 3–4). A drastic example would be a potion that brings a dead person back to life. Since we know that the probability of coming back to life without this magic potion is zero ($p = 0$; an impossible p value in our usual statistical analyses), we can conclude with certainty (!) that the potion was responsible for the effect.

As soon as there is variation and uncertainty in how clients will develop, only probabilistic statements are possible. That is, we can never conclude with 100 % certainty and we need repeated observations from more than one client to increase the level of certainty (or more precisely, to decrease our uncertainty). The outcome of one client is as uninformative as the result of a single coin toss to determine the probability of the coin showing heads or tails. Intuitively, "a larger sample will offer some benefits, because the sampling variability is reduced with increases in the sample size" (Berger 2005, pp. 4–5; see also Sect. 26.4). In a *case series* or *cohort study*, a series or cohort of consecutive patients with a similar type of problem all receive the same intervention, and their outcome is observed. Such a design helps to "ascertain preliminary indications of efficacy" (p. 5) and are therefore used both in the development of drugs (phase II studies) and in psychotherapy studies.

However, it can be argued that any evaluation of an intervention is necessarily comparative in nature. Implicitly or explicitly, one will assume that the intervention is being compared to either the absence of the intervention or to some other intervention or strategy. Case series and single-case studies share the same weakness in this respect, that any comparison must remain implicit. *Historical controls* are one simple way of providing such a comparison more explicitly. The historical control design entails comparing a current cohort of clients who receive the intervention with earlier patients before the intervention was available. (Note that this could either mean before it was invented or before it was made available at a certain place.) Obvious types of bias include shifts in the population and shifts in the care provided. The design is

Table 26.1 An overview of research designs

Design	Definition	Strengths	Weaknesses
Single-case study	Applying the intervention to a single participant and noting change	Simple; close to clinical practice	Sufficient only if changes in the absence of the intervention are known with certainty
Case series	A series of similar clients receive the same intervention	Sampling variability is reduced as sample size increases; ascertains preliminary indications of efficacy	No explicit comparison with the absence of the intervention
Historical controls	Comparing a current cohort to an earlier cohort before the intervention was available	Establishes an explicit comparison	Services and characteristics of the population may have changed
Parallel controls—matching	Choosing control subjects that are matched on known confounding factors	Rules out historical shifts	Difficult to achieve balance; impossible to control for unknown confounders
Parallel controls—randomisation	One sample is divided randomly into different interventions	Can create balance on known and unknown confounders	Clinicians who make decisions about inclusion will try to undermine random assignment
Parallel controls—randomisation with allocation concealment	Randomisation sequence is kept concealed from clinicians	Creates balance on known and unknown confounders, preventing subversion	Clinicians may still attempt to guess the next assignment

not too common in psychotherapy research. It should just be noted that bias can occur in any direction: For example, new treatments (other than the treatment of interest) may have emerged, leading to a bias in favour of the current cohort, or expensive but beneficial treatments may have been discontinued in managed care, leading to a bias in favour of the historical cohort.

Designs with *parallel control groups* avoid these sources of bias, but can still suffer from self-selection bias. For example, a comparison of today's smokers with today's non-smokers to compare their health outcomes will likely be confounded with other lifestyle factors such as alcohol consumption or eating habits. In *matched designs*, one tries to balance such factors, either on a group level or on an individual level, by choosing control subjects that are matched on known confounding factors. This is most feasible when a large pool of control subjects are available. It is then also possible to match several control subjects to one experimental subject, which will improve statistical precision and test power (see Sect. 26.4). However, with an increasing number of such covariates to be considered, matching quickly becomes difficult if not impossible to do practically. Even with advanced statistical methods for improving the matching on several variables (such as propensity score methods), one very substantial problem remains: It is never possible to match on unmeasured variables, but some of the most important confounding factors may well be unmeasured in practice or even unmeasurable in principle. Any matching strategy, however advanced, always relies on the untestable assumption that the groups are balanced on all confounding variables, including those that are unmeasured.

This leads to designs using *randomisation*, a process which "aims to ensure similar levels of all risk factors in each group; not only known, but also unknown, characteristics are rendered comparable, except for either the play of chance or a real effect of the intervention(s)" (Berger 2005, p. 9).

How can it be that a process of randomisation creates a balance that seems impossible to achieve by using other methods? We may understand this intuitively or mathematically: Intuitively, if you play, say, roulette once, you don't know if you will get an odd or an even number; but if you play it many times, you know that odd numbers will appear about equally as often as even numbers. The same is true for high versus low, red versus black, thirds and for any given number of the roulette game. Mathematically, the law of large numbers and the central limit theorem describe exactly how close the balance will be - the larger the sample size, the closer. Note that there is no corresponding "law of small numbers"!

Practically, randomisation is today most often done with a computer-generated list of random numbers, but it is equally valid to draw lots or to toss coins, as long as there is "no opportunity for the subject to select a treatment, and no opportunity for the investigator to assign a treatment based on subject characteristics" (Berger 2005, p. 9). The interest and zeal of researchers, clinicians and patients to subvert this random assignment should not be underestimated. *Allocation concealment* (as discussed in Sect. 26.9 of this chapter) is commonly used to prevent the subversion of randomisation. However, "selection bias may occur even in properly randomized trials" (Berger 2005, p. 15), and in some studies there is evidence that it has occurred, for example, because clinicians successfully guessed the next allocation in some of the cases (pp. 37–84). It is therefore important to be careful even in this most rigorous design (Table 26.1).

26.2.3 Limits of the Hierarchy of Evidence

This evolution of research designs is analogous to reading the hierarchy of evidence from bottom to top. It shows how each next, more advanced design aims to prevent the possible biases from each previous, more basic design. Therefore, the logical reasoning behind the hierarchy of evidence is very clear, even if certain biases can still occur with even the most advanced designs. However, one needs to keep in mind that the hierarchy of evidence is not about the quality of research per se. Qualitative researchers, for example, sometimes feel that the hierarchy of evidence devalues qualitative research by placing RCTs on the top, but that is an over-interpretation of the pyramid. The hierarchy of evidence only ranks the reliability of research designs for one specific purpose—for questions of treatment effects. As Roth and Fonagy (2005, p. 18) note, the hierarchy "should not be misunderstood as indicating the clinical utility of different research designs; depending on the research question being asked, methodologies lower in the hierarchy may be completely appropriate". In practice, the choice of a design also "represents a compromise reflecting the intents, interests, and resources of investigators" (p. 18). It is also true that the hierarchy only reflects the internal validity of studies. It does not say anything about their external validity or about the quality of the clinical work.

26.2.4 Systematic Reviews and Meta-analyses

Systematic reviews (SRs) and meta-analyses—the two terms are often used interchangeably—are both a category within and across the levels of evidence. In hierarchies of evidence they are usually listed just above the design of the studies that are included—for example, an SR of RCTs would be placed above a single RCT. The reason for that is that generalisability is improved when studies carried out in different places, by different investigators, in different contexts but focusing on a similar population and intervention, have found similar results. Meta-analysis is the statistical technique to combine such studies in an analysis (Higgins and Green 2008; The Cochrane Collaboration 2005; see Chap. 28 for an example). The obvious advantage is increased power (see Sect. 26.4) because the total sample size is larger than the sample sizes of each primary study. A less obvious challenge is heterogeneity across studies. *Clinical heterogeneity* is the degree to which study characteristics such as clients, interventions and outcome measures differed; it is to some extent a subjective category and should be considered before deciding what studies to combine in a meta-analysis. In contrast, the extent to which results vary across studies can be measured. To distinguish from the variation between participants within a study (i.e. variance), between-study variation is commonly termed *statistical heterogeneity*. Inferential and descriptive measures have been developed to measure it (Higgins and Green 2008).

A note is warranted about the history of meta-analyses and SRs as a research culture. The earliest meta-analyses, in psychotherapy and other fields, lumped many studies with considerable variation in clients, interventions, outcome measures and study designs. The sheer number of included studies was sometimes used as an argument for the validity of their conclusions. More recently, clinical homogeneity has received more emphasis, leading to smaller and more narrowly focused reviews (and at the same time, the term "systematic review" has become more prevalent, emphasising more the selection process than the statistical analysis part). For example, many Cochrane reviews only include a handful of carefully selected studies; but if these show convincing results, that can be a stronger finding than a larger but more diverse meta-analysis. An additional purpose that such SRs can fulfil is to identify gaps in the research literature. For this reason, it is sometimes recommended to do a SR before designing a new study.

26.3 Do We Really Need Randomised Controlled Trials in Psychotherapy Outcome Research?

There has been a lively discussion in psychotherapy research about whether or not RCTs are necessary and whether or not they are adequate. To some extent the same questions have also been raised within mainstream medicine. For example, Black (1996) argued, quite aptly, that there are situations where RCTs are either unnecessary, inappropriate, impossible or inadequate and that observational studies therefore should have a place in the evaluation of health care. Those situations, however, are highly specific: "Insulin in insulin-dependent diabetes" and "anaesthesia for surgical operations" (Black 1996, p. 1215) are two drastic examples where RCTs are unnecessary. A more hypothetical example, as entertaining as enlightening, is the use of parachutes when jumping off an airplane (Smith and Pell 2003). So the discussion in medicine is really about whether observational studies should be seen as sufficient in "exceptional circumstances" (Smith and Pell 2003, p. 1460). In psychotherapy there seem to be many who question whether RCTs are necessary or adequate at all. In this discussion, some legitimate concerns of how RCTs are carried out in practice are mixed with some misunderstandings and overgeneralisations about the nature of RCTs in principle.

Among the most well-known voices sceptical of RCTs, Seligman (1995) has argued eloquently and provocatively for using uncontrolled survey methods as the best method to evaluate the effectiveness of psychotherapy. Although thought-provoking in many ways, the paper inappropriately equated effectiveness studies with observational studies (see Sect. 26.6) and RCTs with "manualised, fixed duration treatment" (p. 965; see Sect. 26.5). The central element to RCTs is randomisation to two or more different interventions; this does not automatically imply anything about the nature of these interventions (such as the use of manuals or a fixed duration) or participants (such as a medical diagnosis).

As another well-known example in the psychotherapy literature, Howard et al. (1986) conducted a review about the "dose-effect relationship in psychotherapy". Their findings (similarly reproduced for illustrative purposes in Fig. 26.1) suggested that the percentage of patients improved increased with the number of psychotherapy sessions. The curve was steeper at the beginning, resembling a logarithmic curve. A control group was not considered; the actual data were about *changes* during treatment, not *effects* of treatment, in spite of the word "effect" in the title of the paper. There is an important difference between these two words. How these changes can be interpreted is not independent of the question on what changes would have

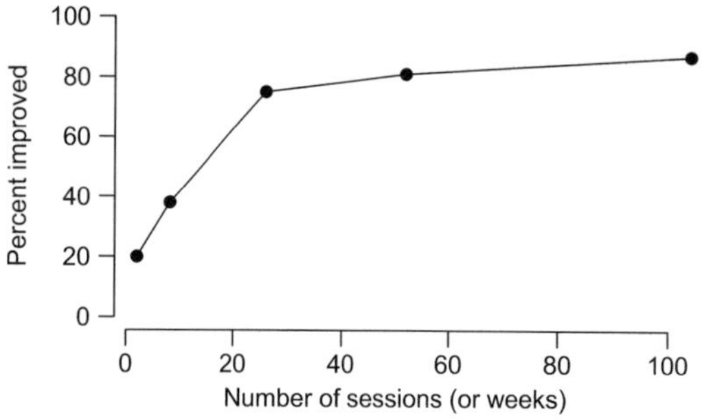

Fig. 26.1 Relation of number of sessions of psychotherapy and percentage of patients improved. *Note*. This figure is similar to Fig. 1 in Howard et al. (1986). The label of the x-axis has been changed from "Number of sessions" to "Number of sessions (or weeks)" to show the implied time dimension explicitly. The numbers shown are similar to Howard's numbers for "objective ratings at termination" but may not be exactly reproduced from the original graph

occurred in the absence of treatment. It is of course reassuring for anyone who cares about psychotherapy clients that they improve over time; however, while this is an interesting finding about psychotherapy *clients*, it is not in itself a finding about *psychotherapy* unless we also consider the counterfactual: How would these clients have changed without psychotherapy? (It should be noted here that the paper by Howard et al. did consider the confounding between time passed and number of sessions received. The limitations of the review, as well as extraneous evidence to support the findings, were discussed. The paper is also notable in its unusually thoughtful discussion of theoretical issues, such as the limitations of "session" as an imperfect proxy measure for psychotherapy's active ingredients.)

Figure 26.2 shows several possible scenarios of what might have been the case. Scenario A is the very unlikely event where nobody would have improved without psychotherapy. Unrealistic as it might be, this would be the implicit assumption when equating changes with effects. Most likely, at least some people will improve over the course of time. Depending on their severity and chronicity and many other factors (such as support from friends or relatives), this rate might be rather low, as in scenario B, or it might be almost as high as with psychotherapy, as in scenario C. It is impossible to know which is correct, but the conclusions would be rather different. Scenario B would suggest a rather dramatic effect, scenario C a much more modest effect. Probably scenario C is more realistic. It might even be that scenario D is correct. This would suggest a harmful effect of psychotherapy: Even though many improved in psychotherapy, there were even more who improved without it. It might be an implausible assumption, but it is possible. It is always easy to find explanations post hoc: Perhaps therapy entrenched them in their role as victims and as helpless and dependent on others? The last two scenarios show more complex interactions of treatment effect and time: There might be an early effect that vanishes over time (scenario E, possibly explained by clients' expectation of improvement and the reinstallation of hope?) or a late onset of effects (scenario F, possibly due to being confronted with conflicts?). More scenarios would be possible to imagine; few could be discarded a priori. This shows the importance of control groups that are, at the outset, similar to the intervention group (such as in a randomised design; see Sect. 26.2.2).

As a play of thought, one might consider a negative event as an outcome. For some reason, such outcomes are not too common in psychotherapy research, but they do have relevance in mental health and are used in the broader field of mental health services research. For example, relapse, attempted suicide or death might be considered. The outcome might either be displayed as a time-to-event curve showing a changing percentage over time (similar to Fig. 26.1, but with reversed signs) or as a percentage at a given time point. What would such a result indicate if only a group receiving psychotherapy was considered? We would hardly conclude that the clients committed suicide as a result of psychotherapy. In terms of treatment effects, the result makes little sense unless we also consider a comparison group receiving some other type of care. Without such a comparison, it would be interesting in terms of the prognosis of clients but not in terms of treatment effects.

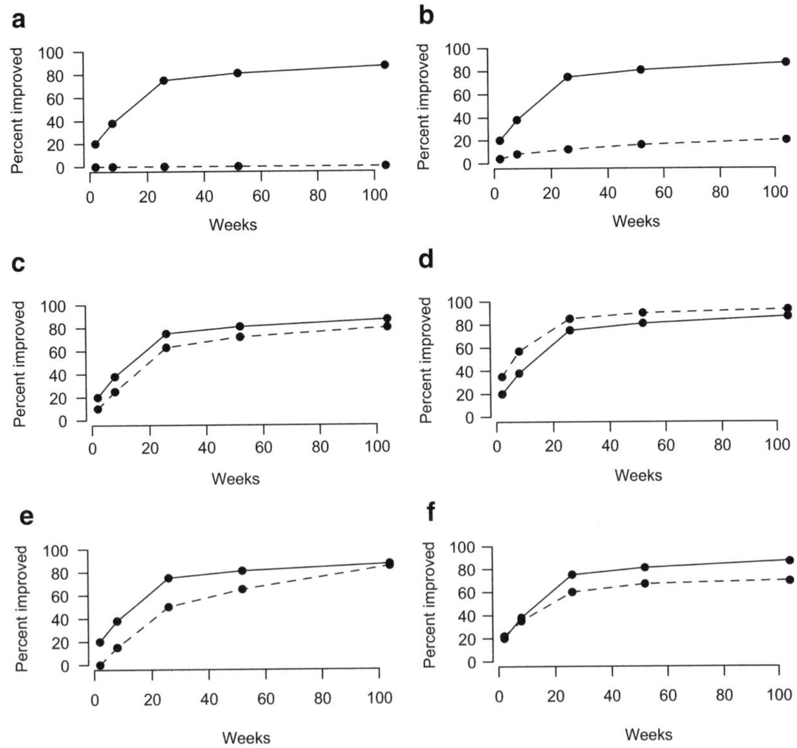

Fig. 26.2 Data from Fig. 26.1 with hypothetical control group added: six possible scenarios. *Note.* The *dashed lines* show the development of a hypothetical control group without psychotherapy

Studies based on large databases of psychotherapy clients continue to emerge and certainly have their appropriate place. However, regardless of how impressively large the patient pools may be, such studies cannot replace a controlled trial. RCTs are needed to understand the effects of psychotherapy, as of any other treatment; but this does not imply anything about how psychotherapy should be delivered or how client groups should be defined.

26.4 Why Are Large Sample Sizes Important?

Put simply, large sample sizes are needed because treatment effects are subtle and because patients are different. If treatment effects are dramatic (e.g. everyone dies without the treatment but survives when offered the treatment), it is not necessary to collect data from many patients to come to a definite conclusion. However, there are very few treatments that have such extreme effects (Smith and Pell 2003). Most treatments, psychotherapy or other, have subtle effects: Some get better with the treatment, but also some without. Some get worse without the treatment and some also with the treatment. The purpose of taking a sample is to be able to generalise to a population. It is intuitively clear that any estimates of a quantity in a population becomes more precise as information from more people becomes available. We always see it on the evening after an election day: The estimates become more precise towards the end of the evening when more votes have been counted. It can also be seen relatively easily from the mathematical formulas.

The standard error of the mean (SEM; may also be abbreviated as SE) describes how far an estimated mean (the mean in a sample) typically deviates from the true mean (the mean in the population). Calculation is based on the standard deviation (SD) of the quantity of interest and the number of cases (n) where this quantity was observed. The formula is $SEM = SD/\sqrt{n}$ [see any statistics textbook or the Wikipedia article on "Standard error (statistics)"]. From this formula one can see several things:

- Having n in the denominator means that the more n increases, the more SEM decreases, or in other words, the more precise the estimate becomes.
- Because the square root of n is involved, this means that the gain in precision with every new participant is smaller when n is already larger. The gain when going from 20 to 21 participants is greater than from 1,000 to 1,001.
- Having SD in the nominator means that the estimate also becomes more precise when SD becomes smaller. This is one reason why researchers often try to select homogeneous samples. For example, a depression questionnaire may have SD = 10 in a population of depressed outpatients but SD = 15 when outpatients and inpatients are combined. (This relationship is somewhat masked when effects are expressed in terms of effect sizes, which are already standardised by their SD.)

SEM is the basis for many statistical tests, and therefore the considerations above can be extended to applications like t-tests (a test to compare two means), ANOVAs (a test to compare three or more means) and many others: An increase in sample size will mean increased precision and thus greater test power. The SEM is also very useful to calculate confidence intervals (CIs). A CI is "a measure of the uncertainty around the main finding of a statistical analysis" (The Cochrane Collaboration 2005). A 95 % CI indicates, in simple terms, that we can have 95 % confidence in it: Only 5 % of the possible samples we could take would be outside this range. CIs have a direct correspondence to a statistical test, while also retaining the descriptive information, and are therefore becoming increasingly common in clinical research. Like the SEM, the CI will also become smaller as sample size increases. Figure 26.3 shows the relationship between n and the 95 % CI. One can see clearly how precision improves as n increases, and one can also see that the gains are greater at the beginning than when n is already large. In a comparative study, the question is not about one quantity, but about comparing two quantities (e.g. the mean in an experimental and a control group). But the issues are the same: one needs a reasonably precise estimate of both means in order to make a statement about their difference.

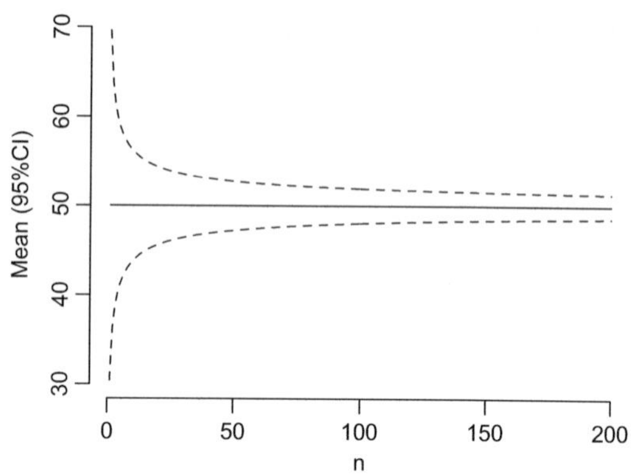

Fig. 26.3 Relationship between sample size (n) and precision. *Note*. This figure shows the mean (*solid line*) and 95 % confidence interval (*dashed line*) as a function of n for a hypothetical quantity (e.g. the sum score of a standardised questionnaire) with $M = 50$ and SD = 10

While it is interesting and important to know this relationship, the question that researchers want to know most is perhaps not just that "the more, the better" but "how many do I need"? This touches the issue of test power, a full discussion of which is beyond the scope of this chapter. Useful descriptions with practical solutions can be found in Indrayan (2008, pp. 370–371, 380–392) and Altman (1991, p. 456). As a rule of thumb, a small clinical trial will have around 30 participants per group (most trials in psychotherapy fall into this category), a medium-sized trial around 100 per group and a large trial around 300 per group (Indrayan 2008, p. 392). The largest samples are needed when

- Treatment effects are small (e.g. when comparing two similar interventions, rather than one active intervention to a no-treatment condition).
- The population is heterogeneous (i.e. SD is large).

– The study should provide a definite answer (i.e. low chance of type I and type II errors or low alpha level and high test power), as opposed to an exploratory pilot study in a new area.

Large samples are difficult to achieve, yet it is important to invest all possible efforts to achieve a reasonably large sample. There is little that can compensate for a too small *n*. A homogeneous sample and a strong treatment effect are two other important aspects that have been mentioned. There is one more thing that can be done to improve power and precision with a limited sample and that is to measure the same outcomes repeatedly in the same subjects. Thereby one increases the number of data points instead of the number of individuals. However, repeated measurements in the same individual are usually correlated, which means that advanced statistical techniques are required and that the gains are more limited than when increasing the number of participants (see Sect. 26.11).

A final cautionary note to conclude this section: Large samples have smaller *random* error than smaller samples, but not necessarily smaller *systematic* error. It is sometimes said that with increasing sample size, the random error does not converge to zero; rather, it converges to the systematic bias. Systematic bias can only be reduced through careful study design. If the study design does not preclude systematic bias, a large sample does not only fail to help against it. It may even be dangerously misleading as it may create the impression of a high precision which is in fact spurious precision.

26.5 Do RCTs Always Involve Therapy Manuals?

26.5.1 Research Rigour Versus Therapeutic Flexibility

Some of the reservation about RCTs in the psychotherapy literature is due to a notion that RCTs have to involve manuals, which are seen by many to restrict the therapist and the patient and to overstructure the therapy. This raises some questions, such as: How did the demand for manuals come up? Who demands that they should be used? What are the pros and cons of using manuals? Are there other solutions?

Psychotherapy manuals were first used for cognitive therapy some 30 years ago, but have more recently also been developed and applied for other approaches. As Cooper (2008, p. 152) writes, "the term 'manual' may conjure up images of minute-by-minute set instructions", but "most manuals are broader guides to treatment", describing principles and techniques of an approach and giving concrete examples. In this way, a manual is not entirely unlike what used to be called simply a textbook (Kächele 2010). Two purposes of a manual can be identified: one purpose is to ensure replicability of the study and a second one might be to guide practitioners who wish to apply the approach in usual practice (outside of a research study). There is a consensus that the form of therapy applied in a study must be described with sufficient clarity to ensure replication and to judge the study's applicability for one's practice. Controversies exist, however, as to how much of a predefined structure such descriptions should impose on the therapy process. This has become more a political than a scientific issue, especially in the USA where approaches not using manuals have been considered unacceptable in principle. Wampold (2001) suggested an RCT comparing psychotherapy with a manual to the same form of therapy without a manual to determine the effects of manuals (p. 213), but added that such a study "would not be funded under current policy" because manuals are not used in all treatments investigated (p. 214). From a scientific perspective, the challenge could be formulated as one of describing the therapy with sufficient clarity without changing it to something else (i.e. replicability vs. generalisability; see also Sect. 26.6). At least in some forms of psychotherapy, the therapist's (and client's) freedom to choose working modalities flexibly and adaptively is an important part of the process. Some have argued that "unpredictability is an intended part of the process" so that there is not only a need to control but also a need *not* to control the process of therapy (Piper and Ogrodniczuk 1999, cit. in Rolvsjord et al. 2005). Others have argued that essential common factors such as the therapist's warmth are at risk when applying manuals too rigidly (Wampold 2001).

From this discussion it becomes clear that the question of manuals is not as much an either-or situation but more a question of degree: To what degree should the therapy be standardised or practised flexibly? How can the best balance between research rigour and therapeutic flexibility be achieved? Some manuals are more prescriptive, while others are more descriptive; some focus more on adherence, others more on competence and some more on overarching principles and attitudes, others more on concrete techniques (Rolvsjord et al. 2005). The right answer to these questions depends on the aims of the research and the type of therapy investigated; it cannot be the same for all studies. A study can be high or low in the hierarchy of evidence (see Sect. 26.2) regardless of whether or not a manual is used. As noted before (see Sect. 26.1.3), powerful EBM organisations such as the Cochrane Collaboration (Higgins and Green 2008) have no opinion on this matter. Another consideration is that pragmatic trials of effectiveness can be characterised by more leeway and flexibility for the therapist than explanatory trials of efficacy (Thorpe et al. 2009).

26.5.2 Related Issues: Beyond the Horse Race

Having opened up the relationship between RCTs and the "medical model" (Wampold 2001) of psychotherapy by showing that RCTs can be valid without manuals, one may want to go a step further in thinking about interesting but less conventional applications of RCTs in the field. RCTs in psychotherapy cannot only be understood as a "horse race" between different schools of thought. It can be worthwhile to consider studies where randomisation is to other things than to schools of psychotherapy:

- Dosage: As Feaster et al. (2003) note, there have been very few studies randomising to different "doses" of psychotherapy, in spite of an abundance of observational studies addressing the topic. Studies could randomise either to different treatment durations or to different frequencies of sessions (the latter even with open-ended duration, as long as measurement time points are independent of treatment duration). Such studies are common in drug development, often called "dose-finding" trials, and would also be beneficial in psychotherapy, addressing a question that is both policy-relevant and relevant for practitioners.
- Variants within the same school: Within each school of thought there may be different approaches whose relative merits are worth examining. One such example—the same therapy with or without using a manual—has been mentioned before. The results of such trials would be directly relevant to practitioners. Such studies would however have to be planned with particular care, as differences in effect are likely small, thus necessitating a large sample (see Sect. 26.4 above).
- Therapist: There are indications from observational studies, as well as from observational data within RCTs, that the person of the therapist may account for a considerable proportion of the effects of psychotherapy (Roth and Fonagy 2005, p. 447ff; Wampold 2001, p. 184ff.). However, to my knowledge no RCT has been conducted where patients were randomised to therapists rather than to therapy methods. It has been argued that such a trial would be unlikely to receive funding (Roth and Fonagy 2005, p. 448), but it would address a scientifically relevant question, particularly in relation to the contextual model of psychotherapy (Wampold 2001). If conducted, such a trial should not focus on the performance of individual therapists but model the degree of variation between them.

These are just some examples of how the scientifically most rigorous design can be applied creatively to address questions that may be more relevant and appealing to practitioners than traditional, "horse-race"-type comparative studies.

26.6 What Is the Difference Between Efficacy and Effectiveness?

It is generally accepted that efficacy is the effect of a treatment under ideal circumstances, whereas effectiveness is its effect under "real-world" circumstances. Less known in the psychotherapy community is the fact that the distinction is not about research design per se, but about the focus of the research question. RCTs can address effectiveness or efficacy, depending on how they are designed. Ten domains—including how participants, interventions, comparisons and outcomes are defined—reflect the degree to which a trial addresses either efficacy or effectiveness (Thorpe et al. 2009).

For example, the glossary of the Cochrane Collaboration (The Cochrane Collaboration 2005) defines efficacy as follows: "The extent to which an intervention produces a beneficial result under ideal conditions. Clinical trials that assess efficacy are sometimes called explanatory trials and are restricted to participants who fully co-operate". In contrast, effectiveness is defined as "the extent to which a specific intervention, when used under ordinary circumstances, does what it is intended to do. Clinical trials that assess effectiveness are sometimes called pragmatic or management trials. See also intention-to-treat".

These definitions make it clear that RCTs can address both types of questions. The design would however vary in many elements: Patients would be less selected in an effectiveness or "pragmatic" trial, in order to more adequately represent typical clinical populations. In efficacy or "explanatory" trials, in contrast, it would be more accepted to have long lists of exclusion criteria, which serve to specify a selected and homogeneous population for which a new treatment is supposed to work, but at the expense of also creating an artificially selected sample that is unlikely to match "real-world" patients. Likewise, the treatment is typically more rigorously defined in an efficacy study than in an effectiveness study. For example, extensive training and selection of therapists before the study, close supervision during the study, treatment manuals (see Sect. 26.5) with assessments of treatment fidelity and relatively low caseloads of therapists all tend to represent an efficacy study. Less selected therapists practising therapy "as usual" according to their professional training, in a clinic with pressure of higher caseloads, tend to be found in effectiveness studies. This list is not exhaustive but merely intended to provide some examples of how "real-world" therapy may differ from "laboratory" therapy. It should also be noted that these are differences of degree, not absolute qualities. A study of humans can never be as "pure" or "ideal" as the definition may suggest, and any study where researchers attempt to observe and analyse outcomes can also never be fully representative of "ordinary circumstances". The definitions of efficacy and effectiveness are probably best understood as prototypical, with many grey zones in between. Psychotherapy researchers have put much emphasis on the distinction between efficacy and effectiveness. As noted before, there is an agreement that the terms differentiate "ideal" from "ordinary" circumstances, but sometimes this is mingled with questions of study design, randomised versus others. One prominent example is Seligman's (1995) report about the "effectiveness" of psychotherapy. Along the lines of ideal versus ordinary circumstances, the author writes that "I came to see that deciding whether one treatment, under highly controlled conditions, works better than another treatment or a control group is a different question from deciding what works in the field" (p. 966). Therefore, he observes, quite in agreement with the definitions above, that "the efficacy study is the wrong method for empirically validating psychotherapy as it is actually done, because it omits too many crucial elements of what is done in the field" (p. 966). He also lists up some important limitations of efficacy studies: For example, psychotherapy as practised in the field is "not of fixed duration" but "keeps going until the client is markedly improved or until he or she quits"; it is "self-correcting" in terms of the techniques used instead of "confined to a small number of techniques, all within one modality and manualised to be delivered in a fixed order" and clients have "multiple problems" rather than being selected "by a long set of exclusion and inclusion criteria" (all on p. 967). What the author did not note, however, was that effectiveness RCTs can be designed to allow for all of these variations. Instead, this much-cited paper went on to suggest a retrospective survey as the ideal alternative. This study design is listed very low in the hierarchy of evidence because many sources of bias are possible. As noted above, the hierarchy of evidence does not devalue any research designs per se but only ranks them with respect to their reliability in answering one type of research question, namely, that of intervention effects (the term "effects" here includes efficacy as well as effectiveness). A survey can be a valuable, even the best, design for many research questions, but not for evaluating treatment effectiveness. For evaluating treatment effectiveness, a survey can produce interesting hypotheses that may be worth examining further. Seligman did acknowledge that a survey could not be the only method or provide the final answer on psychotherapy's effectiveness. However, for many readers, this and similar studies have served to confuse the difference between effectiveness and efficacy on one side and controlled and uncontrolled studies on the other. It is important to be aware that researchers outside the psychotherapy community will expect "pragmatic" RCTs, not observational studies, when questions concerning the effectiveness of psychotherapy are to be addressed.

26.7 What Is a Relevant Outcome Measure?

Much has changed since the early review by Eysenck (1952) (see Sect. 26.1) when researchers in mental health could only rely on a psychiatrist's or other mental health practitioner's subjective and relatively undefined judgment of "improved" or "not improved". Concrete and testable criteria for outcome measures such as objectivity, reliability and validity have been elaborated and used, and many measures have been developed that meet these criteria. In fact, there are today so many different measures that some have raised the question whether this represents "diversity or chaos" (Hill and Lambert 2004, p. 107). 1,430 different measures were found in a review of psychotherapy studies and still 98 measures in studies on agoraphobia only (p. 107). In a review of schizophrenia trials, 640 different instruments were found (Thornley and Adams 1998, p. 1182), and many measures were used only once. While some diversity is certainly necessary and welcome, it seems very unlikely that there are hundreds or thousands of entirely different outcome domains that researchers may want to measure. Several general recommendations can be given when choosing a measure for a new study:

– Is the measure relevant for patients? Is it sensitive to the therapy method (i.e. does it measure what the therapy intends to do)? These are two separate but somewhat complementary questions. The most relevant measure for the patient may not be the most sensitive one for the type of therapy and vice versa, but both criteria should ideally be met. While some psychotherapy methods are targeted directly at symptom reduction, others are not. The broader the population included in a study and the broader the goals of therapy, the more difficult it may be to find a measure that meets both criteria. A related consideration concerns the times when measures are taken: What time points after the beginning of therapy are most relevant from both perspectives? Also, the closer the time point is to the therapy session, the more sensitive the measure may be, but for the patient it may matter more how sustainable these changes are. Behaviour counts in the therapy situation, for example, may not necessarily be indicative of the therapy's effect on the patient's everyday life (Hill and Lambert 2004, pp. 115–116). It should be noted that a smaller effect on a highly relevant outcome may be more *clinically significant* than a bigger effect on a less relevant one. However, the latter might facilitate achieving *statistical significance* (see Chap. 3, Sect. 3.2.4.3). Ideally, there should be measurements before, during and at the end of therapy, as well as at a later follow-up.

- Is it standardised and published? Although "standardised" is a kind of vague term for describing the properties of an instrument, it usually means that efforts have been made to show that it is reliable, objective and valid. It also means usually that it has been published. Unpublished scales may, in addition to having unknown psychometric properties, also be more subjective to manipulation by study investigators. Researchers may, for example, be tempted to exclude items from the scale if that changes the study's results in the desired direction. Whatever the real reason, unpublished scales have been found to be associated with significant findings in RCTs on schizophrenia more than published scales (Marshall et al. 2000).
- Is it feasible with my population, setting and study design? Issues to be considered include who will provide the information (self-report versus independent observer) and how much information can be reasonably collected. An independent observer rating may sometimes be seen as more objective than a self-report (especially when the observer is blinded to the assigned treatment), but a self-report may be more feasible in some settings. Furthermore, some outcomes are subjective in nature. Conversely, some populations may not be able to fill out self-report forms so that one has to choose an independent observer rating. The amount of information also needs to be considered in relation to the population and the measurement schedule. Researchers sometimes tend to choose too many and too long questionnaires in an effort to include everything that might be relevant. Especially when participants are severely disturbed and/or when measurements should be taken frequently, fewer scales with fewer items will improve the study's feasibility. Pilot testing on a few participants can be useful before beginning a full-scale study.
- Is it widely used? Given the very high diversity of existing measures, researchers should check if the scale they intend to use is commonly used. If there are two or more scales that measure the same domain and are equally feasible, the more widespread scale should probably be used to facilitate comparison with other studies.

26.8 What Is a Relevant Comparison Group?

Ideally, a trial should start from a position of equipoise, that is, "a state of uncertainty where a person believes it is equally likely that either of two treatment options is better" (The Cochrane Collaboration 2005; see also Indrayan 2008, pp. 146–147). Realistically it is rarely the case in a given trial that all those involved (the collective of clinicians, the individual clinician and the patient) feel that they are uncertain about which treatment option is better. When a new treatment is tested against standard care, there may be collective clinical equipoise, but therapists practising the method, and probably their clients, will not have equipoise. When two competing therapies are tested against each other, each clinician will be convinced that his or her therapy is better, although in general there may be equipoise.

Basically, three types of strategies can be identified in finding an appropriate comparator: standard care (including no treatment or waiting list), placebo therapy and another treatment. Let's start with the most controversial one, the so-called placebo therapy (it may also be called attention control). A placebo in drug research is a pill (or other form of sham drug) that resembles the active drug as closely as possible, ideally with the same size, shape, colour and taste. The goal of using a placebo is to separate the psychological effects of receiving a drug from the biological effects of the substance in the drug. In psychotherapy, all effects are of psychological nature, and this makes it problematic if not impossible to construct a "placebo" psychotherapy (Wampold 2001). A placebo therapy would have to be "an activity that could be guaranteed to have no therapeutic element that controls for the effect of attention and that is also viewed by patients as being as credible as the active intervention" (Roth and Fonagy 2005, p. 20). In the face of an unfinished discussion about what constitutes the active ingredients of psychotherapy, one may also argue that "research on placebo effects would be better conceptualized as research on common factors" (Lambert and Ogles 2004, p. 151). Consequently, "many authors entirely reject the placebo concept in psychotherapy research" (Lambert and Ogles 2004, p. 150), but others continue to support it. It might be worthwhile to read the arguments of the earliest proponents of placebo therapy to understand the debate. Rosenthal and Frank (1956) acknowledged that effects of psychotherapy had been demonstrated by studies not using placebo therapies, but noted that these "depend to an undetermined extent on factors common to many types of relationship between patient and therapist" (p. 294). This, they stated, posed a problem "for proponents of various specific forms of psychotherapy who are convinced that their successes result from their particular theory or technique" (p. 294). In other words, placebos are needed only if the aim of the study is to demonstrate psychotherapy's *specific* effects, not its effects per se.

In the pragmatic age of EBM, less emphasis is put on the question *why* a certain approach works, as long as it can be demonstrated *that* it works. For policy makers, the important comparison is between realistic alternatives, such as providing a therapy or not. This leads us to a much more simple option: "Standard care" (or "treatment as usual") can be "a sensible control in many settings" (Roth and Fonagy 2005, p. 20). It is by definition a heterogeneous category—some participants may receive different kinds and doses of medication; some may participate in other psychosocial interventions; others may receive no treatment. This can make it "harder to attribute differences in outcome" because "a number of confounds are possible" (p. 20). In an RCT, one can however assume that the amount of other treatments will be balanced between the groups at baseline (see Sect. 26.2.2). At follow-up, it may be wise to ask participants about any changes in other treatments, as it may be that they either compensated for the lack of therapy in some way or that they required less other treatment as a result of the therapy offered. However, all of these may equally occur in placebo-controlled trials. A practical problem is that equipoise is not likely to exist, at least not among therapists who offer the therapy and clients who intend to participate. One common solution is to use waiting lists, so that those assigned to standard care may receive the therapy later. However, this strategy will make the study more expensive and also makes any later follow-up assessments difficult to interpret.

Finally, one may choose an alternative treatment as comparison, for example, another type of psychotherapy, a drug or another "dosage" (i.e. duration or frequency) of the same therapy (see Sect. 26.5.2). It may be argued that comparing to a "treatment with best-established efficacy" constitutes a "powerful test of a treatment efficacy" (Roth and Fonagy 2005, p. 20). Furthermore, such a comparison is clearly also policy relevant. However, sample sizes in such studies would have to be much larger than for studies comparing to standard care, because effect sizes would be expected to be smaller (see Sect. 26.4). Therefore, such a design would be most reasonably considered at an advanced stage of investigation about a particular type of therapy, i.e. when several RCTs have already demonstrated superiority to standard care.

26.9 What Is Allocation Concealment?

Allocation concealment (AC) is "a critical mechanism [in RCTs] that prevents foreknowledge of treatment assignment and thus shields those who enrol participants from being influenced by this knowledge" (Consort Statement item 9, www.consort-statement.org). Once an unpredictable randomisation sequence has been created, it is important to ensure that it remains unpredictable for those who make inclusion decisions with individual patients, until such a decision has been made. It has been mentioned before in this chapter that clinicians as well as researchers may feel tempted to influence the allocation. For example, in a wait-list design they may want give therapy to those who they think need it most urgently or who they think will benefit most from it or who it will be easiest to work with. All of these efforts undermine the purpose of randomisation to create balanced groups. AC is the effort to prevent such manipulations. In all research on humans and perhaps especially in psychotherapy, AC is therefore arguably more important than the precise way in which the randomisation list is generated (i.e. simple or stratified block randomisation or other strategies; Berger 2005). For this reason, studies in which AC was clearly not used risk being excluded from systematic reviews such as Cochrane reviews. Regrettably, it seems to be a somewhat neglected issue in psychotherapy research (e.g. the current edition of the *Handbook of Psychotherapy and Behavior Change* does not include such an index entry).

Practically, AC is best done by an external person or institute that has exclusive access to the randomisation sequence. Investigators contact this randomisation office once a patient has been enrolled and receive the treatment allocation for this patient (identified with a number and some minimal information such as sex and age). Alternatively, when such external involvement is not feasible, other means such as sequentially numbered, opaque, sealed envelopes can be used, but these may carry a somewhat higher risk of being manipulated.

AC is different from blinding (masking) because it only concerns the concealment until a patient is enrolled, whereas blinding concerns concealment also after that (until outcomes have been assessed). It is therefore that it "can always be successfully implemented" (Consort Statement item 9), at least in principle. In practice, inappropriate or incomplete concealment can occur (Berger 2005). But AC is clearly more feasible than blinding in psychotherapy studies. If done properly, it helps to ensure balanced groups and also clarifies the roles of clinicians and researchers, thus saving the involved clinicians from the temptation to manipulate the allocation sequence.

26.10 What Is an Intention-to-Treat Analysis?

Not all studies are as explicit as they should be with regard to how many participants were enrolled and randomised, how many received the intervention, how many completed the outcome assessment and how many were actually used in the analysis. Intention-to-treat (ITT) analysis refers to analysing "all participants according to their original group assignment, regardless of what subsequently occurred" (Consort Statement item 16, www.consort-statement.org), i.e. according to the treatment that was intended. The opposite of this is known as a "per-protocol" or sometimes "on-treatment" analysis: this means that participants are analysed according to which treatment they actually received. The two types of analysis answer two different questions. Especially when there are many who stop treatment early, the answers can be quite different. Some have argued that ITT answers a more policy-relevant question, because policy makers want to know the effect of offering treatment to a population, not the effect of receiving it for those who happen to complete it. ITT is sometimes said to be related more to effectiveness, whereas per-protocol relates more to efficacy (Thorpe et al. 2009). ITT is most often (though not necessarily) the more conservative analysis, because it avoids the bias of selecting responders from the original sample. Another argument for ITT is that it retains the balance created in the randomisation, whereas a per-protocol analysis may distort this balance and make room for confounding variables to influence the results.

As simple as this sounds in principle, as difficult it is to apply in practice. One or more of the following situations may emerge:

- Some participants may have stopped treatment early but still completed the assessment of outcome. These should be included in an ITT analysis.
- Some may have switched to the alternative treatment due to unforeseen circumstances (e.g. because they found this treatment elsewhere or due to an error or due to an emergency). In an ITT analysis, these should be analysed in the group to which they were originally assigned, whereas a per-protocol analysis would allow for analysing them with the treatment they actually received (the protocol they followed).
- A participant may later be found to be ineligible and was apparently included in error. Should this participant be excluded? The ITT principle (strictly interpreted) says no—even though this might seem counterintuitive at first. The argument is again that the balance created in the randomisation would be at risk, and this weighs stronger than the inclusion and exclusion criteria. (Also, researchers might be more zealous to find reasons for excluding nonresponders in the treatment group they favour most, so the strict interpretation of ITT also guards against this form of bias.)
- A difficult but very common situation is when participants dropped out of the study completely, i.e. outcome measurements are not available for them. According to ITT, they should be included, but how can this be done practically? There is no consensus as to what should be done in this situation. When the outcome is dichotomous, one recommendation is to assume the negative outcome where it is missing. When it is continuous, one might insert the last available value (this is known as "last observation carried forward"), a procedure which is common but not uncontroversial. Advanced methods such as "multiple imputation" exist, but analyses have shown that they are not useful for missing data in outcomes unless good auxiliary variables (e.g. other outcomes that are highly correlated with the unobserved outcome) are available (Allison 2002, pp. 54, 70). The simplest solution for continuous outcomes is to disregard the missing values. Some may still call this type of analysis an ITT analysis. Whatever the choice, it is important to be clear and transparent in what has been done.

A review of published RCTs (Hollis and Campbell 1999) showed that there is considerable variation in how exactly ITT is applied. However, much is gained already if authors make the flow of participants through the study and their analysis choices fully transparent. A flow chart showing the numbers available at each stage can be very useful in this respect (Consort Statement item 13, www.consort-statement.org). Sometimes it may also be useful to analyse the data in different ways; this is sometimes referred to as a "sensitivity analysis". If an ITT analysis and a per-protocol analysis lead to the same conclusions, one may have more confidence in the results than if only one type of analysis is presented.

26.11 How Should RCTs *Not* Be Analysed Statistically?

The analysis of an RCT (and many other types of quantitative studies) should usually include some *descriptive statistics* and some *inferential statistics*. The descriptive statistics may be shown using either tables or figures, or both. For continuous outcomes, these should normally include means and standard deviations, perhaps also effect sizes. Dichotomous or other discrete outcomes may be displayed using cross tables and statistics based on them, such as odds ratio, relative risk, risk difference and number needed to treat. Inferential statistics may include confidence intervals (see Sect. 26.4), basic statistical tests (e.g. t-tests, chi-squared tests, one-way ANOVAs) and/or more advanced statistical models (e.g. multiple regression for including more than one predictor of outcome and linear mixed-effect models, hierarchical linear modelling, generalised estimating equations (GEE) or similar approaches for longitudinal data; see also the discussion in Sect. 26.4). There are many different ways in which an RCT may be analysed, which are all equally valid. To review them all would be well beyond the scope of this chapter. However, there are some ways in which RCTs should *not* be analysed (but which are still sometimes encountered in published or submitted papers):

- Presenting only inferential statistics: Some papers show only the results of statistical tests, sometimes with lots of calculation details. This is not very useful as it fails to show the magnitude of any difference that was found. This error may also sometimes be indicative of an inappropriate trust that the results of such a test would show some kind of absolute truth. One needs to keep in mind that a test result can be wrong. It can—occasionally—show an effect where there is none ("type I error"), and it can—more commonly, especially in small samples—fail to show an effect where there is one ("type II error"). A descriptive statistical analysis is an important first step in the analysis that helps to find out what went on in the sample before considering any inferences about the population from which it was drawn. Luckily, this error seems to have become less common lately, and descriptive statistics are now more regularly encountered in published papers. Confidence intervals are an elegant way of combining descriptive and inferential statistics and are also becoming more common (Indrayan 2008; Higgins and Green 2008, pp. 369–371; see Sect. 26.4).
- Testing for changes within each group separately, rather than for between-group differences: Some reports of controlled studies attempt to show a treatment effect by demonstrating that the experimental group changed significantly (from pretest to posttest) and the control group did not. This line of reasoning may be appropriate when examining descriptive statistics, but as soon as statistical tests are used, it is not. The reason lies again in the nature of statistical tests. Whether a test shows a significant result depends on many things, such as sample size and variability within the sample but most importantly chance. It is impossible to assess whether a just-significant change in one group is reliably greater than an almost-but-just-not-significant change in another group, unless these two groups are directly compared to each other. In contrast, calculating the change in each individual and testing for a between-group difference of these change scores (sometimes labelled "difference-in-difference"; Indrayan 2008, pp. 142, 478) are statistically valid and can be more sensitive than comparing only the end points of each group.

It is however also important to keep in mind that good study design should be considered first. When a study is completed, it is still possible to change the statistical calculations, but problems in the design of the study cannot be changed anymore. With a well-designed study, statistical analysis decisions will almost fall into place by themselves and will tend to be much simpler than when attempting to salvage a poorly designed study with a sophisticated analysis.

Summary and Conclusion

This chapter has highlighted some of the basic issues to be considered in designing, conducting, analysing and interpreting quantitative outcome research in psychotherapy. Some of these have been "hot topics" in the psychotherapy research community for a long time; others have received less attention in this community although they are considered important in EBM. The methodology of outcome research has developed rapidly during the last decades and continues to do so. It can be challenging for beginning researchers (as well as for more experienced ones) to stay abreast of these innovations. Furthermore, some controversies will continue to exist, and no ideal solution that would fit for all situations can be recommended. It is hoped that the discussions presented here will help readers to think creatively about designing outcome studies in psychotherapy and to make informed decisions to design studies in ways that are both clinically meaningful and methodologically sound.

References

Allison PD (2002) Missing data. Series: quantitative applications in the social sciences. Sage, Thousand Oaks, CA

Altman DG (1991) Practical statistics for medical research. Chapman & Hall, London

Berger VW (2005) Selection bias and covariate imbalances in randomized clinical trials. Wiley, Chichester

Black N (1996) Why we need observational studies to evaluate the effectiveness of health care. BMJ 312:1215–1218

Cooper M (2008) Essential research findings in counselling and psychotherapy: the facts are friendly. Sage, Thousand Oaks, CA

Else B, Wheeler B (2010) Music therapy practice: relative perspectives in evidence-based reviews. Nord J Music Ther 19(1):29–50. doi:10.1080/08098130903377407

Eysenck HJ (1952) The effects of psychotherapy: an evaluation. J Consult Psychol 16:319–324

Feaster DJ, Newman FL, Rice C (2003) Longitudinal analysis when the experimenter does not determine when treatment ends: what is dose–response? Clin Psychol Psychother 10(6):352–360

Higgins JPT, Green S (eds) (2008) Cochrane handbook for systematic reviews of interventions. Wiley-Blackwell, Chichester

Hill C, Lambert MJ (2004) Methodological issues in studying psychotherapy processes and outcomes. In: Lambert MJ (ed) Bergin and Garfield's handbook of psychotherapy and behavior change, 5th edn. Wiley, New York, NY, pp 84–135

Hollis S, Campbell F (1999) What is meant by intention-to-treat analysis? Survey of published randomised controlled trials. BMJ 319:670–674

Howard KI, Kopta SM, Krause MS, Orlinsky DE (1986) The dose-effect relationship in psychotherapy. American Psychologist 41(2):159–164

Indrayan A (2008) Medical biostatistics, 2nd edn. Chapman & Hall/CRC, Boca Raton, FL

Kächele H (2010) Therapie-Manual: Forschungsmethode und/oder Praxisrealität? [Therapy manual: research method or practice reality?]. Zeitschrift für Individualpsychologie 35(3):239–248

Lambert MJ (ed) (2004) Bergin and Garfield's handbook of psychotherapy and behavior change, 5th edn. Wiley, New York, NY

Lambert MJ, Ogles BM (2004) The efficacy and effectiveness of psychotherapy. In: Lambert MJ (ed) Bergin and Garfield's handbook of psychotherapy and behavior change, 5th edn. Wiley, New York, NY, pp 139–193

Luborsky L, Diguer L, Seligman DA, Rosenthal R, Krause ED, Johnson S, Halperin G, Bishop M, Berman JS, Schweizer E (1999) The researcher's own therapy allegiances: a "wild card" in comparisons of treatment efficacy. Clin Psychol Sci Pract 6 (1):95–106

Marshall M, Lockwood A, Bradley C, Adams C, Joy C, Fenton M (2000) Unpublished rating scales: a major source of bias in randomised controlled trials of treatments for schizophrenia. Br J Psychiatry 176:249–252

Piper WE, Ogrodniczuk JS (1999) Therapy manuals and the dilemma of dynamically oriented therapists and researchers. Am J Psychother 53(4):467–482

Rolvsjord R, Gold C, Stige B (2005) Research rigour and therapeutic flexibility: rationale for a therapy manual developed for a randomised controlled trial. Nord J Music Ther 14(1):15–32. doi:10.1080/08098130509478122

Rosenthal D, Frank JD (1956) Psychotherapy and the placebo effect. Psychol Bull 53(4):294–302

Roth A, Fonagy P (2005) What works for whom? A critical review of psychotherapy research, 2nd edn. Guilford, New York, NY

Sackett DL, Rosenberg WMC, Gray JAM, Haynes RB, Richardson WS (1996) Evidence based medicine: what it is and what it isn't. BMJ 312:71–72

Seligman MEP (1995) The effectiveness of psychotherapy: The Consumer Reports study. American Psychologist 50(12):965–974

Smith CS, Pell JP (2003) Parachute use to prevent death and major trauma related to gravitational challenge: systematic review of randomised controlled trials. BMJ 327:1459–1461. doi:10.1136/bmj.327.7429.1459

The Cochrane Collaboration (2005) Glossary of terms in the Cochrane Collaboration (Version 4.2.5). Retrieved from http://www.cochrane.org/training/cochrane-handbook

Thornley B, Adams C (1998) Content and quality of 2000 controlled trials in schizophrenia over 50 years. BMJ 317:1181–1184

Thorpe KE, Zwarenstein M, Oxman AD, Treweek S, Furberg CD, Altman DG, Tunis S, Bergel E, Harvey I, Magid DJ, Chalkidou K (2009) A pragmatic-explanatory continuum indicator summary (PRECIS): a tool to help trial designers. J Clin Epidemiol 62:464–475. doi:10.1016/j.jclinepi.2008.12.011

Wampold BE (2001) The great psychotherapy debate: models, methods and findings. Lawrence Erlbaum Associates, Mahwah, NJ

Qualitative Methods in Psychotherapy Outcome Research

27

Brian Rodgers and Robert Elliott

Contents

B. Rodgers (✉)
University of Queensland, Brisbane, Australia
e-mail: research@drbrianrodgers.com

R. Elliott
University of Strathclyde, Glasgow, UK

Abstract

This chapter highlights the potential and variety of qualitative methods that can be applied to counselling and psychotherapy outcome research. The chapter's main focus is on outlining the various forms of qualitative data collection methods that are available to researchers. This is followed by an overview of the various qualitative analysis methods that can be utilised for interpreting the data. Finally, the limitations of qualitative outcome research are discussed, including a number of approaches evaluating the credibility of such research.

27.1 Introduction

At first glance, psychotherapy outcome appears to be a natural for quantitative research: We implicitly think of client distress or symptoms as a kind of fever, something that can be measured by quantitative outcome measures, which provide metaphorical thermometers or psychological pain rulers. Thought of in this way, client change over the course of therapy seems naturally to be a quantitative concept, more a matter of *how much* than of *what* or *how* or *why*. If symptoms or distress decreases by enough, that is a good outcome. What place, then, is there for qualitative methods in

O.C.G. Gelo et al. (eds.), *Psychotherapy Research*,
DOI 10.1007/978-3-7091-1382-0_27, © Springer-Verlag Wien 2015

psychotherapy outcome research? That is the question we will address in this chapter.

We will start with a brief, prima facie case for qualitative outcome research: Compared to the quantitative outcome methods discussed in other chapters of this book (see Chaps. 26, 28, 29 and 30), qualitative research methods operate out of an alternative research paradigm or methodology. Crucially, qualitative methods bring a different set of questions to bear on therapy outcome (Barker et al. 2002). Some of these are questions that are logically prior to quantitative measurement, such as 'What do we mean by outcome?' (=definition) or 'What aspects, kinds or varieties of outcome are there?' (=description). Other questions build on the quantification of client change but seek deeper understanding or explanation, such as 'How does change come about in therapy?' and 'Why did this particular client change over the course of therapy?' These are questions that don't readily lend themselves to quantification and point to an important, but generally overlooked, role for qualitative research on therapy outcome.

Rather than imposing a predefined set of outcome criteria, qualitative outcome research attempts to access the participants' own views and reflections on what has changed for the client over therapy. This offers the potential to reveal new knowledge about the participants' experiences of psychotherapy or counselling (we will use the terms interchangeably here), and the impact this has had on the client in particular. Given this potential, surprisingly few studies have adopted this approach. A decade ago, McLeod (2000b) was able to locate only six published qualitative studies on counselling or psychotherapy outcome. Though additional qualitative outcome studies have been published since (e.g. Rodgers 2002; Klein and Elliott 2006), this approach continues to be underresearched, even as qualitative psychotherapy process research has flourished (see Part II of this book).

This situation is unfortunate, given the foundational nature of basic definitional and descriptive qualitative research questions, which logically should have been carried out *before* undertaking quantitative outcome research: It is always good to know *what* something is before you try to measure *how much* of it is present. This suggests that psychotherapy outcome may have been prematurely quantified, prior to careful definitional and descriptive research. Perhaps because of this, it can be argued that standard quantitative approaches to outcome research (see Chap. 26) have reached the limits of their ability to expand our understanding of the outcomes of counselling and psychotherapy (McLeod 2001a). The drive to gain scientific credibility has tended to limit outcome research to the proof of efficacy rather than the discovery of new knowledge. This has artificially narrowed the scope of psychotherapy outcome to a relatively small range of variables, with no assurance that we are even measuring the right things. Sadly, although several authors have challenged this situation (Levitt et al. 2005; e.g. McLeod 2000a; McLeod 2001a; Rodgers 2003; Slife 2004), these critiques have not yet led to a significant uptake of alternative methods.

In a provocative challenge of the status quo, Slife (2004) outlined several areas in which adopting a positivistic approach has constrained our understanding. He asserts that rather than imposing structure onto and manipulating the data, a qualitative approach invites researchers to come into a much more intimate relationship with the data. Further, Slife suggests that we need a change in orientation of therapy outcome research to look not just at feeling better, but to include more existential dimensions such as having more purpose, understanding things more or helping others. Similarly, there is a need to contextualise outcomes within people's lived worlds, where they act as interdependent, fundamentally social beings in relation to other individuals and to their community and culture. Additionally, rather than looking at single variables, outcome researchers should look for patterns of change among experiences, meanings, relationships, etc.

Such an approach would be relevant not only to groups of individuals (nomothetic research) but also to particular clients' experiences over time (idiographic research). Although quantitative research can be idiographic and qualitative research can be nomothetic, we argue that qualitative methods lend themselves more readily to in-depth studies of an individual's experiences of psychotherapy or counselling. In addition, as McLeod (2001b) contended, qualitative outcome research is more consistent with the practices and values of counselling and psychotherapy, which emphasise human agency, reflexivity and emotion, collaborative and dialogical forms of meaning making, the role of language in constructing realities and the validity of sacred experience.

The purpose of the current chapter is thus to highlight the potential and variety of qualitative methods that can be applied to counselling and psychotherapy outcome research. The chapter's main focus will be on outlining the wide range of qualitative data collection methods available to researchers. This will be followed by an overview of relevant qualitative analysis options. We conclude with a consideration of some of the limitations of qualitative outcome research and how these can be handled.

27.2 Qualitative Outcome Data Collection Methods

Qualitative outcome data collection methods can shed light on the richness and diversity of individual client change (see Table 27.1). Rather than restrict description of client change to discrete, predetermined categories or rating scales, such as problems or symptoms, these approaches access client and therapist's perspectives on client changes over the course of therapy. They offer participants an opportunity to describe changes in a more expansive, open-ended format, thus opening the door to rich, in-depth narratives about client change.

27.2.1 Perspective of Observation

A good starting point in thinking about collecting qualitative data on outcome is the perspective of observation (Elliott 1991), that is, who to ask: client, therapist or outside observer? It is clear from the existing literature that most researchers prefer to ask clients, on the grounds that the client is the person likely to have the most direct information about the changes they have experienced, including aspects of their private experience that might not be apparent to others, including the therapist. This is also our personal view and will be the focus of this chapter.

However, it is worth considering briefly the other possibilities, the most obvious of which is to ask therapists about the changes they have seen in their clients. For one thing, therapists are likely to have more highly differentiated language and perceptual training for discerning changes that clients might not be aware of or notice. They also can typically draw on experience with a broad range of clients, sensitising them to possible changes, some of whom may be quite difficult for clients to access. For example, Traynor et al. (2011) interviewed therapists about their views of the helpful aspects and effects of their work with clients with psychotic processes; unexpectedly, the therapeutic change described most often was not decreased thought disturbance or self-harm but rather increased social adjustment. Finally, it is worth pointing out that therapy affects therapists as well as clients, and a logical place to begin the study of therapist outcomes would be to ask therapists.

Yet another possibility is to use observers, either researchers or significant others, as sources of open-ended data about client outcome. For example, Dreier (2008) had researchers observe clients in their daily lives between sessions. Alternatively, although difficult for both practical and ethical reasons, significant others can be interviewed about changes they may have noticed in the client. (One of us once interviewed a research client's adult daughter, who declared the therapy a failure because her mother now made her do her own laundry.)

Of course, client, therapist and observer perspectives are each fraught with difficulties, some of which we will discuss later on, but asking the client does appear to be the logical starting point. For now, we will simply point out that there are other, rarely considered options for collecting data about client (and therapist) outcome.

Table 27.1 Summary of qualitative outcome data collection methods

Interview-based methods	Ad hoc post-therapy qualitative interviews
	Standardised, semi-structured change interviews: • Change interview • Narrative assessment interview
Other verbally based qualitative data collection methods	Qualitative questionnaires
	Personal documents as qualitative data : • Diaries, journals and personal logs • Letter to a friend • Autobiographical and personal accounts of therapy • Auto-ethnography
Visual approaches to qualitative data collection	Photos and video
	Projective drawings
	Timelines and lifelines
	Mapping techniques

27.2.2 Interview-Based Qualitative Data Collection

The most common method for collecting qualitative data on the outcomes of counselling and psychotherapy entails some form of recorded interview. Typically, this approach uses an interview guide consisting of a list of questions or topics that a participant is generally free to respond to in their own way. This allows the person to voice the aspects or dimensions of therapy outcome that are most personally significant for them. Qualitative interviews assessing outcome include ad hoc and standardised formats.

27.2.2.1 Ad Hoc Post-therapy Qualitative Interviews

We begin by considering one-shot interview schedules designed for use in a single study. This approach involves the researcher interviewing several clients at some period after the completion of therapy, typically using a semi-structured interview schedule designed by the researcher for the specific aims of a particular study. Typically, interviews are recorded and transcribed and then analysed using some form of qualitative analysis (see Sect. 27.3 of this chapter).

McLeod's (2000b) review of qualitative outcome research found that studies that adopt this approach (e.g. Howe 1989, 1996) demonstrate that clients possess their own criteria for evaluating therapy, that clients are able to differentiate between change attributed to therapy and change attributed to other life factors and that it is possible to make confident statements of success or failure on the basis of qualitative data. Additionally, Rodgers (2003) argues that this approach to researching the outcomes of therapy not only yields interesting results but also allows researchers to identify the reasons behind the results. For example, in the study by Howe (1989) cited above, in addition to finding that therapy was not as successful as expected, researchers were able to identify several reasons for clients' discontent about the results of their therapy, which then allowed actual changes in practice to be implemented. As such, studies that utilise this method offer the opportunity to provide practitioners with valuable feedback into how their practice is actually being received by clients.

This approach offers the opportunity for clients to express in detail their retrospective reflections on the significance of the changes from before until after therapy. Further, the researcher is able to dialogue with participants in order to check out their understanding and to explore things at greater depth (Kvale 1996). This offers the potential for a rich set of results that more fully capture each individual's experience, including the nuances and subtleties of change. It also offers the client the opportunity to reflect on and consolidate any changes that may have occurred during therapy and to identify any areas that may still need attending to. In this sense, well-conducted post-therapy interviews, in any format, can be seen to offer clients a research procedure aligned to and compatible with their therapy, making it an example of evaluation research that supports rather than detracts from the intervention it evaluates (Patton 1997). Thus, a good ad hoc post-therapy qualitative interview includes specific questions relevant to the researcher's key interests, helps participants provide specific detail about their experiences, goes beyond superficial description to provide understanding, offers practitioners useful feedback and helps clients consolidate therapeutic benefits.

27.2.2.2 Standardised, Semi-structured Change Interviews

Standardising research procedures increases opportunities for comparing results across studies and for building cumulative knowledge. Standardised semi-structured interviews focusing on the client's perceptions of the outcomes of counselling and psychotherapy allow this possibility. Here the approach taken is not so much to ask questions about a specific research topic but rather to collect a general set of qualitative data that can be used in various ways.

27.2.2.2.1 The Change Interview

The Change Interview (Elliott 1999) is a good example of this approach to qualitative outcome data collection. The protocol guides a 60- to 90-min interview that can be administered at the end of therapy and at regular intervals throughout therapy. The interview questions attempt to explore the changes that a person has noticed since therapy began, what the person attributes these changes to, and the helpful and unhelpful aspects of therapy. In the current version of the interview (Elliott and Rodgers 2008), clients are also asked about what resources (personal strengths or things in their life situation) that they feel have helped them to make use of the therapy, as well as any limitations (personal weaknesses or difficulties in their life situation) that have made it harder for them to make use of therapy. The interview also includes questions about the research.

This broad-spectrum approach potentially offers participants more opportunity to tell their story compared to interview schedules that focus on a specific research question. Further, the interview schedule specifically focuses on the participant's attributions of any changes, allowing for change factors outside of therapy to be differentiated from those within therapy. Additionally, the questions on the resources and limitations of a person's life situation allow a more contextualised view of therapy outcomes to be obtained.

Clearly, clients' views of the outcome of their therapy are only one aspect of the Change Interview. However, this aspect is central to the Change Interview: First, outcome is operationalised in terms of 'changes since therapy started'. Second, a set of follow-up questions is used to encourage clients to reflect in detail and at length, including liberal use of the 'Anything else?' question. Third, negative or missing changes are specifically inquired about. Here is the relevant section of the interview schedule, including interviewer instructions:

> 2a. What changes, if any, have you noticed in yourself since therapy started?
>
> *(Interviewer: Reflect back change to client and write down brief versions of the changes for later. If it is helpful, you can use some of these follow-up questions: For example, Are you doing, feeling, or thinking differently from the way you did before? What specific ideas, if any, have you gotten from therapy so far, including ideas about yourself or other people? Have any changes been brought to your attention by other people?)*
>
> 2b. Has anything changed for the worse for you since therapy started?
>
> 2c. Is there anything that you wanted to change that hasn't since therapy started?

This approach to qualitative research allows a standard set of data to be collected at different stages of therapy. By undertaking interviews at various mid-therapy points (e.g. after every 10 sessions), problems associated with both data loss due to dropout and retrospective recall are reduced.

A further benefit of this standardised approach is that it allows similar information to be obtained across different clients, research projects, settings or even different cultures. For example, comparative studies could be undertaken comparing the similarities and differences between a North American university setting and a German outpatient clinic. The key point here is that the structured approach offers the opportunity for researchers to utilise the data in different ways at different times, rather than being restricted to a single study intended to answer a specific research question as with ad hoc qualitative interviews. Researchers can effectively recycle collected data from one study to the next, rather than it going to waste once a study is completed. Additionally, later researchers can retrospectively mine the data for their specific research interests. This reusability factor offers a significant benefit particularly for settings such as university research clinics whereby many researchers can form a shared data collective rather than needing to recruit participants individually.

27.2.2.2.2 The Narrative Assessment Interview: A Pre-post Qualitative Interview

Post-therapy qualitative interviews require clients to implicitly compare their pre- and post-therapy psychological states in order to identify changes. However, retrospective data collection is subject to fading of memory and schema-based shifts and distortions of memories over time. One way around these problems is to conduct qualitative interviews at the beginning of therapy and to compare these to similar interviews conducted after therapy is completed.

The Narrative Assessment Interview (NAI) is an extension of the Change Interview that assesses the outcomes of therapy in terms of changes in the client's macro-narrative or self story (Hardtke and Angus 2004). This approach differs from the standardised, semi-structured interview approach taken with the Change Interview in that the content of the pre-therapy interview can be actively used in the post-therapy interview as a point of reference for the participant to reflect on any changes that have occurred.

NAI protocol consists of three stages: (a) a brief, semi-structured interview conducted after the first session of therapy, (b) a summary of the main aspects of this initial interview and (c) a post-therapy reflection interview. The first-stage interview is intended to be a collaborative exploration of the client's story about self and the views they hold about others' perceptions of them. To facilitate this exploration, three questions are asked:

- How would you describe yourself?
- How would someone who knows you really well describe you?
- If you could change something about who you are, what would you change?

The first two questions are accompanied by an empathic exploration of what emerges, along with a request for recent examples from the person's life to illustrate the points raised. The final question is intended to gain an understanding of what the client hopes to change over the course of therapy and to provide a concrete pre-therapy reference point for the participant to reflect upon at the end of therapy. In the second stage of the protocol, the recording of the initial interview is comprehensively summarised by the researcher to provide a written record of key descriptors. During the final post-therapy interview stage of the protocol, clients are asked to read and critically reflect upon the summary of their initial research interview, in order to facilitate a critical inquiry into their experiences of any change during therapy.

A significant advantage of this approach compared to other qualitative interview protocols is that it offers the field of counselling and psychotherapy outcome research a qualitative approach to a pre-post therapy design. Rather than relying on the client's retrospective recollection of change since therapy began, data are collected at the pre-therapy stage providing the equivalent of a baseline measure. These data can then be directly compared to the client's post-therapy self-descriptions. Additionally, clients are able to define their own criteria about what they are looking to change in therapy and are able to evaluate the significance of changes based on their own perception of the difference in their self-statements. This provides a truly client-oriented approach to assessing the outcomes of therapy and the opportunity to self-evaluate change based on explicit pre-therapy statements rather than having to rely on retrospective recall alone. In this way, the method can be seen as a form of assisted reflexivity (Rodgers 2010).

This key advantage does, however, introduce a number of complexities. In the protocol as described above, the client is reliant on the researcher's summary of the key points of the pre-therapy interview, with the potential for significant loss of content and verbal nuance. Further, this process is highly labour intensive and time critical for the researcher, who must ensure the transcription and summary are completed before therapy finishes. Whilst this may be easily managed in a focused, time-limited research project, it is likely to be more difficult to use more broadly.

27.2.2.3 Summary of Findings of Interview-Based Qualitative Outcome Research

Only qualitative interview studies of therapy outcome exist in sufficient numbers to allow any sort of summary to be made. Timulak and Creaner (2010) have recently published a qualitative meta-analysis of eight studies of client post-therapy changes in humanistic psychotherapy (the topic of most of the existing literature). They reviewed the categories (see Sect. 27.3.2 below) identified in these studies, grouping them into 11 meta-categories shared across studies. These meta-categories fell into three larger meta-categories: *appreciating experiences of self, appreciating experience of self in relation to others, and changed view of self/others*. Their broad division of client post-therapy outcomes into changes in internal self processes vs. changes in self in relation to others replicates an earlier qualitative meta-analysis of a smaller number of qualitative outcome studies (Elliott 2002b). One of Timulak and Creaner's categories occurred in almost all (7 out of 8) of the studies reviewed, *feeling empowered*, making it potentially a key constituent of client outcome. Five other categories also occurred in at least half of the studies, suggesting that they are typical of client post-therapy changes: *smoother and healthier emotional experience, appreciating vulnerability, experience of self-compassion, self-insight/self-awareness* and *enjoying interpersonal encounters*.

27.2.3 Other Verbally Based Qualitative Data Collection Methods

Although interviews are the most common source of qualitative data, numerous other methods exist that have the potential to provide alternative views on the outcomes of therapy. The following section outlines a variety of verbally or linguistic-based methods that utilise language as the primary mechanism for both requesting and recording qualitative data.

27.2.3.1 Qualitative Questionnaires

The simplest alternative to interviews is the use of questionnaires that include some form of open-response questions that allow respondents to reply more fully than in the predetermined format of purely quantitative questionnaires. This approach typically asks more specific questions than in a semi-structured interview schedule whilst at the same time providing more limited opportunity for a client to respond. As this type of questionnaire is relatively simple to construct and cost-effective to implement, this approach is often used by counselling organisations as part of an ad hoc programme evaluation process to gain qualitative information about client benefits of services offered (e.g. Bende and Crossley 2000). However, due to the limits of space and lack of ability to interact with the respondent to check out and request elaboration of client responses, this approach typically produces thin protocols and is thus of limited use for systematic qualitative investigations into the outcomes of therapy. Despite this, the use of qualitative questionnaires alongside standardised outcome measures would seem to be useful in routine service evaluation, given that it offers clients a chance to have their voice heard more directly.

27.2.3.2 Personal Documents as Qualitative Data

The use of personal documents as qualitative data offers a number of potential benefits for researching the outcomes of counselling and psychotherapy. Allport (1942), for example, contended that the use of personal documents in psychological research provides a touchstone for the results of other methods, a more common sense, naturalistic and idiographic approach that can counter the focus on abstract findings derived from nomothetic methods. In particular, qualitative personal documents allow researchers to access a person's subjective experience contextualised within their everyday life, rather than being limited to data collected within a research or therapeutic setting. This sets them apart from qualitative interviews, which are typically conducted in the researcher's territory (either physically or psychologically). Similarly, personal documents allow researchers to see into a person's lived world as it is experienced, rather than as it is recalled in a research interview, and in this way offer a solution to the problem of retrospective recall (Bolger et al. 2003). Further, when utilised in a longitudinal design (such as with diaries), personal documents offer a method for the researcher to gain a more fine-grained access to complex, self-regulating processes, allowing them to watch the course of development and change over time (Schmitz and Wiese 2006).

27.2.3.2.1 Diaries, Journals and Personal Logs

Qualitative personal documents with potential for studying therapy outcome include diaries, journals and personal logs, methods that involve data collection carried out at regular intervals over time. This approach asks a participant to maintain a written account of their experiences, either in a structured manner (e.g. behaviour log) or more free-form manner (e.g. personal diary). These methods can be utilised to gather data at a specific interval (*interval contingent*. e.g. the end of the day), on a predetermined signal (*signal contingent,* e.g. a phone call from the researcher) or after a defined event (*event contingent,* e.g. after a panic attack) (Wheeler and Reis 1991). Recent advances in technology have even enabled researchers to automate the data collection process in the form of ecological momentary assessment (EMA) (Stone and Shiffman 1994; Shiffman et al. 2008). This entails the moment-to-moment recording of data on a pocket computer or PDA in real-world settings such that details like current date, time, location, etc. are recorded along with more qualitative data such as what the person is feeling, thinking or experiencing at that moment.

Though structured diaries, journals and logs have become a popular method for client self-monitoring within behavioural approaches in psychology (Korotitsch and Nelson-Gray 1999), surprisingly few researchers have employed diaries to gather more detailed qualitative data for their therapy research. In a review of qualitative diary studies in psychotherapy research, Mackrill (2008) was only able to identify four published accounts, all largely verbatim reports from clients which had not been formally analysed in any systematic way. Mackrill contrasts these unsolicited diary reports with solicited diaries used in other forms of social science research. Here, participants are specifically requested to write about an area of interest relevant to the research being undertaken, rather than whatever spontaneously arises. This provides a focus for the diary content, allowing a systematic analysis similar to that undertaken with qualitative interviews discussed above.

27.2.3.2.2 Letter to a Friend

An interesting example of the use of personal documents for qualitative psychotherapy outcome data collection is a study by Burnett (1999; Burnett and Van Dorssen 2000). Burnett utilised a 'letter to a friend' method adapted from the Structure of Observed Learning Outcome (SOLO) taxonomy used for the assessment of learning in an educational context (Boulton-Lewis 1995). Burnett's (1999) adaptation of this protocol was a tentative attempt to explore the utility of the letter to a friend (LTF) technique in combination with the SOLO taxonomy to assess the structure of learning gained from counselling. The protocol requested clients to write a letter to a friend describing in as much detail as possible what they had learned and how they had gained or benefited from counselling. This innovative data collection method appears to have yielded in-depth responses from clients enabling a detailed qualitative analysis and evaluation of the outcomes of therapy.

27.2.3.2.3 Autobiographical and Personal Accounts of Therapy

Though typically not intended as a direct source of qualitative data on the outcomes of counselling and psychotherapy, client autobiographical and personal accounts potentially offer a unique insight into what individuals have got out of their therapy. Books such as Alexander's (1995) '*Folie a deux: An experience of one-to-one therapy*' and Sands' (2000) '*Falling for therapy: Psychotherapy from a client's point of view*' along with journal articles such as Bassman (2000, 2001) and Tenney (2000) would seem to offer a valuable insight into clients' changes over the course of therapy. The potential here is that such accounts can be searched in order to hear what people are saying spontaneously about what they got out of psychotherapy. For example, the account by Tenney (2000) argues that what consumers want is recovery-focused mental health services that go beyond symptom reduction and offer 'the sense of empowerment, and the problem-solving skills that gear people toward recovery' (p. 1441).

Similarly, the use of personal accounts of therapy in the form of internet discussion groups, chat room dialogue, web logs (blogs) and social network sites such as Facebook and MySpace offers a wealth of naturalistic texts spanning a significant duration of time, thus giving a more longitudinal perspective on outcomes than is traditionally considered (Murray and Sixsmith 2002).

27.2.3.2.4 Auto-ethnography

Though the above sources of personal accounts do not yet seem to have been utilised in qualitative psychotherapy research, a similar approach, in the form of auto-ethnography, has. Auto-ethnography is a blend of ethnography and autobiography (Scott-Hoy 2002) offering the potential for clients as researchers to tell their own story within the context of formal research. It entails the client-researcher performing some form of narrative analysis on their own lived experience in order to explicate a phenomenon of interest (McIlveen 2008). The aim is to extend and enhance both the client-researcher's and the reader's understanding of the issue being investigated (Sparkes 2000). An example of this approach in the field of counselling is a study by Etherington (2005) into the experiences of people who have suffered childhood trauma. Etherington gathered 10 participants' stories (including her own) showing how they had made sense of childhood trauma and the ways they had found to heal. This study demonstrates the potential to hear detailed, reflective accounts of client's situated experiences of healing, which could be used to help inform us of beneficial and problematic outcomes of therapeutic interventions, as well as contextualising these within a wider set of resources.

27.2.4 Visual Approaches to Qualitative Data Collection

Though verbal or linguistic approaches such as interviews and personal documents seem the most obvious method for collecting qualitative data, visual methods offer an intriguing alternative that is not solely reliant on or limited to the spoken or written word. Sperry (1973) argued that science, and indeed modern society in general, has tended to favour linguistic and symbolic functioning associated with the left hemisphere of the brain at the expense of other, more holistic forms of functioning. Deacon (2000) contends that this traditional privileging of numbers and words over other forms of data has inherently limited our ability to study complex, dynamic systems. In contrast, Oster and Gould Crone (2004) propose that visual methods offer a form of communication with a richness, uniqueness, complexity and spontaneity that is not usually available through words alone. Further, Przyborski and Slunecko (2012) argue that images inherently structure how we perceive the world around us, and by embracing this, radical new approaches to data collection and analysis methods may become available which are not constrained by traditional language-based methodologies.

27.2.4.1 Photos and Video

The use of photos and video as a qualitative data collection method has gained increasing acceptance and usage within several fields (e.g. anthropology, health and nursing studies; Knoblauch et al. 2008). In particular, participatory approaches to visual data collection have been conducted with participants taking photos Kaplan 2008) and compiling video footage (Haw 2008) from their own perspective in order to give researchers a different picture, literally through a different lens. As a potential tool for counselling and psychotherapy outcome research, however, it is not clear how well these methods can give access the participants' inner worlds. Whilst photos and video are convenient for recording the world around us, they do not directly capture the thoughts, feelings and emotions that accompany the recorded scene. These issues may explain the lack of uptake of this approach in counselling and psychotherapy outcome research. At this time, no studies have been found that attempt to use these visual self-report methods of data collection.

27.2.4.2 Projective Drawings

In contrast to documentary use of photos and video, the use of projective drawings or art products offer a clearer route for gaining access to the hidden inner world of participants. The basic premise of projective techniques is that everyone to some degree projects their own traits, attributes or subjective processes onto what they perceive or express (Semeonoff 1976). Projective techniques attempt to make use of this, typically by providing relatively unstructured or ambiguous stimuli or tasks and then observing how an individual perceives, interprets or structures these. An example of this approach is Buck's (1949) House-Tree-Person technique, which simply asks a person to draw a picture of a house, a tree and a person. The instructions are left purposefully vague so as to facilitate the projection of the participant onto the task.

Anastasi (1988) suggests that projective techniques may work best as a supplement to qualitative interviewing. Used in this way, they may act to break the ice during the initial contact with a researcher, by providing a more interesting and entertaining method for engaging participants than standardised questionnaires. Further, Begley and Lewis (1998) propose that this approach may be especially valuable in facilitating communication with participants with reduced language comprehension and expression abilities. Further, projective drawings constitute a permanent sample of a participant's behaviour that can be used for comparison in longitudinal studies. Seen from this perspective, projective techniques would appear to offer a valuable adjunct to qualitative research interviews and could be utilised in a pre-post design offering a method for comparing the qualities of a client's responses from before to after therapy (see Flitton and Buckroyd 2002, for an example of a study which utilises this approach).

27.2.4.3 Timelines and Lifelines

In contrast to projective drawings that generally attempt to reveal the unconscious meaning of pictures, drawing techniques can also be utilised in a more straightforward, direct manner as tools to help research participants provide information. For example, methods such as timelines and lifelines offer a way for researchers to facilitate a structured recall of a sequence of previous events, particularly within the context of qualitative interviews. These methods are especially useful for gathering information of a longitudinal nature, such as a life history, rather than focusing on isolated or single events (Deacon 2000). The method typically uses some form of line with linear markings to represent events of interest (Tracz and Gehart-Brooks 1999). Depending on the participant's drawing style and the nature of the research task, lines can be straight (e.g. Brott 2004) or more curved and 'windy' (e.g. Guenette and Marshall 2009). Events may be marked using simple cross marks with labels, or with diagrammatic and pictorial representations (Tracz and Gehart-Brooks 1999). Guenette and Marshall (2009) propose that timelines are particularly useful when research involves participants recalling sensitive or emotionally charged material. Here the timeline can act as a representational anchor, allowing sensitive topics to first be tentatively marked on the line before being discussed at greater depth.

Within the field of counselling and psychotherapy research, McKenna and Todd (1997) used timelines to investigate how people accessed therapy at different times in their lives. Participants were asked to construct a timeline of their contact with various mental health services. Following this, semi-structured interviews were used for a detailed discussion of each event. Transcripts of these interviews were then analysed in order to extract the dominant themes within and across individuals. In terms of the use of the timeline method, the researchers were able to elicit rich individual accounts that provided detailed narrative examples of the various types of therapy episode. These included *exposure* to the possibility of help before shopping around or *discriminating* a suitable service. Participants also described later *formation* episodes where significant and lasting change took place, followed by *consolidation* and *holding* episodes. This study demonstrates a very different view of outcome than is traditionally considered and demonstrates that individuals look for different types of outcome at different stages in their lives.

27.2.4.4 Mapping Techniques

Similar to timelines and lifelines, mapping techniques provide a method of representation that can be used to help participants to structurally organise and recall information. Whereas timelines provide a method for linearly representing longitudinal data, maps are 'graphic representations that facilitate a spatial understanding of things, concepts, conditions, processes, or events in the human world' (Harley and Woodward 1987, p. xvi). Various mapping techniques have been used in the fields of social work, family therapy and elsewhere where representing the individual as part of a wider system is recognised as important. These techniques include ecomaps (Hartman 1995), social network maps (Tracy and Whittaker 1990), node-link maps (Dees et al. 1994) and various other structured and unstructured approaches such as flow charts, floor plans and life space maps (Peavy 1997, 2004).

Rodgers (2010) recently developed the approach of life space mapping (LSM) to explicitly investigate the outcomes of counselling and psychotherapy. Using this technique, participants are asked to complete an LSM before and after therapy. Participants start with a blank sheet of paper onto which they represent themselves and their personal world, including their present situation. The person is encouraged to use lines, images, colours, words, sentences and symbols to construct a visual representation of their feelings, thoughts, actions and situational details that have meaning in relation to their current concern. After completing their post-therapy LSM, clients are presented with their pre-therapy LSM and asked to reflect on any differences between their maps. This approach has been found to offer an evocative point of reference for participants to reconnect with their pre-therapy life situation. This is significant as participants reported 'forgetting how bad it was' and having lost sight of the reasons they initially came to therapy. Further, the mapping technique tended to decentralise the significance of therapy as a change factor, allowing participants to recall 'what is different from then until now' rather than 'what has changed since therapy began'. Participants also reported that the method allowed them to identify less conscious aspects of change. These points indicate the value of utilising a visual approach as a different culturally based tool (Peavy 1999) for investigating the outcomes of counselling and psychotherapy, allowing different stories to be told by participants and heard by the researcher than would be possible using a purely verbal approach.

27.3 Qualitative Outcome Data Analysis

One of the biggest challenges to qualitative outcome research is the analysis of the rich data sets provided by the data collection methods discussed above. It is not unusual for a qualitative interview to last 60 to 90 minutes, with the resulting transcription of at least 30 pages. Similarly, personal diaries and other documents may amount to hundreds of pages over time. Even more challenging is the analysis of visual forms of data. Given these challenges, it is easy to see why quantitative measures have been favoured, as they provide an elegant method for efficiently reducing potentially vast amounts of data into simple to comprehend results.

There is nothing unique about qualitative outcome data that requires them to be analysed differently from qualitative process data, which means that the options will be generally the same as those described in Part II of this book (see Chap. 20 and 21 for an overview). Most commonly, standard qualitative analysis methods are used, such as varieties of grounded theory (Chap. 22), or conversation/discourse analysis (Chaps. 24 and 25). In addition, a promising approach to interpreting and synthesising rich qualitative outcome data is the interpretive case study method (e.g. Elliott et al. 2009). Here we will focus on the main research questions that are commonly addressed to qualitative outcome data and the analyses that lend themselves to answering those research questions (see Table 27.2).

27.3.1 Descriptive Analyses of Rates or Frequencies: Quantitative Content Analysis

Although qualitative in form, it is not difficult to analyse client descriptions of the effects of therapy using predefined categories or rating scales, a method usually referred to as content analysis. Content analysis (Krippendorff 2003) typically uses predefined categories and then counts the number of occurrences of that category in the data. For example, client open-ended descriptions of what has changed over the course of therapy can be subjected to content analysis to identify frequencies of predefined concepts. For example, Klein and Elliott (2006) used a simple framework of domains of life functioning developed in previous research (Barkham et al. 1996) to classify the content of client post-therapy changes. Traditionally, content analysis has involved assignment of units of text to mutually exclusive and exhaustive categories (e.g. Klein and Elliott 2006: mood symptoms vs. relationships, etc.). However, a more sensitive approach is to treat the concepts as separate rating scale items rather than categories: One or more concepts can be rated for degree of presence on a simple 4-point rating scale: 0 = 'clearly absent', 1 = 'probably absent', 2 = 'probably present', 3 = 'clearly present'. Elliott et al. (1985) used this approach to rate the effects of significant therapy events (within-session outcome) for insight, problem solution, reassurance, etc. This approach makes it possible to work with more complex qualitative descriptions.

Quantitative content analysis can also be useful for working with visual data. For example, the Formal Elements Art Therapy Scale (FEATS) devised by Gantt and Tabone (Gantt 1998; Gantt and Tabone 2003) utilises rating scales that describe the content of a drawing along predefined artistic criteria. Using this approach, drawings can be rated according to prominence of colour, implied energy, space, integration, logic, realism, problem-solving, level of detail, line quality, etc. For example, prominence of colour is rated on a 5-point scale from 'colour used for outlining only' (0) to 'colour used to fill all available space' (5), whilst line quality is rated from 'broken, damaged lines' (0) to 'fluid, flowing lines' (5). Similarly, the video transcription system MoVIQ (Movies and Videos in Qualitative Social Research) provides a systematic method for film and video interpretation

Table 27.2 Summary of qualitative data analysis methods

Descriptive analyses of rates or frequencies	e.g. Quantitative content analysis
Exploratory analyses of kinds or aspects	e.g. Grounded theory and variants
Interpretive case studies/credibility analysis	e.g. Hermeneutic single-case efficacy design

(Hampl 2008). Like the FEATS system for drawings, this approach aims to analyse the formal structure of visual data, in this case moving pictures. For example, segments of video may be categorised in terms of their formal composition such as planimetric composition, perspective projection and scenic choreography.

This form of content analysis thus converts qualitative raw data into quantitative rates or frequencies, which lend themselves to comparison over time and can be used for assessing pre-post change. More importantly, however, this makes it possible to compare data from case to case, across types of therapy or settings or even across studies if the same coding strategy is employed. Much larger amounts of data can be summarised and compared in this way.

27.3.2 Exploratory Analyses of Kinds or Aspects: Grounded Theory and Variants

Often, when faced with a body of qualitative descriptions of outcome, a therapy researcher does not necessarily want to be restricted to a pre-existing set of concepts such as is required for content analysis discussed above. This is particularly the case with new kinds of psychotherapy or counselling (e.g. motivational interviewing) or applications to new client populations (e.g. social anxiety) or in new settings (e.g. groups). Here, the researcher wants to get a broad picture of the *kinds* or *aspects* of client change that are possible. For example, in addition to doing a content analysis of client descriptions of change, Klein and Elliott (2006) also carried out a grounded theory analysis, using the open-coding procedure described by Strauss and Corbin (1998). They found a hierarchical set of categories, with five categories nested within two broader domains: changes within the self (affective change, self-improvement, experiential processing) and changes in life situation (general life functioning, interpersonal relationships); each of the five categories had 2–5 subcategories that defined them in richer detail and went far beyond the generalities of the parallel content analysis they also conducted.

Grounded theory and related methods of qualitative analysis, such as interpretative phenomenological analysis (IPA: Smith et al. 2009) and consensual qualitative analysis (CQR: Hill et al. 1997), require a deeper, more careful reading and a creative process of constructing categories that capture the data nicely. They are therefore more time-consuming than the content analysis procedures described above but produce much richer, more textured accounts of how clients change in therapy, pointing towards new understandings. Even closer readings are possible with discourse or conversation analysis, as illustrated by Elliott's (2006) analysis of how clients construct accounts of having attained insight in therapy, which identified a set of linguistic markers (e.g. 'realise/real'), metaphors (e.g. external force: 'it *makes* me feel good') and contents (e.g. interpersonal patterns vs. specific emotions).

Exploratory methods for analysing visual data are yet to be fully utilised in the field of counselling and psychotherapy outcome research. At present, studies have tended to focus on an exploratory analysis of what images have meant to the client. For example, Rodgers (2010) analysed the qualities of perceived change from therapy using life space maps (LSMs) and found this visual data evoked dimensions of reflexivity such as 'spatiality', 'metaphor' and 'imagery' that other purely verbal methods may not have. Clearly there is potential here to utilise visual data more fully in the analysis process, for example, by requiring the researcher to attend to what the data evoke in them and including this in the process of category formation.

27.3.3 Interpretive Case Studies/ Credibility Analysis

A recent application of qualitative outcome research is within the context of an interpretive case study such as Hermeneutic Single-Case Efficacy Design (HSCED: Elliott 2002a; Elliott et al. 2009). HSCED studies offer an alternative to randomised clinical trials for single therapy cases. Qualitative outcome data play a critical role in the first aspect of HSCED studies, determining whether a client has changed over therapy, and are routinely included in the form of the Change Interview transcripts and excerpts. HSCED also illustrates the importance of incorporating qualitative outcome data within a mixed method or pluralistic research approach (Klein and Elliott 2006). Rich case studies are able to bring together different forms of evidence to present a coherent narrative of individual change. In this way, the different forms of data collection methods discussed above can be brought together, potentially including more traditional quantitative measures.

The HSCED method follows a legalistic model of research, in which two perspectives—affirmative and sceptic—are systematically brought to bear on the available quantitative and qualitative outcome data. In this context, qualitative outcome data from the Change Interview, described earlier in this chapter, are used to interrogate the validity of the quantitative outcome data, and vice versa. In addition to comparing and contrasting qualitative and quantitative outcome data, the manner and content of qualitative client outcome descriptions are examined closely for evidence of attempts to please the research team or therapist (deference) or to convince themselves that they have changed in the absence of actual change. Thus, researchers look carefully for evidence of exaggeration of change or downplaying of continuing difficulties or disappointments; they also look for the presence of idiosyncratic descriptions of change that go beyond vague assertions ('Yeah, a lot has changed, you know') or shared cultural stereotypes about the nature of psychotherapeutic change ('lots of insights into myself'). Often, the verdict of the judges to whom the affirmative and sceptic cases are submitted turns on the credibility of the client as a witness to their own outcome, as evidenced in their qualitative accounts of change (e.g. Stephen et al. 2011).

27.4 Limitations and Credibility of Qualitative Outcome Research

Although qualitative methods offer a rich and in-depth approach to investigating the outcomes of counselling and psychotherapy, they also pose several challenges and limitations. In this section, we briefly review some of these limitations and how they can be addressed.

27.4.1 Reliance on Retrospective Recall

Probably the most critical concern with most qualitative outcome methods is their reliance on the client's retrospective recall of the changes that have occurred over the course of therapy. Especially for studies conducted in real-world settings, where therapy may last for several months or even years, accurately recalling what life was like before therapy began may be problematic. In these instances, qualitative methods place a heavy burden on the participant to try to recall what life was like before therapy and to identify changes that have come about during this particular time period, which may not be particularly distinct in the client's mind. Further, the process of therapy may well alter the participant's fundamental views of themselves and their world, even leading them to reinterpret their life before therapy, which may now seem like looking at a different person.

Utilising mid-therapy interviews such as with the Change Interview may reduce the scale of the problem, as clients are asked to recall changes over a shorter duration (usually 6–10 sessions). However, only by using pre-post interviews such as with the Narrative Assessment Interview can this limitation truly be addressed. Unfortunately, this approach introduces its own complexities in the form of requiring significant analysis and processing of pre-therapy data by the researcher prior to the end of therapy interview. The use of visual methods such as life space mapping may help overcome this limitation, by providing clients with a visual framework to stimulate recall, without relying on researcher interpretation. Nevertheless, the problem of unreliable retrospective recall remains.

27.4.2 Researcher-Centric Focus

In addition, qualitative outcome methods are also limited by the researcher's selection of interview and research questions, regardless of whether these are ad hoc or standardised. Studies are typically designed to satisfy researcher curiosity, not to help clients express their perceptions of therapy outcome. For example, the researcher will usually inform the participant of the aims of the study beforehand and have a set of questions designed to match their central research question. This also comes into play in the analysis of the interviews, as a matter of necessity: All forms of qualitative analysis entail a reduction of data across interviews, dependent on the interests of the researcher and what they choose to extract from the interview. These factors inherently shift the focus towards the researcher's perspective and away from the client's, so that the participant's experience is inevitably filtered by the researcher.

Personal documents do allow a more client-centric view. Here the client is largely writing for themselves rather than for the researcher; the researcher is just another reader of the material. This means the client is more in control of how much and what they choose to write about. Further, there is some evidence that people find it less threatening to reveal personal and sensitive material in writing compared to a face to face interview, especially online (Murray and Sixsmith 2002). Additionally, such material is often available in the public domain (in the form of published books or online discussion forums), so that researchers do not overtly intrude into the person's life in accessing the data. Although undoubtedly subject to self-presentation biases, this form of data collection could be seen as the least problematic for clients, as they are not directly involved with the research.

Perhaps the most client-centric form of qualitative outcome research, which does not subsume the client's voice at all, is that of auto-ethnography, where the researcher's voice and that of the client are one and the same. Here the author is much more aware of and in control of the potential implications of their involvement. Within the mental health professions, this method can also be seen as professionally beneficial with regard to furthering self-awareness as a reflective practitioner, in terms of greater self knowledge, and understanding of one's own thoughts, feelings and experiences (Foster et al. 2006).

27.4.3 Isolated Findings

As noted earlier, qualitative investigations of client-perceived outcomes have generally been governed by the idiosyncratic interests of different researchers, leading to a disparate and difficult-to-synthesise research literature. The tendency has been for each study to employ different research questions and forms of analysis. Although this approach offers a rich diversity of results and can give us a detailed insight into different aspects of therapy, the overall picture is not coherent or cumulative, resulting in a fragmented field that is difficult to interpret in any unified way (McLeod 2001c). Though it can be argued that this approach contributes to local knowledge specific to the individual setting and context of each study (McLeod 1999), it also means that policy makers cannot incorporate the results in standards and guidelines for practice. This raises the ethical question of whether it is justifiable to conduct research that may be of greater benefit for the researcher than for the wider field.

27.4.4 Confidentiality Issues

Because qualitative data are by nature much richer, issues of confidentiality and informed consent become more complex. For this reason extra care needs to be taken at all points in the research process: with the informed consent, with the storing and processing of data and with the presentation of quoted or summarised material in scientific presentations and publications. For example, procedures are needed for disguising or anonymising data during collection, storage and write-up. Whilst quantitative data are naturally anonymised, qualitative data are naturally identifying.

Storage of data over months or years as part of large archival data sets presents particular challenges to securing the confidentiality of client data. For example, digital recordings of Change Interviews need to be secured and encrypted on whatever computer media they are held, whilst the data themselves may be used for different purposes than originally conceived. A potential concern for clients participating in such studies, however, is the very longevity of the data archive that makes it advantageous to researchers. Rather than the data collected being used for a specific purpose and then destroyed, it may instead be archived and reused for purposes very different from those proposed in the original research study where the data were collected. For example, the researcher may have originally planned to map types of helpful therapy factors via grounded theory but later find themselves carrying out a discourse analysis about the moral dimension of participating in research or, alternatively, engaging in a legalistic scrutiny of credibility of descriptions of post-therapy changes with an adjudicated case study.

Careful attention to wording of information sheets and consent forms is therefore essential to ensure that participants have sufficient understanding of the consequences of their participation. However, even the most diligent of consent processes cannot allow for the unknown of the future. What may have been fine for a participant to express during the initial research interview may take on a very different significance and meaning at a later date. The general consent given previously with good intentions may become obsolete and invalid from the participant's perspective in years to come. Hence it would seem important to implement ethical practices such as requiring future researchers to seek explicit additional consent for further uses of the collected data.

A further and highly complicated ethical issue is raised by case study research, which as a matter of standard practice needs to provide enough significant detail about the client to make the case come alive. Doing this requires that researchers hide or disguise key facts about the client that could reveal their identity to others. But what about the possibility that the client might recognise themselves in a publication, from a particularly memorable turn of phrase or a drawing? It appears to us virtually impossible to ensure against client self-recognition in case study write-ups. What should be done in such cases? McLeod (2010) now argues that case study research requires specific rather than generic consent. The additional steps include explicit prior permission for use of client material in case studies, and, going beyond this, asking clients to review descriptions of themselves in articles prior to publication, or even before submission for possible publication.

27.4.5 Reactivity: Influence on the Therapeutic Process

The methods we have described also have the potential to affect therapy. Rather than being a neutral event, research interviews in particular may alter expectations of the therapy or the therapist or directly affect the content of future sessions. For example, after experiencing a structured research interview approach, a client may wish their therapist to become more structured in the therapy sessions. Alternatively, a participant may have had a difficult experience with their researcher and request time during therapy sessions to process what went on. Whilst these events may have the potential to enhance the therapeutic process, they may also act as a distraction from the original intent that a client had when entering therapy.

Furthermore, Mackrill (2007) reported that therapy clients used weekly diaries as a reflective medium to help them make sense of aspects of their lives and to discover new aspects of themselves. This sometimes took the form of participants reflecting in real time as they wrote their diary, thus extending the therapeutic process outside of the therapy room. Along this line, Burnett and Meacham (2002) highlight the many claims of the value of learning and reflective journals for participants, such as providing a tool for critical reflection, allowing a different perspective to be formed and facilitating catharsis or self-expression.

From this perspective, Fischer (1994, 2000, 2006) argues that all research, be it quantitative or qualitative, is most valid when conducted in a collaborative manner, such that the researcher and participant 'co-labour' together to develop a productive understanding of what is being investigated. Rather than attempting to be neutral or objective and potentially ending up being experienced as hindering, researchers are encouraged to embrace the inevitable reactive nature of their interaction with participants such that it is most likely to be experienced as constructive and beneficial (Fischer 1994). Fischer (2006) contends that 'We are least likely to be abusive, and most likely to be useful, when we regard our participants as coassessors and coresearchers. In short, collaboration in both undertakings is likely to be most constructive for all parties and to yield the most believable and useful findings' (p. 354).

27.4.6 Higher Demands on Participants

Qualitative data collection methods place a higher demand on the client. It is relatively easy to fill in a quantitative questionnaire; it is much more demanding to undertake a 60–90 min in-depth interview, not only at the end of therapy but every 10 sessions and perhaps even prior to beginning therapy.

As for client diaries, Bolger et al. (2003) note that the effective use of this research method potentially necessitates considerable training of participants on the research protocol in order to ensure clarity of what is to be recorded and when. Keeping regular and accurate diary entries places a high burden on the participant, requiring a commitment and dedication rarely required in other types of research. Mackrill (2008) highlights the potential for significant variations between participants in both quantity and quality of response, and the potential for a diarist to go off track in their entries. Further, both Mackrill (2008) and Burnett (1999) acknowledge that a certain level of language and writing ability is assumed, which may be problematic for some participants with literacy problems, physical impairments or cultural differences.

This is even more the case for visual methods such as life space mapping. Asking participants to engage in 'art' can be much more problematic than interviewing, with potential negative connotations/associations. Further, if a participant is more familiar and comfortable with working in a cognitive, verbal way, the request to be more creative may be quite daunting or be experienced as too revealing, odd or even threatening (Deacon and Piercy 2001).

Conclusion

The purpose of this chapter has been to highlight the potential and variety of qualitative methods that can be applied to the relatively neglected topic of outcome research on counselling and psychotherapy. We have tried to make a case for broadening the range of methods for studying outcome to incorporate the routine use of qualitative data collection and analysis. Our main focus has been on outlining the various method options available to researchers. We offered an overview of qualitative methods for collecting and analysing rich qualitative data about the effects of therapy on clients, also briefly touching on several options for data analysis as well.

We have been candid about what we see as the limitations of qualitative outcome research; however, in our view quantitative outcome methods suffer from an equally problematic set of difficulties. Many of the limitations of quantitative research overlap with those of qualitative research: reliance on retrospective recall, being dominated by researchers' interests, fragmentation of results due to lack of standardisation and reactivity. However, quantitative methods suffer from additional difficulties specific to them, including thinness of data, decontextualisation and lack of relevance to clients' lives and therapists' practice.

It seems to us that it is not a matter of either/or but of both/and: qualitative outcome methods can complement, enrich, deepen or interrogate quantitative outcome methods in order to provide a more balanced, complete and useful picture of how our clients benefit from psychotherapy and counselling. They deserve a place of equal honour at the banquet of psychotherapy outcome research.

References

Alexander R (1995) Folie A Deux: an experience of one-to-one therapy. Free Association Books, London

Allport GW (1942) The use of personal documents in psychological science. Social Science Research Council, New York, NY

Anastasi A (1988) Psychological testing, 6th edn. Macmillan, New York, NY

Barker C, Pistrang N, Elliott R (2002) Research methods in clinical psychology: an introduction for students and practitioners, 2nd edn. John Wiley, Chichester

Barkham M, Rees A, Stiles WB, Shapiro DA, Hardy GE, Reynolds S (1996) Dose-effect relations in time-limited psychotherapy for depression. J Consult Clin Psychol 64:927–935. doi:10.1037/0022-006X.64.5.927

Bassman R (2000) Agents, not objects: our fights to be. J Clin Psychol 56(11):1395–1411. doi:10.1002/1097-4679(200011)56:11<1395::AID-JCLP3>3.0.CO;2-W

Bassman R (2001) Whose reality is it anyway? Consumers/survivors/ex-patients can speak for themselves. J Humanistic Psychol 41(4):11–35. doi:10.1177/0022167801414002

Begley A, Lewis A (1998) Methodological issues in the assessment of the self-concept of children with down syndrome. Child Psychol Psychiatry Rev 3(1):33–40. doi:10.1017/S1360641797001457

Bende B, Crossley D (2000) Psychotherapy patients' views of treatment: on learning from the patient. Psychiatr Bull 24:453–456. doi:10.1192/pb.24.12.453

Bolger N, Davis A, Rafaeli E (2003) Diary methods: capturing life as it is lived. Annu Rev Psychol 54:579–616. doi:10.1146/annurev.psych.54.101601.145030

Boulton-Lewis GM (1995) The SOLO taxonomy as a means of shaping and assessing learning in higher education. Higher Educ Res Dev 14(2):143–154. doi:10.1080/0729436950140201

Brott PE (2004) Constructivist assessment in career counseling. J Career Dev 30(3):189–200. doi:10.1023/B:JOCD.0000015539.21158.53

Buck J (1949) The H-T-P technique. J Clin Psychol 5:37–74. doi:10.1002/1097-4679(194901)5:1<37::AID-JCLP2270050104>3.0.CO;2-9

Burnett PC (1999) Assessing the structure of learning outcomes from counselling using the SOLO taxonomy: an exploratory study. Br J Guid Counsel 27 (4):567–580. doi:10.1080/03069889908256291

Burnett PC, Meacham D (2002) Learning journals as a counselling strategy. J Counsel Dev 80(4):410–415. doi:10.1002/j.1556-6678.2002.tb00207.x

Burnett PC, Van Dorssen L (2000) What do clients learn from counseling? Int J Adv Counsel 22(3):171–254. doi:10.1023/A:1005611704610

Deacon SA (2000) Creativity within qualitative research on families: new ideas for old methods. Qual Rep 4 (3&4), available from http://www.nova.edu/ssss/QR/

Deacon SA, Piercy FP (2001) Qualitative methods in family evaluation: creative assessment techniques. Am J Fam Therapy 29(5):355–373. doi:10.1080/01926180127627

Dees SM, Dansereau DF, Simpson DD (1994) A visual representation system for drug abuse counselors. J Subst Abus Treat 11(6):517–523. doi:10.1016/0740-5472(94)90003-5

Dreier O (2008) Psychotherapy in everyday life. Cambridge University Press, Cambridge

Elliott R (1991) Five dimensions of therapy process. Psychother Res 1:92–103. doi:10.1080/10503309112331335521

Elliott R (1999) Client change interview protocol. http://www.experiential-researchers.org/instruments/elliott/changei.html. Accessed 8 Sep 2014

Elliott R (2002a) Hermeneutic single case efficacy design. Psychother Res 12(1):1–21. doi:10.1080/713869614

Elliott R (2002b) Render unto Caesar: quantitative and qualitative knowing in person-centered/experiential therapy research. Person-Centered and Experiential Psychotherapy 1:102–117. doi:10.1080/14779757.2002.9688281

Elliott R (2006) Decoding insight talk: discourse analyses of insight in ordinary language and in psychotherapy. In: Castonguay LG, Hill CE (eds) Insight in psychotherapy. APA, Washington, DC, pp 167–185

Elliott R, Rodgers B (2008) Client change interview schedule (v5). http://www.drbrianrodgers.com/research/client-change-interview. Accessed 8 Sep 2014

Elliott R, James E, Reimschuessel C, Cislo D, Sack N (1985) Significant events and the analysis of immediate therapeutic impacts. Psychotherapy 22:620–630. doi:10.1037/h0085548

Elliott R, Partyka R, Wagner J, Alperin R, Dobrenski R, Messer SB et al (2009) An adjudicated hermeneutic single-case efficacy design of experiential therapy for panic/phobia. Psychother Res 19:543–557. doi:10.1080/10503300902905947

Etherington K (2005) Researching trauma, the body and transformation: a situated account of creating safety in unsafe places. Br J Guid Counsel 33(2):299–313. doi:10.1080/03069880500179400

Fischer CT (1994) Individualizing psychological assessment, vol 1. Lawrence Erlbaum Associates, Mahwah, NJ

Fischer CT (2000) Collaborative, individualized assessment. J Pers Assess 74(1):2–14. doi:10.1207/S15327752JPA740102

Fischer CT (2006) Qualitative psychological research and individualized/collaborative psychological assessment: implications of their similarities for promoting a life-world orientation. Hum Psychol 34(4):347–356. doi:10.1207/s15473333thp3404_4

Flitton B, Buckroyd J (2002) Exploring the effects of a 14 week person-centred counselling intervention with learning disabled children. Emotional and Behavioural Difficulties 7(3):164–177. doi:10.1080/13632750200507014

Foster K, McAllister M, O'Brien L (2006) Extending the boundaries: autoethnography as an emergent method in mental health nursing research. Int J Ment Health Nurs 15:44–53. doi:10.1111/j.1447-0349.2006.00402.x

Gantt L (1998) Talk, talk, talk, when do we draw? Research. Am J Art Ther 37(2):57–65

Gantt L, Tabone C (2003) The formal elements art therapy scale and "draw a person picking an apple from a tree". In: Malchiodi CA (ed) Handbook of art therapy. Guildford, New York, NY, p 420

Guenette F, Marshall A (2009) Time line drawings: enhancing participant voice in narrative interviews on sensitive topics. Int J Qual Methods 8(1):85–92

Hampl S (2008) Film and video interpretation with the documentary method. Paper presented at the 7th international conference on social science methodology, Naples, Italy

Hardtke K, Angus L (2004) The narrative assessment interview: assessing self-change in psychotherapy. In: Angus LE, McLeod J (eds) The handbook of narrative and psychotherapy: practice, theory, and research. Sage, London, pp 247–262

Harley JB, Woodward D (1987) The history of cartography, vol 1. University of Chicago Press, Chicago, IL

Hartman A (1995) Diagrammatic assessment of family relationships. Fam Soc 76(2):111–122

Haw K (2008) 'Voice' and video: seen, heard and listened to? In: Thomson P (ed) Doing visual research with children and young people. Routledge, London, pp 95–112

Hill CE, Thompson BJ, Williams EN (1997) A guide to conducting consensual qualitative research. Counsel Psychol 25:517–572. doi:10.1177/0011000097254001

Howe D (1989) The consumer's view of family therapy. Gower, Aldershot

Howe D (1996) Client experiences of counselling and treatment interventions: a qualitative study of family views of family therapy. Br J Guid Counsel 24 (3):367–375. doi:10.1080/03069889608253021

Kaplan I (2008) Being 'seen' being 'heard': engaging with student on the margins of education through participatory photography. In: Thomson P (ed) Doing visual research with children and young people. Routledge, London, pp 95–112

Klein MJ, Elliott R (2006) Client accounts of personal change in process-experiential psychotherapy: a methodolofically pluralistic approach. Psychother Res 16(1):91–105. doi:10.1080/1050330050009099

Knoblauch H, Baer A, Laurier E, Petschke S, Schnettler B (2008) Visual analysis. New developments in the interpretative analysis of video and photography. Forum Qualitative Sozialforschung/Forum: Qualitative Social Research 9(3), doi:10.1167/8.16.10

Korotitsch WJ, Nelson-Gray RO (1999) An overview of self-monitoring research in assessment and treatment. Psychol Assess 11(4):415–425. doi:10.1037/1040-3590.11.4.415

Krippendorff K (2003) Content analysis: an introduction to its methodology, 2nd edn. Sage, Thousand Oaks, CA

Kvale S (1996) Interviews: an introduction to qualitative research interviewing. Sage, Thousand Oaks, CA

Levitt HM, Stanley CM, Frankel Z, Raina K (2005) An evaluation of outcome measures used in humanistic psychotherapy research: using thermometers to weigh oranges. Hum Psychol 33(2):113–130. doi:10.1207/s15473333thp3302_3

Mackrill T (2007) Using a cross-contextual qualitative diary design to explore client experiences of psychotherapy. Counsel Psychother Res 7(4):233–239. doi:10.1080/14733140701722455

Mackrill T (2008) Solicited diary studies of psychotherapy in qualitative research – pros and cons. Eur J Psychother Counsel 10(1):5–18. doi:10.1080/13642530701869243

McIlveen P (2008) Autoethnography as a method for reflexive research and practice in vocational psychology. Aust J Career Dev 17(2):13–20. doi:10.1177/103841620801700204

McKenna PA, Todd DM (1997) Longitudinal utilization of mental health services: a timeline method, nine retrospective accounts, and a preliminary conceptualization. Psychother Res 7(4):383–395. doi:10.1080/10503309712331332093

McLeod J (1999) Practitioner research in counselling. Sage, London

McLeod J (2000a) The contribution of qualitative research to evidence-based counselling and psychotherapy. In: Rowland N, Goss S (eds) Evidence-based counselling and psychological therapies: research and applications. Routledge, London

McLeod J (2000b) Qualitative outcome research in psychotherapy: issues and methods. In: Society for psychotherapy research annual conference, Chicago

McLeod J (2001a) An administratively created reality: some problems with the use of self-report questionnaire measures of adjustment in counselling/psychotherapy outcome research. Counsel Psychother Res 1 (3):215–226. doi:10.1080/14733140112331385100

McLeod J (2001b) Developing a research tradition consistent with the practices and values of counselling and psychotherapy: why counselling and psychotherapy research is necessary. Counsel Psychother Res 1 (1):3–11. doi:10.1080/14733140112331385188

McLeod J (2001c) Qualitative research in counselling and psychotherapy. Sage, London

McLeod J (2010) Case study research in counselling and psychotherapy. Sage, London

Murray CD, Sixsmith J (2002) Qualitative health research via the internet: practical and methodological issues. Health Inform J 8(47):47–53. doi:10.1177/146045820200800109

Oster GD, Gould Crone P (2004) Using drawings in assessment and therapy, 2nd edn. Brunner-Routledge, New York, NY

Patton MQ (1997) Utilization-focused evaluation: the new century text. Sage, Thousand Oaks, CA

Peavy RV (1997) Sociodynamic counselling: a constructivist perspective. Trafford, Victoria, BC

Peavy RV (1999) An essay on cultural tools and the sociodynamic perspective for counselling. http://www.sociodynamic-constructivist-counselling.com/archives/1990s/an_essay_on_cultural_tools.pdf. Accessed 8 Sep 2014

Peavy RV (2004) Sociodynamic counselling: a practical approach to meaning making. Taos Institute, Chargrin Falls, OH

Przyborski A, Slunecko T (2012) Learning to think iconically in the human and social sciences: iconic standards of understanding as a pivotal challenge for method development. Integr Psychol Behav Sci 46 (1):39–56. doi:10.1007/s12124-011-9159-6

Rodgers B (2002) An investigation into the client at the heart of therapy. Counsel Psychother Res 2 (3):185–193. doi:10.1080/14733140212331384815

Rodgers B (2003) An exploration into the client at the heart of therapy: a qualitative perspective. Person-Centered and Experiential Psychotherapies 2 (21):19–30. doi:10.1080/14779757.2003.9688290

Rodgers B (2010) Life space mapping: developing a visual method for investigating the outcomes of counselling and psychotherapy from the client's frame of reference. University of Abertay, Dundee

Sands A (2000) Falling for therapy: psychotherapy from a client's point of view. Macmillan, London

Schmitz B, Wiese BS (2006) New perspectives for the evaluation of training sessions in self regulated learning: time-series analyses of diary data. Contemp Educ Psychol 31:64–96. doi:10.1016/j.cedpsych.2005.02.002

Scott-Hoy K (2002) The visitor: juggling life in the grip of the text. In: Bochner AP, Ellis C (eds) Ethnographically speaking: autoethnography, literature, and aesthetics. AltaMira, Oxford, pp 274–294

Semeonoff B (1976) Projective techniques. John Wiley, London

Shiffman S, Stone AA, Hufford MR (2008) Ecological momentary assessment. Annu Rev Clin Psychol 4:1–32. doi:10.1146/annurev.clinpsy.3.022806.091415

Slife BD (2004) Theoretical challenges to therapy practice and research: the constraint of naturalism. In: Lambert MJ (ed) Bergin and Garfield's handbook of psychotherapy and behavior change, 5th edn. John Wiley, New York, NY, pp 44–83

Smith JA, Flowers P, Larkin M (2009) Interpretative phenomenological analysis: theory, method and research. Sage, London

Sparkes AC (2000) Autoethnography and narratives of self: reflections on criteria in action. Sociol Sport J 17(1):21–43

Sperry RW (1973) Lateral specialization of cerebral function in the surgically separated hemispheres. In: McGuigan FJ, Schoonover RA (eds) The psychophysiology of thinking. Studies of covert processes. Academic, New York, NY

Stephen S, Elliott R, Macleod R (2011) Person-centred therapy with a client experiencing social anxiety difficulties: a hermeneutic single case efficacy design. Counsel Psychother Res 11(1):55–66. doi:10.1080/14733145.2011.546203

Stone AA, Shiffman S (1994) Ecological momentary assessment in behavioral medicine. Ann Behav Med 16:199–202

Strauss AL, Corbin J (1998) Basics of qualitative research: techniques and procedures for developing grounded theory, 2nd edn. Sage, Thousand Oaks, CA

Tenney LJ (2000) It has to be about choice. J Clin Psychol 56(11):1433–1445. doi:10.1002/1097-4679(200011)56:11<1433::AID-JCLP6>3.0.CO;2-5

Timulak L, Creaner M (65) Qualitative meta-analysis of outcomes of person-centred-experiential psychotherapies. In: Cooper M, Watson JC, Hölldampf D (eds) Person-centred and experiential therapies work: a review of the research on counseling, psychotherapy and related practices. PCCS Books, Ross-on-Wye, pp 65–90

Tracy EM, Whittaker JK (1990) The social network map: assessing social support in clinical practice. Fam Soc 71:461–470

Tracz SM, Gehart-Brooks DR (1999) The lifeline: using art to illustrate history. J Fam Psychother 10(3):61–63. doi:10.1300/J085v10n03_05

Traynor W, Elliott R, Cooper M (2011) Helpful factors and outcomes in person-centered therapy with clients who experience psychotic processes: therapists' perspectives. Person-Centered and Experiential Psychotherapies 10(2):89–104. doi:10.1080/14779757.2011.576557

Wheeler L, Reis HT (1991) Self-recording of everyday life events: origins, types, and uses. J Pers 59(3):339–354. doi:10.1111/j.1467-6494.1991.tb00252.x

Outcome Research on Disorder-Specific Treatments: The Case of Grief Therapy 28

Robert A. Neimeyer and Joseph M. Currier

Contents

Abstract

In a sense, every psychotherapeutic intervention targets a specific set of problems, symptoms, or disorders—those brought in by a specific client. In contrast, much of psychotherapy research examines the outcome of more general interventions, sometimes modified slightly to accommodate a particular set of problems (e.g., CBT for depression versus anxiety). In this chapter we consider research on the outcome of one class of disorder-specific therapies, those concerned with improving adaptation to bereavement, and reflect on both what it may teach us about intervention for more intense and disabling forms of grief and implications for psychotherapy research on other conditions. Drawing on a comprehensive analysis of over 60 controlled outcome studies, we attempt to offer a definitive view of the efficacy of current psychosocial treatments for those who have lost loved ones and discuss moderators associated with more effective interventions. Finally, we conclude by considering a handful of theoretically informed approaches that hold promise for the further refinement of evidence-based therapies for bereavement complications and offer some recommendations for outcome studies on other disorder-specific treatments as well.

Copies of relevant papers and information on other resources can be accessed at http://tinyurl.com/neimeyer

R.A. Neimeyer (✉)
Department of Psychology, University of Memphis, Memphis, TN, USA
e-mail: neimeyer@memphis.edu

J.M. Currier
Department of Psychology, University of South Alabama, 307 University Blvd. North, Mobile, AL 36688, USA

O.C.G. Gelo et al. (eds.), *Psychotherapy Research*,
DOI 10.1007/978-3-7091-1382-0_28, © Springer-Verlag Wien 2015

28.1 Case Vignette

Some 18 months after the death of her husband, Mary, age 62, describes herself as "drowning in a sea of grief." Far from moving toward some form of recovery, she experiences herself as "stuck" in a futile protest against the impossibility of living without Jack, who had been the "compass" for her life for the past two decades. Without the special caring, attunement, and structure he provided her, Mary feels "disoriented" and "unreal," as if his death is "just some sort of terrible joke." Jack's relatively fast demise from an aggressive cancer gave her little time to adapt to the harsh reality of his impending loss, but Mary confesses that she spent the majority of this "warning period" actively resisting the knowledge of his eventual death, just as she continues to resist the full emotional implications of his absence. Now, she feels deeply lonely and "cut off" from others, with the exception of her adult daughter, who has grown increasingly concerned by her mother's preoccupation with and anger about the loss, which have begun to erode her relationships with both friends and work colleagues. Tearfully, Mary describes how she has "no purpose for living" since Jack's death, and although she is not actively suicidal, she finds herself wishing that it were she, rather than he, who had died.

Viewed through a wide-angle lens, grief may be the one human problem that can be considered universal in its relevance. Indeed, bereavement may be distinguished among all major life event stressors not only by its near inevitability but also by the high likelihood that we will experience it repeatedly across the course of a normal life span. By later life, loss of grandparents, parents, siblings, spouses, friends, and sometimes children becomes a recurrent theme, even if the circumstances of death and its timing remain unpredictable (Neimeyer et al. 2008). Understanding how people respond to such losses and how psychotherapy can assist when this process is impeded therefore becomes a high priority.

Our goal in the present chapter is to consider the current evidence base regarding the outcome of grief therapy, understood as a disorder-specific treatment of high relevance to many clients. We will begin by describing briefly how adaptation to bereavement can become complicated for a substantial minority of mourners and how effective psychotherapy has proven to be in reducing distress following the death of a loved one. In doing so we will summarize what is known about the efficacy of bereavement interventions, paying special attention to possible moderators of its therapeutic effect. We will then review several recent programs of outcome research on specially tailored grief therapies, highlighting their common features and the models that underpin them. Finally, we will reflect on what the study of these disorder-specific grief therapies might suggest about disorder-specific treatment research for other conditions [e.g., dialectical behavior therapy (DBT) for borderline conditions (e.g., Linehan et al. 2006), interpersonal psychotherapy (IPT) for depression (de Mello et al. 2005), cognitive processing therapy (CPT) for trauma (e.g., Resick and Schnicke 1992)]. In summary, our goal in concentrating on the relatively recent emergence of grief therapies is to complement and reinforce the focus on more general psychotherapy research efforts documented and analyzed elsewhere in this volume.

28.2 When Grief Is Complicated

Although the majority of people either respond to loss in a resilient fashion, experiencing only transitory distress, or follow an adaptive course of adjustment, beginning to recover baseline levels of functioning following the first 6 months, longitudinal research documents substantial and sustained bereavement-related difficulties for many people (Bonanno et al. 2002, 2004). As a consequence, the death of a loved one carries with it significant risks for physiological irregularities and sleep disruption (Hall and Irwin 2001; Hardison et al. 2005), acute separation anxiety (Parkes 1996), disbelief, anger and depression (Holland and Neimeyer 2010; Maciejewski et al. 2007), and even elevated mortality (Center for the Advancement of Health 2004).

Most worrisome is recent evidence that 10–15 % of the bereaved struggle to adapt to their loss over a period of many months or years (Ott 2003; Shear et al. 2011a), with some vulnerable groups like bereaved parents (Keesee et al. 2008) and those who lose loved ones to violent death (McDevitt-Murphy et al. 2012) experiencing three times the incidence of such complication. Like Mary in the clinical vignette with which this chapter opened, mourners who experience complicated or prolonged grief reactions are characterized by intense and persistent yearning for the deceased, intrusive and troubling thoughts regarding the death, a sense of inner emptiness and hopelessness about the future, trouble accepting the reality of the loss, and various other difficulties moving on with life (Lichtenthal et al. 2004). When left untreated, such complicated grief symptoms have been shown to increase vulnerability to functional impairment, high blood pressure, cardiac events, substance abuse, and suicidal ideation over the long term (Prigerson et al. 2009; Shear et al. 2011b), although the psychological and physiological mechanisms responsible for these effects require further study (Center for the Advancement of Health 2004).

In view of the potentially profound and prolonged impact of bereavement on those left behind, it is not surprising that helping professionals and community organizations have stepped forward to provide counsel and companionship to grieving people, in the hope of promoting their adaptation to a changed life. But how effective are these services? Are there features of the bereaved or of the losses they suffer that can inform us about who will most benefit from available interventions? Are there certain symptoms and problems with which bereavement services are more effective? And are there aspects of grief therapy itself—in terms of its timing, duration, structure, or format—that suggest patterns of practice that are likely to be more helpful for those to whom it is offered?

Our goal in this brief review is to address such questions, building on several independent analyses of the status of the field conducted over the past 10 years. In the aggregate, these prior reviews converge on several conclusions about the efficacy of bereavement interventions:

- The benefits of grief therapy are at best modest and at worst negligible in helping the bereaved surmount the symptoms or problems they report (Forte et al. 2004; Jordan and Neimeyer 2003; Kato and Mann 1999; Schut and Stroebe 2005).
- Interventions that target highly distressed survivors rather than all those who suffered a loss seem to produce better outcomes (Currier et al. 2007; Schut et al. 2001).
- There could be benefits in early intervention in the near aftermath of loss, for both adults and children (Allumbaugh and Hoyt 1999; Currier et al. 2007).
- More definitive research is needed, especially of a kind that attends to practical distinctions between (a) interventions offered to all bereaved people, (b) those that target a particular risk group (e.g., survivors of suicide, children who lose a parent), and (c) those that focus only on bereaved people who show heightened or prolonged distress that compromises their daily functioning (Schut et al. 2001).
- Advances in grief therapy are likely to be built on advances in grief theory and basic research, as new methods are devised and tested that draw on current conceptual and empirical developments in the field (Neimeyer and Currier 2009; Neimeyer et al. 2011; Sandler et al. 2003).

Here, we will consider these conclusions in light of our comprehensive review of controlled studies of bereavement interventions (Currier et al. 2008) and then follow with a few thoughts on emerging developments in grief therapy, attempting to extrapolate lessons learned in the area of bereavement that may have relevance for psychotherapy research in other areas.

28.3 Does Grief Therapy Work? A Meta-analysis

Earlier reviewers of the scientific literature on bereavement interventions have reached varying conclusions about its effectiveness, notwithstanding the generally cautious tone of their endorsement. Some level of disagreement among authors might be expected, as most reviews summarized only a small number of studies—either because few controlled evaluations had been conducted at the time the reviews were written or because many potentially available studies were systematically excluded or simply missed in the process. Moreover, different scholars have used different methods in synthesizing the literature, relying either on a narrative recounting of findings of different studies or meta-analysis, using statistical procedures to integrate the results of several different studies to yield general conclusions. Our approach was the latter: we conducted a meta-analysis of all available controlled outcome research on grief therapies (Currier et al. 2008) to convey the "big picture" about its effectiveness and to examine different factors associated with greater or lesser benefit.

The review was based on 61 outcome studies reported in 64 papers—many more studies than were considered in previous reviews—which included 48 published peer-reviewed articles and 16 unpublished dissertations. We used several criteria to select the studies, the most basic of which was that the therapy tested needed to aim specifically to improve bereavement adaptation and that the study included a group of bereaved persons who did not receive any formal help (that is, a no-intervention control group), in order to rule out the possibility that positive change could simply represent the passage of time or other factors not directly related to the treatment. Although most studies adhered to the "gold standard" of random assignment to treatment or control conditions, for the sake of completeness, we included 14 studies that did not do so and analyzed these separately to see if similar trends held in random and nonrandom studies, in view of the generally greater variability in outcome of the latter (Shadish and Ragsdale 1996).

We had two distinct but interrelated aims for the review. Primarily, we were concerned with evaluating the overall effectiveness of grief therapies and exploring commonalities among studies that generated better (and worse) outcomes. These potential moderators included the targeted population, timing of intervention, method of recruiting bereaved persons, person- (e.g., age, sex) and loss-related (e.g., cause of death, relationship to the deceased) factors, and features of the interventions themselves (e.g., number of sessions, group versus individual format). As practicing clinicians as well as clinical scientists, we believed that the most important information would come less from providing estimates of the overall effectiveness of grief therapies and more from identifying the specific circumstances under which subgroups of studies yielded favorable results. In other words, we were hoping to provide practical as well as scientific clarification regarding who would likely benefit from what the field has to offer at this point and under what circumstances.

Secondarily, we assessed the amount of change over time among intervention recipients and participants in the control groups. This allowed us to address issues that we otherwise could not explore by only relying on the standardized differences between intervention and control groups at a particular time point (i.e., conventional Cohen's d). For example, discouraging outcomes discussed in prior reviews (e.g., Currier et al. 2007; Forte et al. 2004; Kato and Mann 1999; Schut et al. 2001) might have been the result of either *deterioration* among intervention recipients—in other words, therapy "backfiring" by making people worse—or of *improved* adjustment among those who did not receive formal help. Clearly, either one of these patterns would diminish the relative therapeutic gains for treated groups, but each would of course carry quite different implications for interventionists "in the trenches."

Our careful efforts to identify as many available studies as possible yielded a long line of research conducted over the past three decades. Researchers from these studies sampled a diversity of bereaved persons and encompassed several different types of losses. The age of the participants ranged from 8 to 71 years, meaning that we included studies of bereaved individuals from childhood through older adulthood. As is consonant with trends in bereavement research in general, three out of four participants were female (71 %) and Caucasian (74 %). The majority (75 %) of the participants in the studies had lost an immediate family member (i.e., spouse, parent, child, or sibling), with over a quarter (27 %) of these losses occurring by homicide, suicide, or a fatal accident.

On average, interventions were administered 14 months following the loved one's death, a point well beyond when indicators of distress have been observed to decrease for most "normal" grievers (Maciejewski et al. 2007). Most of the interventions used a group modality (63 %), although individual (25 %) and family (12 %) approaches were represented as well. The types of interventions included psychotherapy and counseling (63 %), professionally organized support groups (17 %), crisis intervention (11 %), social activities groups (4 %), writing therapy (3 %), a formal widowed persons visiting service (1 %), and a helper training program (1 %). The mean number of sessions for the interventions was 8, indicating the time-limited nature of most of the therapies tested to date.

28.4 What We Found

Consistent with the majority of smaller-scale reviews, our tests of overall effectiveness also failed to yield a very encouraging picture of grief therapies in the aggregate (see Fig. 28.1). Of the four overall analyses, grief therapies were shown to outperform no-intervention control conditions immediately following the intervention in the randomized ($d = 0.16$) and nonrandom ($d = 0.51$) studies, although the magnitude of the effect of the former more rigorously controlled research was relatively small in absolute terms. However, analyses for follow-up outcomes failed to yield intervention effects that were significantly greater than zero an average of 8 months later (randomized $d = 0.05$; nonrandom $d = 0.04$). These results contrast with meta-analyses of general psychotherapy for other disorders or forms of distress, which typically yield effect sizes of 0.7–0.9 by the end of treatment and show enduring improvement (Lambert and Ogles 2004; Smith et al. 1980; Wampold 2001).

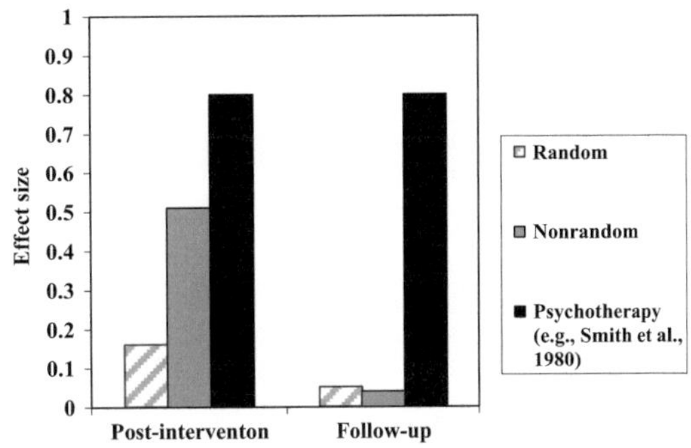

Fig. 28.1 Overall effectiveness of grief therapies compared to general psychotherapy

In contrast, our overall results suggest that the relative benefits of grief therapy are modest and of possibly short duration: on average, on follow-up assessment, recipients of grief therapies are not appreciably less distressed when compared with those who receive no formal help whatsoever. However, beyond this general conclusion, other analyses revealed significant variability for outcomes from each assessment point, with some studies showing little benefit or even negative effects, while other studies suggested impressive effectiveness. This highlighted the need to subdivide the research reports on the basis of clinically and theoretically relevant factors that could account for different results, in a way that we hope will give both researchers and practitioners better guidance as in how to move forward with bereaved clientele.

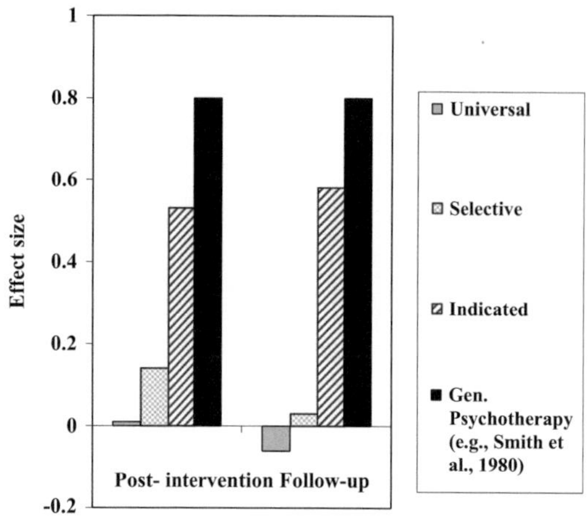

Fig. 28.2 Effectiveness of grief therapies for targeted populations

28.5 Who Do We Help? The Search for Moderators

Of the many potential moderators that we explored, the targeted population emerged as especially critical for researchers and clinicians to consider in their work (see Fig. 28.2). Using the Institute of Medicine categories of interventions, *universal* applications targeting anyone who suffers a loss (e.g., Scruby and Sloan 1989) failed to produce better outcomes than would be expected by the passage of time alone (posttreatment $d = 0.01$; follow-up $d = -0.06$). By comparison, although *selective* interventions with subsets of higher risk grievers (such as parents who lost children to violent death, e.g., Murphy et al. 1998) showed a small effect at posttreatment ($d = 0.14$), these limited benefits were not significant at follow-up ($d = 0.03$). In contrast, for *indicated* interventions that took the further step to assess for difficulties adapting to loss as a requirement for treatment (as in evaluating the presence of complicated grief, as exemplified by Mary's vignette, e.g., Wagner et al. 2006), outcomes were clearly superior and compared favorably with the successes shown for psychotherapy in general (posttreatment $d = 0.53$; follow-up $d = 0.58$).

These specific results reinforce the growing consensus that grief therapies can indeed be effective when clinicians focus on persons who are genuinely in need of professional help. Viewed alongside the growing body of evidence that the passage of time frequently does not alleviate difficulties associated with maladaptive reactions to loss (Prigerson et al. 2009; Shear et al. 2011a), it is encouraging that the subset of studies that targeted distressed grievers consistently yielded benefits. Simply put, for those who are struggling with intense symptomatology over a protracted period, grief therapy appears to be an evidence-based practice that enjoys growing support.

Somewhat to our surprise, however, none of the remaining potential moderators reliably accounted for differences in outcome across the large set of studies. Several of these analyses focused on person- and death-related risk factors and characteristics of the interventions themselves. We found no evidence that grief therapy worked better or worse for children or adults, for men or women, or as a function of the category of relationship (spouse, parent, etc.) one had to the deceased. We also found that the timing of the intervention had little association to outcome, overturning the conclusions of earlier small-scale reviews, including our own with children and adolescents, which had suggested the critical importance of early intervention (Allumbaugh and Hoyt 1999; Currier et al. 2007). Similarly, the source of referral to treatment (i.e., aggressive outreach procedures, simple advertising, or self- or clinical referral) made a difference only at posttreatment, at which time studies intervening with referred clients generated better outcomes than those strictly relying on aggressive outreach. This advantage faded in the coming months, however, again qualifying conclusions of earlier reviewers (Larson and Hoyt 2007; Schut et al. 2001). Nor did the relative success of the interventions vary according to the domain of outcome being assessed. In particular, interventions did no better in reducing grief symptoms than other domains of outcome, such as depression and general psychiatric distress. Viewed affirmatively, these results suggest that grief therapy can be helpful to a wide range of people contending with a wide range of losses, in ameliorating many forms of distress in both the near- and long-term aftermath of bereavement, regardless of how they enter therapy—at least if they are assessed as contending with substantial clinical distress to begin with.

28.6 What Is Going on Here? The Responses of Control Participants

As summarized above, the primary findings of the study tell us more than little, but less than much. That is, without also exploring the amount of change over time for intervention recipients and controls, we cannot fully explain the discouraging picture for interventions for bereaved persons who are not first screened for elevated levels of distress. For this reason we pursued secondary analyses to see what was happening among those assigned to both treatment and no-treatment conditions. It was soon clear that there was no evidence that the average untreated survivor deteriorated (nor did the typical person who was treated, for that matter). Instead, on average, all of the groups, treated and untreated, displayed positive change at post-treatment and follow-up. When favorable treatment effects were observed, these analyses found that they resulted from greater reductions in distress in intervention recipients relative to those who went without formal help. In some cases, it seemed that grief therapies might have accelerated the adjustment process somewhat, although untreated survivors closed the narrow gap in outcome by follow-up. Given other evidence suggesting that the majority of the bereaved tend to regain pre-loss levels of functioning after a transitory period of distress without clinical intervention (e.g., 6–12 months; Bonanno et al. 2002, 2004; Maciejewski et al. 2007), it appeared that most of the control participants had successfully accommodated the experience of loss to varying degrees by the time of their involvement or over the course of the studies. This evidence of human resilience (even in the absence of treatment) is good news for the bereaved, suggesting that clinicians might adopt an attitude of humble appreciation for what many of the bereaved can achieve without professional assistance.

28.7 The Future Horizon

Taken together, the findings of our review reinforce our humility as an interdisciplinary field of bereavement researchers and professionals, but also offer hope that we have much to offer those experiencing the greatest complications in adjusting to bereavement. Recent carefully controlled research completed since our review reinforces these conclusions. For example, an impressive cluster randomized trial of "primary bereavement care" (PBC) in Spain recently assigned 31 family physicians in 19 facilities to receive specialized training in this multifaceted treatment model (e.g., focusing on empathy, active listening, presence, facilitation, psychoeducation, normalization, and strategic grief therapy skills) or to participate in the control condition, without this training (Garcia et al. 2013). Those physicians in the PCB condition then saw 43 widows in the course of their usual practice, applying these grief therapy skills for seven sessions, between 4 and 13 months after the loss, while physicians in the control condition followed a comparable group of widows for the same number of contacts in the context of ordinary medical appointments. Outcome was assessed at 4, 10, 16, and 24 months using a variety of measures. Significantly, no benefits were observed for the PBC treatment group across the course of the study, and in fact control patients showed greater improvement on somatization, general health, and emotional outcomes. Such findings underscore cautions about the advisability of grief therapy dispensed to all bereaved people, without screening for levels of risk for or manifestations of complication.

Beyond this, however, there is a clear need for more research to establish and extend the efficacy of carefully crafted therapies for the subset of the bereaved who struggle to move forward with their lives. Sandler et al. (2003) suggest that programmatic research to construct coherent interventions would do well to work from a clear theoretical base and to design strategies to address modifiable behaviors, attitudes, and skills with a demonstrated relevance to therapeutic outcomes, an advocacy with which we concur (Neimeyer et al. 2011). Fortunately, several relevant theories bearing on neurophysiological, psychological, behavioral, attachment-related, and social processes in bereavement have developed sufficient sophistication and support to guide such efforts (Stroebe et al. 2007).

One classic conceptualization that has proven valuable in shaping contemporary grief therapies is attachment theory (Bowlby 1980), as growing evidence suggests that individuals who experience insecure styles of attachment are more prone to chronic grief trajectories (Bonanno et al. 2004; van der Houwen et al. 2010), especially when bereavement-related challenges are severe and more avoidant styles of coping may break down (Meier et al. 2013). Other useful theories posit a dialectical process in grief adaptation, such as the Dual Process Model (Stroebe and Schut 1999), which captures the typical oscillation the bereaved experience over time between processing the loss and adapting to a changed life, or the Two-Track Model (Rubin 1999), which focuses not only on the biopsychosocial functioning of the bereaved but also their ongoing processing of their evolving relationship to the deceased. Research on both models is benefiting from the recent development of measures to assess their central mechanisms (Caserta and Lund 2007; Rubin et al. 2009).

In addition, a focus on meaning reconstruction as a centrally relevant process in grieving (Neimeyer 2001; Neimeyer and Sands 2011; Park 2008) has yielded a good deal of evidence that an inability to make sense of loss in spiritual, secular, or practical terms can play a pivotal role in adaptation to bereavement, accounting for greatly more of the intensity of persistent grief symptomatology than objective factors such as the cause of death or the passage of time (Keesee et al. 2008) and perhaps even mediating the impact of violent death on complicated grief responses (Currier et al. 2006). The related cognitive-behavioral formulation of complicated grief by Boelen and his colleagues (Boelen et al. 2006) similarly posits a struggle on the part of the bereaved to integrate the reality of loss into autobiographical memory as a key factor in the disorder. Both of these latter two perspectives lend themselves to research on the role of loss in challenging or positively transforming the self-narrative of the griever (Neimeyer 2006a, b), as well as to the refinement of narrative interventions in the context of grief therapy (Neimeyer 2012). Each is also likely to benefit from the recent validation of a measure of its theoretically central concept, namely, the integration of stressful life experiences in a way that promotes their comprehensibility and the mourner's "footing" or grounding in a world transformed by loss (Holland et al. 2010, 2014).

Finally, our optimism about the field of grief counseling is reinforced by the burgeoning collaboration between clinicians and researchers in developing and documenting new models of treatment for complicated grief that are demonstrably effective in randomized controlled studies. One such is the complicated grief therapy (CGT) devised by Shear and her colleagues (Shear et al. 2005), which draws on the Dual Process Model of Stroebe and Schut (1999) to foster accommodation of the loss and promote restoration of life goals and roles. The former entails procedures for revisiting or retelling the story of the death in evocative detail, while promoting cognitive and emotional mastery of the experience, engaging in imaginal conversations to rework the attachment relationship to the deceased, and writing about and reviewing both pleasant and troubling recollections related to the deceased to help the client consolidate a more positive memory of their life together. In addition, in keeping with the restoration focus of the DPM, clients review and revise life goals to align them with the changed circumstance of their lives. Sixteen sessions of CGT were found to be far more effective than interpersonal psychotherapy in alleviating complicated grief symptomatology, although clients showed improvement in both conditions (Shear et al. 2005).

Likewise, Boelen and his associates (Boelen et al. 2007) drew on a cognitive-behavioral model of complicated grief to formulate a two-phase treatment featuring cognitive restructuring and sustained exposure exercises. Cognitive interventions used familiar procedures to identify, challenge, and change negative automatic thoughts in the course of grieving. Exposure treatment entailed inviting clients to tell the story of their loss in detail followed by a homework assignment to write down all of the internal and external stimuli—ranging from specific memories to people and places—that they tended to avoid and used the results to construct a hierarchy of situations that were confronted imaginally and behaviorally in the remaining sessions. Results indicated that 12 sessions of treatment in the cognitive-behavioral conditions outperformed the supportive condition and that exposure interventions were especially effective in ameliorating grief symptomatology. A recent meta-analysis of the literature on interventions using similar CBT methods supports their general efficacy, although it is unclear whether they are more effective than other existing therapies when investigator allegiance is taken into account (Currier et al. 2010).

Recently, Lichtenthal and Cruess conducted a controlled trial of a narrative intervention for bereavement, drawing on meaning-oriented models that emphasize the role of sense-making and benefit finding in the wake of loss (Lichtenthal and Cruess 2010). Randomizing participants to one of four conditions—emotional disclosure (ED), sense-making (SM), benefit finding (BF), or a control (CC) condition—they requested that bereaved participants write for three, 20-min sessions over the course of a week about either their deepest thoughts and emotions related to their loss (ED), making sense of the event by exploring its causes and place in their lives (SM), any positive life changes that came about as a result of their loss experience (BF), or simply the room in which they were seated (CC). They found evidence that writing about the loss experience was more efficacious in reducing grief complication 3 months post-intervention than writing about a neutral topic. The novel BF meaning-making intervention appeared especially beneficial. Significant treatment effects on depressive and PTSD symptoms also emerged, especially among those in the BF condition. An additional randomized controlled trial of an Internet-mediated writing therapy featuring prompts for perspective taking regarding the loss reinforced these general conclusions (Wagner et al. 2006). Because nondirective expressive writing about loss is of uncertain benefit as a treatment for bereavement (Neimeyer and Currier 2009), these results are hopeful in suggesting that narrative procedures that prompt positive meaning making about the loss could play a constructive role either as a homework assignment in the context of bereavement support or grief counseling or as a stand-alone treatment. Several such narrative and meaning-oriented interventions have been formalized to permit their clinical use with clients as well as their further empirical evaluation and refinement (Neimeyer 2012).

Finally, Kissane and his associates have devised a family-focused grief therapy (FFGT), practiced as a brief 4–8 session intervention for distressed relatives of patients receiving end-stage treatment in palliative care settings (Kissane and Bloch 2002). As an alternative to the individualistic orientation of the other research-tested therapies described above, theirs is based on an assessment of family functioning, defined in terms of members' self-reported levels of cohesiveness, expressiveness, and capacity to deal with conflict. Importantly, Kissane and his colleagues offered professional therapy only to those families whose family processes placed them "at risk" for poor bereavement outcomes, "supportive" families that enjoyed high cohesion, and "conflict resolving" families that dealt with problems through effective communication were judged as inappropriate for intervention. Therapy concentrated on telling the story of the illness and related grief while enhancing communication and conflict resolution. Although a large randomized comparison of FFGT with treatment-as-usual produced equivocal effects, significantly greater improvement in general distress and depression, though not social adjustment, was shown by the 10 % of FFGT-treated family members who were most troubled at the outset of treatment. Importantly, members of "sullen" families characterized by muted anger and a desire for help showed the most improvement in depression as a result of FFGT. In contrast, "hostile" families marked by high conflict actually did worse in FFGT than in the control condition (Kissane et al. 2006). Results therefore suggest the utility of family-level bereavement intervention, but only when discretion is exercised in the recruitment of those most likely to benefit (highly distressed and sullen families) and to avoid offering treatment to those who would fare as well or better without it (functional and hostile families).

In summary, a variety of experiential, cognitive-behavioral, narrative, and family-focused methods are being developed and hold promise in the treatment of bereavement-related distress. Common features of these demonstrably effective treatments include (a) their grounding in contemporary, research-informed models of grief; (b) their tendency to screen for significant levels of distress or complicated grief; (c) inclusion of oral or written "retelling" of the loss experience, often in evocative detail; and typically (d) the prompting of some form of meaning making, in the form of consolidation of positive memories, cognitive restructuring of fatalistic thoughts, or integration of the loss into one's self-narrative (Shear et al. 2011b). Our hope is that such common factors, in combination with novel procedures featured in some of the therapies (e.g., directed imaginal dialogues with the deceased or writing of letters to the loved one or to hypothetical others who have experienced a similar loss), will continue to inspire experimentation with new models and methods in order to enrich and deepen the scope and focus of grief therapy.

28.8 Disorder-Specific Grief Therapy and the Broader Field of Psychotherapy Research

As a theoretically informed and evidence-based approach to grief therapy has begun to emerge, what lessons might it carry for the refinement of other therapies that target specific disorders or for the field of psychotherapy research as a whole? Perhaps the most basic response to this question is that there seems to be a clear place for interventions that include, but also supplement, a "common factors" approach to therapy by drawing on research that implicates unique factors in particular disorders and uses this evidence to construct specialized treatments for those who struggle with them. That is, beyond such general factors as the cultivation of a strong working alliance, the practice of accurate empathy, and the instillation of hope, some specific intervention methods may be called for to address particular dimensions of a given disorder or difficulty. In the domain of grief therapy, for example, themes of severed attachment, challenges to the survivor's system of meaning, and the need to reorganize life goals and roles loom large, suggesting the relevance of interventions to reorganize the bond with the deceased, find significance in both the death of the loved one and in one's changed life as a survivor and project new purposes and connections appropriate to an altered future. That is, for many conditions, optimal treatment may consist of a felicitous pairing of common and unique factors tailored to the challenges represented by a given disorder. As evidence from several research programs suggests that grief therapies fitting this description could outperform more generic treatments for depression or distress (Boelen et al. 2007; Lichtenthal and Cruess 2010; Shear et al. 2005), psychotherapy researchers focused on other forms of disorder should be encouraged to design and evaluate theory-guided interventions that transcend more general approaches to psychotherapy. One relevant design, for example, might compare a "common factors" approach to treatment for a specific condition that provides a credible rationale, instills hope, and offers relational and ritual supports for change to an enhanced model that also integrates specialized interventions relevant to the disorder being treated (e.g., exposure, meaning-based or family systems interventions). Such a design would presumably be more informative than a simple attention-placebo-controlled study, suggesting the additional relevance of specific treatment components beyond those associated with a common factors model. In the field of grief research, the investigation by Shear et al. (2005) most approximates this design recommendation to this point.

A second clear implication arises from our finding that grief therapy only demonstrated clinically substantial effects when it was restricted in application to *indicated* (that is, clinically distressed) populations, whereas treating *selected* "at risk" groups produced very modest gains, and *universal* application of grief therapy to anyone who had suffered a loss showed essentially no noticeable effects immediately after intervention or on follow-up (Currier et al. 2008). One inference that could be drawn from this finding is that the psychotherapy research field might benefit from a clear emphasis not only on *what therapy* is being evaluated but also on *to whom* it is being offered. This advocacy is of course in line with that of other reviewers of psychotherapy research who have collaborated to identify transdiagnostic client characteristics (e.g., client reactance, therapy preferences, culture, and spirituality) that have been empirically associated with differential response to particular therapies (Norcross and Wampold 2010). Many programs of outcome research routinely do something of the sort through careful assessment of prospective clients for "goodness of fit" to diagnostic criteria prior to randomization to conditions, but such attention is typically limited to the evaluation of symptoms associated with the diagnosis itself, rather than client characteristics that go beyond diagnostic criteria. For example, in the field of bereavement, research has begun to identify a significant correlate or outcome of complicated grief, in terms of a spiritual crisis that leaves religiously inclined mourners feeling estranged from God and their spiritual community (Burke et al. 2011; Neimeyer and Burke 2011). One implication of this finding is that those bereaved persons evidencing such spiritual struggle might benefit from tailored interventions that target fundamental challenges to their belief systems, their sense of secure connection to the divine, and social conflicts with others in their faith community (Burke and Neimeyer 2011). Likewise, in other specific therapy contexts, it could be prudent to assess whether potential clients display indications that they would benefit from a specialized treatment that attends to their unique struggles, coping styles or treatment preferences.

Third, the recent development of measures of theoretically crucial constructs featured in leading models of bereavement adaptation (Caserta and Lund 2007; Holland et al. 2010; Rubin et al. 2009) bodes well for future research on mechanisms of change in grief therapy. By extension, research on other specific therapies could benefit from the construction and validation of procedures for evaluating those processes theorized to be central to the disorder on which they focus, the remediation of which is the ultimate goal of treatment. Likewise, beyond remediation of distress per se, psychotherapy researchers might give greater attention to *positive* changes engendered by treatment, such as those associated with client resilience. In the field of bereavement research, for example, recent evidence (Currier et al. 2012) suggests that significant (though not overwhelming) levels of grief are associated with greater posttraumatic growth, defined in terms of greater personal strength, appreciation of life, compassion for others, and deepened spirituality (Calhoun and Tedeschi 2006). This highlights the relevance of measuring such outcomes in treatments that target emotion regulation, meaning making, and relational renewal as therapeutic goals. Although the outcome of any given psychotherapy is likely to be shaped by myriad factors, some specific to that treatment and some common to the majority of approaches, the identification of particular mechanisms of change and associated positive outcomes will likely enhance the efficacy of future interventions.

Finally, our study of grief therapy underscores the importance of evaluating changes in the control group as well as in those who are being actively treated. Our finding that controls showed considerable improvement over time seemed to account for much of the poor showing of universally applied bereavement interventions (Currier et al. 2008) is in one sense cautionary, suggesting that professional treatment is required only by a minority of survivors. But at another level it is inspirational, demonstrating the active self-healing efforts of the bereaved in adapting to life without the physical presence of their loved one. Whether the seeming resilience of untreated candidates for treatment is unique to grief (which for many may follow a natural course toward improved adjustment) or whether successful attempts to come to terms with their symptoms or problems characterize other control groups in psychotherapy research deserves further attention.

In conclusion, our study of the outcome of bereavement interventions gives us cause for both humility and hope—humility, because it is clear that not all professional interventions for the bereaved are as substantial in their effects as one might wish, but also hope, because recent theory and research seems to be identifying several active ingredients of interventions that prove efficacious for those, like Mary, who most need them. We hope that our analysis and interpretation of these findings is of benefit to other psychotherapy scholars studying and seeking to ameliorate other forms of human suffering.

References

Allumbaugh DL, Hoyt WT (1999) Effectiveness of grief therapy: a meta-analysis. J Couns Psychol 46:370–380. doi:10.1037//0022-0167.46.3.370

Boelen P, van den Hout M, van den Bout J (2006) A cognitive-behavioral conceptualization of complicated grief. Clin Psychol Sci Pract 13:109–128. doi:10.1111/j.1468-2850.2006.00013.x

Boelen PA, de Keijser J, van den Hout M, van den Bout J (2007) Treatment of complicated grief: a comparison between cognitive-behavioral therapy and supportive counseling. J Clin Consult Psychol 75:277–284. doi:10.1037/0022-006X.75.2.277

Bonanno GA, Wortman CB, Lehman DR, Tweed RG, Haring M, Sonnega J et al (2002) Resilience to loss and chronic grief: a prospective study from preloss to 18-months postloss. J Pers Soc Psychol 83:1150–1164. doi:10.1037//0022-3514.83.5.1150

Bonanno G, Wortman CB, Nesse RM (2004) Prospective patterns of resilience and maladjustment during widowhood. Psychol Aging 19:260–271. doi:10.1037/0882-7974.19.2.260

Bowlby J (1980) Attachment and loss: loss, sadness, and depression, vol 3. Basic, New York, NY

Burke LA, Neimeyer RA (2011) Spirituality and health: meaning making in bereavement. In: Cobb M, Puchalski C, Rumbold B (eds) The textbook on spirituality in healthcare. Oxford University Press, Oxford

Burke LA, Neimeyer RA, McDevitt-Murphy ME, Ippolito MR, Roberts JM (2011) In the wake of homicide: spiritual crisis and bereavement distress in an African American sample. Int J Psychol Relig 21:289–307

Calhoun L, Tedeschi RG (eds) (2006) Handbook of posttraumatic growth. Lawrence Erlbaum, Mahwah, NJ

Caserta MS, Lund DA (2007) Toward the development of an inventory of daily widowed life (IDWL): guided by the dual process model of coping with bereavement. Death Stud 28:489–575. doi:10.1080/07481180701356761

Center for the Advancement of Health (2004) Report on bereavement and grief research. Death Stud 28:489–575

Currier JM, Holland JM, Neimeyer RA (2006) Sense making, grief and the experience of violent loss: toward a mediational model. Death Stud 30:403–428. doi:10.1080/07481180600614351

Currier JM, Holland JM, Neimeyer RA (2007) The effectiveness of bereavement interventions with children: a meta-analytic review of controlled outcome research. J Clin Child Adolesc Psychol 36:1–7. doi:10.1080/15374410701279669

Currier JM, Neimeyer RA, Berman JS (2008) The effectiveness of psychotherapeutic interventions for the bereaved: a comprehensive quantitative review. Psychol Bull 134:648–661. doi:10.1037/0033-2909.134.5.648

Currier JM, Holland JM, Neimeyer RA (2010) Do CBT-based interventions alleviate distress following bereavement? A review of the current evidence. Int J Cogn Ther 3:79–95. doi:10.1521/ijct.2010.3.1.77

Currier JM, Holland JM, Neimeyer RA (2012) Prolonged grief symptoms and growth in the first two years of bereavement: evidence for a non-linear association. Traumatology 18:65–71

de Mello MF, de Jesus MJ, Bacaltchuk J, Verdeli H, Neugebauer R (2005) A systematic review of research findings on the efficacy of interpersonal therapy for depressive disorders. Eur Arch Psychiatry Clin Neurosci 255:75–82. doi:10.1007/s00406-004-0542-x

Forte AL, Hill M, Pazder R, Feudtner C (2004) Bereavement care interventions: a systematic review. BMC Palliat Care 3:3, http://www.biomedcentral.com/1472-684X/3/3/. Accessed 17 March 2007

Garcia JA, Landa V, Grandes G, Pombo H, Mauriz A (2013) Effectiveness of "Primary Bereavement Care" for widows: a cluster randomized trial involving family physicians. Death Stud 37(4):287–310

Hall M, Irwin M (2001) Physiological indices of functioning in bereavement. In: Stroebe MS, Hansson R, Stroebe W, Schut H (eds) Handbook of bereavement research. American Psychological Association, Washington, DC, pp 473–491

Hardison HG, Neimeyer RA, Lichstein KL (2005) Insomnia and complicated grief symptoms in bereaved college students. Behav Sleep Med 3:99–111. doi:10.1207/s15402010bsm0302_4

Holland JM, Neimeyer RA (2010) An examination of stage theory of grief among individuals bereaved by natural and violent causes: a meaning-oriented contribution. Omega 61:105–122. doi:10.2190/OM.61.2.b

Holland JM, Currier JM, Coleman RA, Neimeyer RA (2010) The integration of stressful life experiences scale (ISLES): development and initial validation of a new measure. Int J Stress Manag 17:325–352. doi:10.1037/a0020892

Holland JM, Currier JM, Neimeyer RA (2014) Validation of the integration of stressful life experiences scale in a bereaved sample. Death Stud 38(1–5):234–238

Jordan JR, Neimeyer RA (2003) Does grief counseling work? Death Stud 27:765–786. doi:10.1080/713842360

Kato PM, Mann T (1999) A synthesis of psychological interventions for the bereaved. Clin Psychol Rev 19:275–296. doi:10.1016/S0272-7358(98)00064-6

Keesee NJ, Currier JM, Neimeyer RA (2008) Predictors of grief following the death of one's child: the contribution of finding meaning. J Clin Psychol 64:1145–1163. doi:10.1002/jclp.20502

Kissane DW, Bloch S (2002) Family focused grief therapy. Open University Press, Buckingham

Kissane DW, McKenzie M, Bloch S, Maskowitz C, McKenzie DP, O'Neill I (2006) Family focused grief therapy: a randomized, controlled trial in palliative care and bereavement. Am J Psychiatry 163:1208–1218. doi:10.1176/appi.ajp.163.7.1208

Lambert MJ, Ogles BM (2004) The efficacy and effectiveness of psychotherapy. In: Lambert MJ (ed) Bergin and Garfield's handbook of psychotherapy and behavior change. Wiley, New York, NY, pp 139–193

Larson DG, Hoyt WT (2007) What has become of grief counseling? An evaluation of the empirical foundations of the new pessimism. Prof Psychol Res Pract 38:347–355. doi:10.1037/0735-7028.38.4.347

Lichtenthal WG, Cruess DG (2010) Effects of directed written disclosure on grief and distress symptoms among bereaved individuals. Death Stud 34:475–499. doi:10.1080/07481187.2010.483332

Lichtenthal WG, Cruess DG, Prigerson HG (2004) A case for establishing complicated grief as a distinct mental disorder in *DSM-V*. Clin Psychol Rev 24:637–662. doi:10.1016/j.cpr.2004.07.002

Linehan M, Comtois M, Murray KA, Brown AM, Gallop MZ, Heard HL et al (2006) Two-year randomized controlled trial and follow-up of dialectical behavior therapy vs. therapy by experts for suicidal behaviors and borderline personality disorder. Arch Gen Psychiatry 63:757–766. doi:10.1001/archpsyc.63.7.757

Maciejewski PK, Zhang B, Block SD, Prigerson HG (2007) An empirical examination of the stage theory of grief. J Am Med Assoc 297:716–723. doi:10.1001/jama.297.7.716

McDevitt-Murphy ME, Neimeyer RA, Burke LA, Williams JL (2012) Assessing the toll of traumatic loss: psychological symptoms in African Americans bereaved by homicide. Psychol Trauma 4(3):303–311

Meier AM, Carr DR, Currier JM, Neimeyer RA (2013) Attachment anxiety and avoidance in coping with bereavement: two studies. J Soc Clin Psychol 32:315–334. doi:10.1521/jscp.2013.32.3.315

Murphy SA, Johnson C, Cain KC, Das Gupta A, Dimond M, Lohan J, Baugher R (1998) Broad-spectrum group treatment for parents bereaved by the violent deaths of their 12-to 28-year-old children: a randomized controlled trial. Death Stud 22:209–235

Neimeyer RA (ed) (2001) Meaning reconstruction and the experience of loss. American Psychological Association, Washington, DC

Neimeyer RA (2006a) Re-storying loss: fostering growth in the posttraumatic narrative. In: Calhoun L, Tedeschi RG (eds) Handbook of posttraumatic growth: research and practice. Lawrence Erlbaum, Mahwah, NJ

Neimeyer RA (2006b) Widowhood, grief and the quest for meaning: a narrative perspective on resilience. In: Carr D, Nesse RM, Wortman CB (eds) Spousal bereavement in late life. Springer, New York, NY, pp 227–252

Neimeyer RA (ed) (2012) Techniques of grief therapy: practices for creating meaning. Routledge, New York

Neimeyer RA, Burke LA (2011) Complicated grief in the aftermath of homicide: spiritual crisis and distress in an African American sample. Religions 2:145–164. doi:10.3390/rel2020145

Neimeyer RA, Currier JM (2009) Grief therapy: evidence of efficacy and emerging directions. Curr Dir Psychol Sci 18:252–256. doi:10.1111/j.1467-8721.2009.01666.x

Neimeyer RA, Sands DC (2011) Meaning reconstruction in bereavement: from principles to practice. In: Neimeyer RA, Winokuer H, Harris D, Thornton G (eds) Grief and bereavement in contemporary society: bridging research and practice. Routledge, New York, NY

Neimeyer RA, Holland JM, Currier JM, Mehta T (2008) Meaning reconstruction in later life: toward a cognitive-constructivist approach to grief therapy. In: Gallagher-Thompson D, Steffan A, Thompson L (eds) Handbook of behavioral and cognitive therapies with older adults. Springer, New York, NY, pp 264–277

Neimeyer RA, Winokuer H, Harris D, Thornton G (eds) (2011) Grief and bereavement in contemporary society: bridging research and practice. Routledge, New York, NY

Norcross JC, Wampold BE (2010) What works for whom: tailoring psychotherapy to the person. J Clin Psychol 67:127–132. doi:10.1002/jclp.20764

Ott CH (2003) The impact of complicated grief on mental and physical health at various points in the bereavement process. Death Stud 27:249–272. doi:10.1080/07481180302887

Park CL (2008) Testing the meaning-making model of coping with loss. J Soc Clin Psychol 27:970–994. doi:10.1521/jscp.2008.27.9.970

Parkes CM (1996) Bereavement, 2nd edn. Routledge, London

Prigerson HG, Horowitz MJ, Jacobs SC, Parkes CM, Aslan M, Goodkin K, Raphael B et al (2009) Prolonged grief disorder: psychometric validation of criteria proposed for DSM-V and ICD-11. PLoS Med 6:1–12. doi:10.1371/journal.pmed.1000121

Resick PA, Schnicke MK (1992) Cognitive processing therapy for sexual assault victims. J Consult Clin Psychol 60:748–756. doi:10.1037//0022-006X.60.5.748

Rubin S (1999) The two-track model of bereavement: overview, retrospect and prospect. Death Stud 23:681–714. doi:10.1080/074811899200731

Rubin SS, Malkinson R, Koren D, Michaeli E (2009) The two-track model of bereavement questionnaire (TTBQ): development and validation of a relational measure. Death Stud 33:305–333. doi:10.1080/07481180802705668

Sandler IN, Ayers TS, Wolchik SA, Tein JY, Kwok O, Haine RA et al (2003) The family bereavement program: efficacy evaluation of a theory-based prevention program for parentally bereaved children and adolescents. J Consult Clin Psychol 71:587–600. doi:10.1037/0022-006X.71.3.587

Schut H, Stroebe MS (2005) Interventions to enhance adaptation to bereavement. J Palliat Med 8:140–147. doi:10.1089/jpm.2005.8.s-140

Schut H, Stroebe MS, van den Bout J, Terheggen M (2001) The efficacy of bereavement interventions: determining who benefits. In: Stroebe MS, Hansson RO, Stroebe W, Schut H (eds) Handbook of bereavement research. American Psychological Association, Washington, DC, pp 705–738. doi:10.1037/10436-029

Scruby LS, Sloan JA (1989) Evaluation of bereavement intervention. Can J Public Health 80:394–398

Shadish WR, Ragsdale K (1996) Random versus nonrandom assignment in controlled experiments: do you get the same answer? J Consult Clin Psychol 64:1290–1305. doi:10.1037//0022-006X.64.6.1290

Shear K, Frank E, Houch PR, Reynolds CF (2005) Treatment of complicated grief: a randomized controlled trial. J Am Med Assoc 293:2601–2608. doi:10.1001/jama.293.21.2601

Shear K, Boelen P, Neimeyer RA (2011a) Treating complicated grief: converging approaches. In: Neimeyer RA, Harris D, Winokuer H, Thornton G (eds) Grief and bereavement in contemporary society: bridging research and practice. Routledge, New York, NY, pp 139–162

Shear MK, Simon N, Wall M, Zistook S, Neimeyer RA et al (2011b) Complicated grief and related bereavement issues for DSM-5. Depress Anxiety 28:103–117. doi:10.1002/da.20780

Smith ML, Glass GV, Miller TI (1980) The benefits of psychotherapy. The Johns Hopkins University Press, Baltimore, MD

Stroebe M, Schut H (1999) The dual process model of coping with bereavement: rationale and description. Death Stud 23:197–224

Stroebe M, Hansson R, Schut H, Stroebe W (eds) (2007) Handbook of bereavement research and practice. American Psychological Association, Washington, DC

van der Houwen K, Stroebe M, Stroebe W, Schut H, van den Bout J, Wijngaards-de Meij L (2010) Risk factors for bereavement outcome: a multivariate approach. Death Stud 34:195–220. doi:10.1080/07481180903559196

Wagner B, Knaevelsrud C, Maercker A (2006) Internet-based cognitive-behavioral therapy for complicated grief: a randomized controlled trial. Death Stud 30:429–454. doi:10.1080/07481180600614385

Wampold BE (2001) The great psychotherapy debate. Earlbaum, Mahwah, NJ

Outcome Research: Methods for Improving Outcome in Routine Care

29

Michael J. Lambert

Contents

M.J. Lambert (✉)
Department of Psychology, Brigham Young University, Provo, UT 84602, USA
e-mail: michael_lambert@byu.edu

Abstract
The current review targets efforts to use outcome measures in routine care for the purpose of enhancing patient outcome, particularly for patients whose positive outcome is in doubt. The review first provides a brief historical context that justifies this particular form of outcome assessment, and its role in reducing negative treatment outcomes. The place of outcome measures in solving the negative effects problem is emphasized with a narrow focus on one set of measures that are relatively well advanced in their clinical utility. Other measures are then briefly reviewed before turning to future directions.

29.1 Outcome Research: Methods for Improving Outcome in Routine Care

The current review targets efforts to use outcome measures in routine care for the purpose of enhancing patient outcome, particularly for patients whose positive outcome is in doubt. The review first provides a brief historical context that justifies this particular form of outcome assessment, and its role in reducing negative treatment outcomes. The place of outcome measures in solving the negative effects problem is emphasized with a narrow focus on one set of measures that are relatively well advanced in

O.C.G. Gelo et al. (eds.), *Psychotherapy Research*,
DOI 10.1007/978-3-7091-1382-0_29,

their clinical utility. Other measures are then briefly reviewed before turning to future directions.

By the early 1970s, outcome research established that various forms of psychotherapy had an overall positive effect on patient outcome. The same evidence showed that a small and consistent percentage of people deteriorated while in care (Bergin 1971). The deterioration was mostly connected to patient characteristics, but specific therapist behaviors were also implicated (Lambert et al. 1977). These findings were based on extensive measurement of patient functioning in controlled research where, on average, patients were evaluated on an average of five different scales and from multiple perspectives (Hill and Lambert 2004). Hundreds of outcome measures were employed with no consensus on a core battery (Froyd et al. 1996). Sadly, the findings on negative change were almost entirely ignored by the field with research efforts principally directed to the study of "brand name" treatments and demonstrating the superiority of specific therapies in comparative outcome studies (Lambert et al. 2004a; Wampold 2001).

Interest in the phenomenon of outcome measurement in routine care grew in the late 1980s with the emergence of cost containment efforts. Managed care entities, for example, scrambling to control or even cut costs, had to show that reducing services did not diminish the effectiveness of treatments (Brown and Minami 2010). Assessing outcome was seen as a way of examining whether more could be accomplished with less or at least prove that brief, efficient services could be as effective as intensive, long-term care. The emergence of cost considerations as a major interest of managed care and government-sponsored mental health services in the United States spawned the use of outcome measurement in routine care, but without the comprehensive measurement practices that characterized clinical trials research. Managed care companies were slow to unite the idea of preventing negative outcome with outcome assessment and instead largely relied on implementing "best practices" as proven by clinical trial research. During the 1990s these companies were at least considering the value of using outcome assessment data to reduce negative effects making outcome measurement a routine part of care.

A review of psychotherapy outcome by Lambert and Ogles (2004) estimated that about 5–10 % of adult patients participating in clinical trials also leave treatment worse off than they were when treatment began. In routine care, patient deterioration is more problematic. Hansen et al. (2002) examined outcome in *routine practice settings* ranging from employee assistance programs to community mental health centers. Outcomes for these unselected naturalistic samples totaling more than 6,000 patients suggest the patients did not fare nearly as well as those in clinical trials, with only about one-third showing improvement or recovery and 3–14 % deteriorating.

The situation for child and adolescent outcome in routine care is even more sobering than with adult populations. The small body of outcome studies in community-based usual care settings has yielded an overall mean effect size near zero (Weiss et al. 1999; Weisz et al. 2006; Weisz et al. 1995), yet millions of youth are served each year in these systems of care (National Advisory Mental Health Council 2001; Ringel and Sturm 2001). In a comparison of children being treated in community mental health ($N = 936$) or through managed care ($N = 3{,}075$), estimates of deterioration were 24 % and 14 %, respectively (Warren et al. 2010). Furthermore, increased attention to deterioration in treatment may be warranted given the high rates of treatment dropout observed in clinical practice. It is estimated that 40–60 % of children and adolescents discontinue treatment prematurely (Kazdin 1996; Wierzbicki and Pekarik 1993); many of these dropouts are likely due to perceived lack of benefit from treatment. With regard to measuring treatment response in child and adolescent psychotherapy, Kazdin (2005) noted that "such information would be enormously helpful if used to monitor and evaluate treatment in clinical practice" (p. 555); however, very little research has evaluated the feasibility and utility of using a patient-focused paradigm for monitoring child and adolescent treatment progress and identifying cases that may be at risk for negative outcome.

Evidence-based practice in psychology (EBPP) has been defined as the "integration of the best available research with clinical expertise in the context of patient characteristics, culture, and preferences" (APA 2006, p. 273). Evidence-based practice includes the regular monitoring of patient outcome such that treatment can be adjusted if suitable progress is not observed (APA 2006; Institute of Medicine 2006). One way to accomplish this is with regular monitoring or tracking outcomes with standardized scales throughout the treatment process and providing clinicians with patient progress feedback. The basic rationale behind the concept of providing feedback makes practical sense. If clinicians get information about what seems to be working, and perhaps more importantly what is not working, our performance will improve. In many situations performance and feedback are intertwined and obvious; in others a certain degree of blinding occurs, such that the association is not so temporally connected and the effects of performance are harder to discern (such as in psychotherapy), making it much more difficult to learn and improve. In obvious, as well as more subtle situations, providing feedback to improve performance has been studied quite extensively in a variety of areas and confirms our common sense expectations that feedback is helpful in maximizing the impact of treatments.

Even when an empirically supported treatment (EST) is offered to individuals who have the same disorder and see therapists who have been carefully selected, monitored, and supervised, 30–50 % of patients fail to respond to treatment (Hansen et al. 2002). This means that even if there were a right treatment or "best practice" for an individual, we would need to identify patients who are failing to respond to this treatment. *The major assumptions of this practice is that we can, in fact, identify poorly responding patients in a timely fashion and then take timely actions that will benefit them.* Considerable doubt exists about the ability of clinicians to recognize and predict treatment response, especially with patients that worsen in the course of treatment.

29.2 Measuring Treatment Response

A cornerstone of behavior therapies is the identification of behaviors that need to be modified, counting the frequency of such behaviors, and observing (monitoring) changes as a consequence of treatment. While these methods work especially well with specific behaviors and with children, they are not entirely satisfactory with the broad range of individuals whose psychopathology is much more complex. Nevertheless, what we have learned from behaviorism can be extended to routine care by using general measures of mental health in the place of counting specific behaviors.

The Outcome Questionnaire-45 (OQ-45; Lambert et al. 2004b) was created specifically to measure and assess real-time change in adult psychotherapy which could then be used by therapists to identify deterioration and improve patient outcome prior to treatment termination. It is a 45-item self-report measure designed for repeated administration throughout the course of treatment and at termination. In accordance with several reviews of the literature (e.g., Lambert 1983), the OQ-45 was conceptualized and designed to assess three domains of patient functioning: symptoms of psychological disturbance (particularly anxiety and depression), interpersonal problems, and social role functioning. Consistent with this conceptualization of outcome, the OQ-45 provides a Total Score, based on all 45 items, as well as Symptom Distress, Interpersonal Relations, and Social Role subscale scores. Each of these subscales contains some items related to the *positive* quality of life of the individual. There is also a shortened version of the OQ-45, the Outcome Questionnaire-30 that is in general use with adult patients.

The Youth Outcome Questionnaire (Y-OQ; Burlingame et al. 2005) is a 64-item parent/guardian report measure of treatment progress for children and adolescents (ages 4–17) receiving mental health intervention. Similar in its intent to the OQ-45, the Y-OQ is meant to track actual change in functioning as opposed to assigning diagnoses. The Y-OQ is composed of 64 items that comprise six separate subscales designed to tap diverse elements of healthy behavior. The subscales include Interpersonal Distress (ID), Somatic (S), Intrapersonal Relations (IP), Critical Items (CI), Social Problems (SP), and Behavioral Dysfunction (BD). The Youth Outcome Questionnaire Self-Report (Y-OQ-SR) is the equivalent self-report measure completed by youth ages 12–17. In addition, a shorter form, the Y-OQ-30, is available for parents, clinicians, and youth.

In short, the OQ and Y-OQ are brief measures of psychological disturbance that are reliable, valid, and sensitive to changes patients make during psychotherapy. They are well suited for tracking patient status during and following treatment and provide clinicians with a mental health vital sign. The measures have been extensively reviewed elsewhere (Burlingame et al. 2005; Lambert et al. 2004b; www.oqmeasures.com).

29.3 Prediction of Negative Change

29.3.1 The Surprising Failure of Clinicians to Accurately Predict Negative Outcome

Prior to discussing the accuracy of methods for predicting patient deterioration, it may be helpful to understand how well clinicians can do this task based on their clinical wisdom and experience with patients. After all, why develop elaborate means of predicting negative outcome if clinicians can do the task? In order to examine therapist predictive accuracy, Hannan et al. (2005) examined therapist accuracy by asking 40 therapists (20 trainees and 20 experienced professionals), at the end of each session with each of their patients, if they believed the patient would leave treatment in a deteriorated state and, in addition, if the patient was worse off at this particular session than when they entered treatment. We expected that experienced clinicians, given their extensive contact with patients over the years, would be more accurate in their judgments than trainees (who ranged from first-year graduate students to intern-level providers).

During a 3-week period predictions were made for 550 patients who participated in therapy sessions. In some cases therapists made three predictions, two predictions, or a single prediction based on the number of sessions a patient attended over the 3 weeks. In every other way treatment continued as usual and patients' progress was followed until they terminated treatment, at which time their intake OQ-45 score could be compared with their end of treatment OQ-45 score. While 40 patients were deteriorated at the termination of treatment, only 3 of 550 patients (0.01 %) were predicted by their therapist to leave treatment worse off than when they began, one of whom actually deteriorated. In general, patients' eventual deterioration was not forecast by clinicians who were attempting to do so. Rather than experienced clinicians being more able to predict the phenomenon, they did not identify a single patient who deteriorated—the only accurate prediction out of the three that were made was made by a trainee. In contrast 36 of the 40 (90 %) patients who deteriorated were predicted to do so based on actuarial methods applied to data from the same time period.

The actual deterioration rate for this sample was 7.3 %, very close to the 8 % we expected and informed therapists of at the inception of the study. Despite being armed with base rate information and having familiarity with the outcome measure utilized in the study, therapists showed an inability (unwillingness?) to accurately forecast negative outcome. Their predictions would have improved markedly if they had simply used their judgment that a patient was worse off relative to their intake status at any particular session (16 such patients), but they did not interpret their perception of patient worsening in this way. One might hope that the results of this study are limited to a single clinic consisting of poor or below average therapists—but it seems unlikely that this could explain these results. The therapists were well trained and, as a group, demonstrate patient outcome that are on a par with other treatment centers.

Collaborating information has been found in a related study that applied a different methodology. Hatfield et al. (2010) using an archival database from Midwestern University identified cases that had deteriorated during routine care offered by 13 licensed professionals, nearly half of whom had a Ph.D. with the remaining having a master's degree or completing a predoctoral internship. Outcome was measured with the OQ-45 and the selected patients were in the clinical range and seen by the same therapists from intake through treatment termination. No feedback was given to therapists in a systematic way although session-by-session scores were present in many patient files. The deterioration rate at the center among patients in the clinical range was 9 % (4,253/386). Two hundred fourteen of these cases were randomly selected and further reduced by eliminating patients who had seen more than one therapist, leaving 70 cases whose case files were examined to see if therapists made any note indicating they had worsened from the time they entered treatment. The files that were rated corresponded to those sessions in which the OQ-45 score had increased by 14 points or more (the reliable change index). Case notes were classified as either mentioning change or not, and if worsening was noted. For those where worsening was noted, the actions of therapists were recorded.

Deterioration was noted by therapists in 15 of the 70 patients (21 %) with no mention of progress occurring in 41 (59 %) of the cases. The OQ-45 score was referred to in 9 % of cases. Two (3 %) of the patients were rated as improved. With regard to new treatment decisions for the patients whose negative change was noted by the therapist and those who mentioned the OQ-45 score ($n = 21$), many were noted in the record. The most common actions were referral for medication (24 %), continue treatment as usual (24 %), and change treatment implementation (19 %).

Further examination of the most severe cases of negative change was undertaken by only looking at cases whose negative change was 30 or more points, an extreme negative deviation from entry levels of distress. Among 41 (4.4 % of those entering treatment) patients who met this criterion, deterioration was recorded in a case note in 32 % of the cases. In contrast to the Hannan et al. (2005) study in which therapists were asked to predict the eventual outcome of treatment and virtually never imagined it happening, the Hatfield et al. (2010) study estimated awareness of negative change as indicated in written notes. In this latter instance, even in situations involving very serious symptom worsening, therapists made no mention of it in about 70 % of the cases, and even when it was noted did not bring up supervision/consultation as an appropriate action in a single instance, although changing strategies and referral for medications were noted.

These results are similar to results in Hannan et al. (2005) with regard to asking therapists to judge patient status after specific sessions. Of 55 patients who were identified by the OQ-45 as signal-alarm cases at a specific session, 21 were judged by their therapist as "recovered" or "improved." The Hannan et al. (2005) study provides evidence that therapists not only cannot predict final *negative* outcome but saw nearly 40 % of patients as in an improved state when they were reporting more self-reported symptoms than they had when they started treatment.

In reflecting about the therapist's perception of patient worsening, it seems clear that therapists are overly optimistic about their positive effects on patients. Therapists typically estimate that 85 % of their clients have positive outcomes, but also that they see themselves as well above average in relation to their peers with regard to benefiting their patients (Walfish et al. 2012). The results are consistent with, if not more extreme than, findings from hundreds of studies comparing clinical prediction with actuarial methods. Examples regarding the limitation of clinician ability to make accurate judgments without feedback are plentiful. For example, a review comparing human judgment/diagnosis abilities versus statistical methods consistently shows that statistical methods are much more accurate (Grove et al. 2000). Despite the evidence suggesting that clinical decision-making may not always be accurate, professionals are typically very confident about their eventual clinical decisions (Garb 1998). Owing to the extant research documenting the superiority of actuarial over clinical methods in making such predictions (Garb 2005), there is little doubt that the greatest predictive success will come through real time clinic-based application of computer-assisted actuarial methods. Indeed, we predict that in the future, such psychological "lab test" or "vital sign" data will be as common and important in behavioral health as in medicine.

29.3.2 Empirical Methods for the Prediction of Patient Deterioration

An empirically derived signal-alarm system was developed to alert clinicians to potential treatment failures. This system plots a statistically generated expected recovery curve for differing levels of pretreatment distress on the OQ-45 and uses this as a basis for identifying patients who are not making expected treatment gains and are at risk of having a poor outcome. This empirical or purely statistical method of prediction became possible after repeatedly assessing patients with the OQ-45 following sessions of treatment.

Finch et al. (2001) used the PROC MIXED functions of the Statistical Analysis System (SAS) to apply HLM to a large database consisting of 11,492 patients treated in a variety of settings including employee assistance programs, university counseling centers, outpatient clinics, private practice, and a clinical psychology training clinic. An initial graphical analysis of the data revealed decelerating growth curves similar to those identified in dose-response studies—a lawful linear relationship between the log of the number of sessions and the normalized probability of patient improvement, again illuminating the tendency for larger and larger doses (number of sessions) in order to find a higher percentage of recovered patients.

The resulting groups of data were analyzed to generate a linear model for recovery curves. Administrations of the OQ-45 were nested within an individual patient, who was nested within a specific therapist, who was nested within a specific treatment site, and so forth. This linear model allowed comparisons of individuals even when OQ-45 scores were missing at different sessions, and even when the ultimate number of sessions, length of time between sessions, and overall length of therapy was different between patients. Essentially, a separate regression line and error estimate was generated for each patient in the analysis.

It was possible to establish the upper and lower bounds of tolerance intervals for each of the recovery curves. The tolerance interval is a quality control protocol often used in engineering applications. Tolerance intervals determine the probability that a given OQ-45 score at a given session will fall within a specified interval. The tolerance intervals allowed for the identification of OQ-45 total score values that have an established probability of falling outside of the upper and lower limits of the tolerance interval. Specifically, this means that the tolerance intervals calculated in this model allowed for the identification of the 10 (red signal) and 15 (yellow signal) percent of patients in a given sample whose rate and trajectory of progress deviated significantly from what was the predicted course of recovery for others entering therapy with a similar intake score.

The tolerance intervals created were primarily aimed at identifying this 10 % of the patient population who deviate from the recovery track. These coefficients and tolerance intervals formed the core of the "empirical warning system" by providing table values and charts of predicted therapeutic gains, against which any given patient could be compared at any session of psychotherapy. After an individual has completed a given OQ-45 administration, the total score can then be compared to the corresponding session value for others beginning therapy with a comparable pretreatment score. If, at any session following intake, the OQ-45 total score for a patient does not exceed the tolerance interval, then therapy is judged as proceeding as anticipated for this particular patient, and a green message can be given as feedback for the therapist to proceed as they have been. If the same OQ-45 score falls outside of the upper 15 % and does not surpass the upper bound of the 10 % tolerance interval, the patient is considered to be deviating by greater than one standard deviation from what is expected of a typical person at this point in therapy, and the therapist would receive a yellow message as a warning to attend to this patient's progress. If this same OQ-45 score falls above the upper limits of the 10 % interval, then the patient is deviating significantly in a negative direction from what is predicted for patients at this point in therapy. The 10 % boundary is consistent with the estimate that about 10 % of patients deteriorate following psychotherapy (Lambert and Ogles 2004). At this point the therapist would receive a red warning message that therapy may be heading toward an unsuccessful conclusion and that the therapist may need to consider an alternative course of action. In our program of research, we consider patients whose treatment response crosses either the yellow or red boundary to be alarm-signal or "not-on-track" cases. Such patients are predicted to leave treatment deteriorated unless preventive actions are taken.

Abbreviated messages associated with predictions are as follows:

White Feedback	"The patient is functioning in the normal range. Consider termination."
Green Feedback	"The rate of change the patient is making is in the adequate range. No change in the treatment plan is recommended."
Yellow Feedback	"The rate of change the patient is making is less than adequate. Recommendations: consider altering the treatment plan by intensifying treatment, shifting intervention strategies, and monitoring progress especially carefully. This patient may end up with no significant benefit from therapy."
Red Feedback	"The patient is not making the expected level of progress. Chances are he/she may drop out of treatment prematurely or have a negative treatment outcome. Steps should be taken to carefully review this case and consider a new course of action such as referral for medication or intensification of treatment. The treatment plan should be reconsidered. Consideration should also be given to seeking supervision on this case."

29.3.3 Accuracy of Predicting Treatment Failure with Adults

In contrast to clinician prediction of patient deterioration, the accuracy of the above actuarial methods has been evaluated in a number of empirical investigations (Ellsworth et al. 2006; Lambert et al. 2002a; Lutz et al. 2006; Percevic et al. 2006; Spielmans et al. 2006), and they appear to be successful at predicting which patients will have negative treatment outcome. It is important to note that the signal-alarm system is highly sensitive in that it is able to accurately predict deterioration in 85–100 % of cases that actually end with a negative outcome and is also far superior to clinical judgment in its ability to identify patients who are at risk of having a negative treatment outcome (Hannan et al. 2005). These studies vary with regard to patient populations and methods, and the findings are reviewed briefly below.

Lambert et al. (2002a) examined predictive accuracy of both the rational and empirical methods with 492 patients who were in treatment at a university counseling center. Of these cases, 36 (7.3 %) were reliably worse/deteriorated at termination. The empirical method correctly identified all 36 (100 %), most of whom (86 %) were identified by the third treatment session. The empirical method was highly effective at identifying patients who went on to deteriorate and such a prediction could be predicted very early (although in this setting about 90 % of patients have left treatment by the 15th session). At the same time, the empirical method misidentified 83 (18 %) patients as likely to deteriorate (not on track) when they had not deteriorated at treatment termination. The outcome of these misidentified cases (false alarms/positives) was further studied and contrasted with the outcome of patients who were not identified as signal-alarm cases (predicted positive outcome). Of the 83 misclassified signal-alarm cases, 18 % improved or recovered at termination, while 74 % showed no reliable change. In contrast, of the 373 cases that the empirical method did not identify as signal-alarm cases, 50 % recovered or improved and 50 % showed no reliable change. These findings offer further support for the signal-alarm method in that they suggest that even the false alarms have a poorer outcome than cases that are not identified as likely treatment failures. That is, if an alarm (red or yellow warning) is given, the patient has less than a one in five chance of having a positive outcome, compared to a 50/50 chance if no signal alarm is generated.

Further analyses explored the difference between red and yellow warnings: What was the relative outcome for patients receiving a red versus a yellow signal? Outcome for these patients was classified into three categories: reliably improved/recovered, no reliable change, and deteriorated. Of the 36 deteriorated cases, the empirical method's red alarm picked up 34 of the 36 deteriorated cases, while the yellow signal picked up the remaining two deteriorated cases. The red alarm is indeed a more serious indicator for deterioration, one that should generate greater cause for concern to clinicians than the yellow signal.

In a replication of this study, Spielmans et al. (2006) examined the predictive accuracy of the rational and empirical methods in two treatment centers, a state university counseling center ($n = 216$) and a university-based graduate student training clinic ($n = 83$), where psychotherapy was provided to community members. When reliable worsening (a detrimental change of 14 or more points on the OQ-45) was used as the negative outcome criteria, the empirical method was accurate in 81 % of cases. Of the 16 (5 %) patients who reliably worsened, the empirical method identified 13. When deterioration (leaving treatment in the clinical range and worsening by 14 or more points) was used as the negative outcome criteria, 10 of 13 cases were correctly identified.

When transformed into a standardized mean difference effect size (*ES*; intake OQ-45 score—endpoint OQ-45 score/pooled standard deviation of intake and endpoint OQ-45 scores), those patients predicted to fail by the empirical method improved by an *ES* of .17, which is slightly less than the *ES* of .20 widely considered to represent a small effect size (Cohen 1988). This indicates that little improvement, on average, occurred for those patients who were identified as not on track (signal alarms) by the empirical method. Patients predicted to have a nonnegative outcome (i.e., *not* to have a negative response to treatment) showed positive outcome on average ($ES = .90$). In contrast to the original study which had an identification rate of 100 %, this study showed less accuracy (81 %). A likely reason for this is the amount of missing data. Although HLM can model recovery with missing data, it is more difficult to identify cases that may be in trouble if data is not collected often. Such was the case in the Spielmans et al. (2006) study.

In another evaluation of patient deterioration, Lutz et al. (2006) modeled recovery in 4,365 patients using a variation of calculating the expected treatment response called the nearest neighbor methodology. This rather creative approach had been applied in avalanche research (Brabec and Meister 2001) to predict future avalanches—a fitting metaphor for deterioration in psychotherapy—where patients can undergo serious decomposition. In avalanche prediction research, the best predictors are characteristics of the snow that surrounds an avalanche. Lutz et al. (2005) found this methodology worked well to predict rate of change although they did not examine deterioration itself. In the Lutz et al.'s (2006) study, deterioration, as measured by the OQ-30, was predicted with patient responses to the 15 items ("nearest neighbors") that make up the rest of the OQ-45. In essence the method uses the intake scores of previously treated patients to make predictions about subsets of similar patients. Predictions based on this model were compared to predictions made using the rational method.

Three questions were addressed: (a) How well do the rationally derived and empirically derived decision rules predict outcome? (b) How early in treatment can the decision rules identify negative developments and which method is better? (c) Is the number of warning signals provided from these decision rules predictive of therapy outcome? Unlike past research on prediction from our research group, the authors aggregated reliable improvement and clinically significant change as positive outcome and no change and reliable negative change as negative outcome. Our past predictive studies have only examined the ability to predict negative reliable change, with all other categorizations of patient change considered "positive" (i.e., nonnegative).

Results showed that the nearest neighbor (NN) technique had a specificity of 86 % but sensitivity of only 41 % at the 90 % level of confidence, while the rational method had 66 % specificity and sensitivity of 57 %. (The analysis allows for differing levels of confidence to be specified, the advantage of which is the clinician can choose how sure to make the prediction.) The NN also identified a significantly greater proportion of patients sooner than the rational method. Multiple alarm signals given to individual patients indicated a greater likelihood that the patient would deteriorate. It should be noted that these results suggest the NN method far exceeds clinical judgment but the hit rates are not comparable to our usual studies where deterioration is the predicted state of interest. Counting those who do not reliably change as having a negative outcome makes logical sense, as psychotherapy is intended to provide measurable positive change (except in some clinical circumstances where preventing deterioration is all that can be expected), but it is a difficult task.

29.3.4 Treatment Failure in Children and Adolescents

Predicting treatment failure in children undergoing psychotherapy is more difficult than it is for adults. One reason for this is that in children's services there are more missing data. Often the schedule for administration of the measures is less frequent than weekly. In addition, in outpatient settings the child may be accompanied to their session by a person who did not bring the child to intake, such as a father or sister instead of the mother. Prediction is dependent on tracking change with a single informant, such as an adolescent, or in many cases the mother. These difficulties are unfortunate, as the problem of deterioration in youth is double or triple that found in adults (Warren et al. 2010). Progress in predicting treatment failure and in improving outcomes is being made through the use of the Youth Outcome Questionnaire (Y-OQ; Bishop et al. 2005; Bybee et al. 2007; Warren et al. 2009). Alerts have been developed, their accuracy tested but no studies of feedback effects have been completed.

29.4 Going Beyond Alerting Therapists to Potential Treatment Failure: The Provision of Clinical Support Tool Feedback

Once a patient takes the OQ-45(or Y-OQ), commences treatment, but signals as "not on track," further assessment of the client can be initiated in order to bring to the forefront possible causes for negative change. A Clinical Support

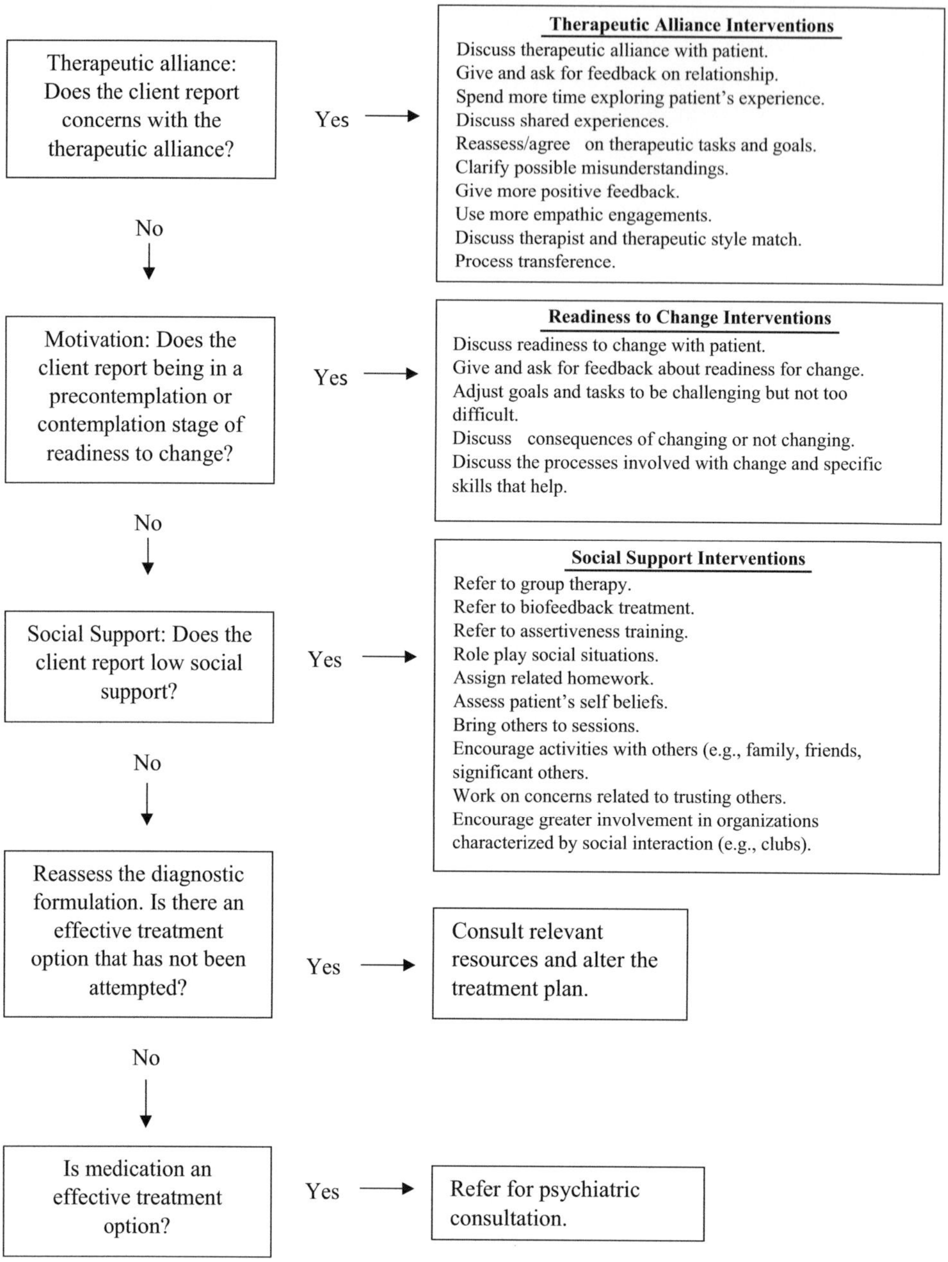

Fig. 29.1 Clinical Support Tool (CST) problem-solving decision tree

Tool Manual (Lambert et al. 2004c) was developed to standardize this procedure and test its effects. The Clinical Support Tool (CST) intervention is driven by a decision tree that organizes clinician problem-solving as well as a brief measure, the Assessment for Signal Cases (ASC). Figure 29.1 depicts the CST problem-solving decision tree provided to therapists treating adult cases in which patients are predicted to have a poor outcome. As can be seen the constructs embedded in the decision tree focus the therapist's attention on the quality of the therapeutic alliance, patient motivation, and patient perceptions of social support, as well as the possible need to reconsider the diagnosis and seek a consultation for medication. The ASC is a 40-item measure that provides subscale score feedback and individual item feedback for therapists to consider as they progress through the decision tree: i.e., the ASC provides some of the information necessary to go through the decision tree.

The first 11-items of the ASC require the patient to reflect on the therapeutic relationship and report his or her perceptions. Items that fall below an empirically based cut score (about one standard deviation from the mean therapist rating on the item) are brought to the therapist's attention along with a list of suggested interventions for repairing alliance ruptures. The ASC contains 11 items aimed at assessing the client's perception of their social support network with particular emphasis on relationships with family and friends. The ASC also contains nine items assessing aspects of patient motivation and expectations for treatment. And finally nine items call for the patient to report on critical life events that may be the source of their deteriorating condition.

29.5 Impact of Feedback on Psychotherapy Outcome in Practice

Enough evidence has now accumulated on the effects of measuring, monitoring, and feeding back this information to establish an empirical basis for claiming it as an effective practice. Some of this evidence is now presented.

29.5.1 Summary of a Recent Meta-analytic Review of the OQ Quality Assurance System

In the most recent meta-analytic and mega-analytic review of the OQ system, Shimokawa et al. (2010) re-analyzed a combined dataset ($N = 6{,}151$) from the six major OQ feedback studies published to date (Harmon et al. 2007; Hawkins et al. 2004; Lambert et al. 2001, 2002b; Slade et al. 2008; Whipple et al. 2003). Each of the studies required about 1 year of daily data collection and evaluated the effects of providing feedback about an individual patient's improvement through the use of progress graphs and warnings about patients who were not demonstrating expected treatment responses (signal-alarm cases).

The six studies shared many things in common: (a) each included consecutive cases seen in routine care regardless of patient diagnosis or comorbid conditions (rather than being disorder specific); (b) random assignment of patient to experimental conditions (various feedback interventions) and treatment-as-usual conditions (no feedback) was made in four of the six studies, while reasonable measures were taken in two studies ensure equivalence in experimental and control conditions at pretreatment; (c) psychotherapists provided a variety of theoretically guided treatments, with most adhering to cognitive behavioral and eclectic orientations and fewer representing psychodynamic and experiential orientations; (d) a variety of clinicians were involved—postgraduate therapists and graduate students each accounted for about 50 % of patients seen; (e) *therapists saw both experimental (feedback) and no feedback cases, thus limiting the likelihood that outcome differences between conditions could be due to therapist effects;* (f) the outcome measure as well as the methodology rules/standards for identifying "signal" of "not-on-track" patients (failing cases) remained constant; (g) the length of therapy (dosage) was determined by patient and therapist rather than by research design or arbitrary insurance limits; and (h) patient characteristics such as gender, age, and ethnicity were generally similar across studies and came from the same university counseling center, with an exception of Hawkins et al. (2004) study which was conducted in a hospital-based outpatient clinic.

In their quantitative review, Shimokawa et al. (2010) conducted intent-to-treat (ITT) and efficacy analyses on the effects of various feedback interventions in relation to treatment as usual (TAU). These two distinct sets of analyses

Table 29.1 Effect sizes of feedback interventions in comparison to TAU (efficacy analysis)

		Posttreatment score		Reliable improvement		Deterioration	
Feedback system	k	Hedges's g [95 % CI]	r	OR [95 % CI]	r	OR [95 % CI]	r^a
OQ system[a]							
NOT Fb	4	0.53*** [0.28, 0.78]	0.25	2.55*** [1.64, 3.98]	0.23	0.44* [0.23, 0.85]	−0.21
NOT P/T Fb	3[c]	0.55*** [0.36, 0.73]	0.25	2.87*** [1.93, 4.27]	0.27	0.68** [0.42, 1.13]	−0.10
CST Fb	3[d]	0.70*** [0.52, 0.88]	0.33	3.85*** [2.65, 5.60]	0.34	0.23*** [0.12, 0.44]	−0.37

Note. k = number of studies; r = correlation r; CI = confidence interval; NOT Fb = not-on-track clients whose therapists received client progress feedback; NOT P/T Fb = not-on-track clients where both clients and therapists received client progress feedback; CST Fb = not-on-track clients whose therapists received client progress feedback and Clinical Support Tools feedback

$^*p < 0.05$; $^{**}p < 0.01$; $^{***}p < 0.001$

[a]Negative correlations indicate greater effect in reducing treatment failure at termination

[b]Effect sizes (Hedges's g and OR) of OQ system-based feedback interventions were meta- and mega-analytically calculated and reported in Shimokawa et al. (2010)

[c]Original data from three studies employing the P/T Fb groups were aggregated and compared to the aggregated TAU data from four studies, using a mega-analytic approach

[d]Original data from three studies employing the CST Fb groups were aggregated and compared to the aggregated TAU data from four studies, using a mega-analytic approach

were performed to investigate the amount of effects expected for each feedback intervention based on treatment assignment alone, which represent the amount of effects expected when each intervention is implemented as a policy in routine care (ITT analysis) and the amount of effects expected among patients who are more likely to have been beneficiaries of the experimental treatments (efficacy analysis). Furthermore, the authors investigated the incremental benefits of newer feedback interventions, provision of formal progress feedback directly to both patients and therapists (patient/therapist feedback; P/T Fb), and provision of formal progress feedback to therapists combined with Clinical Support Tools feedback (CST Fb). In the following sections, we present a summary of a portion of exhaustive meta-analytic findings based on the efficacy analysis.

In these analyses, only those who met the minimum criteria to allow treatment effects to be measured were compared to the TAU, which employed only the minimum criterion to be identified as "not on track" (NOT). The summary of effect sizes is presented in Table 29.1.

Treatment Effects of OQ Progress Feedback (Fb) with at Risk Patients When the NOT Fb group was compared to NOT TAU, the effect size for mean posttreatment OQ score difference was $g = 0.53$, $p < 0.001$, 95 % CI [0.28, 0.78]. These results suggest that the average patient in the NOT Fb group, who stays in treatment until the therapist has received feedback, is better off than approximately 70 % of patients in the NOT TAU group. In terms of the clinically significant classification at termination, 9 % of those in NOT Fb deteriorated, while 38 % achieved clinically significant improvement. In contrast, among patients in NOT TAU, 20 % deteriorated while 22 % clinically significantly improved. When the odds of deterioration and clinically significant improvement were compared between the two groups, results indicated those in the NOT Fb group had less than a half the odds of experiencing deterioration (OR = 0.44, $p < 0.05$, 95 % CI [0.23, 0.85]) while having approximately 2.6 times higher odds of experiencing reliable improvement (OR = 2.55, $p < 0.001$, 95 % CI [1.64, 3.98]).

Treatment Effects of Patient/Therapist Feedback (P/T Fb) on at Risk Patients The effect size of mean posttreatment OQ score comparison in efficacy analysis was reported to be $g = 0.55$, $p < 0.001$, 95 % CI [0.36, 0.73]—effects very similar to that of the NOT Fb group. However, the P/T Fb intervention appeared to have had polarizing effects, resulting in deterioration rate and odds comparable to NOT TAU. The rates of deterioration and clinically significant improvement among NOT P/T Fb were 15 % and 45 %, respectively. The results suggest that patients in the P/T Fb group have approximately 0.7 times the odds of deterioration, OR $= 0.68, p = 0.134$, 95 % CI [0.42, 1.13], while having approximately three times higher odds of achieving clinically significant improvement, OR $= 2.87$, $p < 0.001$, 95 % CI [1.93, 4.27]. These results suggest that, although the average patient in the NOT P/T Fb group was better off than 71 % of patients in NOT TAU, there may have been moderators that facilitated outcome enhancement in some patients while failing to prevent, or possibly contributing to, outcome worsening.

Treatment Effects of Clinical Support Tools Feedback (CST Fb) on at Risk Patients When the outcome of the CST Fb group was compared to the NOT TAU, the effect size for the difference in mean posttreatment OQ scores was $g = 0.70$, $p < 0.001$, 95 % CI [0.52, 0.88]. These results indicate that the average patient in the CST Fb group, who stays in treatment to experience the benefit of this intervention, is better off than 76 % of patients in NOT TAU. The rates of deterioration and clinically significant improvement among the CST Fb group were 5.5 % and 53 %, respectively. The results suggest that patients in the CST Fb group have less than a fourth the odds of deterioration, OR $= 0.23$, $p < 0.001$, 95 % CI [0.12, 0.44] , while having approximately 3.9 times higher odds of achieving clinically significant improvement.

The above findings from the OQ system-based feedback studies indicate that three forms of feedback interventions in the OQ system are effective in enhancing the treatment effects of patients who are at risk of leaving therapy reliably worse off than when they entered treatment. Effects of feedback interventions in terms of mean OQ scores are graphically presented in Fig. 29.2. Table 29.2 displays clinically significant change and reliable change in order to make the impact of feedback more clear. As can be seen, reduction of deterioration and increases in positive outcome are rather dramatic in relation to treatment as usual even though the same therapists offered both interventions. Tracking adult patients' progress in therapy, predicting treatment failure, and providing feedback to therapists have consistently been associated with improved recovery rates in adult patients and have been listed by the APA Task Force on Evidence-Based Practice (2006) as showing great promise as an evidence-based method. The Task Force also indicates that one of the "most pressing research needs" includes this particular type of research, which they summarize as "providing clinicians with real-time patient feedback to benchmark progress in treatment and clinical support tools to adjust treatment as needed." Much less is known about how progress feedback will affect youth and their families.

29.6 Some Alternative Measures

Several psychotherapy outcome management systems that provide progress feedback based on standardized scales have been developed and implemented in clinical service delivery settings worldwide. Though the specific procedures employed in each of these quality management systems vary, a common feature across all of them is the monitoring of patient treatment response and reporting it to clinicians. Among the most important of these is the CORE system widely used in the United Kingdom (Barkham et al. 2001) and the TOPS system developed by Kraus et al. (2005). In general, these two systems have emphasized the administrative use of data rather than feedback to therapists during the course of psychotherapy. Administrative use allows managers of mental health services to examine the periodic and final outcome of interventions and compare outcome to appropriate benchmarks.

Of special note is the Partners for Change Outcome Management System (PCOMS; Miller et al. 2005) which employs two ultra brief scales (four items each). The Outcome Rating Scale (ORS; Duncan and Miller 2008) focuses on mental health functioning, modeled after the domains of outcome measured by subscales of the Outcome Questionnaire-45. The Session Rating

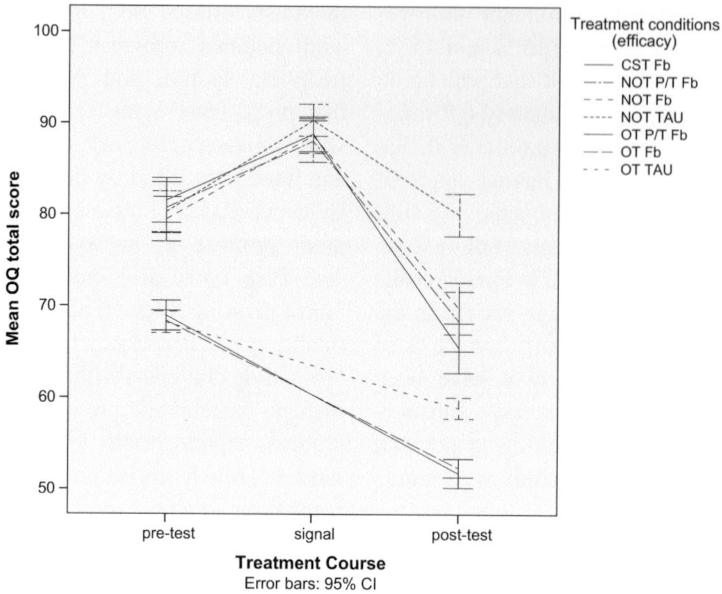

Fig. 29.2 Change from pre- to posttesting of not-on-track (signal alarm) and on-track patients. *Note*: CST Fb = signal-alarm cases whose therapist got feedback and used the Clinical Support Tools; NOT P/T Fb = signal-alarm cases who were assigned to receive feedback and whose therapist also received feedback; NOT Fb = signal-alarm cases whose therapist got a *red* or *yellow* signal, indicating they were at risk for treatment failure; NOT TAU = signal-alarm cases whose therapist got no signal or message; OT-NFb = clients who were making satisfactory progress and whose therapist never received any information about their progress; OT-Fb = clients whose therapist got a *green* or *white* signal and message and who were predicted to have a positive outcome; pretest = OQ-45 administration at intake; signal = average client score on the OQ-45 at the point at which a client qualified for a *yellow* or *red* message (the time of warning varied across patients); posttest = average client OQ-45 score at the session they terminated treatment (number of sessions until termination occurred varied)

Table 29.2 Percent of not-on-track (signal-alarm) cases meeting criteria for clinically significant change at termination summed across six studies (efficacy sample)

Outcome classification	CST Fb[a], *n* (%)	P/T Fb[b], *n* (%)	Fb[c], *n* (%)	TAU[d], *n* (%)
Deteriorated[e]	12 (5.5)	26 (14.7)	24 (9.1)	64 (20.1)
No change	91 (41.9)	71 (40.1)	140 (53.2)	183 (57.5)
Reliable/clinically significant change[f]	114 (52.5)	80 (45.2)	99 (37.6)	71 (22.3)

[a]CST Fb = patients who were not on track and whose therapist received feedback and used clinical support tools
[b]P/T Fb = patients who were not on track and both patients and their therapist received feedback
[c]Fb = patients who were not on track and whose therapist received feedback
[d]TAU = patients who were not on track and whose therapist was not given feedback
[e]Worsened by at least 14 points on the OQ from pretreatment to posttreatment
[f]Improved by at least 14 points on the OQ or improved and passed the cutoff between dysfunctional and functional populations

Scale (SRS; Miller and Duncan 2004) is aimed at assessing the therapeutic alliance. Because of its brevity this system is very clinician friendly and ensures discussion of assessment results by the patient and therapist at each session because rating of mental health status and therapeutic alliance are normally collected in the presence of the therapist.

Two studies investigating the effects of the PCOMS have been published to date (Reese et al. 2009; Anker et al. 2009). Reese et al. (2009) conducted an examination of two samples comparing the treatment outcome of patients receiving the PCOMS feedback intervention and those receiving no feedback. The authors reported an effect size of $d = .54$ when the feedback group and TAU were compared on the basis of ORS total scale scores. They further reported that 80 % of patients in the feedback group experienced reliable change, while 54 % of patients in TAU achieved the same criteria. This was contrasted with 4 % of those in the feedback group meeting the criteria for deterioration, while 13 % of their TAU counterparts meeting the same. The second sample came from a graduate training clinic. The authors reported an effect size of $d = .49$ when comparing the feedback group and TAU on the basis of the ORS scores. The authors of the study reported 16 patients (36 %) in the feedback group and 11 patients (38 %) in TAU were identified as "not progressing," therefore at risk of poor outcome. In terms of clinical significance, 67 % of those in the feedback condition achieved reliable change status, while 4 % deteriorated. This was contrasted to 41 % of patients in TAU achieving reliable change, while 3 % ($n = 1$) deteriorating.

Anker et al. (2009) conducted a randomized controlled study investigating the effects of PCOMS-based feedback intervention on patients in couple's therapy at a community family counseling clinic in Norway. The authors of the study reported an effect size of $d = .50$ when comparing the posttreatment ORS scores after controlling for pretreatment scores. The authors reported posttreatment outcome classification (based on the notion of clinical significance) of couples at posttreatment. It is important to point out that the reported n and percentage of outcome classification were based on couples where *both* individuals in the couple met the same outcome classification. Based on these inclusion criteria, 66 % of couples in the feedback group and 50 % of couples in the TAU were included in the analyses. The outcome classifications at the individual level were not reported. Of those included in the analysis, the authors reported 51 % of couples in the feedback condition achieving either clinically significant change or reliable change, while 2 % deteriorated. In contrast, 23 % of couples in the TAU group reached either clinically significant change or reliable change and 4 % experienced deterioration.

The preceding two studies obtained results similar to those found with the OQ system, suggesting that progress feedback can be effective across systems and lends support to the value of using outcome measures as a means of enhancing treatment effects.

Summary and Conclusions

Consistent findings suggest a deterioration rate of 5–10 % across samples of adult patients undergoing psychotherapy. The negative change problem is even more serious among child and adolescent patients who seem to deteriorate at rates closer to 12–24 % depending on the population. There are serious problems with clinicians' ability to recognize which of their patients are likely to leave treatment worse off and also which might be having notable worsening at a particular time in treatment. Both awareness problems can be overcome through the use of *outcome measures* and actuarial/statistical prediction methods, increasing the probability that therapists could provide better care. Final deterioration can be predicted before it occurs through the use of information about the patient's *initial level of disturbance* and their *treatment response* following sessions of psychotherapy. Several studies were presented that illustrated methods for predicting treatment failure and their success. With regard to prediction it appears that clinicians err on the side of being overly optimistic, while actuarial methods produce a good share of false positives, with the ratio of false alarms to correct identification hovering around 2 to 1.

With children/adolescents predictive accuracy is not as high. The predictive systems are able to identify closer to 70 % of those who deteriorate (with a range of 54–85 %) and produce rates of false alarm similar to adults. It may be that it is just more difficult to make these predictions with children, but it is also true that the data used to model child expected treatment response is based on fewer sessions and has more missing data. Importantly, adolescent self-reported psychological and social functioning proved to be as accurate at identifying negative outcome as parent-based data.

The algorithms we have developed show that if a patient never signals "red" or "yellow," it is almost certain that they will not deteriorate. At the same time the negative predictive power (the proportion of people who are predicted not to deteriorate in treatment who in fact, do not deteriorate in treatment) typically is around 0.90+. The quality of the positive predictive power values is much lower, somewhere around 0.20. There is about a 20 % increase (over baseline rates of 8 % in adults) in ability to predict treatment failure by using the predictive system (in children it is closer to 0.30–0.40). These results are consistent with validity coefficients that can be expected when base rates (such as in suicide) are very low (Steiner 2003).

Unlike some medical decisions where the cost of over identification of signal cases may result in intrusive and even health-threatening interventions such as surgery, the "signal" or "not-on-track" prediction in psychotherapy merely alerts the therapist to the need for reconsidering the value of ongoing treatment, rather than mandating specific changes. Thus, we see the signal alarm as supporting clinical decision-making, rather than supplanting it. Since the signal-alarm alerts therapists to the possible need for action, rather than triggering a negative chain of events such as termination or referral, the current level of misidentification would seem to be tolerable.

Meta-analysis of six large-scale feedback studies using the QO system (informing clinicians of patients predicted to have a negative treatment response and providing Clinical Support Tools to assist in problem-solving) resulted in improved patient outcome with effect sizes of $g = 0.53$ (therapist feedback condition) and $g = 0.55$ (patient/therapist feedback condition) as compared to TAU. Furthermore, when feedback is augmented with the Assessment for Signal Cases and Clinical Support Tools, 53 % of those predicted to deteriorate showed clinically significant improvement at the end of treatment (an effect size of $g = 0.70$ compared to TAU). Such effects sizes are surprisingly large when one considers an average effect for comparative studies (active treatments) typically falls between 0.00 and 0.20 (Lambert and Ogles 2004) and is widely considered important enough to lead to a recommendation of "best practice." A feedback system utilizing the Y-OQ for child and adolescent treatments which is based on the OQ-45 methodology has been developed and awaits future study and evaluation.

Finally, surveys show that practitioners question the role of information technology in improving patient care (with only 10 % classified as "eager-adopters") (Meredith et al. 2000). Even so, with the widespread availability and power of computers, it is now possible for providers to obtain outcome data about the success of individual patients in real time. The findings cited above make it clear that without timely feedback about patient progress, practitioners will grossly underestimate negative outcome. Consequently, they will be less likely to make the adjustments necessary to forestall negative or, for that matter, improve positive outcome rates.

References

Anker MG, Duncan BL, Sparks JA (2009) Using client feedback to improve couple therapy outcomes: a randomized clinical trial in a naturalistic treatment setting. J Consult Clin Psychol 77:693–704

APA Presidential Task Force on Evidence-Based Practice (2006) Evidence-based practice in psychology. Am Psychol 61:271–285

Barkham M, Margison F, Leach C, Lucock M, Mellor-Clark J, Evans C, Benson L, Connell J, Audin K, McGrath G (2001) Service profiling and outcomes benchmarking using the CORE_OM: toward practice-based evidence in the psychological therapies. J Consult Clin Psychol 69:184–196

Bergin AE (1971) In: Bergin AE, Garfield SL (eds) Handbook of psychotherapy and behavior change. Wiley, New York, NY

Bishop MJ, Bybee TS, Lambert MJ, Burlingame GM, Wells MG, Poppleton LE (2005) Accuracy of a rationally derived method for identifying treatment failure in children and adolescents. J Child Fam Stud 14:207–222

Brabec B, Meister R (2001) A nearest-neighbor model for regional avalanche foresting. Ann Glaciol 32:130–134

Brown GS, Minami T (2010) Outcomes management, reimbursement, and the future of psychotherapy. In: Hubble MA, Duncan BL, Miller SD (eds) The heart and soul of change: what works in therapy, 2nd edn. American Psychological Association, Washington, DC, pp 267–298

Burlingame GM, Cox JC, Wells MG, Lambert MJ, Latkowski M, Ferre R (2005) The administration and scoring manual of the youth outcome questionnaire. American Professional Credentialing Services, Salt Lake City, UT

Bybee TS, Lambert MJ, Eggett D (2007) Curves of expected recovery and their predictive validity for identifying treatment failure. Dutch J Psychother 33:419–434

Cohen J (1988) Statistical power analysis for the behavioral sciences, 2nd edn. Erlbaum, Hillsdale, NJ

Duncan BL, Miller SD (2008) The outcome and session rating scales: the revised administration and scoring manual, including the child outcome rating scale. Institute for the Study of Therapeutic Change, Chicago, IL

Ellsworth JR, Lambert MJ, Johnson J (2006) A comparison of the Outcome Questionnaire-45 and Outcome Questionnaire-30 in classification and prediction of treatment outcome. Clin Psychol Psychother 13:380–391

Finch AE, Lambert MJ, Schaalje BG (2001) Psychotherapy quality control: the statistical generation of expected recovery curves for integration into an early warning system. Clin Psychol Psychother 8:231–242

Froyd JE, Lambert MJ, Froyd JD (1996) A review of practices of psychotherapy outcome measurement. J Ment Health 5:11–15

Garb HN (1998) Studying the clinician: judgment research and psychological assessment. American Psychological Association, Washington, DC

Garb HN (2005) Clinical judgment and decision making. Annu Rev Clin Psychol 55:13–23

Grove WG, Zald DH, Lebow B, Snitz B, Nelson C (2000) Clinical versus statistical prediction: a meta-analysis. Psychol Assess 12:19–30

Hannan C, Lambert MJ, Harmon C, Nielsen SL, Smart DW, Shimokawa K, Sutton SW (2005) A lab test and algorithms for identifying clients at risk for treatment failure. J Clin Psychol 61:155–163

Hansen NB, Lambert MJ, Forman EM (2002) The psychotherapy dose-response effect and its implications for treatment delivery services. Clin Psychol Sci Pract 9:329–343

Harmon SC, Lambert MJ, Smart DW, Hawkins EJ, Nielsen SL, Slade K, Lutz W (2007) Enhancing outcome for potential treatment failures: therapist/client feedback and clinical support tools. Psychother Res 17:379–392

Hatfield D, McCullough L, Plucinski A, Krieger K (2010) Do we know when our clients get worse? An investigation of therapists' ability to detect negative client change. Clin Psychol Psychother 17:25–32

Hawkins EJ, Lambert MJ, Vermeersch DA, Slade K, Tuttle K (2004) The effects of providing patient progress information to therapists and patients. Psychother Res 14:308–327

Hill CE, Lambert MJ (2004) Methodological issues in studying psychotherapy processes and outcomes. In: Lambert MJ (ed) Bergin & Garfield's handbook of psychotherapy and behavior change, 5th edn. Wiley, New York, NY, pp 84–135

Institute of Medicine (2006) Improving the quality of health care for mental and substance-use conditions: quality chasm series. National Academies Press, Washington, DC

Kazdin A (1996) Combined and multimodal treatments in child and adolescent psychotherapy: issues, challenges, and research directions. Clin Psychol Sci Pract 3:69–100

Kazdin AE (2005) Parent management training: treatment for oppositional, aggressive, and antisocial behavior in children and adolescents. Oxford University Press, New York, NY

Kraus DR, Seligman D, Jordan JR (2005) Validation of a behavioral health treatment outcome and assessment tool designed for naturalistic settings: the treatment outcome package. J Clin Psychol 61:285–314

Lambert MJ (1983) Introduction to assessment in psychotherapy outcome: historical perspective and current issues. In: Lambert MJ, DeJulio SS, Christensen ER (eds) The assessment of psychotherapy outcome. Wiley-Interscience, New York, NY

Lambert MJ, Ogles BM (2004) The efficacy and effectiveness of psychotherapy. In: Lambert MJ (ed) Bergin & Garfield's handbook of psychotherapy and behavior change, 5th edn. Wiley, New York, NY, pp 139–193

Lambert MJ, Bergin AE, Collins JL (1977) Therapist induced deterioration in psychotherapy patients. In: Gurman AS, Razin AM (eds) Effective psychotherapy: a handbook of research. Pergamon, New York, NY, pp 452–481

Lambert MJ, Whipple JL, Smart DW, Vermeersch DA, Nielsen SL, Hawkins EJ (2001) The effects of providing therapists with feedback on client progress during psychotherapy: Are outcomes enhanced? Psychother Res 11:49–68

Lambert MJ, Whipple JL, Bishop MJ, Vermeersch DA, Gray GV, Finch AE (2002a) Comparison of empirically derived and rationally derived methods for identifying clients at risk for treatment failure. Clin Psychol Psychother 9:149–164

Lambert MJ, Whipple JL, Vermeersch DA, Smart DW, Hawkins EJ, Nielsen SL, Goates MK (2002b) Enhancing psychotherapy outcomes via providing feedback on client progress: a replication. Clin Psychol Psychother 9:91–103

Lambert MJ, Garfield SL, Bergin AE (2004a) Overview, trends, and future directions. In: Lambert MJ (ed) Bergin & Garfield's handbook of psychotherapy and behavior change, 5th edn. Wiley, New York, NY, pp 805–821

Lambert MJ, Morton JJ, Hatfield D, Harmon C, Hamilton S, Reid RC, Shimokowa K, Christopherson C, Burlingame GM (2004b) Administration and scoring manual for the outcome questionnaire-45. American Professional Credentialing Services, Orem, UT

Lambert MJ, Whipple JL, Harmon C, Shimokawa K, Slade K, Christopherson C (2004) Clinical support tools manual. Department of Psychology, Brigham Young University, Provo, UT

Lutz W, Leach C, Barkham M, Lucock M, Stiles WB, Evans C, Noble R, Iveson S (2005) Predicting change for individual psychotherapy clients based on their nearest neighbors. J Consult Clin Psychol 73 (5):904–913

Lutz W, Lambert MJ, Harmon SC, Stulz N, Tschitsaz A, Schürch E (2006) The probability of treatment success, failure and duration – what can be learned from empirical data to support decision making in clinical practice? Clin Psychol Psychother 13:223–232

Meredith RL, Bair SL, Ford GR (2000) Information management for clinical decision making. In: Stricker G, Troy WG, Shueman SA (eds) Handbook of quality management in behavioral health. Kluwer/Plenum, New York, NY, pp 53–94

Miller SD, Duncan BL (2004) The outcome and session rating scales: administration and scoring manual. Authors, Chicago, IL

Miller SD, Duncan BL, Sorrell R, Brown GS (2005) The partners for change outcome system. J Clin Psychol 61:199–208

National Advisory Mental Health Council (2001) Blueprint for change: research on child and adolescent mental health. A report by the National Advisory Mental Health Council's Workgroup on Child and Adolescent Mental Health Intervention Development and Deployment. National Institutes of Health/ National Institute of Mental Health, Bethesda, MD

Percevic R, Lambert MJ, Kordy H (2006) What is the predictive value of responses to psychotherapy for its future course? Empirical explorations and consequences for outcome monitoring. Psychother Res 16:364–373

Reese RJ, Norsworthy L, Rowlands S (2009) Does a continuous feedback system improve psychotherapy outcome? Psychother Theory Res Pract Train 46:418–431

Ringel JS, Sturm R (2001) National estimates of mental health utilization and expenditures for children in 1998. J Behav Health Serv Res 28:319–333

Shimokawa K, Lambert MJ, Smart DW (2010) Enhancing treatment outcome of patients at risk of treatment failure: meta-analytic and mega-analytic review of a psychotherapy quality assurance system. J Consult Clin Psychol 78:298–311

Slade K, Lambert MJ, Harmon SC, Smart DW, Bailey R (2008) Improving psychotherapy outcome: the use of immediate electronic feedback and revised clinical support tools. Clin Psychol Psychother 15:287–303

Spielmans GI, Masters KS, Lambert MJ (2006) A comparison of rational versus empirical methods in prediction of negative psychotherapy outcome. Clin Psychol Psychother 13:202–214

Steiner DL (2003) Diagnostic testing: using and administering diagnostic and screening tests. J Pers Assess 81:209–219

Walfish S, McAlister B, O'Donnell P, Lambert MJ (2012) An investigation of self-assessment bias in mental health providers. Psychol Rep 110(2):639–644. doi:10.2466/02.07.17

Wampold B (2001) The great psychotherapy debate. Lawrence Erlbaum, Mahwah, NJ

Warren JS, Nelson PL, Burlingame GM (2009) Identifying youth at risk for treatment failure in outpatient community mental health services. J Child Fam Stud 18:690–701

Warren JS, Nelson PL, Baldwin SA, Mondragon SA, Burlingame GM (2010) Predicting negative outcomes in youth psychotherapy: community mental health vs. managed care settings. J Consult Clin Psychol 78:144–155

Weiss B, Catron T, Harris V, Phung TM (1999) The effectiveness of traditional child psychotherapy. J Consult Clin Psychol 67:82–94

Weisz JR, Donenberg GR, Han SS, Weiss B (1995) Bridging the gap between laboratory and clinic in child and adolescent psychotherapy. J Consult Clin Psychol 63:688–701

Weisz JR, Jensen-Doss A, Hawley KM (2006) Evidence-based youth psychotherapies versus usual clinical care: a meta-analysis of direct comparisons. Am Psychol 61:671–689. doi:10.1037/0003-066X.61.7.671

Whipple JL, Lambert MJ, Vermeersch DA, Smart DW, Nielsen SL, Hawkins EJ (2003) Improving the effects of psychotherapy: the use of early identification of treatment failure and problem solving strategies in routine practice. J Couns Psychol 58:59–68

Wierzbicki M, Pekarik G (1993) A meta-analysis of psychotherapy dropout. Prof Psychol Res Pract 24 (2):190–195

30 Psychotherapy Outcome Research and Neuroimaging

Roberto Viviani, Magdalena Nagl, and Anna Buchheim

Contents

Abstract

We review here neuroimaging studies that attempted to detect the neurobiological changes associated with the psychotherapy of depression, phobia, anxiety, posttraumatic stress disorder, and obsessive–compulsive disorder. Most studies were carried out to verify the hypothesis of a rebalancing of limbic reactivity and prefrontal control through therapy. Even in the heterogeneity of reported findings, there appears to be some convergence between studies for the normalisation of limbic activity in depression and in panic disorder and for changes in the basal ganglia on obsessive–compulsive disorder. The evidence on the role of prefrontal cortex is at present less conclusive.

30.1 Introduction

One of the aims of neuroimaging approaches to psychotherapy outcome research is the identification of a neural substrate indexing symptomatic remission during treatment. The scientific importance of this substrate depends on the relative lack of specificity of symptomatic improvement. The hope is that, by indexing symptomatic improvement in terms of changes in the function of neural circuits, one may be able to characterise the modes of operation of different psychotherapy approaches and their impact

R. Viviani (✉)
Institute of Psychology, University of Innsbruck, Bruno-Sander-Haus, Innrain 52, 6020 Innsbruck, Austria

Department of Psychiatry and Psychotherapy III, University of Ulm, Leimgrubenweg 12, 89075 Ulm, Germany
e-mail: roberto.viviani@uni-ulm.de

M. Nagl • A. Buchheim
Institute of Psychology, University of Innsbruck, Bruno-Sander-Haus, Innrain 52, 6020 Innsbruck, Austria

O.C.G. Gelo et al. (eds.), *Psychotherapy Research*,
DOI 10.1007/978-3-7091-1382-0_30,

on the processes involved in cognition and emotion (Roffman et al. 2005). In this respect, the role of neuroimaging is similar to the one envisaged in other settings where the observed behaviour, traits, or the inferred mental states of an individual appear to be too general to be effectively associated with the variable of interest (Gottesmann and Gould 2003), as in genetics (Meyer-Lindenberg and Weinberger 2006), in the identification of markers for individually targeted pharmacotherapy (Kirchheiner et al. 2010), or in psychiatric diagnosis (Insel et al. 2010). In all these fields of application, the rationale for the adoption of neuroimaging techniques is a more specific characterisation of differences in mind functioning than the one obtainable by observing behavioural variables.

In this introduction to the application of functional neuroimaging approaches to psychotherapy outcome research, we will first briefly review the principles underlying the detection of brain activations in experiments. We will consider aspects of study design that are important to assess existing studies and evaluate the prospects of a study during planning. We will then briefly review and summarise the existing literature on the effect of psychotherapy on common mental disorders.

30.1.1 Functional Neuroimaging Approaches to the Study of Brain Activity

The first brain imaging studies were carried out in the early eighties using positron emission tomography (PET) techniques (Posner and Raichle 1994). Imaging of brain activity is made possible by detecting radiation produced by annihilating positrons emitted by radioisotopes of common elements, such as oxygen-15. A three-dimensional image is reconstructed using axial tomography techniques, analogous to those in use for X-ray scans. Unlike X-ray scans, which are used only to obtain information on brain structure, PET allows drawing inference on brain function by injecting in the subject's arm a substance labelled with the positron-emitting radioactive isotope that is involved in brain physiology. In water-PET, for example, the use of labelled water allows reconstructing images of brain flow. Glucose-PET is a technique to obtain images of the brain's metabolic activity.

A relatively simple application of PET techniques is imaging brain blood flow or metabolism at rest. In these studies, the subject is not engaged in any task or receives any stimulation during the acquisition of the scan but is simply asked to rest quietly without falling asleep. A more sophisticated application is the demonstration of changes in activity in neural networks associated with specific mental functions indirectly through the accompanying changes in metabolic requirements. Increased glucose consumption can be detected directly with glucose-PET. Increased neural activity can also be detected by measuring increases in local blood flow. In these studies, an image of the neural networks involved in a specific brain activity is obtained by subtracting images obtained while subjects were instructed to perform an operation and a carefully selected control condition. For example, subtracting images obtained while fixing a screen of stationary dots from those obtained when dots were moving leads to identifying the parts of the brain that are involved in the visual representation of motion.

Changes in blood flow also underlie the signal detected by a more recent, non-invasive neuroimaging technique based on the magnetic resonance properties of the protons of water molecules [functional magnetic resonance imaging (fMRI)]. The brain vessels adapt to oxygen consumption by locally overcompensating the arterial supply, thus increasing the fraction of oxygenated haemoglobin (Logothetis 2002). This change results in a modification of the local magnetic properties of tissues, to which magnetic resonance technique is sensitive (blood-oxygen-level-dependent signal, BOLD; Chen and Ogawa 1999).

Modern high-throughput scanners generate information on changes in the local magnetic field with high temporal and spatial resolution (a brain scan with a resolution of about 2 mm may be generated every 1.7–1.8 s). Each scan delivers a three-dimensional snapshot of the brain (*volume*), captured by a discrete set of values corresponding to each *voxel* (the three-dimensional analogue of a pixel in an image). An fMRI experiment consists in controlling the participant's exposure to stimuli or directing the activity of the participant through instructions at specific times, while scanner data are collected (Friston et al. 1995). Similar to the subtraction technique of PET studies, these instructions or changes in the stimuli constitute an experimental manipulation, like treatment and control conditions in standard experiments. For example, to investigate the participant's reaction to emotional stimuli, the experiment may be set up as an alternation of stimuli with and without emotional valence, corresponding to a one-way ANOVA with two levels. This could be realised by showing images with and without emotional valence to participants while fMRI data are acquired. As one would in an ordinary experiment, the effect of emotion in the stimulus would be estimated by a planned contrast between the emotional and the neutral condition. Instead of heart rate, skin conductance levels, or induced mood, the dependent variable in an fMRI experiment is the BOLD signal indirectly reflecting changes in brain activity, demonstrating the existence of brain areas sensitive to the emotional valence of the stimulus.

30.1.2 Application of Neuroimaging Techniques to Psychotherapy Outcome Research

The taxonomy of experimental designs in neuroimaging studies of the effect of psychotherapy is analogous to that of studies about therapeutic outcomes conducted with more traditional approaches. To demonstrate the existence of an effect, a longitudinal design is vastly preferable to a cross-sectional one. To demonstrate the effect of treatment, it is necessary to include a treatment and a control group, often consisting of a treatment-as-usual condition. Finally, neuroimaging studies are characterised by the choice of a set of stimuli or tasks administered during the scan, which elicits the psychological process of interest, usually conceptually tied to the construct used to assess pathology.

The feasibility of longitudinal studies in functional neuroimaging is documented by the reliability of the activation patterns detected in an individual over time (Gountouna et al. 2010). However, while technically feasible, longitudinal designs are demanding in terms of the resources required to execute studies. This may be especially the case for neuroimaging studies due to the cost of scans and the difficulties to allocate time in the scanner, which add to the problems ensuing from recruiting adequate cases and the losses at follow-up.

The existence of a control group is required to demonstrate the specificity of the intervention effects. Existing studies vary in the composition of the control group. An important difference between study designs is the random allocation to treatment and control groups. As shown in the second part of this review (Sect. 30.2), in the current fMRI literature on the effect of therapy, very few studies randomise the allocation to the treatment and control groups.

The choice of the task for an fMRI study of psychotherapy change requires selecting an experimental paradigm that presumably indexes state changes in the disorder under study. To identify and understand changes in mental disorders, neuroimaging studies often refer to a model of the mind that emphasises the progression of emotional processing from the initial perceptual phase (appraisal, Lazarus 1991) to its elaboration at later stages (Phillips et al. 2003) and the existence of individual variations in reappraisal strategies (Ochsner and Gross 2005). This model distinguishes between relatively automatic reactions to emotional stimuli in the early phase, localisable in the limbic system, and cognitive control processes for coping and reappraisal, located in the prefrontal lobes (Phillips et al. 2003). The neurobiological correlates of mental disorders, therefore, are sought at the stations of the chain of emotional processing from limbic to prefrontal networks and their interaction. Mental disorder is envisaged as an unbalance between automatic reaction to emotional stimuli and its elaboration, modelled as enhanced activity of the limbic system coupled with a failure of control in cognitive networks or of their connectivity. Correspondingly, the question of the effects of therapy, be it pharmacological or psychological, is asked in terms of where the change takes place in this chain. According to the hypothesis generated by this model, therapy may act by diminishing reactivity to emotional stimuli in the limbic system or by improving recruitment of top-down control processes (DeRubeis et al. 2008; Roffman et al. 2005).

In the following sections, we will summarise the main studies that have been carried out on the effects of the psychotherapy on depression, anxiety, and obsessive–compulsive disorder (OCD). Details on these studies are available in accompanying tables. Studies were retrieved through a systematic search in medical search engines (PubMed, "Web of Science") using alternating combinations of keywords referring to the imaging method (fMRI, MRI, PET, SPECT), the psychotherapy (cognitive behaviour psychotherapy, interpersonal psychotherapy, psychodynamic psychotherapy, or just psychotherapy), and the mental disorder [depression, OCD, anxiety disorders, and posttraumatic stress disorder (PTSD)]. Among the studies thus identified, we selected those that conducted both a pre- and a post measurement. Studies were excluded when symptomatic improvement could not be demonstrated.

30.2 Neuroimaging Changes in the Psychotherapy of Mental Disorders

30.2.1 Depression

Most studies of depression have investigated the changes after therapy at rest using PET or SPECT techniques (Table 30.1). The studies of Brody et al. (2001a) report several changes in metabolism in the prefrontal and temporal cortices common to treatment with paroxetine and interpersonal psychotherapy. Changes specific to psychotherapy were reductions in the metabolism of the ventral cingulus and anterior insula, while the signal from the dorsal cingulus and dorsolateral prefrontal cortex increased. The study by Martin et al. (2001) in patients treated with venlafaxine or interpersonal therapy detected an increase of signal in posterior cingulus.

The study by Goldapple et al. (2004) involved therapy with paroxetine and cognitive behavioural therapy. Here, reductions in metabolic activity were predominant, affecting the prefrontal cortex in both dorsal and ventral regions (in the ventrolateral area) and in the temporal and parietal cortex. The medial prefrontal cortex was also affected by reductions in activity in the inferior and posterior region, while the dorsal cingulus was among the few areas showing increases. In a study with venlafaxine and cognitive behavioural therapy, Kennedy et al. (2007) reported decreases in the posterior cingulus in the psychotherapy group, while metabolic activity in the ventral cingulus increased.

Fu et al. (2008) is the only study to date to use cognitive behavioural therapy in a functional study in which participants were challenged with an emotionally arousing stimulus. This study reported decreases in the stimulus-bound activity in the amygdala and anterior hippocampus and in the posterior cingulus and the precuneus. Increases of response signal were noted in the prefrontal cortex and in the posterior cingulus. The study by Buchheim et al. (2012) is the only study to date to investigate the effect of psychodynamic psychotherapy on recurrent depression. After 1 year of therapy, hyperreactivity of the amygdalar-anterior hippocampal region to stimuli related to attachment themes had normalised. Unlike Fu et al. (2008), activity in the prefrontal cortex also showed a decrease relative to beginning of therapy.

Dichter et al. (2009) investigated the effect of behavioural activation therapy for depression (BATD; Hopko et al. 2003) on the signal evoked by reward. Signal increases and decreases were reported that differentiated between different phases of the task, which included perception, anticipation, and feedback on decisions involving possible rewards to the participants. The effect of BATD on cognitive control was investigated in Dichter et al. (2010).

Table 30.1 Studies of psychotherapy of depression

Author	Psychotherapy	Neuroimaging technique	Neurobiological effects: Decrease in activation	Neurobiological effects: Increase in activation	Clinical effects
Brody et al. (2001a)	Interpersonal psychotherapy/ paroxetine	FDG-PET	**Interpersonal psychotherapy and paroxetine—group**: Bilateral PFC Right dorsal caudate nucleus Left thalamus **Interpersonal psychotherapy**: Right ventrolateral PFC Right dorsolateral PFC Left anterior cingulate cortex	**Interpersonal psychotherapy and paroxetine—group**: Left insula Inferior temporal lobe (bilateral) **Interpersonal psychotherapy**: Anterior insula Left temporal lobe	**Significant improvements**: *Interpersonal psychotherapy*: HAM-D score: pre 20.5 ± 5.3, post 12.6 ± 4.7 *Paroxetine* HAM-D score: pre 17.8 ± 5.5, post 5.8 ± 2.1 **Nonsignificant changes**: HAM-A Y-BOCS GAF
Brody et al. (2001b)	Interpersonal psychotherapy/ paroxetine	FDG-PET	The improvement in symptom factors anxiety/somatisation and psychomotor inhibition correlates positively with a decrease in metabolism in the *ventral*, as well as *dorsal frontal lobe*. The improvement in factor anxiety/ somatisation correlates positively with a decrease in activation in the *ventral ACC*, as well as in the *anterior insula*	Improvement of psychomotor inhibition shows a significant correlation with the increase in activation of metabolism in the right *dorsal ACC*. Improvement in the symptom factor cognitive impairment correlates significantly with the increase in activation in the *dorsolateral PFC*. Contrary to the original assumption, the correlation between symptomatic improvement and the anterior medial temporal metabolism proved to be in the negative direction	**Significant improvements**: HAM-D POMS
Martin et al. (2001)	Interpersonal psychotherapy/ venlafaxine	SPECT	None	**Venlafaxine and interpersonal psychotherapy patients**: Right basal ganglia **Interpersonal psychotherapy specific**: Right cingulate cortex posterior **Venlafaxine specific**: Right temporal lobe posterior	**Significant improvements**: *Interpersonal psychotherapy group*: HAM-D score: pre 22.7 ± 2.7, post 16.2 ± 7.1 BDI score: pre 27.9 ± 8.9, post 18.0 ± 10.8 HAM-A *Venlafaxine group*: HAM-D score: pre 22.4 ± 3.1, post 10.9 ± 8.6

(*continued*)

Table 30.1 (continued)

Author	Psychotherapy	Neuroimaging technique	Neurobiological effects Decrease in activation	Increase in activation	Clinical effects
					BDI score: pre 26.3 ± 6.2, post 12.0 ± 7.7 HAM-A
Goldapple et al. (2004)	Cognitive behavioural therapy/post hoc comparison with paroxetine effects	FDG-PET	**Cognitive behavioural Therapy group**: Dorsolateral PFC Ventrolateral PFC Medial frontal areas (superior, inferior) Posterior cingulate cortex Inferior parietal and Inferior temporal cortex *Post hoc* comparison with *paroxetine* effects: consistency in the ventrolateral PFC	**Cognitive behavioural Therapy group**: Hippocampus Dorsal cingulate cortex	**Significant improvements**: *Cognitive behavioural therapy group*: 9/14 responder (HDRS score reduction > 50 %) Due to the small sample size also nonresponders were included (HDRS score reduction <50 % but >35 %) *HDRS score*: pre 20 ± 3, post 6.7 ± 4 *Paroxetine group*: clinical effects similar
Lehto et al. (2008)	Psychodynamic psychotherapy	SPECT	None	**Atypical depressives**: increase of the density of serotonin transporters in the mesencephalon; not found in *non-atypical depression*	**Significant improvements**: *Atypicals*: HAM-D-29 score: pre 19.30 ± 9.32, post 20.00 ± 13.00 HAM-D-21 score: pre 19.13 ± 3.94, post 12.50 ± 6.82 *Non-atypicals*: HAM-D-29: pre 27.36+/-9.26, post 15.18+/-9.57 HAM-D-21: pre 22.18+/-7.45, post 10.64+/-7.00
			No changes of the dopamine transporter concentration in the striatum; no correlations between neurobiological and clinical effects		
Kennedy et al. (2007)	Cognitive behavioural therapy/venlafaxine	FDG-PET	**Cognitive behavioural therapy and venlafaxine group**: OFC (bilateral) Left dorsolateral medial PFC **Cognitive behavioural therapy specific**: Left posterior cingulate cortex **Venlafaxine specific**: Left inferior temporal cortex Left subgenual ACC (only responders)	**Cognitive behavioural therapy and venlafaxine group**: Right inferior occipital cortex **Cognitive behavioural therapy specific**: Left inferior temporal cortex Subgenual ACC Ventromedial PFC **Venlafaxine specific**: Left posterior cingulate cortex (only responders)	**Significant improvements**: *Cognitive behavioural therapy*: 7 (out of 12) responder HAM-D score: pre 20.6 ± 3.5, post 9.8 ± 3.8 *Venlafaxine*: 9 (out of 12) responder HAM-D score: pre 20.3 ± 3.2, post 7.4 ± 1.1

Fu et al. (2008)	Cognitive behavioural therapy	fMRI	*Overall decrease in activity*: Right amygdala Hippocampal structures *Linear load response*: Fusiform and lingual gyrus Left lateral temporal and inferior parietal cortex Posterior cingulate cortex Precuneus, cerebellum	*Overall increase in activity*: ACC Gyrus frontalis superior Posterior cingulate cortex Inferior parietal cortex Precuneus	**Significant improvements**: BDI score: pre 38.0 ± 11.7, post 14.5 ± 15.4 HRSD score: pre 20.9 ± 1.9, post 6.4 ± 5.2
			Therapy predictors: low baseline activity in the area of the right gyrus frontalis inferior/insula and left putamen/globus pallidus; high baseline activity in the gyrus frontalis superior		
Dichter et al. (2009)	Behavioural activation therapy for depression (BATD)	fMRI	*During selection phase*: left amygdala, left gyrus frontalis superior, left superior occipital cortex, left gyrus postcentralis, right gyrus supramarginalis, right gyrus temporalis inferior *During anticipation phase*: gyrus temporalis inferior anterior *During feedback phase*: gyrus paracingularis, left posterior cingulate cortex, left nucleus caudatus, left gyrus postcentralis	*During selection phase*: gyrus paracingularis ($p = .06$), left putamen, right gyrus supramarginalis, posterior temporal fusiform cortex *During anticipation phase*: left nucleus caudatus, left gyrus cingularis, left superior occipital cortex, right insula, right precuneus, right temporal fusiform cortex, bilateral gyrus precentralis, temporal poles (bilateral) *During feedback phase*: *In winning trials*: right occipital cortex superior, right temporal fusiform cortex *In no winning trials*: e.g. left OFC	**Significant improvements**: 9 (out of 12) responders (HAM-D score <6) HAM-D score: pre 23.8 ± 2.3, post 8.7 ± 9.4 **Nonsignificant changes**: JAM BAS/BIS
Dichter et al. (2010)	Behavioural activation therapy for depression (BATD)	fMRI	Gyrus paracingularis Right OFC Right frontal pole Left gyrus postcentralis		**Significant improvements**: 9 out of 12 responders (HAM-D score <6) HAM-D score: pre 23.8 ± 9.4, post 8.7 ± 9.4 BDI score: pre 27.1 ± 5.1, post 11.6 ± 8.7
			Therapy predictors: significant negative correlation between the baseline activity of the paracingulate gyrus and the improvement of the BDI scores		

(*continued*)

Table 30.1 (continued)

Author	Psychotherapy	Neuroimaging technique	Neurobiological effects: Decrease in activation	Neurobiological effects: Increase in activation	Clinical effects
Buchheim et al. (2012)	Psychodynamic at one year	fMRI	Amygdala/anterior hippocampus Subgenual cortex Anteromedial prefrontal cortex		**Significant improvements**: BDI score: pre 24.4 ± 9.5, post 12.9 ± 8 2GSI score: pre 1.35 ± 0.75, post 0.69 ± 0.36

FDG-PET ^{18}F-fluorodeoxyglucose positron emission tomography, *SPECT* single-photon emission computed tomography, *fMRI* functional magnetic resonance imaging, *BAS/BIS* behavioural activation/behavioural inhibition scale, *BDI* Beck Depression Inventory, *GAF*, Global Assessment of Functioning, *GSI* Global Severity Index, *HAM-A* Hamilton Rating Scale for Anxiety, *HAM-D* 17-item Hamilton Depression Rating Scale, *HRSD/HDRS* Hamilton Rating Scale for Depression/Hamilton Depressive Rating Scale, *JAM* Jackson Appetitive Motivation Scale, *POMS* profile of mood states, *Y-BOCS* Yale-Brown Obsessive–Compulsive Scale, *ACC* anterior cingulate cortex, *OFC* orbitofrontal cortex, *PFC* prefrontal cortex

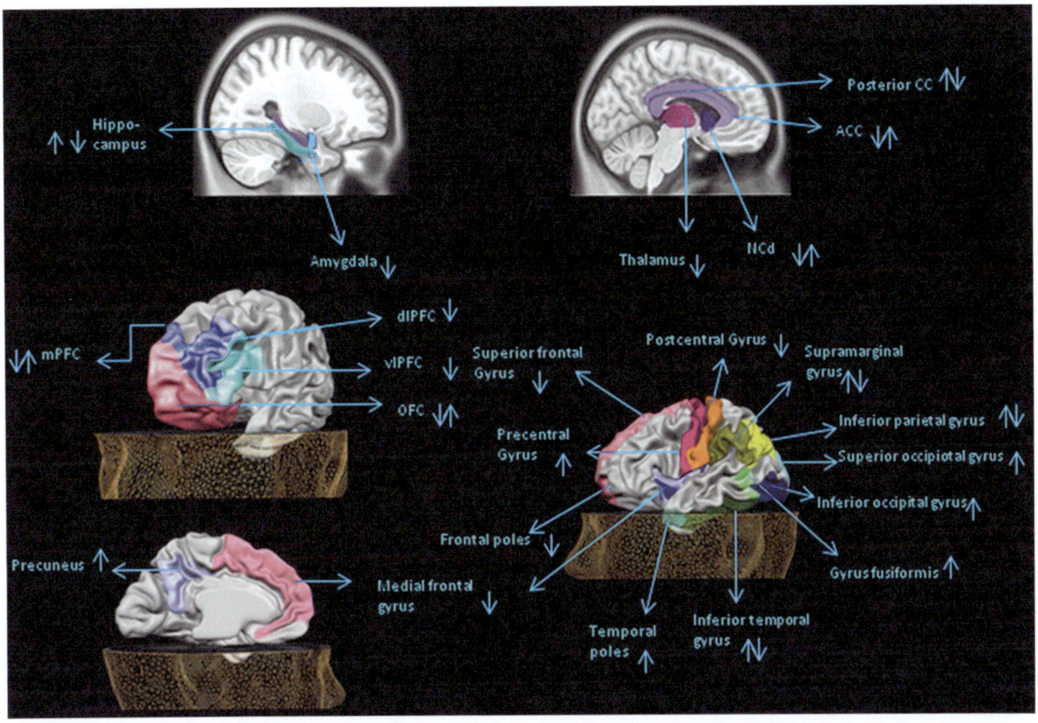

Fig. 30.1 Schematic illustration of brain regions involved in studies of the psychotherapy of depression. *ACC* anterior cingulate cortex, *dlPFC* dorsolateral prefrontal cortex, *mPFC* medial prefrontal cortex, *NCd* caudate nucleus, *OFC* orbitofrontal cortex, *vlPFC* ventrolateral prefrontal cortex; *upward pointing arrow*, increase in activation; *downward pointing arrow*, decrease in activation

Details of neuroimaging studies of the psychotherapy of depression are in Table 30.1 and are summarised in Fig. 30.1.

30.2.2 Phobia and Anxiety Disorders

Studies of the effect of cognitive behavioural therapy on specific phobias have most often adopted a symptom provocation design (Table 30.2). Studies by Paquette et al. (2003), Goosens et al. (2007), and Schienle et al. (2007) reported reduction of the activation elicited by the phobic stimulus in the amygdala and hippocampus, associated with symptom improvement. Several studies also report reductions of activation in the insula (Goosens et al. 2007; Straube et al. 2006; Schienle et al. 2007, 2009). No changes in these areas were found in a study by Johanson et al. (2006). Reported changes in the prefrontal cortex are less consistent in localisation and sign. Of these studies, those of Straube et al. (2006) and Schienle et al. (2007) adopted a randomised design.

Two PET studies of activity at rest investigated the effect of CBT on panic disorder. Prasko et al. (2004) found diffuse reductions of signal in the right hemisphere in the prefrontal and temporal lobes, accompanied by increases in left hemisphere. Sakai et al. (2006) found a correlation between reduction of symptoms and increase of metabolic activity in the left medial prefrontal cortex. A study on the effect of short-term psychodynamic psychotherapy in an inpatient setting reported normalisation of hyperactivity in the amygdala and anterior hippocampus, analogously to studies on specific phobias (Beutel et al. 2010).

A study of the effect of CBT on social phobia reported reductions of the activity in the limbic system (amygdala and the adjacent hippocampal structures) at exposure, common to both the CBT and pharmacologically treated group (citalopram; Furmark et al. 2002).

Table 30.2 Studies of psychotherapy of anxiety disorders/phobia

Author	Psychotherapy	Neuroimaging technique	Neurobiological effects: Decrease in activation	Neurobiological effects: Increase in activation	Clinical effects
Furmark et al. (2002)	Cognitive behavioural therapy/ citalopram	PET (oxygen-15 labelled water)	**Cognitive behavioural therapy and citalopram therapy groups**: Amygdala Hippocampus Rhinal, parahippocampal, and periamygdaloid cortex **Cognitive behavioural therapy**: Periaqueductal grey **Citalopram specific**: Left thalamus Left frontal cortex Inferior	**Cognitive behavioural therapy group**: Right cerebellum	**Significant improvements**: *Cognitive behavioural therapy—group*: STAI-S SPS PCRS distress and anxiety rating *Citalopram—group*: SPS GAF No significant differences between both therapy groups 67 % responders in both therapy groups
Paquette et al. (2003)	Cognitive behavioural therapy	fMRI	Dorsolateral PFC Parahippocampal gyrus	Middle occipital gyrus Superior parietal lobe Left inferior occipital gyrus Left gyrus fusiformis Right inferior frontal gyrus	**Significant improvements**: AAS: pre 6.3/8 ± 1.2, post 0.1/8 ± 0.3 Intensity of anxiety during symptom provocation
Prasko et al. (2004)	Cognitive behavioural therapy/ various SSRI/SNRIs	FDG-PET	**Cognitive behavioural therapy group**: Right inferior temporal gyrus Right inferior and superior frontal gyrus **Antidepressant group**: Right inferior, middle, and superior frontal gyrus Right superior and middle temporal gyrus	**Cognitive behavioural therapy group**: Left inferior frontal gyrus Left middle temporal gyrus Left insula **Antidepressant group**: Left middle frontal gyrus Left middle temporal gyrus	**Significant improvements**: *Cognitive behavioural therapy group*: PDSS: pre 16.5 ± 5.05; post 2.3 ± 2.34 HAM-A: pre 21.5 ± 3.99; post: 3.8 ± 2.93 (reported as significantly better improvement than in the psychopharmacological group) CGI *Antidepressant group*: PDSS: pre 16.7 ± 1.21; post 5.8 ± 4.07 HAM-A: pre 25.3 ± 3.63; post 10.7 ± 6.06 CGI

Straube et al. (2006)	Cognitive behavioural therapy	fMRI	ACC Insula Left thalamus Dorsomedial PFC	Right cuneus	**Significant improvements**: SPQ score: pre 22.69 ± 2.95, post 7.69 ± 5.38 Anxiety rating
Sakai et al. (2006)	Cognitive behavioural therapy	FDG-PET	Right hippocampus Left ACC Left cerebellum Pons Significant positive correlation between changes of second subscale and subscale of PDSS (anticipatory anxiety and agoraphobic symptoms) and changes of metabolism in the left mPFC	Bilateral medial PFC	**Significant improvements**: PDSS State Scale of STAI HAM-D Frequency of panic attacks **Nonsignificant changes**: Trait Scale of STAI Only one patient nonresponder; excluded from study
Johanson et al. (2006)	Cognitive therapy	XE-13 rCBF	*Patients without panic symptoms*: Right PFC (pre, hyperactivity of PFC)	*Patients with panic symptoms*: Right PFC (pre, hypoactivity of PFC)	**Significant improvements**: STAI-S scores : pre 60 ± 12, post 30 ± 7 Systematically collected specific psychophysiological variables, emotions, and cognitions during confrontation **Nonsignificant changes**: STAI-T scores: pre 41 ± 7, post 36 ± 8
Schienle et al. (2007)	Cognitive behavioural therapy	fMRI	Right insula Parahippocampal gyrus Significant positive correlation between the improvement of somatic panic symptoms during the symptom provocation and the decrease in activity in the right amygdala as well as in the insula	Medial OFC (bilateral)	**Significant improvements**: SPQ score: pre 21.9 ± 1.7; post 5.6 ± 3.6 Behavioural test (holding spider in the hand) Anxiety rating/rating of somatic panic symptoms during provocation of symptoms (9-level scale)
Goosens et al. (2007)	Cognitive behavioural therapy	fMRI	Left amygdala Bilateral ACC Insula Significant positive correlation between amygdala-activation and SPQ as well as VAAS scales (pre and post)		**Significant improvements**: SPQ score: pre 23.31 ± 0.74; post 12.63 ± 1.34 VAAS

(*continued*)

Table 30.2 (continued)

Author	Psychotherapy	Neuroimaging technique	Neurobiological effects: Decrease in activation	Neurobiological effects: Increase in activation	Clinical effects
Leutgeb et al. (2009)	Cognitive behavioural therapy	EEG	Against hypothesis: no reduction of P300 and early as well as late LPP amplitudes	Increase of the late LPP amplitude	**Significant improvements**: SPQ score: from pre 20.4 ± 3.7 to post 8.6 ± 4.0 Behavioural test (behaviour avoidance test): patient could hold spider in the hand (maximum number of points reached) Anxiety rating during provocation of symptoms **Nonsignificant changes**: STAI BDI QADS
Schienle et al. (2009) (follow-up of Schienle et al. 2007)	Cognitive behavioural therapy	fMRI	Insula Lateral OFC (bilateral)	Medial OFC (bilateral)	Improvements in clinical data remained stable in the therapy group (see Schienle et al. 2007)
Beutel et al. (2010)	Psychodynamic psychotherapy, inpatient setting	fMRI	Amygdala Anterior hippocampus	Ventrolateral PFC	**Significant improvements**: STAI-S ACQ (agoraphobic cognitions questionnaire) BSQ (bodily sensations questionnaire)

PET positron emission tomography, *FDG-PET* ^{18}F-fluorodeoxyglucose positron emission tomography, *fMRI* functional magnetic resonance imaging, *rCBF* regional cerebral blood flow, *EEG* electroencephalography, *AAS* Anxiety Analogue Scale, *BDI* Beck Depression Inventory, *CGI* Clinical Global Impression severity scale, *GAF* global assessment of functioning, *HAM-A* Hamilton Rating Scale for Anxiety, *HAM-D* 17-item Hamilton Depression Rating Scale, *PCRS* the personal on confidence as a speaker, *PDSS* Panic Disorder Severity Scale, *POMS* profile of mood states, *QADS* Questionnaire for the assessment of disgust sensitivity, *SPQ* Spider Phobia Questionnaire, *SPS* Social Phobia Scale, *SSRI/SNRI* selective serotonin reuptake inhibitors/serotonin norepinephrine reuptake inhibitors, *STAI* State–Trait Anxiety Inventory, *STAI-T* State–Trait Anxiety Inventory, trait subscale, *STAI-S*, State–Trait Anxiety Inventory, state subscale, *TPQ* Therapy Process Questionnaire, *ACC* anterior cingulate cortex, *OFC* orbitofrontal cortex, PFC prefrontal cortex

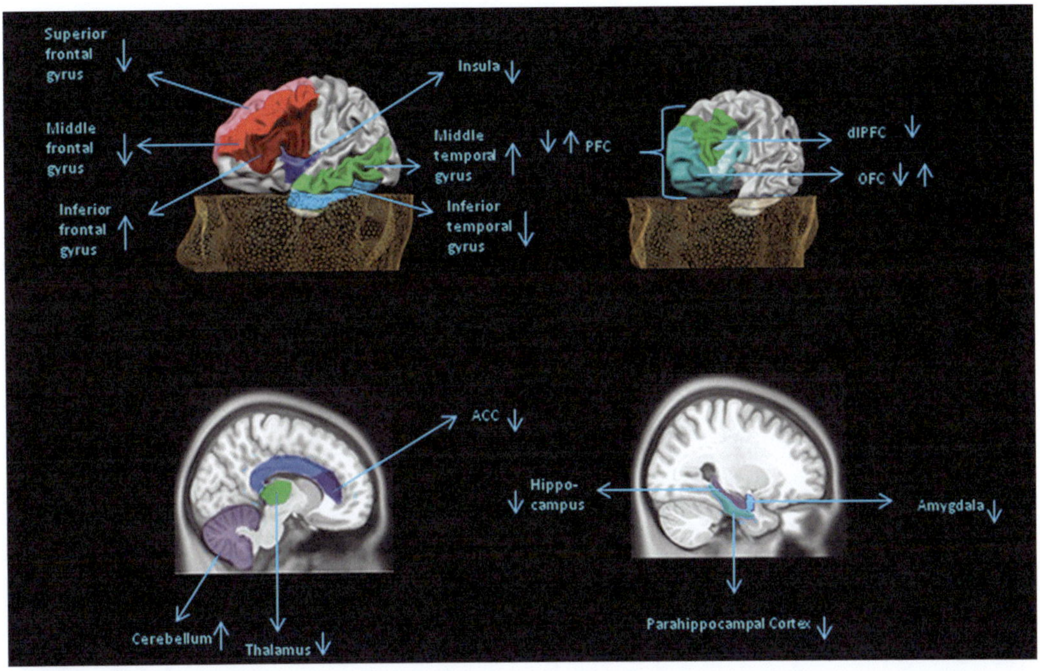

Fig. 30.2 Schematic illustration of brain regions involved in studies of the psychotherapy of phobia and anxiety disorders. *ACC* anterior cingulate cortex, *dlPFC* dorsolateral prefrontal cortex, *OFC* orbitofrontal cortex, *PFC* prefrontal cortex; *upward pointing arrow*, increase in activation; *downward pointing arrow*, decrease in activation

Details on this group of studies and the main involved areas are in Table 30.2 and Fig. 30.2.

30.2.3 Posttraumatic Stress Disorder

Neuroimaging studies of the effect of psychotherapy on PTSD are more heterogeneous in psychotherapeutic technique and the functional network elicited by the task in the scanner. Two studies examined the effect of CBT. Farrow et al. (2005) had participants carry out social cognition tasks during the scan, such as empathy or moral decision tasks, finding increased signal in the left middle temporal gyrus in the former and in the posterior cingulus in the latter. This study, however, did not examine the same patients before and after therapy but different groups. Felmingham et al. (2007) used presentation of facial expression (commonly used to elicit amygdalar activation), finding both increases and decreases of activation in the temporal lobe after therapy. Activation increased in the anterior cingulus.

Pagani et al. (2007) used a symptom provocation design to study the effect of the eye movement desensitisation and reprocessing technique (EMDR; Shapiro 1995), finding no significant changes in the patient group as a whole, but some evidence of normalisation of fronto-limbic activity in responders. This study, however, did not test the interaction of time and group directly. Lindauer et al. (2008) investigated the effect of Brief Eclectic Psychotherapy (BEP; Gersons et al. 2004), reporting a significant correlation between symptomatic improvement and changes in the frontotemporal circuit.

Several studies have shown PTSD pathology to be associated with volumetric reductions of the hippocampus (Rauch et al. 2006; Woon et al. 2010). A study has investigated the effect of psychotherapy on the size of this region using structural imaging (Lindauer et al. 2005), without detecting significant results.

Details on neuroimaging studies of PTSD are in Table 30.3. Figure 30.3 summarises the changes in the areas involved in these studies.

Table 30.3 Studies of psychotherapy of PTSD

Author	Psychotherapy	Neuroimaging technique	Neurobiological effects: Decrease in activation	Neurobiological effects: Increase in activation	Clinical effects
Levin et al. (1999), single case study	Eye movement desensitisation and reprocessing (EMDR)	[99mTc] HMPAO SPECT	None	ACC Left frontal lobe	**Significant improvements**: CAPS: pre 62, post 31 DTS: pre 57, post 30 IES: pre 33, post 13 Hypervigilance index
Farrow et al. (2005)	Cognitive behavioural therapy	fMRI	None	*During an empathy task*: Left middle temporal gyrus *During a forgiving task*: Posterior gyrus cinguli	**Significant improvements**: CAPS: *intrusions*, pre 16 ± 6; post 6 ± 4; *Avoidance*: pre 19 ± 8; post 7 ± 6; *Hyperarousal*: pre 19 ± 5; post 7 ± 4
Lindauer et al. (2005)	Brief eclectic psychotherapy	Structural MRI	Significant lower hippocampal volume of patients before psychotherapy in comparison to traumatised control participants; no significant change of the hippocampi in the context of psychotherapy		**Significant improvements**: 7 (out of 9) responders SI-PTSD score: pre 11.8 ± 2.0, post 4.1 ± 5.0.
Bossini et al. (2007), single case study	Eye movement desensitisation and reprocessing (EMDR)	Structural MRI		Increase in hippocampal volume, bilateral	**Significant improvements**: CAPS score: no more indication of PTSD DTS score: pre 51, post 8
Felmingham et al. (2007)	Cognitive behavioural therapy	fMRI	Right postcentral gyrus Right middle temporal gyrus Left superior temporal gyrus	Bilateral rostral ACC Left middle temporal gyrus Right inferior temporal gyrus Left parietotemporal gyrus Right hippocampus	**Significant improvements**: CAPS score: pre 78.1 ± 20.0, post 28.9 ± 20.3 (corresponds to an average reduction of 30 %)
			Significant positive correlation between the symptom recovery (CAPS score) and the increase in activation of the rostral ACC Significant negative correlation between the activity of the bilateral amygdala and the symptom recovery		
Lindauer et al. (2008)	Brief eclectic psychotherapy	[99mTc] HMPAO SPECT	Right middle frontal gyrus	No	**Significant improvements**: 8 (out of 10) responders PTSD score: pre 11.7 ± 1.6, post 3.7 ± 4.9 No significant changes: STAI-S score
			Significant positive correlation between the improvement of the PTSD score and the rCBF changes in the left superior temporal gyrus and the middle frontal gyrus		

Pagani et al. (2007)	Eye movement desensitisation and reprocessing (EMDR)	[99mTc] HMPAO SPECT	No significant change at the pre-/post-comparison in patients	No significant change at the pre-/post-comparison in patients	**Significant improvements**: 11 of 15 patients were considered responders after no longer satisfying DSM-IV criteria for diagnosis
			Comparison responders vs. nonresponders: Changes in frontal, parietooccipital, occipital cortex, and in the hippocampus Normalisation of global CBF in responders		
Peres et al. (2007)	Exposition in combination with cognitive restructuring	SPECT	Left amygdala	Left parietal lobe Left PFC Left hippocampus Thalamus (bilateral)	**Note**: light symptomatology
			Significant positive correlation between the activity in the left PFC and the left thalamus as well as the left parietal lobe; correlations between clinical data and the rCBF values: significant positive correlation between the CAPS score and the left PFC and significant negative correlation between the CAPS score and the left amygdala		

SPECT single-photon emission computed tomography, *fMRI* functional magnetic resonance imaging, *MRI* magnetic resonance imaging, *rCBF* regional cerebral blood flow, *CBF* cerebral blood flow, *CAPS* Clinician-Administered PTSD Scale, *DTS* Davidson Trauma Scale, *IES* Impact of Event Scale, *SI-PTSD* structural interview for PTSD, *STAI-S* State–Trait Anxiety Inventory, state subscale, *ACC* anterior cingulate cortex

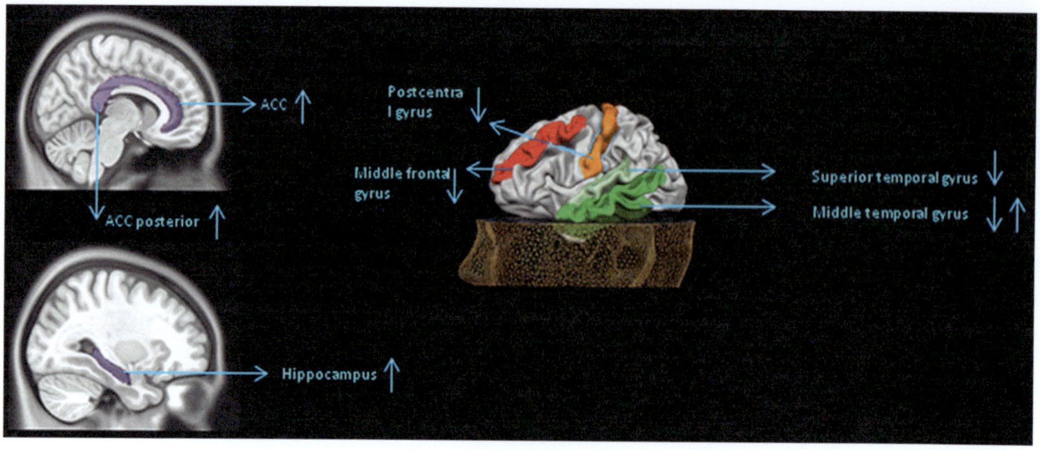

Fig. 30.3 Schematic illustration of brain regions involved in studies of the psychotherapy of PTSD. *ACC* anterior cingulate cortex; *upward pointing arrow*, increase in activation; *downward pointing arrow*, decrease in activation

30.2.4 Obsessive–Compulsive Disorder

The first neuroimaging studies on the effect of psychotherapy on OCD were carried out by Baxter et al. (1992). As in a group treated with fluoxetine, they showed an effect of treatment in the nucleus caudatus, with weaker evidence for an involvement of the thalamus and the medial prefrontal cortex. These results were further substantiated in a subsequent study (Schwartz et al. 1996). The involvement of the basal ganglia, especially the caudatus, and the orbital and medial prefrontal cortex in changes after therapy found broad confirmation in a second series of studies (Freyer et al. 2011; Nabeyama et al. 2008; Nakao et al. 2005; Nakatani et al. 2003; Saxena et al. 2009; Yamanishi et al. 2009). Considerable evidence from other studies implicates these structures in obsessive-–compulsive disorder (Whiteside et al. 2004), suggesting that OCD symptoms are mediated by hyperactivity in orbitofrontal–subcortical circuit, which normalises in symptomatic remission after therapy (Saxena et al. 2001).

Details on studies on OCD are in Table 30.4. Figure 30.4 schematically shows the changes in the brain regions involved in these studies.

30.3 Discussion

An important model of therapeutic change in neurobiological research involves a change in the relative activation of prefrontal and limbic structures, independently from the mental illness or the treatment approach. Prefrontal cortical areas (especially DLPFC) are usually activated not only by the execution of demanding cognitive tasks but also during emotion suppression and regulation (Ochsner and Gross 2005). For this reason, the participation of prefrontal structures in mechanisms of control and inhibition is of particular interest for psychotherapy (Messina et al. 2013). In this interpretive framework, increased recruitment or increased efficiency of prefrontal function may be understood as an increased ability to solve problems in emotionally difficult, stress-inducing events (Frewen et al. 2008; Messina et al. 2013). Besides the DLPFC, other subregions of the PFC have also been repeatedly involved in studies of emotion. Some of them, like the ventrolateral and dorsomedial prefrontal cortex, are associated with various strategies of affect- and self-regulation (Ochsner et al. 2002, 2004).

Table 30.4 Studies of psychotherapy of obsessive–compulsive disorder (OCD)

Author	Psychotherapy	Neuroimaging technique	Neurobiological effects: Decrease in activation	Neurobiological effects: Increase in activation	Clinical effects
Baxter et al. (1992)	Cognitive behavioural therapy/fluoxetine	FDG-PET	*Responders*: **Cognitive behavioural therapy and fluoxetine groups**: Right caudate nucleus **Fluoxetine group only**: Right anterior cingulate Left thalamus **Significant positive correlations** between improvement in percent of the Y-BOCS score and activity reduction in the caudate nucleus in the fluoxetine group. In the cognitive behavioural therapy group, this correlation is not significant		**Significant improvements**: *Cognitive behavioural therapy*: 6 responders out of 9 patients Y-BOCS score: pre 22.3 ± 4.1; post 13.5 ± 4.0 *Fluoxetine*: 7 responders out of 9 patients Y-BOCS score: pre 25.8 ± 3.7; post 13.0 ± 2. **Nonsignificant changes**: *Cognitive behavioural therapy*: HAM-D *Fluoxetine*: HAM-A, GAS
Schwartz et al. (1996)	Cognitive behavioural therapy/fluoxetine	FDG-PET	**Both samples combined** (present study and Baxter et al. 1992): *Responders*: Bilateral nucleus caudate		**Significant improvements**: (only sample of present study): 6 responders out of 9 patients Y-BOCS score: pre 24.3 ± 2.7; post 12.5 ± 2.0 **Nonsignificant changes**: GAS
Nakatani et al. (2003)	Behavioural therapy/ clomipramine	rCBF measurement with Xe-CT	Right nucleus caudatus Significant negative correlation between GAF score and the activity of the right caudatus Significant positive correlation between the Y-BOCS score and the left thalamus Significant negative correlation between change of the GAF score and change of the right caudatus There could not be detected any corresponding correlation between Y-BOCS score and nucleus caudatus though	None	**Significant improvements**: Y-BOCS score: pre 77 ± 5,30, post 12.09 ± 4.68; this corresponds to a reduction of 55.9 % HAM-D GAF

(*continued*)

Table 30.4 (continued)

Author	Psychotherapy	Neuroimaging technique	Neurobiological effects: Decrease in activation	Neurobiological effects: Increase in activation	Clinical effects
Nakao et al. (2005)	Behavioural therapy/ fluvoxamine	fMRI	*Symptom provocation*: Bilateral ACC Right putamen Left insula Bilateral temporal and occipital cortex Bilateral cerebellum Bilateral OFC	*Stroop test*: Bilateral dorsolateral PFC Right ACC Bilateral insula Bilateral temporal and parietal cortex Bilateral cerebellum	**Significant improvements**: Y-BOCS score: pre 29 ± 3.59; post 14.60 ± 9.22. MOCI score STAI HDRS CGI-S and GAF 2 (out of 10) patients showed no improvements on Y-BOCS score (both in the fluvoxamine group)
			Significant negative correlation between baseline rCBF within bilateral OFC and reduction of the Y-BOCS score Significant negative correlation between the change of the rCBF within the right OFC and the change of the Y-BOCS score		
Nabeyama et al. (2008)	Behavioural therapy	fMRI	Bilateral cerebellum Right parietal lobe	Right OFC Left middle frontal gyrus Left gyrus fusiformis Bilateral parahippocampal gyrus Left parietal lobe	**Significant improvements**: Y-BOCS score: pre 29 ± 3.59; post 14.60 ± 9.22; this corresponds to a reduction of 58.99 % CGI-S and GAF **Nonsignificant changes**: HDRS HAS STAI
Saxena et al. 2009	Behavioural therapy	FDG-PET	Bilateral thalamus	Right dorsal ACC (dACC)	**Significant improvements**: Y-BOCS score: pre 25.2 ± 3.3, post 11.0 ± 5.1 HDRS HAS GAS 9 (out of 10) responders
			Significant positive correlation between improvement on Y-BOCS score and increase of glucose metabolism within the right dorsal ACC.		

Yamanishi et al. (2009)	Behavioural therapy	SPECT (99mTc-ECD)	Left middle frontal gyrus Right medial PFC Right inferior frontal cortex Right OFC Significant negative correlation between baseline rCBF within the bilateral OFC and reduction of the Y-BOCS score Significant negative correlation between the rCBF of the right OFC and the changes of the Y-BOCS scores	Right fusiform gyrus Angular gyrus Right cuneus	33 responders; 12 nonresponders **Significant improvements**: *Responders* Y-BOCS score: pre 33.6 ± 4.5, post 16.2 ± 3.7; this corresponds to a reduction of 51.4 ± 7.1 % STAI score **Nonsignificant changes**: *Responders and nonresponders* BDI *Nonresponders* Y-BOCS STAI
Freyer et al. (2011)	Cognitive behavioural therapy	fMRI	Increased activity for patients over the course of therapy in the caudate nucleus	Decreased responsiveness before treatment of the orbitofrontal cortex and right putamen during strategy change at a reversal learning task in patients compared with healthy subjects	**Significant improvements**: Y-BOCS: pre 25.4 ± 4.81, post 14.2 ± 6.18 **Nonsignificant changes**: HAM-D: pre 6.3 ± 5.48, post 4.7 ± 5.10

FDG-PET ^{18}F-fluorodeoxyglucose positron emission tomography, *rCBF* regional cerebral blood flow, *SPECT* single-photon emission computed tomography, *fMRI* functional magnetic resonance imaging, *BDI* Beck Depression Inventory, *CGI-S* Clinical Global Impression severity scale, *GAF* global assessment of functioning, *GAS* Global Assessment Scale, *HAM-A* Hamilton Rating Scale for Anxiety, *HAM-D* 17-item Hamilton Depression Rating Scale, *HAS* Hamilton Anxiety Scale, *HDRS* Hamilton Depression Rating Scale, *MOCI* Maudsley Obsessional Compulsive Inventory, *STAI* State–Trait Anxiety Inventory, *Y-BOCS*, Yale-Brown Obsessive–Compulsive Scale, *ACC* anterior cingulate cortex, *OFC* orbitofrontal cortex, *PFC* prefrontal cortex

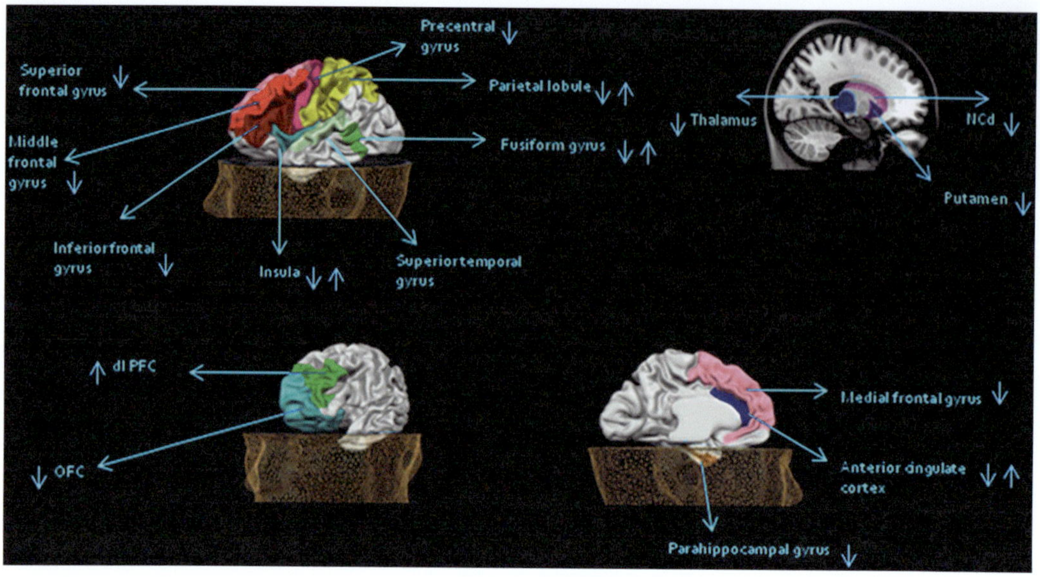

Fig. 30.4 Schematic illustration of brain regions involved in studies of the psychotherapy of obsessive–compulsive disorders. *dlPFC* dorsolateral prefrontal cortex, *NCd* caudate nucleus, *OFC* orbitofrontal cortex; *upward pointing arrow*, increase in activation; *downward pointing arrow*, decrease in activation

DeRubeis et al. (2008) and Roffman et al. (2005) proposed that the specific mechanism through which psychotherapy acts involves less directly the primarily hyperresponsive limbic regions but rather a reinforcement of the frontal inhibition activity. Enhanced prefrontal activation eventually leads indirectly to a more adequate control of negative emotionality, represented by the activation in the limbic system. Thus, remission after psychotherapy would be associated with a healthier balance between emotional and cortical functions.

Many studies appear to converge in detecting changes in the limbic system (amygdala or anterior hippocampus) in emotional disorders characterised by anxiety, especially phobia (Linden 2006; Roffman et al. 2005; Whalen et al. 2002). The normalisation of limbic activity in depression and in panic disorder was also reported by the two existing studies of the effect of psychodynamic psychotherapy (Buchheim et al. 2012; Beutel et al. 2010). The therapy of obsessive–compulsive disorder (ODC) reports changes in the basal ganglia, a structure specifically associated with this disorder. Much less consistent is the picture regarding the correlates of other mental disorders in the prefrontal cortex (Thomas and Elliott 2009). As it has been noted, not all studies have observed changes in prefrontal cortex consistent with a reinforcement of the circuits associated with cognitive control, as would be expected by the prefrontal vs. limbic function model (Linden 2006; Taylor and Liberzon 2007).

There are several aspects of this finding that are worth mentioning. Firstly, detection of changes in the limbic system can be more easily accomplished in the necessarily small sample sizes that are obtainable in this type of studies. As we have noted in the Introduction, a major difficulty in drawing statistical inference from neuroimaging data is the relative lack of power ensuing from the necessity of carrying out a correction for the large number of hypotheses tested. When a specific region is tested, however, this number of hypotheses can be greatly reduced, thus increasing the detection power of the study. The regions that are typically hypothesised to be involved in emotional processing are often very circumscribed (the amygdala, the subgenual cingulus), allowing the formulation of regionally very specific tests. In contrast, the prefrontal cortex is a very large region with relatively variable landmarks and boundaries. This makes verifying a hypothesis on prefrontal cortex functioning comparatively more difficult.

Secondly, there appears to be a systematic difference in the coupling between disorder and stimuli used in the studies. Specifically, studies on phobias can make use of very specific stimuli that are very tightly linked to the symptoms experienced by patients. Here, changes in reactivity to such activating stimuli, improvement in symptom severity, and changes in brain signals are united by a coherent and univocal interpretive framework. In contrast, interpretation and modelling of changes may be more difficult in a multidimensional disorder such as depression.

Finally, note should be taken of the methodological shortcomings of the majority of studies in this field. Small sample sizes and inadequate control groups are issues that compound the problem of creating a placebo condition when the treatment condition is psychotherapy. Because of issues arising with repeated measurements in neuroimaging (habituation and training effects) or the possibility of spontaneous recovery over the time, only the use of control groups, such as healthy controls groups and/or a waitlist control group, allows excluding possible confounds from the observed changes. Many of the discussed studies used a healthy control group (Baxter et al. 1992; Nakatani et al. 2003; Nakao et al. 2005; Nabeyama et al. 2008; Saxena et al. 2009; Paquette et al. 2003; Straube et al. 2006; Schienle et al. 2007, 2009; Goosens et al. 2007; Leutgeb et al. 2009; Brody et al. 2001b; Fu et al. 2008; Dichter et al. 2009, 2010; Farrow et al. 2005; Lindauer et al. 2005, 2008; Pagani et al. 2007) and some also a waitlist control group (Furmark et al. 2002; Straube et al. 2006; Schienle et al. 2007; Leutgeb et al. 2009; Lehto et al. 2008; Lindauer et al. 2005, 2008).

When looking at the perspectives for future research, several tasks appear to need addressing. Some are of methodological nature, such as minimal requirements of studies, and the creation of a meta-analytic framework through which results could be objectively assessed. Other issues concern the nature of brain circuits that may be involved by complex disorders. The existing literature strongly suggests that involvement and reactivity of the limbic system, its specificity within the symptoms treated by psychotherapy, and its capacity to index change constitute a candidate biological marker of psychotherapeutic change. The empirical status of the prefrontal cortex as the site of control processes appears to be empirically less univocal.

References

Baxter LR, Schwartz JM, Bergman KS, Szuba MP, Guze BH, Mazziotta JC, Alzraki A, Selin CE, Ferng HK, Munford P, Phelps ME (1992) Caudate glucose metabolic rate changes with both drug and behaviour therapy for obsessive-compulsive disorder. Arch Gen Psychiatry 49:681–689. doi:10.1001/archpsyc.1992.01820090009002

Beutel ME, Stark R, Pan H, Silbersweig D, Dietrich S (2010) Changes of brain activation pre- post short-term psychodynamic inpatient psychotherapy: an fMRI study of panic disorder patients. Psychiatry Res 184:96–104. doi:10.1016/j.pscychresns.2010.06.005

Bossini L, Fagiolini A, Castrogiovanni P (2007) Neuroanatomical changes after EMDR in PTSD. J Neuropsychiatry Clin Neurosci 19:457–458

Brody AL, Saxena S, Stoessel P, Gillies LA, Fairbanks LA, Alborzian S, Phelps ME, Huang SC, Wu HM, Ho ML, Ho MK, Au SC, Maidment K, Baxter LR (2001a) Regional brain metabolic changes in patients with major depression treated with either paroxetine or interpersonal therapy: preliminary findings. Arch Gen Psychiatry 58:631–640. doi:10.1001/archpsyc.58.7.631

Brody AL, Saxena S, Mandelkern MA, Fairbanks LA, Ho ML, Baxter R (2001b) Brain metabolic changes associated with symptom factor improvement in major depressive disorder. Biol Psychiatry 50:171–178. doi:10.1016/S0006-3223(01)01117-9

Buchheim A, Viviani R, Kessler H, Kächele H, Cierpka M, Roth G, George C, Kernberg OF, Bruns G, Taubner S (2012) Changes in prefrontal-limbic function in major depression after 15 months of long-term psychotherapy. PLoS One 7:e33745. doi:10.1371/journal.pone.0033745

Chen W, Ogawa S (1999) Principle of BOLD-functional MRI. In: Moonen CTW, Bandettini PA (eds) Functional MRI. Springer, Berlin. doi:10.1007/978-3-642-58716-0_10

DeRubeis RJ, Siegle GJ, Hollon SD (2008) Cognitive therapy versus medication for depression: treatment outcomes and neural mechanisms. Nat Rev Neurosci 9:788–796. doi:10.1038/nrn2345

Dichter GS, Felder JN, Petty C, Bizzell J, Ernst M, Smoski MJ (2009) The effects of psychotherapy on neural responses to rewards in major depression. Biol Psychiatry 66:886–897. doi:10.1016/j.biopsych.2009.06.021

Dichter GS, Felder JN, Smoski MJ (2010) The effects of brief behavioral activation therapy for depression on cognitive control in affective contexts: an fMRI investigation. J Affect Dis 126:236–244. doi:10.1016/j.jad.2010.03.022

Farrow TFD, Hunter MD, Wilkinson ID, Gounea C, Fawbert D, Smith R, Lee KH, Mason S, Spence SA, Woodruff PWR (2005) Quantifiable change in functional brain response to empathic and forgivability judgments with resolution of posttraumatic stress disorder. Psychiatry Res 140:45–53. doi:10.1016/j.pscychresns.2005.05.012

Felmingham K, Kemp A, Williams L, Das P, Hughes G, Peduto A, Bryant R (2007) Changes in anterior cingulate and amygdala after cognitive behaviour therapy of posttraumatic stress disorder. Psychol Sci 18:127–129. doi:10.1111/j.1467-9280.2007.01860.x

Frewen PA, Dozois DJA, Lanius RA (2008) Neuroimagingstudies of psychological interventions for mood and anxiety disorders: empirical and methodological review. Clin Psychol Rev 28:228–246

Freyer T, Klöppel S, Tüscher O, Kordon A, Zurowski B, Kuelz AK, Speck O, Glauche V, Voderholzer U (2011) Frontostriatal activation in patients with obsessive-compulsive disorder before and after cognitive behavioural therapy. Psychol Med 41:207–216. doi:10.1017/S0033291710000309

Friston KJ, Holmes AP, Worsley KJ, Poline JP, Frith CD, Frackowiak RSJ (1995) Statistical parametric maps in functional imaging: a general linear approach. Hum Brain Mapp 2:189–210. doi:10.1002/hbm.460020402

Fu CHY, Williams SCR, Cleare AJ, Scott J, Mitterschiffthaler MT, Walsh ND, Donaldson C, Suckling J, Andrew C, Steiner H, Murray RM (2008) Neural responses to sad facial expressions in major depression following cognitive behavioural therapy. Biol Psychiatry 64:505–512. doi:10.1016/j.biopsych.2008.04.033

Furmark T, Tillfors M, Marteinsdottir I, Fischer H, Pissiota A, Langsträm B, Fredrikson M (2002) Common changes in cerebral blood flow in patients with social phobia treated with citalopram or cognitive-behavioural therapy. Arch Gen Psychiatry 59:425–433. doi:10.1001/archpsyc.59.5.425

Gersons BPR, Carlier IVE, Olff M (2004) Manual brief eclectic psychotherapy (BEP) for posttraumatic stress disorder. Academic Medical Centre, Amsterdam

Goldapple K, Segal Z, Garson C, Lau M, Bieling P, Kennedy S, Mayberg H (2004) Modulation of cortical-limbic pathways in major depression. Arch Gen Psychiatry 61:34–41. doi:10.1001/archpsyc.61.1.34

Goosens L, Sunaert S, Peeters R, Griez ELL, Schruers KRJ (2007) Amygdala hyperfunction in phobic fear normalizes after exposure. Biol Psychiatry 62:1119–1125. doi:10.1016/j.biopsych.2007.04.024

Gottesmann II, Gould TD (2003) The endophenotype concept in psychiatry: etymology and strategic intentions. Am J Psychiatry 160:636–645. doi:10.1176/appi.ajp.160.4.636

Gountouna VE, Job DE, McIntosh AM, Moorhead TWJ, Lymer GCL, Whalley HC, Hall J, Waiter GD, Brennan D, McGonigle DJ, Ahearn TS, Cavanagh J, Condon B, Hadley DM, Marshall I, Murray AD, Stelle JD, Wardlaw JM, Lawrie SM (2010) Functional magnetic resonance imaging (fMRI) reproducibility and variance components across visits and scanning sites with a finger tapping task. Neuroimage 49:552–560

Hopko DR, Lejuez CW, Ruggiero KJ, Eifert GH (2003) Contemporary behavioral activation treatments for depression: procedures, principles, and progress. Clin Psychol Rev 23:699–717. doi:10.1016/S0272-7358(03)00070-9

Insel T, Cuthbert B, Garvey M, Heinssen R, Pine DS, Quinn K, Sanislow C, Wang P (2010) Research domain criteria (RDoC): toward a new classification framework for research on mental disorders. Am J Psychiatry 167:748–751. doi:10.1176/appi.ajp.2010.09091379

Johanson A, Risberg J, Tucker DM, Gustafson L (2006) Changes in frontal lobe activity with cognitive therapy for spider phobia. Appl Neuropsychol 13:34–41

Kennedy SH, Konarski JZ, Segal ZV, Lau MA, Bieling PJ, McINtyre RS, Mayberg HS (2007) Differences in brain glucose metabolism between responders to CBT and Venlafaxine in a 16-week randomized controlled trial. Am J Psychiatry 164:778–788. doi:10.1176/appi.ajp.164.5.778

Kirchheiner J, Seeringer A, Viviani R (2010) Pharmacogenetics in psychiatry. A useful clinical tool or wishful thinking for the future? Curr Pharm Des 16:136–144. doi:10.2174/138161210790112728

Lazarus RS (1991) Emotion and adaptation. Oxford University Press, Oxford

Lehto SM, Tolmunen T, Joensu M, Saarinen PI, Valkonen-Korhonen M, Vanninen R, Ahola P, Tiihonen J, Kuikka J, Lehtonen J (2008) Changes in midbrain serotonin transporter availability in atypically depressed subjects after one year of psychotherapy. Prog Neuropsychopharmacol Biol Psychiatry 32:229–237

Leutgeb V, Schäfer A, Schienle A (2009) An event-related potential study on exposure therapy for patients suffering from spider phobia. Biol Psychol 82:293–300. doi:10.1016/j.biopsycho.2009.09.003

Levin P, Lazrove S, van der Kolk B (1999) What psychological testing and neuroimaging tell us about the treatment of posttraumatic stress disorder by eye movement desensitization and reprocessing. J Anxiety Dis 13:159–172

Lindauer RJL, Vlieger EJ, Jalink M, Olff M, Carlier IVE, Majoie CBLM, den Heeten GJ, Gersons BPR (2005)

Effects of psychotherapy on hippocampal volume in out-patients with post-traumatic stress disorder: a MRI investigation. Psychol Med 35:1421–1431. doi:10.1017/S0033291705005246

Lindauer RJL, Booij J, Habraken JBA, van Meijel EPM, Uylings BHM, Olff M, Carlier IVE, den Heeten GJ, van Eck-Smit BLF, Gersons BPR (2008) Effects of psychotherapy on regional cerebral blood flow during trauma imagery in patients with post-traumatic stress disorder: a randomized clinical trial. Psychol Med 38:543–554. doi:10.1017/S0033291707001432

Linden DEJ (2006) How psychotherapy changes the brain. The contribution of functional neuroimaging. Mol Psychiatry 11:528–538. doi:10.1038/sj.mp.4001816

Logothetis MK (2002) The neural basis of the blood-oxygen-level-dependent functional magnetic resonance imaging signal. Philos Trans R Soc Lond B Biol Sci 357:1003–1037. doi:10.1098/rstb.2002.1114

Martin SD, Martin RMN, Rai SS, Richardson MA, Royall R, Eng IEE (2001) Brain blood flow changes in depressed patients treated with interpersonal therapy or venlafaxine hydrochloride: preliminary findings. Arch Gen Psychiatry 58:641–648

Messina I, Sambin M, Palmieri A, Viviani R (2013) Neural correlates of psychotherapy in anxiety and depression: a meta-analysis. PLoS One 8(9): e74657

Meyer-Lindenberg A, Weinberger DR (2006) Intermediate phenotypes and genetic mechanisms of psychiatric disorders. Nat Rev Neurosci 7:818–827. doi:10.1038/nrn1993

Nabeyama M, Nakagawa A, Yoshiura T, Nakao T, Nakatani E, Togao O, Yoshizato C, Yoshioka K, Tomita M, Kanba S (2008) Function MRI study of brain activation alterations in patients with obsessive-compulsive disorder after symptom improvement. Psychiatry Res 163:236–247

Nakao T, Nakgawa A, Yoshiura T, Nakatani E, Nabeyama M, Yoshizato C, Kudoh A, Tada K, Yoshioka K, Kawamoto M, Togao O, Kanba S (2005) Brain activation of patients with obsessive-compulsive disorder during neuropsychological and symptom provocation tasks before and after symptom improvement: a functional magnetic resonance imaging study. Biol Psychiatry 57:901–910. doi:10.1016/j.biopsych.2004.12.039

Nakatani E, Nakgawa A, Ohara Y, Goto S, Uozomi N, Iwakiri M, Yamamoto Y, Motomura K, Iikura Y, Yamagami T (2003) Effects of behavior therapy on regional cerebral blood flow in obsessive-compulsive disorder. Psychiatry Res 124:113–120. doi:10.1016/S0925-4927(03)00069-6

Ochsner KN, Gross JJ (2005) The cognitive control of emotion. Trends Cogn Sci 9:242–249. doi:10.1016/j.tics.2005.03.010

Ochsner KN, Bunge SA, Gross JJ, Gabrieli JDE (2002) Rethinking feelings: an fMRI study of the cognitive regulation of emotion. J Cogn Neurosci 14:1215–1229

Ochsner KN, Ray RD, Cooper JC, Robertson ER, Chopra S, Gabrieli JDE, Gross JJ (2004) For better or for worse: neural systems supporting the cognitive down- and up-regulation of negative emotion. Neuroimage 23:483–499

Pagani M, Högberg G, Salmaso D, Nardo D, Sundin JC, Soares J, Aberg-Wistedt A, Jacobsson H, Larsson SA, Hällström T (2007) Effects of EMDR psychotherapy on ^{99m}Tc-HMPAO distribution in occupation-related post-traumatic stress disorder. Nucl Med Commun 28:747–765. doi:10.1097/MNM.0b013e3282742035

Paquette V, Lévesque J, Mensour B, Leroux JM, Beaudoin G, Bourgouin P, Beauregard M (2003) "Change the mind and you change the brain": effects of cognitive-behavioral therapy on the neural correlates of spider phobia. Neuroimage 18:401–409. doi:10.1016/S1053-8119(02)00030-7

Peres JFP, Newberg AB, Mercante JP, Simao M, Albuquerque VE, Peres MJP, Nasello AG (2007) Cerebral blood flow changes during retrieval of traumatic memories before and after psychotherapy: a SPECT study. Psychol Med 37:1481–1491. doi:10.1017/S003329170700997X

Phillips ML, Drevets WC, Rauch SL, Lane R (2003) Neurobiology of emotion perception I: the neural basis of normal emotion perception. Biol Psychiatry 54:504–514. doi:10.1016/S0006-3223(03)00168-9

Posner MI, Raichle ME (1994) Images of the mind. Freeman, New York, NY

Prasko J, Horácek J, Záleský R, Kopecek M, Novák T, Paskova B, Skrdlantová L, Belohlávek O, Höschl C (2004) The change of regional brain metabolism (^{18}FDG PET) in panic disorder during the treatment with cognitive behavioral therapy or antidepressants. Neuroendocrinol Lett 25:340–348

Rauch SL, Shin LM, Phelps EA (2006) Neurocircuitry models of posttraumatic stress disorder and extinction: human neuroimaging research – past, present, and future. Biol Psychiatry 60:376–382. doi:10.1016/j.biopsych.2006.06.004

Roffman JL, Marci CD, Glick DM, Dougherty DD, Rauch SL (2005) Neuroimaging and the functional neuroanatomy of psychotherapy. Psychol Med 35:1385–1398. doi:10.1017/S0033291705005064

Sakai Y, Kumano H, Nishikawa M, Sakano Y, Kaiya H, Imabayashi E, Ohnishi T, Matsuda H, Yasuda A, Sato A, Diksic M, Kuboki T (2006) Changes in cerebral glucose utilization in patients with panic disorder treated with cognitive-behavioural therapy. Neuroimage 33:218–226. doi:10.1016/j.neuroimage.2006.06.017

Saxena S, Bota RG, Brody AL (2001) Brain-behavior relationships in obsessive-compulsive disorder. Semin Clin Neuropsychiatry 6:82–101. doi:10.1053/scnp.2001.21833

Saxena S, Gorbis E, O'Neill J, Baker SK, Mandelkern MA, Maiment KM, Chang S, Salamon N, Brody AL, Schwartz JM, London ED (2009) Rapid effects of brief intensive cognitive-behavioural therapy on brain glucose metabolism in obsessive-compulsive disorder. Mol Psychiatry 14:197–205. doi:10.1038/sj.mp.4002134

Schienle A, Schäfer A, Hermann A, Rohrmann S, Vaitl D (2007) Symptom provocation and reduction in patients suffering from spider phobia. An fMRI study on exposure therapy. Eur Arch Psychiatry Clin Neurosci 257:486–493. doi:10.1007/s00406-007-0754-y

Schienle A, Schäfer A, Stark R, Vaitl D (2009) Long-term effects of cognitive behaviour therapy on brain activation in spider phobia. Psychiatry Res 172:99–102. doi:10.1016/j.pscychresns.2008.11.005

Schwartz JM, Stoessel PW, Baxter LR, Martin KM, Phelps ME (1996) Systematic changes in cerebral glucose metabolic rate after successful behaviour modification treatment of obsessive-compulsive disorder. Arch Gen Psychiatry 53:109–113. doi:10.1001/archpsyc.1996.01830020023004

Shapiro F (1995) Eye movement desensitization and reprocessing: basic principles, protocols, and procedures. Guilford, New York, NY

Straube T, Glauer M, Dilger S, Mentzel HJ, Miltner WHR (2006) Effects of cognitive-behavioural therapy on brain activation in specific phobia. Neuroimage 29:125–135. doi:10.1016/j.neuroimage.2005.07.007

Taylor SF, Liberzon I (2007) Neural correlates of emotion regulation in psychopathology. Trends Cogn Sci 11:413–418. doi:10.1016/j.tics.2007.08.006

Thomas EJ, Elliott R (2009) Brain imaging correlates of cognitive impairment in depression. Front Hum Neurosci 3:30. doi:10.3389/neuro.09.030.2009

Whalen PJ, Shin LM, Somerville LH, McLean AA, Kim H (2002) Functional neuroimaging studies of the amygdala in depression. Semin Clin Neuropsychiatry 7:234–242. doi:10.1053/scnp.2002.35219

Whiteside SP, Port JD, Abramowitz JS (2004) A meta-analysis of functional neuroimaging in obsessive-compulsive disorder. Psychiatry Res 132:69–79. doi:10.1016/j.pscychresns.2004.07.001

Woon FL, Sood S, Hedges DW (2010) Hippocampal volume deficits associated with exposure to psychological trauma and posttraumatic stress disorder in adults: a meta-analysis. Prog Neuropsychopharmacol Biol Psychiatry 34:1181–1188. doi:10.1016/j.pnpbp.2010.06.016

Yamanishi Y, Nakaaki S, Omori IM, Hashimoto N, Shinagawa Y, Hongo J, Horikoshi M, Tohyama J, Akechi T, Some T, Iidaka T, Furukawa TA (2009) Changes after behavior therapy among responsive and nonresponsive patients with obsessive-compulsive disorder. Psychiatry Res 172:242–250. doi:10.1016/j.pscychresns.2008.07.004

Index

O.C.G. Gelo et al. (eds.), *Psychotherapy Research*,
DOI 10.1007/978-3-7091-1382-0, © Springer-Verlag Wien 2015

MIX
Papier aus verantwortungsvollen Quellen
Paper from responsible sources
FSC® C105338

If you have any concerns about our products,
you can contact us on
ProductSafety@springernature.com

In case Publisher is established outside the EU,
the EU authorized representative is:
Springer Nature Customer Service Center GmbH
Europaplatz 3, 69115 Heidelberg, Germany

Printed by Libri Plureos GmbH
in Hamburg, Germany